Dr JL Berry,
University Department of Medicine,
Manchester Royal Infirmary,
Oxford Road,
Manchester
M13 9WL.

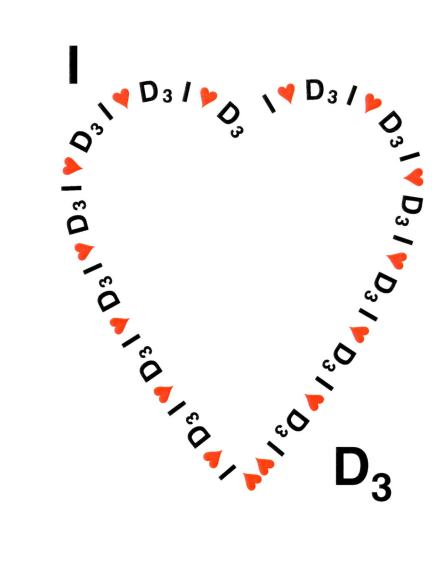

Vitamin D
Endocrine
System
Structural, Biological, Genetic and Clinical Aspects

Proceedings of the Eleventh Workshop on Vitamin D
Nashville, Tennessee, USA - May 27 – June 1, 2000

Editors
Anthony W. Norman, Roger Bouillon, Monique Thomasset

Printing and Reprographics
University of California, Riverside

Editors
Anthony W. Norman, Professor, Ph.D.
Department of Biochemistry
University of California-Riverside
Riverside, CA 92521, USA

Roger Bouillon, Professor, M.D., Ph.D., FRCP
Katholieke Universiteit Leuven
Laboratorium voor Experimentele
    Geneeskunde en Endocrinologie
Onderwijs en Navorsing
Gasthuisberg
B-3000 Leuven, Belgium

Monique Thomasset, Docteur des Sciences
INSERM Unité 438
Hôpital Robert Debré
48 Bd Sérurier
75019 Paris, France

With 540 figures and 104 tables

Library of Congress Cataloging-in-Publication Data

Workshop on Vitamin D (11th: 2000: Nashville, TN, USA.)
Vitamin D endocrine system: structural, biological, genetic and clinical aspects:
proceedings of the Eleventh Workshop on Vitamin D, Nashville, TN, USA - May 27 -
June 1, 2000 / Editors, Anthony W. Norman, Roger Bouillon, Monique Thomasset
Riverside (Calif.) : University of California, Printing and Reprographics, 2000.
xliv, 1014 p. : ill. : 24 cm.
Includes bibliographical references and indexes.
ISBN 1-891168-04-5
1. Vitamin D--Congresses. 2. Vitamin D--Therapeutic use--Congresses. 3.
Vitamin D in the body--Congresses. 4. Steroid hormones--Congresses. I.
Norman, A.W. (Anthony W.) 1938 -   . II. Bouillon, R. (Roger) 1943 -   , III.
Thomasset, M. (Monique) 1942 -   . IV. Title
    QP772.V53W67 2000

Library of Congress card number: 00-107310

FOREWORD

The Eleventh Workshop on Vitamin D was held at the Opryland Hotel and Convention Center in Nashville, Tennessee, USA from May 27 to June 1, 2000. A total of 376 registered delegates from 30 countries were in attendance. These included representatives from Argentina (15), Australia (9), Austria (8), Belgium (15), Brazil (2), Bulgaria (1), Canada (12), Colombia (1), Denmark (16), Finland (3), France (20), Germany (14), India (1), Israel (6), Italy (2), Japan (40), Korea (1), Mexico, (2), Monaco (2), Norway (1), Poland (4), Saudi Arabia (1), Serbia (1), South Africa (1), Spain (7), Sweden (3), Switzerland (2), The Netherlands (9), United Kingdom (25), and the United States (154).

The substantial attendance at the Nashville Workshop reflected the continuing high level of world-wide interest in research developments related to vitamin D. Tabulated below are the dates and attendance, as well as the number of talks given at the eleven Vitamin D Workshops that have now been held.

Workshop Number	Date	Number of Delegates	Number of Countries Represented	Number of Presentations Talks	Posters	Presentations per Delegate
I	October 1973 West Germany	56	3	5	0	0.09
II	October 1974 West Germany	221	22	84	0	0.39
III	January 1977 California, USA	332	20	45	124	0.51
IV	February 1979 West Germany	402	26	80	205	0.76
V	February 1982 Virginia, USA	455	25	95	298	0.86
VI	March 1985 Italy	474	27	77	380	0.96
VII	April 1988 California, USA	381	24	82	292	0.98
VIII	July 1991 France	595	32	76	415	0.82
IX	May 1994 Florida, USA	502	31	91	348	0.89
X	May 1997 France	571	37	87	358	0.78
XI	May 2000 Tennessee, USA	376	30	83	239	0.86

The formal program of the Eleventh Workshop on Vitamin D included verbal presentations by 48 invited speakers and 35 promoted free communications, as well as 239 poster presentations.

A very important feature of the Eleventh Workshop was the presentation of three 40-minute plenary lectures by distinguished scientists who have not actively been conducting research specifically related to vitamin D. This included the opening lecture of the Workshop on Sunday morning that focused on orphan receptors and was entitled "New insights from new nuclear hormone receptors" by Professor David Moore (Houston, Texas, USA). On Monday morning, Professor Robert E. Kingston (Boston, Massachusetts, USA) presented a lecture entitled "Structure and function of chromatin". On Wednesday, Professor Gregory R. Mundy's (San Antonio, Texas, USA) lecture was entitled "The use of vitamin D metabolites in the treatment of bone disease". This talk was an overview of recent developments in bone biology and the implications for clinical applications.

The scientific program was prepared by the Program Committee and implemented by the Advisory Committee. The members of the Program Committee were: D. D. Bikle (USA), L. Binderup (Denmark), B. D. Boyan (USA), P. Brachet (France), A. J. Brown (USA), C. Carlberg (Germany), S. Christakos (USA), K. W. Colston (UK), A. R. deBoland (Argentina), P. J. De Clercq (Belgium), M. B. Demay (USA), J. A. Eisman (Australia), D. Feldman (USA), L. P. Freedman (USA), M. Garabedian (France), F. H. Glorieux (Canada), M. R. Haussler (USA), H. L. Henry (USA), M. Hewison (UK), M. F. Holick (USA), B. W. Hollis (USA), R. L. Horst, (USA), S. Ishizuka (Japan), C. S. Johnson (USA), G. Jones (Canada), S. Kato (Japan), H. P. Koeffler (USA), N. Kubodera (Japan), P. N. MacDonald (USA), P. H. Mäenpää (Finland), E. B. Mawer (UK), A. Mouriño (Spain), W. H. Okamura (USA), S. Peleg (USA), M. Peterlik (Austria), J. M. Pettifor (South Africa), J. W. Pike (USA), G. H. Posner (USA), G. S. Reddy (USA), I. Schuster (Austria), Y. Seino (Japan), J. Silver (Israel), E. Slatopolsky (USA), R. St-Arnaud (Canada), G. S. Stein (USA), T. Suda (Japan), M. R. Uskokovic (USA), J.P.T.M. van Leeuwen (The Netherlands), and J. Welsh (USA). The Program Committee members collectively reviewed the 274 submitted Free Communication abstracts, which were candidates for verbal presentation, and provided scores for 30-40 abstracts that were related to their general areas of research expertise. This allowed formulation of a rank ordered list of the average scores for all the abstracts so that ultimately 35 abstracts were selected for verbal ten-minute presentations at the Workshop.

This book presents the published Proceedings of the Eleventh Vitamin D Workshop and is organized by general topics. The Table of Contents is presented at two levels of organization. First appears a Summary Table of Contents that identifies the major sections amongst which the individual chapters are grouped. This is followed by a Detailed Table of Contents that enumerates the complete titles and names of all authors for each of the 203 chapters that comprise this Proceedings. Within each topic the first series of chapters are written by the Invited or Plenary Speakers (usually 8 pages) followed by the Free Communications (4 pages). This Proceedings book (the tenth in our series) also includes a section of chapters concerning vitamin D nutrition.

The quality and diversity of the science presented at the Eleventh Workshop were again at an exceptionally high level. Remarkable progress continues to be made in research areas related to the vitamin D endocrine system; these include chemistry, biochemistry and biology, and clinical applications.

A highlight of the verbal presentations of the Eleventh Workshop was the fascinating Special Lecture presented by Dr. Dino Moras, Strasbourg, France entitled "Ligand binding to the nuclear receptor for vitamin D". This talk was of high interest to all of the delegates because it provided for the first time the molecular details of the nuclear receptor for $1\alpha,25(OH)_2D_3$, which was based on his team's x-ray crystal structure of the VDR to a resolution of 1.8 Å. This long awaited development will provide fundamental information to many aspects of current research on vitamin D including the chemical design of new analogs of $1\alpha,25(OH)_2D_3$, a detailed understanding of the working of the nuclear VDR and, as well, insight into the molecular basis for a variety of diseases which result from dysfunction of the VDR.

The major focus of the Eleventh Workshop on Vitamin D concerned the molecular biology and biochemistry of the nuclear receptor from $1\alpha,25(OH)_2D_3$ and the details of its interactions with the various promoters of the genes which are either induced or repressed. Three verbal sessions presented on different days were devoted to this topic; in addition there was an additional poster session related to molecular biology of the VDR. No less than 23 chapters concerning the VDR are presented in these Proceedings, while an additional 9 chapters focus on the molecular biology of the VDR.

A number of presentations focused on identifying the specific molecular bases of interaction between the various functional groups of the $1\alpha,25(OH)_2D_3$ molecule with the interior surface of the ligand binding domain of the nuclear VDR. The studies were based on preparation of molecular models of the VDR and, as well, the availability of the coordinates derived from the x-ray crystal structure of the VDR. Also, there were a number of presentations that evaluated the $1\alpha,25(OH)_2$–20-epi-D_3 analogs, which are more potent with respect to transactivation of the VDR, in terms of their detailed molecular interactions with the ligand binding domain of the VDR. Studies of this type also are related to understanding how the nuclear VDR forms heterodimers with RXR and, in turn, more complex assemblies that involve other coactivators so as to generate a competent transcriptional complex. Finally, a notable contribution was the identification of an analog of $1\alpha,25(OH)_2D_3$, (23S)-25-dehydro-1α-OH-D_3-26,23-lactone, which has been found to be the first well-defined antagonist of the nuclear VDR.

An important aspect of understanding the nuclear VDR has been a fuller description of the consequences of a gene knock out (KO) of this protein, which had been first reported in 1997 at the 10th Workshop on Vitamin D. Several fascinating presentations focused on describing the physiological and biological significance of the VDR and to profiling the phenotype that emerges when the VDR protein is not expressed. One of the most remarkable developments has been the appreciation that, in spite of decades of research emphasizing the importance of the VDR to calcium homeostasis, gene knock-out of the nuclear VDR does not result in bone abnormalities as long as a high dietary intake of calcium has been maintained. The most significant consequences of the VDR KO have to do with the development of alopecia reflecting abrogation of important VDR actions in the skin or keratinocytes and reduced infertility in both female and male mice.

Innovative chemical developments, which have been a hallmark of Vitamin D Workshops over the past 15 years, continued; no less than 25 chapters of vitamin D chemistry are included in these Proceedings. The thrust of the presentations continues to be the creation of new analogs that provide insights into the biochemical mode of action of both new and old analogs of $1\alpha,25(OH)_2D_3$ and their potential application to clinical uses. It is clear that, with the acquisition of all of the coordinates of the atoms of the nuclear VDR from the VDR x-ray crystal structure, it becomes increasingly possible to carry out rational drug design of new analogs which may have selective biological actions.

A continuing topic of high importance of the Vitamin D Workshop was the aspect of the biology and mode of action of $1\alpha,25(OH)_2D_3$ in terms of its application to cancer. There were two cancer sessions at the Eleventh Workshop on Vitamin D, yielding 16 chapters on the basic science aspect of cell differentiation and 19 chapters focused on various aspects of cancer, both basic and clinical. In the basic arena, a continuing arena of focus concerned the topics of identifying how $1\alpha,25(OH)_2D_3$ acts on the cell cycle and on the induction of apoptosis. Important cancer presentations included breast cancer, prostate cancer, and colorectal cancer. It is clear that progress is being made on these fronts. The clinical studies have now progressed beyond the Phase I setting and preliminary results were presented on the use of the analogs of $1\alpha,25(OH)_2D_3$ in the treatment of prostate cancer and lymphatic cancers.

Many other advances and topics related to vitamin D were also covered at the Workshop. These included, at the molecular level, a preliminary presentation of the x-ray structure of the vitamin D binding protein (DBP). It is anticipated that in the near future a full three-dimensional structure of this important vitamin D related protein will be available. Two fascinating reports were presented (from Leuven and Milan) concerning the involvement of $1\alpha,25(OH)_2D_3$ and related analogs in the immune system. It is clear that this is an unusually complex field, where $1\alpha,25(OH)_2D_3$ seems to affect all actors of the immune system in a coherent fashion so that one looks forward with anticipation to the likely development of selective analogs of $1\alpha,25(OH)_2D_3$ for the prevention or treatment of autoimmune diseases or graft rejection. The $1\alpha,25(OH)_2D_3$ rapid action session described further progress supporting cross-talk between rapid signaling transduction pathways (MAP kinase) and the genomic pathway of $1\alpha,25(OH)_2D_3$ action through the nuclear VDR. A more detailed understanding of the molecular basis of vitamin D mediated intestinal calcium absorption is emerging because of the discovery and cloning of a vitamin

D-induced calcium channel present in the brush border membrane of the intestinal epithelial cells. The Leuven group presented convincing evidence that there is a microcosm of the vitamin D endocrine system present in keratinocytes. The keratinocyte cell is capable of conversion of 7-dehydrocholesterol into vitamin D with its subsequent metabolism into both $25(OH)_2D_3$ and $1\alpha,25(OH)_2D_3$. This may be reflective of the important autocrine and paracrine system of vitamin D endocrinology present in the setting of the skin. The Leo group then presented the results of a technologically difficult assay involving a liquid chromatography tandem mass spectrometry procedure that can be used for the determination of the concentration of various metabolites and analogs of $1\alpha,25(OH)_2D_3$.

An important presentation of the Eleventh Workshop was a Round Table on Vitamin D Nutrition. The question focused on by all the participants was "What is the optimal level of circulating $25(OH)D_3$ for human health?" This session was co-chaired by Professor Roger Bouillon, from the Department of Endocrinology, Katholieke Universiteit in Leuven, Belgium and Professor Barbara Mawer from the Department of Medicine, University of Manchester, UK. The session included Dr. Bess Dawson-Hughes (USA), Dr. John M. Pettifor (South Africa), Dr. Pierre J. Meunier (France) and Dr. Michael F. Holick (USA). Following their presentations a general discussion ensued. All of these presentations are summarized in the Nutrition section of this Proceedings volume and provide an important milestone describing the importance of adequate vitamin D nutrition in our modern world.

The Eleventh Workshop on Vitamin D continued its tradition of the Awards Ceremony. The Leo Foundation of Copenhagen, Denmark, provided a generous gift of $10,000 to support sixteen travel awards to Young Investigators under the age of 35 who had submitted a meritorious abstract to the Workshop. The recipients are listed on page XII.

Five Vitamin D Workshop Career Recognition Awards were given to distinguished scientists to honor their significant and continuing contributions to the field of vitamin D research during their careers: these included Dr. Pekka H. Mäenpää (Finland), Dr. E. Barbara Mawer (UK), Dr. Pierre J. Meunier (France), Dr. Eduardo Slatopolsky (USA), and Dr. Tatsuo Suda (Japan). The recipients for this Eleventh Workshop, as well as the recipients for the Tenth, Ninth and Eighth Workshops, are listed on page XIV.

The Advisory Committee as well as the Program Committee acknowledge the financial support of the many sponsors of the Eleventh Workshop on Vitamin D. A tabulation of them appears on page XI. Without the generous multi-corporate financial support, it would have been impossible to have had a vitamin D workshop that included such a comprehensive program and world-wide attendance.

The setting for the Workshop was the spacious and modern Opryland Hotel and Convention Center in Nashville, Tennessee. The hotel, with its 2900 rooms, is the world's largest combined hotel/convention center under one roof in the world, with the hotel portion covering approximately 50 acres.

The presentation of the Eleventh Workshop on Vitamin D in Nashville would not have been possible without the dedicated and highly professional contributions of Mrs. Marian Herbert, Workshop Secretary (has attended and assisted in the last three consecutive Workshops), Ms. June E. Bishop, Workshop Coordinator (has attended and assisted in the last nine consecutive Workshops), Ms. Linda B. Johnson, Mrs. Lean Gill, Mr. Craig Bula and Mr. Brett Holmquist.

A very important adjunct to the successful presentation of the Eleventh Workshop on Vitamin D was the preparation and publication of a 237-page Abstract Book. Ms. June E. Bishop (Riverside) monitored and shepherded the preparation of this highly detailed book in a very short interval of time. The Abstract Book was indispensable to the delegates in keeping track of the scheduling of the 239 posters and the 83 verbal presentations.

The Advisory Committee invites interested scientists to the next, the Twelfth Workshop on Vitamin D, which will be held in Maastricht, The Netherlands from July 6-10, 2003. We look forward to meeting you in Maastricht.

Roger Bouillon, Leuven
Anthony W. Norman, Riverside
Monique Thomasset, Paris

June 2000

Official Sponsors and Donors of the
Eleventh Workshop on Vitamin D

LEADERSHIP SPONSOR

Leo Pharmaceutical Products Ltd. A/S. -- Denmark

SPONSORS

Abbott Laboratories -- USA

Bone Care International -- USA

Chugai Pharmaceutical Co., Ltd.
Japan

Procter & Gamble Pharmaceuticals
France

Solvay Pharmaceuticals
The Netherlands

Teijin Limited -- Japan

DONORS

ASTA Medica -- Austria

DiaSorin Inc. -- USA

F. Hoffmann-La Roche Ltd.
Switzerland

IDS Limited -- UK

ILEX Systems, Inc. -- USA

**Laboratory Dr. Limbach, Prof.
Schmidt-Gayk & Colleagues**
Germany

Novo Nordisk Pharma Ltd.
Japan

Pharmacia & Upjohn
Japan

Roche Products Pty. Ltd
Australia

Schering AG -- Germany

Théramex -- Monaco

ELEVENTH WORKSHOP ON VITAMIN D
LEO PHARMACEUTICALS YOUNG INVESTIGATOR TRAVEL AWARDS

MAY 27 – JUNE 1, 2000
NASHVILLE, TENNESSEE

Frank Barletta
UMDNJ – New Jersey Medical School
Dept of Biochemistry & Molecular Biology
Newark, New Jersey, USA

Craig M. Bula
Department of Biochemistry
University of California-Riverside
Riverside, California, USA

Mihwa Choi
Institute of Biomaterials and Bioengineering
Tokyo Medical and Dental University
Tokyo, Japan

Christina S. Clark
Department of Human Biology
    and Nutritional Sciences
University of Guelph
Guelph, Ontario, Canada

Mark A. English
Department of Medicine
Queen Elizabeth Hospital
Birmingham, United Kingdom

Ali Gardezi
University of Texas
MD Anderson Cancer Center
Houston, Texas, USA

Michaela Herdick
Institute für Physiologische Chemie I
Heinrich-Heine-Universität
Düsseldorf, Germany

Brett Holmquist
Biochemistry Department
University of California-Riverside
Riverside, California, USA

Kirsten Prüfer
National Institutes of Health
NIDDK, LCBB
Bethesda, Maryland, USA

Tim Raemaekers
LEGENDO, Katholieke Universiteit
Leuven, Belgium

Karen Sooy
Endocrine Unit, Harvard Medical School
Massachusetts General Hospital
Boston, Massachusetts, USA

Hisashi Tokumaru
Department of Pharmacology
Case Western Reserve University
Euclid, Ohio, USA

Sophie Van Cromphaut
LEGENDO, Katholieke Universiteit
Leuven, Belgium

Christel Verboven
Lab Anal. Chem.
Leuven, Belgium

Marcos Vidal
Renal Division
Washington University School of Medicine
St. Louis, Missouri, USA

Daniel Zehnder
Department of Medicine
Queen Elizabeth Hospital
Birmingham, United Kingdom

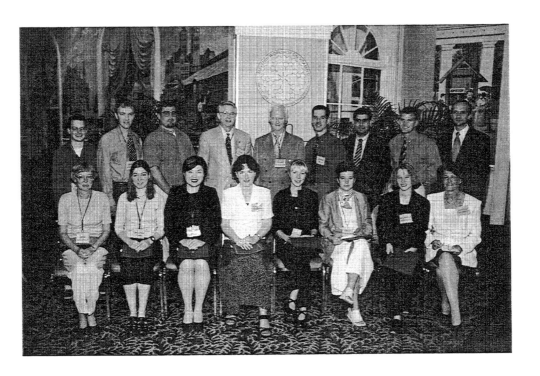

Eleventh Workshop on Vitamin D recipients of the Young Investigator Travel Award, sponsored by Leo Pharmaceutical Products, Ltd.
Front row: Dr. Lise Binderup, Leo Pharmaceutical; Christina S. Clark; Mihwa Choi; Dr. Kirsten Prűfer; Sophie van Cromphaut; Dr. Christel Verboven; Michaela Herdick; Dr. Monique Thomasset, Workshop Advisory Committee.
Back row: Dr. Mark A. English; Daniel Zehnder; Frank Barletta; Dr. Anthony W. Norman, Workshop Advisory Committee; Dr. Roger Bouillon, Workshop Advisory Committee; Craig Bula; Dr. Ali Gardezi; Brett Holmquist; Tim Raemaekers.
Not shown: Dr. Karen Sooy, Hisashi Tokumaru, Marcos Vidal.

RECIPIENTS OF OUTSTANDING CAREER AWARDS
for vitamin D-related research.

Eleventh Workshop on Vitamin D
(Nashville, Tennessee, USA 2000)

Dr. Pekka H. Mäenpää (Finland)	Vitamin D Actions
Dr. E. Barbara Mawer (United Kingdom)	Vitamin D Nutrition & Actions
Dr. Pierre J. Meunier (France)	Osteoporosis & Vitamin D Nutrition
Dr. Eduardo Slatopolsky (USA)	Renal Osteodystrophy
Dr. Tatsuo Suda (Japan)	Vitamin D Actions

Tenth Workshop on Vitamin D
(Strasbourg, France 1997)

Dr. Norman H. Bell (USA)	Clinical Studies on Vitamin D
Dr. Tadashi Kobayashi (Japan)	Vitamin D Nutrition & Action
Dr. Yasuho Nishii (Japan)	Vitamin D Drug Development
Dr. Jeffrey L. H. O'Riordan (United Kingdom)	Clinical Studies on Vitamin D
Dr. Maurits E. Vandewalle (Belgium)	Vitamin D Chemistry

Ninth Workshop on Vitamin D
(Orlando, Florida, USA 1994)

Dr. Angelo Caniggia (Italy)	Osteoporosis Research
Dr. Jack W. Coburn (USA)	Renal Osteodystrophy
Dr. Nobuo Ikekawa (Japan)	Chemistry of Vitamin D
Dr. B. Lawrence Riggs (USA)	Osteoporosis Research
Dr. Robert H. Wasserman (USA)	Calcium Binding Proteins

Eighth Workshop on Vitamin D
(Paris, France 1991)

Dr. Sonia Balsan (France)	Pediatrics
Dr. Livia Miravet (France)	Rheumatology
Dr. B. E. C. Nordin (Australia)	Osteoporosis Research
Dr. Milan R. Uskoković (USA)	Chemistry of 1,25-Dihydroxyvitamin D_3

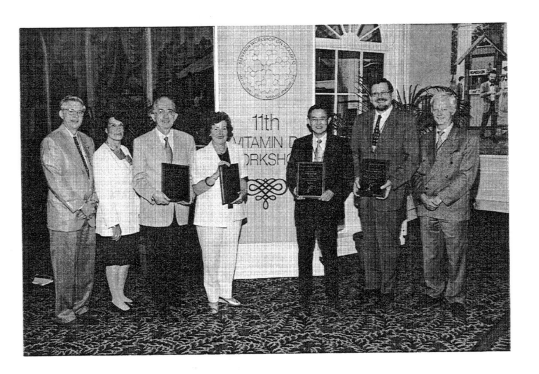

Outstanding Career Award recipients for the Eleventh Workshop on Vitamin D.
Left to right: Dr. Anthony W. Norman, Workshop Advisory Committee;
Dr. Monique Thomasset, Workshop Advisory Committee; Dr. Pierre J. Meunier,
Dr. E. Barbara Mawer, Dr. Tatsuo Suda, Dr. Pekka H. Mäenpää, Dr. Roger
Bouillon, Workshop Advisory Committee.
Not shown, Dr. Eduardo Slatopolsky.

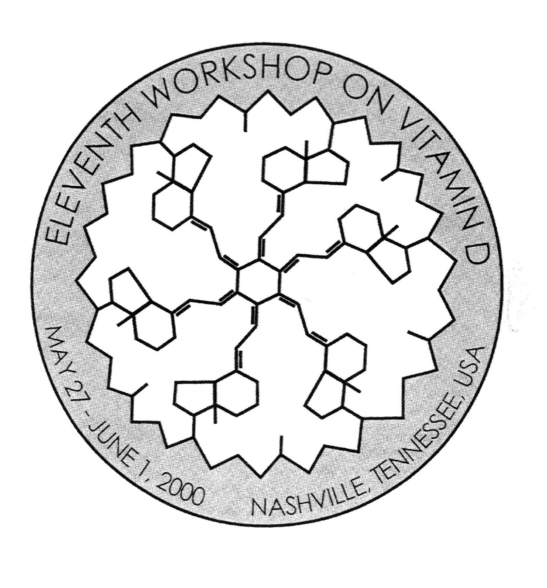

Table of Contents

Table of Contents

CHEMISTRY AND STRUCTURE / FUNCTION ANALYSIS

CONCEPTUALLY NEW 20-EPI-22-OXA-26-SULFONE SYNTHETIC ANALOGS OF THE NATURAL HORMONE 1α,25-DIHYDROXYVITAMIN D₃

Gary H. Posner,* Kenneth Crawford, Department of Chemistry, School of Arts and Sciences, The Johns Hopkins University, Baltimore, MD 21218; Sara Peleg, Department of Medical Specialties, The University of Texas, M.D. Anderson Cancer Center, Houston, TX 77030; Patrick Dolan, and Thomas W. Kensler, Department of Environmental Health Sciences, School of Hygiene and Public Health, The Johns Hopkins University, Baltimore, MD 21205

Introduction   Conventional wisdom requires the presence of **both** the 1α- and the 25-hydroxyl groups for the natural hormone 1α,25-dihydroxyvitamin D₃ (1,25D₃, calcitriol, **1**) to elicit its characteristically potent and diverse physiological responses in humans (1,2). In 1994, however, we showed for the first time that hybrid analog **2** bearing an unnatural 1β-hydroxymethyl group and also a potentiating side-chain with a tertiary hydroxyl group [*cf.* Leo Pharmaceutical Company's promising drug candidate KH-1060 (**3**)], was able to match the antiproliferative/prodifferentiating potency of the natural hormone but importantly without causing hypercalcemia (3). Recently, we showed for the first time that some synthetic 16-ene 24- and 25-*tert*-butyl sulfones, with natural 1α,3β hydroxyl groups but lacking a side-chain tertiary hydroxyl group, also have powerful but selective biological activities *in vitro* as well as nontoxic properties *in vivo* (4). Also we have reported that the 16-ene functionality, introduced and popularized by Hoffmann-La Roche researchers (5), is not required for a side-chain sulfone to be therapeutically desirable (6). Thus, 20-epi-22-oxa-26-sulfone **4a** is powerfully antiproliferative and transcriptionally active *in vitro* but noncalcemic *in vivo* (6). The high potency but low toxicity of oxasulfone **4a** reinforces and broadens our recent claim (4) that side-chain *t*-butyl sulfones, even though lacking the traditional side-chain tertiary hydroxyl group, represent a conceptually new class of calcitriol analogs having considerable potential as sensitive molecular probes of ligand-receptor interactions and as pharmacologically valuable new chemical entities. To explore the relationship of chemical structure with biological activity in this side-chain 22-oxa-26-sulfone series, we report here chemical synthesis and initial biological evaluation of 25-difluorinated oxasulfones **5**.

Results and Discussion   25-Difluorinated 26-sulfones **5a** and **5b**, synthesized as outlined in Scheme I, were rationally designed based on the following three major considerations: 1. the fluorine atoms should protect these 1,25D₃ analogs from enzymatic hydroxylation (*i.e.* catabolism) adjacent to the 26-sulfonyl group, a side-chain position typical of metabolite formation in many 1,25D₃ analogs (7), 2. the corresponding non-fluorinated analog **4a**, but not its 1β,3α diastereomer **4b**, is powerfully antiproliferative and transcriptionally active *in vitro* but desirably noncalcemic *in vivo* (6), and 3. some of our side-chain fluorinated hybrid analogs of 1,25D₃ are highly effective and safe for preventing mouse skin carcinogenesis (8).

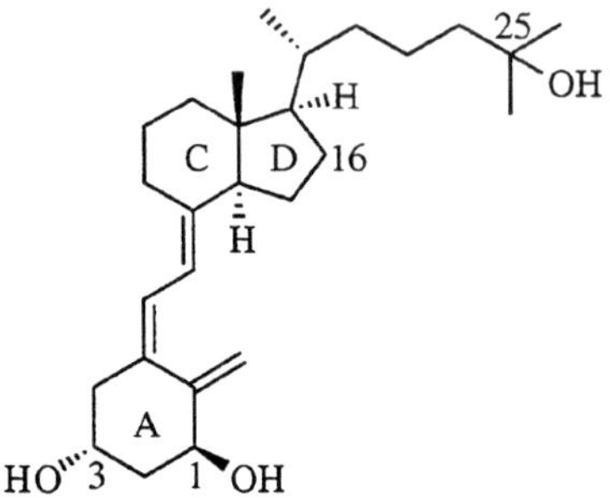

4

1α,25-dihydroxyvitamin D$_3$
(1,25D$_3$, calcitriol, **1**)

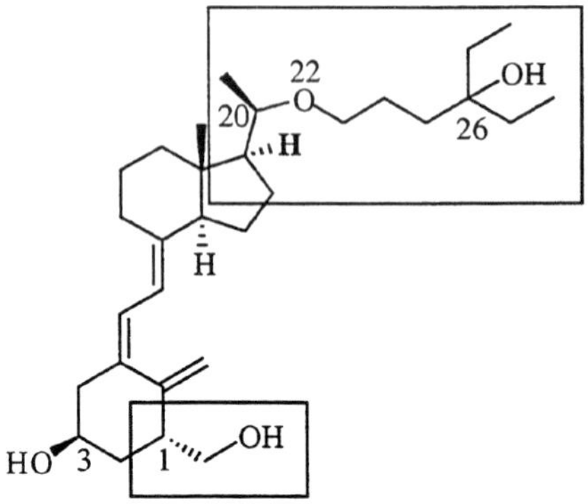

2 (MCW-YB)

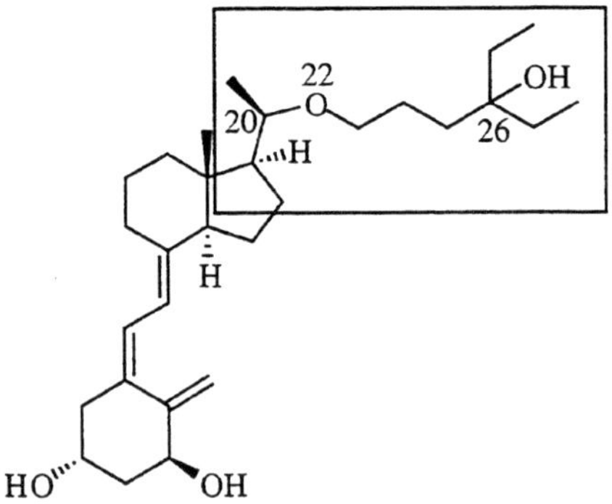

3 (KH-1060)

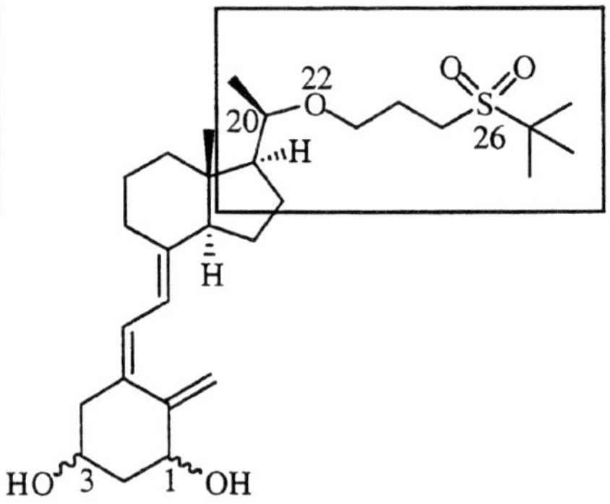

(–)-**4a** (1α,3β), KRC-20-epi-22-oxa-26-SO$_2$-1
(–)-**4b** (1β,3α), KRC-20-epi-22-oxa-26-SO$_2$-2

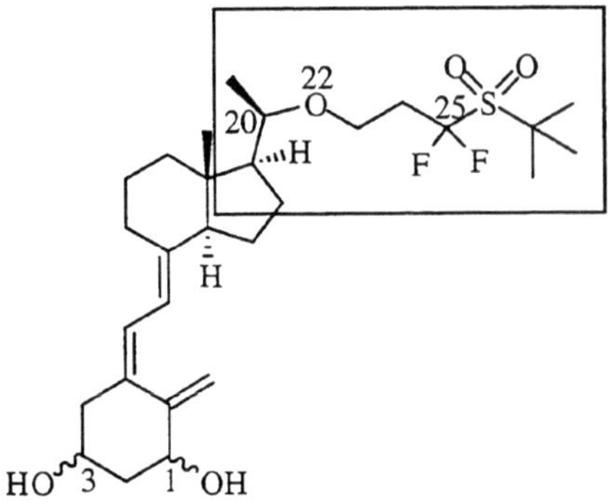

(–)-**5a** (1α,3β), KRC-20-epi-22-oxa-25-F$_2$-26-SO$_2$-1
(–)-**5b** (1β,3α), KRC-20-epi-22-oxa-25-F$_2$-26-SO$_2$-2

Scheme I

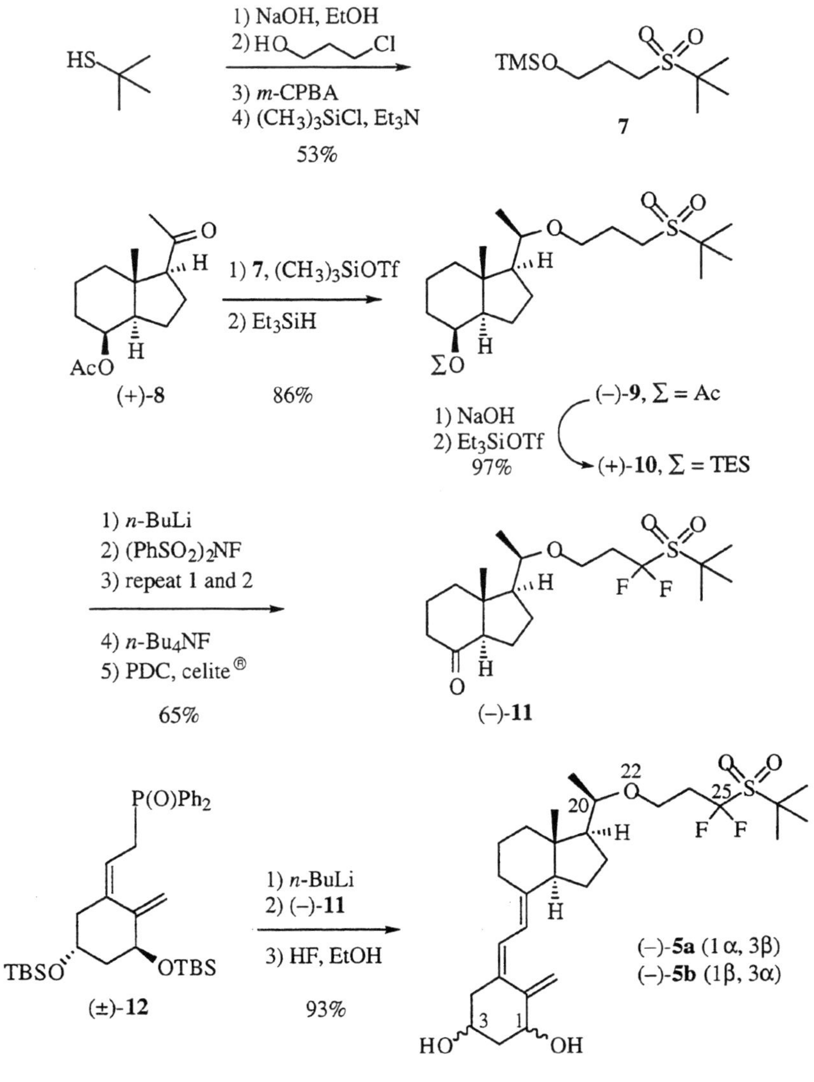

Noteworthy features of the synthesis of 25-fluorinated sulfones **5** (Scheme I) are as follows: 1. smooth reductive etherification (9) of ketone **9** without interference by the side-chain sulfonyl group, and 2. exceptionally high yields in both the final convergent coupling step and the HF-promoted desilylation step.

Antiproliferative efficacy *in vitro,* using our previously described murine keratinocyte protocol (10), showed 25-fluorinated sulfone **5a** with natural 1α,3β (OH)₂ stereochemistry to inhibit cell growth much more than its diastereomer **5b** but significantly less than natural 1,25D₃ (Fig. 1).

6

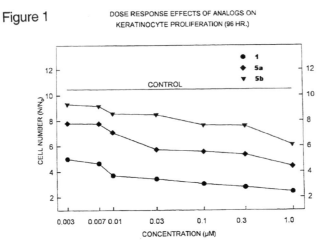

Figure 1   DOSE RESPONSE EFFECTS OF ANALOGS ON
KERATINOCYTE PROLIFERATION (96 HR.)

The vitamin D receptor (VDR)-mediated transcriptional potencies of fluorosulfones **5a** and **5b**, determined *in vitro* using a previously described protocol in rat osterosarcoma ROS 17/2.8 cells (11), were as follows: **5a**, ED_{50} = 0.2 nM; **5b**, ED_{50} = 100 nM. For comparison in this assay, $1,25D_3$ has ED_{50} = 0.4 nM, and non-fluorinated sulfone **4a** has ED_{50} = 1.6 nM (6).

25-Fluorinated sulfone **5a** is virtually noncalcemic even when administered to mice at 20 times higher concentration than $1,25D_3$ (Fig. 2).

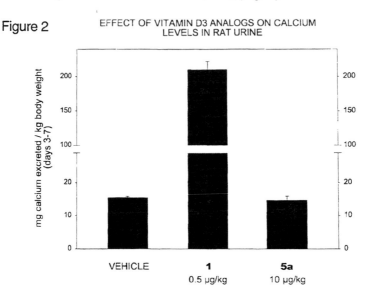

Figure 2   EFFECT OF VITAMIN D3 ANALOGS ON CALCIUM
LEVELS IN RAT URINE

In conclusion, 25-fluorinated *t*-butyl sulfone **5a** showed desirable antiproliferative and transcriptional activities *in vitro* and lack of calcemic activity *in vivo*. Thus, 25-fluorinated sulfone **5a** joins its parent non-fluorinated analog **4a** as a useful and sensitive new molecular proble of ligand-receptor interactions and as a pharmacologically valuable new chemical entity.

Experimental Section

General. Unless otherwise noted, all reactions were performed in oven-dried glassware stirred under an atmosphere of ultra-high-purity Ar. THF was distilled from Na/benzophenone ketyl immediately prior to use. TMSCl, CH_2Cl_2, and Et_3N were distilled from CaH_2. *m*-CPBA was washed with aqueous phosphate buffer (pH 7.5) and vacuum dried prior to use. N-Fluorobenzenesulfonimide (NFSI) was recrystallized from toluene:Et_2O prior to use. Organolithiums were titrated prior to use following known methods (12). All other reagents were used as received from commercial suppliers. Analytical TLC analysis was conducted on precoated glass-backed silica gel plates (Merck Kieselgel 60 F_{254}, 250 μm thickness) and visualized with *p*-anisaldehyde or $KMnO_4$ stains. Column chromatography was performed using short path silica gel (particle size < 230 mesh) or flash silica gel (particle size 230–400 mesh). HPLC was carried out using a Rainin HPLX system equipped with two 25-mL/min preparative pump heads using Rainin Dynamax 10-mm x 250-mm (semipreparative) columns packed with 60 Å silica gel (8 μm pore size) as C-18-bonded silica and a Rainin Dynamax UV-C dual-beam variable-wavelength detector set at 264 nm. Yields are reported for pure products (>95% based on their chromatographic and spectroscopic homogeneity) and are unoptimized. Melting points were determined in open capillaries using a Mel-Temp metal-block apparatus and are uncorrected. Optical rotations were measured at the Na line using a Perkin-Elmer 141 Polarimeter. NMR spectra were obtained on a Varian XL-400 spectrometer, operating at 400 MHz for ^{1}H, 376 MHz for ^{19}F, and 100 MHz for ^{13}C. Chemical shifts are reported in ppm (δ) and are referenced to $CHCl_3$ (7.26 ppm for ^{1}H and 77.0 ppm for ^{13}C) and $CFCl_3$ (0.00 ppm for ^{19}F). IR spectra were obtained using a Perkin Elmer 1600 Series FT-IR instrument. HRMS were obtained with electronic or chemical ionization (EI or CI) either at (1) Johns Hopkins University on a VG Instruments 70-S spectrometer run at an ionizing voltage of 70 eV for EI and run with ammonia (NH_3) as a carrier gas for CI or (2) University of Illinois at Urbana– Champaign on a Finnigan-MAT CH5, a Finnigan-MAT 731, or a VG Instruments 70-VSE spectrometer run at an ionizing voltage of 70 eV for EI and run with methane (CH_4) as a carrier gas for CI. Elemental analyses were performed by Atlantic Microlab Inc., Norcross, GA.

***t*-Butyl 3-(Trimethylsilyloxy)-propyl Sulfone 7.** To a solution of *t*-butyl 3-hydroxypropyl sulfone (13) (1.01 g, 5.60 mmol) in CH_2Cl_2 (25 mL) was added Et_3N (1.17 mL, 8.40 mmol) and TMSCl (0.78 mL, 6.16 mL). The resulting solution was stirred for 1 h, cooled to 0 °C, and quenched with saturated aqueous $NaHCO_3$ (5 mL). After warming, the reaction mixture was diluted with H_2O (10 mL), extracted with CH_2Cl_2 (3 x 15 mL), dried over solid Na_2SO_4, filtered, and concentrated to a red oil. Rapid column chromatography (25% EtOAc/hexanes) afforded the desired product **7** as a clear, colorless oil [0.75 g, 53% from 2-methyl-2-propanethiol (13)]: ^{1}H NMR ($CDCl_3$) δ 3.73 (t, *J* = 6.0 Hz, 2H), 3.02 (m, 2H), 2.09 (m, 2H), 1.42 (s, 9H), 0.11 (s, 9H); ^{13}C NMR ($CDCl_3$) δ 60.7, 58.8, 42.5, 23.8, 23.3, -0.63; IR (neat, cm^{-1}) 2959, 2906, 2875,

1478, 1463, 1301–1249, 1113, 947, 841; HRMS: calcd for $C_{10}H_{24}O_3SSi$ 252.1215, found 252.1285.

Acetoxy Sulfone (–)-9. To a cooled (–78 °C) solution of ketone (–)-**8** (6) (250 mg, 1.05 mmol) and **7** (356 mg, 1.36 mmol) in CH_2Cl_2 (11 mL) was added TMSOTf (0.190 mL, 1.05 mmol) via syringe and the resulting solution stirred at –78 °C for 1 h. Triethylsilane (0.168 mL, 1.05 mmol) was added via syringe and the reaction mixture quickly brought to rt. After 4 h, the reaction was ceased by cautious addition of a saturated aqueous $NaHCO_3$ solution (2 mL). This mixture was diluted with H_2O (10 mL), extracted with CH_2Cl_2 (3 x 10 mL), dried ($MgSO_4$), filtered, concentrated, and passed through flash silica gel (25–30% EtOAc/hexanes) to afford (–)-**9** as a clear, colorless oil (364 mg, 86%): $[\alpha]_D$ –5.7 (c 2.8, $CHCl_3$); ^1H NMR ($CDCl_3$) δ 5.14 (m, 1H), 3.69 (dt, $J = 9.2, 6.0$ Hz, 1H), 3.35 (dt, $J = 9.2, 6.0$ Hz, 1H), 3.30 (m, 1H), 3.04 (t, $J = 7.8$ Hz, 2H), 2.13 (m, 2H), 2.03 (s, 3H), 1.83 (m, 1H), 1.41(s, 9H), 1.05 (d, $J = 6.0$ Hz, 3H), 0.88 (s, 3H); ^{13}C NMR ($CDCl_3$) δ 170.8, 77.7, 71.1, 65.8, 58.8, 56.6, 50.9, 43.2, 41.8, 40.0, 30.6, 24.7, 23.4, 22.8, 21.7, 21.4, 18.1, 17.8, 13.7; IR (neat, cm^{-1}) 2942, 2873, 1732, 1304, 1279, 1247, 1115; HRMS: calcd for $C_{21}H_{38}O_5S$ + H 403.2518, found 403.2521.

Triethylsilyloxy Sulfone (+)-10. An aqueous solution of NaOH (1.0 mL, 10 M) was added to a stirred solution of acetoxy sulfone (–)-**9** (114 mg, 0.283 mmol) in EtOH (12 mL). After 8 h the resulting solution was diluted with EtOAc (10 mL) and cautiously neutralized with aqueous HCl (10%). Upon extracting the aqueous layer with EtOAc (3 x 10 mL), the combined organics were washed with brine (25 mL), dried ($MgSO_4$), filtered and concentrated to a clear oil which solidified upon cooling. This solid was dissolved in THF (10 mL), cooled to –78 °C, and treated with 2,6-lutidine (86.0 µL, 0.741 mmol) and TESOTf (77.0 µL, 0.342 mmol). Additional TESOTf (38.0 µL) was added to drive the reaction to completion. After quenching with H_2O, the solution was warmed to rt, extracted with EtOAc (3 x 10 mL), dried, filtered and concentrated. Flash column chromatography (5–10% EtOAc/hexanes) afforded the desired triethylsilyloxy sulfone (+)-**10** as a pale yellow oil [130 mg, 97% from (–)-**9**]: $[\alpha]_D$ +3.7 (c 4.7, $CHCl_3$); ^1H NMR ($CDCl_3$) δ 4.02 (m, 1H), 3.69 (dt, $J = 9.2, 6.0$ Hz, 1H), 3.30 (m, 2H), 3.03 (m, 2H), 2.10 (m, 2H), 1.97 (m, 1H), 1.39 (s, 9H), 1.03 (d, $J = 6.0$ Hz, 3H), 0.92 (t, $J = 8.0$ Hz, 9H), 0.90 (s, 3H), 0.53 (q, $J = 8.0$ Hz, 6H); ^{13}C NMR ($CDCl_3$) δ 77.7, 69.1, 65.8, 58.7, 57.0, 52.6, 43.3, 41.9, 40.7, 34.7, 24.9, 23.3, 23.1, 21.7, 18.1, 17.6, 14.2, 6.87, 4.86; IR (neat, cm^{-1}) 2949, 2874, 1456, 1371, 1304, 1281, 1166, 1116, 1079, 1018; HRMS: calcd for $C_{25}H_{50}O_4SSi$ – H 403.3121, found 403.3120.

Keto _gem_-Difluorinated Sulfone (–)-11. n-BuLi (0.976 mL, 1.6 M in hexanes) was added dropwise to a cold (–78 °C) solution of sulfone (+)-**10** (353 mg, 0.743 mmol) in THF (3.7 mL) and stirred 30 min. Then a solution of NFSI (492 mg, 1.56 mmol) in THF (7.8 mL) was added and the resulting solution warmed to rt over 1h. Upon aqueous workup, extraction (3 x 10 mL Et_2O), drying, and concentration, this procedure was repeated. The resulting yellow oil was filtered through a 1" plug of silica (Et_2O) and concentrated. A portion of the resulting syrup (102 mg) was dissolved in THF (5.0 mL), treated with TBAF (0.499 mL, 1.0 M in THF) for 16 h, concentrated, filtered through a 1" plug of silica (Et_2O) and concentrated to a pale yellow oil. A portion of this resulting oil (51 mg) was dissolved in CH_2Cl_2 (6.0 mL), treated with PDC and celite® (70 mg each) for 16 h, filtered through celite and concentrated to a brown oil. Flash column chromatography (15% EtOAc/hexanes) gave the desired _gem_-

difluorinated sulfone (−)-**11** as a white solid [35 mg, 65% from (+)-**10**]: mp 53–56 °C; [α]$_D$ −33.3 (c 2.2, CHCl$_3$); ^{1}H NMR (CDCl$_3$) δ 3.86 (dt, J = 9.4, 7.0 Hz, 1H), 3.52 (dt, J = 9.4, 7.0 Hz, 1H), 3.35–3.27 (m, 1H), 2.66–2.52 (m, 2H), 2.45 (dd, J = 11.4, 7.4 Hz, 1H), 2.32–2.16 (m, 3H), 1.52 (s, 9H), 1.11 (d, J = 6.0 Hz, 3H), 0.64 (s, 3H); ^{13}C NMR (CDCl$_3$) δ 212.0, 128.2 (t, J = 289 Hz), 77.8, 77.2, 63.2, 61.4, 60.0, 56.6, 49.7, 41.1, 38.7, 31.4 (t, J = 19.4 Hz), 25.0, 24.1, 19.3, 18.0, 12.9; ^{19}F NMR (CDCl$_3$) δ −96.8 (q, J = 19.8 Hz); IR (neat, cm^{-1}) 2962, 2876, 1713, 1371, 1321, 1225, 1184, 1134, 1105; HRMS: calcd for C$_{19}$H$_{32}$F$_2$O$_4$S + H 395.2067, found 395.2070.

20-Epi-22-oxa-25-difluoro-26-*tert*-butyl Sulfone Analogs 5a and 5b. Racemic phosphine oxide (±)-**12** (14) (70 mg, 0.12 mmol) was dissolved in 1.2 mL of THF and cooled to −78 °C under argon. To this solution was added 80 μL of *n*-BuLi (0.12 mmol, 1.53 M in hexanes) dropwise *via* syringe. The deep red solution was stirred for 1 h, at which time a cold (−78 °C) solution of C,D-ring ketone (−)-**11** (24 mg, 0.061 mmol) in 1.0 mL of THF was added dropwise *via* cannula. The resulting solution was stirred at −78 °C in the dark for approximately 3 h, then slowly warmed to −40 °C over 2 h. The reaction mixture was quenched with H$_2$O (1 mL), warmed to rt, extracted with Et$_2$O (3 x 10 mL), washed with brine, dried over MgSO$_4$, filtered, concentrated and purified by silica gel column chromatography (5–40% EtOAc/hexanes) to afford 43 mg of the coupled product as a clear oil. This oil was immediately dissolved in 3.0 mL of EtOH. To this solution was added 100 μL of an aqueous HF solution (49% wt) dropwise *via* syringe. The reaction mixture was stirred for 4 h in the dark, which, after general aqueous workup and column chromatography (75% EtOAc/hexanes), yielded 30 mg [93% from (−)-**11**] of a mixture of diastereomers **5a** and **5b**. This diastereomeric mixture was purified by reversed-phase HPLC (C-18 semipreparative column, 49% MeCN/H$_2$O, 3 mL/min) giving 10 mg (31%) of **5a** (1α, 3β, t_R 111 min) and 3.0 mg (9%) of **5b** (1β, 3α, t_R 105 min): **5a** (1α, 3β): [α]$_D$ −53.4 (c 9.0, CHCl$_3$); ^{1}H NMR (CDCl$_3$) δ 6.38 (d, J = 11 Hz, 1H), 5.99 (d, J = 11 Hz, 1H), 5.32 (m, 1H), 4.99 (m, 1H), 4.45–4.39 (m, 1H), 4.26–4.17 (m, 1H), 3.84 (m, 1H), 3.51 (m, 1H), 3.31 (m, 1H), 2.82 (dd, J = 16, 4.3 Hz, 1H 1H), 2.60 (m, 3H), 2.31 (dd, J = 18, 8.8 Hz, 1H), 1.52 (s, 9H) 1.09 (d, J = 5.6 Hz, 3H), 0.54 (s, 3H); ^{13}C NMR (CDCl$_3$) δ 147.6, 143.1, 132.8, 125.0, 116.9, 111.7, 78.6, 70.8, 66.8, 60.0, 56.6, 55.8, 45.8, 45.2, 42.8, 40.2, 31.5, 29.1, 25.1, 24.1, 23.5, 22.4, 18.1, 12.5; ^{19}F NMR (CDCl$_3$) δ −96.8 (quintet, J = 18.3 Hz); IR (neat, cm^{-1}) 3636–3104 (b), 2934, 2875, 1372, 1322, 1135, 1106, 1055, 755; HRMS: calcd for C$_{28}$H$_{44}$F$_2$O$_5$S 530.2878, found 530.2877; **5b** (1β, 3α): [α]$_D$ −55.0 (c 9.0, CHCl$_3$); ^{1}H NMR (CDCl$_3$) δ 6.40 (d, J = 12 Hz, 1H), 5.98 (d, J = 12 Hz, 1H), 5.31 (m, 1H), 5.00 (m, 1H), 4.44 (m, 1H), 4.23 (m, 1H), 3.85 (m, 1H), 3.52 (m, 1H), 3.31 (m, 1H), 2.82 (dd, J = 16, 4.3 Hz, 1H 1H), 2.59 (m, 3H), 2.29 (dd, J = 18, 8.8 Hz, 1H), 1.52 (s, 9H) 1.09 (d, J = 6.0 Hz, 3H), 0.54 (s, 3H); ^{13}C NMR (CDCl$_3$) δ 147.3, 143.2, 132.7, 125.0, 116.9, 112.5, 78.6, 71.4, 66.8, 60.1, 56.6, 55.8, 45.8, 45.5, 42.8, 40.2, 31.5, 29.1, 25.1, 24.1, 23.5, 22.4, 18.1, 12.6; ^{19}F NMR (CDCl$_3$) δ −96.8 (quintet, J = 18.3 Hz); IR (neat, cm^{-1}) 3789–3001 (b), 2943, 1370, 1321, 1134, 1107, 1058; HRMS: calcd for C$_{28}$H$_{44}$F$_2$O$_5$S 530.2878, found 530.2877.

Acknowledgment

We thank the NIH for support of this research (CA 44530 to G.H. Posner and T.W. Kensler, and DK 50583 to S. Peleg).

References and Notes

1. Feldman, D., Glorieux, F., Pike, J.W. *Vitamin D*, Academic Press, San Diego, CA, (1997).
2. Bouillon, R., Okamura, W. H., Norman, A. W. (1995) *Endocrine Reviews*, 16, 200-257.
3. Posner, G.H., White, M.C., Dolan, P., Kensler, T.W., Yukihiro, S., Guggino, S.E. (1994) *Bioorg. Med. Chem. Lett.*, 4, 2919-2924.
4. Posner, G.H., Wang, Q., Han, G., Lee, J.K., Crawford, K., Zand, S., Brem, H., Peleg, S., Dolan, P., Kensler, T.W. (1999) *J. Med. Chem.*, 42, 3425-3435.
5. Uskokovic, M. R., Studzinski, G. P., Gardner, J. P., Reddy, S. G., Campbell, M. J., Koeffler, H. P. (1997) *Curr. Pharm. Design*, 3, 99-123.
6. Posner, G.H., Crawford, K., Siu-Caldera, M.-L., Reddy, G.S., Sarabia, S.F., Feldman, D., van Etten, E., Mathieu, C., Gennaro, L., Vouros, P., Peleg, S., Dolan, P., Kensler, T.W. (2000) *J. Med. Chem.*, submitted.
7. Dilworth, F.J., Williams, G.R., Kissmeyer, A.-M., Nielsen, J.L., Binderup, E., Calverley, M.J., Makin, H.L.J., Jones, G. (1997) *Endocrinol.*, 138, 5485-5496.
8. Kensler, T.W., Dolan, P.M., Gange, S.J., Lee, J.-K., Wang, Q., Posner, G.H. (2000) *Carcinogenesis*, 21, No. 7, in press.
9. Hatakeyama, S., Ikeda, T., Irie, H., Izumi, C., Mori, H., Uenoyama, K., Yamada, H., Nishizawa, M. (1995) *J. Chem. Soc., Chem. Commun.*, 1959-1960.
10. Posner, G.H., Nelson, T.D., Guyton, K.Z., Kensler, T.W. (1992) *J. Med. Chem.*, 35, 3280-3287.
11. Posner, G. H., Lee, J. K., Wang, Q., Peleg, S., Burke, M., Brem, H., Dolan, P., Kensler, T. W. (1998) *J. Med. Chem.* 41, 3008-3014.
12. Suffert, J. (1989) *J. Org. Chem.* 54, 509-510.
13. Aberkane, O., Mieloszyndki, J. L., Robert, D., Born, M., Paquer, D. (1993) *Phosphorus, Sulfur, and Silicon*, 79, 245-256.
14. Posner, G. H., Dai, H. (1994) *Synthesis*, 1383-1398.

CONSTITUTIONAL AND CONFORMATIONAL ISOMERS OF 1α,25-DIHYDROXYVITAMIN D₃ AND ITS METABOLITES

William H. Okamura*, Steven Do*, Hoim Kim*, Edwin Tan*, Fook Tham*,
S. Jeganathan*, Miguel Ferrero*, and Anthony W. Norman[#]

Department of Chemistry* and Department of Biochemistry[#],
University of California, Riverside, California 92521, USA

Introduction. The steroid hormone 1α,25-dihydroxyvitamin D_3 (**1**, 1,25-D3) is a highly conformationally dynamic steroid hormone (1). As shown by the 13 curved arrows in the top panel of Figure 1, this hormone can assume an infinite array of topologies by carbon-carbon single bond (conformational) rotations. This dynamic flexibility is also characteristic of other metabolites (middle panel of Figure 1) such as vitamin D_3 (**3**, D3), 25-hydroxyvitamin D_3 (**4**, 25-D3) and 24R,25-dihydroxyvitamin D_3 (**5**, 24R,25-D3). This paper focuses on studies of conformational snapshots of the chair-chair equilibrium characteristic of the A-ring, but most particularly on the matter of the 6,7-single bond orientation of the seco-B ring. Attempts to mimic conformational 'snapshots' of these rotamers have focussed on chemically synthesized constitutional isomers of 1,25-D3. The constitutional isomers of interest are molecules with the same molecular formula as 1,25-D3 but have different atom connectivities and are neither conformational isomers nor configurational (stereo) isomers.

The most well known constitutional isomer of 1,25-D3 is 1α,25-dihydroxyprevitamin D_3 (**2**, 1,25-PreD3), also known as analog **HF** (Figure 1, middle panel) (2). The equilibrium formation of **HF** almost certainly occurs via a reversible antarafacial [1,7]-sigmatropic hydrogen shift (3) involving the intermediate 6-s-cis conformer of 1,25-D3, namely **1'** (2a). In solution, 1,25-D3 is believed to exist almost entirely (>99%) as 6-s-trans- 1,25-D3 (**1**) (4) wherein its 6,7-single bond rotamer 6-s-cis-1,25-D3 (**1'**) is spectroscopically invisible. Nevertheless, the latter (**1'**) must be present in kinetically competent amounts since it mediates the known equilibration of **1** (95%) with **2** (5%) (2a).

There are a large number of other constitutional isomers of 1,25-D3. We deal in this paper with only the eight selected constitutional isomers **6** to **12** (Figure 1, lower panel) as well as 1,25-PreD3 (**2**, **HF**) shown in the upper panel. It should be noted that in the Riverside laboratories, one or two letter codes (**C**, **HF**, **JB**, etc) are used to additionally identify analogs and metabolites to avoid cumbersome systematic chemical names. The analog **JB** results from the treatment of **HF** with catalysts such as iodine while analogs **JN** and **JM** results from photochemical irradiation of the same precursor **HF** (2e). In contrast, vinylallene analogs **JV** and **JW** (5) as well as the suprasterol analogs **8** and **9** are known skeletal types previously recognized as photoisomers of the parent D3 (**3**) and, in part, 25-D3 (**4**) (6).

The Solid State Conformation of Vitamin D. X-ray crystallographic studies (7) have nicely provided snapshots of specific vitamin D conformers and, in all cases, the sterically more stable 6-s-trans conformer has been observed, typicallly within ± 10° of planarity (Figures 2 and 3). A highly interesting finding is that both D3 and the related vitamin D_2 (D2, shown as a line drawing in Figure 3) crystallize as a 'pseudo-homo-dimer' wherein a 1:1 hydrogen bonded complex of opposite chair forms of the A-ring, the so called α-chair with an equatorial 3-hydroxyl and the β-chair with an axial orientation of the same hydroxy, are observed (7a-c). The metabolite

25-D3 however crystallizes only as the α-chair conformer (7d). In stark contrast, the parent hormone 1,25-D3 crystallizes with its A-ring in just the opposite chair, the β-chair (7e). The 'extra' hydroxyl of 1,25-D3 at the C-1 position is equatorial.

Figure 1. Conformational isomerism of 1,25-D3 (top panel), metabolic pathway leading to 1,25-D3 and its tautomerism to 1,25-PreD3 (middle panel), and the structures of selected constitutional isomers of 1,25-D3 (bottom panel).

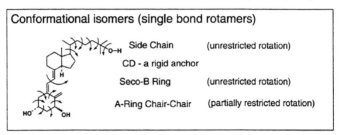

Figure 2. X-Ray Crystallographic Snapshots of Vitamin D Conformers

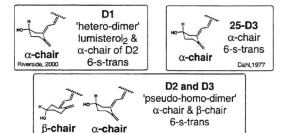

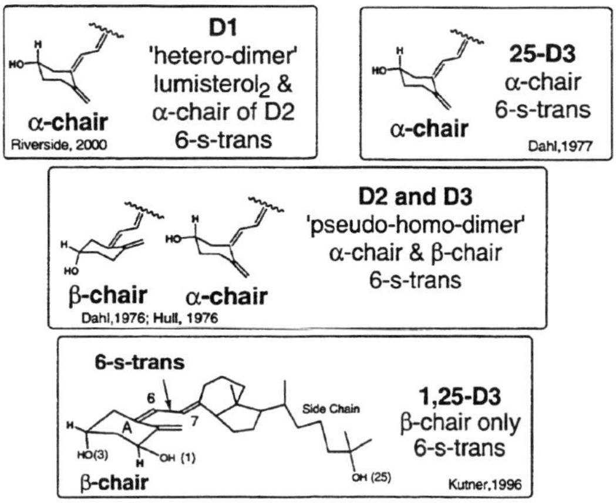

A historically fascinating finding is that the very first anti-rachitic factor, vitamin D₁ (D1), proved to be a mixture of two compounds. In 1931, Windaus (8) first identified this substance as a sharp melting solid but this substance was later shown to be a mixture of two photoproducts of ergosterol, namely D2 and lumisterol₂ (Lumi2) whose line bond formulas are shown in Figure 3. Recently, the subtleties of the conformational features of D1 was established by this laboratory through single crystal x-ray investigations of material produced by co-crystallization of a mixture of Lumi2 and D2. Unlike the pseudo-homo-dimeric crystal structure of D2 alone, the D2 portion of D1 exists only as an α-chair. This fills in a missing gap in the detailed structural understanding of the calciferols.

Figure 3. Vitamin D₁ (Windaus, 1931) is a 1:1 heterodimer containing a vitamin D₂ α-chair and a lumisterol₂. Note that in the x-ray structure (panel), the A-ring of D2 is oriented upside down, just the opposite that shown in Figure 2.

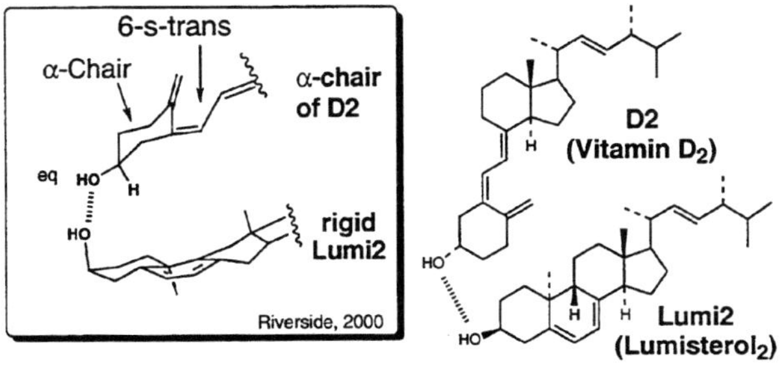

The Solution Structure of Vitamin D. The solution structures of vitamin D compounds have been most extensively studied by NMR spectroscopy (1c). Figure 4 depicts schematically the now well known α-chair / β-chair equilibrium for the A-ring of D3 (and also for D2 and 25-D3). Our laboratory as well as the LaMar group at the University of California, Davis reported in 1974 that the ratio of these A-ring conformers in solution was 55/45 (4a-c). Studies in other laboratories later revealed that in more polar, hydroxylic solvents, this ratio shifts to ~85/15, favoring the α-chair (9). Our laboratory has recently shown (1c, 10) that in SDS-micelles, this equilibrium shifts essentially completely to the α-chair. This medium dependence is not seen for the natural hormone 1,25-D3 (Figure 5) wherein the A-ring is distributed between near

Figure 4. Vitamin D3: the A-ring α- and β-chair ratio is medium dependent, but invariably 6-s-trans. In SDS-micelles (water), D3 exists only in the α-chair conformer. There are differences in organic solvents as follows: ethanol or methanol solution--85/15 α / β ratio (Havinga, DeLuca); chloroform solution--55/45 α / β ratio (Riverside, Davis)

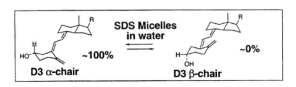

equimolar amounts of conformers irrespective of non-polar (chloroform) or polar (methanol) solvents, or even in micelles. However, it has been suggested by Eguchi and Ikekawa (8c) that the β-chair is replaced by a half-chair conformer at low temperatures in methanol. Thus, the A-ring distribution of conformers is dynamic and quite different from that in the solid state. Regarding the seco-B conformation, the 6,7-single bond orientation is 6-s-trans and planar within experimental error of NMR measurements of vicinal scalar coupling constants.

Figure 5. 1,25-D3 consists of a ~1:1 ratio of A-ring conformers and is invariably 6-s-trans. The ratio of A-ring conformers is essentially independent of medium including SDS-micelles. A half-chair conformer has been detected.

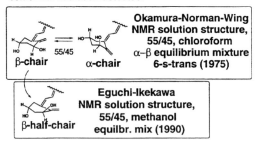

The Solid State Structure of 1,25-D3 Bound to the VDR-LBD. In 1974, we proposed (4d) that the hormone 1,25-D3 requires the 1α-hydroxyl equatorial chair conformer (the β-chair) for optimal biological activity. This was based on the finding that dihydrotachysterol₃ (DHT), one of four diasteromeric '10,19-dihydrovitamin Ds', was the most biologically active stereoisomer. DHT was shown by NMR spectroscopy (4a,e, f) to contain the highest population of the β-conformer (with its pseudo-1α-hydroxyl equatorially oriented) as in the recent x-ray structure of 1,25-D3 bound to its nuclear receptor. In a seminal paper, the Strasbourg group (11) has recently reported the first x-ray crystallographic study of a vitamin D ligand bound to protein, namely that of 1,25-D3 bound to a nuclear vitamin D receptor-ligand binding domain protein (VDR-LBD). The solid state structure (Figure 6, upper panel) of a doubly truncated 118-425(Δ[165-215]) VDR-LBD revealed that the ligand exhibited some of the same conformational features as the free ligand itself (Figure 2, lower panel). Most notably, the A-ring assumes the β-chair conformer both in the bound and free states (11a, 7e). There were notable differences. Key differences include the northerly orientation of the side chain and the ~30° twisted 6-s-trans conformation of the intercyclic diene that connects the A- and C-rings in the VDR-LBD structure. An edge on view (upper panel of Figure 6) reveals a 'bowl' shaped structure with the A-ring and side chain tilted upwards with the bottom of the bowl being the CD ring plane.

Figure 6. The Rochel et al (2000) x-ray structure of the 1,25-D3, 118-425(Δ[165-215]) VDR-LBD (upper panel) reveals an A-ring in the β-chair conformation with the 1-OH equatorial and the 3-OH axial, a "330°" (-30°) twisted 6-s-cis conformation of the seco-B ring and a northerly orientation of the side chain. The oxygen-1 to the oxygen-25 distance is 12.99 angstrons. The lower panels compare molecular mechanics displays (PC Model, Serena Software) including several key structural parameters for two constitutional isomers of 1,25-D3, Analogs JB and JN.

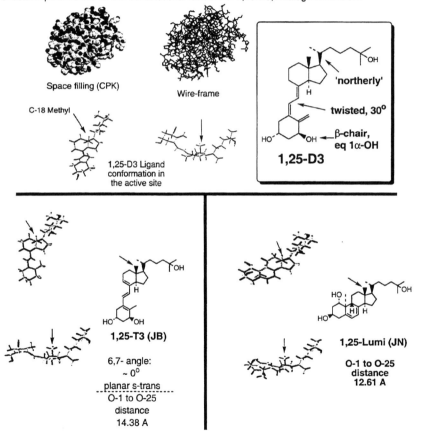

It is known that 1,25-D3 fully exerts both genomic and rapid actions (1a). We earlier reported that the 6-s-cis conformationally locked mimics (**HF** and **JN**) of the 6-s-cis conformer of 1,25-D3 (see Figure 1) are as active as the natural hormone 1,25-D3 in stimulating its rapid actions (2). The behavior of **HF** and **JN** as conformationally locked mimics of a 'spectroscopically invisible' conformer (**1'** in Figure 1) was intriguing and suggested studies of other constitutional isomers (lower panel, Figure 1). It was also intriguing that **HF** and **JN** exhibited weak genomic actions and that the 6-s-trans locked analog **JB** exhibited neither genomic nor rapid actions (2e). These observations collectively suggested the possibility that a twisted 6-s-cis conformer of 1,25-D3 might be responsible for genomic actions and a more planar 6-s-cis conformer of this same hormone was responsible for rapid actions. On the contrary, the Strasbourg crystallographic result suggests that a 6-s-trans (albeit twisted) conformer is responsible for genomic actions. In an elegant evaluation (11a), the Strasbourg group attributes the genomic inactivity of **JB** (2e) to the inability of this analog to twist across the 6,7-bond (because of the presence of the planar double bond at this position). The lower left panel of Figure 6 gives an energy minimized, molecular mechanics (12) representation of **JB** (using the same CD side chain orientation as in the x-ray structure (PDB file 1DB1)). In addition to the Strasbourg explanation, we note with interest that the distance between oxygen-1 (C-1 OH) and O-25 (C-25 OH) are quite different for 1,25-D3 (~13 angstroms) and **JB** (14.4 angstroms). This provides an alternative rationale for the lack of a genomic effect observed for **JB**. The lower right panel of Figure 6 depicts a similar energy minimized structure (12) of **JN**. The residual genomic effect observed (2e) for this 6-s-cis locked conformational mimic is difficult to rationalize but it is interesting to note that the O-1 to O-25 distance for **JN** (12.6 angstroms) is not all that dissimilar to that for 1,25-D3 (13 angstroms). This would however require some conformational 'wiggle' room in the active site of the VDR-LBD. Although the shape of **JN** is quite different from that of the receptor bound form of 1,25-D3 (Figure 6), further attempts should be made to assess the ability of **JN** to dock into the active site of the VDR-LBD (13).

Vinylallenes and Suprasterols as Orthogonal 6,7-Rotamer Mimics of 1,25-D3. Figure 7 is a circle diagram whose perimeter corresponds to the 6,7-torsion angle from 0 to 360 degrees as the A-ring is rotated clockwise about the 6,7-bond with the CD ring stationary. The captions inside the circle point to specific compounds and their experimental or predicted 6,7 single bond torsion angles. For example, the planar 6-s-trans angle found for free 1,25-D3 by NMR (4a, 4b) and by x-ray crystallography (7e) corresponds to snapshot #1 and has been arbitrarily set to 0°.

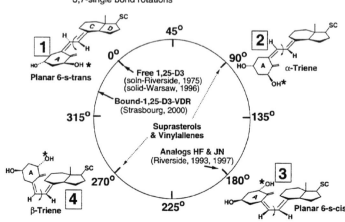

Figure 7. 1,25-D3: Snapshots of conformers via 6,7-single bond rotations

This position also corresponds to the biologically impotent analog **JB** (2e). A 180° clockwise rotation of the 6,7-single bond leads to snapshot position #3, the planar 6-s-cis conformer of 1,25-D3. A slightly twisted s-cis planar form corresponds to that found in the 6-s-cis analogs **HF** and **JN**. It seems that 180° analogs are selective for the rapid actions of 1,25-D3. It also appears that since the Strasbourg crystal structure of 1,25-D3 bound to the VDR-LBD resides at the counterclockwise 6-s-trans 330° position, this angle should correspond to analogs with selective genomic actions. It became intriguing to consider two other extreme snapshot analogs, namely vitamin D compounds that might mimic 90° and 270° topologies #2 and #4, respectively. We have identified two types of analogs which might fulfill this requirement, namely suprasterols and vinylallenes.

Suprasterols and vinylallenes are well known photoproducts in the D3 and D2 series (Figure 8) (6), but prior to our work they were unknown in the 1,25-D3 series (5, 10). The major photoproducts of D3 are suprasterol-I$_3$ (S-I) and suprasterol-II$_3$ (S-II), but the equally desirable topologically related compounds 6β-vinylallene$_3$ (6β-VA or S-III) and 6α-vinylallene$_3$ (6 α-VA or S-IV) are produced in impractical amounts as evidenced by the low yields shown (Figure 8). As summarized in Figure 9, an efficient, convergent synthesis of 1,25-6β-VA (**11**, analog **JV** in Figure 1) and 1,25-6α-VA (**12**, analog **JW** in Figure 1) has been reported by this laboratory (5). Like **HF** and **JN**, **JV** and **JW** are constitutional isomers of 1,25-D3. We have shown that all possible geometric isomers of 1,25-D3 including the parent hormone can be accessed from these 1,25-vinylallenes as well (5). The two vinylallene stereoisomers can be converted to 1,25-S-I and 1,25-S-II in a completely new synthetic route as illustrated for the more easily available 1,25-vinylallene **11** (analog **JV**). Oxidation of **11** afforded via selective allylic oxidation the vinylallenone **13**. The latter in turn undergoes a triplet sensitized photoisomerization to a mixture of suprasterol ketones **14** and **15**. We have speculated that this isomerization proceeds via a C-H insertion reaction of an intermediate cyclopropylcarbene (10). Sodium borohydride reduction of either suprasterol ketone affords carbon-1 epimeric mixtures of the 1,25-S-I or 1,25-S-II, with the desired 1α-isomer being the minor stereoisomer as expected. Efforts are underway to improve the stereoselectivity of this reduction.

Figure 8. UV radiation of vitamin D$_3$ produces six constitutional isomers and one stereoisomer (Windaus, Dauben, Havinga and others).

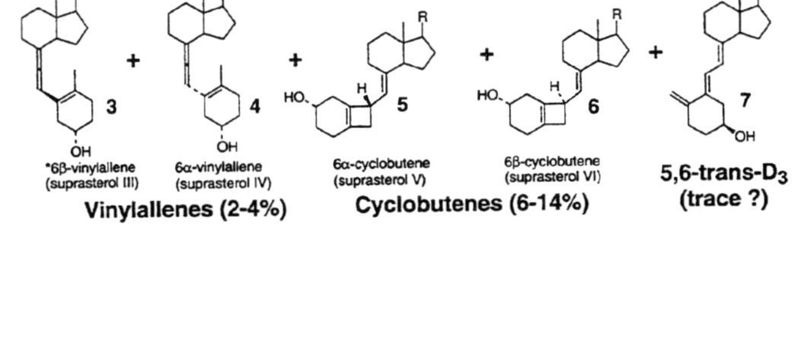

18

Figure 9. Suprasterols and Vinylallenes, 90° and 270° conformationally locked mimics of 1,25-D3, have been synthesized in a convergent route from separate CD and A-ring fragments. The suprasterols of all of the main metabolites of vitamin D are available by direct photochemical irradiation of D3, 25-D3 and 1,25-D3.

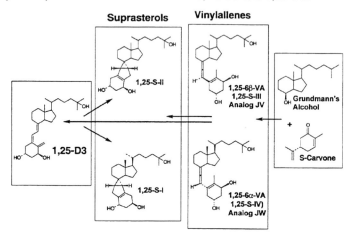

Figure 10. Synthesis of 1,25-Suprasterols from a vinylallenone

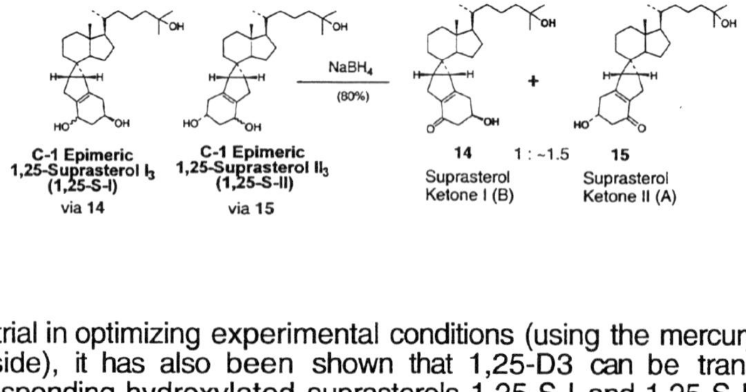

After some trial in optimizing experimental conditions (using the mercury lamps available in Riverside), it has also been shown that 1,25-D3 can be transformed directly to the corresponding hydroxylated suprasterols 1,25-S-I and 1,25-S-II (lower panel of Figure 11). Prior to these optimization studies, we carried out extensive photochemical optimization studies of the parent D3 similar to those depicted in Figure 8 (6) and our results are summarized in the upper panel of Figure 11. Our focus was entirely directed towards optimization of the production of S-I and S-II so no attempt

Figure 11. Direct photolysis of D3, 25-D3 and 1,25-D3 lead to suprasterols I and II.

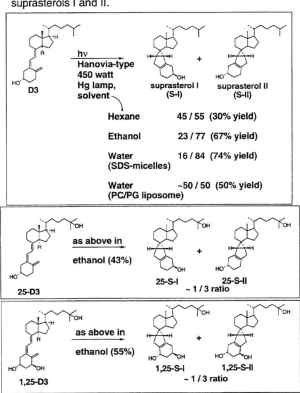

Figure 12. Analogs **JW** and **JV** resemble the 90° and 270° rotamer snapshots, respectively (the left pair of panels), of 1,25-D3. The hormone 1,25-D3 possesses a relative competitive index (RCI) of 100 (by definition) for both chick intestinal VDR binding as well as for human serum vitamin D carrier protein (DBP) binding. Vinylallenes bind poorly to the nuclear VDR but bind effectively to the serum DBP when compared to 1,25-D3. Binding is enchanced for the 1-deoxy analog series.

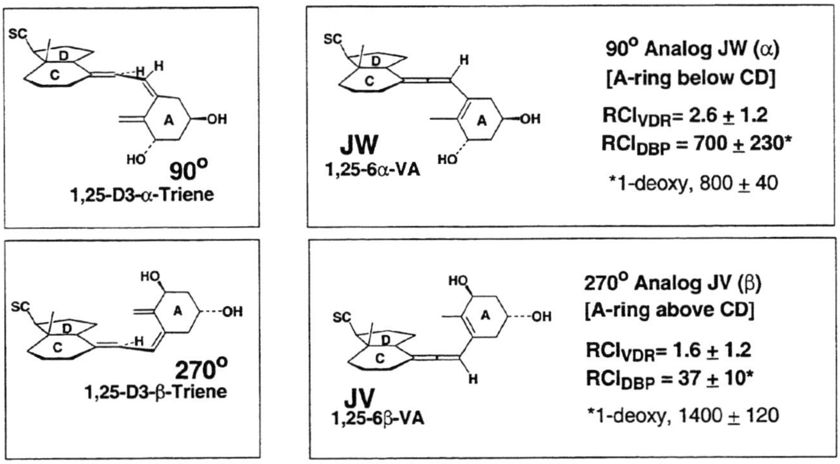

was made towards quantifying the minor photoproducts. It is evident that the highest stereoselectivity and yield was obtained using D3 in SDS-micelles in water (recall from Figure 4 that the D3 A-ring exists as a single chair conformer). However, the most practical results were obtained using ethanol as solvent. Similar results were obtained with 25-D3 leading to 25-S-I and 25-S-II (middle panel, Figure 11), which has been previously reported (14).

As summarized in Figure 12, neither the 90° nor the 270° analogs, **JW** and **JV**, respectively, bound the chick intestinal VDR particularly well, although somewhat more effectively than did the 0° analog **JB** (RCI_{VDR} = 0.0046 $\pm$ 0.019). By contrast, **JV** and particularly **JW** had good affinity towards human DBP in comparison to 1,25-D3 (15). A casual inspection of drawings, or a more detailed comparison of Dreiding molecular models, of **JW** and **JV** with the corresponding 90° twisted snapshots of 1,25-D3 (compare the left hand panel of structures with those to the immediate right in Figure 12) reveals a less than perfect match. In spite of this mismatch, it is remarkable that these vinylallenes whose A-ring is forced perpendicular to the CD ring bind so effectively to DBP.

By contrast to the vinylallenes, molecular modeling reveals that the suprasterols represent better topological mimics of the 90° and the 270° rotamers of 1,25-D3 (Figure 13). 1,25-S-II (**10**) seems to be a particularly good conformationally locked mimic of the carbon skeleton of the 270° snapshot of 1,25-D3; 1,25-S-I (**9**) would appear to match up slightly less effectively with the carbon skeleton of the 90° snapshot of the hormone. It would also appear however that repositioning of the 1α- and 3β-hydroxyls of 1,25-S-II to the 2α- and 4β-positions would render the match even better. It remains for future experiments to evaluate the potential of these perpendicular snapshot analogs.

Figure 13 1,25-S-II resembles the 270° rotamer snapshot of 1,25-D3 (1,25-S-I is not as similar to the 90° rotamer)

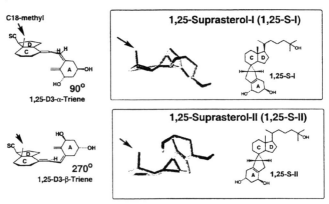

Summary. Constitutional isomers of 1,25-D3 may serve as useful snapshots of higher energy conformers of the hormone for structure-function studies. The utility of some of these analogs as biochemical research tools has already been demonstrated. These include, for example, **HF** (1,25-PreD3), **JN** (1,25-Lumi), **JM** (1,25-DHC), and

JB (1,25-T3). Effective synthesis routes to 1,25-vinylallenes (**JV** and **JW**) have previously been developed in our laboratories and now all of the suprasterols related to D3, 25-D3, and 1,25-D3 have become available. It is anticipated that the 1,25-vinylallenes (**JV** and **JW**) and the 1,25-suprasterols (1,25-S-I and 1,25-S-II) will also provide useful structure-function information. Structural studies such as the recent solution of the detailed D1 structure will continue along other areas.

Acknowledgments

This work was supported by United States Public Health Service Grants DK-16595 (to W.H.O) and DK-09012 (to A.W.N.), and an Omnibus UCR Academic Senate Grant (to W.H.O.),. We also acknowledge Cambridge Isotopes Laboratory, Hoffmann-LaRoche, Leo Pharmaceuticals and Solvay Pharmaceuticals for generous gifts of chemicals. This paper includes the combined content of an invited lecture (W.H.O.) and a poster presentation (S.D.). We thank the Advisory Committee of the 11th Vitamin D Workshop for this opportunity. Finally, we are most grateful to Professor M. Mark Midland for providing advice (12) on the molecular modeling aspects of this project.

References

(1) (a) Bouillon, R., Okamura, W. H., and Norman, A. W. (1995) Endocrine Reviews **16**, 200-257. (b) Zhu, G.-D., and Okamura, W. H. (1995) Chemical Reviews **95**, 1877-1952. (c) Okamura, W. H., and Zhu, G.-D. "Vitamin D" (1997) (Feldman, D.; Glorieux, F. H.; Pike, J. W., eds.); Academic Press: Chapter 57.

(2) (a) Curtin, M. L., and Okamura, W. H., (1991) J. Am. Chem. Soc., **113**, 6958-6966. (b) Okamura, W. H., Midland, M. M., Hammond, M. W., Abd. Rahman, N., Dormanen, M. C., Nemere, I., and Norman. A. W. (1995) J. Steroid Biochem. Molec. Biol. **53**. 603-613. (c) Norman, A. W., Okamura, W. H., Farach-Carson, M. C., Allewaert, K., Branisteanu, D., Nemere, I., Muralidharan, K. R., and Bouillon, R. (1993) J. Biol. Chem., **268**, 13811-13819. (d) Nemere, I., Dormanen, M. C., Hammond, M. W., Okamura, W. H., and Norman, A. W. (1994) J. Biol. Chem. **269**, 23750-23756. (e) Norman, A. W., Okamura, W. H., Hammond, M. W., Bishop, J. E., Dormanen, M. C., Bouillon, R., van Baelen, H., Ridall, A., Daane, E., Khoury, R., and Farach-Carson, M. C. (1997) Molec. Endrocin. **11**, 1519-1531.

(3) Hoeger, C. A., Johnson, A. D., and Okamura, W. H., (1987) J. Am. Chem. Soc., **109**, 4690-4698.

(4) (a) Wing, R. M., Okamura, W. H., Pirio, M. R., Sine, S. M., and Norman, A. W. (1974) Science, **186**, 939-941. (b) Wing, R. M., Okamura, W. H., Rego, A., Pirio, M. R. and Norman, A. W. (1975) J. Am. Chem. Soc., **97**, 4980-4985. (c) LaMar, G. N. and Budd, D. L. (1974) J. Am. Chem. Soc., **96**, 7317-7324. (d) Okamura, W. H., Norman, A. W., and Wing, R. W. (1974) Proc. Natl. Acad. Sci. USA, **71**, 4194-4197. (e) Okamura, W. H., Hammond, M. L., Rego, A., Norman, A. W., and Wing, R. M. (1977) J. Org. Chem., **42**, 2284-2291. (f) Mourino, A. and Okamura, W. H. (1978) J. Org. Chem., **43**, 1653-1656.

(5)   Van Alstyne, E. M., Norman, A. W. and Okamura, W. H. (1994) <u>J. Am. Chem. Soc.</u>, **116**, 6207-6216.

(6)   (a) Havinga, E. (1973) <u>Experientia</u>, **29**, 1181-1316. (b) Windaus, A., Gaede, J., Köser, J. and Stein, G. (1930) <u>Justus Liebigs Ann. Chem.</u> **483**, 17-30. (c) Dauben, W.G. and Baumann, P. (1961) <u>Tetrahedron Lett.</u> 565-572. (d) Westerhof, P. and Keverling Buisman, J.A. (1956) <u>Rec. Trav. Chim.</u> **75**, 1243-1251. (e) Saunderson, C.P. and Crowfoot Hodgkin, D. (1961) <u>Tetrahedron Lett.</u> 573-578. (f) Bakker, S.A., Lugtenburg, J. and Havinga, E. (1972) <u>Rec. Trav. Chim.</u> **91**, 1459-1464. (h) Kobayashi, T., Yoshimoto, S. and Yasumura, M. (1977) <u>J. Nutr. Sci. Vitaminol.</u> **23**, 291-298. (l) Dauben, W.G. and Kellogg, M.S. (1972) <u>J. Am. Chem. Soc.</u>, **94**, 8951-8953.

(7)   (a) Trinh-Toan, DeLuca, H. F. and Dahl, L. F. (1976) <u>J. Org. Chem.</u>, **41**, 3476-3478. (b) Hull, S. E., Leban, I., Main, P., White, P. S. and Woolfson, M. M. (1976) <u>Acta Cryst.</u> **B32**, 2374-2381. (c) Leban, I., DeGraaff, R. A. G., DeGelder, R., Turkenburg, J., Wilson, K. S. and Dauter, Z. (1994) <u>Interline Pub.</u> Bangalore, India. **111**, 43-51. (d) Trinh-Toan, Ryan, R. C., Simon, G. L., Calabraese, J. C. and Dahl, L. F. (1977) <u>J.C.S. Perkin II.</u>, 393-401. (e) Suwinska, K. and Kutner, A. (1996) <u>Acta Cryst.</u> **B52**, 550-554.

(8)   (a) Windaus, A., Lüttringhaus, A. and Deppe, M. (1931) <u>Ann.</u> **489**, 252. (b) Askew, F. A., Bourdillon, R. B., Bruce, H. M., Callow, R. K., Philpot, J. St. L. and Webster, T. A. (1932) **B109**, 488-506.

(9)   (a) Helmer, B., Schnoes, H. K and DeLuca, H. F. (1985) <u>Archives of Biochem. Biophys.</u> **241**, 608-615. (b) Gielen, J. W. J. (1981) Ph.D. Thesis. State University of Leiden, Leiden, The Netherlands. (c) Eguchi, T. and Ikekawa, N. (1990) <u>Bioorg. Chem.</u> **18**, 19-29.

(10)   Okamura, W. H., Do, S., Kim, H., Jeganathan, S., Vu, T., Zhu, G-D. and Norman, A. W. (2000) <u>Steroids</u> (in press).

(11)   (a) Rochel, N., Wurtz, J. M., Mitschler, A., Klaholz, B. and Moras, D. (2000) **5**, 173-179. (b) Juntunen, K., Rochel, N., Moras, D. and Vihko, P. (1999) <u>Biochem. J.</u> **344**. 297-303.

(12)   PC Model, Serena Software.

(13)   Norman, A . W., Adams, D., Collins, E. D., Okamura, W. H. and Fletterick, R. J. (1999) <u>J. Cellular Biochem.</u> **74**, 323-333.

(14)   Vroom, E. M. and Jacobs, H. J. C. Vitamin D: Gene regulation, structure-function analysis and clinical application. (1991) (Norman, A. W., Bouillon R., Thomasset, M., eds); Walter de Gruyter and Co., Berlin. 196-197.

(15)   Bishop, J. E., Collins, E. D., Okamura, W. H., and Norman, A. W. (1994) <u>J. Bone and Mineral Res.</u> **9**, 1277-1288.

DEVELOPMENT OF CD-RING MODIFIED ANALOGS OF 1α,25(OH)₂D₃ WITH CONSTRAINED SIDE-CHAIN ORIENTATION.

Pierre De Clercq[a], Xiaoming Zhou[a], Gui-Dong Zhu[a], Stefan Gabriëls[a], Y.-J. Chen[a], Ibrahim Murad[a], Dirk Van Haver[a], Maurits Vandewalle[a], Annemie Verstuyf[b], Roger Bouillon[b].
[a] Department of Organic Chemistry, Ghent University; [b] Laboratorium Experimental Medicine and Endocrinology (LEGENDO), KULeuven, Belgium.

Introduction The last decade has witnessed a very active search for analogues of 1α,25-dihydroxyvitamin D₃ (**1**, further abbreviated as 1,25(OH)₂D₃), the hormonally active form of vitamin D (1). Next to its classical calciotropic activity, 1,25(OH)₂D₃ (**1**) has been shown to possess immunosuppressive activity, to inhibit cellular proliferation and to induce cellular differentiation. Its therapeutic utility in the treatment of certain cancers and skin diseases is however limited since effective doses provoke calcemic side effects such as hypercalcemia, hypercaliuria and bone decalcification. This has stimulated the development of analogues of the natural hormone in which the calcemic activity and the antiproliferative and/or prodifferentiating activities are dissociated (2). In this context various successful structural modifications have already been introduced, such as e.g. 19-*nor* (3), 22-oxa (4), 23-yne (5), 20-*epi* (**2**) (6) derivatives and combinations thereof. Whereas above modifications are located in the flexible parts of the molecule, i.e. the side-chain and the A-ring, our laboratory has focussed in recent years on the development of analogues that vary in the structure of the central CD-ring system (7). A typical example is analogue **3**, the structure of which is characterized by the absence of the six-membered C-ring and by the presence of an enlarged D-ring, so a formal 8,9-*seco*-9,11-bis*nor*-15-*homo* derivative (7f). For the sake of simplicity and clarity we will further use "6D analogues" as descriptive term. Furthermore, the carbon atoms of the modified vitamin D skeleton will be referred to according to the conventional steroid numbering.

Table 1. Selected biological activities of **1-3**.[a]

Entry	Binding		Differentiation	Calcium
	VDR(pig)	DBP (human)	HL-60	Ca serum (mice)
1	100	100	100	100
2	88	0.2	3000	800
3	125	80	90	4

[a] The activities are presented as relative values, the reference value of $1,25(OH)_2D_3$ (**1**) being defined as 100%.

The comparison of some relevant biological activities for compounds **1-3** shown in Table 1 illustrates the possibility of discrimination of the various actions of vitamin D. It is hereby striking how with similar affinities for the vitamin D receptor (VDR), the 20-epimer **2** is several orders of magnitude more potent than the natural hormone **1** both in prodifferentiating and calcemic activity, whereas 6D analogue **3** is much less calcemic.

Results The present study fits into a project aiming at the development of analogues possessing side-chains with biased spatial orientations. In particular 6D analogues **4** are presented here so that, depending on the relative orientation of the methyl substituents at C13 and C16, the side-chain at C17 would adopt different and distinct conformations. The three selected configurations **a,b** and **c** constrain the mobility in the segment C17-C20-C22 in a way that is further illustrated below. For each of these configurations is (are) shown the preferred conformation(s) on the basis of: (1) a chair conformation for the six-membered D-ring possessing the two larger substituents on C14 and C17 in equatorial position; (2) the four-carbon C17- C20-C22-C23 chain adopting conformations in which steric interactions are minimized, in particular in which *syn*-pentane interactions are avoided.

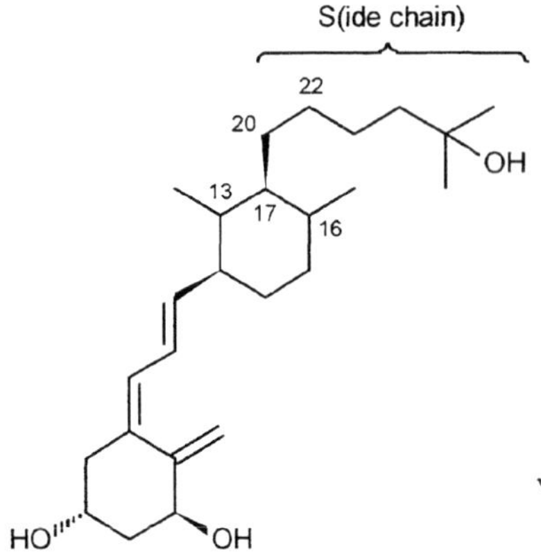

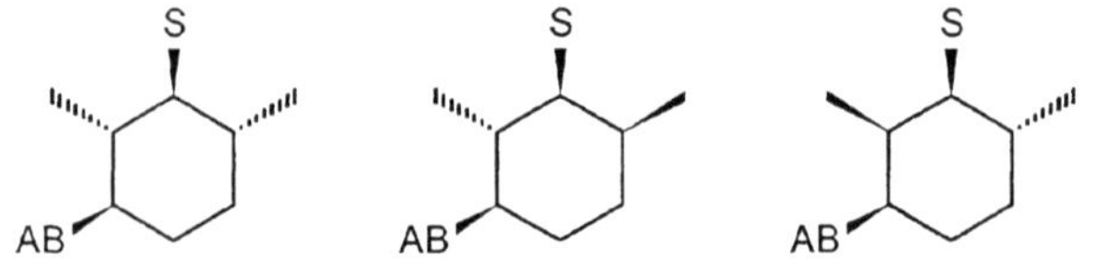

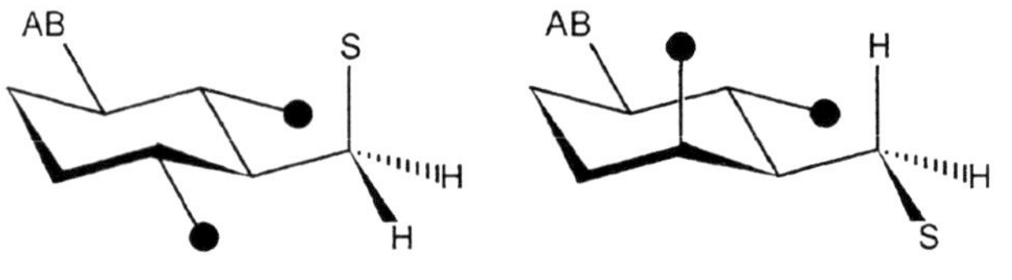

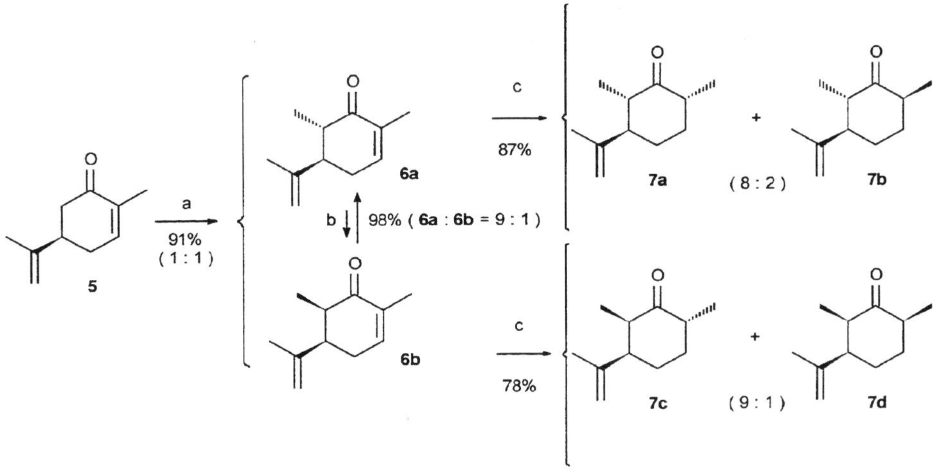

Scheme 1. Reaction conditions: a) LDA, THF; MeI, DMPU. b) NaOMe, MeOH-THF. c) Na₂S₂O₄, Adogen 464, NaHCO₃, toluene-H₂O.

The enantioselective preparation of analogues **4a,4b** and **4c** is outlined in the synthetic Schemes 1-4 (8). The introduction of the methyl group at C13 involves a classical alkylation reaction on (R)-(-)-carvone (**5**) which led to a separable 1:1 mixture of **6a** and **6b** (Scheme 1). The configurational assignment of both isomers at this stage follows from the observation that isomerization in base (sodium methoxide) leads to an equilibrium mixture in favor of the more stable isomer **6a** (**6a:6b** = 9:1) (9). Further conjugate reduction of **6a** and **6b** with sodium dithionite under phase transfer conditions led to mixtures of ketones **7** in which diastereomers **7a** and **7c**, respectively, predominate (10). The confirmation of the configuration of the three required ketones **7a**, **7b** and **7c** follows from inspection of the ¹H NMR spectral data.

The introduction of the ethoxycarbonylmethyl substituent with the required configuration at C17 (cf. **13**) is performed in two stages (Scheme 2): appendage of the two-carbon chain as α,β-unsaturated ester (**8a**, **11b** and **12c**, respectively), followed by dissolving metal reduction to afford esters **13a**, **13b** and **13c**, respectively (11). Whereas the direct Peterson olefination proved unsuccessful, a two-stage process involving addition of the Grignard derivative derived from ethoxyethyne, followed by sulfuric acid hydrolysis, afforded the required unsaturated derivatives (12). In the case of **7a** this reaction led to a separable 1:1 mixture of the desired unsaturated ester **8a** (as an unseparable E,Z-mixture) and the tertiary alcohol **9a**. Elimination of the latter through subsequent formation of the corresponding acetate **10a** led to a further portion of **8a**. In contrast with the a-series, reaction of **7b** and of **7c** directly led to the desired unsaturated ester derivatives in a single isomeric form, i.e. E-**11b** and Z-**12c**, respectively. Again the configurational assignment of both compounds rests on the detailed analysis of the relevant ¹H NMR spectral data. It is symptomatic how in both cases the ester group has lodged itself in the open space that is available through the axial disposition of one of the methyl groups. The subsequent conjugate reduction of the α,β-unsaturated esters **13** proved quite instructive. Indeed, whereas the lithium-liquid ammonia reduction led in each series selectively to the more stable diastereomer, i.e. **13a**, **13b** and **13c**, respectively, the magnesium in methanol reduction afforded in each case a mixture of **13** and **14**, the two possible stereoisomers at C17.

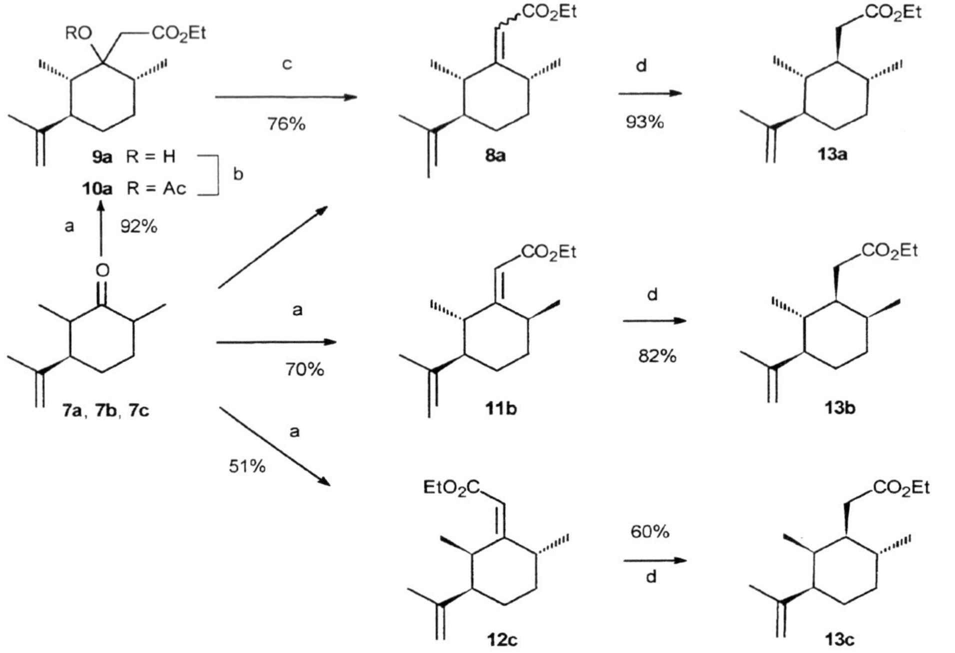

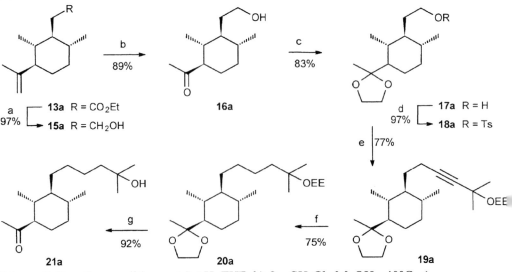

9a R = H
10a R = Ac
a 92%
b
7a, 7b, 7c
c 76%
8a
d 93%
13a
a 70%
11b
d 82%
13b
a 51%
12c
60% d
13c

<u>Scheme 2:</u> a) Ethoxyethynyl-MgBr, toluene-THF; dil. H$_2$SO$_4$, THF. b) AcCl, PhNMe$_2$, CHCl$_3$. c) KO*t*Bu, *t*BuOH. d) Li, l.NH$_3$, *t*BuOH, Et$_2$O.

13a R = CO$_2$Et
a 97%
15a R = CH$_2$OH
b 89%
16a
c 83%
17a R = H
d 97%
18a R = Ts
e 77%
19a
f 75%
20a
g 92%
21a

<u>Scheme 3.</u> Reaction conditions: a) LAH, THF. b) O$_3$, CH$_2$Cl$_2$-MeOH, -40°C. c) HO(CH)$_2$OH, HC(OMe)$_3$, *p*TsOH. d) *p*TsCl, CH$_2$Cl$_2$, Et$_3$N, DMAP. e) NaH, DMSO; OEE-protected 2-methyl-3-butyn-2-ol, DMSO. f) 5% Rh-Al$_2$O$_3$, H$_2$, EtOAc. g) PPTS, acetone-H$_2$O.

The followed sequence for the further conversion of esters **13a**, **13b** and **13c** into the corresponding ketones **21a**, **21b** and **21c** is described in detail for the **a**-series (Scheme 3). After reduction of ester **13a** to the corresponding alcohol **15a**, oxidative cleavage (ozone in dichloromethane-methanol) of the propenyl double bond led to ketone **16a**. After protection of the carbonyl through acetalisation to **17a** and conversion of the alcohol to the corresponding tosylate **18a**, substitution with the sodium salt of 2-methyl-3-butyn-2-ol, protected as ethoxyethyl ether, afforded alkyne **19a** in good yield (13). Catalytic hydrogenation to **20a**, followed by acid hydrolysis, further led to methyl ketone **21a**.

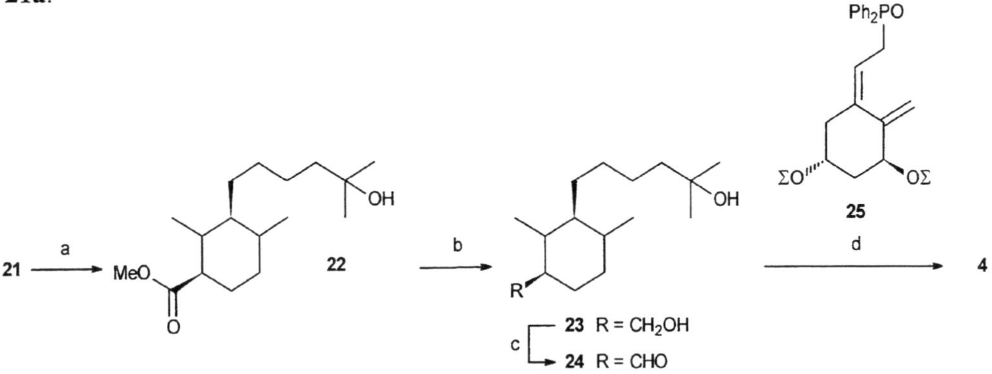

Scheme 4: Reaction conditions: a) NaBr, MeOH, Pt-electrode, 20-30 V. b) LAH, THF. c) PCC, CH$_2$Cl$_2$. d) nBuLi, **25**, THF; TBAF.

The final conversion of the methyl ketones **21a**, **21b** and **21c** into the vitamin D analogues **4a**, **4b** and **4c**, respectively, is outlined in Scheme 4. The transformation of ketone **21** into the required aldehyde **24** for subsequent attachment of the *seco*-B,A-ring portion of the vitamin D molecule involved three steps: (1) the electrochemical oxidation of **21** into ester **22** (14), (2) lithium aluminumhydride reduction to **23**, and (3) oxidation with pyridinium chlorochromate supported on alumina to **24** (15). The first step is the electrochemical variant of the classical bromoform reaction: two platinum electrodes are immersed in a solution of ketone **21** and of sodium bromide as electrolyte in methanol and submitted to a 20-30 V tension. For reasons that remain unclear, in the **a**-series the yield was deceivingly low: 28% of **22a**, compared to 46% of **22b** and 76% of **22c**. Finally, treatment of the aldehydes **24a**, **24b**, and **24c** with the anion derived from the known phosphine oxide **25** (16), followed by in situ silylether deprotection with tetrabutylammonium fluoride (TBAF), led to the analogues **4a**, **4b** and **4c** in fair yield.

The biological evaluation of analogues **4a-c** includes the determination of (1) the binding affinity for the porcine intestinal VDR, (2) the antiproliferative activity in vitro on breast cancer MCF-7 cell, (3) the cell-differentiating activity in vitro on a leukemic HL-60 cell line, and (4) the calcemic activity in vivo in vitamin D-replete normal NMRI mice. Results are shown in Table 2. The 6D analogue **4a** displayed 20% of the VDR affinity compared to 1,25 (OH)$_2$D$_3$. The two epimers **4b** and **4c** demonstrated only 2% of the affinity for the VDR. The 6D analogue **4a** has equipotent prodifferentiating activity when compared with the activity of 1,25(OH)$_2$D$_3$ on HL-60 cells while this analogue was 2 times more potent to inhibit the proliferation of MCF-7 cells. **4b** and **4c** were less potent to inhibit the MCF-7 cell proliferation or to stimulate the HL-60 cell differentiation compared to 1,25 $(OH)_2D_3$ whereas both analogues had poor calcemic effects in vivo (< 0.25% compared to 1,25$(OH)_2D_3$).

Table 2. Selected biological activities of **4a-c**.[a]

Entry	Binding	Cell differentiation and proliferation		Calcium
	VDR(pig)	HL-60	MCF-7	Ca serum (mice)
1	100	100	100	100
4a	20	90	200	4
4b	2	9	30	<0.25
4c	2	8	70	<0.25

[a] The activities are presented as relative values, the reference value of 1,25$(OH)_2D_3$ (**1**) being defined as 100%.

When vitamin D expresses its activity via the genomic pathway. the hormone binds with the intracellular vitamin D receptor (VDR) so as to regulate gene transcription and the synthesis of new proteins that are more directly responsible for the biological response. In view of this mechanism the geometry of the VDR-1,25$(OH)_2D_3$ complex is crucial. Until recently, no precise information about the active shape of the hormone was known because of problems encountered in obtaining a detailed crystal structure of the liganded nuclear receptor (17). So indirect means had to be developped. The determination of the active shape of the vitamin D hormone is intrinsically difficult because of its flexible nature. Indeed, flexible ligands are known to undergo substantial distortions away from their preferred geometry in order to achieve optimal binding with the receptor. Since a greater preorganization of the active geometry is expected to result in enhanced binding, it is logical to conceive analogues that are characterized by reduced mobility in the flexible parts of the molecule. With regard to the side chain this may consist in constraining one or several of the rotatable carbon-carbon bonds along the C17-C25 chain. Whereas this goal can be achieved by the introduction of unsaturated moieties within the side chain, a more subtle way may consist in changing the substitution pattern in this part of the molecule. The present work has been performed in this particular context. Central in this and related work is the use of conformational maps to describe the preferred geometries of the side chain. The concept of dot maps in this area was first introduced by Okamura and Midland (18). In this approach force field calculations are performed so as to generate within a given energy window all possible local minimum energy conformations that the side chain may adopt. The orientation in space of each found conformation is further defined by a dot that corresponds to the position of the 25-oxygen atom in that particular conformation. Subsequently, volume maps have been used in our laboratory in order to optimize the visualization aspect of the procedure (19).

Volume maps corresponding to the side-chain conformations of **4a-c** are presented in Figure 1. Note that these have been generated for model derivatives that lack the A-ring. From inspection of the figure it is readily apparent that with each configuration **a**, **b** and **c** fits a specific and different side-chain orientation. Prior to this work four conformationally restricted 22-methyl substituted analogues of $1\alpha,25(OH)_2D_3$ (**1**), diastereomeric at C20 and C22, have been studied by Yamada *et al*, with the aim of studying the three-dimensional structure of vitamin D that is involved in the binding to the receptor (20). Interestingly, one among those was found to posses a markedly higher binding affinity for the VDR; moreover, the same diastereomer was substantially more potent than the natural hormone **1** in inducing differentiation of HL-60 cells. In a more recent study dealing with structure-function relationship as related to the orientation of the side chain, the same group identified particular regions, the preferred occupation of which by the 25-hydroxy group would correspond with increased cell-differentiating potency (21). Following this active space group concept five main regions designated as A, G, EG, EA and F were indentified and a correlation was proposed between the cell-differentiating potency of numerous analogues and the regions in space occupied by the vitamin D side-chain. As an important result it was observed that the preferred side-chain orientations of almost all potent analogues were distributed among the EA region. This region corresponds fairly well with the relative activity volume that was generated on the basis of the conformational profiles of the most and least active diastereomers among the four 22-methyl substituted analogues developped by Yamada. The applied procedure has been described in detail (19). The occupation of this volume by the 25-hydroxy group of the side chain was calculated to correspond to 63%, 6% and 5% for **4a**, **4b** and **4c**, respectively. It is also interesting to note that the biological activity of the 6D analogue **3** is quite similar to the one observed for **4a**, in particular the differentiation of HL-60 cells and calcemic activity are identical (7g). Furthermore, the conformational profile of the side chain **3** is analogous to the one calculated for **4a**; in particular the occupation of the same relative activity volume by the 25-hydroxy group of **3** corresponds to 69%. This further confirms the existence of a (qualitative) correlation between side-chain orientation and cell-differentiating potency.

References

(1) See the nine volumes of the consecutive Proceedings of Vitamin D Workshop; Walter De Gruyter: Berlin, 1974-1997.
(2) R. Bouillon, W. Okamura, A. W. Norman, Endocrinol Rev. 1995, 16, 200-257.
(3) K. L. Perlman, R. R. Sicinski, H. K. Schnoes, H. F. DeLuca, Tetrahedron Lett. 1990, 31, 1823-1824.
(4) J. Abe, T. Nakano, Y. Nishii, T. Matsumoto, E. Ogata, K. Ikeda, Endocrinology 1991, 129, 832-837.
(5) S. J. Yung, Y. Y. Lee, S. De Vos, E. Elstner, A. W. Norman, J. Green, . Uskokovic, H. P. Koeffler, Leuk. Res. 1994, 101, 713-718.

(6)   L. Binderup, S. Latini, E. Binderup, C. Bretting, M. Calverley, K. Hansen, Biochem. Pharmacol. 1991, 42, 1569-1575.

(7)   a) R. Bouillon, P. De Clercq, P. Pirson, M. Vandewalle, Novel Structural Analogues of Vitamin D. Patent PCT/EP 93.202037.3; priority date 09-07-1993; b) K. Sabbe, C. D'Halleweyn, P. De Clercq, M. Vandewalle, R. Bouillon, A. Verstuyf, Bioorg. Med. Chem. Lett. 1996, 6, 1697-1702; c) G.-D. Zhu, Y. Chen, X. Zhou, M. Vandewalle, P. J. De Clercq, R. Bouillon, A. Verstuyf, Bioorg. Med. Chem. Lett. 1996, 6, 1703-1708; d) Y. J. Chen, P. De Clercq, M. Vandewalle, Tetrahedron Lett. 1996, 37, 9361-9364; e) Y. Wu, C. D'Halleweyn, D. Van Haver, P. De Clercq, M. Vandewalle, Bioorg. Med. Chem. Lett. 1997, 7, 923-928; f) B. Linclau, P. De Clercq, M. Vandewalle, Bioorg. Med. Chem. Lett. 1997, 7, 1461-1468; g) A. Verstuyf, L. Verlinden, S. Ling, Y. Wu, C. D'Halleweyn, D. Van Haver, G.-D. Zhu, D. Zhu, Y. Chen, X. Zhou, H. Van Baelen, P. De Clercq, M. Vandewalle, R. Bouillon, J. Bone Miner. Res. 1998, 13, 549-558; h) X. Zhou, G.-D. Zhu, D. Van Haver, M. Vandewalle, P. J. De Clercq, A. Verstuyf, R. Bouillon, J. Med. Chem. 1999, 42, 3539-3556; i) A. Verstuyf, L. Verlinden, E. Van Etten, L. Shi, Y. Wu, C. D'Halleweyn, D. Van Haver, G.-D. Zhu, Y.-J. Chen, X. Zhou, M. R. Haussler, P. De Clercq, M; Vandewalle, H. Van Baelen, C. Mathieu, R. Bouillon, J. Bone Miner. Res. 2000, 15, 237-252.

(8)   For a comprehensive review on synthetic strategies in the vitamin D area, see: G.-D. Zhu, W. Okamura, Chem. Rev. 1995, 95, 1877-1952.

(9)   a) R. M. Cory, R. M. Renneboog, J. Org. Chem. 1984, 49, 3898-3904; b) J.-P. Gesson, J.-C. Jacquesy, B. Renoux, Tetrahedron 1989, 45, 5853-5866; c) T. K. M. Shing, Y. Tang, Tetrahedron 1990, 46, 2187-2194.

(10)   F. Camps, J. Coll, J. Guitart, Tetrahedron 1986, 42, 4603-4609.

(11)   For the application of a similar strategy in a related project, see: S. Gabriëls, D. Van Haver, M. Vandewalle, P. De Clercq, D. Viterbo, Eur. J. Org. Chem. 1999, 1803-1809.

(12)   G. E. Arth, G. I. Poos, R. M. Lukes, F. M. Robinson, W. F. Johns, M. Feurer, L. H. Sarett, J. Am. Chem. Soc. 1954, 76, 1715-1722.

(13)   A. Fuerst, L. Labler, W. Meier, Helv. Chim. Acta 1982, 65, 1499-1521.

(14)   G. Nikishin, M. N. Elison, I. Makhova, Tetrahedron 1991, 47, 895-905.

(15)   Y. S. Cheng, W. L. Lin, S. Chen, Synthesis 1980, 223.

(16)   E. G. Baggiolini, J. A. Incobelli, B. M. Hennesy, A. D. Batcho, J. F. Sereno, M. R. Uskokovic, J. Org. Chem. 1986, 51, 3098-3108.

(17)   N. Rochel, J. N. Wurtz, A. Mitschler, B. Klaholz, D. Moras, Molecular Cell 2000, 5, 173-179.

(18)   a) W. H. Okamura, J. A. Palenzuela, J. Plumet, M. M. Midland, J. Cell. Biochem. 1992, 49, 10-18; b) M. M. Midland, J. Plumet, W. H. Okamura, Bioorg. Med. Chem. Lett. 1993, 3, 1799-1804.

(19)   D. Van Haver, P. J. De Clercq, Bioorg. Med. Chem. Lett. 1998, 8, 1029-1034.

(20)   K. Yamamoto, W. Y. Jun, M. Ohta, K. Hamada, H. F. DeLuca, S. Yamada, J. Med. Chem. 1996, 39, 2727-2737.

(21)   S. Yamada, K. Yamamoto, H. Masuno, M. Ohta, J. Med. Chem. 1998, 41, 1467-1475.

SYNTHESIS AND ANTITUMOR ACTIVITY OF 1,25(OH)$_2$-23E-ENE-26,27F$_6$-19-NOR-20-CYCLOPROPYL VITAMIN D$_3$, RO 27-0574

M.R. Uskokovic', P. Manchand, M. Koike, K. Koshizuka, H. Kawabata, R. Yang, H. Taub, J. Said, N. Tsuruoka and H.P. Koeffler
Hoffmann-La Roche, Inc., Nutley, N.J. and Cedars-Sinai Research Center, Los Angeles, C.A.

Structural modifications of 1α,25-Dihydroxy vitamin D$_3$ [1,25(OH)$_2$D$_3$] have been systematically investigated with main focus on improvement of its cancer cell growth inhibitory activity and induction of cancer cell differentiation. Significant improvement of these activities has been accomplished by optimization of the side chain configuration using the structural modifications at C$_{17}$ and C$_{20}$ positions, i.e., insertion of C$_{16}$-C$_{17}$ double bond (1), or inversion of the configuration at C$_{20}$ position (2). Further improvements resulted from prevention of the side chain degradation initiated by metabolic hydroxylations at C$_{23}$, C$_{24}$ and C$_{26}$. This was accomplished by incorporation of C$_{23}$ and C$_{24}$ into double or triple bonds, and by the replacement of C$_{26}$ and C$_{27}$ hydrogens with fluorine. Additional gain in these activities have been attained by prevention of the inactivating metabolic 3-epimerization using the 19-nor ring A modification. An assembly of all these structural changes of the 1,25(OH)$_2$D$_3$ molecule has produced one of the most potent analog, 1α,25-dihydroxy-16,23E-diene-26,27-hexafluoro-19-nor vitamin D$_3$ (Ro 25-9022). This analog is 10 to 10,000 times more active than 1,25(OH)$_2$D$_3$ in induction of HL-60 myeloid leukemia cells differentiation, and growth inhibition of MCF-7 and ZR-75 breast cancer cell lines, and prostate cancer cell lines LNCaP, PC-3 and DU-145.

Scheme 1

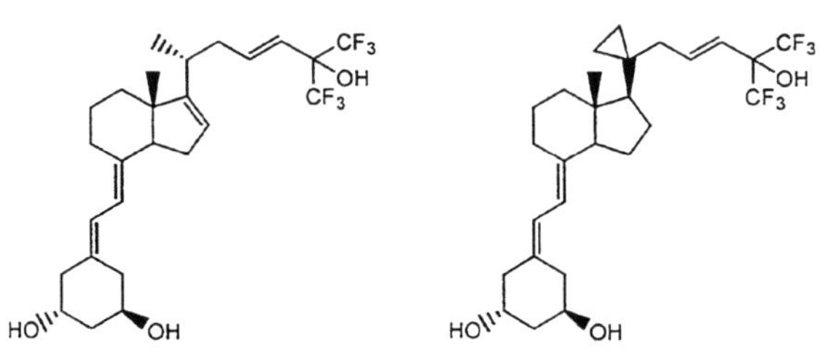

Ro 25-9022   Ro 27-0574

Subsequently we investigated other modifications that were meant to optimize the side chain configuration of 1,25(OH)$_2$D$_3$ in respect to antiproliferative and cell differentiation activities. One of these modifi-cations involved installation of the cyclopropyl group at C$_{20}$. This has produced the analog 1,25-dihydroxy-23E-ene-26,27-hexafluoro-19-nor-20-cyclopropyl vitamin D$_3$, Ro 27-0574 (3), exhibiting a similar activity profile to that of Ro 25-9022 (Scheme 2).

Scheme 2

	ED$_{50}$ (M) HL-60 cells Differentiation		ED$_{50}$(M) Cell Growth Inhibitory activity			
			MCF-7	LNCaP	PC-3	DU-145
1,25(OH)$_2$D$_3$	8×10^{-9}		1×10^{-7}	NR	8×10^{-7}	NR
Ro 25-9022	3×10^{-10}		3×10^{-10}	2.5×10^{-11}	7.5×10^{-10}	1×10^{-9}
Ro 27-0574	2×10^{-10}		4×10^{-10}	3×10^{-10}	9×10^{-10}	8×10^{-7}

NR indicates that no ED$_{50}$ was reached with 1×10^{-7}M concentration.

Effect on the cell cycle of LNCaP prostate cancer cell was determined after a 72 hour exposure to 10^{-7}M Ro 27-0574. An increase in the G$_0$/G$_1$ phase of the cell cycle from 72% to 88% occurred with a concomitant decrease in the percent of cells in S phase from 22% to 6%. CDK inhibitors p21^{Wafl} and p27^{Kip1} levels in LNCaP cell line increased by several folds after exposure to the 10^{-7}M of analog Ro 27-0574 for 3 days (3).

The 1,25(OH)$_2$D$_3$ response element (VDRE) was placed in front of a thymidine kinase promoter of the reporter gene CAT. This construct was transfected into PC-3 cells. In the absence of the analog Ro 27-0574, almost no CAT activity was detected. The analog increased CAT activity in a dose dependent manner. At 10^{-7}M Ro 27-0574 CAT activity increased 12.5 fold (3).

Three groups of 5 mice each received 300 rads whole body irradiation prior to being bilaterally, s.c. injected with 3×10^6 PC-3 cells/tumor in 0.1 ml matrigel. One group of mice served as control. The two other groups received Ro 27-0574 analog intraperitonealy every other day, 0.005 µg/mouse and 0.01 µg/mouse, except Saturday and Sunday, for six weeks. Administration of Ro 27-0574 retarded tumor growth for 40%. Tumors in control group showed infiltrating poorly differentiated adenocarcinoma, until tumors from the mice that received Ro 27-0574 were almost entirely necrotic with scattered nuclear fragments. The analog did not elevate serum calcium (3).

Synthesis of Ro 27-0574 starts from the Inhoffen Lythgoe diol **1** which is converted to the allylic alcohol **4** via an *ene* extension of the elimination product **3** with formaldehyde. The allylic alcohol **4** is then efficiently converted to the cyclopropyl alcohol **5**. A completion of the full length side chain proceeds via aldehyde **6** and acetylene **7**, and incorporates hexafluoroacetone at the final stage **7 - 8**. Triple bond is reduced stereospecifically to the *trans* double bond **9**, and the remainder of the synthesis followed a standard procedure for making the 19-nor vitamin D$_3$ analogs as shown in Scheme 3.

Scheme 3

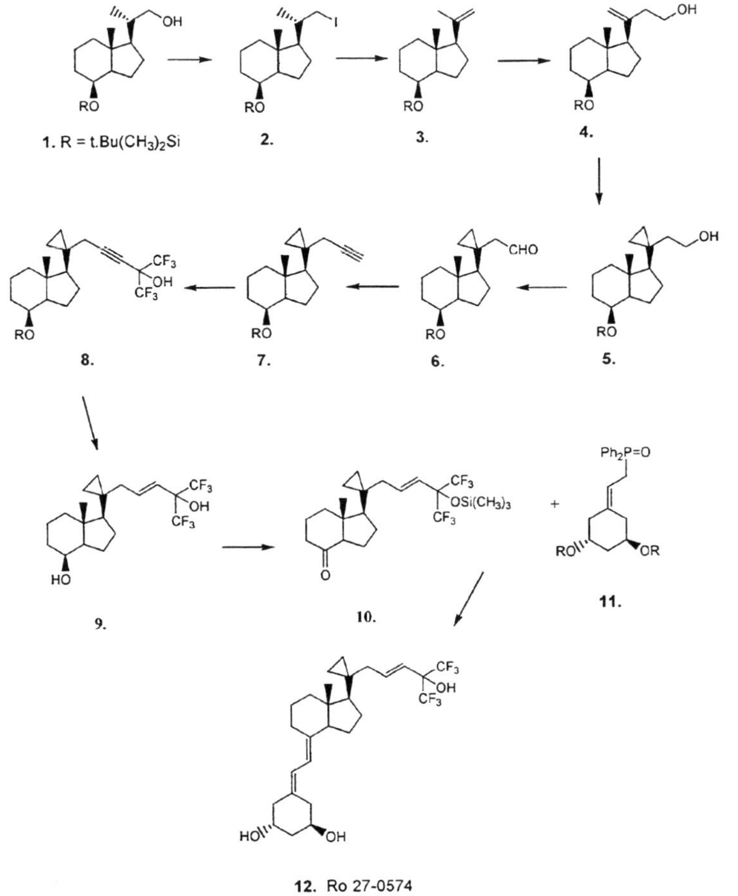

12. Ro 27-0574

REFERENCES:

(1)   Uskokovic', M.R., Studzinski, G.P., and Reddy, S.G. (**1997**) *Vitamin D*, Edited by D. Feldman, F.H. Glorieux, and J.W. Pike. Academic Press 1045-1070.

(2)   Binderup, L., Latini, S., Binderup, E., Bretting, C., Calverley, M., and Hansen, K. (**1991**). *Biochem. Pharmacol.* 42, 1569-1575.

(3)   Koike M., Koshizuka, K. Kawabata, H., Yang, R., Taub, H.E., Said, J., Uskokovic', M., Tsuruoka, N., and Koeffler, H.P. (**1999**). *Anticancer Res.* 19, 1689-1698.

STUDIES ON ANALOGS OF 1α,25-DIHYDROXY-VITAMIN D₃ LACKING A CHIRAL CENTER AT C-20: STEREOSELECTIVE SYNTHESES OF THE NEW 17(20)-DEHYDRO-DERIVATIVES

M. J. Calverley, F. Björkling, L. K. A. Blæhr, C. Bretting, G. Grue-Sørensen, and W. von Daehne   Department of Medicinal Chemistry, Leo Pharmaceutical Products, DK-2750 Ballerup, Denmark

The recently published crystal structure of the VDR LBD with its bound natural ligand (1), reveals an active side chain conformation of calcitriol (1) that is also accessible to the 20-epimer (2). On the other hand, limited protease digestion studies (2) (in which the bound ligands stabilize different fragments of the receptor) suggest that the side chains of the 20-normal and 20-epi compounds have different contact sites within the LBD, and that a unique location for the hydroxyl group is therefore not a requirement for receptor activation. Indeed there is evidence that the receptor-active "double side chain" analog (3), containing both the normal *and* the 20-epi side chains in one molecule (3,4), interacts differently from either 1 or 2 (3). In one attempt to restrict the conformational freedom of the side chains in 3 we formally tied them together by incorporation into a strain-free cyclohexane, thereby essentially locking the locus of the 25-*O*. These simplest "re-converging" double side chain analogs (the *cis* and *trans* isomers of 21,24-methano-1α,25-dihydroxyvitamin D₃, 4, **MC 2108**, and **MC 2110**, *respectively*) (5) were however markedly less potent than the parent compounds 1, 2, and 3 in a cell proliferation test, indicating that an agonistic LBD interaction of the side chain hydroxyl group is essentially "locked out" in these "snapshot" versions of side chain geometries accessible to both the normal and epi parents (1 and 2).

In further pursuit of analogs having an active, but at the same time conformationally restricted, side chain, we have considered other simple modifications that like compounds 3 and 4 lack a chiral center at C-20. The 17(20)-dehydro derivatives 5 and 6 which fall into this category, present two, quite different, fixed C-22 locations together with fewer degrees of rotational freedom for the calcitriol side chain (6). An indication that the 17Z series would indeed be biologically active is to be found in the report by one of us on a series of 22-yne analogs including the first 17(20)-ene calciferols (7). The 17(20)-dehydro-side chain of cholesterol itself in both its *E* and *Z* configurations (8,9), and the *Z*-configurated 25-hydroxy-cholesterol side chain in tetracyclic steroidal intermediates for vitamin D synthesis (10,11) have been described in the literature. There is thus ample precedence for the establishment of the tetra-substituted olefin moiety in 5 and 6. One common method is dehydration of a tertiary C-20 alcohol. This dehydration reaction had been shown in the cholesterol series to be non-selective (giving in fact the undesired

20(22)E-ene as the major product). This is in contrast to the situation in the 22-yne series (7), where largely the 17Z-17(20)-ene was produced. The difficulty of separating the regio- and stereo-isomers encountered in all these cases prompted us to look for stereoselective approaches.

In connection with work on a 16-ene series of calcitriol analogs, an efficient route to the aldehyde intermediate 7 was devised (12). We argued that base treatment, under conditions used for the equilibration of the 20-formyl-seco-pregnane ("protected vitamin D C$_{22}$-

7   NaOH, TBA$^+$Br$^-$ / H$_2$O, CH$_2$Cl$_2$, r.t. / 1 h / E:Z = 1:19   8

aldehydes") (13), the 16-ene would migrate into conjugation with the carbonyl function, and this was indeed the case. An unanticipated and welcome benefit of this reaction was the high Z-selectivity encountered. Apparently the stereoselectivity is a result of kinetic control, since the E-isomer (in experiments performed on the model compound (11), vide infra) was found to be stable under the same conditions. With the key intermediate 8 in hand, the way was open to a series of 17(20)Z-ene vitamin D analogs. For the synthesis of the parent title compound in this series (6), the key step in the elaboration of the 25-hydroxylated side chain was displacement of an allylic ester function with the requisite Grignard reagent. The use here of pivalate as leaving group is a modification to the original conditions (acetate) (14) for this copper-catalyzed coupling method employed by us in order to minimize deacylation (attack of Grignard on the carbonyl), a major competing reaction for this evidently sterically hindered substrate. The remainder of the synthesis (triplet-sensitized photo-isomerization and deprotection) followed our well-established protocol (15).

Although limited amounts of the corresponding intermediates in the 17(20)E-series were available from aldehyde 7, a stereoselective synthesis of the other title compound (5) was desirable. For this purpose we adapted the methodology worked out for the synthesis of 17(20)E-dehydro-cholesterol (9), but in order to facilitate entry into the vitamin D seco-sterol series, we elected to work on CD-ring (des-AB-ring) intermediates. A key to the success of this sequence is the isolation of the epimerically pure cyanohydrin (9) after acid-catalysed deprotection of the 20R-O-trimethylsilyl ether, formed kinetically with high (Felkin-Anh) diastereoselectivity. Dehydration under the literature conditions then afforded the E-nitrile (10) as the only product. After DIBAL reduction (with hydrolytic work-up) to the key intermediate, aldehyde 11, the construction of the side chain proceeded as before. Completion of the synthesis of (5) followed the Hoffmann-LaRoche protocol involving Horner-Wittig coupling (of 12) with the ring-A building block (13) (16).

Biological screening of the 17(20)-ene derivatives **5** and **6** revealed that both the receptor binding and the potent *in vitro* (cancer cell proliferation) and *in vivo* (elevation of calcium excretion in normal rats) activities of calcitriol reside only with the Z-isomer (**6**), suggesting that an active conformation of the side chain is excluded in the *E*-isomer (**5**). Molecular modeling studies (17) indicate a high degree of conformational flexibilty for the side chains (approx. 110 conformers, with their associated "parking zones" for the side chain oxygen, within a 3 kcal/mol energy window from the global minimum for each analog), with a distribution both above and below the "plane" of the CD-ring system. Selective destabilization of particular accessible regions in other systems has been achieved by incorporating a substituent (oxy (18,19) or methyl (20)) on C-22. To investigate this effect (if any) in the 17(20)Z-ene series, the aldehyde (**8**) was treated with organometallic reagents to generate the epimeric 22-hydroxy-compounds which were separated by chromatography. The NMR-spectra of the two series of epimers showed significant diagnostic differences. Thus, in the *more polar* series. the 18-H_3 singlet consistently appeared 0.06-0.07 ppm up-field of the corresponding signal in the less polar series; and, in the ^{13}C-NMR, C-17 resonated 1.2-1.8 ppm down-field. The conclusion is that one and the same C-22 configuration is associated with this series. That this configuration is in fact *R* was proven by chemical correlation of the **14**, R= Me compound in the more polar series, *via* the ketone derived by ozonolysis of the *tert-*

38

butyldimethylsilylated side chain. This ketone had the *opposite* optical rotation (α_D^{20} = +7.1°) to the compound derived from ethyl *S*-lactate (21) The vitamin D analogs derived in the more polar series were found to be the more active. Molecular modeling studies indicate a parallel with the published studies on 20-normal and 20-epi series, the "active" configuration of the 22-substituent selectively destabilizing the conformations associated with the below-plane orientation of C-23 and *vice versa*. Indeed, structures very close in energy to the refined global minimum for the compound **15** can be aligned closely with the "active" conformer of calcitriol extracted from the Moras structure (1)

We thank Drs. L. Binderup, C. Mørk Hansen, P. Kaae Holm and M. Winkel Madsen for the biological screening.

References

1. Rochel, N., Wurtz, J. M., Mitschler, A., Klaholz, B., and Moras, D. (2000) *Mol. Cell* **5**, 173-179
2. Liu, Y., Collins, E. D., Norman, A. W., and Peleg, S. (1997) *J. Biol. Chem.* **272**, 3336-3345
3. Uskokovic, M. R., Manchand, P. S., Peleg, S., and Norman, A. W. (1997) in *Vitamin D* (Norman, A. W., Bouillon, R., and Thomasset, M. eds) pp. 19-21, University of California, Riverside (Calif.)
4. Kurek-Tyrlik, A., Makaev, F. Z., Wicha, J., Zhabinskii, V., and Calverley, M. J. (1997) in *Vitamin D* (Norman, A. W., Bouillon, R., and Thomasset, M. eds) pp. 30-31, University of California, Riverside (Calif.)
5. Calverley, M. J. (1999) First International Conference on Chemistry and Biology of Vitamin D Analogs,September 26-28, Providence, R.I., USA; *Steroids*, in press
6. For the synthesis of 21-nor-**5** and -**6**, see: Martinez Perez, J. A., Sarandeses, L., Granja, J., Palenzuela, J. A., and Mouriño, A. (1998) *Tetrahedron Lett* **39**, 4725-4728
7. Bretting, C., Mørk Hansen, C., and Rastrup Andersen, N. (1994) in *Vitamin D - A pluripotent steroid hormone: Structural studies, molecular endocrinology and clinical applications* (Norman, A. W., Bouillon, R., and Thomasset, M. eds) pp. 73-74, Walter De Gruyter, Berlin
8. Chaudhuri, N. K. and Gut, M. (1965) *J. Am. Chem. Soc.* **87**, 3737-3744
9. Nes, W. R., Varkey, T. E., Crump, D. R., and Gut, M. (1976) *J. Org. Chem.* **41**, 3429-3433
10. Segal, G. M. and Torgov, I. V. (1982) *Sovj. J. Bioorg. Chem.* **7**, 242-247
11. Takayama, H., Ohmori, M., Yamada, S., and Takano, Y. (1988) in *Vitamin D: molecular, cellular and clinical endocrinology* (Norman, A. W., Schaefer, K., Grigoleit, H.-G., and Herrath, D. v. eds) pp. 64-65, De Gruyter, Berlin
12. von Daehne, W., Mørk Hansen, C., Hansen, D., and Mathiasen, I. S. (1997) in *Vitamin D* (Norman, A. W., Bouillon, R., and Thomasset, M. eds) pp. 81-82, University of California, Riverside (Calif.)
13. Calverley, M. J. and Binderup, L. (1993) *BioMed. Chem. Lett.* **3**, 1845-1848
14. Fouquet, G. and Schlosser, M. (1974) *Angew. Chem.* **86**, 50-51
15. Calverley, M. J. (1987) *Tetrahedron* **43**, 4609-4619
16. Baggiolini, E. G., Iacobelli, J. A., Hennessy, B. M., Batcho, A. D., Sereno, J. F., and Uskokovic, M. R. (1986) *J. Org. Chem.* **51**, 3098-3108
17. Using the dot-map methodology described by: Midland, M. M., Plumet, J., and Okamura, W. H. (1993) *BioMed. Chem. Lett.* **3**, 1799-1804
18. Eguchi, T., Yoshida, M., and Ikekawa, N. (1989) *Bioorg. Chem.* **17**, 294-307
19. Calverley, M. J., Bretting, C., and Grue-Soerensen, G. (1994) in *Vitamin D - A pluripotent steroid hormone: Structural studies, molecular endocrinology and clinical applications* (Norman, A. W., Bouillon, R., and Thomasset, M. eds) pp. 85-86, Walter De Gruyter, Berlin
20. Yamamoto, K., Ooizumi, H., Umesono, K., Verstuyf, A., Bouillon, R., DeLuca, H. F., Shinki, T., Suda, T., and Yamada, S. (1999) *Bioorg. Med. Chem. Lett* **9**, 1041-1046
21. Denmark, S. E. and Stavenger, R. A. (1998) *J. Org. Chem.* **63**, 9524-9527

AN INDUSTRIAL ENANTIOSELECTIVE SYNTHESIS OF KEY A-RING PRECURSORS FOR 19-NOR VITAMIN D ANALOGUES.

Yurui Zhao,[a] Yusheng Wu,[a] Pierre De Clercq,[a] Maurits Vandewalle,[a,*] Philippe Maillos[b] and Jean-Pierre Pascal[b]
[a] Laboratory of Organic Synthesis, Department of Organic Chemistry, University of Ghent, Krijgslaan 281 S4, B-9000 GENT, Belgium
[b] Théramex S.A., 4-6 Avenue du Prince Héréditaire Albert, F-98007 Monaco

Introduction The importance of 19-nor 1α,25-dihydroxyvitamin D analogues (1) in the separation of calcemic activity from cellular differentiation activities is now well established. This selective activity toward differentiation has first been demonstrated by DeLuca *et al* (1). Our interest (2,3,4) in such analogues has led in the past to several synthetic approaches for substituted bicyclo [3.1.0] hexanes (such as 2) as 19-nor A-ring precursors (5,6,7). These are intermediates in the "cyclovitamin strategy" (8) which involves coupling with the lithiated derivative of 3 and subsequent acid catalyzed solvolysis of the cyclopropane ring. This concept is an alternative for Lythgoe's classical coupling process and has been developed by Wilson (9) and Uskokovic (10) for natural A-ring analogues.

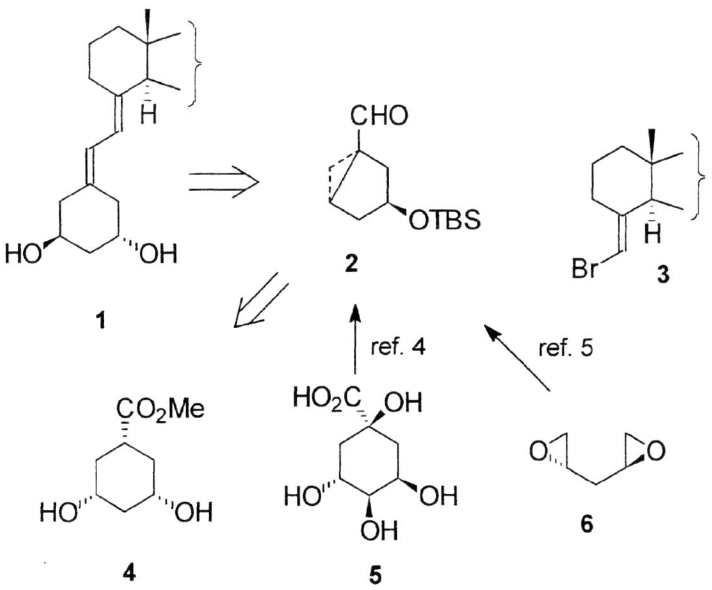

Scheme 1

Next to intrinsic biological properties a 19-nor A-ring is also of crucial importance for the development of analogues, which, due to other structural modifications such as a 6C-ring (3) or 14-epi-analogues (6), would be prone to shift to a previtamin structure.

Results Presently we want to report a practical synthesis, applicable to large scale production, of the bicyclo [3.1.0]-cyclohexane precursor 2. Our previously described syntheses showed several drawbacks for upscaling (Scheme 1). In a first approach (4), which started from (-) quinic acid (5), the Barton-McCombie deoxygenation process for removal of the 1- and 4-hydroxyl groups, via the bis-thiocarbonyl imidazolide, was unpracticable on large scale. On the other hand the approaches starting from 6 (5) or 3-cyclopentenol (6) involved oily or quite volatile intermediates and difficult purifications. Therefore, an important aim of the present synthesis consisted in the formation of crystalline intermediates together with a minimum of purifications.

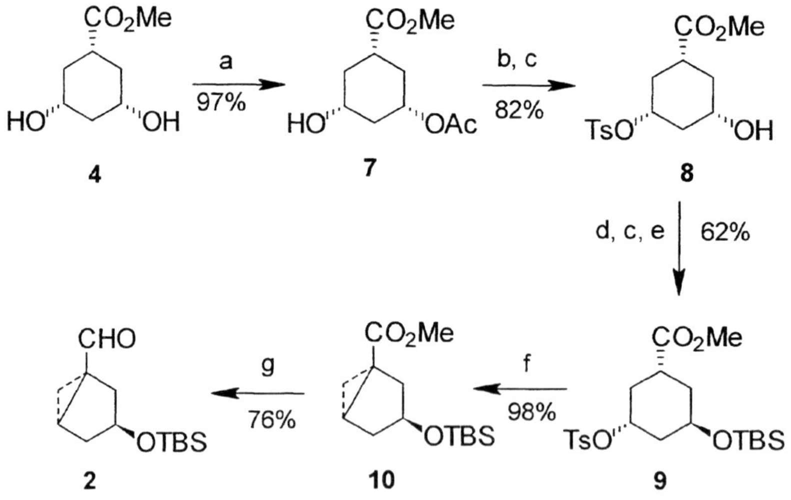

(a): PPL, vinyl acetate, 2d, rt; (b): TsCl, Et$_3$N, CH$_2$Cl$_2$, cat.DMAP, 24h, rt; (c): K$_2$CO$_3$, MeOH, 1h, rt; (d): AcOH, (Ph)$_3$P, DEAD, Tol., 1.2h, rt; (e): TBSCl, imid., cat.DMAP, DMF, 1.5h, rt; (f): t-BuOK, t-BuOH, 60°C, 1.2h; (g): i) DIBAL, Tol., -78°C, 1.5h, ii) PCC, CH$_2$Cl$_2$, 12h, 1h.

Scheme 2

The present synthesis centers around cis, cis-3,5-dihydroxy-1-(methoxycarbonyl) cyclohexane (4), possessing the 3 essential functions, as starting material. Transfor-mation of 4 to 2 involves 3 key-steps (i) asymmetrization, (ii) inversion of the 3-hydroxyl group (iii) cyclopropane ring formation. Product 4 was obtained upon catalytic hydrogenation of commercially available 3,5-dihydroxybenzoic acid. Asymmetrization of 4, catalyzed by PPL (hog pancreas lipase) was performed via vinyl acetate mediated acylation and afforded enantiopure 7 in almost quantitative yield (Scheme 2).

Subsequent to facile transformation of **7** into **8**, Mitsunobu inversion followed by acetate hydrolysis and hydroxy group protection gave **9**.

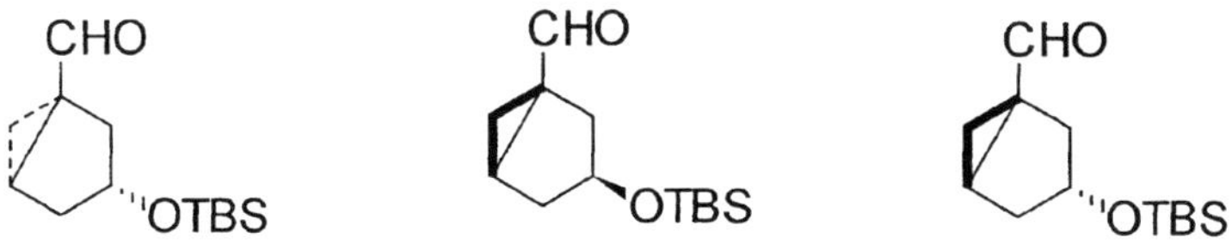

2-*epi*-**2**   3a, 4a-*bisepi*-**2**   *ent*-**2**

Scheme 3

The stage was now set for the third key-step; intramolecular alkylation of the ester-enolate of **9** gave the bicyclic product **10**. The ester was converted in aldehyde **2** *via* a 2-step reduction-oxidation procedure. The overall yield of the 9 step sequence, starting from 800 g of **4**, is 36 %; only 4 purifications are needed and intermediates **4**, **7**, **8** and **9** are crystalline. An important feature of the approach is the fact that it allows easy access to the stereoisomers of **2**, respectively 2-*epi*-**2**, 3a,4a-*bisepi*-**2** and *ent*-**2**, upon changing the order of the reaction sequence shown in (Scheme 2). For the first two no inversion is needed; they are precursors for A-ring epimers of 19-nor vitamin D analogues.

References
1. (a) Perlman, K.L., Sicinski, R.R., Schnoes, H.K., DeLuca, H.F. (1990) Tetrahedron Lett. 31, 1823-1824; (b) Perlman, K.L., Swenson, R.E., Paaren, H.E., Schnoes, H.K., DeLuca, H.F. (1991) Tetrahedron Lett. 32, 7663-7666.
2. Bouillon, R., Sarandeses, A., Allewaert, K., Zhao, J., Mascareñas, J., Mouriño, A., Vrielynck, S., De Clercq, P., Vandewalle, M. (1993) J. Bone & Mine. Res. 8, 1009-1115.
3. Zhou, X., Zhu, G.-D., Van Haver, D., Vandewalle, M., De Clercq, P.J., Verstuyf, A., Bouillon R. (1999) J. Med. Chem. 42, 3539-3556.
4. Verstuyf, A., Verlinden, L., Van Etten, E., Shi, L., Wu, Y., D'Halleweyn, C., Van Haver, D., Zhu, G.-D., Chen, Y., Zhou, X., Haussler, R., De Clercq, P., Vandewalle, M., Van Baelen, H., Mathieu, C., Bouillon, R. (2000) J. Bone & Min. Res. 15, 237-252.
5. Huang, P.Q., Sabbe; K., Pottie, M., Vandewalle, M. (1995) Tetrahedron Lett. 36, 8299-8302.
6. Zhou, S.Z., Anné, S., Vandewalle, M. (1996) Tetrahedron Lett. 37, 7637-7640.
7. Yong, W., Vandewalle, M. (1996) Synlett. 9, 911-912.
8. Sheves, M., Mazur, Y. (1976) Tetrahedron Lett., 2987-2990.
9. Wilson, S.R., Vankatesan, A.M., Augelli-Szafran, C.E., Yasmin, A. (1991) Tetrahedron Lett. 32, 2339-2342.
10. Kabat, M., Kiegiel, J., Cohen, N., Toth, K., Wovkulich, P.M., Uskokovic, M.R. (1991) Tetrahedron Lett. 32, 2343-2346.

Synthesis and Biological Evaluation of A-ring Diastereomers of 1α,25-Dihydroxy-22-oxavitamin D3 (OCT)

Susumi Hatakeyama[a], Toshio Okano[b], Junji Maeyama[a], Yoshiharu Iwabuchi[a], Kimie Nakagawa[b], Keiichi Ozono[c], Akira Kawase[d], and Noboru Kubodera*[d]. [a]Faculty of Pharmaceutical Sciences, Nagasaki University, Nagasaki 852-8521, Japan, [b]Department of Hygienic Sciences, Kobe Pharmaceutical University, Kobe 658-8558, Japan, [c]Department of Environmental Medicine, Osaka Medical Center for Maternal and Children Health, Osaka 594-1101, and [d]Chugai Pharmaceutical Co., Ltd., Tokyo 104-8301, Japan

Various analogs of 1,25(OH)2D3 (**1**) have been synthesized to separate differentiation-induction and antiproliferation activities from calcemic activity with the aim of obtaining useful analogs for the medical treatment of psoriasis, cancer, etc., without risk of hypercalcemia. 1α,25-Dihydroxy-22-oxavitamin D3 (OCT)(**2**) was obtained in such synthetic studies and (**2**) has been shown to be highly potent in stimulating monocytic differentiation of human promyelocytic leukemic HL-60 cells but less calcemic than 1,25(OH)2D3 (**1**).[1,2] OCT (**2**) is now under the process of approval as an injection for the treatment of secondary hyperparathyroidism underlying renal insufficiency and as an ointment for skin disease, psoriasis.

Recently, the epimerization of the 3-hydroxy group of vitamin D3 compounds has bee reported. 3-Epi-1α,25-dihydroxyvitamin D3 (3-epi-1,25(OH)2D3) was also found in the serum of rats treated with 1,25(OH)2D3. In the case of 24,25-dihydroxyvitamin D3 (24,25-(OH)2D3), the other major natural metabolite of vitamin D3, 3-epi-24,25-dihydroxyvitamin D3 was recently identified in the bile of rats administered with 24,25(OH)2D3. Although the biological characterization of the epimerized vitamin D3 compounds at 3-position has yet remained to be clarified, we have been interested in the new metabolic pathway of vitamin D3 compounds at the A-ring part in addition to the classic metabolic pathway at the side chain. It is a matter of no little interest to us to synthesize putative A-ring metabolites of OCT (**2**) and investigate their biological characters.

As A-ring diastereomers of OCT (**2**), 3-epi-1α,25dihydroxy-22-oxavitamin D3 (3-epiOCT) (**3**) and 1,3-diepi-1α,25-dihydroxy-22-oxavitamin D3 (1,3-diepiOCT) (**4**) were synthesized by the convergent method (Fig. 2). Their *in vitro* binding affinity for vitamin D receptor (VDR) and vitamin D binding protein (DBP), differentiation-inducing activity on HL-60 cells, and transcriptional activity using rat 24-hudroxylase gene and human osteocalcin gene, were evaluated as the preliminary biological evaluation of synthesized A-ring diastereomers in comparison with 1,25(OH)2D3 (**1**), OCT (**2**), and 1-epi-1α,25-dihydroxy-22-oxavitamin D3 (1-epiOCT) (**5**) consist of all possible A-ring diastereomers of OCT (**2**) (Fig. 1).

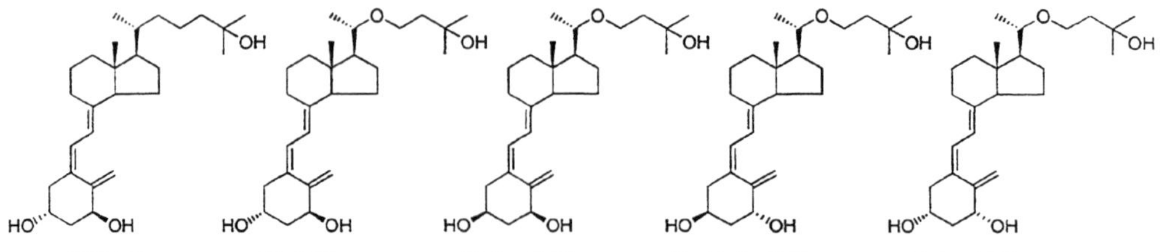

Fig. 1   Structures of active vitamin D3 and OCT analogs

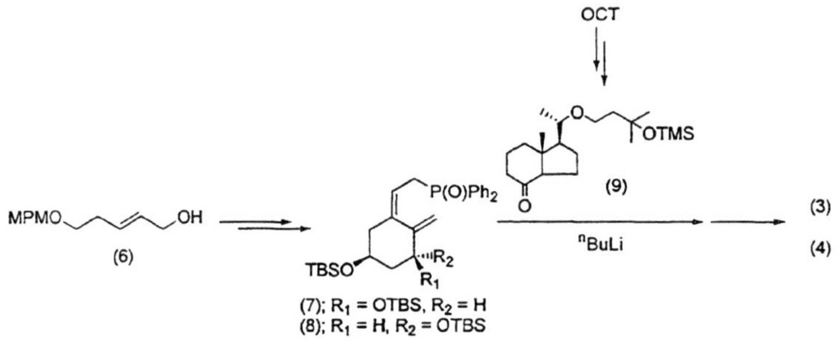

Fig. 2   Convergent synthesis of A-ring diastereomers of OCT

Table 1.   Biological evaluation of A-ring diastereomers of OCT

	DBP	VDR	HL-60	Rat 24-Ohase	Human Osteocalcin
1,25(OH)$_2$D$_3$ (1)	100	100	100	100	100
OCT (2)	N.B	5.1	130	433	422
3-EpiOCT (3)	N.B.	<0.1	5	19	10
1,3-DiepiOCT (4)	7.2	<0.1	<1	<1	<1
1- EpiOCT (5)	0.9	N.B.	<1	<1	<1

References

1.   *Chem. Pharm. Bull.*, **1986**, *34*, 4410.

2.   *Chem. Pharm. Bull.*, **1992**, *40*, 1494.

3.   *Bioorg. Med. Chem. Lett.*, **1994**, *4*, 1523.

A-RING CONFORMATION AND BIOLOGICAL ACTIVITY: BASED ON THE STUDIES OF FLUOROVITAMIN D ANALOGS

M. Shimizu, A. Ohno, Y. Iwasaki, S. Yamada, H. Ooizumi,[§] and H. F. DeLuca,[¶] Institute of Biomaterials and Bioengineering, Tokyo Medical and Dental University, 2-3-10, Surugadai, Kanda, Chiyoda-ku, Tokyo 101-0062, Japan; [§]Kyoto University; [¶]University of Wisconsin-Madison

Introduction $1\alpha,25$-Dihydroxyvitamin D_3 [$1\alpha,25$-$(OH)_2D_3$; **1**] exerts its hormonal effects on intestine, bone, kidney, and parathyroid glands, where it plays a crucial role in calcium homeostasis, the prevention of rickets and bone mineralization. Moreover, **1** has been shown to inhibit cell growth, to induce differentiation in malignant cells, and to induce apoptosis in human cancer cells. Vitamin D receptor (VDR) belongs to the superfamily of steroid receptors that regulate gene expression in response to binding of their specific ligands. Ligand binding changes the conformation of the receptors enabling transactivation and results in either gene activation or repression depending on the target gene.

Fig. 1.

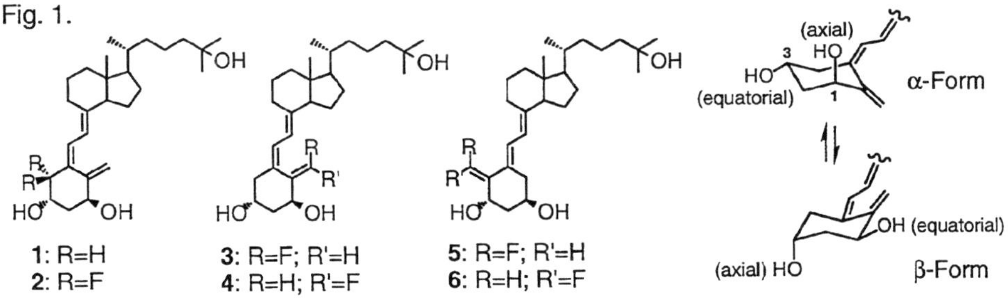

1: R=H
2: R=F

3: R=F; R'=H
4: R=H; R'=F

5: R=F; R'=H
6: R=H; R'=F

$1\alpha,25$-$(OH)_2D_3$ **1** is highly mobile and can adopt a number of conformations around the A-ring, seco-B-ring, and side chain. We have focused on the A-ring whose conformation is thought to be essential for the recognition of the active site of VDR ligand cavity. In solution, the vitamin D A-ring exists predominantly in two chair conformation, designated as α (1α-OH in axial; 3β-OH in equatorial) and β (1α-OH in equatorial; 3β-OH in axial), according to ^{1}H NMR and X-ray analysis (Fig. 1). In a series of studies on conformation-function relationship of vitamin D, we proposed a three-dimensional model of a liganded VDR in conjunction with mutation studies to substantiate the model (1). Recently the crystal structure of a deletion mutant (Δ 165-215) of holo-VDR-ligand binding domain (LBD) was reported. In the crystal structure it was revealed that the A-ring of the natural ligand **1** adopts β-conformation (2).

    In our studies, to directly elucidate the A ring conformation in the vitamin D-VDR complex by ^{19}F NMR spectroscopy, we synthesized 4,4-difluoro- and 19-

fluoro-1α,25-dihydroxyvitamin D_3 (**2**, **3** and **4**) as probe compounds (Fig. 1) (3, 4, 5). In this paper, biological activities of these analogs were evaluated and the A-ring conformation in the fluorovitamin D bound to VDR was analyzed.

Conformational analysis of fluorovitamin D derivatives by NMR spectroscopy

We investigated the variable temperature ^1H and ^{19}F NMR spectra of the fluorovitamin D analogs **2**, **3** and **4**, and the results are shown in Fig. 2 and Table 1 (4, 5).

Fig. 2.

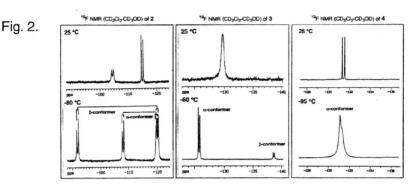

Table 1. A-Ring conformation of 1α,25-(OH)₂D₃ and fluorovitamin D analogs in various solvents

Compounds	Conformer ratio in each solvent		
	THF α : β	CDCl₃ α : β	CD₃OD α : β
1	38 : 62	45 : 55	46 : 54
2	34 : 66	ND	54 : 46
3	69 : 31	71 : 29	77 : 23
4	100 : 0	100 : 0	100 : 0

In the low temperature ^{19}F NMR spectra of both **2** and **3** (in CD_3OD, CD_3OD-CD_2Cl_2 and THF), ^{19}F signals of the two A-ring conformers were well-separated (**2**: α–form = -122.2 & -111.0 ppm and β-form = -122.2 & -94.1 ppm; **3**: α-form = -127.0 & β–form = -139.3 ppm). The protons at C(1) and C(3) in the two conformers of **3** were also observed separately at -95 °C. (*10Z*)-Isomer **4** did not show any separated fluorine signals of the two A-ring conformers at the temperature down to -95 °C. Each conformer of **2**, **3** and **4** was assigned based on the analysis of the observed coupling constants of the 3α-proton or the geminal fluorine atoms (5). 4-Fluoro-analog **2** consists of approximately 1:1 mixtures of the α- and β-conformers, whereas isomeric 19-fluoro-analogs **3** and **4** exist preferentially or exclusively in the α-conformer. The ratio of conformers in these fluoro-analogs was slightly affected by solvent and the proportion of the β-conformer increased with decreasing solvent polarity.

On the basis of the dynamic NMR studies, the energy barrier ($\Delta G^{\ddagger}$) for the interconversion of α- and β-conformers was estimated to be 9.8 kcal mol^{-1} for **2** and 10.8 kcal mol^{-1} for **3**. The $\Delta G^{\ddagger}$ at coalescence of **2** and **3** is high by 0.3 and 1.3 kcal mol^{-1}, respectively, compared with that of **1** (9.5 kcal mol^{-1}). The somewhat large increase in the $\Delta G^{\ddagger}$ for **3** is probably due to the steric repulsion between 7-H and 19-F at the transition state of the ring A inversion.

Biological evaluation of fluorovitamin D analogs Five fluorovitamin D analogs were tested for their binding affinity for bovine thymus VDR and in VDR-mediated transcriptional potency compared with the natural ligand **1** (Table 2).

Table 2. VDR affinity and transcriptional activity

Compounds	VDR Binding	Transactivation
1	100	100
2	1	42
3	8	53
4	9	27
5	0.14	19
6	0.35	14

CV-1 cells were cotransfected with a luciferase reporter plasmid in combination with a GAL-DBD and VDR-LBD fusion plasmid. The cells were treated with 10^{-8}M of vitamin D compounds in DMEM containing 10% FBS.

All the fluorinated analogs decreased binding activity (9~0.1%) for VDR. The 4-fluoro-analog **2** was 100-fold less potent and the 19-fluoro-analogs **3** and **4** were about 10-fold less effective than the natural hormone **1**. The dramatic decrease in the binding affinity of **2** for VDR can be explained as followes: The gem-difluoro group in **2** probably causes the steric repulsion with the residues in the LDB. Interestingly, all the tested compounds were only 7 to 2 times less active in transcriptional assay than the native ligand at concentrations of 10^{-8} M: They diplayed higher activity than expected from the potency of their VDR binding. We have no sufficient data which explain the discrepancy between VDR affinity and transcriptional activity. Since **1** led to a higher transcriptional activity in the absence of FBS than in the presence of FBS, one possibility is that DBP-associated processes might be involved.

^{19}F NMR spectra of the fluorinated vitamin D ligand and VDR complex
We investigated direct interaction of the fluorovitamin D analog with VDR-LBD by ^{19}F NMR. The rat VDR-LBD (amino acids 115-423) was expressed as an amino-terminal His-tagged protein in E. coli expression system and purified on a

48

Ni-NTA and a SP HiTrap column chromatography. The molecular weight of the purified VDR-LBD protein based on sequence was 37400 Da and the dissociation constant (K_d) was 0.3 nM (6). We first examined the ^{19}F NMR of (10E)-19-fluorovitamin D **3** to probe the A-ring conformation of the ligand bound to VDR, since **3** exhibits only one set of fluorine signals derived from α- and β-conformers, the chemical shift difference between two conformers (~13 ppm) is larger, and **3** has highest VDR affinity. Purified VDR-LBD (ca. 30 mg by protein assay) dissolved in 20 mM NaH_2SO_4 (pH 7) and 100 mM NaCl was concentrated to a small volume (~0.5 mL) and the fluorinated ligand **3** (1.5 equiv.) and D_2O were add. The ^{19}F NMR spectrum of the complex solution is shown in Fig. 3 compared with that of free **3**. A new broad signal (~ -126 ppm) probably due to a VDR-bound ligand was observed in a lower field than the free-ligand signal. The chemical shift of observed bound signal appears at nearly identical as that of the α-conformer of **3**. Thus, the present study suggests that the 19-fluorovitamin D **3** bound to VDR adopts α-conformer at the A-ring. More detailed ^{19}F NMR studies including a ligand-VDR binding stoichiometry are progressing .

Fig. 3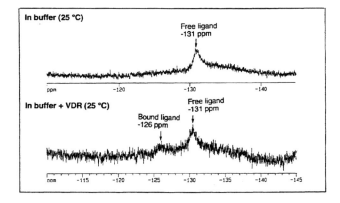

References

1. Yamamoto, K., Masuno, H., Choi, M., Nakashima, K., Taga, T., Ooizumi, H., Umesono, K., Sicinska, W., VanHooke, J., DeLuca, H.F. and Yamada, S. (2000) *Proc.Natl. Acad. Sci. USA* **97**, 1467-1472.

2. Rochel, N., Wurtz, J.M., Mitschler, A., Kaholz, B. and Moras, D. (2000) *Mol. Cell.* **5**, 173-179.

3. Iwasaki, Y., Shimizu, M., Hirosawa, T. and Yamada, S. (1996) *Tetrahedron Lett.* **37**, 6753-6754.

4. Shimizu, M., Iwasaki, Y., Ohno, A. and Yamada, S. (1997) in *Vitamin D: Chemistry, Biology and Clinical Applications of the Steroid Hormone* (Norman, A.W., Bouillon, R. and Thomasset, M., Eds.) p.24-25, University of California, Riverside.

5. Shimizu, M., Iwasaki, Y. and Yamada, S. (1999) *Tetrahedron Lett.* **40**, 1697-1700.

6. Strugnell, S.A., Hill, J.J., McCaslin, D.R., Bridgette, A., Wiefling, B.A., Royer, C.A. and DeLuca, H.F. (1999) *Archieves Biochem. Biophys.* **364**, 42-52.

FACILE SYNTHESIS OF 2α-(HYDROXYALKOXY)-1α,25-DIHYDROXYVITAMIN D$_3$

Atsushi Kittaka,[a] Yoshitomo Suhara,[a] Hitoshi Takayanagi,[a] Toshie Fujishima,[a] Masaaki Kurihara,[b] and Hiroaki Takayama*[a]

[a] Faculty of Pharmaceutical Sciences, Teikyo University, Sagamiko, Kanagawa 199-0195, Japan and [b] National Institute of Health Sciences, Kamiyoga, Setagaya-ku, Tokyo 158-8501, Japan

Introduction Recently, we have synthesized C2-methylated 1α,25-dihydroxyvitamin D$_3$ [1α,25(OH)$_2$D$_3$] derivatives and found that the 2α-isomer showed higher potency than the native hormone in terms of binding affinity to vitamin D receptor (VDR), elevation of rat serum Ca concentration, and induction of HL 60 cell differentiation (1). Further modification of the 2α-methyl group, especially, introduction of the 2α-(3-hydroxypropyl) group into the C2α position of 1α,25(OH)$_2$D$_3$ brought about 500 times higher potency in calcium-mobilizing activity (2). On the other hand, 2β-(3-hydroxy-propoxy)-1α,25(OH)$_2$D$_3$ (ED-71) has been developed by Chugai Pharmaceutical Co. as a promising candidate for the treatment of osteoporosis (3). Most of the biological actions of 1α,25(OH)$_2$D$_3$ are considered to be mediated by the vitamin D receptor (VDR), which belongs to the nuclear receptor superfamily acting as a ligand-dependant transcription factor with coactivators (4). In accordance with these facts, we planed to synthesize new analogs (1a-c) having the ω-hydroxyalkoxy group at the C2α-position to understand detail structure-activity relationships particularly on the A-ring (Figure 1). We wish to present here a new efficient synthetic route to 2α-(ω-hydroxyalkoxy)-1α,25(OH)$_2$D$_3$ analogs (1a-c), and their higher binding activity to VDR than that of the native hormone.

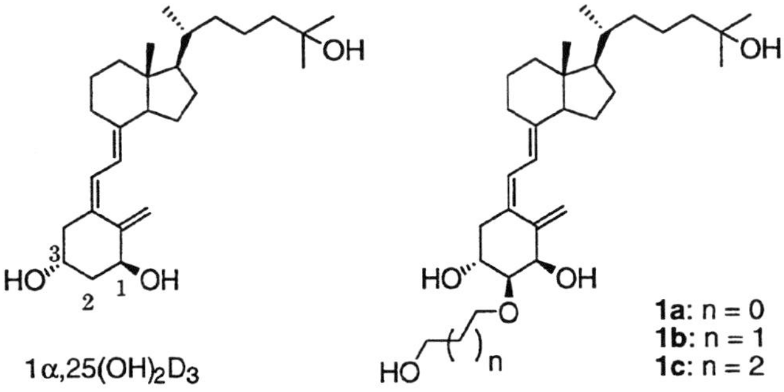

1α,25(OH)$_2$D$_3$

1a: n = 0
1b: n = 1
1c: n = 2

Figure 1. Structures of 1α,25(OH)$_2$D$_3$ and its 2α-hydroxyalkoxylated analogs **1a-c**.

Results and Discussion To create 1α,2α,3β–stereochemistry on the ring A of the target vitamin D$_3$ analogs (1a-c), the readily available crystalline epoxide 2 from methyl α-D–glucoside was chosen as the chiral template (5). The regiospecific ring opening by a suitable alkanediol (3a) at the C3 position has proceeded to afford altrose configuration, in which C2, C3, and C4 asymmetric centers satisfy the corresponding desired 3β–, 2α–, and 1α–stereochemistries of **1a-c**, respectively.

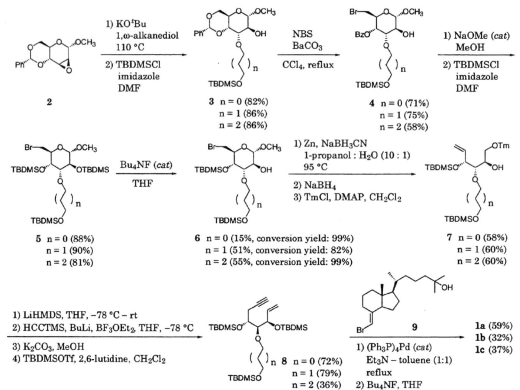

Scheme 1. Synthesis of 2α-(ω-hydroxyalkoxy)-1α,25(OH)$_2$D$_3$ analogs (**1a-c**).

As illustrated in Scheme 1, for example, **2** was heated with 1,3-propanediol in a basic condition to yield methyl α-D–3-O-(3-hydroxypropyl)altropyranoside (n = 1). After the selective protection of the primary alcohol, treatment of the benzylidene acetal **3** with NBS (6) gave the bromide **4**. Exchange of the protecting group on the C4 hydroxyl group was accomplished through mild solvolysis of the benzoate, persilylation, and selective deprotection of the C2 hydroxyl group to obtain the bis-O-silylated **6** in a good yield (7). Reaction of the bromide **6** with activated zinc powder generated an aldehyde, which was directly reduced to the alcohol (8). Sulfonylation of the primary alcohol gave **7** and LiHMDS treatment afforded epoxide, to which was subsequently introduced the acetylene unit with ring opening. Removal of the terminal TMS group and the protection of the secondary alcohol with TBDMS provided 1,7-enyne **8** in a high yield, which was the suitable A-ring precursor for the following Trost-Dumas palladium-catalyzed coupling reaction (9). The other A-ring precursors **8** (n = 0 and 2) were also prepared by the same procedure using ethylene glycol and butanediol. The coupling reaction with the known bromoolefin **9** of the CD fragment (9) and subsequent deprotection furnished the aimed 2α-(ω-hydroxyalkoxy)-1α,25(OH)$_2$D$_3$ (**1a-c**) in 32-59% yields.

The relative binding affinity of **1a-c** to VDR was evaluated (10), and the results are summarized in Table 1. Interestingly, the highest binding affinity of this series was recognized in **1b** (n = 1) as 1.8 times higher one than that of $1\alpha,25(OH)_2D_3$.

Table 1. Relative binding affinity of the series of **1** for bovine thymus $1\alpha,25$-dihydroxyvitamin D_3 receptor (VDR).

compounds	affinity to VDR[a]
$1\alpha,25(OH)_2D_3$	100
1a (n = 0)	120
1b (n = 1)	180
1c (n = 2)	40

[a] The potency of $1\alpha,25(OH)_2D_3$ is normalized to 100.

Very recently, the three-dimensional structure elucidation of the $1\alpha,25(OH)_2D_3$ docking VDR ligand binding domain has been in progress (11). Around the C2 position, there is a rather hydrophobic cavity surrounded by Phe-150, Tyr-143, Tyr-147, and Tyr-236. At the end of this long cavity, Asp-144 exists. The potent VDR affinity of **1a** and **1b** would be explained by molecular mechanics calculation based on the crystal structure established by Moras *et al.* (11a). In the preliminary calculation (12), the C2α-terminal hydroxyl group of **1b** reaches to Asp-144 to form a new hydrogen bond. This hydroxyl group is also likely to create an additional hydrogen bond with Tyr-236. On the other hand, the C2α-terminal hydroxyl group of **1a** probably forms a hydrogen bond with Arg-274. Formation of the new hydrogen bonds should be one of the reasons for the high affinity. Further information from the calculation is that the 2α-substituted A-ring, except a 2α-methyl case, fits in the α-conformation in the cavity to minimize steric repulsion. In such a case, the 1α-hydroxyl group retains hydrogen bonding to Ser-237. We have reported that the binding activity of 2α-(3-hydroxypropyl)-$1\alpha,25(OH)_2D_3$ showed 3 times higher than $1\alpha,25(OH)_2D_3$ itself (2). The distance between the C2-atom and the terminal hydroxyl group of 2α-(3-hydroxypropyl)-$1\alpha,25(OH)_2D_3$ is almost same as compound **1a**. Different binding activity of these two analogs would be considerable by matching of the hydrophobicity just around the C2 position.

Conclusion We have developed the efficient synthetic route to the new biologically active 2α-(ω-hydrokyalkoxy)-$1\alpha,25(OH)_2D_3$ (**1a-c**) in major three key steps: 1) the readily available epoxide **2** from D-glucose was converted to bromide **4** after reaction with alkanediol followed by NBS bromination, 2) Zn-mediated reduction provided olefin **7**, and 3) elongation of the acetylene unit gave the A-ring precursor enyne **8**, which was ready to couple with bromoolefin **9** having the CD-ring moiety. It has been found that VDR binding affinity of **1b** is 1.8 times higher than that of the native hormone. This remarkable affinity was elucidated by molecular mechanics calculation based on the crystal structure of VDR bound to its natural ligand reported by Moras *et* *al.* (11a). We believe this synthetic strategy is applicable to a wide range of the novel 2α-substituted 1α,25(OH)$_2$D$_3$ derivatives that satisfy medicinal needs. Further synthetic studies in this area are currently in progress in our laboratory.

Reference and notes
1. (a) Konno, K., Maki, S., Fujishima, T., Liu, Z. –P., Miura, D., Chokki, M. and Takayama, H. (1998) Bioorg. Med. Chem. Lett. 8, 151-156. (b) Nakagawa, K., Kurobe, M., Ozono, K., Konno, K., Fujishima, T., Takayama, H. and Okano, T. (2000) Biochem. Pharmcol. 59, 691-702.
2. Suhara, Y., Nihei, K. –I., Tanigawa, H., Fijishima, T., Konno, K., Nakagawa, K., Okano, T. and Takayama, H. (2000) Bioorg. Med. Chem. Lett. in press.
3. (a) Miyamoto, K., Murayama, E., Ochi, K., Watanabe, H. and Kubodera, N. (1993) Chem. Pharm. Bull. 41, 1111-1113. Biological activities of a series of 2β-substituted analogs, see: (b) Tsugawa, N., Nakagawa, K., Kurobe, M., Ono, Y., Kubodera, N., Ozono, K. and Okano, T. (2000) Biol. Pharm. Bull. 23, 66-71. Syntheses of 19-nor and 2-(4-hydroxybutyl) analogs of ED-71 were also reported, see: (c) Sicinski, R. F., Perlman, K. L. and DeLuca, H. F. (1994) J. Med. Chem. 37, 3730-3738. (d) Posner, G. H. and Johnson, N. (1994) J. Org. Chem. 59, 7855-7861.
4. (a) Umesono, K., Murakami, K. K., Thompson, C. C. and Evans, R. M. (1991) Cell 65, 1255-1266. (b) DeLuca, H. F. and Zierold, C. (1998) Nutr. Rev. 56, 54-75. (c) Takeyama, K. –I., Masuhiro, Y., Fuse, H., Endoh, H., Murayama, A., Kitanaka, S., Suzawa, M., Yanagisawa, J. and Kato, S. (1999) Mol. Cell. Biol. 19, 1049-1055. (d) Yanagisawa, J., Yanagi, Y., Masuhiro, Y., Suzawa, M., Watanabe, M., Kashiwagi, K., Toriyabe T., Kawabata, M., Miyazono, K. and Kato, S. (1999) Science 283, 1317-1321.
5. Wiggins, L. S. (1963) Methods Carbohydr. Chem. 2, 188-191.
6. Hanessian, S. (1972) Methods Carbohydr. Chem. 6, 183-189.
7. In the case of n = 1, recovered 5 (23%) and a mixture of diols (15%), which could be quantitatively recycled to the tris-*O*-TBDMS derivative 5, were obtained. Then, the conversion yield of this step was 82%.
8. Bernet, B. and Vasella, A. (1979) Helv. Chim. Acta 62, 1990-2016.
9. Trost, B. M., Dumas, J. and Villa, M. (1992) J. Am. Chem. Soc. 114, 9836-9845.
10. Imae, Y., Manaka, A., Yoshida, N., Ishimi, Y., Shinki, T., Abe, E., Suda, T., Konno, K., Takayama, H. and Yamada, S. (1994) Biochim. Biophys. Acta 1213, 302-308.
11. (a) Rochel, N., Wultz, J. M., Mitschler, A., Klaholz, B. and Moras, D. (2000) Molecular Cell 5, 173-179. (b) Yamamoto, K., Masuno, H., Choi, M., Nakashima, K., Taga, T., Ooizumi, H., Umesono, K., Sicinska, W., VanHooke, J., DeLuca, H. F. and Yamada, S. (2000) PNAS 97, 1467-1472.
12. Calculated by MacroModel® ver. 6.5 (Schrodinger, Inc.) on SGI O2 Workstation.

NEW ANALOGS OF 1α,25-DIHYDROXY-19-NORVITAMIN D₃: SYNTHESIS, CONFORMATIONAL ANALYSIS, AND BIOLOGICAL ACTIVITY OF 2-ETHYL AND 2-ETHYLIDENE DERIVATIVES

Rafal R. Sicinski and Hector F. DeLuca, Department of Biochemistry, University of Wisconsin-Madison, Madison, WI 53706, USA.

Introduction. The discovery of the hormonally active form of vitamin D₃, 1α,25-dihydroxyvitamin D₃ (1α,25-$(OH)_2D_3$, calcitriol, **1**, Figure 1), has greatly stimulated research into its physiology and chemistry (1,2). Recently, the chemistry of vitamin D

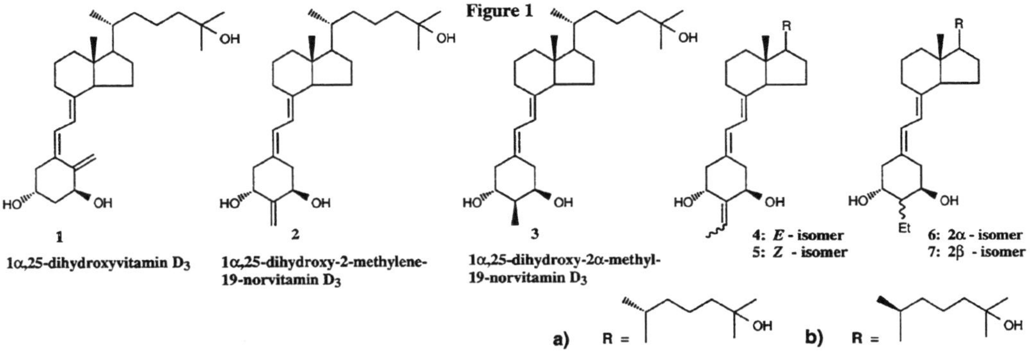

Figure 1

1
1α,25-dihydroxyvitamin D₃

2
1α,25-dihydroxy-2-methylene-19-norvitamin D₃

3
1α,25-dihydroxy-2α-methyl-19-norvitamin D₃

4: *E* - isomer
5: *Z* - isomer

6: 2α - isomer
7: 2β - isomer

a) R =   b) R =

focused on the design and synthesis of such analogs that can exert selective biological actions. In our continuing investigation of the structure-activity relationship of the vitamin D molecule, we prepared an analog of the natural hormone **1** with transposed exocyclic methylene group, i.e., 1α,25-dihydroxy-2-methylene-19-norvitamin D₃ (**2**), and 2α-methyl analog **3** that was obtained by selective hydrogenation of **2** (3). Both analogs were characterized by significant biological potency, enhanced especially in their isomers in the 20*S*-series. In the search for biologically active vitamins we have prepared novel 19-nor analogs of **1**, substituted at C-2 with ethylidene (**4a,b** and **5a,b**) and ethyl (**6a,b** and **7a,b**) groups.

Chemistry. The strategy of our synthesis was based on Lythgoe type Wittig-Horner coupling (4). Since the corresponding C,D-ring ketones were available, we focused our attention on the synthesis of the phosphine oxide A-ring synthons (Scheme 1). Configurations of the ethylidene unit at C'-4 in compounds **16-18**, were determined by analysis of their ¹H NMR spectra and NOE measurements.

The Wittig-Horner reaction of the conjugate base of **18** with the Grundmann's ketone **20** produced the 19-norvitamin D compound **21** in a very high yield (Scheme 2), but an analogous coupling of the isomeric phosphine oxide **19** was considerably less efficient. Considering this fact and low yield of the Wittig reaction of the cyclohexanone **13**, an alternative synthetic approach to 2-ethylidene-19-norvitamins **4a** and **5a** was sought.

Scheme 1

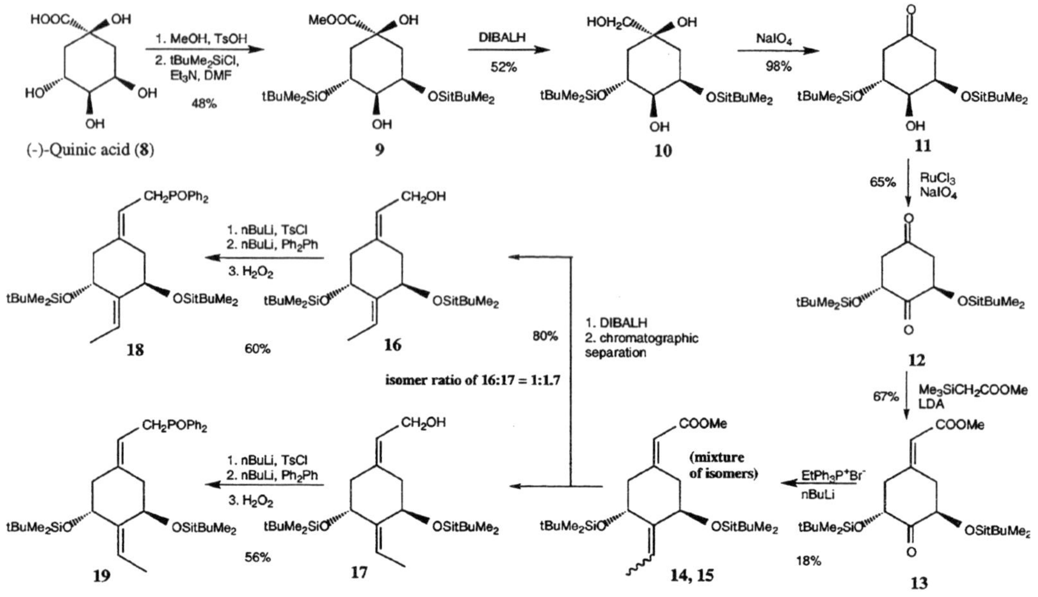

HOOC,,, OH — (-)-Quinic acid (**8**) — HO, OH, OH

1. MeOH, TsOH
2. tBuMe₂SiCl, Et₃N, DMF
48%

MeOOC,,, OH — tBuMe₂SiO, OSitBuMe₂, OH — **9**

DIBALH 52%

HOH₂C,,, OH — tBuMe₂SiO, OSitBuMe₂, OH — **10**

NaIO₄ 98%

tBuMe₂SiO, OSitBuMe₂, OH — **11**

65% RuCl₃ NaIO₄

tBuMe₂SiO, OSitBuMe₂ — **12**

67% Me₃SiCH₂COOMe LDA

CH₂POPh₂ — tBuMe₂SiO, OSitBuMe₂ — **18**

1. nBuLi, TsCl
2. nBuLi, Ph₂Ph
3. H₂O₂
60%

CH₂OH — tBuMe₂SiO, OSitBuMe₂ — **16**

80%
1. DIBALH
2. chromatographic separation

isomer ratio of 16:17 = 1:1.7

COOMe (mixture of isomers) — tBuMe₂SiO, OSitBuMe₂ — **14, 15**

EtPh₃P⁺Br⁻ nBuLi

COOMe — tBuMe₂SiO, OSitBuMe₂ — **13**
18%

CH₂POPh₂ — tBuMe₂SiO, OSitBuMe₂ — **19**

1. nBuLi, TsCl
2. nBuLi, Ph₂Ph
3. H₂O₂
56%

CH₂OH — tBuMe₂SiO, OSitBuMe₂ — **17**

Scheme 2

20 + CH₂POPh₂ — tBuMe₂SiO, OSitBuMe₂ — **18**

OSiEt₃

PhLi 91%

OSiEt₃ — tBuMe₂SiO, OSitBuMe₂ — **21**

nBu₄NF 64% → **4a**

CH₂POPh₂ — tBuMe₂SiO, OSitBuMe₂ — **19**

20, PhLi 13%

OSiEt₃ — tBuMe₂SiO, OSitBuMe₂ — **22**

nBu₄NF 56% → **5a**

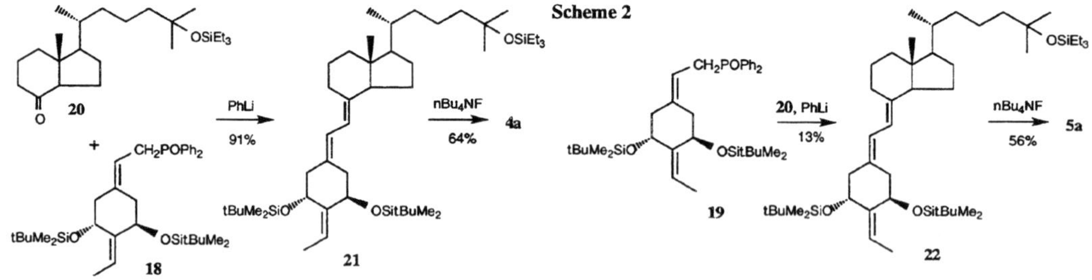

Thus, the carbonyl group in **13** was protected as O-trimethylsilyl hemimethyl-thioketal (**5**) and the corresponding phosphine oxides **25** were efficiently synthesized (Scheme 3). Coupling of their anions with the hydrindanone **26** afforded the protected 19-norvitamin D compound **27** in a high yield. This, after deprotection of the 2-oxo group, the Wittig reaction and subsequent hydrolysis was converted to (20S)-2-ethylidene-19-norvitamins **4b** and **5b**. The selective catalytic hydrogenation of 2-ethylidene analogs **4a,b** and **5a,b** (Scheme 4) provided the corresponding 2-ethyl-19-norvitamins **6a,b** and **7a,b**, which were easily separated by HPLC.

The stereochemistry at C-2 in the synthesized vitamin D compounds was tentatively assigned on the basis of conformational analysis, molecular modeling studies, and 500 MHz ¹H NMR spectroscopy.

Conformational Analysis. It has been established (6) that vitamin D compounds in solutions exist as a mixture of two rapidly equilibrating A-ring chair conformers. In the synthesized 2-ethylidene-19-norvitamin D compounds a strong $A^{(1,3)}$-strain

Scheme 3

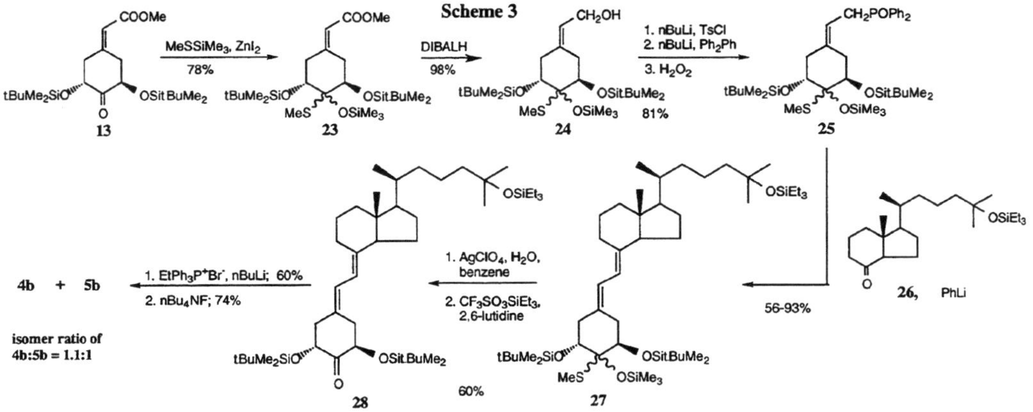

Scheme 4

| 4a: 20R | (Ph₃P)₃RhCl, H₂ | 6a: 20R | + | 7a: 20R | 5a: 20R | (Ph₃P)₃RhCl, H₂ | 6a: 20R | + | 7a: 20R |

$$4a: 20R \xrightarrow[\text{ca. 45\%}]{(Ph_3P)_3RhCl, H_2} 6a: 20R + 7a: 20R$$

(or 4b: 20S)   (or 6b: 20S) (or 7b: 20S)

isomer ratio of 6:7 = 3:1

$$5a: 20R \xrightarrow[\text{ca. 45\%}]{(Ph_3P)_3RhCl, H_2} 6a: 20R + 7a: 20R$$

(or 5b: 20S)   (or 6b: 20S) (or 7b: 20S)

isomer ratio of 6:7 = 3:1

interaction (7) is involved, existing between the methyl group from the ethylidene moiety and equatorial hydroxyls at C-1 or C-3. It results in the significant bias toward conformers with an axial orientation of this hydroxyl to which the methyl group from ethylidene fragment is directed. Presence of bulky 2-alkyl substituents, characterized by large conformational free energy *A* values, shifts the A-ring conformational equilibrium of the obtained 2-ethyl-19-norvitamins toward the conformers with the equatorial C(2)-substituents. The preferred, energy minimized

Figure 2

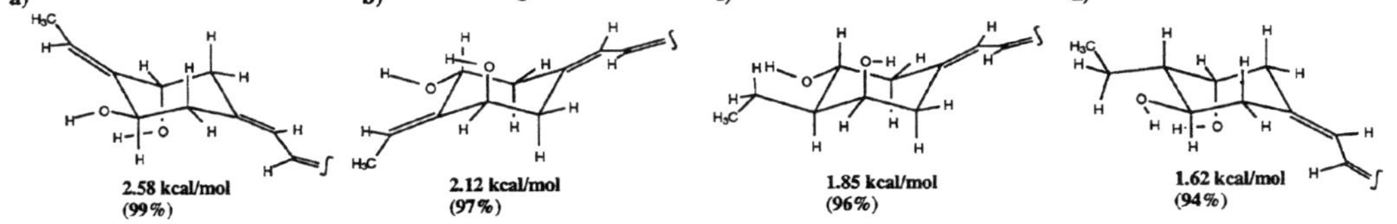

a) 2.58 kcal/mol (99%) b) 2.12 kcal/mol (97%) c) 1.85 kcal/mol (96%) d) 1.62 kcal/mol (94%)

(PC MODEL 6.0, *Serena Software*) A-ring conformations of the synthesized analogs: **4a,b** (a), **5a,b** (b), **6a,b** (c) and **7a,b** (d) are shown in <u>Figure 2</u>. The steric energy differences between the preferred conformers and their partners with the inverted chair forms (calculated for model compounds lacking side chain) are given. The corresponding percentage populations (in parentheses) of conformers are given for room temperature (25 °C).

<u>Biological Evaluation.</u> The synthesized vitamins were tested for their ability to bind the porcine intestinal vitamin D receptor. It was established that 2-ethylidene-19-norvitamins, possessing methyl group from ethylidene moiety directed toward C-3, i.e. *trans* in relation to C(6)-C(7) bond (*E* isomers **4a,b**), are more active than 1α,25-(OH)₂D₃ in binding to VDR. Among their counterparts with *cis* relationship between ethylidene methyl substituent and C(7)-H group (*Z* isomers), the analog **5b** with

"unnatural" stereochemistry of the methyl group at C-20 has equivalent activity with the natural hormone **1**, while the 20*R*-isomer **5a** is 12-fold less active. The competitive binding analysis also showed that 2α-ethyl-19-norvitamins bind the receptor better than their isomers with 2β-ethyl substituents. Among the former analogs 20*R*-isomer **6a** has similar binding affinity for receptor as 1α,25-(OH)$_2$D$_3$ whereas 20*S*-compound **6b** is 2-fold more active. Their 2β-substituted counterparts **7a** and **7b** are 100- and 6-fold less effective than hormone. In the next assay, the cellular activity of the synthesized compounds was established by studying their ability to induce differentiation of human promyelocyte HL-60 cells into monocytes. Both isomers (*E* and *Z*) of (20*S*)-2-ethylidene-19-norvitamin D$_3$ **4b** and **5b**, and both 2α-ethyl-19-norvitamins **6a,b** are more potent (6 - 22 times) than 1α,25-(OH)$_2$D$_3$ in this assay, whereas the remaining tested compounds are equivalent to the hormone **1** or slightly less potent. Both *E* isomers of 2-ethylidene-19-norvitamins **4a,b**, when tested *in vivo* in rats exhibited very high calcemic activity, the 20*S*-compound being especially potent. On the contrary, isomeric *Z* compounds are significantly less active. 2-Ethyl-19-norvitamins have some ability to mobilize calcium from bone but not to the extent of the hormone **1**, while being inactive in intestine. The only exception is 2α-ethyl isomer from 20*S*-series (**6b**) that shows strong calcium mobilization response and marked intestinal activity.

References

(1) (a) DeLuca, H.F., Burmester, J., Darwish, H., and Krisinger, J. (1991) In Comprehensive Medicinal Chemistry (Hansch, C., Sammes, P.G., Taylor, J. B., Eds.), Pergamon Press: Oxford, Vol. 3, pp. 1129-1143. (b) DeLuca, H.F. (1974) Fed. Proc. *33*, 2211-2219.

(2) (a) Norman, A.W., Bouillon, R., and Thomasset, M., Eds. (1994) *Vitamin D, a pluripotent steroid hormone: Structural studies, molecular endocrinology and clinical applications.* Walter de Gruyter: Berlin. (b) Norman, A.W., Ed., *Vitamin D, the calcium homeostatic steroid hormone.* Academic Press: New York, 1979.

(3) Sicinski, R.R., Prahl, J M., Smith, C.M., and DeLuca, H.F. (1998) J. Med. Chem. 41, 4662-4674.

(4) (a) Lythgoe, B.(1981) Chem. Soc. Rev. 449-475. (b) Lythgoe, B., Moran, T.A., Nambudiry, M.E.N., Tideswell, J., and Wright, P.W. (1978) J. Chem. Soc., Perkin Trans. 1, 590-595. (c) Lythgoe, B., Moran, T.A.; Nambudiry, M.E.N., and Ruston, S. (1976) J. Chem. Soc., Perkin Trans. 1, 2386-2390.

(5) Evans, D.A., Truesdale, L.K., Grimm, K.G., and Nesbitt, S.L. (1977) J. Am. Chem. Soc. 99, 5009-5017.

(6) (a) Okamura, W.H., Midland, M.M., Hammond, M.W., Abd.Rahman, N., Dormanen, M.C., Nemere, I., and Norman, A.W. (1995) J. Steroid. Biochem. Molec. Biol. 53, 603-613. (b) Havinga, E. (1973) Experientia 29, 1181-1316.

(7) (a) Johnson, F. (1968) Chem. Rev. 68, 375-413. (b) Johnson, F. and Malhotra, S. K. (1965) J. Am. Chem. Soc. 87, 5492-5493.

DEVELOPMENT OF CE-RING MODIFIED ANALOGS OF 1,25(OH)$_2$D$_3$ WITH VARYING RING SIZES.

H. Van Dingenen,[1] X. Q. Xu,[1] C. D'Halleweyn,[1] D. Van Haver,[1] M. Vandewalle, P. De Clercq,[1] A. Verstuyf[2] and R. Bouillon[2] [1] Department of Organic Chemistry, Ghent University; [2] Lab. Exp. Med. & Endocrinology (LEGENDO), KU Leuven, Belgium.

Introduction. In recent years, research in the vitamin D$_3$ area has grown exponentially owing to the discovery that 1,25(OH)$_2$D$_3$, the hormonally active form of vitamin D$_3$, has a much broader spectrum of activities than originally thought, such as promoting cell differentiation and inhibiting cell proliferation in addition to its classical roles of regulating calcium and phosphorus metabolism (1). This has resulted in a very active search for analogs in which the calcemic activity and the other activities are dissociated. Indeed, the therapeutic utility of the natural hormone in the treatment of certain cancers and skin diseases is severely limited because effective doses provoke hypercalcemia. To date, a number of structurally modified analogs with potent cell differentiation and proliferation without causing hypercalcemia, have been subjected to preliminary clinical studies. In particular, several side-chain modified analogs have been developed which are promising with respect to the above differentiation potential, such as 23-yne, 22-oxa, 20-epi derivatives, homo derivatives (i.e., 24-homo,...) and combinations thereof (2,3).

1,25(OH)$_2$D$_3$

Results. In the context of the study of structure-function relationship, our laboratory has been focusing on the development of 1α,25(OH)$_2$D$_3$ analogs possessing a modified CD-ring system (4).
In the present study we'll describe the synthesis of analogs characterized by a trans-decalin CE-ring skeleton containing an unnatural E-ring.

58

In general, the synthesis of these vitamin D analogs occurs in three stages. First, the bicyclic CE-ring skeleton is build up, on which the side chain is appended in a second step. At last, the CE intermediate is coupled to the A-ring phosphine oxide in a Horner Wittig reaction (5). The construction is best carried out in this order since the triene system of the A-ring is chemically not very stable.

An ideal precursor for the central CE-fragment is the bicyclic enone **3**. It was obtained from the cyclohexanone **1** in 4 steps including a Michael addition (6). After hydrolysis of the imine function, Michael adduct **2** was subjected to a base induced Robinson annelation. After recrystallisation, the desired enone **3** was obtained in 50% overall yield and in 87 % ee.

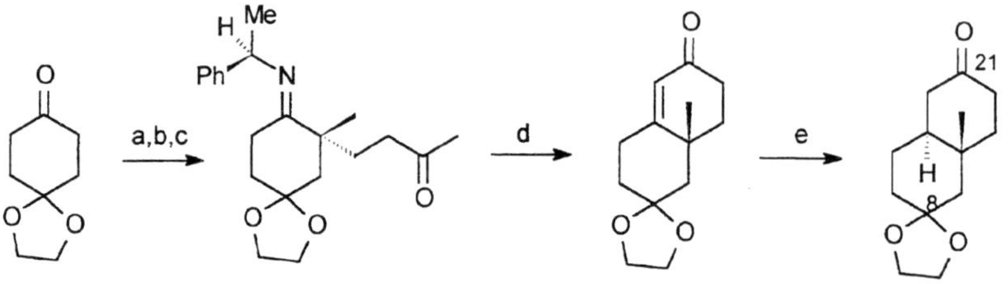

1   2   3   4

Scheme 2. Reaction conditions: (a) LDA, $C_6H_{12}NO_3B$, MeI, DMF, -30°C, (80%); (b) α-(+)-methylbenzyl amine, Dean Stark; (c) methyl vinyl ketone, 40°C; (d) MeOH, KOH, 60°C, (50% overall yield, 87% ee); (e) Li/NH$_3$, t-BuOH, -30°C, (85%).

For the synthesis of the first series of analogs, bearing the side chain on C-21, enone **3** was reduced with lithium in liquid ammonia to the *trans*-fused decalone **4**. Construction of the analogs **10** to **16** involves (i) attachment of the side chain via the carbonyl function on C-21 and (ii) appending the A-ring on the carbonyl function at C-8 via a Horner-Wittig reaction (6).

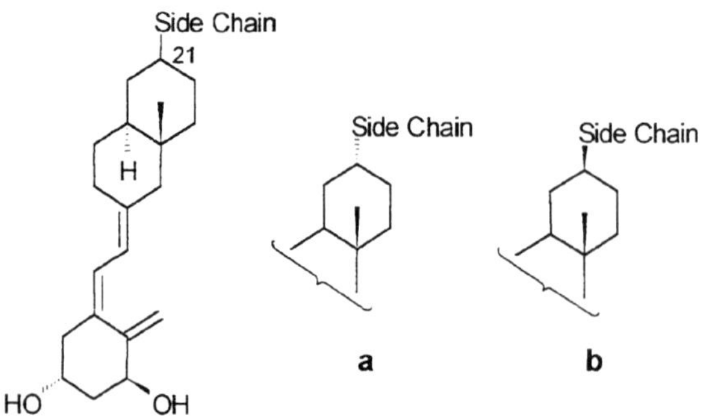

	Side Chain
10 b	-OCH$_2$CH$_2$C(OH)Me$_2$
11 a	-OCH$_2$CH$_2$C(OH)Me$_2$
12 b	-CH$_2$C(OH)Me$_2$
13 b	-C≡CC(OH)Me$_2$
14 b	-CH$_2$CH$_2$C(OH)Me$_2$
15 b	-CH$_2$CH$_2$CH$_2$C(OH)Me$_2$
16 a	-CH$_2$CH$_2$CH$_2$C(OH)Me$_2$

Selective reduction of the carbonyl function in **4**, gave rise to the axial or the equatorial alcohol, depending on the reaction conditions. These were further transformed to the CE intermediates **5a** and **5b**, followed by the Lythgoe coupling with the A-ring phosphine oxide **9** to form the oxa-analogs **10b** and **11a**. After introduction of a methylene function by a Wittig reaction on ketone **4**, a hydroboration resulted in the alcohol mixture **6a** and **6b**, which could be separated. Further functionalisation of the side chain, removal of the acetal protective group and coupling of the obtained ketones **7** and **8** with **9** leads to the analogs **13b** and **14b**, as well as to the 24-homo analogs **15b** and **16a**.

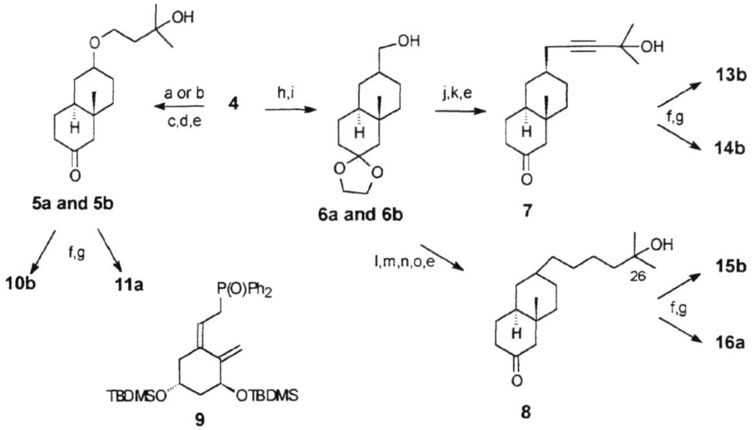

Scheme 3. Reaction conditions: (a) Li/NH$_3$, t-BuOH, -78°C, (80%); (b) LS-Selectride, THF, -78°C, (80%); (c) NaH, 4-chloro-2-methyl-2-butene, DMF, (70%); (d) Hg(OAc)$_2$, H$_2$0, NaOH, NaBH$_4$, THF, (60%); (e) pTsA, H$_2$O, acetone, (90%); (f) **9**, n-BuLi, THF, (65%); (g) TBAF, THF, rt, (87%); (h) Ph$_3$PBrCH$_3$, n-BuLi, THF, rt, (85%); (l) BH$_3$, H$_2$O$_2$, NaOH, (94%); (j) TsCl, Et$_3$N, DMAP, CH$_2$Cl$_2$, (88%); (k) NaH, 3-ethoxy-3-methyl-1-butyn, DMSO, (93%, for analog **14b** followed by hydrogenation); (l) Py.SO$_3$, DMSO, CH$_2$Cl$_2$, -10°C, (99%); (m) (EtO)$_2$POCH$_2$CHCHCOOEt, LDA, THF, -78°C, (70%); (n) Rh/Al$_2$O$_3$, EtOAc, H$_2$, rt, (92%); (o) MeMgBr, THF, -78°C, (87%).

The second series includes analogs containing the side chain on the C-20 or C-12' position, i.e. where the side chain is appended on the vicinal carbon in comparison with the former series. Therefore, a 1,2-carbonyl transposition is carried out starting from the CE-intermediate **3**, followed by a selective reduction to the desired axial alcohol. Attachment of the side chain was performed by a Williamson ether synthesis, followed by the introduction of the hydroxyl function. After the deprotection of the acetal function on C-8, the obtained ketones **19** and **23** were each subjected to the usual Horner-Wittig conditions that led to the oxa-analogs **20** and **24**.

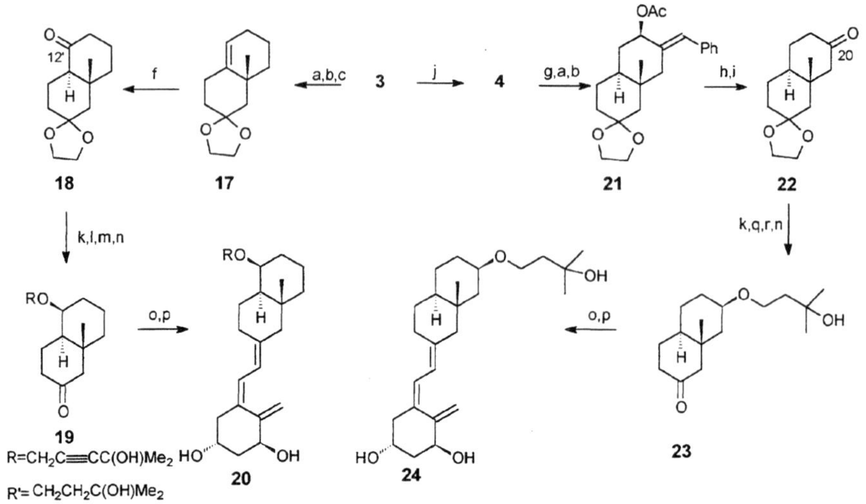

Scheme 4. Reaction conditions: (a) NaBH₄, CeCl₃, MeOH, rt, (86%); (b) Et₃N, Ac₂O, rt, (94%); (c) Li/NH₃, Et₂O, reflux, (96%); (d) BH₃, NaOH, H₂O₂, THF, (87%); (e) TPAP, NMMO, molecular sieves, CH₂Cl₂, rt, (84%); (f) Epimerisation: MeONa, MeOH, rt (93% after 3 cycli); (g) PhCHO, NaOH, EtOH, H₂O, -30°C, (80%); (h) KMnO₄, NaIO₄, H₂O, THF, (80%); (i) Li/NH₃, THF, -78°C, (85%); (j) Li/NH₃, t-BuOH, THF, -78°C, (84%); (k) NaBH₄, MeOH, rt, (93%); (l) NaH, propargyl bromide, THF/DMF, (50%, recuperation starting material); (m) n-BuLi, acetone, -30°C, (79%); (n) pTsA, acetone, H₂O, rt, (90%); (o) **9**, n-BuLi, -78°C to rt, (62%); (p) TBAF, THF, ty, (90%); (q) NaH, 4-chloro-2-methyl-2-butene, DMF, (70%); (r) Hg(OAc)₂, H₂O, NaOH, NaBH₄, THF, (60%).

Acknowledgements: Financial support to the laboratory by THERAMEX S.A. is gratefully acknowledged. HVD thanks the IWT for a scholarship.

References:
(1)   DeLuca, H.F., Burmester, J., Darwish, H., Krisinger, J. (1990) Comprehensive Medicinal Chemistry, Pergamon Press, New York, vol.3, 1129.
(2)   Bouillon, R.; Okamura, W.H.; Norman, A.W. (1995) Endocrine Reviews, 16, 200.
(3)   Okamura, W.H.; Palenzuela, A.J.; Plumet, J.; Midland, M.M (1992) J.Cellular Biochem., 49, 10.
(4)   De Clercq, P.J.; D'Halleweyn, C.; Gabriels, S.; Linclau, B.; Sabbe, K.; Sas, B.; Sebastian, S.; Van Dingenen, H.; Van Haver, D.; Chen, Y.; Ling, S.; Xu, X.; Wu, Y.; Wu; Y, Zhao, X.; Zhoa, X.; Zhu, G.; Vandewalle, M (1997) Proceedings of the tenth workshop in vitamin D, Strasbourg, France (may 24-29)
(5)   Lythgoe, B.; Moran, T.A.; Nambudiry, M.E.N.; Tideswell, J.; Wright, P.W. (1978) J.Chem.Soc., Perkin Trans I, 591; Kocienski, P.J.; Lythgoe, B (1978) J.Chem.Soc., Perkin Trans I, 1290.
(6)   Pfau, M.; Jabin, I.; Revial, G. (1993) J.Chem.Soc., Perkin Trans I, 1935.

EFFICIENT SYNTHESES AND BIOLOGICAL EVALUATION OF NOVEL 2α-SUBSTITUTED 1α,25-DIHYDROXYVITAMIN D₃ ANALOGS: REMARKABLE POTENCY FOR CALCIUM-REGULATING EFFECT

Yoshitomo Suhara, Ken-ichi Nihei, Hirokazu Tanigawa, Toshie Fujishima, Katsuhiro Konno, Kimie Nakagawa[a] Toshio Okano,[a] Masaaki Kurihara,[b] and Hiroaki Takayama*
Faculty of Pharmaceutical Sciences, Teikyo University, Sagamiko, Kanagawa 199-0195, Japan. [a]Department of Hygenic Sciences, Kobe Pharmaceutical University, Higashinada-ku, Kobe 658-8558, Japan. [b]National Institute of Health Sciences, Kamiyoga, Setagaya-ku, Tokyo 158-8501, Japan

Introduction In order to investigate the A-ring conformation-activity relationships, we synthesized all the A-ring diastereomers of 2-methyl-1,25-dihydroxyvitamin D₃ and found that the 2α-methyl isomer (**2**) showed higher potency than **1** in terms of VDR binding affinity, elevation of rat serum Ca concentration, and induction of HL-60 cell differentiation.[1] Furthermore, the combination of this 2α-methyl substitution with 20-epimerization, *i.e.*, double modification, produced a much more potent analog.[2] These results prompted us to design new analogs with further modification of the 2α-methyl group. We anticipated that if the 2α-methyl group were replaced by a longer 2α-alkyl or the 2α-hydroxyalkyl group, the resulting analogs would provide insight into the biological significance of the 2α-methyl substitution. We report here the synthesis of several new analogs, **3-7**, and their biological evaluation.

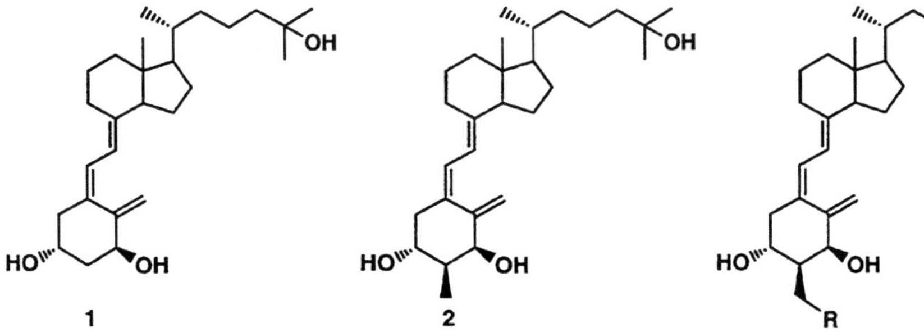

3: R = CH₃
4: R = CH₂CH₃
5: R = OH
6: R = CH₂OH
7: R = CH₂CH₂OH

Chemical Synthesis Our synthetic strategy is shown below. As shown in Scheme 1, we chose a D-xylose derivative (**8**) for stereoselective synthesis of A-ring portions of the title compounds (**3**)-(**7**).[3] After a hydroxymethyl group was introduced to the *C*-3 position of D-xylofuranose derivative (**8**), the furanose ring was opened by Wittig reaction. The *C*-5 hydroxy group was converted to ethynyl group followed by the selective pivaloyl protection, MOM deprotection and silyl protection to afford the fully protected triol **17** in good yield. Finally, further protecting group manipulation through **18** gave the desired A-ring synthon **19** in high yield.

Elongation of the 2α-substituent of the A-ring synthon was carried out in a conventional manner as shown in Scheme 2. Sequential sulfonylation, cyanide addition and reduction from the alcohol **18** furnished the single-carbon-elongated alcohol **20** in good overall yield, and this was protected to

62

Scheme 1

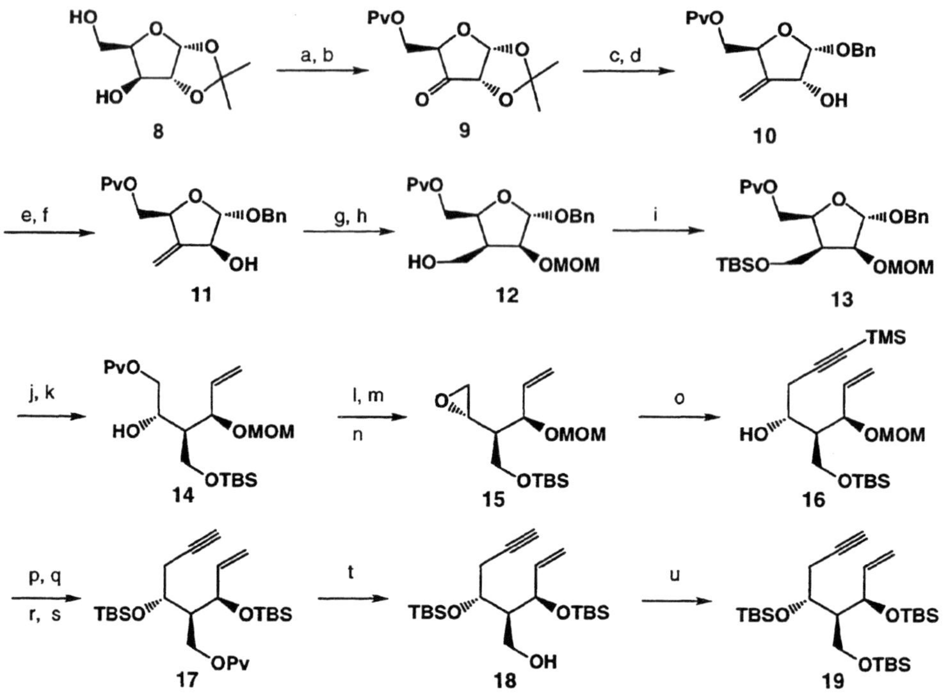

(a) PvCl, Py, 86%; (b) PCC, MS 4A, CH$_2$Cl$_2$, 98%; (c) Ph$_3$P$^+$CH$_3$Br$^-$, KHMDS, THF, 85%; (d) 1 N HCl, BnOH, 1,4-dioxane/toluene, 58%; (e) p-nitrobenzoic acid, Ph$_3$P, DEAD, THF; (f) 10 mM NaOH, H$_2$O/MeOH, 84% (2 steps); (g) MOMCl, DIPEA, TBAI, CH$_2$Cl$_2$, 88%; (h) 9-BBN, THF, then 3 M NaOH, 30% H$_2$O$_2$, 85%; (i) TBSCl, imidazole, DMF, 99%; (j) H$_2$, Pd(OH)$_2$, EtOH; (k) Ph$_3$P$^+$CH$_3$Br$^-$, LiHMDS, THF, 79% (2 steps); (l) DIBAL-H, CH$_2$Cl$_2$, 84%; (m) TmCl, DMAP, CH$_2$Cl$_2$; (n) LiHMDS, THF, 86% (2 steps); (o) TMSC≡CH, n-BuLi, BF$_3$·OEt$_2$, THF, 80%; (p) TBAF, THF, 99%; (q) PvCl, Py/CH$_2$Cl$_2$, 85%; (r) PPTS, t-BuOH, 74%; (s) TBSOTf, 2,6-lutidine, CH$_2$Cl$_2$, 99%; (t) DIBAL-H, CH$_2$Cl$_2$, 96%; (u) TBSCl, imidazole, DMF, 88%.

Scheme 2

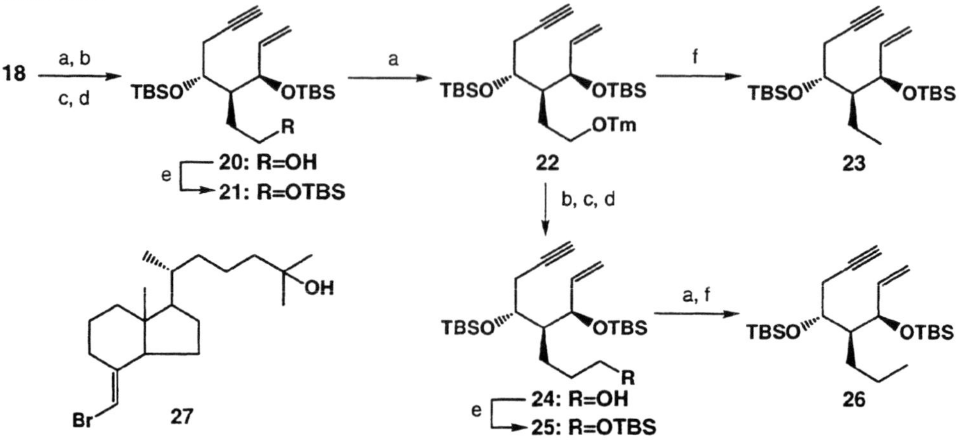

(a) TmCl, DMAP, CH$_2$Cl$_2$; (b) NaCN, DMSO, 61%-82% (2 steps); (c) DIBAL-H, CH$_2$Cl$_2$, 85%-89%; (d) NaBH$_4$, MeOH, 82-98%; (e) TBSCl, imidazole, DMF, 78-83%; (f) LAH, Et$_2$O, 80% (2 steps).

A-ring synthon **21**. The alcohol **20** was further converted to the 2α-ethyl substituent through the tosylate **22**. In the same manner, the double-carbon-elongated synthons **25** and **26** were prepared from **22** through **24**. Finally, palladium-catalyzed coupling of the A-ring synthons **19**, **21**, **23**, **25**, and **26** with the CD-ring portion **27**,[3] followed by deprotection with camphorsulfonic acid (CSA) in MeOH gave the 2α-alkyl and 2α-hydroxyalkyl analogs **3-7**.[4]

Biological Evaluation   The results of biological evaluation are summarized in Table 1, in comparison with those of 1α,25-dihydroxyvitamin D_3 (**1**) and 2α-methyl-1α,25-dihydroxyvitamin D_3 (**2**). First of all, we examined the receptor binding in an assay using bovine thymus VDR. The 2α-alkyl analogs **3** and **4** showed much lower binding affinity than the 2α-methyl analog **2**; in other words, the shortest-chain analog has the highest affinity among the 2α-alkyl analogs. In contrast, the 2α-hydroxypropyl analog **7**, bearing the most elongated chain, showed the highest binding affinity, 3-fold higher than that of **1**, among the 2α-hydroxyalkyl analogs.[5]

Table 1. Relative potency of the synthesized analogs.[a]

Compound	VDR[b] binding affinity	DBP[c] binding	HL-60 cell[d] differentiation	Ca mobilization[e]
1 (1α,25-(OH)$_2$VD$_3$)	100	100	100	100
2 (2α-methyl)	400	44	444	658
3 (2α-ethyl)	40	48	106	68
4 (2α-propyl)	20	21	44	636
5 (2α-hydroxymethyl)	20	95	10	124
6 (2α-hydroxyethyl)	70	74	86	372
7 (2α-hydroxypropyl)	300	362	240	50866

(a) The potency of 1α,25-(OH)$_2$VD$_3$ is normalized to 100 in each case. (b) Bovine thymus. (c) Rat serum. (d) Cell differentiation was assessed in terms of expression of antigen CD11b. (e) Rat serum Ca level.

The affinity for vitamin D binding protein (DBP) was tested using rat serum DBP. The binding affinity was decreased in the 2α-alkyl analogs including **2**, whereas it was largely retained or even increased in the 2α-hydroxyalkyl analogs.

The rank order of potency for inducing differentiation in HL-60 cells was parallel to that of VDR binding; that is, as the chain length became longer, the potency decreased in 2α-alkyl analogs, whereas it increased in the 2α-hydroxyalkyl analogs. Only compounds **2** and **7** showed much higher activity than 1α,25-dihydroxyvitamin D_3 in this experiment.

Most of the new analogs exhibited higher calcium-mobilizing activity than **1**, in particular, the analog **7** showed 500 times higher potency, and this remarkably high activity is unique among vitamin D analogs reported to date. Therefore, this 2α-hydroxypropyl analog **7** may provide clues to achieving separation of the biological functions of vitamin D.

Conformational Analysis   We investigated the three-dimensional structure of the 2α-hydroxypropyl analog **7**, which had exhibited exceptionally potent calcium-regulating activity, docking VDR ligand binding domain. Very recently, Moras *et al.* reported molecular mechanics calculation based on the crystal structure of VDR.[6] Then we evaluated the binding-state of **7** using the Moras' VDR ligand conformation in the preliminary calculation as shown below.[7] In this study, the 1α-hydroxyl group retains hydrogen bonding to Ser-237, and an additional hydrogen bonding was observed between the C-2α terminal hydroxyl group of **7** and Arg-274. In addition, the alkyl chain of hydroxypropyl group of **7** would make a role of hydrophobic interaction to the cavity surrounded by Phe-150, Tyr-143, Tyr-147, and Tyr-236. These facts should be one of the reasons for the high binding affinity to VDR.

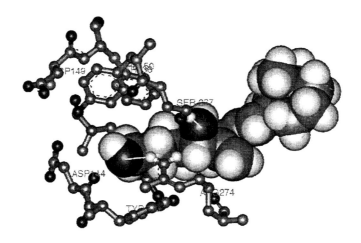

Conclusion   Thus, the activity profiles of the synthesized analogs are high structure-sensitive, in that even a single-carbon chain difference greatly alters the profile. Consequently, these analogs should be useful for studies on the action mechanism of vitamin D, and also as lead compounds for developing therapeutic agents. Further studies, however, are needed to elucidate fully the activity profiles and modes of action of these analogs.

References and Notes
1. Konno, K., Maki, S., Fujishima, T., Liu, Z.-P., Miura, D., Chokki, M., Takayama, H. (1998) Bioorg.Med.Chem.Lett. 8, 151-156.
2. Fujishima, T., Liu, Z.-P., Miura, D., Chokki, M., Ishizuka, S., Konno, K., Takayama, H. (1998) Bioorg.Med.Chem.Lett. 8, 2145-2148.
3. Trost, B.M., Dumas, J. and Villa, M. (1992) J.Am.Chem.Soc. 114, 9836-9845.
4. Suhara, Y., Nihei, K., Tanigawa, H., Fujishima, T., Konno, K., Nakagawa, K., Okano, T., Takayama, H. Bioorg.Med.Chem.Lett., in press.
5. Posner *et al.* previously reported that a 2α-hydroxybutyl-1α,25-dihydroxyvitamin D$_3$ analog had virtually no affinity for VDR. Posner, G. H.; Johnson, N. (1994) J.Org.Chem. 59, 7855-7861.
6. Rochel, N., Wurtz, J.M., Mitschler, A., Klaholz, B., Moras, D. (2000) Molecular Cell 5, 173-179.
7. Calculated by MacroModel® ver.6.5 (Schrodinger, Inc) on SGI O2 Workstation.

1α,25-DIHYDROXYPREVITAMIN D₃ AND ITS ANALOGS

Rena Hayashi and William H. Okamura*
Department of Chemistry, University of California, Riverside, California 92521, USA

Introduction. The steroid hormone 1α,25-dihydroxyvitamin D_3 (1,25-D3, **1**), the active form of vitamin D_3, back equilibrates with ~5% of 1α,25-dihydroxyprevitamin D_3 (1,25-PreD3, **2**) at 37 °C via a [1,7]-H shift through 6-s-cis-1,25-D3 (**3**) as shown in Figure 1. Earlier studies from this laboratory resulted in the synthesis of 9,14,19,19,19-pentadeuterio-1,25-PreD3 in order to evaluate the kinetic details of [1,7]-sigmatropic shifts. In addition, these earlier studies were directed towards an assessment of the biological activities of these previtamins (1,2).

Figure 1. 1,25-PreD3 undergoes a slow hydrogen migration to 6-s-cis-1,25-D3 which rapidly rotates to its more stable conformation, 6-s-trans-1,25-D3. 1,25-D3 back equilibrates with ~5% of 1,25-PreD3, which exhibits minimal genomic actions but is as active as 1,25-D3 towards rapid responses.

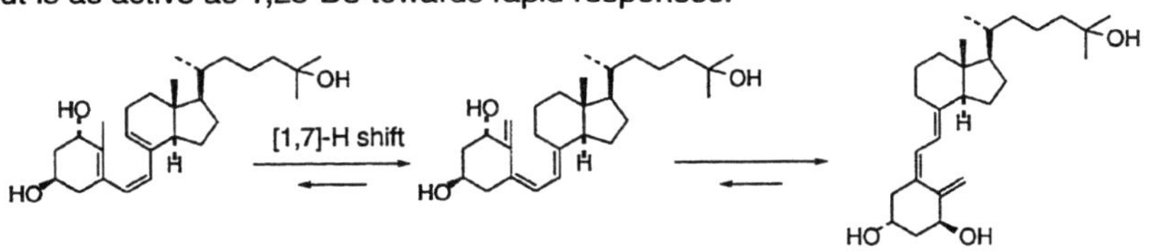

2
(~ 5%)

3
6-s-cis (< 1%)

1
6-s-trans (~ 95%)

1,25-PreD3

1,25-D3

It is known that 1,25-D3 induces genomic responses by initially binding to nuclear receptors (n-VDR) and rapid responses by binding to putative membrane receptors (m-VDR) (Figure 2). Interestingly 1,25-PreD3 was discovered to be equally as active as 1,25-D3 towards rapid responses including transcaltachia but exhibits only weak genomic actions (2, 3, 4).

Figure 2. The steroid hormone 1,25-D3 binds to its nuclear receptor protein (n-VDR) inducing genomic responses. It also induces rapid responses via a putative membrane receptor (m-VDR). 1,25-PreD3 as well as other 6-s-cis locked analogs induce rapid responses but weak or negligible genomic responses.

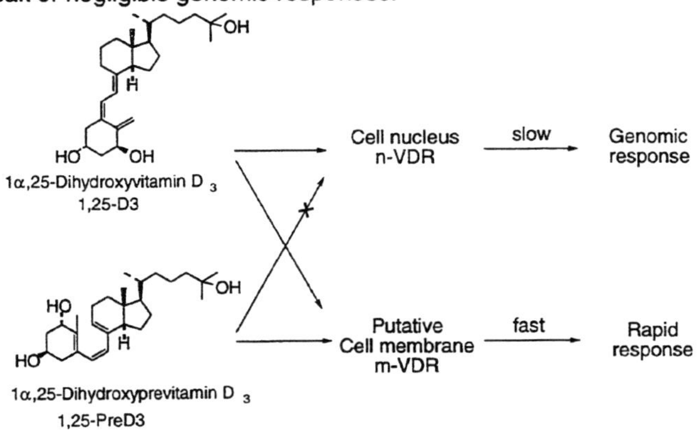

1α,25-Dihydroxyvitamin D₃
1,25-D3

1α,25-Dihydroxyprevitamin D₃
1,25-PreD3

| Cell nucleus n-VDR | slow | Genomic response |

| Putative Cell membrane m-VDR | fast | Rapid response |

In order to more thoroughly evaluate the active conformations involved in inducing both rapid and genomic responses, new 1,25-PreD and 1,25-D analogs are essential. As shown in Figure 3, it became of intense interest to develop a synthesis of 10,19-modified-1,25-PreD3 analogs and a synthesis of isotopically labeled 1,25-PreD3 and 1,25-D3. The latter pair of isotopomers were deemed of interest for direct NMR studies of ligands bound to host proteins and for metabolic investigations using mass spectrometry.

Figure 3. Goal -- Develop a synthesis of 10,19-modified-1,25-PreD3 analogs and a synthesis of isotopically labeled 1,25-PreD3 and 1,25-D3

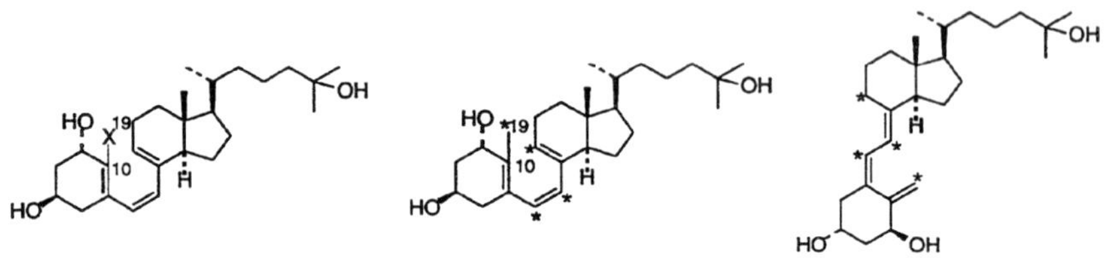

10-Modified-1,25-PreD3 Analog
X=Br, Cl, R

1,25-PreD3

1,25-D3

The previous studies of isotopically substituted 1,25-PreD3 and 1,25-D3 from our laboratory used (S)-carvone as a starting material to obtain a key enyne A-ring fragment, which was then transformed to a labeled A-ring enyne fragment (5). The A-ring enyne was then coupled to labeled CD-ring fragment as per Mouriño et al (6). Yamada and Holick were able to synthesize other 10 and 19-substituted analogs using vitamin D-SO$_2$ adducts as key intermediates (7, 8). In this paper, progress towards developing a new synthetic approach to 10,19-modified-1,25-PreD3 analogs will be described.

Results and Discussion. As given in Figure 4, the synthesis of a new A-ring fragment, the bromo-enoltriflate 9 is described. This bromo-enoltriflate was synthesized from quinic acid (4) via the C$_2$ ketone 7, whose synthesis has been previously reported by DeLuca et al (9). Compound 7 was brominated at the α-position using LiHMDS followed by treatment with bromine. The α-bromoketone 8 was then transformed into the bromo-enoltriflate 9 by the action of KHMDS with HMPA followed by the triflating reagent. It was envisaged that 9 could be cross-coupled in a stepwise manner using transition metal catalysts to a wide variety of electrophiles as an initial step to analogs.

Figure 4. Synthesis of an A-ring bromo-enoltriflate from quinic acid via the C$_2$ ketone 7

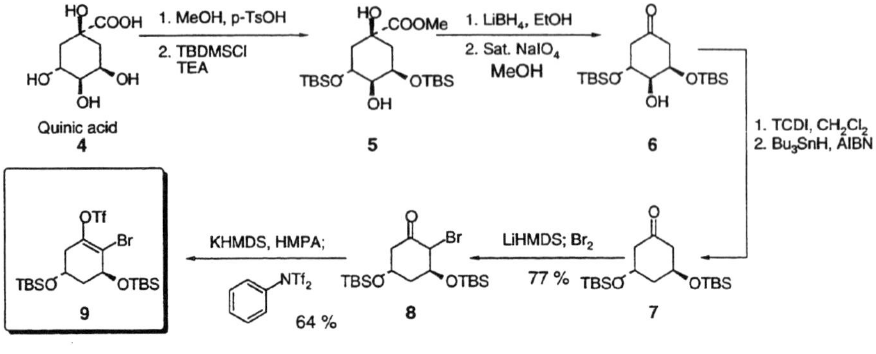

In one successful synthetic approach, the key intermediate **9** underwent selective triflate group substitution via a Stille reaction using tributylvinyltin with tris(dibenzylideneacetone)dipalladium(0), triphenylarsine and lithium chloride in NMP as shown in Figure 5. As shown in Figure 6, coupling of various alkynes using a variety of catalysts, conditions, and substrates were not successful. Parallel experiments using the enol-phosphate analogous to the triflate **9** were also unsuccessful. The vinyl compound **10** however could be cleaved with osmium tetraoxide and sodium periodate to give bromo aldehyde **11** which was then transformed into bromo-enyne in one step using (trimethylsilyl)diazomethane with butyllithium.

Figure 5. A vinylstannane can be coupled to the A-ring bromo-enoltriflate

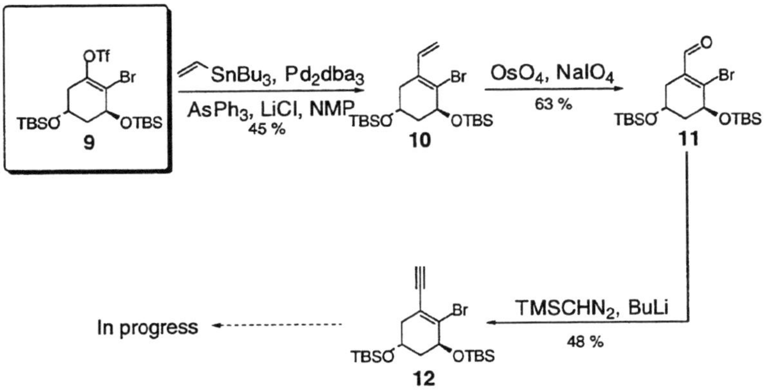

Figure 6. Alkynyl substrates have failed to couple to the A-ring bromo-enoltriflate

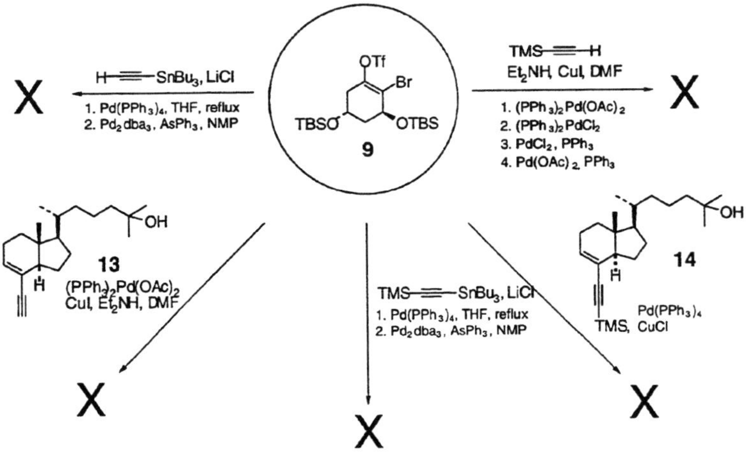

To summarize, bromo-A-ring synthons, compounds **9**, **10**, **11**, and **12**, have been synthesized from quinic acid via the C₂ ketone **7**. Further transformation of these A-ring synthons to 10-modified-1,25-PreD3 analogs (Figure 3) are under active investigations.

68

Acknowledgement. Support under NIH Grant No DK-16595 is acknowledged. Dr. Susana Fernandez is also acknowledged for earlier contributions to this project and Solvay for providing selected starting material.

References.

(1) Curtin, M.L., Okamura, W.H. (1991) J. Am. Chem. Soc. 113, 6958-6966.

(2) Norman, A.W., Okamura, W.H., Farach-Carson, M.C., Allewaert, K., Branisteanu, D., Nemere, I., Muralidharan, K.R., Bouillon, R. (1993) J. Biol. Chem. 268, 13811-13819.

(3) Nemere, I., Dormanen, M.C., Hammond, M.W., Okamura, W.H., Norman, A.W. (1994) J. Biol. Chem. 269, 23750-23756.

(4) Norman, A.W., Okamura, W.H., Hammond, M.W., Bishop, J.E., Dormanen, M.C., Bouillon, R., van Baelen, H., Ridall, A.L., Daane, E., Khoury, R., Farach-Carson, M.C. (1997) Mol. Endo. 11, 1518-1531.

(5) Aurrecoechea, J.M., Okamura, W.H. (1987) Tetrahedron Lett. 28, 4947-4950.

(6) Mascareñas, J.L., Sarandeses, L.A., Castedo, L., Mouriño, A. (1991) Tetrahedron 47, 3485-3498.

(7) Iwasaki, Y., Shimizu, M., Hirosawa, T., Yamada, S. (1996) Tetrahedron Lett. 37, 6753-6754.

(8) Ray, R., Vicchio, D., Yergey, A., Holick, M.F. (1992) Steroids 57, 142-146.

(9) DeLuca, H.F., Schnoes, H.K., Periman, K.L., Swenson, R.E. (1992) European Patent Application, 92304837.5

VITAMIN D₃ ANALOGUES WITH TWO SIDE CHAINS

Yvonne Bury[1], Michaela Herdick[1], Milan R. Uskokovic[2] and Carsten Carlberg[1]

[1]Institut für Physiologische Chemie I and Biomedizinisches Forschungszentrum, Heinrich-Heine-Universität, D-40001 Düsseldorf, Germany, [2]Hoffmann-La Roche Inc., Nutley, NJ 07110, USA

Summary: A $1\alpha,25(OH)_2D_3$ analogue with two side chains (Ro27-2310 or Gemini) was found to stabilize functional $1\alpha,25(OH)_2D_3$ receptor (VDR) conformations and VDR-retinoid X receptor (RXR) heterodimers on a $1\alpha,25(OH)_2D_3$ response element (VDRE) with a slightly lower sensitivity than the natural hormone. A 19-nor derivative of Gemini (Ro27-5646) showed similar sensitivity, whereas 5,6-trans (Ro27-6462), 3-epi (Ro27-5840) and 1α-fluoro (Ro27-3752) derivatives were comparable to each other but approximately 30-times less sensitive than Gemini. A C,D-des derivative of Gemini (Ro28-1909) showed only residual activity at maximal concentrations. In contrast to $1\alpha,25(OH)_2D_3$, Gemini and its derivatives showed a differential preference in stabilizing VDR conformations, which was found to be modulated by DNA, coactivator and corepressor proteins. Gemini was highlighted as an interesting drug candidate, which could not be optimized through obvious chemical modifications in its A-ring.

Introduction: More than 2000 analogues of $1\alpha,25(OH)_2D_3$ have been developed with the goal to improve the biological profile of the natural hormone for a potential therapeutic application (1). The effects of $1\alpha,25(OH)_2D_3$ and its analogues on bone mineralization as well as on cell cycle regulation, i.e. their therapeutic potential in quite different diseases such as osteoporosis, psoriasis and breast cancer, are mediated through the regulation of specific genes by the nuclear receptor VDR. This indicates that the analysis of the gene regulatory potential of a VDR agonist is essential for its evaluation as a candidate drug. Recent understanding of $1\alpha,25(OH)_2D_3$ signalling mechanisms (2) made clear that conformational changes of the ligand binding domain (LBD) of VDR induce the dissociation of nuclear receptor-corepressor com-plexes and facilitate the interaction with coactivator proteins, which consequently results in stimulation of transcriptional activity via various additional protein-protein inter-actions. Conformational changes of DNA-bound VDR-RXR hetero-

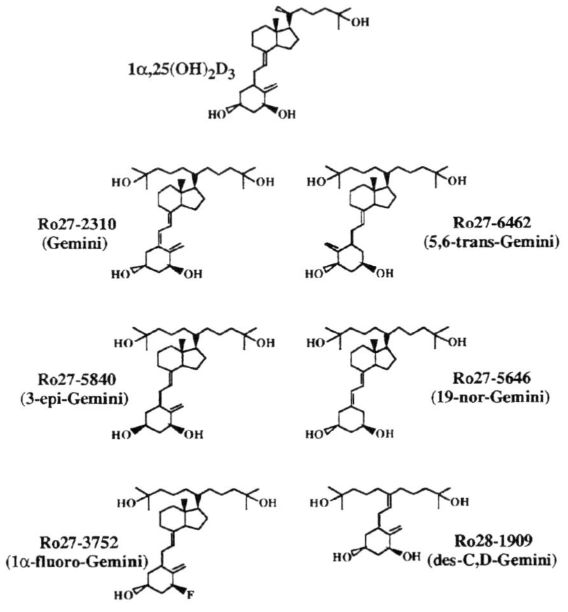

Figure 1: Structure of $1\alpha,25(OH)_2D_3$, Gemini and its derivatives.

dimers are therefore the core of the $1\alpha,25(OH)_2D_3$ molecular signalling switch. Therefore, investigations focus on the interaction of VDR agonists with the receptor via the induction of a conformational change in its LBD. Modern methods, such as limited protease digestion (LPD) and ligand-dependent gel shift (GS) assays, are quite well suited for the *in vitro* evaluation of VDR agonists and allow for an extrapolation of their gene regulatory potential. In this report, the gene regulatory potential of a novel $1\alpha,25(OH)_2D_3$ analogue, called Ro27-2310 or Gemini, which contains two side chains at carbon 20, was studied *in vitro* and *in vivo*. Moreover, obvious chemical modifications of its A-Ring, such as 5,6-trans, 3-epi, 19-nor, 1α-fluoro and des-C,D derivatives were analyzed for their potential to optimize the gene regulatory profile of Ro27-2310.

Results and Discussion: DNA-independent (classical) LPD assays were performed with graded concentrations of $1\alpha,25(OH)_2D_3$ and Ro27-2310 (for structures see Fig. 1) and provided two digestion products, $c1_{LPD}$ and $c3_{LPD}$, which are interpreted as functional VDR conformations (Fig. 2A). In DNA-dependent LPD assays VDR was complexed with RXR on a DR3-type VDRE (Fig. 2B), or additionally incubated with a coactivator protein (TIF2) (Fig. 2C). Interestingly, the RXR-driven complex formation on a VDRE was found to clearly increase the ligand sensitivity of the agonistic VDR conformation $c1_{LPD}$ (10-fold for $1\alpha,25(OH)_2D_3$ and from not detectable to 2 nM for Ro27-2310). An EC_{50}-value

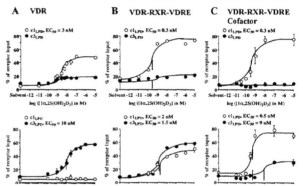

Figure 2: Dose-dependent stabilization of VDR conformations modulated by DNA and cofactor. Limited protease digestion assays were performed by preincubating *in vitro* translated [^{35}S]-labelled VDR or heterodimers of *in vitro* synthesized [^{35}S]-labelled VDR and unlabelled RXR with graded concentrations of $1\alpha,25(OH)_2D_3$ and Gemini. Protein-DNA complexes were then formed on the unlabelled DR3-type VDRE (B, C) from the rat ANF gene promoter in the absence (A, B) or presence (C) of bacterially expressed GST-TIF2$_{646-926}$.

for the non-agonistic VDR conformation $c3_{LPD}$ was only detectable with Ro27-2310 and decreased 6-fold by complex formation of the VDR. DNA-dependent LPD assays in the presence of coactivator did not demonstrate a reasonable effect on ligand sensitivity of $c1_{LPD}$ with $1\alpha,25(OH)_2D_3$ whereas $c1_{LPD}$ was protected with a 4-fold higher sensitivity and $c3_{LPD}$ with a 6-fold lower sensitivity with Ro27-2310. In parallel, at saturating concentrations of Ro27-2310 the $c1_{LPD}/c3_{LPD}$ ratio increased. These results suggest that in contrast to the natural hormone and all presently investigated $1\alpha,25(OH)_2D_3$ analogues, Ro27-2310 appears to differentiate between VDR in solution and DNA-bound VDR (3).

This finding was supported by GST pull-down assays that were performed with GST-TIF2 fusion proteins, *in vitro* translated VDR and graded concentrations of $1\alpha,25(OH)_2D_3$ and Ro27-2310. $1\alpha,25(OH)_2D_3$ mediated a precipitation of 19 % of VDR with an EC_{50}-value of 9 nM (Fig. 3A), whereas Ro27-2310 was only able to precipitate 11 % of VDR input with an EC_{50}-value of 150 nM. The converse GST pull-down assays using GST-VDR fusion protein and *in vitro* translated coactivator proteins SRC-1, TIF2 and RAC3 demonstrated very similar results (3), i.e. that in

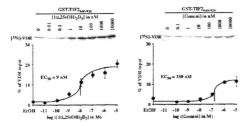

Figure 3: Ligand-triggered VDR-coactivator interaction. GST pull-down assays were performed with *in vitro* translated [^{35}S]-labelled VDR and bacterially expressed GST-TIF2$_{646-926}$. Nuclear receptors were preincubated at room temperature with graded concentrations of $1\alpha,25(OH)_2D_3$ and Gemini.

contrast to $1\alpha,25(OH)_2D_3$, Ro27-2310 was quite ineffective in mediating an *in vitro* interaction of VDR with coactivator proteins in solution. There is growing evidence that VDR not only acts as a DNA-bound transcription factor, but also as a DNA-independent modulator of other nuclear signalling pathways. One example is the repression of IL-2 gene expression by $1\alpha,25(OH)_2D_3$, for which it was suggested that the VDR inhibits the complex formation of the T-cell transcription factor NF-AT on its specific binding site in the IL-2 promoter (4). The selectivity of Ro27-2310 compounds for DNA-dependent $1\alpha,25(OH)_2D_3$ signalling pathways suggests that they would not be able to regulate IL-2 gene expression.

Different derivatives of Ro27-2310 were synthesized that show modifications in the A-ring (for structures see Fig. 1). DNA-dependent LPD assays were performed in order to assess the effect of RXR, DNA and cofactors on the potency of Ro27-2310 and its derivatives. The percentage of stabilized VDR con-formations c1$_{LPD}$ and c3$_{LPD}$ was quantified at saturating ligand con-centrations (10 µM) (Figs. 4A-D). The complex formation of VDR with RXR on the VDRE (Fig. 4B) resulted for all VDR agonists in an increased, selective stabilization of c1$_{LPD}$, whereas the amount of c3$_{LPD}$ did not appear to be significantly affected. Interestingly, the addition of a coactivator protein (SRC-1) to the protein-DNA complex (Fig. 4C) conferred Ro27-2310 and its derivatives with a similar profile to the natural hormone, i.e. a preferential stabilization of c1$_{LPD}$ in relation to c3$_{LPD}$. In contrast, the addition of a corepressor protein (NCoR) to the VDR-RXR-VDRE complex (Fig. 4D) resulted in the inverse effect, for all VDR agonists i.e. a low amount of VDR molecules were stabilized in c1$_{LPD}$, which was for Ro27-2310 and its derivatives even lower than the amount of VDR molecules that were stabilized in c3$_{LPD}$. However Ro28-1909 did not demonstrate a stabilization of c1$_{LPD}$ or c3$_{LPD}$ that was markedly different to that of the solvent control at any of these conditions. Conformations of the VDR bound by graded concentrations

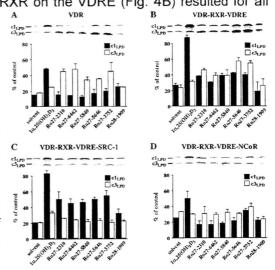

Figure 4: DNA- and cofactor-dependent stabilization of VDR conformations. Limited protease digestion assays were performed by preincubating *in vitro* translated [^{35}S]-labelled VDR alone (A) or in combination with the unlabelled RXR and the unlabelled DR3-type VDRE from the rat ANF gene promoter (B) and bacterially expressed GST-SRC-1$_{596-790}$ (C) or GST-NCoR$_{1679-2453}$ (D) in the presence of saturating concentrations (10 µM) of indicated ligands.

of $1\alpha,25(OH)_2D_3$, Ro27-2310 and its derivatives, were analyzed by DNA-independent LPD assays (Tab. 1). Ligand-dependent GS assays were performed with *in vitro* translated VDR-RXR heterodimers bound to a DR3-type VDRE and graded concentrations of the VDR agonists (Tab. 1). Mammalian one-hybrid assays were performed in HeLa cells that were transiently transfected with an expression vector for a fusion protein containing the DNA binding domain (DBD) of the yeast transcription factor GAL4 and the LBD of the VDR together with a reporter gene construct containing a GAL4 binding site-driven luciferase gene and stimulated with graded ligand concentrations (Tab. 1). Additionally, reporter gene assays were performed in VDR- and RXR-overexpressing Cos-7 cells, in which the luciferase reporter gene was driven by four copies of a DR3-type VDRE (Tab. 1).

Table 1: *In vitro* and *in vivo* evaluation of $1\alpha,25(OH)_2D_3$, Gemini and its derivatives.

Ligands	$1\alpha,25(OH)_2D_3$	Ro27-2310 (Gemini)	Ro27-6462 (5,6-trans-Gemini)	Ro27-5840 (3-epi-Gemini)	Ro27-5646 (19-nor-Gemini)	Ro27-3752 (1α-fluoro-Gemini)	Ro28-1909 (des-C,D-Gemini)	solvent
Limited Protease Digestion Assay (DNA-independent)								
$c1_{LPD}$ (in %)	55	10	10	10	10	10	10	10
$c3_{LPD}$ (in %)	20	60	50	40	40	50	20	10
EC_{50} [nM]	3	10	300	220	30	100	10000	-
Gel Shift Assay with DR3-type VDRE								
Complex formation (in%)	15	13	12	11	13	13	5	5
EC_{50} [nM]	0.2	0.3	4	10	0.6	6	>10000	-
Reporter Gene Assay in HeLa cells transfected with (Gal4)₃-tk-Luc and CMVGal4$_{DBD}$VDR$_{LBD}$								
Maximal fold induction	42	40	20	25	40	40	10	1
EC_{50} [nM]	0.9	0.1	7	6	0.25	10	300	-
Reporter Gene Assay in Cos-7 cells transfected with (DR3)₄-tk-Luc, pSG5-VDR and pSG5-RXR								
Maximal fold induction	12	5	4	6	4	4	1	1
EC_{50} [nM]	1.8	0.04	3	3	0.8	5.5	>10000	-

The *in vitro* and the cell culture assays provided a very similar ranking for Ro27-2310 and its derivatives. Ro27-5646 decreased the sensitivity only by a factor of 2-3, Ro27-6462, Ro27-5840 and Ro27-3752 derivatives were comparable to each other but approximately 30-times less sensitive than Ro27-2310. Ro28-1909 demonstrated only residual activity at maximal concentrations and therefore cannot be considered as a VDR agonist. Taken together, the five obvious A-ring chemical modifications of Ro27-2310 were not able to improve the sensitivity of this novel type of analogue. Future modifications of Ro27-2310 will address the significance of side chains as it was done for most other $1\alpha,25(OH)_2D_3$ analogues (1).

References:
1. Bouillon, R., Okamura, W. H., and Norman, A. W. (1995) *Endocr. Rev.* **16**, 200-257
2. Carlberg, C., and Polly, P. (1998) *Crit Rev Eukaryot Gene Expr* **8**, 19-42
3. Herdick, M., Bury, Y., Quack, M., Uskokovic, M., Polly, P., and Carlberg, C. (2000) *Mol. Pharmacol.* **57**, 1206-1217
4. Alroy, I., Towers, T. L., and Freedman, L. P. (1995) *Mol. Cell. Biol.* **15**, 5789-5799

5,6-*TRANS*-2-METHYL-1,25-DIHYDROXYVITAMIN D$_3$ AND THEIR 20-EPIMERS: SYNTHESIS AND BIOLOGICAL EVALUATION.

Toshie Fujishima, Katsuhiro Konno, Kimie Nakagawa,[a] Maki Tanaka,[a] Toshio Okano[a] and Hiroaki Takayama*
Faculty of Pharmaceutical Sciences, Teikyo University, Sagamiko, Kanagawa 199-0195, Japan. [a]Department of Hygienic Sciences, Kobe Pharmaceutical University, Kobe 658-8558, Japan.

Introduction   In order to study the structure-activity relationships of 1α,25-dihydroxyvitamin D$_3$ (**1**), we have synthesized all eight possible A-ring stereoisomers of 2-methyl-1,25-dihydroxyvitamin D$_3$ and found that the simple introduction of a methyl group yielded analogues with unique activity profiles (1). In particular, 2α-methyl-1α,25-dihydroxyvitamin D$_3$ (**2a**, Chart 1) exhibited 4-fold higher potency than **1** both in VDR binding and in *in vivo* calcium-regulating activity, and 2-fold

Chart 1

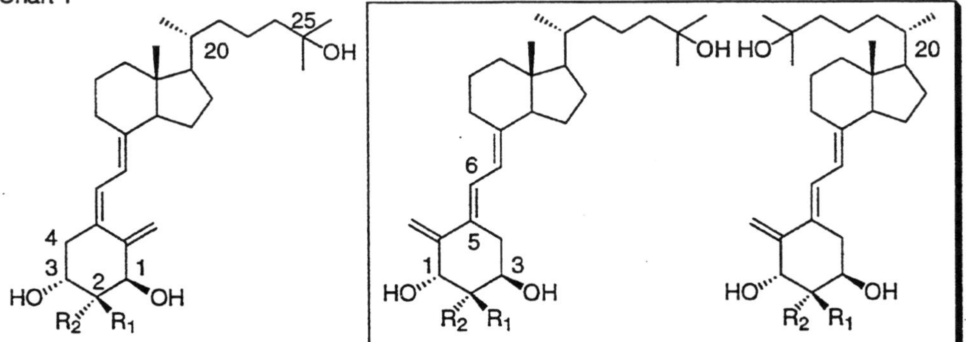

1: R$_1$=R$_2$=H
2a: R$_1$=Me, R$_2$=H
2b: R$_1$=H, R$_2$=Me

3: R$_1$=R$_2$=H
4a: R$_1$=Me, R$_2$=H
4b: R$_1$=H, R$_2$=Me

5a: R$_1$=Me, R$_2$=H
5b: R$_1$=H, R$_2$=Me

higher potency in HL-60 cell differentiation (1a). Our research on 2-methyl-20-*epi* analogues also revealed that combination of the 2α-methyl introduction and 20-epimerization yielded analogues with exceptionally high potency: in the case of the 20-epimer of **2a** , 12-fold higher in VDR binding, 6-fold in *in vivo* calcium-regulating activity and 590-fold in HL-60 cell differentiation (1b). A known geometric isomer of **1**, 5,6-*trans*-1α,25-dihydroxyvitamin D$_3$ (**3**), in which the exocyclic 19-methylene group appears to be transposed to position 4 in a formal sense, has become of interest in connection with potent 19-norvitamin D$_3$ analogues (2). In addition, analogues with the 5,6-*trans* motif, in combination of 16-ene modification, reported to be promising antiproliferative agents quite recently (3). In our present work, we designed all possible A-ring stereoisomers of 5,6-*trans*-2-methyl-1,25-dihydroxyvitamin D$_3$ (**4a-h**) and their 20-epimers (**5a-h**) as novel A-ring analogues with the 5,6-*trans* modification in order to investigate how these combinations affect the biological activity profiles.

Chart 2

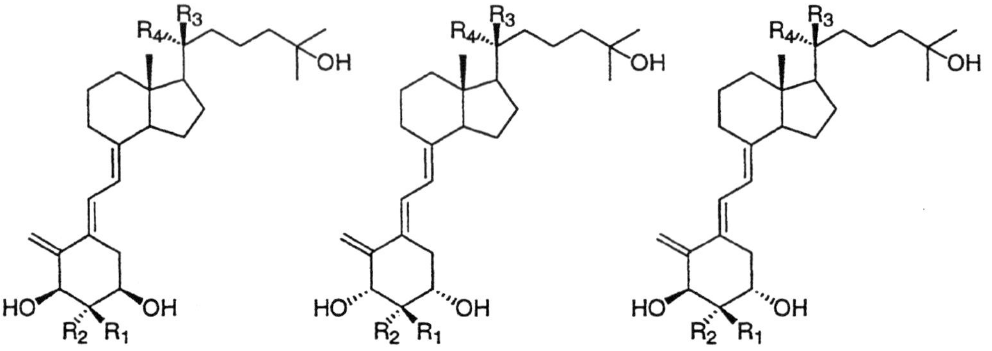

4c: $R_1=R_4=Me$, $R_2=R_3=H$
4d: $R_1=R_3=H$, $R_2=R_4=Me$

5c: $R_1=R_3=Me$, $R_2=R_4=H$
5d: $R_1=R_4=H$, $R_2=R_3=Me$

4e: $R_1=R_4=Me$, $R_2=R_3=H$
4f: $R_1=R_3=H$, $R_2=R_4=Me$

5e: $R_1=R_3=Me$, $R_2=R_4=H$
5f: $R_1=R_4=H$, $R_2=R_3=Me$

4g: $R_1=R_4=Me$, $R_2=R_3=H$
4h: $R_1=R_3=H$, $R_2=R_4=Me$

5g: $R_1=R_3=Me$, $R_2=R_4=H$
5h: $R_1=R_4=H$, $R_2=R_3=Me$

Synthesis The 5,6-*trans* analogues were synthesized from their 5,6-*cis* counterparts via the SO_2 adducts (4). Scheme 1 exemplifies the synthesis of 5,6-*trans*-2β-methyl-1α,25-dihydroxyvitamin D_3 **4a** from the 5,6-*cis* isomer **2b**. Treatment of **2b** with SO_2 gave a 6-epimeric mixture of the adducts **6**. Subsequent removal of SO_2 in **6** by thermolysis in the presence of $NaHCO_3$ afforded **4a** in 66% yield (2 steps). In the case of **4a**, 3β-hydroxyl, 2β-methyl and 1α-hydroxyl groups may act as pseudo 1α-hydroxyl, 2α-methyl and 3β-hydroxyl groups, respectively. The other analogues (**4b-h, 5a-h**) were synthesized by exactly the same sequence of reactions from the corresponding 5,6-*cis* compounds. As a reference compound, 5,6-*trans*-1α,25-dihydroxyvitamin D_3 (**3**) was prepared and its molar absorptivity was determined: UV (ethanol) λ_{max} 274 nm (ε 23500), λ_{min} 230 nm (ε 4900) (5). The hyperchromic effect and red shift observed in **3** compared to **1** would be explained by the change of the triene structure.

Scheme 1

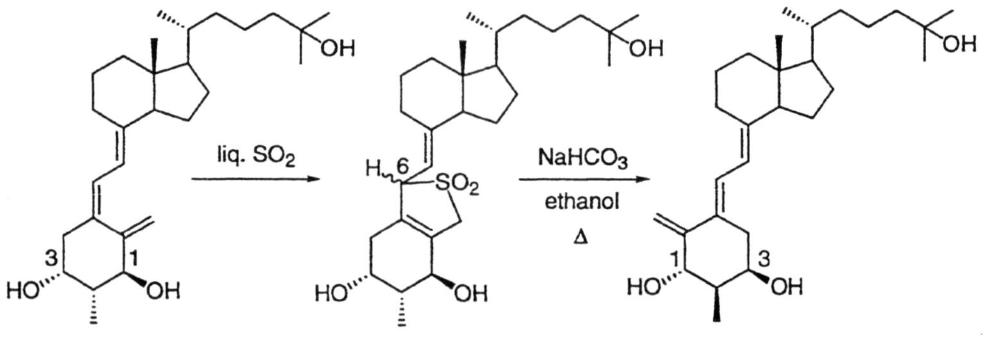

Biological Evaluation   The biological activities of the synthesized analogues were assessed in terms of affinities for vitamin D receptor (VDR) and vitamin D binding protein (DBP) in comparison with the natural hormone 1 and its 5,6-*trans* isomer 3 (Table 1). In the binding assay using bovine thymus VDR, the 5,6-*trans* modification of **1** decreased the activity by approximately 100-fold. Among the 2-methyl analogues with natural (20*R*)-configuration, those having pseudo 1α-hydroxyl and 2α-methyl groups showed a significant activity. A similar trend was found among the 20-*epi* analogues with (20*S*)-configuration. As observed among the 5,6-*cis*-2-methyl analogues (1), 20-epimerization of each isomer elevated the affinity to VDR by approximately 5- to 10-fold. In the binding assay using rat serum DBP, the analogues having the pseudo 1β-hydroxyl configuration were preferred and the 20-epimerization greatly decreased the affinity. Cell differentiation-inducing activity of the analogues towards HL-60 cells at 10^{-8} M was shown in Chart 3. The analogues **4a**, **5a** and **5b** exhibited a comparable or even higher potency than the natural hormone **1**. It is noteworthy that **5e** was significantly active in spite of having pseudo 1β-hydroxyl configuration, which should impart low or no activity.

Summary   All possible A-ring stereoisomers of 5,6-*trans*-2-methyl-1,25-dihydroxyvitamin D_3 and their 20-epimers were designed and efficiently synthesized. Biological evaluation of the 5,6-*trans* analogues revealed that the pseudo 2α-methyl introduction to the parent 5,6-*trans*-1α,25-dihydroxyvitamin D_3 (**3**) enhanced the potency, as in the case of the 2α-methyl introduction to **1**. The combined modification of the pseudo 2α-methyl introduction and 20-epimerization resulted in additive effects on VDR binding and cell differentiation-inducing activity. The analogue **5e** having a significant activity in cell differentiation would make a clue to understand the structure-activity relationships of the 1α,25-dihydroxyvitamin D_3.

Table 1. Relative Binding Potencies of the 5,6-*trans*-2-Methyl Analogues.[a]

(20*R*)	VDR[b]	DBP[c]	(20*S*)	VDR	DBP
1	100	100			
3	0.8	14			
4a	8.6	7.7	5a	45	1.0
4b	0.4	17	5b	1	0.7
4c	0.1	34	5c	0.8	2.1
4d	<0.01	81	5d	0.03	1.8
4e	0.04	6.0	5e	0.5	<0.1
4f	0.013	11	5f	0.2	<0.1
4g	0.03	8.8	5g	0.2	<0.1
4h	<0.01	28	5h	0.08	0.4

[a] The potencies of 1α,25-dihydroxyvitamin D_3 (**1**) are taken as 100.
[b] Bovine thymus. [c] Rat serum.

76

Chart 3. HL-60 cell Differentiation-Inducing Activity of the Analogues.[a]

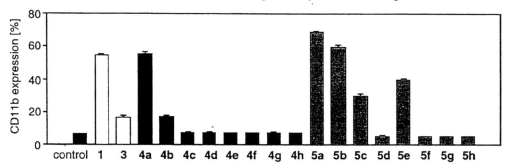

[a] HL-60 cells were treated with 10^{-8} M of 1α,25-dihydroxyvitamin D_3 (1) or the analogues (3, 4a-h, 5a-h) for 72 h. Cell differentiation was assessed in terms of expression of CD11b.

Acknowledgements This work was supported by a Grant-in-Aid from the Ministry of Education, Science and Culture of Japan, and a Grant from the Hayashi Memorial Foundation for Female Natural Scientists.

References and Notes
1. (a) Konno, K., Maki, S., Fujishima, T., Liu, Z.-P., Miura, D., Chokki, M. and Takayama, H. (1998) Bioorg. Med. Chem. Lett. 8, 151-156; (b) Fujishima, T., Liu, Z.-P., Miura, D., Chokki, M., Ishizuka, S., Konno, K. and Takayama, H. (1998) *ibid.* 8, 2145-2148; (c) Nakagawa, K., Kurobe, M., Ozono, K., Konno, K., Fujishima, T., Takayama, H. and Okano, T. (2000) Biochem. Pharmacol. 59, 691-702; (d) Fujishima, T., Konno, K., Nakagawa, K., Kurobe, M., Okano, T. and Takayama, H. (2000) Bioorg. Med. Chem. 8, 123-134.
2. Sicinski, R. R., Prahl, J. M., Smith, M. and DeLuca, H. F. (1998) J. Med. Chem. 41, 4662-4674, and the references cited therein.
3. Hisatake, J., Kubota, T., Hisatake, Y., Uskokovic, M., Yomoyasu, S. and Koeffler, P. (1999) Cancer Res. 59, 4023-4029.
4. (a) VanAlstyne, E. M., Norman, A. W. and Okamura, W. H. (1994) J. Am. Chem. Soc. 116, 6207-6216; (b) Ray, R., Vicchio, D., Yergey, A. and Holick (1992) Steroids 57, 142-146; (c) Yamada, S. and Takayama, H. (1979) Chem.Lett. 583-586; (d) Reischl, W. and Zbiral, E. (1979) Helv. Chim. Acta. 62, 1763-1769.
5. Purification to determine the molar absorptivity was conducted by reversed phase recycle HPLC (acetonitrile: water = 9: 1), followed by recrystalization from ethyl acetate to give analytically pure 3 as colorless fine prisms. Mp 175-176 °C; $[\alpha]_D^{27}$ + 159 (c = 0.059, CHCl$_3$); Anal. Calcd. for $C_{27}H_{44}O_3$·1/4H$_2$O: C, 77.0; H, 10.5. Found: C, 76.91; H,10.43.

NOVEL VITAMIN D KETONES

Andreas Steinmeyer*, Herbert Wiesinger, Gernot Langer,
Marianne Fähnrich, Martin Haberey
Schering AG, Preclinical Drug Research, D-13342 Berlin, Germany

Introduction Vitamin D derivatives are known to exert a variety of biological effects. Especially analogs derived from $1\alpha,25$-dihydroxyvitamin D_3 (calcitriol) have been found to modulate proliferation and differentiation of several cell types such as tumor cells, keratinocytes, cells of the immune system and many other cells.

Most analogs which were synthesized over the years exhibit structural modifications in the side chain. Among these a hydroxy group in a position beyond C-23 seems to be of crucial importance for biological activity. The usefulness of most calcitriol analogs is clearly limited by the occurrence of hypercalcemia in vivo at dosages required for antiproliferative effects in vitro. Thus, structural variations are highly desirable which preserve the desired inhibitory effects on cell growth in vitro and in vivo without induction of hypercalcemia in vivo.

Chemistry In the course of the vitamin D research program at Schering many calcitriol derivatives were synthesized with the overall aim to identify compounds with therapeutic effects in cancer, skin diseases and other disorders of the immune system. By developing a new chemical approach an interesting novel series of vitamin D ketones was accessible. Experience from us (1, 2) and others (3) revealed that the incorporation of a cyclopropyl ring into the side chain may result in distinct, possibly selective, biological activities.

An optimal substrate for the introduction of artificial side chain substructures is the vitamin D aldehyde **1** which was synthesized via the modified Barton-Hesse approach (4). By a photochemically induced isomerization reaction utilizing anthracene as triplett sensitizer aldehyde **2** exhibiting the natural triene system was elaborated (Scheme 1). The sulfones **3** and **4** which were generated starting from ethyl acetoacetate (5) could easily been deprotonated with lithium diisopropylamide and reactions with aldehyde **2** were carried out yielding a diastereomeric mixture of hydroxy sulfones **5**. Julia-olefination with sodium amalgam still proved to be the method of choice to generate the E-olefin **6**. Finally, deprotection was achieved with acidic ion exchange resin to open access to the vitamin D ketones **7-12** (n=1) and **13-18** (n=2). In this reaction the silyl groups and the ketal were cleaved simultaneously.

In summary, a new straight-forward synthesis of side chain modified vitamin D analogs was developed allowing a high degree of structural flexibility. In the present case systematic variations of the overall length of the side chain are discussed.

Scheme 1

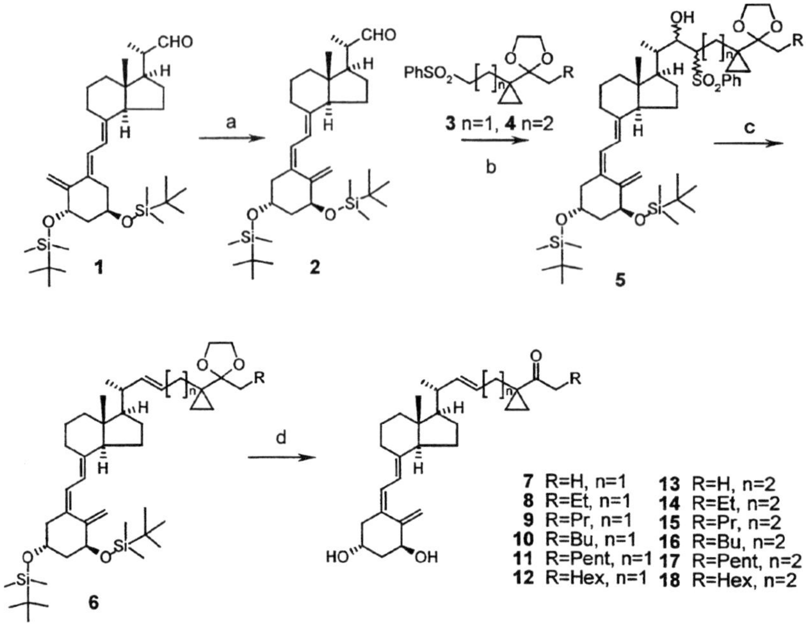

Conditions: a) hv, anthracene, NEt₃, toluene, 25°C; b) LDA, **3** or **4**, THF, -78°C; c) Na/Hg, Na₂HPO₄, CH₃OH, 25°C; d) Dowex, CH₃OH, CH₂Cl₂, 25°C

Biology In the pharmacological screening at Schering the activities of new vitamin D analogs are investigated in cellular assays which are believed to have predictive value for in vivo situations and, hence, for therapeutic applications in humans. Initially, the binding affinities of the compounds for the vitamin D receptor protein (VDR) are examined (6). As a surrogate model for cancer the human leukemia cell line HL 60 is applied (6). Human peripheral blood mononuclear cells (PBMC) are used to investigate activity on immunologic effector cells (lymphocytes) (7). The metabolic stability of the compounds is studied in rat liver microsomes in comparison to calcitriol (7). Since no suitable in vitro model exists for assessing the hypercalcemic nature of new analogs the influences on calcium homeostasis are evaluated in rats in vivo (s.c. administration) compared to calcitriol (6, 7).

Results For all derivatives the binding affinities for the VDR are significantly reduced in comparison to calcitriol (Table 1). However, the derivatives with shorter side chains (**7**, **8**, **9**, **13**, **14** and **15**) bind moderately to the VDR (RBA = 10-20%). The other analogs show very low binding affinities (RBA ≤ 3%). Calcitriol induces differentiation of HL 60 cells to monocytes and macrophages. The analogs **7**, **13** and **14** with rather short side chains have higher potencies than calcitriol in this system, whereas the close derivative **8** is nearly equipotent to the natural vitamin D metabolite. Further extention of the side chain leads to moderately active vitamin D ketones (**9**, **10**, **15** and **16**) while the other analogs having extremely long side chains are nearly inactive. Calcitriol inhibits the phytohemagglutinine (PHA)-

stimulated proliferation of human PBMC. Here again compounds exhibiting short side chains give rise to high potencies (**7**, **8**, **13** and **14**). Similar to the HL 60 assay side chain elongation results in loss of agonistic acitivity. Incubation of the new analogs in rat liver microsomes revealed stabilities in the same range as calcitriol (results not displayed). Single administrations of the vitamin D ketones to rats (s.c.) indicate remarkably reduced effects on calcium homeostasis as compared to calcitriol. The abilities to induce hypercalcemia are 20 to 75 fold reduced for compounds with short side chains (**7**, **8**, **13** and **14**) whereas the derivatives with moderately or extremely elongated side chains are less hypercalcemic by a factor of 100-300.

Table 1

	VDR RBA [%]	HL 60 DR	PBMC DR	Hypercalcemia DR
Calcitriol	100	1	1	1
7	10	0.5	2.5	50
8	10	1.7	4.9	75
9	14	19	47	100
10	3	9	70	300
11	1	>290	360	>300
12	2	>290	nd	>300
13	20	0.5	4.3	20
14	10	0.2	1.4	30
15	10	17	19	100
16	1	24	31	200
17	2	>290	320	>300
18	1	280	nd	>300

RBA = relative binding affinity: IC_{50} Calcitriol / IC_{50} analog x 100
DR HL 60 or PBMC: ED_{50} analog / ED_{50} calcitriol (low values indicate high potencies)
DR Hypercalemia:
dose derivative equipotent to 2 µg/kg Calcitriol / 2 µg/kg Calcitriol (low values indicate high potencies)
nd = not determined

Discussion   By this new synthetic approach two (sub)series of novel vitamin D ketones were accessible. Both series possess a cyclopropyl ring adjacent to the carbonyl group in the side chain and differ only by the distance between that cyclopropyl unit and the double bond. The influence of the total length of the side chain was investigated. The binding affinities for all vitamin D ketones were considerably reduced as compared to calcitriol (RBA ≤ 20%), however, some derivatives with short side chains (**7**, **8**, **13** and **14**) still exerted potent effects in vivo. Interestingly, the potency of the methyl ketones **7** and **13** in HL 60 cells were higher than that of calcitriol while in PBMC both ketones were slightly less active than the natural metabolite. These analogs have significantly lower hypercalcemic activities than calcitriol. As a consequence of the elongation of the side chain biological activities in vitro were substantially reduced. In parallel hypercalcemic effects dropped to the same extent (**9**, **10**, **15** and **16**). The compounds bearing extremely long side chains (**11**, **12**, **17** and **18**) were nearly inactive. It can be concluded that it is not absolutely necessary to incorporate hydroxy groups into the side chains of vitamin D derivatives in order to display biological effects. A keto group as the only heteroatomic function is sufficient to exert remarkable vitamin D activity unless a certain length of the side chain is surpassed. Furthermore, these new compounds show dissociation of regulatory effects on tumor cells or cells of the immune system versus undesired hypercalcemia. Since the novel structures proved to exhibit the same stability in liver microsomes than calcitriol it can be assumed that it is not a rapid metabolic clearance which causes the dissociation.

In summary, two promising novel series of vitamin D ketones have been identified which could potentially be used in treatment of tumor diseases, disorders of the immune system and probably skin diseases. To evaluate the full potential of these compounds, further studies in animal models will be conducted.

References
1) Wiesinger, H., Ulrich, M., Fähnrich, M., Haberey, M., Neef, G., Schwarz, K., Kirsch, G., Langer G., Thieroff-Ekerdt, R. and Steinmeyer, A. (1998) J. Invest. Dermatol. 110, 532.
2) Herdick, M., Steinmeyer, A. and Carlberg, C. (2000) J. Biol. Chem. in print.
3) Binderup, L. (1993) Pharmacol. Toxicol. 72, 240-244.
4) Calverley, M.J. (1987) Tetrahedron 43, 4909-4619.
5) Schering AG WO 99/16745.
6) Steinmeyer, A., Neef, G., Kirsch, G., Schwarz, K., Rach, P., Haberey, M. and Thieroff-Ekerdt, R. (1992) Steroids 57, 447-452.
7) Werz, O., Wiesinger, H., Steinmeyer, A. and Steinhilber, D. (2000) Biochem. Pharmacol. 59, 1597-1601.

SYNTHESIS OF THE ENANTIOMER OF NATURAL 1α,25-DIHYDROXY VITAMIN D₃ AND RELATED STEREOANALOGUES.

A. Przeździecka*, B.Achmatowicz*, S. Marczak*, A. Steinmeyer**, J. Wicha* and U. Zuegel** *Institute of Organic Chemistry, Polish Academy of Sciences, 01-224 Warsaw, Poland, **Schering AG, Institute of Medicinal Chemistry, D-13342 Berlin, Germany

INTRODUCTION Six asymmetric carbon atoms are incorporated in the structure 1α,25-dihydroxyvitamin D₃ (C1, C3, C13, C14, C17, C21). An interesting line of the structure - activity studies is committed to stereoisomers of the natural product. Epimers differing in configuration at C1, C3, C14 and C20 have been studied (1-4). More recently, certain diastereomers of 1α,25-dihydroxyvitamin D₃ differing from the natural product in configuration at two asymmetric carbon atoms have been also investigated (5,6). In light of high activity of some stereoisomers, in particular those with inverted configuration at C20 and, in consequence, "reversed" orientation of the side chain, it appeared of interest to synthesize and evaluate activity of the enantiomer of 1α,25-dihydroxyvitamin D₃ and selected analogues of 1α,25-dihydroxyvitamin D₃ with inverted configuration at the hydrindane rings structural unit.

Scheme 1   **New vitamin D analogues**

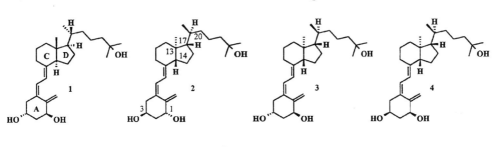

1a,25-dihydroxyvitamin D₃   *ent*-1a,25-dihydroxyvitamin D₃
1S, 3R, 13R, 14R, 17R, 20R   1R, 3S, 13S, 14S, 17S, 20S   1S, 3R, 13S, 14S, 17S, 20S   1S, 3S, 13S, 14S, 17S, 20S

RESULTS AND DISCUSSION Our synthetic plan embraced separate preparation of the ring A and rings CD-side chain precursors and coupling of these building blocks in the Julia's alkenylation reaction.

Synthesis of the ring A building blocks 9 and 13. (See Scheme 2)
Vitamin D₂ related triol **5**(7) was subjected to the Mitsunobu reaction(8) in order to invert the orientation of the oxygen substituent at C-3. The best results were obtained using α-picolic acid(9) as the nucleophile, and diethyl azodicarboxylate (DEAD) . The derivative **6** was oxidized(10) with SeO₂ to give tetrol **7**. After the protecting groups adjustment (that involves hydrolysis of picolate ester mediated by copper(II) acetate), the vicinal diol **8** was cleaved with Pb(OAc)₄ with subsequent reduction of the crude product(11) to give the required ring A precursor **9**.
Well-known ring A building block(12) **10** was protected as a benzoate ester and this derivative was exposed to the reaction with tetrabutylammonium fluoride hydrate (TBAF) in THF to give a mixture of mono- and di-hydroxy products. Chromatography of this product afforded alcohol

11. The hydroxy group in **11** was subjected to the Mitsunobu inversion followed by hydrolysis to give isomer **12**. Protection of the hydroxy group in **12** with the TBS group and reduction of the benzoate function completed the synthesis affording allylic alcohol **13**.

Scheme 2   **Synthesis of the analogues: ring A fragments**

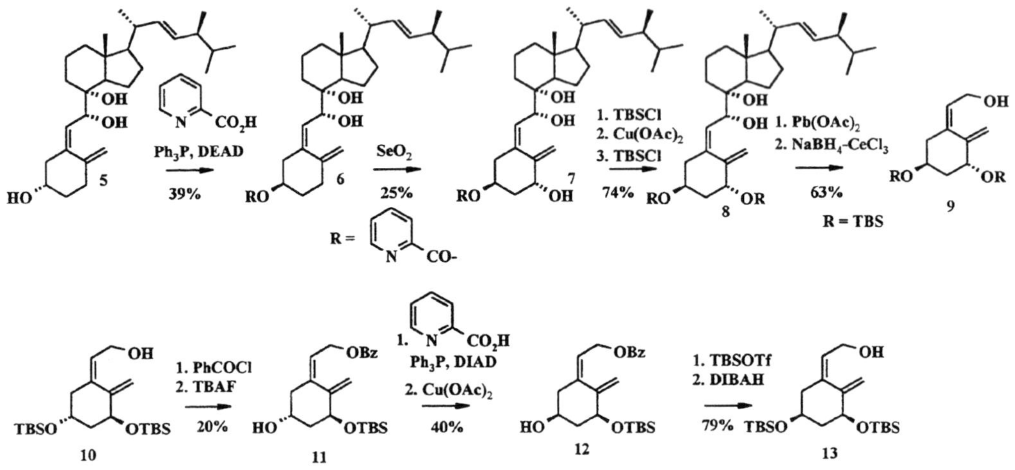

Synthesis of the rings CD - side chain building block (18). (see Scheme 3)
Ester **15** was prepared in six - step synthesis illustrated in Scheme 3, *via* intermediate **14** generated in asymmetric Robinson annulation with the use of phenylsulfanylmethyl vinyl ketone.(13,14) Alkylation of ester **15** with bromide **16** yielded the derivative **17** as the only product.(15) Intermediate **17** was reduced into vitamin D precursor **18** using efficient three-step procedure.

Scheme 3   **Synthesis of *ent*-analogue: CD fragment**

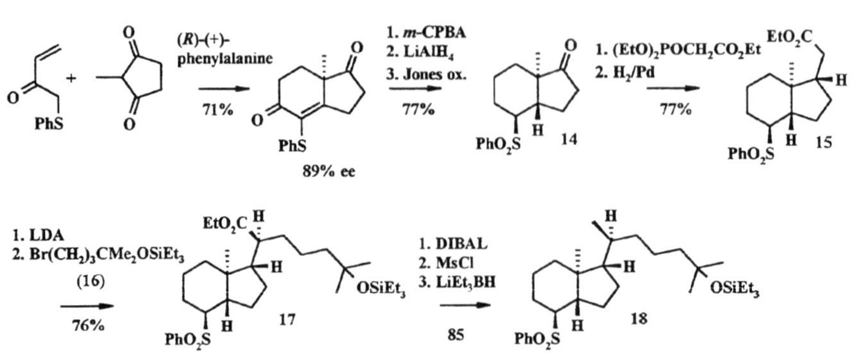

Building blocks coupling reactions (see Scheme 4)
Aldehydes **19**, **20** and **21** were prepared by oxidation of alcohols **10**, **9** and **13**,respectively, with the Dess-Martin reagent.(16) In all cases a mixture of the aldehyde and the respective

pyrones were formed.(11,17) These mixtures were used without purification immediately after preparation. Since aldehydes 21 and, particularly, 19 were more precious components in the coupling reaction, a special small - scale procedure in which the sulfone 18 was used in excess was developed. Although the yields of the products from sulfone 18 were rather low (ca. 20% - 35%) high conversion of aldehydes was secured. Sulfone 18 was treated with butyl lithium and the resulting α-lithio derivative was allowed to react with a respective mixture of aldehyde and pyrone. The diastereomeric adducts were treated *in situ* with acetyl chloride. The intermediate products were isolated by flash chromatography and then subjected consecutively to reduction and desilylation reactions. The reaction products consisted of two major components substantially differing in polarity, each accompanied by its minor satellites. These components were separated by column chromatography on silica gel. The more mobile fraction consisted mainly of 25-acetates (which were eventually hydrolyzed to the respective free alcohols with methanolic KOH). The main fraction provided the required ent -CD analogue and its geometric isomers. HPLC analysis showed that the double bond isomer are present, similarly as it was found in model experiments on vitamin D_4 synthesis.(17)

Scheme 4 **Building blocks coupling reactions**

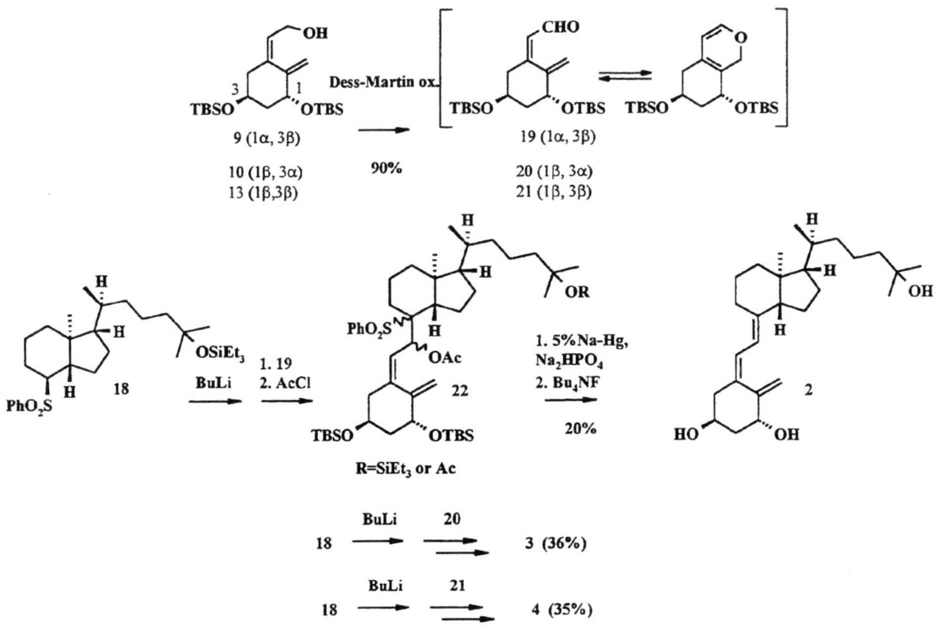

Pure compounds 2, 3 or 4 were isolated and purified by preparative HPLC. The retention times of the synthesised analogues (2, 3 and 4) on the analytical HPLC column matched that of a sample of the natural 1α,25-dihydroxy vitamin D_3 (1). ^{1}H NMR spectrum of 2 and 3 are virtually indistinguishable from that of 1, only a spectrum taken from compound 4 shows small but significant differences, mainly in the A ring protons region. Enantiomeric nature of 2 and 1 and diasteromeric nature of 3, 4 and 1 were clearly confirmed by comparison of their CD spectra.

CONCLUSIONS Vitamin D analogues **2**, **3**, and **4** were synthesized. Compound **3** is a reasonable vitamin D receptor binder with weak activity in inducing the differentiation of HL 60 cells (surrogate model for cancer). On the other hand the proliferation of cells of the immune system (PBMC) is moderately inhibited by the compound, however, the potencies are lower than that of 1α,25-dihydroxyvitamin D_3. In a murine model of contact allergy the immuno suppressive effect is not detectable in the dose of 10 μg/kg/d while slight but not significant elevation of urinary calcium occurs. Thus it could be concluded that ent-CD-vitamin D **3** is a weak 1α,25-dihydroxyvitamin D_3 agonist which is not potent enough to exert considerable activity in vivo. "Natural" configuration of stereogenic centers in the hydrindane rings is not a necessary requirement for biological activity of vitamin D analogues. Results of biological testing of compounds **2** and **4** will be reported in a due course.

ACKNOWLEDGMENT We thank Dr Marek Kabat for bringing to our attention patented work on preparation of compound **7**. We are indebted to Dr. Jadwiga Frelek for the CD measurements Financial support from the Polish State Committee for Scientific Researches, Grant is acknowledged.

REFERENCES:
1. Muralidharan, K. R., Lera, A. R. d., Isaeff, S. D., Norman, A. W., and Okamura, W. H. (1993) *J. Org. Chem.* **58**, 1895-1899
2. Ishida, H., Shimizu, M., Yamamoto, K., Iwasaki, Y., and Yamada, S. (1995) *J. Org. Chem.* **60**, 423-424
3. Jeganathan, S., Jonston, A. D., Kuenzel, E. A., Norman, A. W., and Okamura, W. H. (1984) *J. Org. Chem.* **49**, 2152-2158
4. Binderup, L., Latini, S., Binderup, E., Bertting, C., Calverley, M., and Hansen, K. (1991) *Biochem. Pharmacol.* **42**, 1569-1575
5. Van Gool, M., Zhao, X., Sabbe, K., and Vandewalle, M. (1999) *Eur. J. Org. Chem.*, 2241-2248
6. Fujishima, T., Konno, K., Nakagawa, K., Kurobe, M., Okano, T., and Takayama, H. (2000) *Bioorg. Med. Chem.* **8**, 123-134
7. Toh, H. T., and Okamura, W. H. (1983) *J. Org. Chem.* **48**, 1414-1417.
8. Mitsunobu, O. (1981) *Synthesis*, 1-28
9. Sammakia, T., and Jacobs, J. S. (1999) *Tetraheron Lett.* **40**, 2685-2688
10. Tahara, Y. (1994) in *U. S. Patent 5,283,345 Application, May 6, 1992*
11. Blakemore, P. R., Kocienski, P. J., Marczak, S., and Wicha, J. (1999) *Synthesis*, 1209-1215
12. Hamon, C., Rodriguez, J. D. S., Kalchhauser, H., and Reischl, W. (1997) *Monatsh. Chem.* **128**, 1297-1300.
13. Przezdziecka, A., Stepanenko, W., and Wicha, J. (1999) *Tetrahedron: Asymmetry* **10**, 1589-1598
14. Hajos, Z. G., and Parrish, D. R. (1974) *J. Org. Chem.* **39**, 1615-1621
15. Wicha, J., and Bal, K. (1978) *J. Chem. Soc. Perkin Trans. 1*, 1282-1288
16. Dess, D. B., and Martin, J. C. (1983) *J. Org. Chem.* **48**, 4155.
17. Blakemore, P. R., Grzywacz, P., Kocienski, P. J., Marczak, S., and Wicha, J. (1999) *Polish J. Chem.* **73**, 1209-1217

SYNTHESIS AND BIOLOGICAL EVALUATION OF ACTIVE METABOLITES
OF VITAMIN D$_3$ AND SIDE-CHAIN MODIFIED ANALOGUES OF VITAMIN D$_2$

Michał Chodyński[a], Małgorzata Krupa[a], Jacek Choliński[a], Wanda Wojciechowska[a],
Hanna Fitak[a], Jan Zorgdrager[b], Jan-Paul van de Velde[b], Andrzej Kutner[a]

[a]Pharmaceutical Research Institute, 01-793 Warszawa, Poland,
akutner@pleam.edu.pl
[b]Solvay Pharmaceuticals, 1381 Weesp, The Netherlands

<u>Introduction</u>   The recent results of phase I clinical trials of calcitriol against solid tumours (1,2) indicated that the only dose limiting toxicity is related to calcemic activity of the compound when administered in hyperphysiological doses. This finding has greatly stimulated the search for vitamin D compounds with high cell differentiation activity and substantially lowered calcemic properties. In our search for new vitamin D leads (3,4) we synthesised a group of highly hydroxylated vitamin D$_3$ metabolites, their precursors and diastereomers (**1 – 4**) as well as a group of side-chain modified analogues of vitamin D$_2$ (**5 – 8**). Vitamin D$_3$ metabolites and related compounds hydroxylated at C-24 show a much-lowered calcemic activity compared to calcitriol. To the best of our knowledge these known compounds have not been tested for cell differentiating properties up to now. Our vitamin D$_2$ analogues with extended, rigid and substituted side-chain were designed based on the structure-activity correlation of our previously obtained side-chain unsaturated homoanalogues (5,6,7) and molecular modeling using both molecular mechanics and molecular dynamics platform.

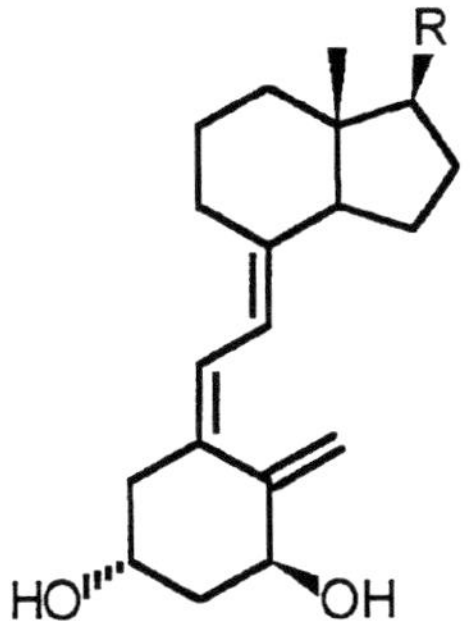

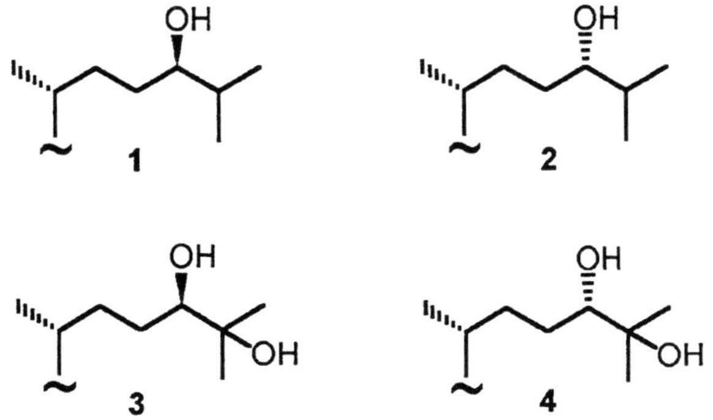

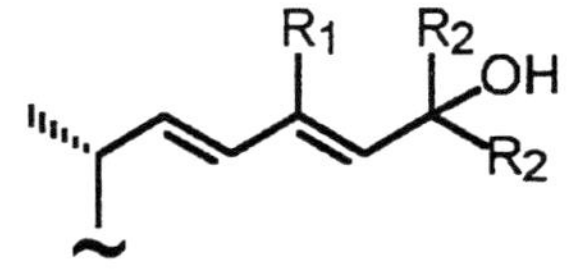

5 R$_1$ = R$_2$ = Me
6 R$_1$ = Me; R$_2$ = Et
7 R$_1$ = Me; R$_2$ = Pr
8 R$_1$ = Me; R$_2$ = n-Bu

<u>Chemistry</u> In our convergent synthetic strategy we used sulfone **9** (Scheme I) as a vitamin D synthon. For the preparation of 1,24*R*-$(OH)_2D_3$ (**1**, tacalcitol, PRI-2191) carbanion of sulfone **9** was used (8) to open (*S*)-oxirane **10**. 1,24*S*-$(OH)_2D_3$ (**2,** PRI-2192) was obtained from (*R*)-oxirane **11**.

Scheme I

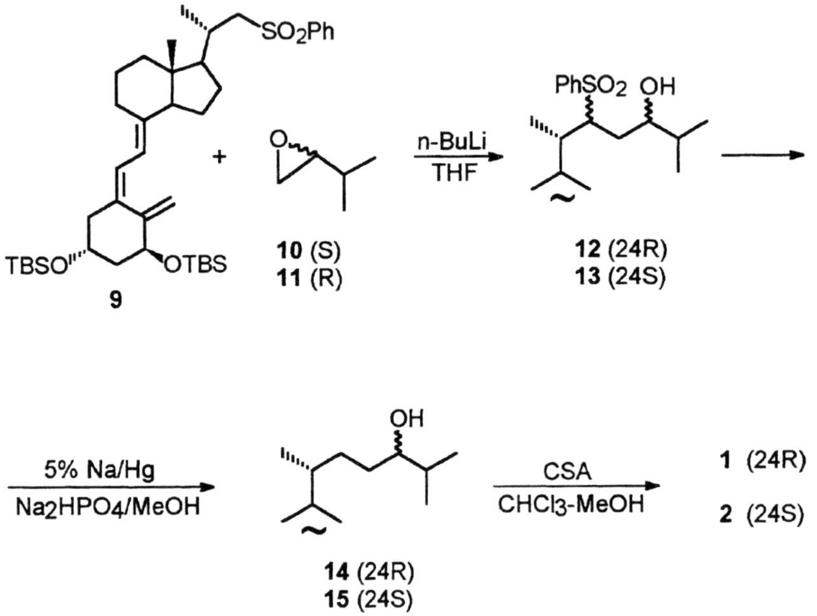
SO2Ph
TBSO
OTBS
9
+
10 (S)
11 (R)
n-BuLi
THF
PhSO2 OH
12 (24R)
13 (24S)
5% Na/Hg
Na2HPO4/MeOH
OH
14 (24R)
15 (24S)
CSA
CHCl3-MeOH
1 (24R)
2 (24S)

The most highly hydroxylated metabolite of vitamin D_3 [**3**, 1,24*R*,25-$(OH)_2D_3$, PRI-2193] and its C-24 diastereomer (**4**, PRI-2194) were obtained by direct asymetric oxidation (4) of enolate derived from the C-25 ester (**16**, Scheme II) with (+)-(2*R*,8a*S*)- and (-)-(2*S*,8a*R*)-(8,8-dichlorocamphorylsulphonyl)oxaziridine (DCO), respectively.

Scheme II

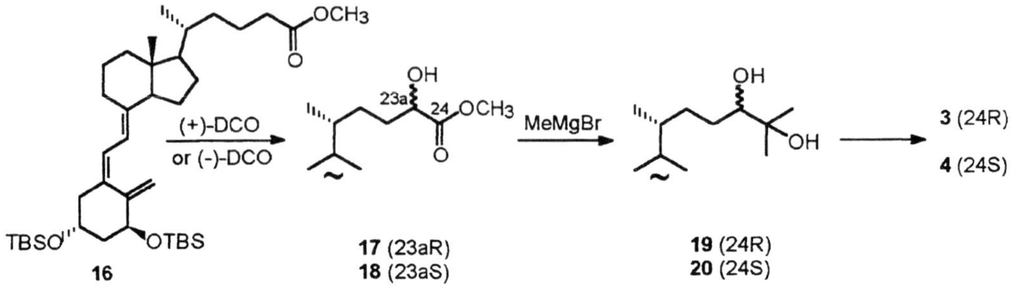
OCH3
O
TBSO
OTBS
16
(+)-DCO
or (-)-DCO
OH
23a
24
OCH3
O
17 (23aR)
18 (23aS)
MeMgBr
OH
OH
19 (24R)
20 (24S)
3 (24R)
4 (24S)

Sulfone **9** was also used in our syntheses of vitamin D_2 analogues **5 – 8** (Scheme III). Julia olefination of **9** with aldehyde **21** resulted in diastereomeric mixture of hydroxysulfones **22**. Grignard or alkyllithium reaction of ester **22** gave diols **23 - 26**. Sodium amalgam desulfonylation, followed by CSA desilylation resulted in a series of analogues **5 – 8** (9). *All-trans* geometry of the side-chain was confirmed by experimental and calculated ^{1}H NMR data.

Scheme III

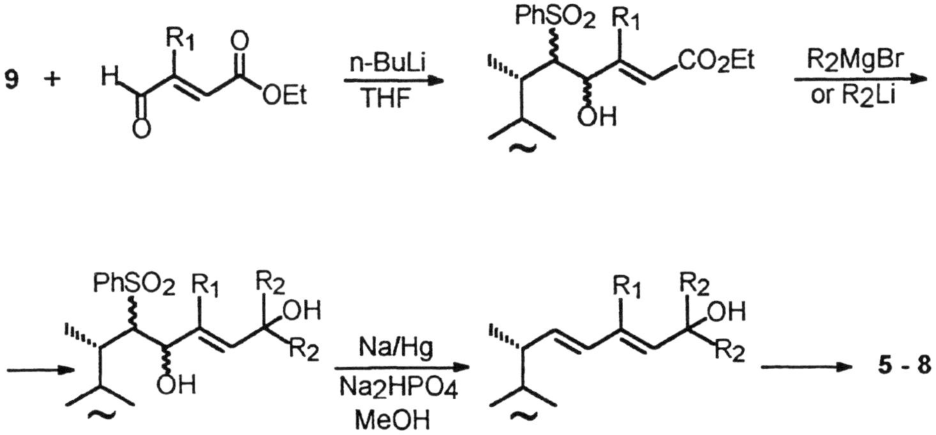

23 - 26   **27 - 30**   **5 - 8**

Molecular modeling   Molecular dynamics was used in order to design the optimal structure of the side-chain of vitamin D_2 analogues and select compounds for further synthesis. Dynamic behaviour of vitamin D2 analogues was correlated with the one of PRI-2171 [24-homo-1,25-$(OH)_2D_3$] used as a model compound.   Point maps were created by transient positions of O(25) atom within a simulation time of $20 – 50$ ps. The high activity of an analogue was well correlated with the well separated areas occupied by terminal O(25) atoms, as seen for **5** (PRI-1906) in both CD plane and in the side-chain view from O(25) to C(20).

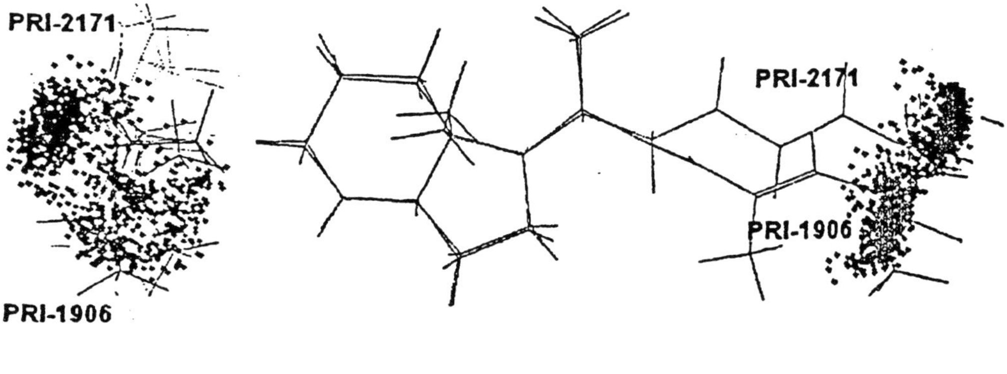

<u>Biological evaluation</u> As expected, the binding affinity of vitamin D_3 metabolites and diastereomers (**1 – 4**) for calf thymus VDR, determined with a Nichol's kit (4) was lower than that of 1,25-$(OH)_2D_3$. However, the affinity of natural (24*R*) compounds **1** and **3** was consistently one order of magnitude higher than that of the respective (24*S*) diastereomers **2** and **4**. Contrary to lowered binding affinity metabolites **1** and **4** showed the antiproliferative activity against human T47D and MCF-7 breast carcinoma and HL-60 leukemia cell lines, using the MTT technique, 5 to 20-times higher or comparable to 1,25-$(OH)_2D_3$, respectively (10,11,12). This seems to be the first indication of potential anticancer activity of **1**, considered, up to the present, as the effective antipsoriatic agent, only. Our 24a-homo analogue of vitamin D_2 (**5**, PRI-1906) showed the antiproliferative activity in human breast and leukemia cell lines 50-100 times higher than that of 1,25-$(OH)_2D_3$. Quite interestingly, the activity of diethyl analogue **6** (PRI-1907) was much lower, similar to that of 1,25-$(OH)_2D_3$ (4).

References
1. Gross, C., Stamey, T., Hancock, S., Feldman, D. (1998) J. Urol. 159, 2035-2040.
2. Smith, D.C., Johnson, C.S., Freeman, C.C., Muindi, J., Wilson, J.W., Trump, D. (1999) Clin. Cancer Res. 5, 1339-1345.
3. Odrzywolska, M., Chodyński, M., Halkes, S.J., Velde van de, J.-P., Fitak, H., Kutner, A. (1999) Chirality, 11, 249-255.
4. Odrzywolska, M., Chodyński, M., Zorgdrager, J., Velde van de, J.-P., Kutner, A. (1999) Chirality, 11, 701-706.
5. Chodyński, M., Kutner, A. (1991) Steroids, 56, 311-315.
6. Chodyński, M., Wojciechowska, W., Halkes, S.J., Velde van de, J.-P., Kutner, A. (1997) Steroids, 62, 546-553.
7. Marcinkowska, E., Kutner, A., Radzikowski, C. (1998) J. Steroid Biochem. Molec. Biol. 67, 71-78.
8. Chodyński, M., Szelejewski, W., Odrzywolska, M., Fitak, H., Kutner, A., Pol. Pat. Appl. Pat. Appl. P- 324274, 1998; PCT Appl. No. PCT/PL98/00051, 1999.
9. Chodyński, M., Odrzywolska, M., Kutner, A., Zorgdrager, J., Velde van de J-P., Pol. Pat. Appl. No. P-331693, 1999.
10. Opolski, A., Wietrzyk, J., Chrobak, A., Marcinkowska, E., Wojdat, E., Kutner, A., Radzikowski, C., (1999) Anticancer Res. 19, 5217-5222.
11. Opolski, A., Wietrzyk, J., Siwińska, A., Marcinkowska, E., Chrobak, A., Kutner, A., Radzikowski, C. (2000) Curr. Pharm Design 6, in press.
12. Majewski, S., Kutner, A., Jabłońska, S. (2000) Curr. Pharm Design, 6 in press.

PRELIMINARY INVESTIGATIONS ON SOLID STATE CONFORMATIONS OF 1-HYDROXY-PREVITAMIN D BY NMR

M. Puchberger[1] and W. Reischl[2]

[1]Department of Chemistry, University of Agricultural Sciences, A-1190 Vienna, AUSTRIA [2]Institute of Organic Chemistry, University of Vienna, A-1090 Vienna, AUSTRIA

Introduction. Previtamin D is like vitamin D a highly flexible molecule. It´s A-ring exist in solution as a dynamic equilibrium of two chair conformations (the 3-OH occupies the equatorial and the axial position). In addition, rotation around the C-5 - C-6 single bond is possible and gives rise to additional sets of s-trans and s-cis conformations. The latter conformations are structural precursors for the transition states of the sigmatoripic [1,7] hydrogen shift to give vitamin D. The preferred geometries of previtamin D and their relative steric energies are still a subject of debate [1-5]. A knowledge of previtamin D flexibility is mandatory in understanding its wavelength depending photochemistry or when using previtamin D analogs with the aim of mimicking the shape of the closed steroidal topology in biochemical investigations [6]. It should be noted that in solution evidence for the existance of s-cis conformations have been found [7]. The aim of our study was to gain some information about the conformations of previtamin D in the solid state by using CP-MAS-13C NMR spectroscopy, since up to now no single crystal x-ray structure determination is available, due to lack of suitable crystals. We have been encouraged by our previous results in studying vitamin D by solid state NMR.

Results. Vitamin D. The CP-MAS 13C [8] spectrum of a crystalline sample of vitamin D is highly resolved in which each sp-3 and sp2- carbon resonance appears as a set of two signals with the exception of C-19 which is a broad singulett. Since it is well known from the x-ray structure of vitamin D [9] that in the crystal unit cell both A-ring chair forms (OH-ax/OH-eq) are present and no polymorph forms of vitamin D crystals are known, the doubling of the carbon resonances in the spectrum arise from the two vitamin D conformers. When a commercial powder sample of vitamin D was measured under the same conditions the sp-3 region of the spectrum was essential the same, but the sp-2 resonance's appeared broad and structureless. Upon cooling the sample stepwise to −40 °C the sp-2 carbon resonaces became narrower and more structured but never gained the high resolution observed earlier. After warming the sample to room-temperature again the signals stayed structured. Therefore, the low temperature annealing caused a reordering effect in the crystals. We attribute this effect to disorders in the arrangement of the carbons of the diene bridge in the solid state.

Previtamin D. The CP-MAS 13C spectrum of 1-hydroxy-previtamin D is in the sp-3 region again highly resolved. Upon deconvolution four lines for each sp3 carbon resonance can be seen, with an estimated relative intensity of approx. 1:1:1:1. The sp-2 region of the spectrum is broad and comparable structureless as the sp-2 region of the vitamin D spectrum. Upon cooling of the sample no change in the sp-2 region of the spectrum was observed.

The presence for the line splitting into a set of four may be either due to four distinct conformers consisting of the two A-ring chairs of the s-cis and the two A-ring chairs of the s-trans form or the existing of polymorphism in the solid state. A recent study by Grant [10] on verbenol where polymorphism is known showed similar behavior in the solid state NMR (splitting of sp-2 and sp-3 resonances). In this case the polymorphism arises from different orientations of verbenol's hydroxyl group causing different hydrogen bond networks in the crystal lattices. In 1-hydroxy-previtamin D, where two hydroxyl groups are present, polymorphism may occur for similar reasons. At the present time of our study we are not able to distinguish between polymorphism and distinct conformers. Further work is in progress.

Nevertheless this present study demonstrates the usefulness of solid state NMR for fast inspection of crystalline samples.

CP/MAS spectrum of vitamin D

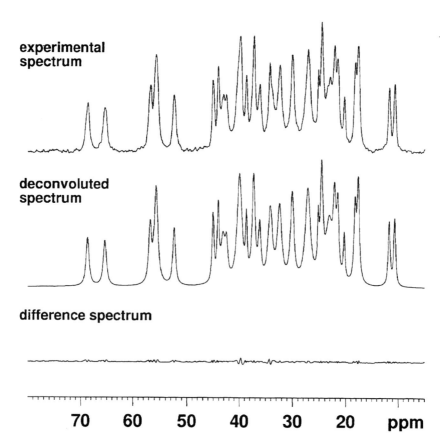

CP/MAS spectrum of previtamin D

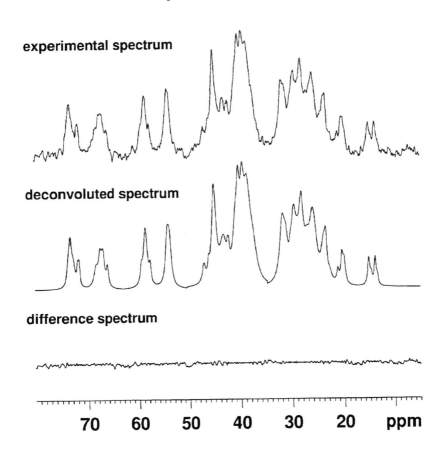

experimental spectrum

deconvoluted spectrum

difference spectrum

70   60   50   40   30   20   ppm

Acknowledgement. Support from Österreichische Nationalbank (Jubiläumsfonds-projekt Nr.:7395 to W.R.) and a generous gift of 1-hydroxy-previtamin D and vitamin D by Dr. J. Zorgdrager (Solvay Pharmaceuticals) is gratefully acknowledged. M. P is grateful to Professor Geoffrey Hunter and Dr. J. A. Chudek from the University of Dundee, Great Britain for introducing him to the fascinating subject of solid state NMR and for funding.by a `Stipendium für kurzfristige wissenschaftliche Arbeiten im Ausland`, from the University of Agriculture .

References

1. Dauben, W.G., Funhoff, D.J.H., J. Org. Chem. 53 (1988) 5070-5075.
2. Dauben, W. G., Disanyaka, B., Funhoff, D.J.H., Kohler, B.E., Schilke, D.E., Zhou, B., J. Am. Chem. Soc. 113 (1991) 8367-8374.
3. Fuß, W. Lochbrunner, S., J. Photochem. Photobiol. A: Chem. 105 (1997) 159-164.
4. Dmitrenko, O.G., Reischl, W., J. Mol. Struc. (Theochem) 431 (1998) 221-236.
5. Dmitrenko, O.G., Tereneskaya, I.P., Reischl, W., J. Photochem. Photobiol. A: Chem. 104 (1997) 113-117.
6. Okamura, W.H., Midland, M.M., Hammond, M.W., Rahman, N.Abd., Dormanen, M.C., Nemere, I., Norman, A.W., J. Steroid. Biochem. Molec. Biol. 43 (1995), 603-613.
7. Dauben, W. G., Funhoff, D.J.H., J. Org. Chem. 53 (1988), 5376-5379.
8. The solid state standart CP/MAS spectra were measured on a 300MHz Chemagnetics spectrometer. Peak deconvolution was done with the Bruker XWin NMR software.
9. Trinh-Toan, DeLuca, H.F., Dahl, L.F., J. Org. Chem. 41 (1976), 3476-3478
10. Harper, J.K, Grant, D.M., J. Am. Chem. Soc. 122 (2000) 3708-3714.

EFFICIENT SYNTHESIS AND BIOLOGICAL EVALUATION OF 1-METHYL-1,25-DIHYDROXYVITAMIN D₃ AND 3-METHYL-1,25-DIHYDROXYVITAMIN D₃

Toshie Fujishima, Yasuhiro Harada, Katsuhiro Konno, Kimie Nakagawa,[a] Maki Tanaka,[a] Toshio Okano[a] and Hiroaki Takayama*
Faculty of Pharmaceutical Sciences, Teikyo University, Sagamiko, Kanagawa 199-0195, Japan. [a]Department of Hygienic Sciences, Kobe Pharmaceutical University, Kobe 658-8558, Japan.

Introduction In order to investigate the structure-activity relationships, we have synthesized 2-methyl and 4-methyl analogues of 1α,25-dihydroxyvitamin D₃ (**1**) and found that the simple introduction of a methyl group to the A-ring moiety yielded analogues with unique activity profiles (1,2). Recent research has revealed that A-ring analogues with "unnatural" hydroxyl configurations, as depicted below in Chart 1 (R₁=R₂=H), have become of interest in connection with metabolic as well as apoptotic studies (3). In the present work, we designed two sets of all four possible 1-methyl-1,25-dihydroxyvitamin D₃ (**2a-d**) and 3-methyl-1,25-dihydroxyvitamin D₃

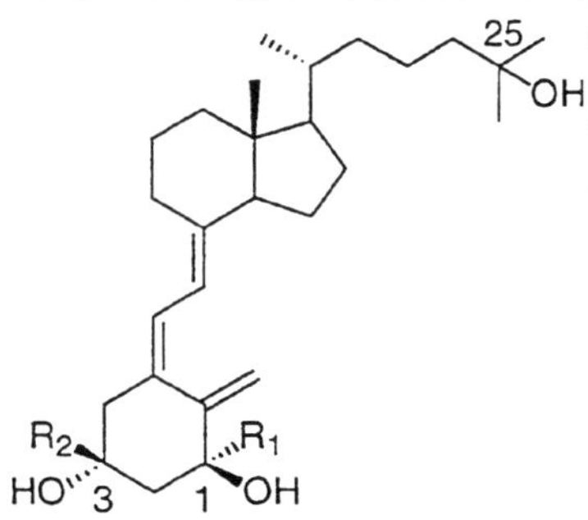

1: R₁ = R₂ = H
2a: R₁ = Me, R₂ = H
3a: R₁ = H, R₂ = Me

(**3a-d**) in order to study the effect of the methyl group upon the A-ring conformation and biological potency (4).

Chart 1

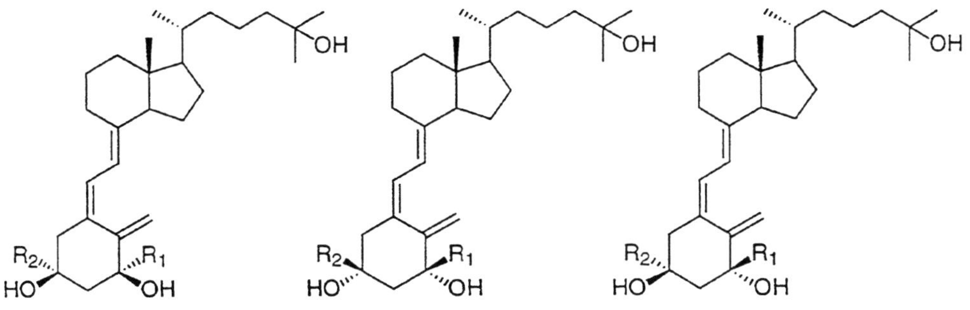

2b: R₁ = Me, R₂ = H
3b: R₁ = H, R₂ = Me

2c: R₁ = Me, R₂ = H
3c: R₁ = H, R₂ = Me

2d: R₁ = Me, R₂ = H
3d: R₁ = H, R₂ = Me

Synthesis The analogues were synthesized by employing the convergent method of Trost et al (5). Scheme 1 outlines the synthetic route to the 1β-methyl-A-ring synthon (**12**) and the 3α-methyl-A-ring synthon (**17**). Both A-ring enynes were prepared via the same synthetic intermediate **6**, starting from 3-methyl-3-buten-1-ol derivative **4** using the Sharpless asymmetric dihydroxylation as a key step. The coupling reaction with the known CD-ring portion (5) using palladium catalyst, followed by deprotection with TBAF gave the 1β-methyl analogues (**2a**, **2b**) and 3α-methy analogues (**3a**, **3c**), from **12** and **17**, respectively, in good yields (combined yield for the 2-step conversion; up to 57%). Oxidation of **4** using AD-mix-β instead of AD-mix-α gave the antipode of **5**, which led to the other stereoisomers, 1α-methyl analogues (**2c**, **2d**) and 3β-methy analogues (**3b**, **3d**). In this way, syntheses of two sets of four stereoisomers of 1-methyl-1,25-dihydroxyvitamin D_3 and 3-methyl-1,25-dihydroxyvitamin D_3 were accomplished.

Scheme 1

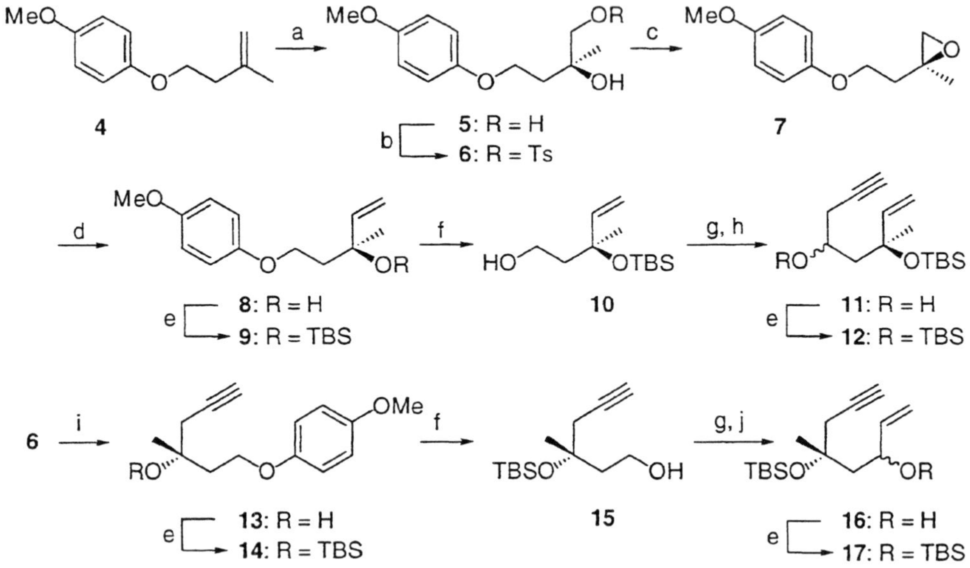

(a) AD-mix-α/ t-BuOH-H_2O, 0 °C, 88%, 95%ee; (b) TsCl/ pyridine, 0 °C, 82%; (c) LiHMDS/ THF, 0 °C, 91%; (d) Me_3Si-n-BuLi/ THF, -10 °C, 80%; (e) TBSOTf, 2,6-Lutidine/ CH_2Cl_2, 0 °C, 86% for **9**, 99% for **12**, 99% for **14**, 99% for **17**; (f) CAN/ MeCN-H_2O, 0 °C, 71% for **10**, 79% for **15**; (g) PDC/ CH_2Cl_2, r.t., 87% for **11**, 72% for **16**; (h) Allenyl MgBr/ ether, -78 °C, 82%; (i) Lithium acetylide-EDA/ DMSO, r.t., 86%; (j) Vinyl MgBr/ toluene, -78 °C, 62%.

Conformational Analysis To gain information on the A-ring conformation-activity relationships, the solution conformations of the A-ring of the synthesized analogues were examined by means of ¹H NMR analyses using $CDCl_3$ as a solvent. The conformational equilibrium of **2a** deduced from the vicinal coupling constant between H3α-H4β (9.2 Hz) showed a ratio of 80: 20 in favor of α-form (4). The usual method for vitamin D compounds using ^3J(H3α-H4β) was not applicable for the 3-methyl analogues because the introduction of a 3-methyl group resulted in a quarternary carbon at position 3. In the case of **3a**, however, the large vicinal coupling constant between H1β-H2α (11.7 Hz) as well as the long range coupling constant between H2β-H4β (2.1 Hz) suggested that the A-ring of **3a** was locked essentially completely in the β-form. This was supported by the NOESY experiment as shown in Chart 2. The J-HMBC experiment allowed us to determine some of the C-H long range coupling constants of **3a** (6). Relatively large magnitude of ^3J(C2-H4β) and ^3J(C4-H2β), which were 5.3 Hz and 4.4 Hz, respectively, also supported the above conclusion.

Chart 2. Conformational Analysis of **3a**.

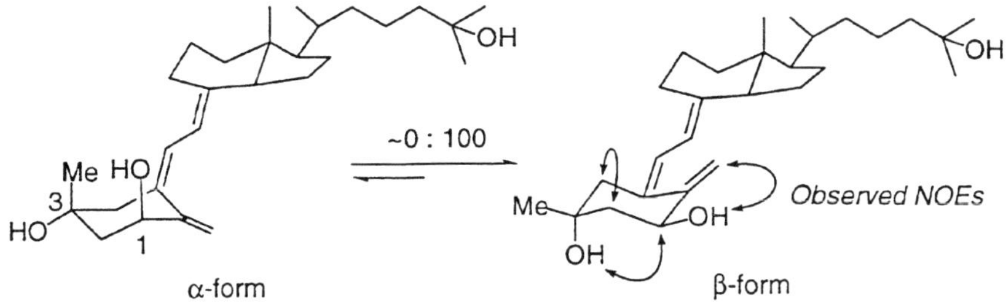

~0 : 100

α-form   β-form

Biological Evaluation The biological activities of the synthesized analogues were assessed in terms of affinities for vitamin D receptor (VDR) and vitamin D binding protein (DBP) in comparison with the natural hormone **1** (Table 1). In the binding assay using bovine thymus VDR, all the 1-methyl compounds showed virtually no affinity to VDR even in the case of **2a**, which has the active hydroxyl configuration of (1α,3β). On the other hand, **3a** and **3b** exhibited a significant binding affinity to VDR. In the binding assay using rat serum DBP, the analogues having the 1β-hydroxyl configuration were preferred as previously reported (3c), except for the case of **2c**. Cell differentiation-inducing activity of **3a** towards HL-60 cells was comparable to that of the natural hormone **1** (Chart 3), while each 1-methyl analogue showed no activity (data not shown).

Summary All possible A-ring stereoisomers of 1-methyl- and 3-methyl-1α,25-dihydroxyvitamin D_3 were efficiently synthesized. The 3-methyl analogue **3a** showed a comparable activity to 1α,25-dihydroxyvitamin D_3 in terms of cell differentiation-inducing activity. These results indicate that analogues which adopt the β-form can essentially bind to VDR and trigger the whole sequence of actions.

Table 1. Relative Binding Potencies of the 1-Methyl and 3-Methyl Analogues.[a]

	VDR[b]	DBP[c]
1	100	100
2a	0.05	6
2b	0.002	12
2c	0.001	15
2d	<0.001	450
3a	5	2
3b	0.2	140
3c	0.05	230
3d	<0.01	190

[a] The potencies of 1α,25-dihydroxyvitamin D_3 (**1**) are taken as 100. [b] Bovine thymus. [c] Rat serum.

Chart 3. HL-60 cell Differentiation-Inducing Activity of the 3-Methyl Analogues.[a]

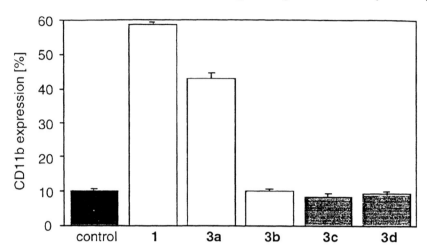

[a]HL-60 cells were treated with 10^{-8} M of 1α,25-dihydroxyvitamin D_3 (1) or the analogues (3a-d) for 72 h. Cell differentiation was assessed in terms of expression of CD11b.

Acknowledgements   We thank Dr. Yukiko Kan (Suntory Institute for Bioorganic Research) for the NOESY and J-HMBC experiments. This work was supported by a Grant-in-Aid from the Ministry of Education, Science and Culture of Japan, and a Grant from the Hayashi Memorial Foundation for Female Natural Scientists.

References and Notes

1. (a) Konno, K., Maki, S., Fujishima, T., Liu, Z.-P., Miura, D., Chokki, M. and Takayama, H. (1998) Bioorg. Med. Chem. Lett. 8, 151-156; (b) Fujishima, T., Liu, Z.-P., Miura, D., Chokki, M., Ishizuka, S., Konno, K. and Takayama, H. (1998) *ibid.* 8, 2145-2148; (c) Nakagawa, K., Kurobe, M., Ozono, K., Konno, K., Fujishima, T., Takayama, H. and Okano, T. (2000) Biochem. Pharmacol. 59, 691-702.

2. Maki, S., Harada, Y., Liu, Z.-P., Fujishima, T., Konno, K. and Takayama, H. (1998) Abstract of the 118th Annual Meeting of Pharma. Soc. Jpn. 2, 171.

3. (a) Nakagawa, K., Kurobe, M., Konno, K., Fujishima, T., Takayama, H. and Okano, T. Biochem. Pharmacol. *in press*; (b) Okano, T., Nakagawa, K., Kubodera, N., Ozono, K., Isaka, A., Osawa, A., Terada, M. and Mikami, K. (2000) Chem. Biol. 7, 171-184; (c) Fujishima, T., Konno, K., Nakagawa, K., Kurobe, M., Okano, T. and Takayama, H. (2000) Bioorg. Med. Chem. 8, 123-134, and the references cited therein.

4. Synthesis of 2a and 2c was reported: Ishida, H., Shimizu, M., Yamamoto, K., Iwasaki, Y. and Yamada, S. (1995) J. Org. Chem. 60. 1828-1833.

5. Trost, B. M., Dumas, J. and Villa, M. (1992) J. Am. Chem. Soc. 114, 9836-9845.

6. Matsumori, N., Kaneko, D., Murata, M., Nakamura., H. and Tachibana, K. (1999) J. Org. Chem. 64, 866-876.

AN EXPEDITIOUS ROUTE TO 25-HYDROXY WINDAUS-GRUNDMANN KETONE

M. Torneiro,[1] Y. Fall,[2] C. Vitale[1] J. Avión[1] and A. Mouriño[1]
[1]Departamento de Química Orgánica y Unidad Asociada al CSIC, Facultad de Química, Universidad de Santiago de Compostela. 15706 Santiago de Compostela, Spain. [2]Departamento de Química Física y Química Orgánica, facultad de Ciencias, Universidad de Vigo. 36200 Vigo, Spain.

Introduction   1α,25-Dihydroxyvitamin D_3 [**1a**, 1α,25-$(OH)_2$-D_3, calcitriol] the hormonally active form of vitamin D_3(1) (**1b**, calciferol) has a much broader spectrum of activities than originally thought and has been used together with its analogues in the treatment of a diverse range of human illness, including osteoporosis (2), psoriasis (3), cancer and AIDS (5). 25-Hydroxy Windaus-Grundmann ketone (**2a**) has proven useful in the convergent synthesis of **1a**(6).

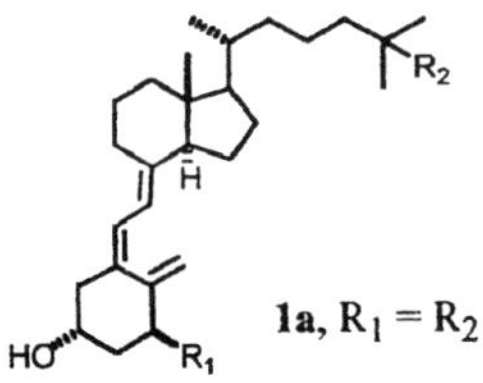

1a, $R_1 = R_2 = OH$

1b, $R_1 = R_2 = H$

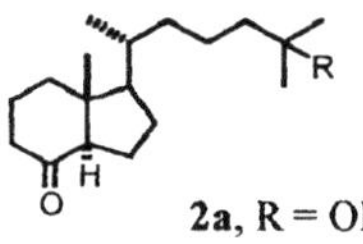

2a, R = OH

2b, R = H

Results Our synthetic approach takes advantage of the readily available Inhoffen-Lythgoe diol **5** (7), direct precursor of aldehyde **4** (Scheme 1). Reaction of ylide **3** with aldehyde **4** gave the expected D22-25-hydroxy compound **6** in 96% yield. Hydrogenation of **6** (H_2, PtO_2, EtOH) afforded alcohol **7** in 99% yield. Removal of the silil protecting group with TBAF gave diol **8** which was oxidized using PDC in dichloromethane at room temperature to afford the target compound **2a** 97% yield. Synthesis of ylide **3** was carried out using cheap and commercially available ethyl 3-bromopropionate. Thus reaction of ethyl 3-bromopropionate with methyl magnesium iodode (2 equiv) followed by reaction with triphenylphosphine in refluxing acetonitrile afforded quantitatively the corresponding phosphonium bromide as a pure and stable salt which on treatment with methyllithium (2 equiv) in ether at −20° C provided ylide **3**.

98

Scheme 1

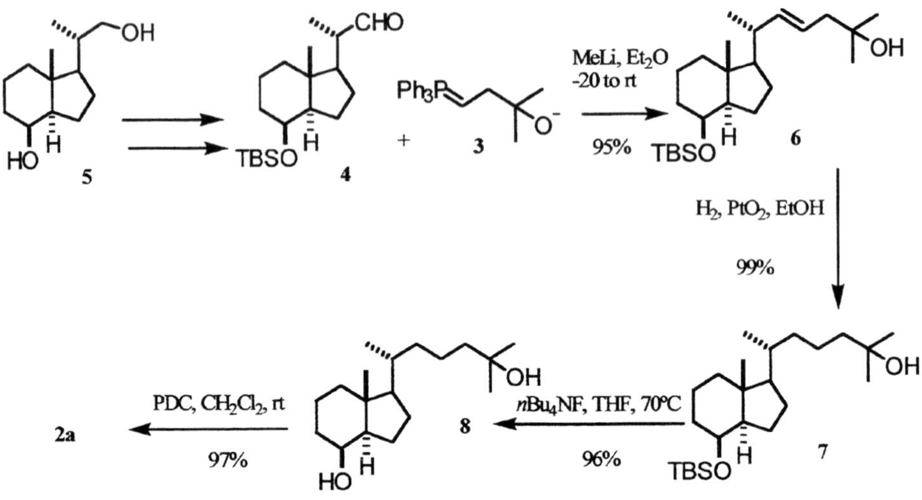

Acknowledgements We are grateful to the DGES (Spain, project PM97-0166) for financial support and Solvay Pharmaceuticals (Weesp, The Netherlands) for the gift of starting material.

References (1) (a) For a leading review on the classical actions of 1,25-(OH)₂-D₃, see: Deluca, H. F.; Burmester, J.; Darwish, H.; Krisinger, J. Molecular Mechanism of the Action of 1,25-Dihydroxyvitamin D₃. In Comprehensive Medicinal Chemistry; Hansch, C.; Sammes, P. C.; Taylor, J. B., Eds.; Pergamon Press: Oxford, **1991**; vol 3, 1129-1143.(b) Norman, A. W.; Litwack, G. *Hormones*; Academic Press: San Diego, **1997**. (c) Feldman, D.; Glorieux, F. H.; Pike, J. W. *Vitamin* D; Academic Press: San Diego, **1997**. (2) (a) Deluca, H. F. FASEB **1987**, 224. (b) Nodin, B. E. C.; Morris, H. A. *J. Cell. Biochem.* **1992**, *49*, 19.(3) (a) Kragballe, K. *J. Cell. Biochem.* **1992**, *49*, 46. (b) van de Kerkhof, P. C. M. *Br. J. Dermatol.* **1995**, *132*, 675 and referencies therein. (4) (a) Munker, R.; Norman, A.; Koeffler, H. P. *J. Clin. Invest.* **1988**, 424. (b) Zhou, J. Y.; Norman, A. W.; Akashi, M.; Chen, D. L.; Uskokovic, M. R.; Aurrecoechea, J. M.; Dauben, W. G.; Okamura, W. H.; Koeffler, H. P. *Blood* **1991**, *78*, 75. (c) Eisman, J. A.; Barkla, D. H.; Jutton, P. J. M. *Cancer res.* **1987**, *47*, 21.(5) Connor, R. I.; Rigby, W. F. C. *Biochem. Biophys. Res. Commun.* **1991**, *176*, 852.. (6) Zhu, G.-D ; Okamura, W. H. Chem. Rev. **1995**, *95*, 1877. (7) (a) Leyes, G. A.; Okamura, W. H. *J. Am. Chem. Soc.* **1982**, *104*, 6099. (b) Sardina, F. J.; Mouriño, A.; Castedo, L. *J. Org. Chem.* **1986**, *51*, 1264.

STEREOSELECTIVE SYNTHESIS OF VITAMIN D3 ANALOGUES WITH CYCLIC SIDE CHAINS

Y. Fall,[1] C. Fernandez,[1] V: Gonzalez,[1] C. Vitale[2] and A. Mouriño[2]
[1]Departamento de Química Física y Química Orgánica, facultad de Ciencias, Universidad de Vigo. 36200 Vigo, Spain.[2]Departamento de Química Orgánica y Unidad Asociada al CSIC, Facultad de Química, Universidad de Santiago de Compostela. 15706 Santiago de Compostela, Spain.

Introduction   The importance of $1\alpha,25$-Dihydroxyvitamin D_3 [Calcitriol, $1\alpha,25$-$(OH)_2$-D_3, **1**] the hormonally active metabolite of vitamin D_3 is presently well recognized[1]. It exhibits control over the expression of various genes which are involved in calcium and phosphorus metabolism, cellular differentiation and regulation of the immune system[2]. $1\alpha,25$-$(OH)_2$-D_3 is a multifunctional hormone[3] which is believed to exert its activities by a mechanism mediated by the nuclear vitamin D receptor (VDR)[4]. In the expression of vitamin D function, two proteins play important roles: The specific nuclear receptor protein (vitamin D receptor, VDR) and the transport protein (vitamin D binding protein, DBP). It is of crucial importance to find out the conformation of $1\alpha,25$-$(OH)_2$-D_3 responsible for the binding to those proteins. For that purpose, Yamada[5,6]designed the synthesis of four new vitamin D analogues (**2a**, **2b**, **3a**, **3b**) with restricted side chain conformation.

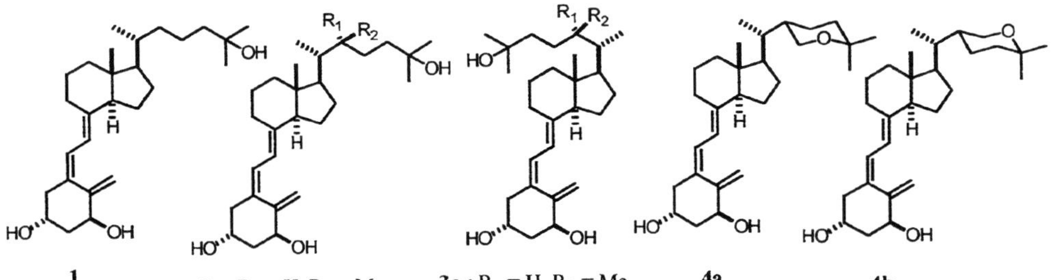

1

2a : R_1 = H, R_2 = Me
2b : R_1 = Me, R_2 = H

3a : R_1 = H, R_2 = Me
3b : R_1 = Me, R_2 = H

4a

4b

Results   Nitrile **6** (7), readily obtained from Inhoffen-Lythgoe diol **5** was deprotonated with two equivalents of LDA in THF at $-78°C$. A solution of bromide **7**

(8) in THF was added and the mixture allowed to reach room temperature affording cyanoalcohol **8** (9) (89%) as a mixture of unseparable diastereoisomers. Reaction of nitrile **8** with Dibal in dichloromethane at −10°C and subsequent acid work up afforded the corresponding aldehyde which was taken up in methanol and reacted with excess of sodium borohydride (10) to afford a 2:1.5 mixture of alcohols **9c** and **9d** which were cleanly separated by flash chromatography (15% EtOAc-hexanes) as colorless oils (64%). At this stage of the synthesis the stereochemistry of both compounds at C22 was unknown. Conventional deprotection of the TES group gave triols **10c** and **10d** in 92% and 90% yield respectively as white solids. Recrystallization of **10c** (11) from dichloromethane-methanol afforded a single crystal which was subjected to X-ray crystallographic analysis that confirmed its structure .

Scheme 1

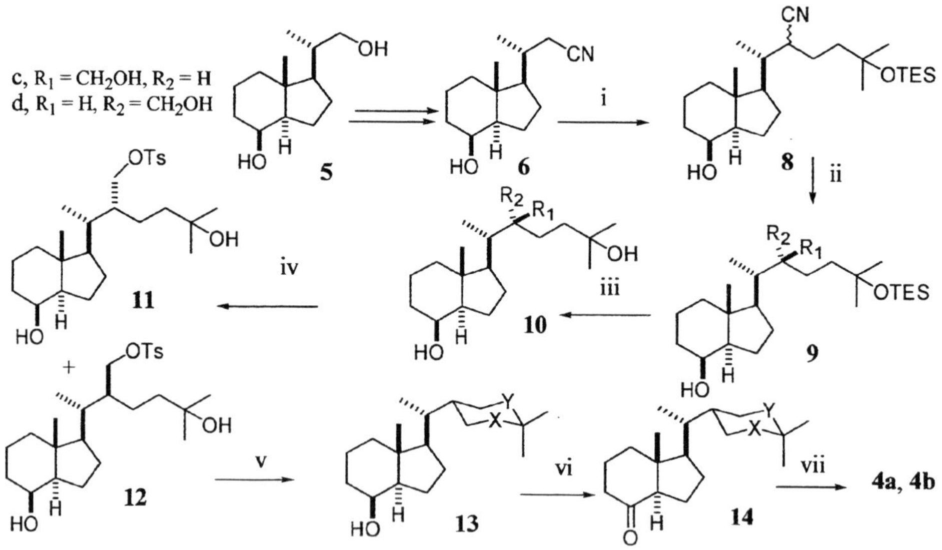

Reagents and conditions: (i) LDA,THF, −78°C; **7** (89%). (ii) Dibal,CH$_2$Cl$_2$, −10°C; HCl; NaBH$_4$, MeOH (64% 2 steps). (iii) nBu$_4$NF,THF rt (90%). (iv) TsCl, Pyr, 0°C, 12h (84%). (v) NaH, DMF, rt (61%). (vi) PDC, CH$_2$Cl$_2$, rt 5h (90%). (vii) a) ringA phosphine oxyde; nBuLi, THF, −78°C, b) nBu$_4$NF, THF rt (75%).

Selective tosylation of the primary alcohol in **10c** and **10d** gave tosylates **11** and **12** in 80% and 84% yield respectively. Tosylates **11** and **12** were individually treated with sodium hydride in DMF at rt to afford alcohols **13** bearing a cyclic side chain.

Pyridinium dichromate oxidation of alcohols **13** afforded ketones **14a** and **14b** in 90% and 95% yield respectively. With these key precursors in hand the stage was set for the Wittig-Horner reaction using the A ring phosphine oxydephosphine oxyde **7**[12]. Coupling reaction of **8a** and **8b** with **7** and subsequent removal of the silyl ptotecting groups afforded the target analogues **4a** (13) and **4b** (14) in 75% and 78% yield respectively.

Acknowledgements We are grateful to the DGES (Spain, project PM97-0166) for financial support and Solvay Pharmaceuticals (Weesp, The Netherlands) for the gift of starting material.

References (**1**)Bouillon, R. ; Okamura, W. H. ; Norman, A. W. *Endocr. Rev.* **1995**, *16*, 200. (**2**) Vitamin D. Feldman, D. ; Glorieux, F. H. ; Pike, J. W., Eds. ; Academic Press, **1979**. (**3**) Reichel, H.; Koeffler, H. P.; Norman, A. W. *New. Engl. J. Med.* **1989**, *320*, 980.. (**4**) (a) Minghetti, P. P.; Norman, A. W. FASEB J. 1988, 2, 3043. (b) Deluca, H. F.; Krisinger, J.; Darwish, H. *Kidney Int. (Suppl.)* **1990**, *38*, 52. (**5**) Yamamoto, K.; Takahashi, J.; Hamano, K.; Yamada, S.; Yamaguchi, K.; Deluca, H. F. *J. Org. Chem.* **1993**, *58*, 2530. (**6**) Yamamoto, K.; Yan Sun, W.; Ohta, M.; Hamada, K.; Deluca, H. F.; Yamada, S. *J. Med. Chem.* **1996**, *39*, 2727. (**7**) (a) Leyes, G. A.; Okamura, W. H. *J. Am. Chem. Soc.* **1982**, *104*, 6099. (b) Sardina, F. J.; Mouriño, A.; Castedo, L. *J. Org. Chem.* **1986**, *51*, 1264. (c) Fall, Y. ; Torneiro, M. ; Castedo, L. ; Mouriño, A. *Tetrahedron* **1997**, *53*, 4703.(**8**) Andrews, D. R. ; Barton, D. H. R. ; Hesse, R. H. , Pechet, M. M. *J. Org. Chem.* **1986**, 51, 4819.(**9**) All new compounds exhibited satisfactory ^{1}H and ^{13}C NMR, analytical, and/ or high resolution mass spectral data. (**10**)Wovkulich, P. M.; Barcelos, F.; Batcho, A. D.; Sereno, J. F.; Baggiolini, E. G.; Hennessy, B. M.; Uskokovic, M. R. *Tetrahedron* **1984**, *40*, 2283.(**11**) The X-ray data for **10c** will be deposited at the Cambridge Data Center.(**12**)Mouriño, A. ; Torneiro, M. ; Vitale, C. ; Fernandez, S. ; Pérez-Sestelo, J. ; Anné, S. ; Gregorio, C. ; *Tetrahedron Lett.* **1997**, *38*, 4713.

Synthesis of Vitamin D₃ Analogues with Semi-Rigid Side-Chains

Miguel Maestro,[1] Ana Fernández-Gacio,[2] Cristian Vitale,[2] Ricardo Riveiros[2] and Antonio Mouriño*[2]

[2]Departamento de Química Orgánica y Unidad Asociada al CSIC, Universidad de Santiago de Compostela, 15706 Santiago de Compostela, Spain. [1]Departamento de Quimica Fundamental, Universidad de A Coruna, Spain.

Introduction

1α,25-Dihydroxyvitamin D₃ [1α,25-(OH)₂-D₃, calcitriol], the hormonally active form of vitamin D₃, besides its important role in calcium homeostasis, also promotes cell differentiation and inhibits cell proliferation of various tumor cells, a fact that suggests its possible use in the treatment of cancer. Unfortunately, the therapeutic value of 1α,25-(OH)₂-D₃ as an antitumor agent found serious limitations due to its potent calcemic effects. For this reason, there is continued and increasing interest aimed at the rational design of new analogs of 1α,25-(OH)₂-D₃ with selective biological functions as possible drugs for medical use. However, the incomplete understanding of the conformation or conformations that the hydroxylated side chain of 1α,25-(OH)₂-D₃ adopt upon binding to its receptor (VDR) or receptors (VDRs) has led to the synthesis of numerous side-chain modified analogs of which only a few have been identified as promising drugs for the treatment of certain cancers and psoriasis.

Figure 1

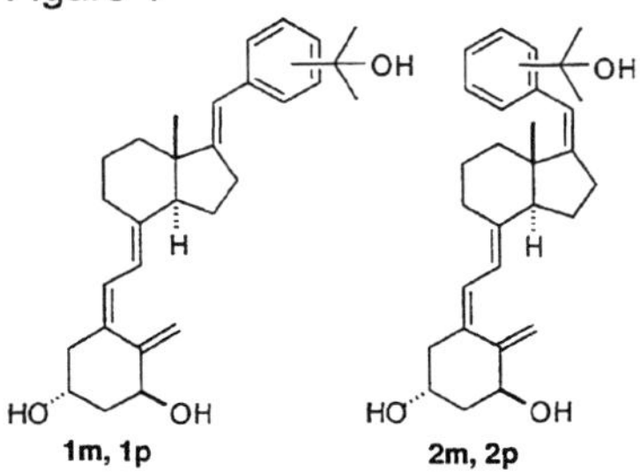

1m, 1p   2m, 2p

As part of our efforts to understand the side-chain conformation of calcitriol in its bioactive form, we recently reported (2, 3) the synthesis and conformational analysis of four side-chain analogs of 1α,25-(OH)₂-D₃. The four compounds in question incorporate conformationally locked units in the form of a double bond or a cyclopropane ring at C17–C20. Here we report the synthesis of four new analogs (**1, 2**, Figure 1) in which the side chain features both an aromatic ring at C20 and a conjugated double bond at C17–C20 (4, 5).

Results and Discussion

The synthesis of analogs **1** (*E* configuration at C20) and **2** (*Z* configuration at C20) (Scheme 1) follows the mild convergent Wittig–Horner approach originally developed by Lythgoe and later improved by the Hoffmann La Roche group. The known ketone **8**, readily prepared from vitamin D₂ (**6**) was separately treated with potassium carbanions of phosphonates **10** to give the *E* olefins **11** (~70%) and the corresponding Z-isomers (~12%). Palladium-catalyzed carbomethoxylation of bromides **11** in MeOH/DMSO under an atmosphere of CO provided the desired esters **12** (~85%).Cleavage of the silyl ether protecting groups to give alcohols **13**

was followed by PDC oxidation to afford the desired ketones **5** (~88% over the two steps). Treatment of the phosphine oxide **9** with butyllithium followed by reaction of the resulting anion with ketones **5** according to known procedures, provided the protected vitamin D analogs (~91%) with a methoxycarbonyl group at C25 for further functionalization. Treatment of these esters with methyllithium and subsequent removal of the silyl groups with tetrabutylammonium fluoride afforded the desired vitamin D analogs **3** (~80% over the two steps, ~33% overall yield from ketone **3**, 7 steps).

Scheme 1

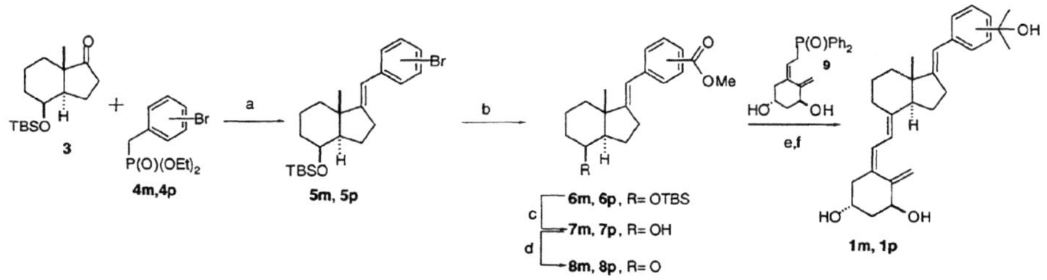

m = *meta*-series, p = *para*-series. (a) KH, THF, Δ . (b) CO, Pd(OAc)$_2$, Et$_3$N, dppp, MeOH, DMSO, Δ. (c) HF, MeCN. (d) PDC, CH$_2$Cl$_2$. (e) *n*-BuLi, THF, —78°C, **9**; **8m** or **8p**. (f) MeLi, THF, —78°C; *n*-Bu$_4$NF, THF .

Scheme 2

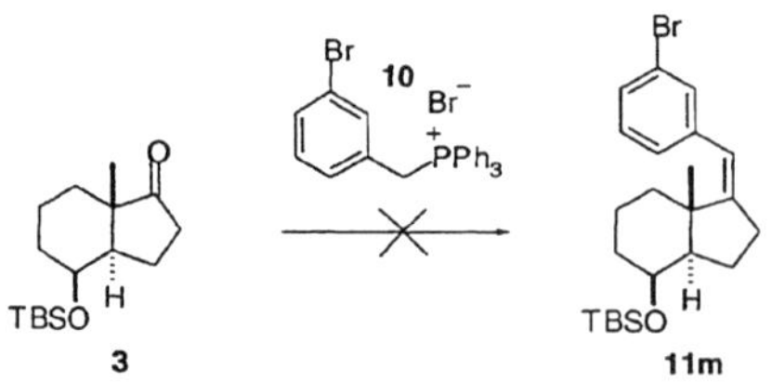

epoxide.

Synthesis of Analogs 2. Initial efforts to introduce the Z geometry by reaction of the ylide prepared from phosphonium salt **10** (KOt-Bu or NaH) with ketone **3** resulted in the recovery of starting material, presumably for steric reasons (Scheme 2). Attempts to isomerize olefin **12** to **19** by employing the Vedejs protocol (7) were unsuccessful due to difficulties in isolating the corresponding

At this point we decided to explore photochemical isomerization as an alternative strategy to obtain the Z analogs. After much experimentation we were pleased to find that direct irradiation (THF, medium pressure-Hg, Pyrex reactor, 90 min) of (E)-ester **6** proceeded cleanly to provide a separable 4:1 mixture of the desired (Z)-ester **12** (~75%) and starting material (17%). Desilylation and oxidation afforded ketones **14** (~96%), which were required for the Wittig–Horner coupling. The remaning steps to vitamin D analogs **2** are similar to those described for the preparation of vitamin D analogs **1** (2 steps, overall yield from ketone **3**, 28%).

Scheme 3

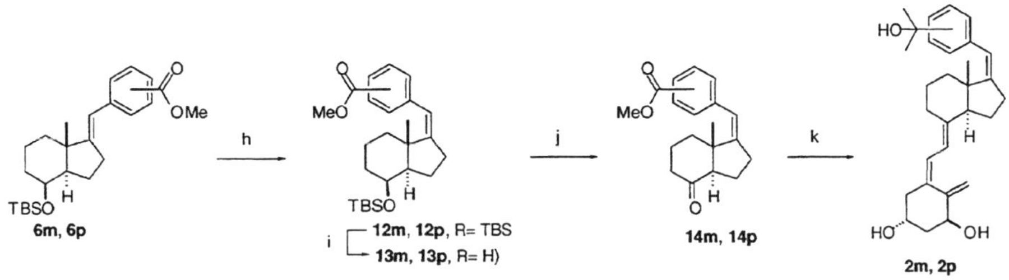

(h) hv, THF. (i) HF, MeCN. (j) PDC, CH$_2$Cl$_2$. (k) n-BuLi, THF, —78 °C,**14m** or **14p**. (l) MeLi, THF, —78°C. (m) n-Bu$_4$NF, THF.

In summary, we used the Lythgoe–Hoffmann La Roche approach to synthesize four new analogs of the hormone 1α,25-(OH)$_2$-D$_3$ with partially locked side chains (7–8 steps, overall yield ~30%). The results of biological testing of the new analogs as well as studies of their conformational analysis will be reported elsewhere.

Acknowledgment. Financial support from the Spanish Ministry of Education and Culture (Grant PM97-0166) is gratefully acknowledged. We thank Drs. J. P. van de Velde, J. Zorgdrager and S. J. Halkes (Solvay Pharmaceuticals B. V.) and R. Suau (Universidad de Málaga) for valuable suggestions. A. F.-G. thanks the Spanish Ministry of Education and Culture for an F. P. U. grant.

References. (1) This work was taken in part from the doctoral thesis of Ana Isabel Fernández-Gacio (Universidad de Santiago de Compostela. 1999). (2) Martínez-Pérez, J. A.; Sarandeses, L.; Granja, J.; Palenzuela, J. A.; Mouriño, A. *Tetrahedron Lett.* **1998**, *39*, 4725. (3) For conformational analysis of non-locked side-chain analogs of 1α,25-(OH)$_2$-D$_3$, see: Yamada, S.; Yamamoto, K.; Masuno, H.; Ohta, M. Conformation-Function Relationship of Vitamin D: Conformational Analysis Predicts Potential Side-Chain Structure, *J. Med. Chem.* **1998**, *41*, 1467 and references therein. (4) For the synthesis and biological evaluation of side-chain analogs of 1α,25-(OH)$_2$-D$_3$ with aromatic units at C22, see: Figadère, B.; Norman, A. W.; Henry, H. L.; Koeffler H. P.; Zhou, J.-Y.; Okamura, W. H. *J. Med. Chem.* **1991**, *34*, 2452. (5) For other analogs of 1α,25-(OH)$_2$-D$_3$, possessing a double bond at C17–C20, see: Bretting, C.; Hansen, C. M.; Anderson, N. R. *Vitamin D, A Pluripotent Steroid Hormone: Structural Studies, Molecular Endocrinology and Clinical Applications.* Norman, A. W., Bouillon, R., Thomasset, M., Eds.; Walter de Gruyter: Berlin, **1994**, pp 73–74. (6) (a) Sardina, F. J.; Mouriño, A.; Castedo, L. *J. Org. Chem.* **1986**, *51*, 1264. (b) Fernández, B.; Martínez-Pérez, J. A.; Granja, J. R.; Castedo, L.; Mouriño, A. *J. Org. Chem.* **1992**, *57*, 3173. (7). **1971**, *93*, 4070.

THE DESIGN AND SYNTHESIS OF 1α,25-DIHYDROXYVITAMIN D₃ DIMERS AS POTENTIAL CHEMICAL INDUCERS OF VITAMIN D RECEPTOR DIMERIZATION

José Pérez Sestelo,[a] Antonio Mouriño[b] and Luis A. Sarandeses[a]

[a] Departamento de Química Fundamental, Universidade da Coruña, E-15071 A Coruña, Spain. [b] Departamento de Química Orgánica y Unidad Asociada al C.S.I.C., Universidade de Santiago de Compostela, E-15706 Santiago de Compostela, Spain.

The biological activity of vitamin D is clearly influenced by the interaction of 1α,25-dihydroxyvitamin D₃ (calcitriol, **1b**), the hormonally active form of vitamin D₃ (**1a**), with the vitamin D protein receptor (VDR).[1] Calcitriol acts through a genomic pathway in the nucleus cell by binding to the VDR, forming a complex that interacts with the DNA-activating signal transduction processes. During the calcitriol interaction the VDR can exist as a homodimer (VDR-VDR) or a heterodimer with the retinoid X receptor (VDR-RXR), although the role of dimeric VDR structures in the activation of gene transcription is not clear.[2]

R = H, Vitamin D₃ (**1a**)
R = OH, 1α,25-(OH)₂-D₃ (**1b**)

2, n=1
3, n=3

1α,25-(OH)₂-D₃ dimers

Recently it has been shown that molecules with the ability to bind two protein receptors simultaneously can induce the receptor's dimerization and lead to the activation of different signal transduction processes. These compounds have been coined as chemical inducers of dimerization (CID's).[3] Important examples

(1) For a general review of vitamin D chemistry and biology see: (a) Vitamin D: Chemistry, Biology and Clinical Applications of the Steroid Hormone; Norman, A. W., Bouillon, R., Thomasset, M., Eds.; Vitamin D Workshop, Inc.: Riverside, CA, 1997. (b) Zhu, G.-D.; Okamura, W. H. (1995) Chem. Rev. 95, 1877–1952.
(2) Freedman, L. P.; Lemon, B. D. In Vitamin D; Feldman, D., Glorieux, F. H., Pike, J. W., Eds.; Academic Press: San Diego, 1997; Chapter 9, pp 127–148.
(3) (a) Driver, S. T.; Schreiber, S. L. (1997) J. Am. Chem. Soc. 119, 5106–5109. (b) Ho, S. N.; Biggar, S. R.; Spencer, D. M.; Schreiber, S. L.; Crabtree, G. R. (1996) Nature 382, 822–826. (c) Spencer, D. M.; Wandless, T. J.; Schreiber, S. L.; Crabtree, G. R. (1993) Science 262, 1019–1024.

of CID's are the dimers of the immunosuppressive agents FK506 (FK1012) and cyclosporin A [(CyA)$_2$].[4]

In the field of vitamin D research we envisioned the synthesis of a calcitriol dimer that could bind the vitamin D receptor doubly with a view to the exploration and possible exploitation of their role in transcription control.[5] The design of the calcitriol dimer took into account the fact that the triene system and the hydroxyl groups at positions 1α and 25 are crucial for the biological activity of calcitriol[6] and that the incorporation of new functional groups alters its biological activity dramatically.[3,7] These considerations, as well as the absence of other functional groups in the vitamin D structure, ruled out direct dimerization and we therefore decided to construct a molecule consisting of two calcitriol moieties linked by an alkyl chain attached to each calcitriol at ring C, which is probably the least active part of the vitamin D structure.

The synthetic plan for 2 and 3 was based on a Wittig–Horner approach[8] between a dimeric ketone (4, 5) containing the upper fragment of the vitamin D structure and the phosphonium oxide 6 containing ring A. The dimeric ketones 4 and 5 would be obtained by an olefin metathesis reaction of 7 or 8,[9] which can be prepared from enone 9 by cuprate addition.

Scheme 1. Retrosynthetic analysis

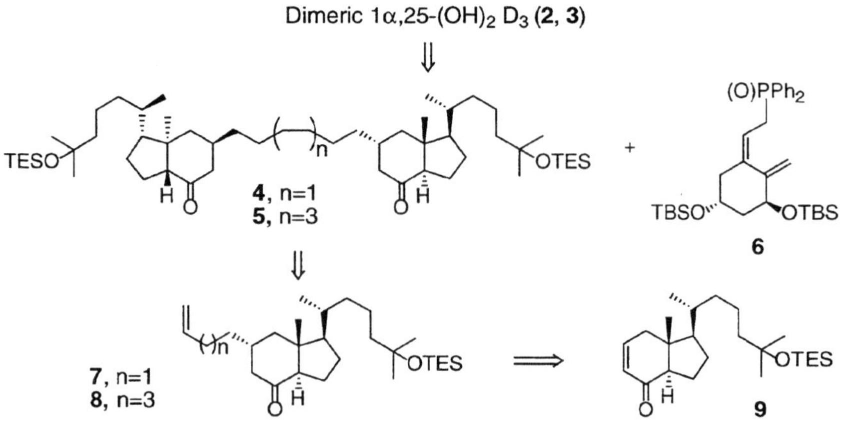

Dimeric 1α,25-(OH)$_2$ D$_3$ (2, 3)

(4) Schreiber, S. L. (1998) Bioorg. Med. Chem. 6, 1127–1152 and references therein.

(5) Pérez Sestelo, J.; Mouriño, A.; Sarandeses, L. A. (1999) Org. Lett. 1, 1005–1007.

(6) Calverley, M. J.; Jones, J. In Antitumor Steroids; Blickenstaff, R. T., Ed.; Academic Press: San Diego, 1992; Chapter 7, pp 193–270.

(7) Bouillon, R; Okamura, W. H.; Norman, A. W. (1995) Endocr. Rev. 16, 200–257.

(8) Lythgoe, B.; Moran, T. A.; Nambudiry, M. E. N.; Ruston, S.; Tideswell, J.; Wright, P. W. (1975) Tetrahedron Lett. 3863–3866.

(9) Olefin metathesis has proved to be useful for homodimerization, see: Clark, T. D.; Gadhiri, M. R. (1995) J. Am. Chem. Soc. 117, 12364–12365 and ref. 3a.

The synthesis began with the known ester **10**.[10] Addition of MeLi (3 equiv) followed by oxidation with PDC and alcohol protection with TESOTf at low temperature afforded ketone **11** in good yield (73% overall). Treatment of **11** under Saegusa conditions[11] led to the α,β-unsaturated ketone **9** in 83% yield. We then proceeded to incorporate the olefinic side chain by cuprate addition at the C-11 position. Addition of the cuprates derived from 4- and 6-bromobutene gave the corresponding 1,4-addition products **7** and **8**, respectively, as the only diastereoisomers, as detected by ¹H NMR, in high yield (90–95%).

Scheme 2. Synthesis of ketones **7** and **8**.

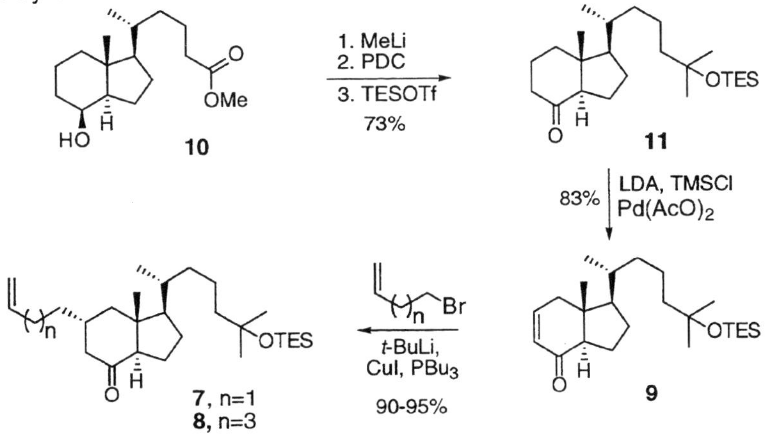

Having obtained ketones **7** and **8** we proceeded to perform the dimerization step using the olefin metathesis reaction. Treatment of **7** and **8** with Grubbs catalyst[12] gave dimers **12** and **13**, respectively, in 40–50% yield as a mixture of alkene isomers in a variable ratio (from 2:1 to 6:1) depending of the reaction conditions. The unreacted ketone (40%) was also recovered. Hydrogenation of **12** and **13** with a rhodium/alumina catalyst (5%) at atmospheric pressure afforded the dimers **4** and **5**, respectively, as single products in quantitative yield.

Wittig–Horner reaction between the dimeric ketones **4** or **5** and the ylide derived from the phosphonium oxide **6**[13] led to the stereoselective formation of protected calcitriol dimers **14** and **15** in excellent yield (85% and 95%). Removal of the six silyl groups with TBAF in THF (rt, 24h) afforded the desired calcitriol dimers **2** (74% yield) and **3** (63% yield).

(10) Mascareñas, J. L.; Pérez Sestelo, J.; Castedo, L.; Mouriño, A. (1991) Tetrahedron Lett. 32, 2813–2816.
(11) Ito, Y.; Hirao, T.; Saegusa, T. (1978) J. Org. Chem. 43, 1011–1013.
(12) Schwab, P.; Grubbs, R. H.; Ziller, J. W. (1996) J. Am. Chem. Soc. 118, 100–110.
(13) Mouriño, A.; Torneiro, M.; Vitale, C.; Fernández, S.; Pérez Sestelo, J.; Anné, S.; Gregorio, C. (1997) Tetrahedron Lett. 38, 4713–4716.

Scheme 3. Synthesis of calcitriol dimers **2** and **3**.

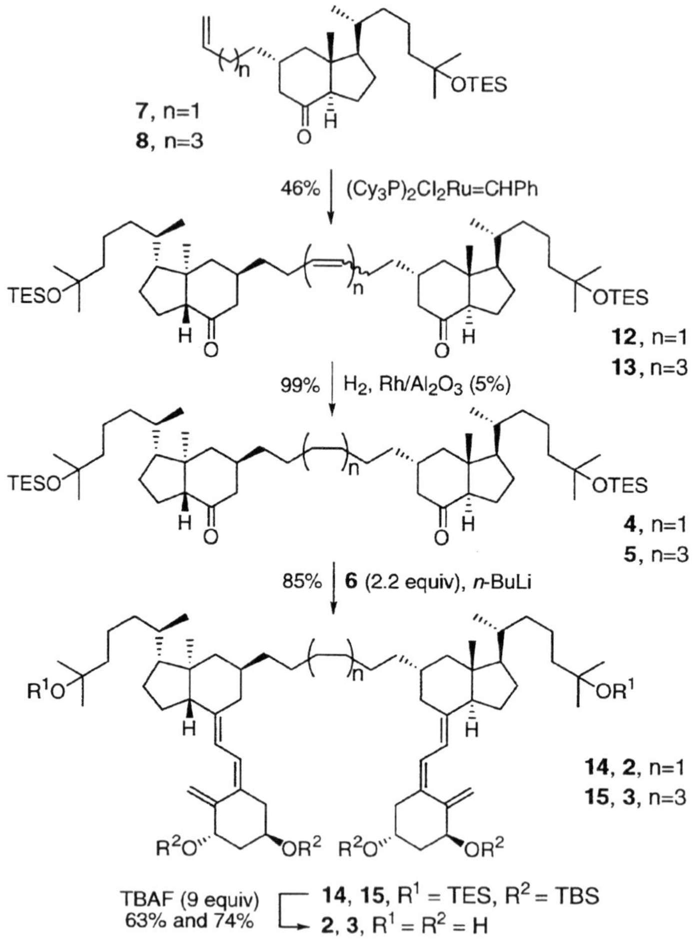

In summary, we have designed the first generation of calcitriol dimers (**2** and **3**) linked through the C-11 position. The dimers link two units of calcitriol with an alkyl chain of six and ten carbons, meaning that the VDR binding region remains unobstructed. The synthesis, which is short and convergent, should allow the preparation of an entire family of calcitriol dimers. Biological studies of dimers **2** and **3** are already in progress and the results will be published in due course.

Acknowledgments. J. P. S. thanks the Spanish Ministry of Education and Culture for a research grant. We thank the DGES (Spain, PM97-0166), Xunta de Galicia (XUGA 10305A98) and University of A Coruña for financial support. We also thank Mrs. Paulina Freire for reproducing some experiments and Mr. Carlos Gregorio for the preparation of an advanced intermediate of the A ring phosphine oxide.

DENSITY FUNCTIONAL STUDIES ON A [1,7]-H SHIFT IN THE THERMAL ISOMERIZATION OF PREVITAMIN D

O. Dmitrenko [1),3)] R. D. Bach [1)] and W. Reischl [2)]

[1)] Department of Chemistry and Biochemistry, University of Delaware, DE 19716, USA, [2)] Institute of Organic Chemistry, University of Vienna, A-1090 Vienna, Austria, [3)] Institute of Surface Chemistry of NASU, Pr.Nauki 31, Kiev, Ukraine

Introduction. The classical sigmatropic [1,7]-H shift in previtamin D (**1**) is the thermal step of the vitamin D synthesis. It has been directly demonstrated through NMR experiments that this process is characterized by antarafacial stereochemistry [1] and that the helical conformation of the previtamin D, which places the A-ring under the CD-ring system (right-handed helix) is preferred for the hydrogen migration by a factor of 2 [2]. The modification of previtamin D by substitution of the α- or β-hydrogen at C11 (according to the standard atom numbering in steroid molecules) for the OH group was found to exert a significant *syn* π-facial directive effect on the helicity of the hydrogen migration process [3]. In particular, it has been demonstrated that 11β-hydroxyl substitution may reverse the characteristic tendency in the previtamin D hydrogen migration in favor of the left-handed helix with the A-ring above the CD-ring plane [3]. This effect is still unclear from a mechanistic point of view. Another feature that needs to be better understood is the high value of the KIE and the temperature dependence for the [1,7]-H shift which is sensitive to the molecular structure and microenvironment, and varies even upon changes of substituents [4]. In this work we have applied the DFT computational method to study in detail the [1,7]-H shift in 3-desoxy-analogs of previtamin D, vitamin D and corresponding transition structures and kinetic isotope effects. Based upon B3LYP/6-31G(d) calculations on 11α- and 11β-OH analogs we attempted also to gain an understanding of the 11-OH directivity effect.

Results. The eight lowest energy ground state conformers of 3-desoxy-previtamin D, four conformers of 3-desoxy-vitamin D [5] and four transition structures (TS) have been fully optimized and characterized at the B3LYP/6-31G(d) level. The transition structures found differ in the conformation of the A-ring (the 3β-H can be axial or equatorial) and the helicity of the triene system (right-handed (**RH**) and left-handed (**LH**)) (Figure 1). There is no energetic difference between axial and equatorial 3β-hydrogen orientations in the corresponding transition structures. The calculated energy difference between these **RH** and **LH** transition structures (**RH-LH** energy gap) is 2.17 kcal/mol which is much larger than is expected based upon an experimental factor of 2:1 (0.4 kcal/mol) indicating an **RH** helical transition structure topography preference [2].The calculated activation enthalpy is in good agreement with experiment (20 vs 19 kcal/mol), but there is a significant difference between calculated and experimental activation entropy (-9 e.u. vs -20 e.u.) [4]. We think that the -11 e.u.

112

may be due to specific solvent organization induced by charge separation accompanying H-shift in the transition structure. This suggestion is consistent with the smaller experimental **RH-LH** energy gap. The **LH** transition structure has the C-18 methyl on the same side as the migrating hydrogen, with respect to the CD-ring plane, and this partially shields the shifting partially positively charged hydrogen atom. Thus, in solvent, the microenvironment is more chaotic in the case of the **LH** transition state, that makes it potentially more stabilized by an entropy contribution than the **RH** transition state.

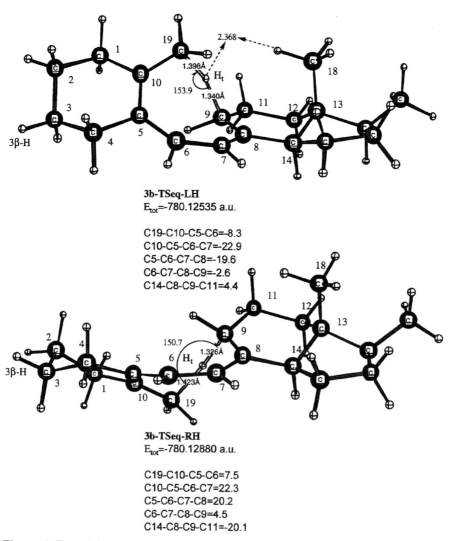

3b-TSeq-LH
E_{tot}=-780.12535 a.u.

C19-C10-C5-C6=-8.3
C10-C5-C6-C7=-22.9
C5-C6-C7-C8=-19.6
C6-C7-C8-C9=-2.6
C14-C8-C9-C11=4.4

3b-TSeq-RH
E_{tot}=-780.12880 a.u.

C19-C10-C5-C6=7.5
C10-C5-C6-C7=22.3
C5-C6-C7-C8=20.2
C6-C7-C8-C9=4.5
C14-C8-C9-C11=-20.1

Figure 1. Transition structures for [1,7]-H shifts in 3-desoxy-previtamin D analogs.

In order to better understand the 11-OH directivity effect [3] we have replaced the 11α (β)-H in transition structures **3-TSeq-LH** and **3-TSeq-RH** with an OH group. Some similarity in accord with experiment is observed: 11α-substitution increases the **RH-LH** energy gap, whereas 11β-substitution results in a decrease. Nevertheless, we did not get a preference for the **LH** helix with the 11β-OH. The calculated charge distribution data indicates that in all cases when the OH-group is on the same side as the migrating hydrogen, the positive charge on this hydrogen is apparently reduced. This charge reduction induced by σ-σ interaction with the C-O bond of the neighboring hydroxyl group may distort (compensate the "charge separation") local organization of the microenvironment thereby increasing the entropy of the whole solute-solvent system. This acts to stabilize the corresponding transition structure (**RH** in case of 11α-OH and **LH** in case of 11β-OH). Thus, we are suggesting that 11-OH directivity involves to a large extent entropy contributions from solute-solvent system re-organization.

For the computation of the kinetic isotope effect (KIE) we used the known expression [6]: KIE=MMI*ZPE*EXC*Q   (1)

where the first three terms are responsible for a semi-classical isotope effect and Q is a tunnel correction. MMI is the mass and moment of inertia effect. It arises from the rotational and translational partition functions:

$$MMI = \prod_{i=1}^{3N-6}(v_D^r/v_H^r)/\prod_{i=1}^{3N^*-7}(v_D^r/v_H^r) \qquad (2)$$

the ZPE term accounts for the zero-point vibrational energies:

$$ZPE = \exp\{(hc/2kT)[\sum_{i=1}^{3N-6}(v_H^r - v_D^r) - \sum_{i=1}^{3N^*-7}(v_H^{\neq} - v_D^{\neq})]\} \qquad (3)$$

The excitation term (EXC) arising from vibrational partition functions is a contribution from any appreciable populations of vibrational states

$$EXC = \prod_{i=1}^{3N-6}\{[1-\exp(-hv_H^r c/kT)]/[1-\exp(-hv_D^r c/kT)]\}/$$

$$/\prod_{i=1}^{3N^*-7}\{[1-\exp(-hv_H^{\neq} c/kT)]/[1-\exp(-hv_D^{\neq} c/kT)]\} \qquad (4)$$

Tunneling corrections were calculated using two approaches, Wigner (5) and Bell (6):

$$Q_W = [1+(hv_H^i c/kT)^2/24]/[1+(hv_D^i c/kT)^2/24] \qquad (5)$$

$$Q_B = \frac{0.5u_t^{\neq}}{\sin(0.5u_t^{\neq})} - \sum_{n=1}^{\infty}(-1)^n\frac{\exp(\frac{u_t^{\neq}-2n\pi}{u_t^{\neq}}\alpha)}{\frac{u_t^{\neq}-2n\pi}{u_t^{\neq}}\alpha} \qquad (6)$$

Where

$$u_t^{\neq} = hc\nu_t^{\neq}/kT,$$

$$\alpha = \Delta E^{\neq}/kT$$

The theoretical data for model **3** are given in Table 1. The Bell equation gives the best results for room temperature KIE which are reasonably close to the experimentally found KIE=11.4 (at 25° C) [3]. Nevertheless, the high temperature (80° C) kinetic isotope effect can not be reproduced either by Bell's approach (KIE$_B$), or Wigner's approximation (KIE$_W$).

Table 1. Calculated Kinetic Isotope Effects (B3LYP/6-31G(d)) for [1,7]-H Shift with $\Delta G(T)^{\neq}$ = 23 kcal/mol.

KIE$_W$		KIE$_B$	
298.15° K	353.15° K	298.15° K	353.15° K
3.88	**3.13**	**15.37**	**3.02**
(3.78)	(3.06)	(11.29)	(2.74)

[a] The numbers in bold are calculated with the scaling factor 0.9804.
[b] The numbers in parenthesis are calculated with the scaling factor 0.9613.

Acknowledgement. Support from Österreichische Nationalbank (Jubiläumsfonds-projekt Nr.:7395 to W.R.) is gratefully acknowledged.

References
1. (a) Hoeger, C.A. and Okamura, W.H. (1985) J. Am. Chem. Soc. 107, 268-270.. (b) Hoeger, C.A.; Johnston, A.D., and Okamura, W.H. (1987) J. Am. Chem. Soc. 109, 4690-4698.
2. Sheves, M., Berman, E., Mazur, Y. and Zaretskii, Z.V.I. (1979) J.Am. Chem. Soc. 101, 1882-1883.
3. (a) Wu, K.-M.and Okamura, W.H. (1990) J.Org.Chem. 55, 4025-4033. (b) Enas, J.D., Palenzuela, J.A. and Okamura, W.H. (1991) J. Am. Chem. Soc. 113, 1355-1363.
4. (a) Okamura, W.H., Hoeger, C.A., Miller, K.J. and Reischl, W. (1988) J. Am. Chem. Soc. 110, 973-974. (b) Okamura, W.H., Elnagar, H.Y., Ruther, M. and Dobreff, S. (1993) J.Org.Chem. 58, 600-610. (c) Curtin, M.L. and Okamura, W.H. (1991) J. Am. Chem. Soc. 113, 6958-6966. (d) Palenzuela, J.A., Elnagar, H.Y. and Okamura, W.H. (1989) J. Am. Chem. Soc. 111, 1770-1773.
5. (a) Dmitrenko, O., Reischl, W., Vivian J.T. and Frederick, J.H. (1999) J.Mol.Struc.(Theochem), 467, 195-210 . (b) Dmitrenko, O., Frederick, J.H. and Reischl, W. (2000) J.Mol.Struc.(Theochem), in press.
6. Melander, L. and Saunders, W.H., Jr. Reaction Rates of Isotopic Molecules; Wiley-Interscience: New York, 1980.

VITAMIN D
BINDING PROTEIN

CRYSTALLIZATION AND PRELIMINARY X-RAY INVESTIGATION OF THE HUMAN VITAMIN D-BINDING PROTEIN IN COMPLEX WITH 25-HYDROXYVITAMIN D_3.

I. Bogaerts[†], C. Verboven[†], A. Rabijns[†], H. Van Baelen[*], R. Bouillon[*], C. De Ranter[†]. [†]Laboratorium voor Analytische Chemie en Medicinale Fysicochemie, Faculteit Farmaceutische Wetenschappen, E. Van Evenstraat 4, B-3000 Leuven and [*]LEGENDO, Onderwijs & Navorsing, Gasthuisberg, B-3000 Leuven, Belgium.

Introduction

Vitamin D-binding protein (DBP) is a 51 300 Dalton glycoprotein present in human plasma. It is the main carrier of vitamin D_3, its metabolites like 1,25-dihydroxyvitamin D_3 ($1,25(OH)_2D_3$), i.e. the active vitamin D_3 hormone, and 25-hydroxyvitamin D_3 ($25(OH)D_3$) and its analogs [1]. DBP binds one mole of vitamin D_3 per mole with high affinity ($K_a = 5 \times 10^8$ M^{-1} for $25(OH)D_3$) [2,3]. $1,25(OH)_2D_3$ not only plays a role in the calcium homeostasis, but newly discovered functions suggest also a role for $1,25(OH)_2D_3$ in the treatment of psoriasis, several cancers and auto-immune diseases. DBP's importance in these clinical applications is not restricted to mere transport, for DBP clearly affects the pharmacokinetics of the vitamin D_3 hormone/analogs. Moreover, all analogs with good dissociation of action (i.e. low calcemic versus high proliferative effects) display low DBP-binding affinity [1,4].

To have better insights in the mechanism of action of vitamin D_3 and its metabolites, characterization of the binding pocket of DBP would be very helpful to design new analogs with selective therapeutic potential. To gain this important information the structure of the DBP:$25(OH)D_3$ complex is studied.

Purification and crystallization

DBP was isolated from pooled human serum by means of affinity chromatography on immobilized anti-DBP antibodies. Further purification was performed with ion-exchange chromatography (HiLoad 16/10, Q SepharoseHP) [5].

Crystals of the complex were obtained by co-crystallization. A mixture of DBP (30 mg/ml) and a two-fold excess of $25(OH)D_3$ was left for 19 hours at 4°C to get complete complexation. Crystallization was performed in VDX plates (Hampton Research) by the hanging drop vapor diffusion method at a temperature of 4°C. The best crystals were

118

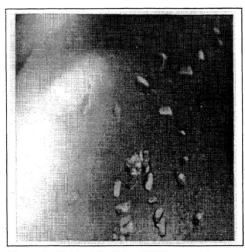

grown from 7.5% polyethylene glycol 400, 0.1M sodium acetate buffer pH 5.2 and 12% ethanol. Drops of 1μl reservoir solution by 1μl protein solution were equilibrated against 750 μl reservoir solution. The drops were streak seeded with a DBP crystal after one week. Crystals of 0.05mm by 0.05mm appeared three weeks after seeding. (Fig. 1)

Figure 1 : Typical DBP-25(OH)D$_3$ crystals.

Data collection and processing

Diffraction data were collected at the EMBL X11 beamline at the Doris storage ring, DESY, Hamburg with a MAR CCD detector. The experiments were performed at 100K using a N$_2$ gas stream to cool the crystals (Oxford cryogenic cooling system). The crystals were cryoprotected by soaking in their crystallization solution with a raised polyethylene glycol 400 concentration of 35%. The data were collected at a wavelength of 0.9091 Å. The crystal to detector distance was 300 mm. The crystal rotation angle per image was 0.5°. The diffraction pattern displays hexagonal symmetry. All data were processed and scaled with the HKL package [6]. The results of the processing are summarized in table 1.

According to the unit cell dimensions, the calculated volume of the unit cell is 1.68x10^6 Å^3. By space-group symmetry, the unit cell must contain six asymmetric units. The observation of a significant peak in the self rotation function supported the assumption of two molecules of 51 300 Dalton in the asymmetric unit. That leads to a Matthews coefficient (V$_M$) of 2.73 Å^3/Da implying a solvent content of the DBP:25(OH)D$_3$ crystals of 55% [7].

Molecular replacement

The molecular replacement method using the DBP-structure as a search probe was suited to solve the structure [8]. The Crystallography

Space group	P6(1)
Cell parameters	$a = b = 124.7$ Å
	$c = 125.1$ Å
	$\alpha = \beta = 90°$
	$\gamma = 120°$
Resolution range	$30.0 - 3.5$ Å
Number of measured reflections	45146
Number of unique reflections	13938
Overall redundancy	3.24
$<I/\sigma(I)>$ overall	9.6
highest resolution shell	2.4
Completeness overall	99.0%
highest resolution shell	95.7%
lowest resolution shell	96.6%
Rsym overall	9%
highest resolution shell	48.1%

Table 1: Data processing results

& NMR System, Version 0.9 was employed for this purpose [9]. After performing a rotation search, a translation search was carried out for all possible spacegroups. The solution for spacegroup $P6_1$ had a significantly higher correlation coefficient than all the others. This solution was further used for the calculation of the electron density maps. The programs MAPMAN and O were used to manipulate and display the maps [10,11].

Biochemical studies have demonstrated that the aminoterminal residues 35 to 49 and 145 are involved in the binding of vitamin D_3 [12,13]. The current electron density map displays at this biochemically identified vitamin D-binding region clear positive electron density. (Fig. 2). These observations suggest that the $25(OH)D_3$ molecule is indeed bound to DBP in the crystals. Moreover, it is the first indication for the three-dimensional architecture of the vitamin D-binding pocket.

Conclusions

Crystals of the DBP:$25(OH)D_3$ complex were obtained which allowed to identify the vitamin D-binding pocket. The resolution of the current electron density map is, however, insufficient to draw firm conclusions. Better diffracting crystals should be grown. Currently other crystallization protocols are tested for this purpose.

120

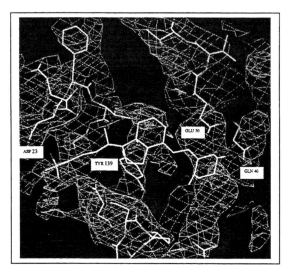

Figure 2 : 2Fo-Fc map of the vitamin D-binding region. Three blobs of positive density (at Asp 23, Gln 46, Glu 50 and Tyr 139) can accommodate the 25(OH)D_3 molecule. The labeled amino acids are those involved in the 25(OH)D_3-binding

References

1. Bouillon, R., Okamura, W.H. and Norman, A.W. (1995) Endocr. Rev. 16, 200-257.
2. Bouillon, R., Van Baelen, H. and De Moor, P. (1980) J. of Steroid Biochem. 13, 1029-1034.
3. Cooke, N.E. and Haddad, J.G. (1997) In : Vitamin D. Feldman, D., Glorieux, F.H. and Pike, J.W., eds., 87-101, Academic Press, Orlando.
4. Pols, H.A.P., Birkenhäger, J.C. and van Leeuwen, J.P.T.M. (1994) Clin. Endocr. 40, 285-291.
5. Verboven, C., De Bondt, H., De Ranter, C., Bouillon, R. and Van Baelen, H. (1995) J. Steroid Biochem. Molec. Biol. 54, 11-14.
6. Otwinowski, Z. and Minor, W. (1997) Meth. Enzymol. 276, 307-326.
7. Matthews, B.W. (1968) J. Mol. Biol. 33, 491-497.
8. Verboven, C. (1998) *Three-dimensional crystal structure determination of the human vitamin D binding protein.* Proefschrift ter verkrijging van de graad van doctor in de farmaceutische wetenschappen.
9. Brunger, A.T., Adams, P.D., Clore, G.M., Delano, W.L., Gros, P., Grosse-Kunstleve, R.W., Jiang, J.-S., Kuszewski, J., Nilges, N., Pannu, N.S., Read, R.J., Rice, L.M., Simonson, T. and Warren, G.L. (1998) Acta Cryst. D54, 905-921.
10. Kleywegt, G.J. and Jones, T.A. (1996) Acta Cryst. D52, 826-828.
11. Jones, T.A., Zou, J.Y., Cowan, S.W. and Kjelgaard, M. (1991). Acta Cryst. A47, 110-119.
12. Haddad, J.G., Hu, Y.Z., Kowalski, M.A., Laramore, C., Ray, K., Robzyk, P. and Cooke N.E. (1992) Biochemistry 31, 7174-7181.
13. Swamy, N., Brisson, M. and Ray, R. (1995) J. Biol. Chem. 270, 2636-2639.

THREE-DIMENSIONAL ARCHITECTURE OF THE VITAMIN D-BINDING PROTEIN-G-ACTIN COMPLEX

N. Swamy[1], D. Weitz[1], M. Caughron[2], J.F. Head[2], and R. Ray[1]
[1]Bioorganic Chemistry & Structural Biology, Vitamin D Laboratory; and [2]Department of Physiology, Boston University School of Medicine, Boston, MA 02118, USA

Introduction: Vitamin D-binding protein (DBP) is a polymorphic serum glycoprotein with multiple functions that include binding of vitamin D metabolites, fatty acids, G-actin and chemotactic agents (1,2). In addition, a post-translational modification of DBP involving its carbohydrate moiety produces DBP-*maf* with potent macrophage- and osteoclast-activating properties (3,4).

Interaction between DBP and G-actin has been subjected to several studies which indicated that DBP plays an important role during injury and cell lysis in depolymerizing actin polymers in circulation with profound implications in cardiac and cerebral stroke (5-7). It has also been observed that this sequestration process is further aided by the rapid clearance of DBP-actin complex.

DBP, similar to serum albumin, has a triple-domained modular structure. Recently it was shown that the actin-binding and vitamin D sterol-binding activities are restricted to Domain III (C-terminal) and Domain I (N-terminal) of DBP respectively (8-14). This suggested that actin-binding and vitamin D sterol-binding activities (by DBP) may be independent of each other.

The object of our present study was to obtain a homogeneous preparation of DBP-G-actin complex in sufficient quantity for crystallization with an ultimate goal to determine the 3-D structure of such a complex by x-ray diffraction analysis.

Preparation and purification of DBP-actin complex by 25-hydroxy-vitamin D$_3$-Sepharose affinity chromatography (Figure 1): Rabbit muscle acetone powder (250 mg) was suspended in 10 ml of 1.0 mM Tris-Cl pH 7.4 and stirred at 4^{0}C for 20 min on a magnetic stirrer. The mixture was filtered, and the clear supernatant was added to 10 ml of human plasma at 4^{0}C. The plasma solution was adjusted to a final concentration of 10 mM Tris.HCl, pH 7.4, 0.1 mM EDTA, 0.5 mM ATP and 0.2 mM CaCl$_2$. The mixture was incubated at 0^{0}C, 60 min.,

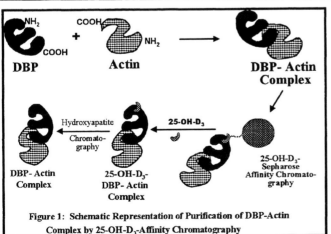

Figure 1: Schematic Representation of Purification of DBP-Actin Complex by 25-OH-D$_3$-Affinity Chromatography

diluted 1:1 with a buffer (10 mM of Tris.HCl, pH 7.4, 0.1 mM EDTA, 0.5 mM ATP 0.2

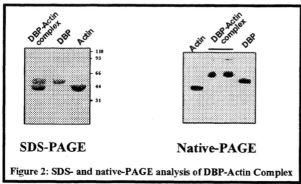

SDS-PAGE   **Native-PAGE**

Figure 2: SDS- and native-PAGE analysis of DBP-Actin Complex

mM $CaCl_2$ and 0.1% Triton X 100) and passed through a 25-$OH-D_3$-Sepharose column at 4^0C (15). The column was washed thoroughly with column buffer, and finally eluted with 25-$OH-D_3$ (2.0 mg in 25 mL of column buffer) at 25^0 C. The fractions containing protein were pooled, and passed through a Hydroxylapatite column, and the protein complex was eluted with 75 mM phosphate buffer, pH 7.4, and concentrated by filtration.

Homogeneity of the complex was determined by analysis on native- and denaturing (SDS)-PAGE (**Figure 2**) which showed that the complex was comprised of two components, which co-migrated with DBP and actin in the gel. In the native-PAGE the two bands coalesced to a slower-moving band (intact complex). Thus, *we have successfully purified DBP-actin complex in a single affinity-purification step.*

25-hydroxyvitamin D_3- binding analysis: Competitive binding assays of native DBP and DBP-actin complex with ^3H-25-OH-D_3 and various concentrations of 25-OH-D_3 were carried out according to published procedure (11). *As shown in* **Figure 3**, *binding curves of DBP and DBP-actin*

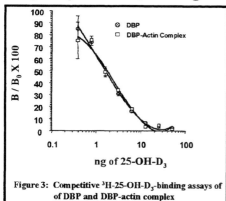

Figure 3: Competitive ^3H-25-OH-D_3-binding assays of of DBP and DBP-actin complex

complex were almost identical, strongly suggesting that vitamin D sterol- and actin-bindings (by DBP) are largely independent of each other.

Stability of DBP-actin complex towards urea and trypsin : The stability of the DBP-actin complex was tested in the presence of different concentrations of

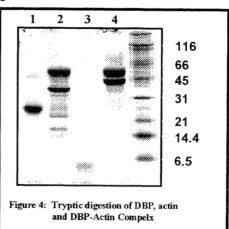

Figure 4: Tryptic digestion of DBP, actin and DBP-Actin Compelx

1: DBP + Trypsin, 2: DBP-Actin Complex +Trypsin, 3: Actin + Trypsin, 4: DBP-Actin Complex

urea and native-PAGE analysis. *We observed that the complex was stable up to 4 M urea at 4°C for 60 days* (results not shown).

Incubation of DBP with trypsin (20:1) resulted in a prominent 25 KDa band on SDS-PAGE (**Figure 4**, **Lane 1**). Under similar condition actin was completely digested (**Lane 3**), but DBP-actin complex ((**Lane 4**) showed two prominent bands (52 and 35 Kda) (**Lane 2**). Sequencing of these bands revealed that the 52 KDa band was from DBP (5 amino acids shorter in N-terminus) and 34 KDa band was from actin (starting from amino acid position 69). *These results indicated that the interaction between DBP and actin largely stabilized each other in tryptic-cleavage.*

Crystallization and x-ray diffraction analysis: Hamptons Crystal screen kit was used to determine the appropriate conditions for crystallization of DBP-actin complex for preliminary screening using hanging drop method. The crystals were transferred into a cryoprotectant solution (mother liquor containing 10% glycerol), and flash frozen in a liquid nitrogen stream. X-ray diffraction data were collected on RAXIS IIc area detector facility at Boston University School of Medicine using DENZO/SCALEPACK which showed the space group to be **primitive orthorhombic** with **unit cell dimensions of a=79.5A, b=87.0A and c=161.1A**. The crystals diffracted to 2.6A and a full data set was collected to **2.8A**. Systematic absences show the **space group** to be **P212121** and Vm calculations indicate a single molecule of the complex in the asymmetric unit (Vm=2.9).

Structure of DBP-actin complex as a molecular replacement model: At this is point our attempts to attempts to obtain diffractable heavy metal derivative/s of the DBP-actin crystal, required for phasing, did not materialize. Hence a molecular replacement (MR) solution to the structure was sought using the known structure of actin derived from the structure of actin-DNase complex (16) and human serum albumin (17), and the program AmoRe. The structure is represented in **Figure 5**.

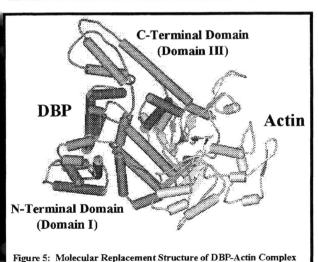

Figure 5: Molecular Replacement Structure of DBP-Actin Complex

DISCUSSION

The salient features of the DBP-actin complex, that can be gleaned from **Figure 5**, are (**a**) DBP is made up of 22 helices (7, 12 and 3 in Domains I-III respectively), and (**b**) Domain III of DBP interacts with actin with interaction phases that include residues 389-392 and 78-81 of DBP and actin respectively. The figure

124

also indicates that there is considerable interaction between Domain I of DBP (166-170) and actin (147-149). A functional proof of such interaction was obtained when we observed that the addition of 25-OH-D$_3$ to the DBP-actin crystal completely destroyed the latter, indicating a large conformational change in the Domain I of DBP (upon 25-OH-D$_3$-binding). This is in apparent contradiction with our results involving affinity-purification of DBP-actin complex using a 25-OH-D$_3$-affinity matrix (**Figure 1**) and binding assays (**Figure 2**). We hypothesize that there may be subtle differences in the crystal and solution structures of the DBP-actin complex which is reflected in our surprising observation.

In conclusion, we have crystallized the DBP-actin complex and determined its unit-cell dimension. We have also developed a molecular replacement model of the complex, refinement of which is currently in progress.

REFERENCES

1.   Cooke, N.E., and Haddad, J.G. (1989) Endo. Rev. 10, 294-307.
2.   Ray, R. (1996) Proc. Soc. Exp. Biol. Med. 212, 305-312.
3.   Yamamoto, N., Homma, S., Millman, I. (1991) J. Immunol. 147,273-280.
4.   Schneider, G.B. Benis, K.A. Flay, N.W. Ireland, R.A. and Popoff, S.N. (1995) Bone. 16, 657-662.
5.   Van Baelen, H., Bouillon, R. and DeMoor, P. (1980) J. Biol. Chem. 255, 2270-2272.
6.   Haddad, J.G. (1982) Arch. Biochem. Biophys. 213, 538-544.
7.   Goldschmidt-Clermont, P.J., Williams, M.H., and Galbraith, R.M. (1987) Biochem. Biophys. Res. Comm. 146, 611-617.
8.   Haddad, J.G., Hu, Y.Z., Kowalski, M.A., Laramore, C., Ray, K., Robzyk, P., and Cooke, N.E. (1992) Biochemistry, 31, 7174-7181.
9.   Ray, R., Holick, S.A., Hanafin, N., and Holick, M.F. (1986) Biochemistry 25, 4729-4733.
10.   Ray, R., Bouillon, R., Van Baelen, H.G., and Holick, M.F (1991). Biochemistry 36, 4809-4813.
11.   Ray, R., Bouillon, R., Van Baelen, H.G., and Holick, M.F. (1991) Biochemistry 30, 7638-7642
12.   Swamy, N., and Ray, R. (1995) Arch. Biochem. Biophys. 319, 504-507.
13.   Swamy, N., Dutta, A., and Ray, R. (1997) Biochemistry 36, 7432-7436.
14.   Swamy, N., Brisson, M., and Ray, R. (1995) J. Biol. Chem. 270, 2636-2639.
15.   Chang, R., Brisson, M., and Ray, R. (1995) Protn. Expressn. Purifn. 6, 185-188.
16.   Kabsch, W., Mannherz, H.G., Suck, D., Pai, E.F., and Holmes, K.C. (1990) Nature 347,37-44.
17.   Sugio, S., Kashima, A., Mochizuki, S., Noda, M., and Kobayashi K. (1999) Protein Eng. 6,439-46.

DBP-*maf* ACTIVATES MACROPHAGES TO PRODUCE TNF-α AND NITRIC OXIDE.

N. Swamy[1], D.G. Alleva[2] and R. Ray[1]   [1]Bioorganic Chemistry & Structural Biology, Vitamin D Laboratory, Boston University School of Medicine, Boston, MA 02118; and [2]Neurocrine Biosciences, Inc., San Diego, CA, USA.

Introduction   Vitamin D binding protein (DBP) is a multi-functional serum glycoprotein that is responsible for binding of vitamin D metabolites, G-actin, fatty acids and chemotactic agents like C5desArg and activation of macrophages and osteoclasts. The macrophage/osteoclast activation property (of DBP) is due to the post-translational modification of DBP. It has been shown that inflammation-induced cell surface sialidase, mannosidase and β-galactosidase of B- and T-lymphocytes deglycosylate DBP in a stepwise manner to generate a potent macrophage activating factor termed DBP-macrophage activating factor (DBP-*maf*) (**Figure 1**). DBP-*maf* was initially identified by its property to stimulate macrophages (MØ) to enhance the Fc-receptor mediated phagocytic activity and superoxide production (1). DBP-*maf* is also known to activate osteoclasts to enhance bone resorption (2).

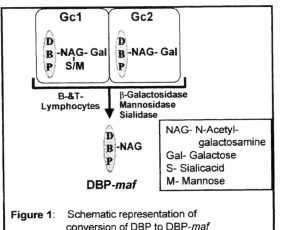

Figure 1:   Schematic representation of conversion of DBP to DBP-*maf*

MØ are leukocytes (white blood cells) which are present in all tissues of the body. They are specialized cells, which engulf large particles such as bacteria, yeast and dying cells by a process called phagocytosis. They secrete signalling molecules called cytokines and chemokines that orchestrate the immune response. Furthermore, MØ secrete and respond to a wide range of inflammatory mediators and play a central role in acute and chronic inflammation. They also secrete proteases and growth factors, which are important in tissue remodelling and in wound repair after injury. Moreover, MØ can present processed foreign antigens to T-lymphocytes allowing the development of a specific immune response (3).

MØ function is modulated by cytokines. MØ also produce cytokines upon stimulation. Cytokines are small proteins, which allow cells of the immune system to communicate with one another via cytokine receptors expressed at the cell surface. The MØ produce super oxide and nitric oxide, which are part of host defense mechanism (3,4). In the present report, we investigated the activation of MØ by DBP-*maf* and studied the generation of TNFα, nitric oxide and superoxide.

Materials and Methods   DBP was isolated from human plasma (5).   DBP was converted to DBP-*maf* using immobilized β-galactosidase, mannosidase and sialidase (6). RAW 264.7 and WEHI-164 cells were cultured in RPMI 1640 containing 5% FBS. Three- to four-week old C57BL/6 male mice (Jackson laboratories, Inc. Bar Harbor, ME) were maintained for one to two weeks after arrival under germ-free conditions in a vivarium.   Thioglycollate-elicited peritoneal exudate MØ were obtained by peritoneal lavage and isolated by adherence to plastic (7). 2×10^5 peritoneal exudate cells were seeded per well in a 96-well flat-bottom tissue culture-treated plates. The cells were allowed to adhere for 2 hours, and non-adherent cells were washed away. MØ were activated with DBP or DBP-*maf* in the presence or absence of IFN-γ for 16-24 hours and culture-conditioned medium was collected, centrifuged and cell-free supernatant were stored at $-20°C$ for assessment of TNFα, NO and super oxide. LPS was used as a positive control. TNFα production by MØ was assessed using the WEHI-164 bioassay. Alamar Blue solution was used to assess WEHI cell-viability, reported as absorbance units (8).   TNFα levels were quantitated by using Cytoscreen^{TM} TNFα ELISA kit (Biosource International, Camarillo, CA). NO production by MØ was assessed by using Griess reagent (9). Superoxide production was followed by monitoring the oxidative burst activity using reduced fluorescin (2',7'-dichlorofluorescin diacetate–DCFH-DA) (10).

Results and Discussion   MØ play an important role in various chronic inflammatory diseases. In addition, MØ also posses the ability to combat the growth of tumors. MØ produce numerous secretory components including monokines (IL-1, IL-6, IL-12, TNF-α), chemokines [i.e., IL-8, Monocyte chemotactic protein-1 (MCP-1), monocyte chemotactic and activation factor (MCAF)], and two sets of inorganic compounds of high reactivity: reactive oxygen intermediates (ROI, superoxide and hydrogen peroxide), and reactive nitrogen intermediates (RNI, NO˙) (3,4).

The role of DBP in inflammation mediated activation of macrophages was established by Yamamoto and coworkers in 1991[1,11]. It was shown that DBP is converted to DBP-*maf* by β-galactosidase and sialidase of the inflammation primed B- and T-lymphocytes. DBP can also be converted to DBP-*maf* by treatment with immobilized β- galactosidase, mannosidase and sialidase to generate DBP-*maf* ex-vivo (6).

Treatment of the peritoneal MØ with DBP-*maf* was earlier shown to increase the superoxide production by the peritoneal macrophages and ingestion of erythrocyte ghosts (1). We used a sensitive fluorimetric assay of Wan and co-workers (10) to determine the oxiburst induced by DBP-*maf* in RAW 264.7 cells, in which reduced fluorescin was oxidized by the reactive oxygen species generated (by RAW 264.7 cells). Treatment of RAW 264.7 cells with 1.0 ng of DBP-*maf* for 3 hours resulted in an increase of the superoxide-production 5 fold over the untreated control. However, DBP (the precursor to DBP-*maf*) failed to show such increase in superoxide production (**Figure 2**). The generation of superoxide by RAW 264.7 cells upon treatment with DBP-*maf* was comparable to that of mouse peritoneal MØ reported by Yamamoto and co-workers (1).

Mouse peritoneal MØ were tested for the production of TNFα upon stimulation by DBP-*maf*. As a first step, the bioactivity of TNFα was tested as cytotoxicity towards WEHI 164.13 cells. Incubation of mouse peritoneal MØ with DBP-*maf* produced TNFα which resulted in marked reduction of viability of WEHI 164.13. The production of TNFα was augmented in the presence of IFN-γ. However, DBP, the precursor to DBP-*maf*, showed only marginal effect on MØ to produce TNFα, which was not influenced by IFN-γ (**Figure 3**). These results strongly indicated that upon stimulation by DBP-*maf*, MØ produced TNFα.

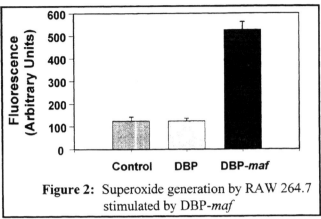

Figure 2: Superoxide generation by RAW 264.7 stimulated by DBP-*maf*

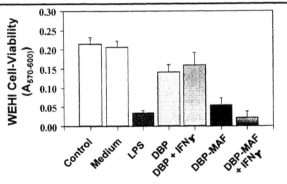

Figure 3: WEHI-164 bioassay for TNFα secretion by peritoneal macrophages

TNFα was further quantified by using mouse TNFα specific ELISA. Treatment of RAW 264.7 cells with increasing amount of DBP-*maf* resulted in increased generation of TNFα in a dose-dependent fashion. However, DBP did not show any such effect. Coactivation with IFN-γ enhanced the amount of TNFα produced upon stimulation by DBP-*maf* and no such effect was observed when DBP was used as a stimulator (**Figure 4**).

Incubation of RAW 264.7 cells with DBP-*maf* produced NO as measured by conversion to nitrite. However, treatment with DBP did not result in the production of NO. Furthermore, IFNγ did not increase the production of NO by MØ when stimulated by DBP-*maf* or DBP (**Figure 5**). These

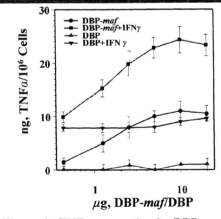

Figure 4: TNFα generation by DBP-*maf* activated RAW 264.7 cells

128

results clearly indicated that DBP-*maf* activated MØ to produce NO.

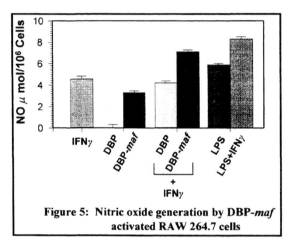

Figure 5: Nitric oxide generation by DBP-*maf* activated RAW 264.7 cells

It is important to note that MØ activation was achieved by only DBP-*maf* and DBP did not activate MØ in each case tested (ROI, RNI and TNFα). NO, is one of the most effective mediators of inflammation. The generation of reactive oxygen species by the process of oxidative burst is considered to be a major mechanism by which MØ and mediate their antimicrobial and tumoricidal functions. TNF-α initiates a cascade of cytokines, which mediate an inflammatory response. Furthermore, TNFα regulates the expression of many genes important for the host response to infection and other functions. We have shown for the first time that MØ activation by DBP-*maf* results in the production of TNF-α and NO (by MØ). The activation of MØ by DBP-*maf* may represent a new biological role for DBP- *maf* as a cytokine. DBP is present in plasma in large abundance (300-500μg/ml). DBP can be found amply in biological fluids like synovial fluid, cerebrospinal fluid and lymph, and conversion of DBP to DBP-*maf*, which is a potent activator of MØ, may implicate yet unknown activities for DBP in different diseases.

References
1. Yamamoto N. Homma S. Millman I. (1991) *J.Immunol.* **147**:273-280.
2. Schneider, G.B. Benis, KA. Flay, NW. Ireland, RA. Popoff, SN. (1995) *Bone.* **16**:657-662.
3. Fedorko ME. (1999) *Med Hypotheses.***53**:107-109.
4. Knight JA. (2000) Free radicals, antioxidants, and the immune system. *Ann Clin Lab Sci.* **30**:145-158.
5. Swamy N. Roy A. Chang R. Brisson M. Ray R. (1995) *Protein Express.Purif.* **6**:185-188.
6. Yamamoto, N. Kumashiro, R. (1993) *J. Immunol.* **151**:2794-2802.
7. Alleva, D.G., S.B. Kaser, D.I. Beller. (1997) *J. Immunol.* **159**:5610-5619.
8. Espevik, T.Nissen-Meyer J. (1986) J. Immunol. Methods **95**:99-105.
9. Green LC, Wagner DA, Glogowski J, Skipper PL, Wishnok JS, Tannenbaum SR. (1982) *Anal Biochem.***126**:131–138.
10. Wan CP, Park CS, Lau BH. (1993) *J Immunol Methods* **162**:1-7.
11. Yamamoto, N. Homma, S. (1991) *Proc. Natl. Acad. Sci.* **88**:8539-8543.

CHARACTERIZATION AND EXPRESSION OF VITAMIN D BINDING PROTEIN (DBP) IN OSTEOPETROTIC AND NORMAL RATS

Fayez F. Safadi[1], Jie Xu[1], Gary B. Schneider[2], Hugo van Baelen[3], Roger Bouillon[3], Motoki Osawa[4] and Steven N. Popoff[1]
[1]Department of Anatomy and Cell Biology, Temple University School of Medicine, Philadelphia, PA 19140, [2]Northeastern Ohio Universities College of Medicine, Rootstown, OH 44272, [3]Catholic University of Leuven, Belgium B-3000, [4]Department of Forensic Medicine, Tokai University School of Medicine, Japan 259-1193

Introduction

Vitamin D binding protein (DBP), also known as group specific component (Gc), is an abundant serum glycoprotein secreted by the liver. DBP has a molecular weight of 58 kDa. It exhibits a single vitamin D sterol binding domain near the N-terminus and a single G-actin binding site near the carboxyl terminus, and therefore, it serves to transport vitamin D sterols and binds to actin monomers sequestering them from polymerization. DBP has also been found to be associated with the IgG Fc receptor on the membranes of subpopulations of T-lymphocytes (1). Recently, we have shown that DBP null mice, when maintained on vitamin D deficient diets, develop osteomalacia and secondary hyperparathyroidism (2). Vitamin D metabolism was also altered, suggesting that DBP markedly prolonged the serum half-life of 25(OH)D and less dramatically prolonged the serum half-life of vitamin D evident by slowing its hepatic uptake and increasing the efficiency of its conversion to 25(OH)D by the liver (2).

The most recent function of DBP involves its ability to activate macrophages and osteoclasts via enzymatic cleavage of sugar moieties from the glycosylation site to yield vitamin D binding protein-macrophage activating factor (DBP-MAF) (3). We have previously reported independent defects in DBP-MAF-primed macrophage activation in two distinct osteopetrotic mutations in the rat, *osteopetrosis* (*op*) and *incisors-absent* (*ia*) (3). The *op* mutation is a lethal mutation characterized by an increase in bone mass associated with a defect in osteoclast-mediated bone resorption (4). The *ia* mutation is a non-lethal mutation with less severe abnormalities in their bone (5). We have shown that treatment with exogenous DBP-MAF resulted in an increase in bone resorption associated with increased osteoclastic activity (6). In this study, we characterized the expression and structural properties of DBP in these two mutations. We also localized DBP in rat primary osteoblast cultures.

Methods

Radial Immunodiffusion (RID) and Isoelectric Focusing:

Five µl undiluted plasma from *op* and *ia* rats were loaded into 3 mm diameter pre-cut wells into solidified matrix and subjected to RID as described previously using antiserum for rat DBP (2). Serum DBP was purified from Wistar, *ia* and *op* rats and subjected to isoelectric focusing on 6% polyacrylamide gels as previously described (7).

RNA Isolation and Northern Analysis:

Liver total RNA was isolated using TRI-zol Ultrapure according to the manufacturer's protocol. Twenty µg total RNA was electrophoresed on 1% agarose-formaldeyde gels. Gels were transferred onto Nytran membranes and blots were hybridized with ^{32}P-labeled DBP cDNA as a probe.

Generation of DBP cDNA Probe and cDNA Sequence Analysis:

Liver total RNA was reverse-transcribed using Super Script^{TM} II RNA reverse transcriptase. First strand cDNA was amplified by PCR using the following primers UP-1 (5'ATGAAGAGGGTTCTGGTTCTCCTGCTGGCCTTAGC-3') and DN-1 (5'-TCAGGACTGCAGGATGTCTCTCATTTCTGCATCAA-3'). PCR was carried out for 30 cycles: 94 °C for 20 sec., 68 °C for 40 sec., 72 °C for 2 minutes. The amplified cDNA was cloned into the PCR-Script Sk$^{(+)}$ vector. Plasmid containing the DBP cDNA was used for Northern analysis and sequencing using the UP-1 and DN-1 primers.

Immunofluorescent Localization of DBP in Primary Rat Osteoblast Cultures:

Neonatal rat calvaria from normal animals were isolated as described previously (8). Cells were cultured for one week, fixed with 4% paraformaldehyde and stained for DBP using a monoclonal anti-DBP primary antibody, followed by fluorescein-conjugated secondary antibody. Cells were examined using fluorescent microscopy.

Results

Serum DBP Levels in Wistar, ia and op Rats

Serum levels of DBP were significantly decreased in mutant *op* (p<0.01) and *ia* (p<0.001) rats when compared with their normal littermates (Figure-1).

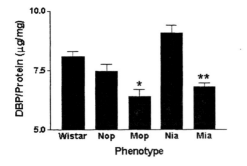

Figure 1: Serum DBP Levels in Wistar, *op* and *ia* Rats

Serum from Wistar, normal *op* (Nop), mutant *op* (Mop), normal *ia* (Nia) and mutant *ia* (Mia) rats was measured by RID assay. Data presented as the mean ± SEM. Using *t*-test, * p<0.01 represents the comparison between Mop and Nop. ** P<.0.001 represents the comparison between Mia and Nia.

Isoelectric Focusing

Wistar rats express two isoforms of DBP, DBP-1 and DBP-2, which represent two alleles for DBP. DBP-1 has a lower pI value (4.9) compared to DBP-2 (5.0). Previous studies have not determined the structural difference between these two isoforms. Normal and mutant rats of *ia* stock only express the DBP-1 isoform, whereas normal and mutant rats of *op* stock express the DBP-2 isoform. Therefore, the *ia* and *op* strains exhibit different isoforms of DBP (Figure-2).

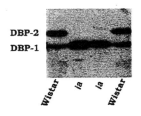 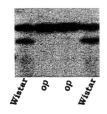

Figure 2: Isoelectric Focusing of Serum DBP from Wistar (control), *ia* **and** *op* **Rats**
Notice that *ia* rats express only DBP-1 and *op* rats express only DBP-2 when compared to Wistar rats that express both isoforms.

cDNA sequence analysis

DBP cDNAs generated from liver of normal and mutant rats of *ia* and *op* strains were sequenced. Comparison between *ia* and *op* strains showed that there are three nucleotide differences, although there were no differences between normal and mutant rats of each stain. The *op* sequence was identical to the published sequence for rat DBP (9). Comparison of the predicted amino acid sequence represents one important difference between rats of *ia* and *op* stocks. The amino acid Lysine (*op*) is substituted with Glutamine (*ia*) and this substitution with a charged amino acid is likely to account for the different isoelectric mobilities (pI) of *ia* and *op* DBP (see Figure-2).

Northern Blot of Liver from 2, 4 and 6 Week Old Normal and Mutant (op and ia) Rats

DBP gene expression was undetectable in the liver of 2 week old *op* mutant rats compared with normal rats. At 4 and 6 weeks, DBP mRNA levels were markedly decreased in *op* mutants when compared with their normal littermates (Figure-3). Northern blot analysis of liver from 2, 4, and 6 week old normal and *ia* mutant rats showed that DBP transcript levels in *ia* mutants were not significantly different compared with their normal, age-matched littermates (data not shown). Northern blot analysis of kidney from normal and *op* mutant rats showed that DBP expression was markedly reduced in *op* mutant when compared with normal rats at all aged examined (data not shown).

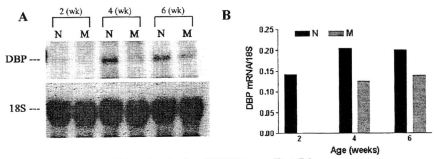

Figure 3: Northern Blot Analysis of DBP in *op* **Rat Liver**
A: Twenty µg of total RNA from normal (N) and mutant (M) *op* liver, at 2, 4 and 6 week old rats, was loaded in each lane and probed for DBP. The blot was stripped and re-hybridized for 18S to serve as a loading control. In normal animals, DBP mRNA level was detected at all ages examined, however, in mutants, DBP mRNA expression was only detected at 4 and 6 week of age.
B: Relative intensity of DBP mRNA message levels corrected for loading differences using 18S RNA.

Immunolocalization of DBP in Primary Rat Osteoblast Cultures

Immunolocalization of DBP in primary rat osteoblast cultures showed that DBP is present in osteoblasts and localized mainly in the nucleus with some staining observed in the cytoplasm. These data suggest that DBP may play an important role to facilitate the entry vitamin D metabolites into target cells and maintain their bioavailability, activation and end-organ responsiveness.

Discussion

DBP and its recently described derivative, DBP-MAF, have been studied for their multifunctional properties. Although the main function of DBP is to bind and transport vitamin D metabolites in the blood to their target cells, it also binds G-actin (1), activates macrophages *in vivo* (2) and mediates osteoclastic bone resorption (10). It has been shown that infusion of DBP-MAF into *ia* and *op* osteopetrotic mutations, improved the skeletal defects by increasing osteoclast numbers and decreasing bone volume (6). In this study, we characterized DBP and evaluated its expression in the *ia* and *op* mutations. Serum DBP levels were significantly decreased in *ia* and *op* mutants when compared to their normal littermates. DBP mRNA levels were markedly reduced in *op* but not in *ia* mutants when compared to their normal littermates. Since it has been shown that TGF-β decreases DBP expression in a dose dependent manner (11) and *op* mutants have increased levels of TGF-β expression (unpublished observation), this could explain the decrease in DBP expression in *op* mutants. DBP cDNA and predicted amino acid sequence analyses of *ia* and *op* stocks showed that there is one amino acid (Lysine in *op* versus Glutamine in *ia*) difference between the two strains. This substitution is likely to account for the different isoelectric mobilities (pI) of the *ia* and *op* DBP. The actions of DBP in bone per se are still not fully understood. We were able to localize DBP in osteoblasts in culture, and these data suggest that DBP may have direct effects in regulating bone cell functions in addition to its role to facilitate the entry and subsequent actions of vitamin D metabolites on osteoblasts.

Reference

1. Cooke, N.E. and Haddad, J.G. (1995) Endocrine Rev. 10, 294-307.
2. Safadi, F.F., Thornton, P., Magiera, H., Hollis, B.W., Gentile, M., Haddad, J.G., Liebhaber, S.A. and Cooke, N.E. (1999) J. Clin. Invest. 103, 239-251.
3. Popoff, S.N. and Schneider, G.B. (1996) Mol. Med. Today. 2, 349-358.
4. Marks, S.C. and Popoff, S.N. (1989) Am. J. Anat. 186, 325-334.
5. Marks, S.C. (1973) Am. J. Anat. 138, 165-190.
6. Schneider, G.B., Benis, A.K., Flay, N.W., Ireland, R.A. and Popoff, S.N. (1995) Bone 16, 657-662.
7. Imawari, M., Kida, K. and Goodman, D.S. (1976) J. Clin. Invest. 58, 514-523.
8. Jie, X., Smock, S.L., Safadi, F.F., Rosenzweig, A.B., Odgren, P.R., Marks, S.C., Owen, T.A. and Popoff, S.N. (2000) J. Cell. Biochem. 77, 103-115.
9. Mc Leod, J.F. and Cooke, N.E. (1989) J. Biol. Chem. 21760-21769.
10. Adebanjo, O.A., Moonga, B.S., Haddad, J.G., Huang, C.L. and Zaidi, M. (1998) 28, 668-671.
11. Guha, C., Osawa, M., Werner, P.A., Galbraith, R.M. and Paddock, G.V. (1995) 21, 1675-1681.

VITAMIN D: HYDROXYLASES AND METABOLISM

NEW APROACHES FOR THE STUDY OF VITAMIN D METABOLISM

Glenville Jones¶, Valarie Byford¶, David Prosser¶, Hugh LJ Makin§, Rene St Arnaud†, Marie Demay‡, Joyce Knutson*, Stephen Strugnell* and Charles W Bishop*

¶ Department of Biochemistry and Medicine, Queen's University, Kingston ON Canada
§ St Bartholomew's and the Royal London Hospital of Medicine and Dentistry, London UK
† Shriner's Hospital & McGill University, Montreal PQ, Canada
‡ Endocrine Unit, Massachusetts General Hospital, Boston MA USA
* Bone Care International, Madison WI USA

Introduction

Over the past decade, enormous progress in molecular biology has led to the cloning of three cytochrome P450s (CYP1α, CYP24 and CYP27) involved in vitamin D metabolism [1]. While there seems to be the potential for discovery of at least one more cytochrome P450, a second 25-hydroxylase, the impending completion of the human genome project makes this ever more unlikely. Nevertheless, the post-genomics era begins with plenty of work still to be completed in the vitamin D metabolism field. Much interest still surrounds:-

a) the substrate specificity of vitamin D hydroxylases;

b) regulation of the vitamin D hydroxylases especially renal and extra-renal 1α-hydroxylases;

c) molecular modelling of vitamin D-related cytochrome P450 has become feasible after the first crystal structure of a mammalian cytochrome P450 was published [2];

d) the physiological role of mitochondrialCYP27 and its presumed microsomal counterpart;

e) the possible development of specific CYP1α, CYP24 and CYP27 inhibitors for use in calcium homeostatic and hyperproliferative conditions.

Consequently, there is a need for development of new and imaginative approaches to the study of vitamin D metabolism and its cytochrome P450's. While the overall strategy has not varied over the past four decades, still requiring selection of 3 components :-

biological system----->assay system------>analytical system

the choices within each component have increased dramatically over that time. This chapter will focus on the new possibilities in these areas citing examples wherever possible to illustrate how this has improved our knowledge and understanding of vitamin D metabolism.

New Strategies for Vitamin D-related cytochrome P450s:

•	Biological System	Normal Wild Type Gene for Enzyme Mutagenised Gene for Enzyme Null or Knockout Gene for Enzyme
•	Assay System	Intact Whole Animal In vitro Cell Systems Isolated recombinant protein systems
•	Analytical Systems	HPLC with Photodiode array detection HPLC with [^{3}H] Detection LC-(Mass Spectrometry)^n

The advent of new possibilities in each of these component parts to a metabolic study gives a plethora of permutations that metabolic biochemists of a decade ago could only dream about.

Cytochrome P450 Gene Manipulation

The cloning of the vitamin D-related cytochromes P450 has necessitated the need for expression systems. While E coli and Baculovirus insect cell expression systems have been tried with some success [3,4], most studies have been performed with mammalian expression systems using commercially available p vector systems and Cos-1 cell transient or stable transfection [5,6]. Recently, my colleagues at Cytochroma and I [6] cloned the extra-renal 1α-hydroxylase from a human lung non-small cell carcinoma and showed it to be identical to the renal enzyme cloned earlier. We transiently transfected extra-renal CYP1α enzyme lacking its upstream promoter sequence into Cos-1 cells and showed it produce a small amount of 1α,25-$(OH)_2D_3$ over a short incubation time detectible by HPLC-[^{3}H]detector(Figure1).Longer term activity measurement of CYP1α in Cos-1 cells is hampered by the presence of CYP24 and its possible induction of CYP24 further by the product of CYP1α. CYP24 has the potential to sequester substrate from CYP1α and also selectively use the product of CYP1α as a substrate. We and others are searching for cells which lack constitutive or inducible CYP24 to act as host for stably transfected CYP1α.

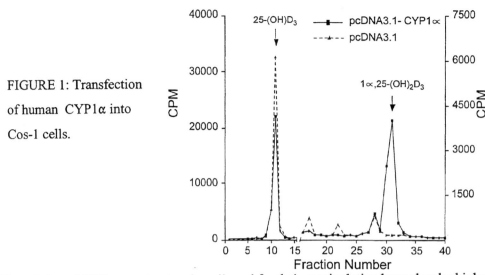

FIGURE 1: Transfection of human CYP1α into Cos-1 cells.

Knowledge of CYP gene structure has allowed for their manipulation by molecular biological techniques. Mice null for CYP24 and CYP27 have been engineered [7,8]; CYP1α knockout mice are expected shortly. Pigs with mutant CYP1α have been available for 20 years but were largely undeveloped. Recently, we have been studying CYP-24 null mice with Rene St Arnaud. As postulated by us over a decade ago [9] and as recently reported in abstract form [10] CYP24-null mice have a block in $1\alpha,25\text{-}(OH)_2D_3$ clearance. We find 20-30-fold higher levels of $1\alpha,25\text{-}(OH)_2D_3$ in the bloodstream of CYP24 null as compared to heterozygote littermates at 24,48 and 96 hrs after a bolus of $[1\beta\text{-}{}^3H]1\alpha,25\text{-}(OH)_2D_3$ indicating the critical importance of CYP24 and 24-oxidation to catabolic processes (Figure 2).

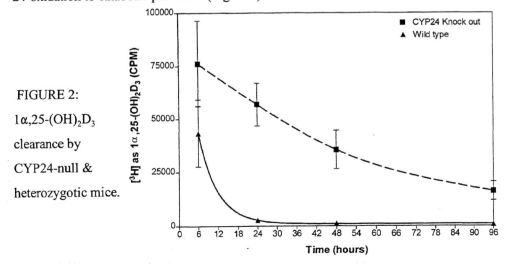

FIGURE 2: $1\alpha,25\text{-}(OH)_2D_3$ clearance by CYP24-null & heterozygotic mice.

138

Because of the inducible nature of vitamin D-target cell CYP24, VDR-null mice[11] represent a "partial CYP24 knockout model". With Marie Demay's lab, we studied primary keratinocytes from VDR-null and wild-type mice incubated with 10μM 1α,25-(OH)$_2$D$_3$ as previously described [in 12], and found significant metabolism to C-24 catabolic products over 24 hr in cells from wild-type mice but much reduced metabolism in cells from VDR-XO mice (Figure 3). The difference illustrates the highly inducible nature of target-cell CYP24.

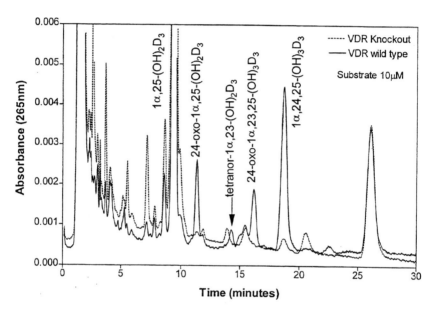

FIGURE 3:Metabolism of 1α,25-(OH)$_2$D$_3$ by primary keratinocytes from VDR-XO & wild type mice

Modelling of Cytochrome P450s

The availability of recombinant CYP27 made transient expression in Cos-1 cells and substrate specificity studies possible [5]. Since CYP27 has been well studied in vitro and human gene defects have been reported in the disease cerebrotendinous xanthomatosis, we felt it desirable to model the protein based upon various X-ray crystal structures and sequence homologies. Our model [13] is depicted in Figure 4 showing the putative active site. Mutagenesis studies have been performed to attempt to validate the model with some success. Interestingly, the ratio of 25:27 hydroxylation products is altered by certain mutated residues at Phe248Met or Leu516Val [13].This implies that changes in the helices bordering on the active site cause subtle changes in the substrate pocket leading to radical changes in hydroxylation site.

Active site of CYP27

FIGURE 4:

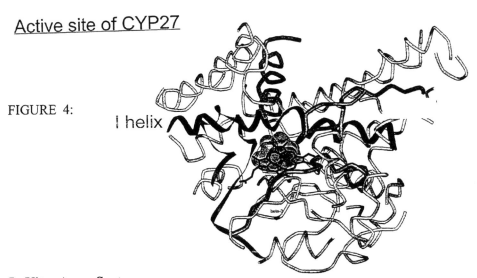

I helix

In Vitro Assay Systems

Cultured keratinocytes have proven to be a valuable tool in elucidating the target cell actions of vitamin D. Various models from freshly isolated primary keratinocytes to keratinocyte cell lines have been used. One cell line with remarkable metabolic activity towards vitamin D is HPK1A-ras.

Developed by Richard Kremer [14], this human keratinocyte-derived cell line shows highly inducible expression of CYP24 as measured by northern analysis or RT-PCR. We have used HPK1A-ras cells to study the metabolism of a variety of vitamin D analogs including MC-903, OCT, EB1089 and KH1060 [15-18]. More recently we have been studying the possible direct hydroxylation of 1α-hydroxylated prodrugs such as 1α-OH-D_2. Gniadecki & Calverley [19] reported the local biological effects of topically administered prodrugs lacking side chain hydroxylation.

They postulated the possibility of side-chain hydroxylation in the skin cells. We recently tested this idea by incubating high concentrations of 1α-OH-D_2 with HPK1A-ras cells and found production of both active dihydroxylated compounds and inactive secondary trihydroxylated catabolites. A typical chromatogram is depicted in Figure 5 showing the clearcut evidence of metabolites of 1α-OH-D_2 and in the process illustrating the remarkable reproducibility that can

140

be obtained from multiwell plate cell culture coupled with modern LC-photo diode array detection.

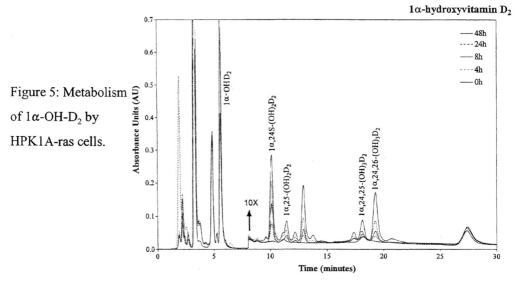

Figure 5: Metabolism of 1α-OH-D$_2$ by HPK1A-ras cells.

Detection Techniques

While LC-PDA is powerful and convenient for vitamin D analysis because of its intense UV chromophore, the technique does not approach the sensitivity offered by other detectors. When radioactive substrates are available a [³H] detector can be of great value permitting detection of compounds into the picomolar range. However, the most promising sensitive and universal detector is based upon mass spectrometry. The emerging fields of LC-MS and LC-MS-MS will permit the current metabolic approaches to be extended over a wider range of substrate concentrations. While present LC-PDA instruments work optimally at substrate concentrations in the 1-10 μM range, the expectation is that current LC-MS-MS machines can allow metabolic studies to be pushed into the picomolar range therefore permitting kinetic studies over the full physiological range of vitamin D. Part of the reason that LC-MS techniques are so valuable is that they require no derivatization as in GC-MS. Whereas we have used a time-consuming method of off-line GC-MS to identify LC peaks in Figure 5, the new technology makes this unnecessary and allows the LC solutes to be separated from mobile phase in effluent and to flow directly into a mass spectrometric detector. The main disadvantage of LC-MS-MS is the loss of information derived from fragments produced in GC-MS.

In LC-MS vitamin D metabolites tend to dehydrate and then fragment [20]. Figure 6 shows LC-MS^3 of a E ring analog KS176 (M Wt= 390) which we found to be highly unstable during conventional GC-MS. One can see in MS1 the molecular ion(MH$^+$ at m/z 391) which is small while the dehydration products predominate at m/z 373 (MH-18), 355 (MH-18-18) and 337 (MH-18-18-18). The successive fragmentation is confirmed by examination of MS2 and MS3 which represent in turn the fragments of m/z 373 (MS2) and m/z 355 (MS3). Selection of successive fragments makes the technique more specific and also more sensitive.

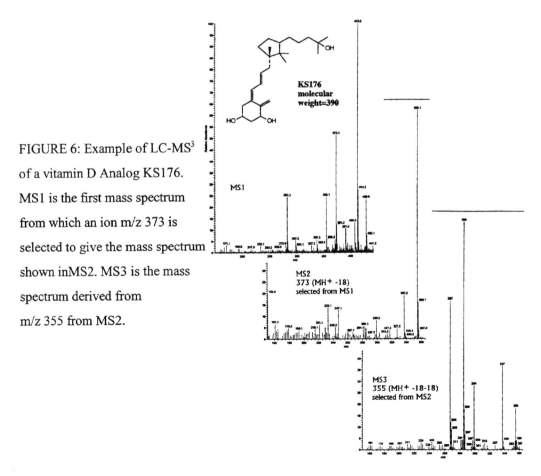

FIGURE 6: Example of LC-MS^3 of a vitamin D Analog KS176. MS1 is the first mass spectrum from which an ion m/z 373 is selected to give the mass spectrum shown inMS2. MS3 is the mass spectrum derived from m/z 355 from MS2.

Conclusions

1. A multifaceted approach blends a variety of biological, assay and analytical systems
2. New biological systems include animals with null and mutant genes for CYPs

3. New In vivo and in vitro systems each offer advantages and disadvantages for extracting the metabolic data required.

4. Newer high sensitivity analytical systems (eg LC-MS) permit a full range of vitamin D concentrations to be used in metabolic studies & permit characterisation of minor products.

Acknowledgements

David Prosser prepared some of the figures used in this paper. The author wishes to acknowledge the continued support and friendship of Hugh LJ Makin, Joyce Knutson, Stephen Strugnell, Charlie Bishop, Martin Calverley and Anne Marie Kissmeyer. Collaborators for some of this work included Martin Petkovich and Jay White of Cytochroma; Roger Bouillon, University of Leuven.

GJ is supported by grants from the Medical Research Council of Canada and Bone Care International.

References

1. Jones G, Strugnell S and DeLuca HF (1998). Physiological Reviews **78**:1193-1231.
2. Williams PA, Cosme J, Sridhar V et al (2000) Mol Cell **5**:121-131
3. Sakaki T, Sawada N, Nonaka Y, Ohyama Y, Inouye K (1999) Eur J Biochem **262**:43-48
4 Beckman MJ, Tadikonda P, Werner E, et al (1996) Biochemistry **35**:8465-8472
5. Guo, Y.D., Strugnell, S., Back, D.W. et al(1993). Proc. Natl. Acad. Sci. USA, **90**:8668-8672.
6. Jones G., Ramshaw H., Zhang A.et al (1999) Endocrinology, **140**: 3303-3310.
7. St Arnaud R.(1999) Bone **25**:127-129
8. Li YC, Pirro AE, Amling M, et al (1997)Proc Natl Acad Sci U S A **94**:9831-5
9. Makin, G., Lohnes, D., Byford, V., Ray, R. and Jones, G. (1989) Biochem. J. **262**:173-180.
10. Barletta F, Arrigo C, Parker G et al (1998) Bone **23**: S185, 1153
11. Ohyama Y, Ozono K, Uchida M et al (1994) J Biol Chem **269**:10545-10550
12. Masuda, S., Strugnell, S., Calverley, M., et al (1994). J. Biol. Chem.**269**:4794-4803
13. Prosser D, Guo Y-D and Jones G (1999) J Bone Min Res **14S**, SU468, p 548, abstract.
14. Henderson J, Sebag M, Rhim J, et al (1991) Cancer Res **51**:6521-8
15. Dilworth, F.J., Calverley, M.J., Makin, H.L.J. et al (1994) Biochem. Pharm.**47**:987-993.
16. Masuda S, Byford V, Kremer R, et al (1996) J Biol Chem **271**:8700-8708.
17. Shankar VN, Dilworth FJ, Makin HLJ,et al (1997) Biochem Pharmacol.**53**:783-793.
18. Dilworth F.J., Williams G.R., Kissmeyer A-M, et al (1997) Endocrinology, **138**: 5485-5496.
19. Gniadecki R, Calverley MJ (1998) Pharmacol Toxicol **82**:173-6
20. Jones G and Makin HLJ (2000) in "Modern Chromatographic Analysis of the Vitamins" 3rd Edition. Eds VanBocxlaer J, Lambert W, De Leenheer A. Marcel Dekker, New York, pp75-141.

CLONING OF VITAMIN D 1α-HYDROXYLASE (P450c1α) AND ITS MUTATIONS CAUSING VITAMIN D-DEPENDENT RICKETS TYPE 1 (VDDR-1)

WALTER L. MILLER* and ANTHONY A. PORTALE[+]
Department of Pediatrics[**], The Metabolic Research Unit*, and Department of Medicine[+], University of California San Francisco, California 94143, USA

Introduction. The principal hormonal regulator bone mineralization is vitamin D. Dietary deficiency of vitamin D and genetic disorders of vitamin D biosynthesis and action can cause rickets. Recent work has elucidated the molecular basis of disorders of vitamin D bioactivation.

The Vitamin D Biosynthetic Pathway. Vitamin D is found in two forms: ergocalciferol (vitamin D_2) produced by plants, and cholecalciferol (vitamin D_3) produced by animal tissues and by the action of near-ultraviolet (290-310 nm) light on 7-dehydro-cholesterol in human skin. Vitamin D is a biologically inactive pro-hormone. In order to acquire the ability to bind to and activate the vitamin D receptor and thus exhibit biological activity, vitamin D must first undergo two successive hydroxylations at carbons #25 and #1. The 25-hydroxylation of vitamin D occurs primarily in the liver, apparently catalyzed by the same mitochondrial cytochrome P450 enzyme that also hydroxylates carbons 26 and 27 to initiate bile acid synthesis. The gene for this enzyme is officially termed CYP27, but is often referred to as P450c25, to connote its hydroxylation of carbon 25. The abundant 25-hydroxylase activity in the liver is not under tight physiologic regulation; most vitamin D is 25-hydroxylated, so that its circulating concentration is about 10^{-7} M. Like vitamin D itself, 25-hydroxyvitamin D (25OHD) has minimal capacity to bind to the vitamin D receptor and elicit a biologic response.

The active form of vitamin D is 1,25-dihydroxyvitamin D [1,25(OH)$_2$D], formed by the 1α-hydroxylation of 25OHD. The 1α-hydroxylase is expressed in the proximal convoluted tubules of the kidney, and circulating concentrations of 1,25(OH)$_2$D primarily reflect its renal synthesis; however, 1α-hydroxylase activity also is found in keratinocytes, macrophages and osteoblasts. Renal 1α-hydroxylase activity is tightly regulated by parathyroid hormone, calcium, phosphorus, and 1,25(OH)$_2$D itself.

The Vitamin D Biosynthetic Enzymes are Mitochondrial Forms of Cytochrome P450. The vitamin D 25-hydroxylase, the 1α-hydroxylase, and the 24-hydroxylase are cytochrome P450 enzymes found in mitochondria. All cytochrome P450 enzymes function as oxidases using electrons from NADPH and molecular oxygen (1,2). There are two forms of cytochrome P450 enzymes. Type I, found in mitochondria and in some bacteria, receives electrons from NADPH via the intermediacy of an electron-transfer chain consisting of two proteins. Ferredoxin reductase, a flavoprotein bound to the inner mitochondrial membrane, receives electrons from NADPH, and then transfers them to ferredoxin, an iron-sulfur protein that may be loosely associated with the inner membrane or may be in solution in the mitochondrial matrix. Ferredoxin then interacts with one of a variety of different P450 moieties, which bind the substrate, receive electrons and molecular oxygen, catalyze the reaction through the intermediacy of a heme group, and release the product. Type II cytochrome P450 enzymes, such as the hepatic enzymes involved in drug metabolism or the steroidogenic 17α-hydroxylase and 21-hydroxylase enzymes, are found in the endoplasmic reticulum, where they receive electrons from a flavoprotein termed P450 oxidoreductase; in some cases, electron transfer from P450 oxido-reductase is allosterically facilitated by cytochrome b_5 (3,4). P450 oxidoreductase is quite different from ferredoxin reductase, and functions without the need of an iron/sulfur intermediate such as ferredoxin. Thus mitochondrial (Type I) and microsomal (Type II) P450 enzymes are substantially different genetically and enzymologically.

Molecular Cloning and Characterization of Human Vitamin D 1α-Hydroxylase. Although the vitamin D 25-hydroxylase (5) and 24-hydroxylase (6) were cloned in 1990 and 1991, the 1α-hydroxylase, which is the rate-limiting and hormonally regulated enzyme, resisted cloning until the second half of 1997, when four independent groups using different approaches succeeded in cloning the mouse, rat, and human vitamin D 1α-hydroxylase, P450c1α (7-12). Several reasons underlay the difficulty in cloning P450c1α, the principal one being that there is very little P450c1α protein in the kidney. Although physiologic induction of the protein, e.g., by raising rats on a D-deficient, low-phosphorus diet in the absence of UV light, provides a significant increase in 1α-hydroxylase activity, efforts to purify a 1α-hydroxylase protein, as had been done before for the 24- and 25-hydroxylases, were consistently unsuccessful. Thus, the direct protein-based immunologic approaches used to clone P450c24 and P450c25 did not work. Here we review our cloning of the human 25-hydroxyvitamin D-1α-hydroxylase and its role in vitamin D dependent rickets, type I.

We solved the problem of the low renal abundance of P450c1α by using a non-renal system, the cultured human keratinocyte (7). Bikle's work in the 1980s had shown that when primary cultures of human keratinocytes are grown in serum-free medium in the presence of low concentrations of calcium, they acquire substantial 1α-hydroxylase activity (13-15). These cells gave us a source of RNA enriched for 1α- hydroxylase mRNA, and had the advantage of permitting us to work directly with a human system. We used several sets of degenerate-sequence primers based on the conserved sequences of the ferredoxin-binding site and heme-binding site to amplify a 300 bp fragment from human keratinocyte cDNA. This cDNA had a unique sequence that resembled other mitochondrial P450s. The 300 bp cDNA was used to clone a 1.9 kb cDNA from a human keratinocyte cDNA library, then the 5' end was obtained by primer extension to yield the full-length 2.4 kb cDNA (7).

Because we had cloned P450c1α from keratinocytes rather than kidney, we provided four lines of evidence that the keratinocyte and renal enzymes are encoded by the same gene (7). First, we showed that our keratinocyte cDNA clone encoded an enzyme that catalyzed the conversion of 25OHD to 1,25(OH)$_2$D, as measured by radioreceptor assay and as shown by co-migration with authentic 1,25(OH)$_2$D standards by HPLC using two different solvent systems (Fig 1A). To prepare the 1,25(OH)$_2$D produced by our enzyme, we expressed our cDNA in mouse Leydig

MA-10 cells. These cells contain abundant ferredoxin and ferredoxin reductase, which are needed by all mitochondrial forms of cytochrome P450 (16); hence, transfection of cDNAs for mitochondrial P450s into these cells yields 100- to 1000-fold more activity than when such P450s are expressed in COS-1 cells (17), as used by others. The use of this cell system permitted us to show that the enzyme had a Km of 2.7×10^{-7} (Fig. 1B), which is similar to the circulating concentration of the 25OHD substrate. Second, we provided definitive chemical proof that our enzyme produced authentic $1,25(OH)_2D$ and not some other related metabolite of vitamin D. The increased 1α-hydroxylase activity we achieved with MA-10 cells permitted us to prepare biochemically useful amounts (230 ng) of the $1,25(OH)_2D$ product and to prove its complete chemical identity by gas chromatography/mass spectrometry of the trimethylsialated derivative. Third, we used reverse transcription/ polymerase chain reaction (RT-PCR) to show that the same sequences we had cloned from keratinocytes were expressed in the human kidney, as well as in other tissues. Finally, we provided genetic proof of the identify of our P450c1α by obtaining keratinocytes from a patient with VDDR-I, cloning cDNA from these, and showing that the patient was a compound heterozygote for two premature translation termination (non-sense) mutations. Primary cultures of keratinocytes from this patient were devoid of 1α-hydroxylase activity (Fig. 1A). These findings provide unambiguous genetic proof that the keratinocyte and renal P450c1α are one and the same, and provided the first proof that VDDR I is caused by mutations in P450c1α (7).

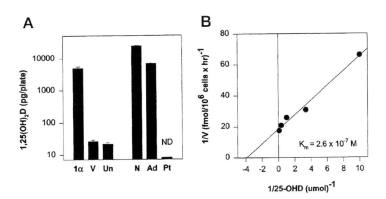

Figure 1. **A.** The three *left* bars depict expression of the keratinocyte P450c1α cDNA in MA-10 cells. 1α-hydroxylase activity, expressed as picograms of $1,25(OH)_2D$ produced per 10 cm plate of cells; the logarithmic y-axis begins at 8 pg, the detection limit per plate. MA-10 cells have a minimal endogenous level of 1α-hydroxylase activity, shown by the level in untransfected cells (Un) or vector-transfected cells (V) of ~25 pg/plate. By contrast, cells expressing the P450c1α cDNA (1α) produced ~5000 pg/plate. The three *right* bars depict 1α-hydroxylase activity of keratinocytes from human neonatal foreskin (N), adult skin (Ad), and skin from a patient with VDDR-1 (Pt). Activity was not detected in the patient. **B.** Lineweaver-Burke plot of 1α-hydroxylase activity of P450c1α expressed in MA-10 cells; the Km was ~2.6×10^{-7} M.

We then cloned and sequenced the human gene for P450c1α, localized it to chromosome 12 by somatic cell hybrid analysis, localized the transcriptional start site, and compared the structures of the genes for the four mitochondrial P450s now available (P450c1α, P450c24, P450scc, P450c11) (8).

The Molecular Genetics of 1α-Hydroxylase Deficiency (VDDR-I). Although our first patient (7) and the subsequent four consanguineous patients of Kitanaka, et al. (18) proved that mutations in P450c1α could cause VDDR-I, several questions remained. It was not yet clear if all patients with the clinical VDDR-I syndrome had the same disease (i.e., vitamin D 1α-hydroxylase deficiency). Furthermore, it was well established that VDDR-I was very common in French Canada, but it was not clear if all these patients had two distinct mutations, as had been indicated by careful linkage analysis of VDDR-I families to microsatellite markers in the 12q13-q14 locus (19,20). Finally, there was no structure/function information about the enzyme.

We studied the P450c1α genes and microsatellite haplotypes of 17 families from multiple ethnic groups, including 5 French Canadians, 3 Poles, 4 Caucasian Americans, 1 Filipino, 1 Chinese, 1 Haitian, 1 Black American and 1 Hispanic (21). All of our patients had typical hormonal findings of 1α-hydroxylase deficiency, including hypocalcemia, hypophosphatemia, high serum alkaline phosphatase and PTH concentrations, normal 25OHD concentrations and low $1,25(OH)_2D$ concentrations. Furthermore, all patients had radiographic evidence of rickets and all responded to physiologic replacement doses of $1,25(OH)_2D$. Because we had found that the P450c1α gene is small and had obtained its complete sequence (8), we developed a procedure for PCR-amplification of the whole gene from genomic DNA as a single 4.2 kb product. This DNA was then subjected to direct sequencing on both strands, identifying mutations in all patients. By sequencing the mutant exons from both parents, we were able to identify the parental origin of all mutations. The inheritance of each mutation was confirmed by performing microsatellite haplotyping of chromosome 12q13 using the markers D12S90, D12S305 and D12S104 in all patients and parents.

By examining these same microsatellite markers, Labuda et al. had previously shown that the French Canadian patients with VDDR-I carried one of two haplotypes. Those whose ancestry could be traced to the Charlevoix-Seguenay-LacSaint Jean area of Quebec (the "Charlevoix" population) carried haplotype 4-7-1, while those whose ancestry could be traced to Eastern Canada (the "Acadian" population) carried the haplotype 6-7-2 (19). Among our 5 French Canadian families, 9 of 10 unique alleles carried the 4-7-1 haplotype and all 9 carried the same mutation, the deletion of a guanosine at position 958 (ΔG958). This mutation lies in codon 88 (in exon 2), changes the reading frame, and leads to premature translational termination, thus ablating all enzyme activity. The mutation deletes the G in the sequence 5' ACGT 3', which is recognized by the endonucleases Tai I and Mae II. This permitted us to design a rapid, accurate PCR-based diagnostic tactic that can detect this mutation in genomic DNA from any source (21). There are several additional Tai I and Mae II sites in the P450c1α gene, including 3 just downstream in exon 3. However, PCR amplification of genomic DNA with a sense oligonucleotide corresponding to bases 42-81 and an anti-sense oligonucleotide corresponding to bases 1612-1638 generates a 1458 bp fragment that contains only the *Tai* I/*Mae* II site affected by the ΔG958 mutation. When unaffected DNA is amplified and digested with *Tai* I or *Mae* II, two fragments of 778 and 680 bp are seen; by contrast, DNA carrying the ΔG958 mutation will remain undigested as the 1458 bp fragment.

Four French Canadian families were also studied by Yoshida et al.; three were homozygous for the ΔG958 mutation and one was homozygous for duplication of a 7 bp sequence in exon 8 (22). Based on the regions of Canada from which each patient originated, these authors inferred that the ΔG958 is the Charlevoix mutation and the 7 bp duplication is the Acadian mutation. However, they did not perform microsatellite haplotyping; hence, it is not known whether the patient who was homozygous for the 7 bp duplication was "Acadian" as defined by carrying the 6-7-2 haplotype (19). We found the 7 bp duplication on seven distinct alleles (Fig. 2). Four of these alleles bore a different haplotype, 9-7-2, but were found in different ethnic groups: Polish, Chinese and Hispanic. The other three alleles carrying the 7 bp duplication carried the haplotypes 9-6-2, 9-3-3 and 6-6-1, and were found among Filipino, Caucasian American and Black American patients. Thus, the 7 bp duplication appears to have arisen *de novo* among different ethnic groups, probably as the result of a slipped-strand mispairing mechanism during meiosis (23). Finally, one of our Polish patients was heterozygous for the "Acadian" 6-7-2 haplotype, but that allele carried the mis-sense mutation P497R rather than the 7 bp duplication. Thus, the identity of the 'Acadian' mutation has not been established.

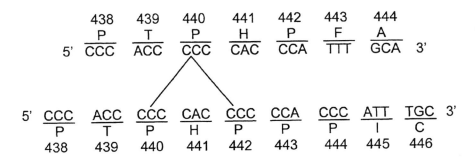

Figure 2. The 7 bp duplication. Upper line: The sequence CCCACCC is normally duplicated in exon 8, which encodes residues 438 to 442 (Pro-Thr-Pro-His-Pro). Lower line: The mutation involves the insertion of a third copy of the CCCACCC sequence, changing the reading frame, beginning with residue 443. The "triplication" is arbitrarily shown as an insert at codon 440 between the two normal copies of the CCCACCC sequence; it is impossible to specify which of the three copies in the mutant sequence is "new."

Among our 17 patients we identified 14 different mutations, of which 7 were amino acid replacement (mis-sense) mutations. By performing site-directed mutagenesis and expressing these mutants in transfected MA-10 cells, we could assess the enzymatic activity of each (21). In this set of experiments, the background level of 1α-hydroxylase activity in MA-10 cells was about 65 pg of 1,25(OH)$_2$D produced per plate, which is only ~4% of the level achieved by expression of the wild-type enzyme; by contrast, the activities of the seven mutants ranged from 45-85 pg (2.9% to 5.6% of control), i.e., levels indistinguishable from the vector control. Thus, none of the mis-sense mutations that we identified had significant 1α-hydroxylase activity. Ten other mis-sense mutations have now been reported by other groups including one patient with rather mild clinical manifestations, but all of these mutants have lacked detectable 1α-hydroxylase activity when tested *in vitro* by a variety of means (24,25). Thus, although a total of 37 patients have now been studied at a molecular genetic level and although 26 distinct mutations, including 17 mis-sense mutations (Fig. 3), have been found, none of these has resulted in an enzyme with decreased, rather than absent activity. This may be because not enough distinct patients have been studied yet; alternatively, it is possible that mutations that decrease 1α-hydroxylase activity may not produce a clinical phenotype.

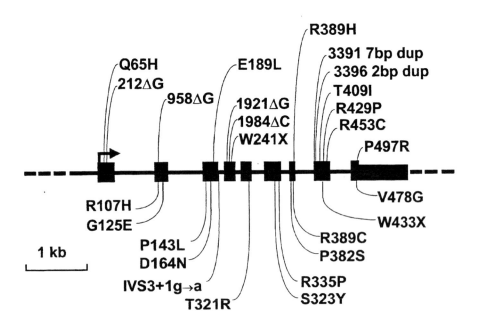

Figure 3. Scale diagram of the intron/exon organization of the human gene encoding P450c1α, as reported by Fu et al. (8). All mutations causing 1α-hydroxylase deficiency reported through mid-1999 are shown. All mutations depicted above the gene are reported

by Wang et al. (21); ΔG958 and 3391 7bp dup, also reported by Yoshida et al. (22); R107H, G125E, R335P, and P382S, reported by Kitanaka et al. (18); S323Y and V478G, reported by Smith et al. (25); P143L, D164N, IVS3+1g→a, T321R, R389C, and W433X, reported by Kitanaka et al. (24).

Acknowledgements. Supported by NIH grants DK37922 (WLM), DK42154 (WLM), DK/AR54433 (AAP), by grants from the March of Dimes Birth Defects Foundation (WLM and AAP), and gifts from the David Carmel Trust (AAP).

References
1. Black, S.D., and Coon, M.J. (1987) *Mol. Biol.* **60,** 35-87
2. Nebert, D.W., and Gonzalez, F.J. (1987) *Annu. Rev. Biochem.* **56,** 945-993
3. Auchus, R.J., and Lee, T.C., and Miller, W.L. (1998) *J. Biol. Chem.* **273**, 3158-3165
4. Geller, D.H., Auchus, R.J., and Miller, W.L. (1999) *Mol. Endocrinol.* **13**, 167-175
5. Usui, E., Noshiro, M., and Okuda, K. (1990) *FEBS Lett.* **262**, 135-138
6. Ohyama, Y., Noshiro, M., and Okuda, K. (1991) *FEBS Lett.* **278**, 195-198
7. Fu, G.K., Lin, D., Zhang, M.Y.H., Bikle, D.D., Shackleton, C.H.L., Miller, W.L., and Portale, A.A. (1997) *Mol. Endocrinol.* **11**, 1961-1970
8. Fu, G.K., Portale, A.A., Miller, W.L. (1997) *DNA Cell Biol.* **16,** 1499-150
9. Monkawa, T., Yoshida, T., Wakino, S., Shinki, T., Anazawa, H., DeLuca, H.F., Suda, T., Hayashi, M., Saruta, T. (1997) *Biochem. Biophys. Res. Commun.* **239,** 527-533
10. Shinki, T., Shimada, H., Wakino, S., Anazawa, H., Hayashi, M., Saruta, T., DeLuca, H. (1997) *Proc. Natl. Acad. Sci. USA* **94,** 12920-12925
11. St-Arnaud, R., Messerlian, S., Moir, J.M., Omdahl, J.L., Glorieux, F.H. (1997) *J Bone Miner. Res.* **12,** 1552-1559
12. Takayama, K., Kitanaka, S. Sato, T., Kobori, M., Yanagisawa, J., and Kato, S. *Science* **277**,1827-1830
13. Bikle, D., Nemanic, M,. Whitney, J., and Elias, P. (1986) *Biochemistry* **25**, 1545-1548
14. Bikle, D., and Pillai, S. (1993) *Endocr. Rev.* **14,** 3-19
15. Bikle, D.D., Nemanic, M.K., Gee, E., Elias, P. (1986) *J. Clin. Invest.* **78**, 557-566
16. Miller, W.L. (1988) *Endocr. Rev.* **9,** 295-318
17. Fardella, C.E., Hum, D.W., Rodriguez, H., Zhang, G., Barry, F., Bloch, C.A., and Miller, W.L. (1996) , *J. Clin. Endocrinol. Metab* **81**, 321-326
18. Kitanaka, S., Takeyama, K., Murayama, A., Sato, T., Okumura, K., Nogami, M., Hasegawa, Y., Niimi, H., Yanagisawa, J., Tanaka, T., Kato, S. (1998) *N. Engl. J. Med.* **338**, 653-661
19. Labuda, M., Labuda, D., Korab-Laskowska, M., Cole, D.E.C., Zietkiewicz, E., Weissenbach, J., Popowska, E., Pronicka, E., Root, A.W., Glorieux, F.H. (1996) *Am. J. Hum. Genet.* **59**, 633-643
20. Labuda, M., Morgan, K., Glorieux, F.H. (1990) *Am. J. Hum. Genet.* **47**, 28-36
21. Wang ,J. Lin, C.J., Burridge, S.M., Fu, G.K., Labuda, M., Portale, A.A., Miller, W.L. (1998) *Am. J. Hum. Genet.* **63,** 1694-1702

22. Yoshida T, Monkawa T, Tenenhouse, H., Goodyer, P., Shinki, T., Suda, T., Wakino, S., Hayashi, M., and Sanuta, T. (1998) Kidney Intl. 54, 1437-1443
23. Levinson, G., and Gutman, G. (1987) *Mol Biol Evol* **4,** 203-221
24. Kitanaka, S., Murayama, A., Sakaki, T., Inouye, K., Seino, Y., Fukumoto, S., Shima, M., Yukizane, S., Takayanagi, M., Niimi, H., Takeyama, K.-I., and Kato, S. (1999). *J Clin Endocrinol Metab*, **84,** 4111-4117
25. Smith, S.J., Rucka, A.K., Berry, J.L., Davies, M., Mylchreest, S., Paterson, C.R., Heath, D.A., Tassagehji, M., Read,A.P., Mee,A..P., & Mawer, E.B. (1999). *J Bone Mineral Res*, **14,** 730-739.

CHROMOSOMAL LOCALIZATION OF THE PORCINE VITAMIN D-25-HYDROXYL-ASE (*CYP25*) GENE

Daniel C. Ciobanu, Rajbir K. Gill,* Max F. Rothschild, and Norman H. Bell.* Department of Animal Science, Iowa State University, Ames, IA, USA. *Department of Medicine, Medical University of South Carolina, Charleston, SC, USA

Introduction Vitamin D itself is biologically inactive and first must undergo conversion to 25-hydroxyvitamin D [25(OH)D] by the enzyme vitamin D-25-hydroxylase (CYP25) to become biologically active (1). The human mitochondrial enzyme CYP27 is involved in metabolism of cholesterol to bile acids and was previously cloned and sequenced and found nonspecifically to 25-hydroxylate vitamin D_3 but not vitamin D_2 (2,3). The enzyme evidently is not of major physiologic importance in vitamin D metabolism since deficiency of the enzyme results in cerebrotendinous xanthoma-tosis, an autosomal recessive lipid-storage disease, and not rickets or osteomalacia (4-6), and serum 25(OH)D is increased rather than decreased in mice with gene knockout of CYP27 (7). Recently, porcine CYP25 cDNA, a microsomal enzyme, was cloned and characterized and found to have 83 percent homology with human CYP2D6 cDNA, an enzyme involved in metabolism of debrisoquine and other drugs (8,9). Purified and recombinant porcine CYP25 were found to convert vitamins D_2 and D_3 to $25(OH)D_2$ and $25(OH)D_3$ equally well, and CYP25 therefore was proposed to be the true vitamin D-25-hydroxylase (8,9). Human CYP2D6 was cloned and characterized and the CYP2D6 gene was located on chromosome 22 (10,11). Mutations of human CYP2D6 are common and are associated with abnormal drug metabolism and not rickets or osteomalacia (12,13). A new disease was recently described in which isolated deficiency of 25(OH)D is associated with rickets and requires treatment with pharmacologic doses of vitamin D (14,15). The disease pre-sumably results from mutations in the *CYP25* gene. Based on these considerations, we conducted a study to determine the chromosomal locus of the porcine *CYP25* gene so that we might relate it by synteny to the locus for the human *CYP2D6* gene.

Methods

Isolation of DNA: DNA was extracted and isolated from porcine peripheral leukocytes by standard methods.

Preparation of DNA fragment: A fragment of porcine genomic DNA was obtained by PCR as follows: PCR primers were designed from the published sequence for porcine CYP25 cDNA (GenBank accession number Y16417). The position of the forward and reverse primers corresponded to 506-530 bp and 830-854 bp, respect-ively, of the porcine cDNA. The primer pair amplified a 348 bp fragment of the cDNA and an 854 bp fragment from the pig genomic DNA. The 854 bp fragment was sub-cloned into a pNoTA vector, and identity was confirmed by sequencing. Genomic DNA sequences from 1-74, 169-329 and 749-854 bp showed 100% homology to the cDNA. Primers derived from the porcine sequences were as follows: forward, 5'-GGG CAA GAA GGG GTC GTT GGA GGA GTC-3', representing bp 506-530 of the cDNA and reverse, 5'-ACT CGA CTA GTG TCT CGT GTT CTA C-3', representing bp

AdvanTaq DNA polymerase (Clontech, Palo Alto, CA), 16mM $(NH)_4SO_4$, 67.5 mM Tris buffer pH 8.8, 100 µM dNTPs, 1.5 mM $MgCl_2$, 0.01% Tween-20 and 50 ng of genomic DNA. Thermocycling was carried out in a Perkin Elmer GeneAmp 9600 PCR System. The PCR cycling conditions included initial denaturation at $95°$ C for 4 min followed by 30 cycles at $95°$ C for 45 sec, $60°$ C for 1 min, $72°$ C for 2 min and final extension at $72°$ C for 10 min. The 854 bp fragment of the porcine *CYP25* gene produced by PCR contained two introns, portions of two exons, and a full exon.

When genomic DNA from frog, chicken, mouse, rat and hamster was used, no PCR product was generated under similar conditions, whereas multiple genomic fragments were generated when human DNA was used. These findings indicated that this primer pair could be used to test the presence of porcine CYP25 genomic DNA in somatic cells and/or radiation hybrids.

Chromosomal Location. The 854 bp fragment of porcine *CYP25* gene was used for fine mapping to amplify the INRA-University of Minnesota Porcine Radiation Hybrid panel (IMpRH) (16).

Results The results shown in Table I indicate that the *CYP25* gene locus is located on pig chromosome 5 near the aconitase (*ACO2*) gene locus. Since the *ACO2* gene locus previously was physically mapped to the pig chromosome 5p14-15 region, the CYP25 gene locus is likely near this location.

Table 1. Mapping the *CYP25* gene by using IMpRH panel – two point analysis

Order	Chromosome	Marker	--	-+	+-	++	p(Break)	Distance (Ray)	LOD
1	5	ACO2	72	4	19	21	0.47	0.64	6.17
2	5	Sw1482	67	9	22	18	0.63	0.63	2.93
3	5	DK	52	25	13	28	0.64	1.03	2.77
4	5	SW152	59	16	20	2	0.67	1.12	2.29

Discussion: A porcine vitamin D-25-hydroxylase previously was cloned and characterized (8,9). The gene codes for a cytochrome P450 microsomal enzyme that is expressed in liver and kidney. Porcine CYP25 cDNA consists of 1,652 bp, and the purified protein consists of 500 amino acids and catalyzes equally the conversion of vitamin D_2 and vitamin D_3 to $25(OH)D_2$ and $25(OH)D_3$, respectively (8,9). Porcine CYP25 therefore was proposed to be the true vitamin D-25-hydroxylase. As indicated already, porcine CYP25 cDNA is 83% homologous with human CYP2D6 cDNA, an enzyme involved in the metabolism of debrisoquine and other drugs (8). Pig liver was found to have no CYP2D6 activity (17), but recombinant or purified CYP25 has not been evaluated in this regard. As indicated in the present report, porcine *CYP25* gene locus maps to pig chromosome 5p14-15, close to the *ACO2* gene locus (18). This region is syntenic to human chromosome 22q12-13 containing the loci for the human *CYP2D6* and *ACO2* genes (10,11). Further studies are

eeded to determine the possible relationship between porcine CYP25 and human
YP2D6, to clone and characterize the gene that modulates 25-hydroxylation of
tamin D, and to characterize mutations of the gene that cause isolated 25(OH)D
eficiency and rickets.

cknowledgements These studies were supported in part by PIC group and the Iowa
griculture and Home Economics Experimental Station, Ames, by Hatch Act and
tate of Iowa funds, and by an institutional grant from the Medical University of South
arolina.

eferences

Ponchon, G., Kennan, A.L., and DeLuca, H.F. (1969) *J. Clin. Invest.* **48**, 2032-2037.

Cali, J.J., and Russell, D.W. (1991) *J. Biol. Chem.* **266**, 7774-7778.

Guo, Y.-D., Strugness, S., Back, D.W., and Jones, G. (1993) *Proc. Natl. Acad. Sci. U.S.A.* **90**, 389-393.

Cali, J.J., Hsieh, C.-L., Francke, U., and Russell, D.W. (1991) *J. Biol. Chem.* **266**, 7779-7783.

Leitersdorf, E., Reshef, A., Neiner, V., Levitzki, R., Schwartz, S.P., Dann, E.J., Berkman, N., Cali, J.J., Klapholz, L., and Berginer, V.M. (1993) *J. Clin. Invest.* **91**, 2488-2496.

Berginer, V.M., Shany, S., Alkalay, D., Berginer, J., Dekel, S., Salen, G., Tint, G.S., and Gazit, D. (1992) *Metab. Clin. Exp.* **42**, 69-74.

Rosen, H., Reshef, A., Maeda, N., Lippoldt, A., Shpizen, S., Triger, L., Effertsen, G., Björkhem, I., and Leitersdorf, E. (1998) *J. Biol. Chem.* **273**, 14805-14812.

Postline, H., Axen, E., Bergman, T., and Wikvall, K. (1997) *Biochem. Biophys. Res. Commun.* **241**:491-497.

Axen, E., Bergman, T., and Wikvall, K. (1994) *J. Steroid Biochem. Molec. Biol.* **51**, 97-106.

). Gonzalez, F.J., Vilbois, F., Hardwick, J.P., McBride, O.W., Nebert, D.W., Gelboin, H.V., and Meyer, U.A. (1988) *Genomics* **2**, 174-179.

. Gough, A.C., Smith, C.A.D., Howell, S.M., Wolf, C.R., Bryant, S. P., and Spurr, N. K. (1993) *Genomics* **15**, 430-432.

. Gough, A.C., Miles, J.S., Spurr, N.K., Moss, K.E., Gaedigk, A., Eichelbau, M., and Wolf, C.R. (1990) *Nature* **347**, 773-776.

. Gerard, M.N., Vincent-Viry, M., Galteau, M.M., Jacqz-Aigrain, E., and Krisna-moorthy, R. (1993) *Br. J. Clin. Pharmacol.* **35**, 161-165.

. Casella, S.J., Reiner, B.J., Chen, T.C., Holick, M.F., and Harrison, H.E. (1994) *J. Pediatr.* **124**, 929-932.

. Nutzenadel, W., Mehls, O., and Klas, G. (1994) *J. Pediatr.* **126**, 676-677.

. Hawken, R. J., Murtaugh, J., Flickinger, G.H., Yerle, M., Robie, A., Milan, D.J., Gellin, J., Beattie, C.W., Schook, L.B., and Alexander, L.J. (1989) *Mamm. Genome* **10**, 824-830.

. Skaanild, M.T., and Friis, C. (1999). *Pharmacol. Toxicol.* **85**, 174-180.

. Yasue H, Hisamatsu, N, Awata, T., Wada, Y., and Kusumoto, H.Y. (1999) *Anim. Genet.* **30**, 161-162.

154

CATABOLISM OF 1,25-DIHYDROXYVITAMIN D$_2$ BY RECOMBINANT HUMAN 1,25-DIHYDROXYVITAMIN D-24-HYDROXYLASE

MJ Beckman, CJ Czuprynski, GS Reddy[†] and RL Horst[*]   Department of Pathobiological Sciences, School of Veterinary Medicine, University of Wisconsin, Madison, WI 53706, [†]Department of Ped., Women and Infants' Hospital of Rhode Island, Brown University School of Medicine, Providence, RI 02905 and [*]USDA-ARS, National Animal Disease Center, Periparturient Diseases of Cattle Research Unit, Ames, IA 50010.

Introduction

The 1,25-dihydroxyvitamin D-24-hydroxylase (P450cc24) is a catabolic enzyme that is induced by 1,25-dihydroxyvitamin D and is involved in the catabolism of 25-OH-D and 1,25-dihydroxyvitamin D to less active metabolites (figure 1)[1,2]. Little is known about the role of P450cc24 in the catabolism of vitamin D$_2$ metabolites and analogs[3], however, vitamin D$_2$ analogs retain biological activity in vivo for longer duration than vitamin D$_3$ analogs[4,5] and thus have greater potential for therapeutic purposes[6]. This project seeks to more thoroughly explore the catalytic properties of the human P450cc24 on vitamin D$_2$ analogs by recombinant eukaryotic expression of the human P450cc24 and its cofactor proteins in *Sf9* insect cells.   The objective of this project was to develop a recombinant human 1,25-dihidroxyvitamin D-24-hydroxylase as a tool in the assessment of vitamin D$_2$ analog metabolism.

Methods

Radiolabled compounds: [26,27-^{3}H]-1,25-(OH)$_2$D$_3$ and [9,11-^{3}H]-1,25-(OH)$_2$D$_2$ were provided by Dr. Ronald Horst. These compounds were purified by HPLC before their use in experiments.

DNA constructs: Adrenodoxin and adrenodoxin reductase cDNAs were generously provided by Dr. Michael Waterman, Vanderbuilt University.   The constructs were separately expressed in a DH5α E. coli strain.   Cells were sonicated to lyse the protein contents and the respective cofactors were chromatographically isolated as previously described[7,8] . The human P450cc24 reading frame was PCR cloned from a human MCF-7 breast cancer cell line following induction by 20 nM 1,25-(OH)$_2$D$_3$ for 6 hours. The P450cc24 cDNA was inserted into the Zeocin resistant plasmid pIZT, Invitrogen.

Cells and handling: *Spodotera frugiperda* (*Sf9*) cells were purchased from Invitrogen. Cells were cultured and sub-cultured as adherent cells in Grace's insect medium, pH 6.2, containing *Trichoplusia ni* Medium-Formulation Hink (TNM-FH) as supplement, 10 µg/ml gentamycin and 10% FBS. A log phase cell viability of 95% and cell doubling time of 24 hr was used as the standard growth parameters prior to any manipulations via transfection, lysis, etc. Cell counts were determined by the trypan blue exclusion method.

Expression of h-P450cc24 in *Sf9* cells: Transient expression of of the plasmid DNA was performed on log phase *Sf9* cells. 2×10^6 *Sf9* cells were seeded in a 60 mm dish and rocked gently side-to-side for 3 minutes to evenly distribute the cells. After attachment, medium containing serum was replaced with serum-free medium and plasmid DNA (10μg) was transfected in the presence of Insectin-Plus, Invitrogen. The cells were rocked side-to-side at room temperature for 4 hrs. Serum was replaced and the cells were returned to the incubator. At 2, 3 and 4 days post-transfection cells were assayed for GFP. Generally, three days was required for full expression of GFP and p450cc24. Mitochondrial proteins from harvested *Sf9* cell extracts were prepared by cellular fractionation and solubilized in 160 mM KPO_4, pH 7.4, containing 0.63% sodium cholate, 1 mM EDTA, and 20% glycerol.

Enzyme assay: Functional P450cc24 activity was reconstituted in the presence of 100 nmol NADP and 1.6 nmol adrenodoxin and 0.1 nmol adrenodoxin reductase cofactors. Reactions were initiated by the addition of either 1 μCi $[26,27-^3H]-1,25-(OH)_2D_3$ or $[9,11-^3H]-1,25-(OH)_2D_2$. The length of the reactions varied by experiment. Reactions were terminated by addition of 1 N acetic acid.

HPLC: Sample extractions and HPLC were performed as previously described[9].

GFP Assay: Serum containing medium was removed from *Sf9* cells. The cells were washed twice with PBS, pH 7.4. Fresh PBS was added and the cells were sloughed off by continuous pipetting of medium over the cell layer until they released. Next, 1×10^3 cells were spotted onto glass cover slips coated with polyornithine and allowed 15 min to attach. Cells were then fixed with 4% paraformaldehyde, washed with PBS, pH 7.4, and mounted cell side down onto glass slides. GFP was monitored by fluorescent microscopy.

Periodate cleavage assay: To monitor for functional P450cc24 activity in *Sf9* cells, a saturated (8% w/v) solution of aqueous sodium periodate ($NaIO_4$) was mixed with mitochondrial enzyme reactions that were initiated with $[26,27-^3H]-1,25-(OH)_2D_3$. The reactions were incubated on ice for 30 min. The $[^3H]$acetone was separated from the labeled substrate and other reaction components by aspirating the reaction mixture through a C-18 cartridge. Reactions were eluted with 1.5 ml ice-cold water and analyzed by liquid scintillation counting.

Results and Discussion
Renal C-28 and C-26 hydroxylations are considered to be important enzymatic steps involved in the inactivation of 1α-25-dihydroxyvitamin D_2 [1α-25$(OH)_2D_2$] under physiological conditions. The enzyme(s) responsible for C-28 and C-26 hydroxylations on vitamin D_2 compounds is not known, but it is speculated that the multicatalytic properties of the 24-hydroxylase (P450cc24) may play a role. To test this, we cloned the human form of P450cc24 from a human MCF-7 breast cancer cell line. Furthermore, we are developing a cDNA construct of human P450cc24 in the Zeocin resistant pIZT/V5-His expression vector to express the

P450cc24 following transient and stable transfection in *Sf9* insect cells. Expression of P450cc24 was monitored by the coexpression of GFP via fluorescent microscopy. By day 3 post-transfection, 95% of the cells expressed intense GFP. Human P450cc24 activity was examined by reconstitution of solubilized *Sf9* mitochondrial protein in the presence of its cofactors and [26,27-^{3}H]-1,25-(OH)$_2$D$_3$, as substrate. The periodate cleavage assay demonstrated functional P450cc24 activity in cells transfected with P450cc24 (p24-OHase) but not in cells transfected with chloramphenicol transferase (pCAT). We plan to generate and compare by HPLC the catalytic products produced from P450cc24 activity on [9,11-^{3}H]-1,24-(OH)$_2$D$_2$ and [9,11-^{3}H]-1,25-(OH)$_2$D$_2$ metabolites. These experiments are not yet completed. A second part of the project is to develop a stably transfected line of *Sf9* cells containing high constitutive expression from a construct consisting of human 24-hydroxylase contiguous with bovine adrenodoxin and bovine adrenodoxin reductase gene products. Furthermore, this system will be developed for the general purpose to rapidly analyze the catalytic properties of P450cc24 on the metabolism of any vitamin D analog.

A.
B.

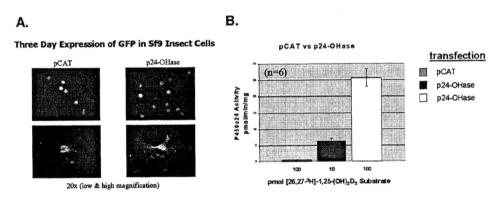

Figure 1. Protein expression of either chloramphenicol transferase or human P450cc24 in *Sf9* cells growing in adherent cultures. Ten µg of plasmid DNA was transfected into 1x10^6 cells. Cells were incubated for 3 days at 28°C. A. Shows the expression of GFP in either control (pCAT) or experimental (p24-OHase) transfection. Results are shown at both low and high power in parafomaldehyde fixed *Sf9* cells. B. Assessment of functional P450cc24 activity in transfected cells. Activity measurements were determined by periodate cleavage of side-chain tritium using [26,27-^{3}H]-1,25-(OH)$_2$D$_3$ as substrate.

References

1. Beckman MJ, Tadikonda P, Werner E, Prahl J, Yamada S and DeLuca HF (1996) Human 25-hydroxyvitamin D$_3$-24-hydroxylase, a multicatalytic enzyme. *Biochemistry* 35:8465-8472.

2.   Akiyoshi-Shibita M, Sakaki T, Ohyama Y, Noshiro M, Okuda K and Yabusaki Y (1994) Further oxidation of hydroxycalcidiol by calcidiol 24-hydroxylase. A study with the mature enzyme expressed in *Escherichia coli. Eur. J. Biochem.* 224:335-343.

3.   Jones G, Byford V, Makin HL, Kremer R, Rice RH, DeGraffenried LA, Knutson JC, Bishop CW (1996). Anti-proliferative activity and target cell catabolism of the vitamin D analog 1alpha,24(S)-(OH)$_2$D$_2$ in normal and immortalized human epidermal cells. *Biochem. Pharmacol.* 52:133-140.

4.   Erben RG, Bante U, Birner H and Stangassinger M (1997).   1α-Hydroxyvitamin D$_2$ partially dissociates between preservation of cancellous bone mass and effects on calcium homeostasis in ovariectomized rats. Calcif. Tissue Int. 60: 449-456.

5.   Gallager JC, Bishop CW, Knutson JC, Mazess RB and DeLuca HF (1994). Effects of increasing doses of 1α-hydroxyvitamin D$_2$ on calcium homeostasis in postmenopausal osteopenic women. J. Bone Min. Res. 9:607-614.

6.   Tan AU, Levine BS, Mazess RB, Kyllo DM, Bishop CW, Knutson JC, Kleinman KS and Coburn JW (1997).   Effective suppression of parathyroid hormone by 1αhydroxyvitamin D$_2$ in hemodialysis patients with moderate to severe secondary hyperparathyroidism. Kidney Int. 51:317-323.

7.   Sagara Y, Hara T, Ariyasu Y, Ando F, Tokunaga N and Horiuchi T (1992). Direct expression in *Escherichia coli* and characterization of bovine adrenodoxins with modified amino-terminal regions. FEBS 300:208-212.

8.   Sagara Y, Wada A, Takata Y, Waterman MR, Sekimizu K and Horiuchi T (1993).   Direct expression of adrenodoxin reductase in *Eschericia coli* and functional characterization. Biol. Pharm. Bull. 16:627-630.

9.   Rao DS. Siu-Caldera ML. Uskokovic MR. Horst RL and Reddy GS. (1999).   Physiological significance of C-28 hydroxylation in the metabolism of 1alpha,25-dihydroxyvitamin D(2). Archives of Biochemistry & Biophysics. 368:319-28.

ANALYSIS OF THE TISSUE DISTRIBUTION OF 1α-HYDROXYLASE INDENTIFIES NOVEL EXTRA-RENAL SITES FOR THE SYNTHESIS OF 1,25-DIHYDROXYVITAMIN D$_3$.

Daniel Zehnder, Rosemary Bland, Susan V Hughes, Ravinder S Chana, Arthur R Bradwell*, Paul M Stewart and Martin Hewison. Division of Medical Sciences, *Immunology and Infection, University of Birmingham, Birmingham B15 2TH, UK

Introduction: 1α-hydroxylase plays a key role in calcium homeostasis by catalysing the synthesis of 1,25-dihydroxyvitamin D$_3$ (1,25(OH)$_2$D$_3$) in the kidneys. Previous reports have shown that 1,25(OH)$_2$D$_3$ is also synthesised in cells from various extra-renal tissues including keratinocytes and activated macrophages[1]. This is particularly evident in granulomatous diseases such as sarcoidosis or tuberculosis, where the associated hypercalcaemia appears to be linked to the ectopic synthesis of 1,25(OH)$_2$D$_3$(2-5). In contrast to the kidney, which supports the systemic, endocrine actions of 1,25(OH)$_2$D$_3$, extra-renal 1α-hydroxylase appears to act in an autocrine or paracrine fashion by modulating cell differentiation and/or function at a local level (6,7). Until recently analysis of the tissue distribution of 1α-hydroxylase relied on relatively insensitive enzyme assays using semi-purified tissue samples. However, in recent studies we have used novel cRNA probes and polyclonal antisera to describe for the first time the precise localisation of 1α-hydroxylase along the nephron (8). In data presented here, we have carried out similar studies using a variety of extra-renal tissues, including pathological samples from patients with psoriasis and sarcoidosis.

Methods: The tissue specimen database from the University of Birmingham was screened for routine surgical samples that were classified as normal. Psoriatic skin and granulomata forming diseases such as sarcoidosis and tuberculosis were also included. A 1α-hydroxylase antibody for the antigenic region of the reported mouse amino acid sequence (9): peptide 266-289 was used for immunohistochemistry on paraffin embedded sections (n=5 for every tissue) and Western blot analysis as described previously(8,10). Control experiments have confirmed cross-reactivity with the human 1α-hydroxylase protein. Human umbilical vein endothelial cells (HUVEC) (n=4) were cultured in 20% foetal calf serum and treated for 24 h with forskolin (10µM), TNFα (30ng/ml) and LPS (1µg/ml). For enzyme activity assays, ^{3}H-25(OH)D$_3$ was used as substrate and conversion to 1,25(OH)$_2$D$_3$ measured by quantitative thin layer chromatography.

Results: Initial studies were carried out using extra-renal tissues, which have been shown previously to be able to produce 1,25(OH)$_2$D$_3$. In normal skin, epidermal 1α-hydroxylase expression was restricted to keratinocytes within the stratum basalis, although the enzyme was also expressed strongly in hair follicles. In contrast, psoriatic skin samples showed widespread expression of 1α-hydroxylase throughout the dysregulated stratum spinosum. In normal lymph nodes, 1α-hydroxylase was widely expressed, but particularly evident in germinal centers.

Similar results were obtained with sections of human tonsil tissue and white pulpa of the spleen. Analysis using lymph tissue from patients with sarcoidosis or tuberculosis showed increased expression of 1α-hydroxylase, specifically in the epitheloid cell granuloma (cells positive for the macrophage cell surface antigen CD68). Heart and liver tissue showed no staining for the enzyme. A variety of other extra-renal tissues were examined as listed in table 1. Western blot analysis showed the presence of a 56kDa protein species corresponding to the predicted size of 1α-hydroxylase in renal and extra-renal tissue (Figure 1). In some sections, renal and extra-renal tissue endothelia also stained for 1α-hydroxylase, particularly in the presence of inflammation of the surrounding tissue. This prompted us to look in more detail at possible inflammatory regulators of 1α-hydroxylase in HUVEC, as an endothelial cell model. Western blot analysis again showed the presence of a 56kDa protein corresponding to 1α-hydroxylase (Figure 2).

Table 1: Expression for 1α-hydroxylase protein in various tissues (levels of expression ranging from low (+) to high (+++):

| | Staining for 1α-hydroxylase protein | |
	positive	negative
Kidney	proximal convoluted tubule + , distal nephron +++	
Skin	basal keratinocytes ++, hair follicle +++, sweat glands ++	
Placenta	decidual cells ++, trophoblastic cells +++	
Pancreas	islets ++	exocrine
Adrenal	medulla +++	cortex
Colon	epithelial cells +++, enteric nervous system (ganglion) ++	myocytes
Brain	purkinje cells in cerebellum ++, other neuronal cells ++	
Lymph node	germination centers +/++, post-capillary cuboidal endothelia +/++	
Endothelium	particularly in an inflammatory environment +/++	
Heart		myocytes
Liver		hepatocytes
Psoriasis	throughout dysregulated stratum spinosum ++, inflammatory infiltrates ++	
Sarcoidosis/ tuberculosis	granulomas (epitheloid cells ++, multinuclear giant cells ++), particularly cells positive for the macrophage marker CD68 ++	

Discussion: Immunohistochemical data presented here show for the first time the distribution of 1α-hydroxylase protein in extra-renal tissues. The expression of 1α-hydroxylase appears to be more widespread than previously thought, suggesting diverse functions for the local production of 1,25(OH)$_2$D$_3$ in peripheral tissues. The expression of 1α-hydroxylase in keratinocytes within the stratum basale is consistent with previous analysis of 1,25(OH)$_2$D$_3$ production by keratinocytes(11). Proliferating keratinocytes showed high levels of 1,25(OH)$_2$D$_3$ synthesis that decreased as the cells differentiated towards cornified cells(11). It was particularly

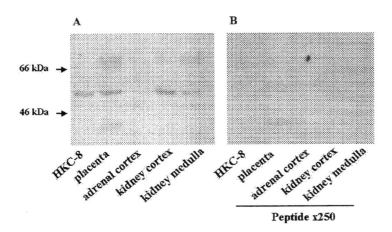

Figure 1: Western blot analysis of renal and extra-renal tissue: (A) an appropriate band for the 1α-hydroxylase protein (56kDa) was detectable in placenta, kidney cortex and medulla. In adrenal cortex, this band is not detectable. Human kidney cell line (HKC-8) was used as positive control. (B)Blocking experiments involving pre-absorption of antiserum with x250 excess of immunising peptide confirmed the specificity of Western blot.

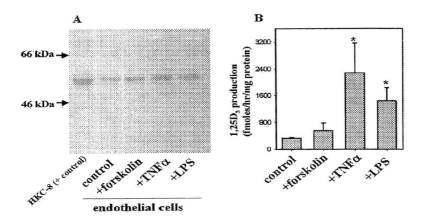

Figure 2: *In vitro* studies on human umbilical vein endothelial cells (HUVEC). (A) Western blot analysis confirmed expression of 1α-hydroxylase protein, which was increased following treatment with LPS. (B) A significant increase of 1,25(OH)$_2$D$_3$ production (±SD) compared to control occurs after 24-h stimulation with TNFα (1054±166) or LPS (1381±88) (*p<0.01).

1,25(OH)$_2$D$_3$ production in psoriasis. Granulomata observed in sarcoidosis and tuberculosis showed expression of 1α- hydroxylase protein, particularly in CD68 positive cells, confirming previous observations, that activated macrophages are able to produce 1,25(OH)$_2$D$_3$(2,3). Immunohistochemical detection of 1α-

interesting to note the widespread expression of 1α-hydroxylase throughout the dysregulated stratum spinosum in psoriatic lesions, suggesting dysregulated hydroxylase in tissue from the placenta bed confirms previous enzyme activity studies, which indicate that 1,25$(OH)_2D_3$, may be produced by decidual and trophoblastic cells(12). The enzyme may contribute to both the materno-fetal transfers of calcium, as well as possible immunomodulatory actions during placentation. The presence of 1α-hydroxylase in pancreatic islet cells provides a further link between vitamin D and insulin secretion, shown recently in studies *in vivo* and *in vitro*(13). The potential role for local synthesis of 1,25$(OH)_2D_3$ as a modulator of secretory function is emphasised by the further observation that 1α-hydroxylase is detectable in other secretory tissues, such as the adrenal medulla. Expression of 1α-hydroxylase was also relatively strong in sweat glands. This, together with the presence of 1α-hydroxylase in colonic epithelial cells and the distal part of the nephron suggests an association between the enzyme and sites of sodium transport and regulation.

Finally, we have shown for the first time, the presence of this enzyme in human endothelia. Our experiments suggest, endothelial cell expression of 1α-hydroxylase may be stimulated during inflammation. We can therefore postulate that up-regulation of the activity of enzyme by inflammatory mediators may play an important role in regulating trafficking of macrophages through the endothelial cell layer.

Reference List

1. Bell, N. H. (1998) *J.Bone Miner.Res.* **13,** 350-353.
2. Papapoulos, S. E., Clemens, T. L., Fraher, L. J., Lewin, I. G., Sandler, L. M., and O'Riordan, J. L. (1979) *Lancet* **1,** 627-630.
3. Barbour, G. L., Coburn, J. W., Slatopolsky, E., Norman, A. W., and Horst, R. L. (1981) *N.Engl.J.Med.* **305,** 440-443.
4. Adams, J. S., Sharma, O. P., Gacad, M. A., and Singer, F. R. (1983) *J.Clin.Invest* **72,** 1856-1860.
5. Adams, J. S. and Gacad, M. A. (1985) *J.Exp.Med.* **161,** 755-765.
6. Walters, M. R. (1992) *Endocr.Rev.* **13,** 719-764.
7. Bouillon, R., Garmyn, M., Verstuyf, A., Segaert, S., Casteels, K., and Mathieu, C. (1995) *Eur.J.Endocrinol.* **133,** 7-16.
8. Zehnder, D., Bland, R., Walker, E. A., Bradwell, A. R., Howie, A. J., Hewison, M., and Stewart, P. M. (1999) *J.Am.Soc.Nephrol.* **10,** 2465-2473.
9. Takeyama, K., Kitanaka, S., Sato, T., Kobori, M., Yanagisawa, J., and Kato, S. (1997) *Science* **277,** 1827-1830.
10. Bland, R., Walker, E. A., Hughes, S. V., Stewart, P. M., and Hewison, M. (1999) *Endocrinology* **140,** 2027-2034.
11. Pillai, S., Bikle, D. D., and Elias, P. M. (1988) *J.Biol.Chem.* **263,** 5390-5395
12. Weisman, Y., Harell, A., Edelstein, S., David, M., Spirer, Z., and Golander, A. (1979) *Nature* **281,** 317-319
13. Bourlon, P. M., Faure-Dussert, A., and Billaudel, B. (1997) *Br.J.Pharmacol.* **121,** 751-758

VITAMIN D METABOLISM IN VITAMIN D RECEPTOR NULL MUTANT MICE IN HYPO- AND NORMO-CALCEMIC CONDITIONS

N. Tsugawa[1], Y. Fukushima[1], C. Ashiwa[1], T. Yoshizawa[2], S. Kato[2] and T. Okano[1], [1]Department of Hygienic Sciences, Kobe Pharmaceutical University, Kobe 658-8558, Japan and [2]Institute of Molecular and Cellular Biosciences, The University of Tokyo, Tokyo 113-8657, Japan

Introduction The vitamin D receptor (VDR) null mutant mice (VDR-KO mice)[1, 2] generated by target gene disruption have severe hypocalcemia, impaired bone formation, growth retardation and alopecia, indicating lack of VDR-mediated action of 1,25-dihydroxyvitamin D_3 (1,25(OH)$_2$D$_3$). The expression and regulation of renal 1α-OHase activity is tightly regulated by plasma levels of Ca, PTH and 1,25(OH)$_2$D$_3$. It has been reported that expression of 24-OHase is strongly induced by 1,25(OH)$_2$D$_3$. However, it remains unclear whether 1,25(OH)$_2$D$_3$ regulates expressions of 25-OHase and 1α-OHase. Recent *in vivo* studies indicated that administration of 1,25(OH)$_2$D$_3$ to normal rats resulted in decreases in serum levels of 25(OH)D$_3$ [3,4]. Moreover, it is also shown that 1,25(OH)$_2$D$_3$ inhibits the production of 25(OH)D$_3$ in the liver [3,5]. Alternatively, other laboratories have shown that administration of 1,25(OH)$_2$D$_3$ to normal rats resulted in significant decrease of plasma 25(OH)D$_3$ levels due to increased metabolic conversion rate of 25(OH)D$_3$ to 24R,25(OH)$_2$D$_3$, not due to inhibition of 25-OHase activity by 1,25(OH)$_2$D$_3$ [4,6]. The molecular basis for the discrepancy between the effects of 1,25(OH)$_2$D$_3$ on 25-OHase remains to be elucidated. Expression of 1α-OHase is known to be up-regulated in low vitamin D/ low Ca state in mammals. It is also generally accepted that both PTH and calcitonin are positive regulators for expression of 1α-OHase. Negative regulation of 1α-OHase by 1,25(OH)$_2$D$_3$ itself is reported [7] and the negative vitamin D response element on promoter of 1α-OHase gene has been proposed [8,9], but that precise mechanism is not well understood. In this study, to further clarify the possible role of the VDR in the regulation of vitamin D metabolism, we examined the plasma levels of calcium (Ca), parathyroid hormone (PTH) and vitamin D metabolites, and mRNA levels of 25-hydroxylase (25-OHase) in the liver, 1α-hydroxylase (1α-OHase), PTH receptor and megalin in the kidney, and PTH in the parathyroid gland (PG) of mice in hypo- and normo-calcemic conditions.

Results and Discussion

Calcium metabolism VDR-KO mice originally raised by Yoshizawa et al. [1] were used in this study. The animals were fed *ad libitum* autoclaved rodent chow F-2 (Oriental Yeast Co.Ltd., Osaka, Japan) containing 0.74% Ca, 0.65%

phosphorus, vitamin D_3 50 ng/g of diet, as normal Ca diet (N-Ca). Newborn mice were housed with their mothers fed normal Ca diet for 21 days, then weaned at 22 days after birth. Two- and 3-weeks-old mice were used as pre-weaning ones and 4- and 7- weeks-old mice were used as post-weaning ones. In another group, animals were fed *ad libitum* autoclaved high Ca (H-Ca) diet (Clea Japan, Inc., Tokyo) containing 2.0% Ca, 1.25% phosphorus, 20% lactose, 50 ng/g vitamin D_3. As shown in Fig. 1, plasma levels of Ca in the VDR-KO mice were within the normal range at the pre-weaning period of age (at 2 and 3 weeks of age), and then they were markedly reduced and reached to severe hypocalcemic levels at the post-weaning period of age (at 4 and 7 weeks of age) in VDR-KO mice fed N-Ca diet. Plasma Ca levels of 7-weeks-old VDR-KO mice fed H-Ca diet were maintained within normal range. These results were consistent well with

those of previous paper [1,2]. Plasma PTH levels of VDR-KO mice were slightly but significantly higher than those of wild-type mice at the pre-weaning period of age, and they markedly increased at post-weaning period of age according to decrease of plasma Ca levels (Fig. 1). Plasma PTH levels of 7-weeks-old VDR-KO mice fed H-Ca diet were lower than those of VDR-KO mice fed normal Ca diet, but not completely recovered to normal range. PTH secretion is regulated by extracellular Ca. To examine the PTH production in parathyroid gland, PTH mRNA levels were measured by real-time quantitive RT-PCR method.

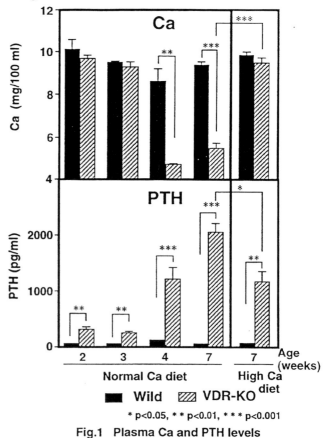

* p<0.05, * * p<0.01, * * * p<0.001

Fig.1 Plasma Ca and PTH levels

Figure 2 shows the relative quantity of PTH mRNA / β-actin mRNA in parathyroid gland. PTH mRNA levels of VDR-KO mice were remarkably higher than those of wild-type mice in normo-calcemic condition. In contrast, those levels were normal in both wild-type and VDR-KO mice fed H-Ca diet, although parathyroid gland was

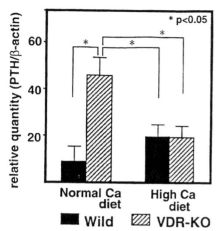

Fig. 2 Expression of PTH mRNA
in Parathyroid gland

still in hyperplasia in the VDR-KO mice fed H-Ca diet. PTH mRNA levels in whole tissue of parathyroid gland of VDR-KO mice were also higher than those of wild-type mice in normal Ca diet, and these levels were partially but not completely reduced, by feeding of H-Ca diet. The result suggests that the VDR have a possible role in proliferation of parathyroid cells.

Vitamin D metabolism Plasma levels of $25(OH)D_3$ in the VDR-KO mice were relatively stable through the pre-weaning period as well as the post-weaning period of age. In contrast, the levels of the wild-type mice were similar to those of the VDR-KO mice at the pre-weaning period of age, thereafter, they increased gradually with age. There was no significant differences in the plasma $25(OH)D_3$ levels between the VDR-KO mice fed either N-Ca diet or H-Ca diet for four weeks after weaning. No significant differences were observed in hepatic 25-OHase (CYP-27) mRNA levels and 25-OHase activity in the both type of mice fed either N-Ca diet or H-Ca diet for four weeks (Fig. 3). There was no significant difference in the mRNA levels of megalin, which is known to mediate the tubular uptake of $25(OH)D_3$ filtered through the glomerulus in the kidney. From these results, 25-OHase activity in the liver may not be regulated directly by $1,25(OH)_2D_3$.

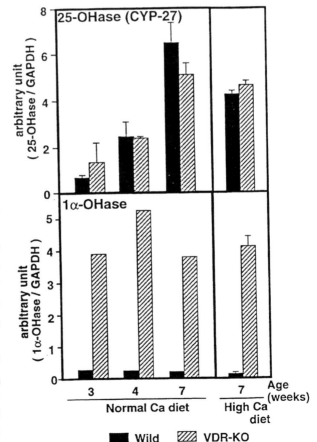

Fig. 3 Expression of hepatic 25-OHase (CYP27)
mRNA and renal 1α-OHase mRNA

Remarkable elevations of plasma $1,25(OH)_2D_3$ levels and renal 1α-OHase mRNA levels were observed in the VDR-KO mice independent of Ca concentrations in diets (Fig. 3). PTH is a positive regulator for expression of 1α-OHase. However, no correlation was observed between the levels of renal 1α-OHase mRNA and plasma PTH in the VDR-KO mice. In the rats, calcitonin stimulates the expression of 1α-OHase mRNA in normocalcemia. However, plasma calcitonin levels of the VDR-KO mice were similar to those of wild-type mice. PTH receptor mRNA levels of the kidney were measured to examine whether high expression of renal 1α-OHase in the VDR-KO mice is related to the alteration of the PTH receptor levels. However, no significant difference was observed in renal PTH receptor mRNA levels between both type of mice, suggesting that the susceptability of PTH in the kidney is not changed in the VDR-KO mice. These results indicate that decreased plasma levels of $25(OH)D_3$ levels of the VDR-KO mice are probably due to high metabolic conversion rate of $25(OH)D_3$ to $1,25(OH)_2D_3$. Moreover, since the 1α-OHase mRNA expression did not differ in the VDR-KO mice with high or normal plasma PTH levels, it would be postulated that the VDR might regulate directly and negatively the 1α-OHase mRNA expression in the kidney.

Reference

1) Yoshizawa T., Handa Y., Uematsu Y., Takeda S., Sekine K., Yoshihara Y., Kawakami T., Arioka K., Sato H., Uchiyama Y., Masushige S., Fukamizu A., Matsumoto T., Kato S. (1997) Nat. Genet. 16, 391-396.

2) Li Y.C., Pirro A.E., Amling M., Delling G., Baron R., Bronson R., Demay M.B. (1997) Proc. Natl., Acad. Sci. USA 94, 9831-9835.

3) Bell N.H., Shaw S., Turner R.T. (1984) J. Clin. Invest. 74, 1540-1544.

4) Halloran B.P., Bikle D.D., Levens, M.J., Castro M.E., Globus R.K., Holton E. (1986) J. Clin. Invest. 78, 622-628.

5) Reinholts G.G., DeLuca H.F. (1998) Arch. Biochem. Biophys. 355, 77-83.

6) Halloran B.P., Castro M.E. (1989) Am. J. Physiol. 256, E686-E-691.

7) Booth B.E., Tsai H.C., Morris R.J. (1985) J. Clin. Invest. 75, 155-161.

8) Murayama A., Takeyama K., Kitanaka S., Kodera Y., Hosoya T., Kato S. (1998) Biochem. Biophys. Res. Commun. 249, 11-16.

9) Kong X.F., Zhu X.H., Pei Y.L., Jackson D.M., Holick M.F. (1999) Proc. Nattl. Acad. Sci. USA 96, 6988-6993.

DIFFERENTIAL REGULATION OF 1,25(OH)$_2$D$_3$ SYNTHESIS ALONG THE NEPHRON: ANALYSIS OF 1α-HYDROXYLASE EXPRESSION AND ACTIVITY IN HUMAN PROXIMAL TUBULE AND COLLECTING DUCT CELL LINES

Rosemary Bland, Daniel Zehnder, Susan V. Hughes, Pierre M. Ronco*, Paul M. Stewart and Martin Hewison. Division of Medical Sciences, The University of Birmingham, Birmingham, B15 2TH, UK. *INSERM U64, Paris, France.

Introduction: The cloning of mouse and human cDNAs for 25 hydroxyvitamin D$_3$,1α-hydroxylase (1α-OHase) [1,2,3] has facilitated a more sensitive analysis of this enzyme. Recent immunohistochemistry and *in situ* hybridization studies by our group have shown that expression of the enzyme is not restricted to the proximal tubule. RNA and protein for 1α-OHase are abundantly expressed in more distal regions of the nephron such as distal convoluted tubules and cortical collecting ducts [4]. Using two human cell lines which express characteristics of proximal convoluted tubules (HKC-8 cells; [5]) and cortical collecting ducts (HCD cells; [6]), the aim of this study was to examine the regulation of 1α-OHase activity in two distinct regions of the nephron.

Methods: *Cell culture*: HKC-8 cells were maintained in DMEM-HamsF12 medium supplemented with 5% fetal calf serum (FCS) and 2mM glutamine. HCD cells were maintained in DMEM-HamsF12 medium supplemented with 2% FCS, 2mM glutamine, 10mM HEPES, transferrin (5µg/ml), sodium selenite (5ng/ml), insulin (5µg/ml) and dexamethasone (5×10^{-8}M). For assessment of enzyme activity, mRNA and protein expression, cells were transferred to defined medium, as described previously [7]. For treatments containing lipopolysaccharide (LPS) cells were treated in FCS containing medium, which was replaced with defined medium for the duration of the enzyme activity assessment. Where indicated cells were incubated in calcium free medium supplemented with CaCl$_2$ to give a calcium concentration of 0.5mM.
RT-PCR: RNA was prepared using a single step extraction method (RNazol B RNA isolation kit, AMS Biotechnology Ltd., UK) according to the manufactures protocol. RT of 1µg of RNA was performed using a Promega reverse transcription system. PCR was performed using primers specific for 1α-OHase and the PTH receptors type 1 and 2.
Western analysis: Total cell lysates were subjected to SDS-PAGE (3 or 10µg/lane) and electroblotted as described previously [7]. Filters were analyzed with (i) specific monoclonal antibodies against the human VDR (Cambridge BioScience, UK), and the human calcium sensing receptor (CaR) (NPS Pharmaceuticals) (ii) polyclonal antiserum to the mouse 1α-OHase sequence (The Binding Site Ltd., UK).
Enzyme activity: 1α- and 24-hydroxylase (24-OHase) activity was assessed by incubating the cells with 25(OH)$_2$D$_3$ (3.75 - 28.75nM) containing a tracer of ^{3}H-25(OH)$_2$D$_3$ for 4 hours. The resulting vitamin D metabolites were separated by

TLC using dichloromethane:isopropanol (9:1) as a running solvent and analyzed using a Bioscan System 200 imaging scanner. Data are reported as production of $1,25(OH)_2D_3$ (1α-OHase activity) or $24,25(OH)_2D_3$ (24-OHase activity). Results are represented as the mean $\pm$ SEM (n = 3 - 8).

Results: RT-PCR and Western blot analysis demonstrated the presence of 1α-OHase mRNA and protein in both the HKC-8 and HCD cells (Figure 1) and both cell lines expressed mRNA encoding 24-OHase (data not shown).

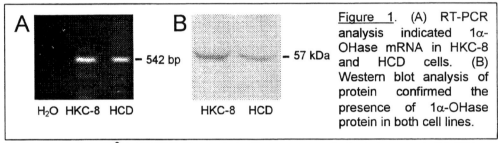

Figure 1. (A) RT-PCR analysis indicated 1α-OHase mRNA in HKC-8 and HCD cells. (B) Western blot analysis of protein confirmed the presence of 1α-OHase protein in both cell lines.

TLC analysis of ^3H-$25(OH)_2D_3$ metabolism demonstrated 1α- and 24-OHase activity in both cell lines. Basal activity of 1α-OHase in HKC-8 cells (360 fmoles/mg/h) was 5 fold higher than that in HCD cells ($\sim$70 fmoles/mg/h). However, 24-OHase activity was 2 fold higher in HCD cells (HCD 1400 fmoles/mg/h vs HKC-8 650 fmoles/mg/h). RT-PCR analyses demonstrated mRNA encoding PTH receptors (type 1 and type 2) in both cell lines. Western blot analysis and $1,25(OH)_2D_3$ binding assays indicated that HKC-8 and HCD cells expressed similar levels of vitamin D receptors (data not shown).

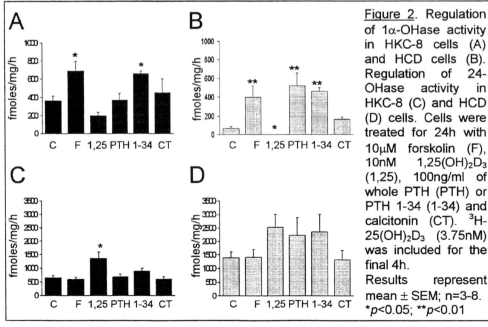

Figure 2. Regulation of 1α-OHase activity in HKC-8 cells (A) and HCD cells (B). Regulation of 24-OHase activity in HKC-8 (C) and HCD (D) cells. Cells were treated for 24h with $10\mu M$ forskolin (F), 10nM $1,25(OH)_2D_3$ (1,25), 100ng/ml of whole PTH (PTH) or PTH 1-34 (1-34) and calcitonin (CT). ^3H-$25(OH)_2D_3$ (3.75nM) was included for the final 4h. Results represent mean $\pm$ SEM; n=3-8. $*p<0.05$; $**p<0.01$

Synthesis of 1,25(OH)₂D₃ was significantly increased by forskolin (10μM, 24h) and bioactive parathyroid hormone (PTH 1-34; 100ng/ml, 24h) and was decreased by 1,25(OH)₂D₃ (10nM, 24h) (Figure 2). Interestingly, whole PTH (100ng/ml) only stimulated 1,25(OH)₂D₃ production in HCD cells. In contrast the activity of 24-OHase was significantly stimulated by 1,25(OH)₂D₃ in HKC-8 cells, but was unaffected by any other treatment in either cell line (Figure 2).

Incubation in medium containing 0.5mM calcium (normal medium calcium concentration = 1mM) significantly up-regulated 1α-OHase activity (Figure 3). In the HKC-8 cells this was a transient response. Maximal stimulation was seen by 4h with levels returning to basal levels after 24h. In contrast, low calcium stimulation of 1α-OHase in HCD cells induced a maximal response at 4h, which was sustained at 24h. Northern and Western blot analyses confirmed the presence of CaR mRNA and protein. In addition to an appropriately sized band of approximately 120 kDa, HCD cells also appeared to express a larger protein species (data not shown).

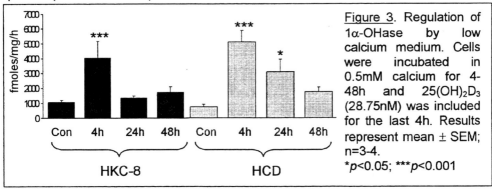

Figure 3. Regulation of 1α-OHase by low calcium medium. Cells were incubated in 0.5mM calcium for 4-48h and 25(OH)₂D₃ (28.75nM) was included for the last 4h. Results represent mean ± SEM; n=3-4.
*$p<0.05$; ***$p<0.001$

The most striking induction of 1α-OHase activity was observed in the HCD cells following incubation with LPS (1μg/ml). Activity was induced 5 fold after 24h incubation and was further elevated to 24 fold after 48h. In contrast LPS elicited only a small (2.5 fold), non-significant induction in HKC-8 cells (Figure 4).

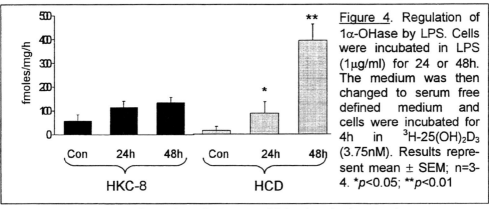

Figure 4. Regulation of 1α-OHase by LPS. Cells were incubated in LPS (1μg/ml) for 24 or 48h. The medium was then changed to serum free defined medium and cells were incubated for 4h in ³H-25(OH)₂D₃ (3.75nM). Results represent mean ± SEM; n=3-4. *$p<0.05$; **$p<0.01$

Discussion: Until recently, analysis of the expression and function of 1α-OHase in the kidney has been limited. We have now demonstrated that as well as expression of 1α-OHase mRNA and protein, 1α-OHase activity can be detected in cells from the distal nephron. This activity was stimulated by PTH and inhibited by 1,25(OH)$_2$D$_3$. Previous studies by our group have demonstrated the direct regulation of 1α-OHase by medium calcium concentration in HKC-8 cells [7]. We have now demonstrated that calciotropic signalling is an important regulator of 1α-OHase activity throughout the nephron. It has been recently shown that the expression of CD14 molecules is greater in the distal nephron, than in the proximal region [8]. As predicted the distal HCD cells were more responsive to LPS, than the HKC-8 cells. The induction of 1α-OHase activity seen in the HCD cells following treatment was striking, with a 24 fold induction after 48h treatment, demonstrating that in addition to calciotropic signalling 1α-OHase activity is also regulated via an immunological pathway.

The precise function of 1α-OHase in different areas of the nephron remains to be determined. However, the lower basal expression of 1α-OHase coupled with the high 24-OHase activity in the distal cells suggests that 1,25(OH)$_2$D$_3$ production is under a much stronger feedback control than in the proximal tubules. We would propose that 1α-OHase activity in the distal nephron maybe involved with local responses rather than the endocrine effects associated with the proximal tubule.

References:
1. Takeyama, K.,Kitanaka, S., Sato, T., Kobori, M., Yanagisawa, J. and Kato, S. (1997) Science 77, 1827-1830.
2. Fu, G.K., Lin, D., Zhang, M.Y., Bikle, D.D., Shackleton, C.H., Miller, W.L. and Portale, A.A (1997) Mol. Endocrinol. 11, 1961-1970.
3. Monkawa, T., Yoshida, T., Wakino, S., Shinki, T., Anazawa, H., DeLuca, H.F., Suda, T., Hayashi, M. and Saruta, T. (1997) Biochem. Biophys. Res. Commun. 239, 527-533.
4. Zehnder, D., Bland, R., Walker, E.A., Bradwell, A.R., Howie, A.J., Hewison, M. and Stewart, P.M. (1999) J. Am. Soc. Nephrol. 10, 2465-2473.
5. Racusen, L.C., Monteil, C., Sgrignoli, A., Lucskay, M., Marouillat, S., Rhim, J.G.S. and Morin, J.P. (1997) J. Lab. Clin. Med. 129, 318-329.
6. Prie, D., Friedlander, G., Coureau, C., Vandewalle, A., Cassingena, R. and Ronco, P.M. (1995) Kidney Int. 47, 1310-1318.
7. Bland, R., Walker, E.A., Hughes, S.V., Stewart, P.M. and Hewison, M. (1999) Endocrinology. 140, 2027-2034.
8. Yang, T., Sun, D., Huang, Y.G., Smart, A., Briggs, J.P., and Schnermann, J.B. (1999) Am. J. Physiol. 276, F10-F16.

Acknowledgements: This work was supported by a Fellowship award from the National Kidney Research Fund to R. Bland.

EVIDENCE THAT 1,25-DIHYDROXYVITAMIN D₃ SYNTHESIS BY HUMAN PLACENTA IS MEDIATED BY A MITOCHONDRIAL CYTOCHROME P450-DEPENDENT STEROID HYDROXYLASE

Lorenza Díaz, Irene Sánchez, Euclides Avila, Ali Halhali, Felipe Vilchis and Fernando Larrea. Department of Reproductive Biology, Instituto Nacional de la Nutrición Salvador Zubirán, Mexico City, Mexico, 14000.

Introduction Synthesis of 1,25-dihydroxyvitamin D3 ($1,25$-$(OH)_2D_3$), or calcitriol, is the result of a renal 25-hydroxyvitamin D_3 1α-hydroxylase (1α-(OH)ase), a mitochondrial cytochrome P_{450} enzyme. The first observation leading to the establishment of an extrarrenal source of 1α-(OH)ase was in pregnant rats (1). In fact, it has been shown that decidual cells synthesize calcitriol during pregnancy (2). Although *in vitro* studies provided evidence that in addition to human decidua, placental trophoblasts produced $1,25$-$(OH)_2D_3$ (1,2), a number of investigators have been unable to demonstrate a consistent and detectable production of calcitriol by these cells (3,4). Hollis et al (5) have suggested that calcitriol produced by human placenta, is the result of a free radical chemistry rather than an enzymatic-driven 1α-hydroxylation reaction. In contrast, and in agreement with earlier observations (6,7), we have recently shown (8) that human syncytiotrophoblast cells in culture were able to synthesize calcitriol from 25OHD₃. This conversion was significantly enhanced by insulin-like growth factor I, and blocked by the protein synthesis inhibitor cycloheximide, which suggested a hormonally regulated, protein-dependent hydroxylation reaction. These findings are of importance, since 1α-(OH)ase gene expression has not yet been detectable in the human placenta (9,10,11). Herein, we report the presence, in cultured human syncytiotrophoblast cells of a 1α-(OH)ase gene transcription product with identical nucleotide sequence to transcripts previously characterized in the human kidney.

Results The trophoblast cell culture technique has proven to be a good experimental model to study placental metabolism *in vitro* (12). In this study, the cell culture used was characterized by it's ability to secrete human chorionic gonadotrophin and to respond to 8-bromo-cAMP stimulation (8). Since initial attempts to identify 1α-(OH)ase gene products from the human placenta were unsuccessful (9,10), we decided to use cultured syncytiotrophoplasts as the source of RNA. Northern blots using a ^{32}P-298 bp 1α-(OH)ase probe, synthesized by PCR from human embryonic kidney (HEK 293) cells, were performed. This approach allowed us to detect a single band similar in size (2.5 kb) to the one obtained from human kidney HEK 293 cells and decidua. (Fig.1).

These results prompted us to enrich RNA by RT-PCR/Southern blot. Fig. 2 shows a 543-bp 1α-(OH)ase RT-PCR product obtained from both syncytiotrophoblast and HEK 293 cells (Fig 2, lane 2 and 4, respectively). These RT-PCR products were further amplified and sequenced. As control for reverse transcription reactions, the ubiquitous cyclophilin mRNA was also amplified. In the absence of RT, none of the RNA samples from syncytiotrophoblast cells gave positive results (Fig. 2, lane 3). Similar data were obtained when human genomic DNA was used instead of RNA (Fig. 2, lane 1).

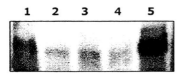

Figure 1. Northern blot analysis of 1α-(OH)ase mRNA from HEK 293 (lane 1), syncytiotrophoblast (lanes 2-4) and decidua cells (lane 5) hybridized with a 1α-(OH)ase probe.

Figure 2. RT-PCR / Southern blot analysis of 1α-(OH)ase mRNA. 1) Genomic DNA, 2) trophoblast cDNA, 3) trophoblast RNA (no RT) and 4) HEK 293 cDNA.

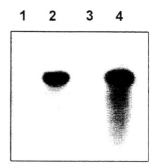

The 543-bp nucleotide sequence was found to be 100% identical, over all the nucleotides flanked by the PCR primers, to the human 1α-(OH)ase cDNA clones contained in the GeneBank (data not shown). The complete 1α-(OH)ase cDNA sequence consists of 2469-bp (10). The fragment reported herein is located within 706- and 1248-bp sections of the full-length cDNA. Identical results were obtained when the 543-bp RT-PCR fragment from HEK 293 cells was sequenced.

In order to study the temporal pattern of expression of 1α-(OH)ase mRNA throughout culture, total cellular RNA was obtained at different times from plating and prepared for Northern blots. As shown in Fig. 3, it was demonstrated that 1α-(OH)ase mRNA is expressed at all culture times, including in the less differentiated Percoll gradient-purified cytotrophoblast cells taken as representatives of day zero of culture. The relative levels of 1α-(OH)ase mRNA expression showed a gradual increase of transcription of the 1α-(OH)ase gene (CYP27B1) up to 96 h of culture (Fig. 3C).

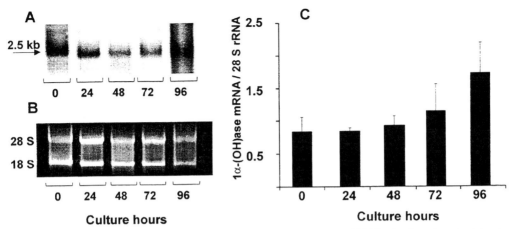

Figure 3. Temporal expression of 1α-(OH)ase mRNA during trophoblast culture. (A) Northern blot. 30 μg of RNA were loaded in 1.2% agarose gel, transferred and hybridized with a 1α-(OH)ase probe. (B) Ethidium bromide stained gel. C) Relative optical density of 1α (OH)ase mRNA vs. 28 S RNA.

Activity of 1α-(OH)ase was also assessed in placental cultures by their ability to convert $[^3H]25OHD_3$ into $[^3H]1,25-(OH)_2D_3$. Cells at various times of plating were incubated in the presence of substrate. Analysis of samples using two-step straight phase HPLC (8) showed the presence of a more polar metabolite that co-eluted as a single peak with authentic unlabeled $1,25-(OH)_2D_3$ (data not shown). As depicted in Fig. 4, the amount of putative $[^3H]1,25-(OH)_2D_3$ formed by syncytiotrophoblasts significantly increased (P < 0.001) at the second and fourth day of culture.

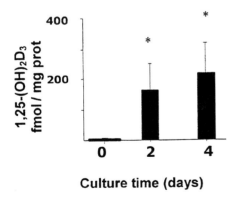

Figure 4. Synthesis of $[^3H]1,25-(OH)_2D_3$ by cultured syncytiotrophoblasts. Cells were incubated in the presence of $[^3H]25OHD_3$ and the conversion products were separated by HPLC. Each bar represents the mean ± SD of three independent cultures. *p<0.001 vs time zero.

Discussion The placental production of $1,25-(OH)_2D_3$ has been clearly established by many investigators; nevertheless, there is a discrepancy regarding the nature of trophoblastic $25OHD_3$ 1α-hydroxylation. In the present study, we were able to detect a specific *CYP27B1* gene product, coding for 1α-(OH)ase in the human trophoblast. The level of transcription correlated with the 1α-hydroxylation enzymatic activity in culture. Taken together, these data establish for the first time the presence of 1α-(OH)ase enzyme in the human trophoblast independently of the cell differentiation stage in culture. The overall data support recent observations from our laboratory suggesting that conversion of [^{3}H]25OHD$_3$ to [^{3}H]1,25-(OH)$_2$D$_3$ in cultured placenta is attributed to an enzymatic 1α-hydroxylation reaction.

Acknowledgments This work was supported by grants from the National Council of Science and Technology (CONACyT, México), and the Special Programme for Research, Development and Research Training in Human Reproduction of the World Health Organization (Geneva, Switzerland).

References

1. Weisman, Y., Vargas, A., Duckett, G., Reiter, E., and Root, A.W., (1978) Endocrinology 103, 1992-1996.
2. Weisman, Y., Harell, A., Edelstein, S., David, M., Spirer, Z., and Golander, A. (1979) Nature 281, 317-319.
3. Delvin, E.E., Arabian, A., Glorieux, F.H., and Mamer, O.A. (1985) J. Clin. Endocrinol. Metab. 60, 880-885.
4. Rubin, L.P., Yeung, B., Vouros, P., Vilner, L.M., and Reddy, G.S. (1993) Pediatr. Res. 34, 98-104.
5. Hollis, B.W., Iskersky, V.N., and Chang, M.K. (1989) Endocrinology 125, 1224-1230.
6. Zerwekh, J.E., and Breslau, N.A. (1986) J. Clin. Endocrinol. Metab. 62, 192-196.
7. Whitsett, J.A., Ho, M., Tsang, R.C., Norman, E.J., and Adams, K.G. (1981) J. Clin. Endocrinol. Metab. 53, 484-488.
8. Halhali, A., Díaz, L., Sánchez, I., Garabédian, M., Bourges, H., and Larrea, F. (1999) Mol. Hum. Reprod. 5, 771-776.
9. Fu, G.K., Lin, D., Zhang, M.Y.H., Bikle, D.D., Shackleton, C.H.L., Miller, W.L. and Portale, A.A. (1997) Mol. Endocrinol. 11, 1961-1970.
10. Monkawa, T., Yoshida T., Wakino, S., Shinki, T., Anazawa, H., DeLuca, H.F., Suda, T., Hayashi, M., and Saruta, T. (1997) Biochem. Biophys. Res. Commun. 239, 527-533
11. Takeyama, K., Kitanaka, S., Sato, T., Kobori, M., Yanagisawa, J., and Kato, S. (1997) Science 277, 1827-1830.
12. Kliman, H.J., Nestler, J.E., Sermasi, E., Sanger, J.M., and Strauss III, J.F. (1986) Endocrinology 118, 1567-1582.
13. Stephanou, A., Ross, R., and Handwerger, S. (1994) Endocrinology 135, 2651-2656.
14. Bouillon, R., Okamura, W.H., and Norman, A.W. (1995) Endocr. Rev. 16, 200-257.

MOLECULAR BASIS OF PSEUDO VITAMIN D-DEFICIENCY RICKETS (PDDR) IN THE HANNOVER PIG MODEL.

L. Chavez, J. Harmeyer, S Choe and J. Omdahl Department of Biochemistry and Molecular Biology, University of New Mexico School of Medicine, Albuquerque, NM USA 87131 and Department of Physiology, School of Veterinary Medicine, 30173, Hannover, Germany.

Introduction

Genetic breading in pigs during the 1960's resulted in the generation of porcine strains that expressed a rachitic phenotype (1,2) that was similar to the human correlate "hereditary rickets" described initially by Prader *et al.*, in 1961 (3). This human genetic disorder was subsequently differentiated into two types of vitamin D resistance. One disorder involved low circulating levels of 1,25-dihydroxyvitamin D3 [$1,25(OH)_2D_3$] that was proposed to be the result of a defective 1-OHase enzyme. The disease was named type I vitamin D-dependency rickets, type I, or pseduo vitamin D-deficiency rickets (PDDR) and localized to chromosome 12q13-14 (4,5). The second genetic disease was associated with target-organ resistance to $1,25(OH)_2D_3$ due to defects in the vitamin D receptor (VDR) transcription factor, and was named vitamin D-dependent rickets, type II, or hereditary vitamin D-resistant rickets (HVDRR) (6).

Studies into the molecular basis of PDDR has been made possible by the recent cloning of the 1-OHase enzyme (5,7-9). Based upon its sequence and functional-domain analysis, the 1-OHase was found to be a member of the mitochondrial cytochrome P450 family of mixed-function oxidases, and was subsequently named cytochrome P450c1 (CYP27B1). Possible mutations in the human P450c1 has been evaluated in different populations of PDDR patients in which numerous point mutations (9-12) and deletions (13) were detected and found to be associated with a dysfunctional enzyme. Based upon the enzyme mutational data and chromosome 12 FISH analysis (5), it was possible to document the basis of PDDR as a functional defect in cytochrome P450c1. A similar molecular approach was used in the current communication to clone the pig P450c1 and use the attendant sequence information to analyze the molecular basis for PDDR in the Hannover piglet model (14,15).

Methods and Procedures

RNA Samples: Total RNA was obtained from quick-frozen tissue that was extracted using TRIzol reagent (Life Technologies). Wild-type tissue was obtained from vitamin D deficient weanling pigs (R. Horst) and PDDR tissues were obtained from three homozygous Hannover PDDR piglets. RNA was quantitated by uv spectrometry and tested for integrity using intactness of the 18S/28S ribosome bands.

RT-PCR and Cloning: RNA samples were reversed transcribed (RT) using AMV-RT (Promega). PCR products were derived from the RT first-strand cDNA product using one forward-primer and two reverse nested-primers that encompassed the full-coding sequence. PCR was conducted using Platinum Taq (Life Technologies) and a hemi-nested protocol. PCR products were cloned into pCR-Script (Stratagene) and positive inserts subcloned into pcDNAIII (Invitrogen) for expression in MA10 cells or pTrcA99 (Pharmacia) for bacterial expression.

Sequence Analysis: Cloned products were PCR amplified with Taq polymerase (Promega) and sequenced using BigDye terminator technology and an ABI Prisim 377 DNA Analyzer (Applied Biosystems). Sequence data for PDDR samples were compared to pig wild-type reference data using the GCG program (Wisconsin Package) and FastA subroutine.

Results

Using RT-PCR technology, a full-length clone was obtained for pig P450c1, which was highly similar to a previously reported sequence (16) with no apparent intraspecies variance. The DNA sequence coded for a 504 amino acid protein with a typical mitochondrial P450 architecture. Estimates of P450c1 mRNA levels for PDDR samples revealed induced expression levels that approximated the values seen in mRNA from vitamin D-deficient pigs highly induced for P450c1 (data not shown).

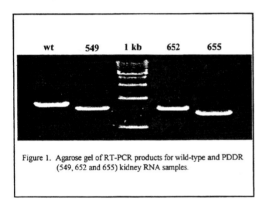

Figure 1. Agarose gel of RT-PCR products for wild-type and PDDR (549, 652 and 655) kidney RNA samples.

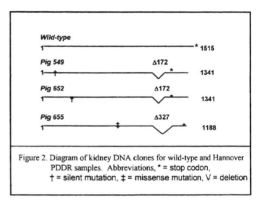

Figure 2. Diagram of kidney DNA clones for wild-type and Hannover PDDR samples. Abbreviations, * = stop codon, † = silent mutation, ‡ = missense mutation, V = deletion

RT-PCR analysis for P450c1 coding sequences in RNA samples from three Hannover pig kidney tissues demonstrated significantly smaller products than obtained with full-length wild type sample (Fig. 1). The PCR products from the Hannover PDDR samples were determined to have two deletion-types, both beginning at nucleotide 950. Two PDDR pigs (549 and 652) had 172 bp deletions between nts 950 and 1123 that gave a 1341 bp PCR product when using the primer sets for full-length P450c1. In a similar manner, the third PDDR pig sample (655) had a 327 bp deletion between nts 950 and 1280 resulting in an 1188 bp PCR product (Fig. 1). In addition to the deletions, two silent mutations were detected in the 1341 bp products and a missense mutation (V223A) in the 1188 bp PCR product (Fig. 2). As a result of the coding-region deletions, a frameshift occurred in each P450c1 coding region that resulted in nonsense *opal* mutations and expression of a premature stop codon. Consequently, the shortened and truncated coding regions gave predicted protein products of 337 aa for the 1341 bp mutant

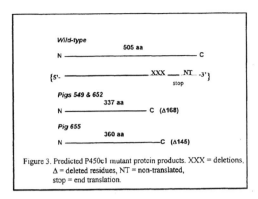

Figure 3. Predicted P450c1 mutant protein products. XXX = deletions, Δ = deleted residues, NT = non-translated, stop = end translation.

and a longer 360 aa product for the shorter 1188 bp deletion product (Fig. 3). The same mutants were observed for bone P450c1 mRNAs obtained from the Hannover PDDR animals (data not shown).

Discussion

To date, mutations associated with human PDDR have involved predominantly missense mutations, although one report has documented an insertion mutation leading to a premature nonsense stop codon (13). However, the current study describes studies in the Hannover PDDR piglet model in which two new deletion mutations were documented for the kidney P450c1 enzyme. Although not detected previously in cytochrome P450c1, deletion mutants have been noted for a dysfunctional form of cytochrome P450c21 (17).

The two deletions in the P450c1 mutants had identical 5'-break points but different 3'-break points. When compared to the human and rat *P450c1* genes, the common break points would be predicted to occur within exon 5 near its 3'- splice site. The 3'-break points for the two deletions would be predicted to occur in exons 6 and 7, with both breaks occurring near their respective 3'-splice sites. It is possible, therefore, that the deletions were derived as a result of erroneous exon:intron splicing reactions. But such a possibility must await genomic studies on the pig *P450c1* gene.

The cytochrome P450c1 enzyme is a highly complex hemoprotein that facilitates the generation of an active oxyferryl heme-center that is used in the specific 1-hydroxylation of a substrate molecule. A single mutation can render the enzyme inactive. Therefore, it is quite reasonable that the truncated PDDR enzyme would lack catalytic function due to its loss of critical domains associated with heme binding, oxygen activation, substrate binding and conformational integrity. Indeed, these animals respond to $1,25(OH)_2D_3$ therapy but not to physiological levels of vitamin D or $25(OH)D_3$. Recognizing the diversity of mutations in P450c1, it is interesting to note that the enzyme's chromosome 12 localization in near the chromosome 12 locus for the *VDR* gene, which also displays a host of mutations. In contrast, no mutations have been documented for cytochrome P450c24 on chromosome 20. Mutations in cytochrome P450c24 would seemingly be documented due to predicted lesions in bone growth and mineralization, which could suggest a low incidence of occurrence. It would be of fundamental interest, therefore, to investigate whether chromosome 12 has a mutational "hot spot" within its q13-14 region

Reference List

1. Plonait, H. (1969) *Zentralbl.Veterinarmed.[A]* 16, 289-316.
2. Meyer, H. and Plonait, H. (1968) *Zentralbl.Veterinarmed.[A]* 15, 481-483
3. Prader, A., Illig, R., and Heierli, E. (1961) Eine bedondere Form der primaren Vitamin D resistenten Rachitis mit Hypocalcamie und autosomal-dominantem Erbgang. Helvetica Paediatrica Acta 16, 452-468.
4. Labuda, M., Fujiwara, T. M., Ross, M. V., Morgan, K., Garcia-Heras, J., Ledbetter, D. H., Hughes, M. R., and Glorieux, F. H. (1992) *J.Bone Miner.Res.* 7, 1447-1453.
5. St Arnaud, R., Messerlian, S., Moir, J. M., Omdahl, J. L., and Glorieux, F. H. (1997) *J.Bone Miner.Res.* 12, 1552-1559.
6. Malloy, P. J., Pike, J. W., and Feldman, D. (1997) Hereditary 1,25-Dihydroxyvitamin D Resistant Rickets. In Feldman, D., Glorieux, F. H., and Pike, J. W., editors. *Vitamin D*, Acadmic Press, San Diego.
7. Nakamura, Y., Eto, T. A., Taniguchi, T., Miyamoto, K., Nagatomo, J., Shiotsuki, H., Sueta, H., Higashi, S., Okuda, K. I., and Setoguchi, T. (1997) *FEBS Lett.* 419, 45-48.
8. Takeyama, K., Kitanaka, S., Sato, T., Kobori, M., Yanagisawa, J., and Kato, S. (1997) *Science* 277, 1827-1830.
9. Fu, G. K., Lin, D., Zhang, M. Y., Bikle, D. D., Shackleton, C. H., Miller, W. L., and Portale, A. A. (1997) *Mol.Endocrinol.* 11, 1961-1970.
10. Kitanaka, S., Takeyama, K., Murayama, A., Sato, T., Okumura, K., Nogami, M., Hasegawa, Y., Niimi, H., Yanagisawa, J., Tanaka, T., and Kato, S. (1998) *N.Engl.J.Med.* **338,** 653-661.
11. Yoshida, T., Monkawa, T., Tenenhouse, H. S., Goodyer, P., Shinki, T., Suda, T., Wakino, S., Hayashi, M., and Saruta, T. (1998) *Kidney Int.* 54, 1437-1443.
12. Wang, J. T., Lin, C. J., Burridge, S. M., Fu, G. K., Labuda, M., Portale, A. A., and Miller, W. L. (1998) *Am.J.Hum.Genet.* 63, 1694-1702.
13. Smith, S. J., Rucka, A. K., Berry, J. L., Davies, M., Mylchreest, S., Paterson, C. R., Heath, D. A., Tassabehji, M., Read, A. P., Mee, A. P., and Mawer, E. B. (1999) *J.Bone Miner.Res.* 14, 730-739.
14. Kaune, R. and Harmeyer, J. (1987) *Acta Endocrinol.(Copenh)* 115, 345-352.
15. Wilke, R., Harmeyer, J., von Grabe, C., Hehrmann, R., and Hesch, R. D. (1979) *Acta Endocrinol.(Copenh)* 92, 295-308.
16. Yoshida, T., Yoshida, N., Nakamura, A., Monkawa, T., Hayashi, M., and Saruta, T. (1999) *J.Am.Soc.Nephrol.* 10, 963-970.
17. Strumberg, D., Hauffa, B. P., Horsthemke, B., and Grosse-Wilde, H. 1992) *Eur.J.Pediatr.* 151, 821-826.p

RESPONSE SPECIFIC EFFECTS OF 24-HYDROXYLATION FOR 1,25-DIHYDROXYVITAMIN D_3 ACTION IN HUMAN OSTEOBLASTS

Gert-Jan C.M. van den Bemd, Cok J. Buurman, Huibert A.P. Pols, Johannes P.T.M. van Leeuwen, Department of Internal Medicine, Erasmus Medical Center Rotterdam, PO BOX 1738, 3000 DR Rotterdam, The Netherlands

Introduction: The effect of the biologically most active vitamin D_3 metabolite, 1,25-dihydroxyvitamin D_3 (1,25$(OH)_2D_3$) on bone resorption is well known. Furthermore, 1,25$(OH)_2D_3$ has multiple stimulatory effects on osteoblasts (e.g. osteocalcin, osteopontin, alkaline phosphatase, transforming growth factor ß). In addition to the indirect effect on bone formation via stimulation of intestinal calcium absorption, 1,25$(OH)_2D_3$ might have direct anabolic effects on bone.

24-Hydroxylation is considered as a major step in the catabolic pathway of 1,25$(OH)_2D_3$. However, there are indications that some of the metabolites of 1,25$(OH)_2D_3$ also have biological potency. In the present study, we investigated the impact of 24-hydroxylation of 1,25$(OH)_2D_3$ by studying the effect of 1,24,25-trihydroxyvitamin D_3 (1,24,25$(OH)_3D_3$) on the growth and differentiation of SV-40 transfected human fetal osteoblasts (SV-HFO).

Materials & methods: SV-HFO were cultured in 10 cm^2 dishes for up to 21 days. Three days after seeding treatment was started with medium replacement and addition of 1,25$(OH)_2D_3$ and/or 1,24,25$(OH)_3D_3$ every two or three days. After 7 (proliferative phase), 14 (matrix maturation phase), and 21 (mineralization phase) days of culture cells were analyzed for: DNA content, alkaline phosphatase activity, calcium deposition in the extracellular matrix, and osteocalcin concentration in the medium. Note: Day 7, 14, and 21 implicates a treatment period of 4, 11, and 18 days, respectively.

180

Results and Discussion:

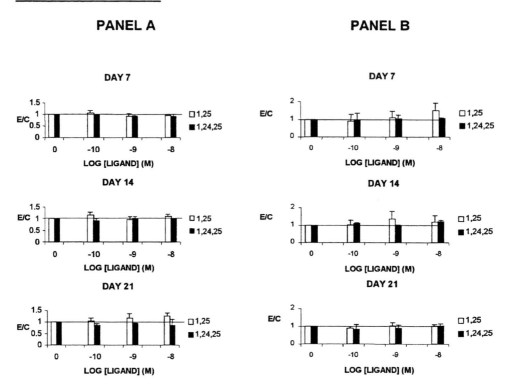

Figure 1: DNA content (Panel A) and alkaline phosphatase activity (Panel B) at 7, 14, and 21 days of culture.

After 18 days of 1,25(OH)$_2$D$_3$ treatment (21 days of culture) the DNA content was slightly increased. 1,24,25(OH)$_3$D$_3$ alone had no effect. In the combination experiments the effect of 1,25(OH)$_2$D$_3$ was not affected by 1,24,25(OH)$_3$D$_3$ (data not shown).

After 7, and 14 days of culture the alkaline phosphatase activity was increased in the 1,25(OH)$_2$D$_3$-treated cells. 1,24,25(OH)$_3$D$_3$ had no effect. In the combination experiments the effect of 1,25(OH)$_2$D$_3$ was not affected by 1,24,25(OH)$_3$D$_3$ (data not shown).

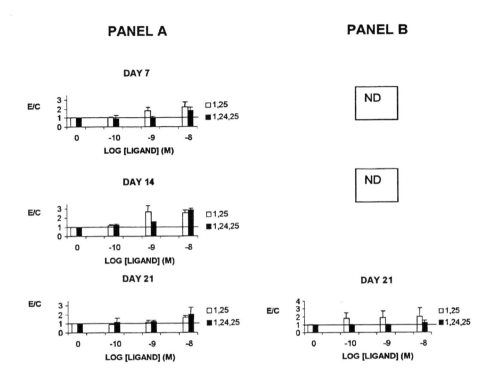

Figure 2: Osteocalcin synthesis (Panel A) and calcium deposition (Panel B).
After 7, 14, and 21 days of culture, osteocalcin secretion was increased in the medium of $1,25(OH)_2D_3$- or $1,24,25(OH)_3D_3$-treated cells. In the combination experiments the effect of $1,25(OH)_2D_3$ was not affected by $1,24,25(OH)_3D_3$ (data not shown).
After 7 and 14 days of culture no mineralization of the extracellular matrix could be observed (ND). After 21 days of culture, calcium deposition was increased in the $1,25(OH)_2D_3$-treated cells. $1,24,25(OH)_3D_3$ had no effect on calcium deposition. In the combination experiments the effect of $1,25(OH)_2D_3$ was not affected by $1,24,25(OH)_3D_3$ (data not shown).

$1,25(OH)_2D_3$ has direct anabolic effects on human osteoblasts: stimulation of alkaline phosphatase activity, stimulation of osteocalcin synthesis, and stimulation of calcification of the extracellular matrix formed. The effects of $1,25(OH)_2D_3$ are dependent on osteoblast differentiation (e.g. alkaline phosphatase activity, mineralization). The 24-hydroxylated metabolite of $1,25(OH)_2D_3$ displays a response-specific activity. It loses its stimulatory activity on alkaline phosphatase activity, DNA, and calcium deposition, while the stimulatory effect on osteocalcin is preserved. This implicates that 24-hydroxylation is not merely a step in the degradation of $1,25(OH)_2D_3$ and that various responses of $1,25(OH)_2D_3$ may be differently affected by 24-hydroxylation.

CONSTITUTIVE ACTIVITY OF 1α-HYDROXYLASE IN PRIMARY HUMAN KERATINOCYTES, REVEALED BY SELECTIVE INHIBITION OF CYP24.

I.Schuster[1], H.Egger[2], G.Herzig[2], G.S.Reddy[3], M.Schüssler[2], G.Vorisek[2]. [1]Institut für Theoretische Chemie und Molekulare Strukturbiologie, University Vienna, A-1090. [2]Novartis Research Institute, A-1235 Vienna. [3]Women&Infant's Hospital, Brown University Providence, RI 02905-2499, USA.

Introduction   Primary cultures of human keratinocytes (PHK) convert 25(OH)D$_3$ to hormonally active 1α,25(OH)$_2$D$_3$ (1,2). 1α,25(OH)$_2$D$_3$ rapidly induces 24-hydroxylase (CYP24) and becomes metabolized by it, yielding a cascade of transient, eventually inactive products (C-24 oxidation pathway (3,4)). On induction of CYP24, generation of 1α,25(OH)$_2$D$_3$ from 25(OH)D$_3$ apparently ceases and hormone levels dramatically decline (2). It is generally assumed that 1α,25(OH)$_2$D$_3$ causes a massive down-regulation of 1α-hydroxylase. Our group intensively worked on a program that aimed at the identification of strong, selective inhibitors of CYP24 (5). Testing several of these compounds in PHK, we surprisingly observed that inhibition of CYP24 led to continuing 1α-hydroxylation of ^{3}H-25(OH)D$_3$ over extended time periods (6). This paper describes a set of experiments designed to study whether 1α,25(OH)$_2$D$_3$ might have a direct regulatory effect on 1α-hydroxylase activity and its expression at the mRNA level.

•Effect of exogenous 1α,25(OH)$_2$D$_3$ on 1α-hydroxylation of ^{3}H-25(OH)D$_3$. In order to test whether 1α,25(OH)$_2$D$_3$ directly inhibited 1α-hydroxylase activity or whether commencing

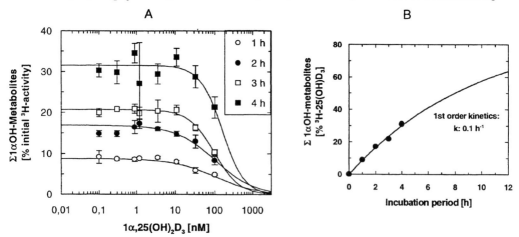

Figure 1. 1α-Hydroxylation of ^{3}H-25(OH)D$_3$ in the presence of exogenous 1α,25(OH)$_2$D$_3$. Incubations with 20 nM [26,27n-^{3}H]-25(OH)D$_3$ were done in KGM at 0.06mM calcium for the indicated time periods. Then, lipophilic incubation extracts were analyzed by HPLC on Zorbax-Sil (5). A: In the presence of cold 1α,25(OH)$_2$D$_3$ (0.1 - 100 nM) only weak inhibition of 1α-hydroxylase was noticed (IC$_{50}$ ≥100 nM; determined by the GRAFIT IC$_{50}$-software). B: Σ1α-hydroxylated metabolites increased according to first order kinetics (curves calculated by the GRAFIT-rate software). Data ±SD (n = 4).

CYP24 induction would be accompanied by down-regulation of 1α-hydroxylase, we incubated PHK with ^{3}H-25(OH)D$_3$ in the presence of unlabeled 1α,25(OH)$_2$D$_3$ (at a range overing and exceeding presumptive physiological concentrations) for 1-4 h. Lipophilic extracts of incubations were analyzed by sensitive HPLC with on-line ^{3}H-activity detection, ccording to (5). Up to 2 h incubation, [3]H-1α,25(OH)$_2$D$_3$ and [3]H-1α,25(OH)$_2$-3-epi-D$_3$ were he predominant products in metabolite profiles, after 3 h sequential products arising from ommencing CYP24 oxidation were identified. For determination of 1α-hydroxylase ctivity, we added all 1α-hydroxylated metabolites (= Σ1αOH-metabolites), according to 5). Figure 1 clearly demonstrates that 1α,25(OH)$_2$D$_3$ did not directly affect 1α-hydroxylase ctivity unless far higher concentrations than presumptive physiological levels (in skin) vere used (IC$_{50}$ = 101.05 ± 3.17 nM (n=8)). Moreover, 1α-hydroxylation continued over he tested incubation period, closely following first order kinetics. Therefore, we could rule ut direct inhibition of 1α-hydroxylase by 1α,25(OH)$_2$D$_3$ and down-regulation of 1α-ydroxylase at starting CYP24 induction.

Selective inhibition of CYP24 reveals persisting 1α-hydroxylation in PHK. HPLC profiles f lipid extracts from incubations with [3]H-25(OH)D$_3$ showed a transient time course of 1α-ydroxylated products (peaking at 2 -3 h), due to their rapid CYP24-catalyzed conversion o polar metabolites (Figure 2). This was revealed by using VID400, a strong, selective nhibitor of CYP24 discovered in our laboratory (IC$_{50}$ around 15 nM, (5)). Inhibition of CYP24 led to an unmasking of lipophilic 1α-hydroxylated products that continued for ≥ 8 , following 1st order kinetics. At the depicted high VID 400 concentrations, impairment of α-hydroxylase activity (by 20% and 60%) was in accordance with the respective IC$_{50}$-alue (616 nM).

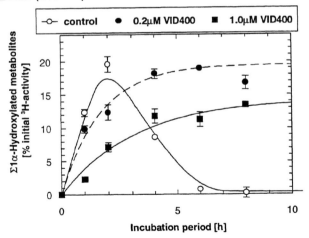

Figure 2. In the presence of VID400, a selective CYP24 inhibitor, 1α-hydroxylation of [3]H-25(OH)D$_3$ continues for ≥ 8 h. Incubations of PHK with 20 nM [26,27n-^{3}H]-25(OH)D$_3$ were done in KGM at 0.06mM calcium for the indicated time periods, in absence and presence of VID400. Then, lipophilic incubation extracts were analyzed by HPLC on Zorbax-Sil (5). In presence of VID400, Σ1α-hydroxylated metabolites increased according to first order kinetics (curves calculated by the GRAFIT-rate software). Representative data ±SD from 1 out of 5 independent studies.

Preincubation with 1α,25(OH)$_2$D$_3$ does not lead to a substantial reduction of 1α-ydroxylase activity in PHK. After proving that 1α,25(OH)$_2$D$_3$ - endogenously produced rom 25(OH)D$_3$ or exogenously added - did not down-regulate 1α-hydroxylase within a eriod of ≥ 8 h, we checked whether a prolonged pre-treatment (24 h) with 20 nM α,25(OH)$_2$D$_3$ might lead to a substantial decrease of 1α-hydroxylase. 1α-hydroxylase ctivity was determined in a subsequent incubation with [3]H-25(OH)D$_3$ for 1 h. Under these onditions, pre-incubation with vehicle resulted in a 12% conversion of [3]H-25(OH)D$_3$ to α,25(OH)$_2$D$_3$ and its 3-epimer (data not shown). After pre-treatment with 1α,25(OH)$_2$D$_3$ an lmost identical extent of 1α-hydroxylation was noticed, however, for still remaining CYP24 activity 1α,25(OH)$_2$D$_3$ levels were reduced in expense of its sequential 24-

hydroxylated metabolites (Figure 3). When CYP24 activity was inhibited by VID400, $1\alpha,25(OH)_2D_3$ levels almost equaled untreated controls; VID400 reduced 1α-hydroxylase only slightly (by 20%, see also Figure 2).

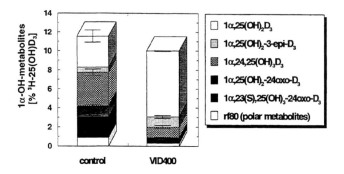

Figure 3..1α-Hydroxylation of ^3H-25(OH)D$_3$ after 24 h pre-treatment with $1\alpha,25(OH)_2D_3$. PHK were pre-treated with 20nM $1\alpha,25(OH)_2D_3$ for 24h, thereafter washed and incubated wih 20nM ^3H-25(OH)D$_3$ in absence and presence of 200 nM VID400 for a further hour. 1α-Hydroxylation was determined from HPLC analyses of lipid extracts. Representative data (±SD) from 1 out of 30 independent studies.

● Rate-determining step of 25(OH)D$_3$ metabolism in PHK. Analyzing the time course of ^3H-25(OH)D$_3$ metabolism, first order kinetics was well-suited to fit experimental data (Figure 4A). In the initial phase (up tp 2 h), ^3H-25(OH)D$_3$ declined with the rate by which $1\alpha,25(OH)_2D_3$ was formed. In order to examine the effect of rising CYP24 activity on subsequent ^3H-25(OH)D$_3$ metabolism, we inhibited CYP24 by VID400, using concentrations that exceeded the IC_{50} for CYP24 (13fold and 65-fold). Compared to control incubations, VID400 caused only a slightly lower rate at 200 nM and about 60% reduction at 1μM. These rates did not reflect the massive suppression of CYP24 (checked

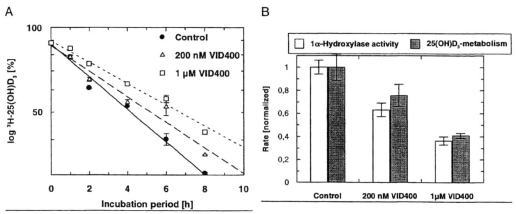

Figure 4. Time course of 20nM ^3H-25(OH)D$_3$ in PHK. Incubations were performed in KGM in the absence and presence of VID400. ^3H-25(OH)D$_3$ was quantified by HPLC-analyses of lipid extracts and its kinetics analyzed by the Grafit-rate software. A) Metabolism follows 1st order kinetics and does not reflect the massive inhibition of CYP24 by VID400, B) Activity of (normalized) 1α-hydroxylase parallels rate of 25(OH)D$_3$ decline. Representative data (±SD) from 1 out of 3 independent studies)

by HPLC-analysis), indicating that 24-hydroxylation was not rate-limiting in 25(OH)D$_3$ metabolism. However, the observed rates were in excellent agreement with the activity of α-hydroxylase in the absence and presence of VID400 (IC_{50} 616 nM (5)), pointing to a ate-determining role of this enzyme in 25(OH)D_3 metabolism.

Effect of pre-treatment with 1α,25(OH)$_2$D$_3$ on 1α-hydroxylase mRNA expression. Quantification of 1α-hydroxylase mRNA expression relative to GAPDH-mRNA was done by the new Real-Time RT PCR technique, as described (7). On treatment with vehicle, 1α-ydroxylase mRNA amounted to 0.67 (±0.06)% of GAPDH-mRNA after 5 h, and decreased to 0.51 (±0.06)% after 20 h. Figure 5 illustrates that extent and time course of α-hydroxylase mRNA expression were only slightly affected (20 -30%) by pre-treatment with 1α,25(OH)$_2$D$_3$. A down-regulation of 1α-hydroxylase mRNA was not observed on pre-treatment with the 1α,25(OH)$_2$D$_3$ precursor 25(OH)D$_3$ and D$_3$ either (7).

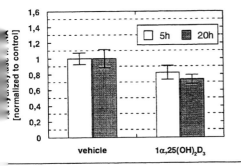

Figure 5. 1α-hydroxylase mRNA expression is not substantially reduced by pre-treatment of PHK with 1α,25(OH)$_2$D$_3$ PHK were incubated in KGM at 0.06 mM calcium with vehicle or 20 nM 1α,25(OH)$_2$D$_3$ for 5 and 20 h. Then, total RNA was extracted by the Trizol method and 500 ng samples subjected to Real-Time RT-PCR, on a ABI PRISM 7700 SDS (Perkin Elmer Applied Biosystem), using specific probes and primers for 1α-hydroxylase and GAPDH as reference (7). Data are means ± SD (n = 3), normalized to GAPDH in vehicle-treated controls.

Conclusions. The experiments decribed in this paper clearly demonstrate that 1α-ydroxylase is not inversely correlated with CYP24 in PHK. At (supra-)physiological evels,1α,25(OH)$_2$D$_3$, exogenously added or generated from 25(OH)D$_3$, did not down-regulate mRNA or activity of 1α-hydroxylase, suggesting its constitutive expression. The apparent decline of 1α-hydroxylated products of 25(OH)D$_3$ could be explained by their very fast 24-hydroxylation to polar products that escaped usual HPLC-analysis of organic xtracts. Effective reduction of CYP24 activity by VID400, a strong selective inhibitor of CYP24 revealed that 1α-hydroxylated metabolites were continuously formed. In a recent paper, we have shown expression of 25-hydroxylase (CYP27) in PHK that also was not modified by vitamin D-metabolites and the presence of 1α-hydroxylase and CYP27 in ntact epidermis too (7). Constitutive expression of both enzymes in skin enables a continuous generation of 1α,25(OH)$_2$D$_3$, suggesting a role as an important local hormone.

References
. Bikle, D.D., Nemanic M.K., Whitney J.O., Elias P.W. (1986) Biochemistry 25, 1545-1548.
. Bikle, D.D., Nemanic M.K., Gee E.A., Elias P.W. (1986) J.Clin.Invest. 78, 557-566.
. Reddy G.S., Tserng K.Y. (1989) Biochemistry 28, 1753-1769.
. Makin G., Lohnes D., Byford V., Ray R., Jones G. (1989) Biochem.J. 262, 173-180
. Schuster I,, Egger H., Bikle D., Herzig G., Reddy G.S., Stuetz A., Stuetz P., Vorisek G. (2000) Steroids, in press
. Schuster I,, Egger H., Astecker N., Herzig G., Schüssler M., Vorisek G. (2000) Steroids, in press
. Schüssler M., Astecker N., Herzig G., Vorisek G., Reddy G.S., Schuster I. (2000) Steroids, in press.

EXPRESSION OF 25-HYDROXYVITAMIN D$_3$-1α-HYDROXYLASE IN CERVICAL TISSUE

Jörg Reichrath[2], Michael Friedrich[1], Tai C. Chen[3], Ingrid Gherson[3], Wolfgang Tilgen[2], Werner Schmidt[1], Michael F. Holick[3]
[1]Department of Gynecology and [2]Dermatology, University of Saarland, D-66421 Homburg/Saar, Germany; and [3]Vitamin D, Skin and Bone Research Laboratory, Boston University Medical Center, 02118 Boston, MA, USA

Introduction: Epidemiological studies have suggested the association of 1,25-dihydroxyvitamin D$_3$ (1,25(OH)$_2$D$_3$) deficiency with an increased risk of various malignancies (1). The molecular mechanisms involved in this phenomenon are still unknown. *In vitro* studies have demonstrated that 1,25(OH)$_2$D$_3$ suppresses proliferation and induces differentiation in various cell types, including epithelial cells (2). It is generally thought that the antiproliferative effect is the result of a vitamin D receptor (VDR) mediated action on the genome (3). There are two principal enzymes involved in the formation of circulating 1,25(OH)$_2$D$_3$ from vitamin D, the hepatic microsomal or mitochondrial vitamin D 25-hydroxylase and the renal mitochondrial enzyme 1α-hydroxylase for vitamin D and 25-hydroxyvitamin D$_3$ (25(OH)D$_3$), respectively (4). These hydroxylases belong to a class of proteins known as cytochrome P450 mixed function monooxidases. Recently, extrarenal activity of 1α-hydroxylase for 25(OH)D$_3$ has been reported in various cell types includuding macrophages and keratinocytes (5). The aim of this study was to analyze the expression of 1α-hydroxylase for 25-hydroxyvitamin D$_3$ in normal cervical tissue and in cervical carcinomas on mRNA-level to evaluate whether cervical tissue possesses the capacity to produce 1,25(OH)$_2$D$_3$ from 25(OH)D$_3$ and whether metastatic cervical carcinomas may be a target for treatment with precursors of biologically active vitamin D analogues.

Materials and Methods: Biopsies from normal cervical tissue (n=4) were obtained from patients that underwent surgery for uterine leiomyomas. Histological examination by a certified pathologist confirmed normality. Biopsies from cervical carcinomas (n=8) were obtained from patients that underwent surgery after the tumour was histologically diagnosed. Usually, a radical abdominal hysterectomy was performed. Biopsies were taken from macroscopically visible tumor areas. Histological examination by a certified pathologist confirmed diagnosis. All cervical specimens were immediately embedded in OCT-Tissue-Tek II (Miles Laboratories, Naperville, Illinois, U.S.A.), snap frozen in melting isopentane, precooled in liquid nitrogen and stored at -80° C. Total RNA was extracted from normal cervical tissue, from cervical carcinomas and from the cervical cancer cell line HeLa using the method of Chomczynski and Sacchi (6). RNA was reverse-transcribed and RNA-levels were semiquantitatively detected by polymerase chain reaction (PCR) using sequence specific primers for human 25-hydroxyvitamin D$_3$-1α-hydroxylase (forward: 5`GGA-AAT-TCT-CGT-GTC-CCA-GA 3`; reverse: 5`AAA-CCA-GGC-

TAG-GGC-AGA-TT 3`) or GAPDH (30 cycles, 94°C-30s/60°C-30s/72°C-1m). RT-PCR products were run on 1% or 1,5% agarose gels.

Results: We detected mRNA of 25-hydroxyvitamin D_3-1α-hydroxylase in more than 50% of cervical carcinomas and normal cervical samples analyzed with no visible difference between both groups (Figure 1). In the cervical cancer cell line HeLa, mRNA of 1α-hydroxylase for 25-hydroxyvitamin D_3 was detected as well (Figure 2). In some samples additional bands could be detected, indicating alternate splice variants.

Figure 1: RT-PCR-products of 25-hydroxyvitamin D_3-1α-hydroxylase in benign cervical tissue and in cervical cancer on agarose gel (1,5 %); at 1,0 kb a specific band for the 1α-hydroxylase for 25-hydroxyvitamin D_3 is detected.

Lane 1-8:   Cervical cancer samples
Lane 9-12: Benign cervical tissue samples

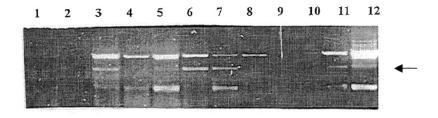

Figure 2: RT-PCR-products of the 1α-hydroxylase for 25-hydroxyvitamin D_3 in Hela-cells on agarose gel (1,5%), at 1,0 kb a specific lane for the 1α-hydroxylase for 25-hydroxyvitamin D_3 is detected.

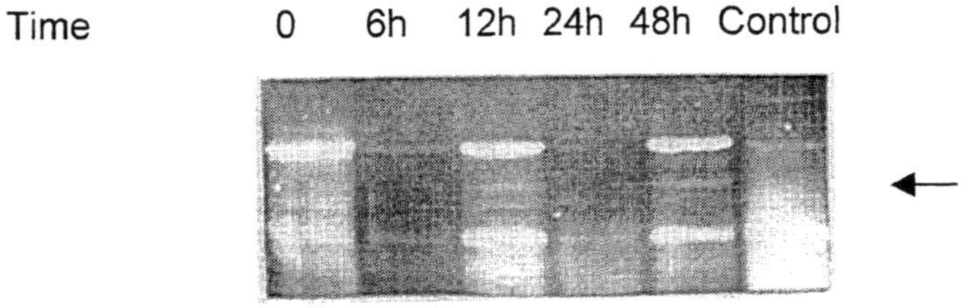

Discussion: Recently, extrarenal activity of 1α-hydroxylase for vitamin D has been reported in various cell types includuding macrophages and keratinocytes (5). This hydroxylase belongs to a class of proteins known as cytochrome P450 mixed function monooxidases. Cytochrome P450 enzymes are involved in the oxidative metabolism of steroids such as vitamin D, retinoids, fatty acids, prostaglandins and leukotrienes and biogenic amines. Additionally, cytochrome P450 enzymes have been shown to metabolize drugs, chemical carcinogens, mutagens, and other environmental agents. This dual functionality thus allows them to be characterized as having "mixed functions" (7). To our knowledge, this is the first report demonstrating expression of 1α-hydroxylase for 25-hydroxyvitamin D_3 in benign cervical tissue and in cervical carcinomas. Interestingly, there were no visual differences in the expression of 1α-hydroxylase for 25-hydroxyvitamin D_3 comparing benign and malignant cervical tissue. However, both in benign cervical tissue and in cervical carcinomas several PCR products were detected indicating multiple variants of the 1α-hydroxylase for 25-hydroxyvitamin D_3 as a result of alternate splicing. We conclude that benign cervical tissue and cervical carcinomas are target tissues for preventive, adjuvant or palliative treatment with precursors of biologically active vitamin D metabolites that exhibit little systemic side effects. At the moment we are doing studies to demonstrate conversion of 25-hydroxyvitamin D to $1,25(OH)_2D_3$ in cervical tissue to confirm the biological significance of our finding.

References:
[1]   Garland, C., Shekelle, R.B., Barrett-Connor, E., Criqui, M.H., and Rossof, A.H. (1985) The Lancet 1, 307-309.
[2]   Smith, E.L., Walworth, N.C., and Holick, M.F. (1986) J. Invest. Dermatol. 86, 709-714.
[3]   Stumpf, W.E., Sar, M., Reid, F.A., Tanaka, Y., and DeLuca, H.F. (1979) Science 206, 1189-1190.
[4]   Henry, H.L. (1992) J. Cell. Biochem. 49, 4-9.
[5]   Bikle, D.D., Nemanic, M.F., Gee, E., Elias, P. (1986) J. Clin. Invest. 78, 557-566.
[6]   Chomczynski, P., Sacchi, N. (1987) Anal Biochem 162, 156-160.
[7]   Nebert, D.W., Gonzalez, F.J. (1987) Ann. Rev. Biochem. 56, 945-993.

EXPRESSION OF 25-HYDROXYVITAMIN D$_3$-1α-HYDROXYLASE IN BREAST TISSUE

Michael Friedrich[1], Jörg Reichrath[2], Tai C. Chen[3], Vin Tanpricha[3], Ingrid Gherson[3], Wolfgang Tilgen[2], Werner Schmidt[1], Michael F. Holick[3] [1]Department of Gynecology and [2]Dermatology, University of Saarland, D-66421 Homburg/Saar, Germany; and [3]Vitamin D, Skin and Bone Research Laboratory, Boston University Medical Center, 02118 Boston, MA, USA

Introduction: Epidemiological studies have suggested the association of 1,25-dihydroxyvitamin D$_3$ (1,25(OH)$_2$D$_3$) deficiency with an increased risk of various malignancies (1). The molecular mechanisms involved in this phenomenon are still unknown. In vitro studies have demonstrated that 1,25(OH)$_2$D$_3$ suppresses proliferation and induces differentiation in various cell types, including epithelial cells (2). It is generally accepted that the antiproliferative effect is the result of a vitamin D receptor (VDR)-mediated action on the genome (3). There are two principal enzymes involved in the formation of circulating 1,25(OH)$_2$D$_3$ from vitamin D, the hepatic microsomal or mitochondrial vitamin D 25-hydroxylase and the renal mitochondrial enzyme 1α-hydroxylase for vitamin D and 25(OH)D$_3$, respectively (4). These hydroxylases belong to a class of proteins known as cytochrome P450 mixed function monooxidases. Recently, extrarenal activity of 1α-hydroxylase for 25(OH)D$_3$ has been reported in various cell types includuding macrophages and keratinocytes (5). The aim of this study was to analyze the expression of 1α-hydroxylase for 25-hydroxyvitamin D$_3$ in normal breast tissue and in breast carcinomas to evaluate whether breast tissue possesses the capacity to produce 1,25(OH)$_2$D$_3$ from 25(OH)D$_3$ and whether metastatic breast carcinomas may be a target for treatment with precursors of biologically active vitamin D analogues.

Materials and Methods: Biopsies from normal breast tissue (n=4) were obtained from patients that underwent surgery for hyperplasia of the breast. Histological examination by a certified pathologist confirmed normality. Biopsies from breast carcinomas (n=8) were obtained from patients that underwent surgery for breast tumours. Usually, a breast preserving surgery was performed. Biopsies were taken from macroscopically visible tumor areas. Histological examination by a certified pathologist confirmed diagnosis. All breast specimens were immediately embedded in OCT-Tissue-Tek II (Miles Laboratories, Naperville, Illinois, U.S.A.), snap frozen in melting isopentane, precooled in liquid nitrogen and stored at -80° C. Total RNA was extracted from normal breast tissue, from breast carcinomas and from MCF-7 cells using the method of Chomczynski and Sacchi (6). RNA was reverse-transcribed and RNA-levels were semiquantitatively detected by polymerase chain reaction (PCR) using several pairs of sequence specific primers for human 1α-hydroxylase for 25-hydroxyvitamin D$_3$ or GAPDH (30 cycles, 94° C-30s/60° C-30s/72° C-1m). RT-PCR products were run on 1% or 1,5% agarose gels. For proliferation analysis, preconfluent MCF-7 cells were starved of serum for 24 hrs and subsequently treated with or without 10^{-7}-10^{-9} M 25(OH)D$_3$ or

190

1,25(OH)$_2$D$_3$ and with and without EGF or 0.1% FBS for 20hrs. Cells were then pulsed with [^{3}H]-thymidine for 3 hrs. Proliferation was estimated by [^{3}H]-thymidine incorporation and measured by beta particle emission with a scintillation counter. Bars in Fig. 3 represent the average of 6 replicates ± SD, $p < 0.005$.

Results: We detected mRNA of 1α-hydroxylase for 25-hydroxyvitamin D$_3$ in more than 50% of samples analyzed in each group with no visible difference between both groups (Figure 1). mRNA for 1α-hydroxylase was detected in the breast cancer cell line MCF-7 as well (Figure 2). When cells were treated with 1,25-dihydroxyvitamin D$_3$, cell proliferation was inhibited (Figure 3).

Figure 1:   RT-PCR-analysis of the 25-hydroxyvitamin D$_3$-1α-hydroxylase in benign breast tissue samples and in breast cancer samples on agarose gel (1,5 %), at 1,0 kb a specific lane for the 25-hydroxyvitamin D$_3$-1α-hydroxylase is detected.

Lanes 1-14:   Breast cancer samples
Lanes 15-21:   Benign breast tissue samples

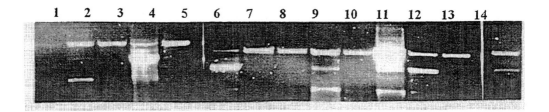

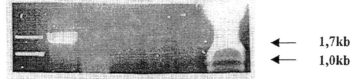

⟵   1,7kb
⟵   1,0kb

Figure 2: RT-PCR-analysis of 25-hydroxyvitamin D_3-1α-hydroxylase in MCF-7 breast adenocarcinoma cells

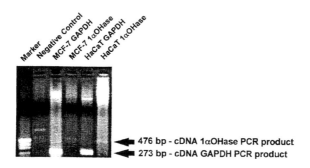

◀ 476 bp - cDNA 1αOHase PCR product
◀ 273 bp - cDNA GAPDH PCR product

Figure 3: Effect of $1,25(OH)_2D_3$ on the proliferation of MCF-7 Breast adenocarcinoma cells

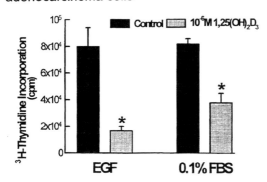

Table 1: Effect of $25(OH)D_3$ or $1,25(OH)_2D_3$ on the proliferation of MCF-7 Breast adenocarcinoma cells

Conc.	$25(OH)D_3$	$1,25(OH)_2D_3$
	% of control	
10^{-9} M	98 ± 5 %	89 ± 5 %
10^{-8} M	95 ± 11 %	97 ± 6 %
10^{-7} M	93 ± 6 %	77 ± 3 %

RESTORATION OF SERUM CALCIUM WITH BISPHOSPHONATE LEADS TO THE ENHANCED EXPRESSION OF 1α-HYDROXYLASE IN A RAT MODEL OF HUMORAL HYPERCALCEMIA OF MALIGNANCY

Toshimi Michigami[*], Hideyuki Yamato[$], Hiroyuki Suzuki[$], Yumiko Nagai-Itagaki[$] and Keiichi Ozono[*]. [*]Department of Environmental Medicine, Osaka Medical Center and Research Institute for Maternal and Child Health, Izumi, Osaka 594-1101, Japan. [$]Kureha Chemical Industry Co., Shinjyuku-ku, Tokyo 169-8503, Japan.

Introduction

Humoral hypercalcemia of malignancy (HHM) is one of the most common paraneoplastic complications, which is associated with the overproduction of parathyroid hormone-related peptide (PTHrP) by the tumor. Although PTHrP exerts its functions through a common receptor with PTH, there is a notable difference in vitamin D metabolism between HHM and primary hyperparathyroidism (1°HPT) (1). The circulating 1,25-dihydroxyvitamin D [1,25(OH)$_2$D] concentration is elevated in a significant number of patients with 1°HPT. In contrast, serum levels of 1,25(OH)$_2$D are reduced in most HHM patients. The reasons for this discrepancy still remain unclear, since administration of synthetic peptides for PTHrP[1-34] or PTHrP[1-36] increases the plasma 1,25(OH)$_2$D concentration as does the administration of PTH[1-34], which is not consistent with the situation in patients with HHM. In the present study, we have investigated the mechanisms underlying the impaired vitamin D metabolism in HHM using a newly-developed animal model where PTHrP-producing human infantile fibrosarcoma (named OMC-1) is inoculated to athymic nude rats (2). To examine whether serum calcium (Ca) level affects the serum 1,25(OH)$_2$D concentration, the effects of bisphosphonate YM529 on OMC-1-bearing rats were also studied.

Results

1. Changes of serum PTHrP, Ca and body weight in OMC-1-bearing rats.

OMC-1 tumor is a PTHrP-producing infantile fibrosarcoma originally obtained from an 8-month-old boy who manifested severe hypercalcemia, and is heterotransplantable to immunocompromised nude mice and nude rats. In the present experiments, we first investigated the changes of serum PTHrP, Ca and body weight in OMC-1-bearing rats. Six weeks after tumor inoculation, the serum levels of PTHrP in OMC-1-bearing rats were elevated to 11.1±2.6 pmol/l, while those in control animals was 1.1±0.0 pmol/l. Seven weeks after inoculation, the PTHrP levels of OMC-1-bearing animals further increased and reached 38.5±3.6 pmol/l. Simultaneously with the rise in the circulating PTHrP concentration, the serum Ca levels began to elevate in OMC-1-bearing rats.

Associated with the elevation of serum Ca and plasma PTHrP levels, OMC-1-bearing rats lost body weight and became cachechitic 6 weeks after the tumor inoculation.

2. Serum concentrations of vitamin D metabolites in OMC-1-bearing rats.

Blood was taken from OMC-1-bearing rats at various stage (5 to 8 weeks after tumor inoculation) or age-matched control rats, and was subjected to the measurement of serum Ca and vitamin D metabolites. The samples from OMC-1-bearing rats were divided into two groups referring to Ca levels; normocalcemia to mild hypercalcemia (<15 mg/dl) and severe hypercalcemia (≥15 mg/dl). The results are shown in Figure 1.

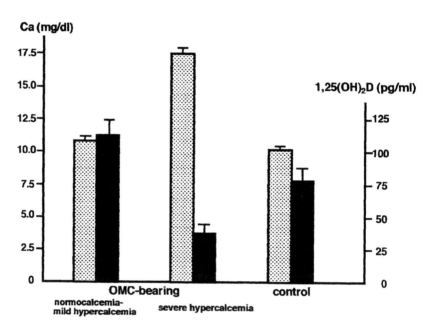

Figure 1. Serum Ca levels (gray bars) and 1,25(OH)$_2$D levels (black bars) in OMC-1-bearing rats and control rats. In OMC-1-bearing rats with mild hypercalcemia, serum levels of 1,25(OH)$_2$D were slightly elevated compared with the values in control rats. In contrast, in OMC-1-bearing rats with severe hypercalcemia, 1,25(OH)$_2$D levels were markedly reduced.

The correlation between serum levels of Ca and 1,25(OH)$_2$D was significant ([1,25(OH)$_2$D]= 21.0 x [Ca] -151.3; R^2=0.778, p<0.005) in the non-tumor-bearing control group and normocalcemia to mild hypercalcemia group of OMC-1-bearing rats. The levels of Ca and 1,25(OH)$_2$D in severe hypercalcemia group in OMC-1-bearing rats did not fit the linear regression curve, and the levels of 1,25(OH)$_2$D were apparently suppressed compared with those in the control group and normocalcemia to mild hypercalcemia group of OMC-1-bearing rats. These results suggested that serum Ca levels might affect the serum $1,25(OH)_2D$ level.

3. Effects of bisphosphonate YM529 in OMC-1-bearing rats.

To further examine whether an increased level of serum Ca was responsible for the impaired vitamin D metabolism, we administered bisphosphonate YM529 (provided by Yamanouchi Pharmaceuticals) to OMC-1-bearing rats. Administration of YM529 (0.1 mg/kg, iv) reduced the serum Ca level in OMC-1-bearing rats from 16.7±0.8 to 10.7±0.5 mg/dl in 4 days (n=4, p<0.001). The serum $1,25(OH)_2D$ level after the treatment with YM529 was markedly elevated (154.5±18.0 pg/ml) compared with that in untreated OMC-1-bearing rats with severe hypercalcemia (29.1±5.9 pg/ml, p<0.0001), and higher even than that in untreated OMC-1-bearing rats with mild hypercalcemia (Figure 2).

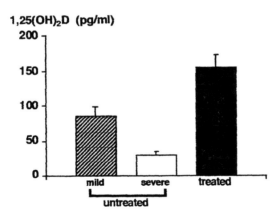

Figure 2. Effect of YM529 on serum $1,25(OH)_2D$ concentrations in OMC-1-bearing rats. Hatched bar, untreated OMC-1-bearing rats with normocalcemia to mild hypercalcemia; white bar, untreated OMC-1-bearing rats with severe hypercalcemia; black bar, OMC-1-bearing rats treated with YM529.

4. Expression of 1α-hydroxylase in kidney in OMC-1-bearing rats.

Expression of 1α-hydroxylase in kidney was examined by reverse transcription-polymerase chain reaction (RT-PCR). In non-tumor-bearing control rats, very faint signals were detected. Kidneys obtained from OMC-1-bearing rats with mild hypercalcemia still retained detectable levels of 1α-hydroxylase. In contrast, kidneys from OMC-1-bearing rats with severe hypercalcemia (≥15 mg/dl) exhibited a reduced expression of the gene. In kidneys from OMC-1-bearing rats treated with YM529, the expression of 1α-hydroxylase was markedly increased. These results suggested that serum Ca levels affected the expression of 1α-hydroxylase in OMC-1-bearing rats, and that PTHrP may stimulate the expression of the gene in normocalcemic state as PTH does.

Conclusion

In the present study, we have investigated the mechanisms underlying the impaired vitamin D metabolism in HHM utilizing OMC-1-bearing rats as an animal model. In these rats, serum Ca levels affected the serum levels of 1,25(OH)$_2$D. Restoration of serum Ca levels with bisphosphonate YM529 resulted in the enhanced 1α-hydroxylase expression.

References

1. Goltzman, D., and Henderson, J. E. (1997) Cancer Treat. Res. 89, 193-215.
2. Michigami, T., Yamato, H., Mushiake, S., Nakayama, M., Yoneda, A., Satomura, K., Imura, K., and Ozono, K. (1996) J Clin. Endocrinol. Metab. 81, 1090-1095.

REGULATION OF VITAMIN D HYDROXYLASE EXPRESSION IN A SMALL CELL LUNG CANCER CELL LINE (NCI-H82) AND A HUMAN KIDNEY CELL LINE (HKC-8).

SE Heys-Jackson, AP Mee and EB Mawer. Musculoskeletal Research Group, University Department of Medicine, Manchester Royal Infirmary, Manchester M13 9WL, UK.

Introduction

The human small cell lung cancer (SCLC) cell line, NCI-H82 constitutively synthesises $1,25(OH)_2D_3$ (1,25D) from $25(OH)D_3$[1] but lacks 1,25D-receptors (VDR) and 24-hydroxylase (24-OHase) activity. Studies have shown that expression of transfected VDR in H82 cells was coupled to a significant reduction in 1,25D production, and induction of 24-OHase activity. The present study aimed to investigate further the effect of VDR expression on $1\propto$- & 24- OHase mRNA expression in H82 cells and renal HKC-8 cells using modulators of vitamin D activity.

Methods.

VDR Transfection. Wild type (WT) H82 cells were transiently transfected using a cationic lipid (DMRIE-C, Gibco BRL) and an EBV episomal expression vector containing a cadmium-inducible metallothionein II promoter (pMEP4) with a sense orientated 2kb cDNA for VDR (kindly donated by M. Hewison). 20µg DMRIE-C and 5µg DNA were incubated with 2×10^6 cells in 1.2ml serum free medium for 4h at 37°C, followed by addition of 2ml RPMI growth medium containing 15% FBS ± the addition of $CdCl_2$ to a final concentration of 2 µM. Cells were assayed for gene expression at 48 h post-transfection. In some experiments, 1,25D (10^{-7} M) was added during the final 24 h incubation.

Gene Expression

Following 24 h treatment with forskolin (Fsk, 25 µM), phorbol ester (PMA, 10^{-7} M) or 1,25D (10^{-7} M), cells were examined for mRNA expression using *in situ* hybridisation (ISH) and VDR protein expression using immunocytochemistry.

Detection of $1\propto$- & 24- OHase mRNA using ISH. A 514bp cDNA probe for $1\propto$-OHase was generated from RT-PCR using H82 mRNA, and cloned into bluescript KS+. Sequencing data revealed 100% identity with the renal $1\propto$-OHase mRNA. Partial length (1.8kb) cDNA for human kidney $P450_{cc24}$ cloned into bluescript KS+ was a gift from J. Ohmdahl and B. May. The plasmids were linearised and the cDNAs used as templates for *in vitro* transcription with $[^{35}S]rUTP\propto S$, from T5 and T7 promoters generating sense and antisense riboprobes respectively. WT H82 and VDR transfected H82 cells, cultured and treated in 6 well plates, were cytospun onto organosilanated glass slides and fixed in 10% formalin/PBS. Renal HKC-8 cells cultured in 4 well glass chamber slides (LabTek) were fixed for 2 min in 10% formalin/PBS. Standard ISH was performed as described elsewhere[2]. Slides were exposed at 4°C for 7 days, developed and counterstained with haematoxylin and eosin, then viewed by light and dark field microscopy.

<u>*Detection of VDR protein expression using immunocytochemistry.*</u>
Following treatments, cells were washed in tris buffered saline (TBS) pH 7.6 and fixed for 10 min in Carnoys. Following permeabilisation, non specific binding was blocked with 10% normal rabbit serum. Cells were then incubated with primary antibody, 9A7g monoclonal antibody raised in rat against chick VDR. Negative control cells were incubated with rat IgG. All samples were incubated with biotinylated rabbit anti-rat antibody, then alkaline phosphatase labelled Avidin Biotin complex (Dako) and developed with new fuschin. Slides were counterstained with toluene blue and viewed by light field microscopy.

Results

<u>*Expression of 1∝-OHase mRNA.*</u>
PMA stimulated 1∝-OHase mRNA expression in WT H82 cells, and 1,25D reduced expression in VDR transfected H82 cells. In renal HKC-8 cells, Fsk stimulated 1∝-OHase mRNA expression compared to control cells.

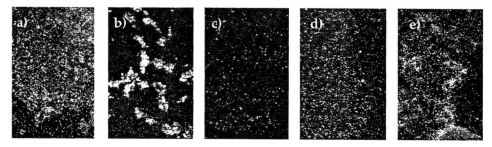

Fig.1. Photomicrographs of H82 and HKC-8 cells showing hybridisation with 1∝-OHase antisense riboprobes following ISH. Dark field views of a) WT H82 cells, b) PMA treated H82 cells, c) VDR transfected H82 cells, d) HKC-8 control cells and e) Fsk treated HKC-8 cells.

<u>*Expression of 24-OHase mRNA*</u>
1,25D induced 24-OHase mRNA expression in VDR transfected H82 cells, but not in WT cells, and stimulated high expression in renal HKC-8 cells compared with control cells.

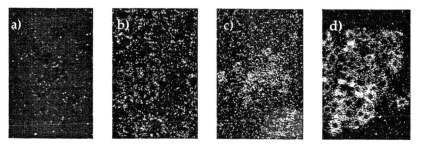

Fig. 2. Photomicrographs of H82 and HKC-8 cells showing hybridisation with 24-OHase antisense riboprobes following ISH. Dark field views of a) WT H82 cells, b) 1,25D treated transfected H82 cells, c) HKC-8 control cells and d) 1,25D treated HKC-8 cells.

Expression of VDR protein.

VDR protein expression was detected in transfected H82 cells stimulated with cadmium, but absent in WT H82 cells. In HKC-8 cells, expression of VDR protein was increased after treatment with 1,25D and PMA.

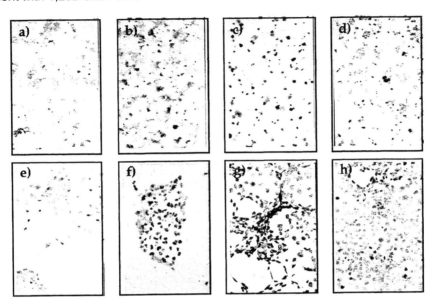

Fig. 3. Photomicrographs of VDR protein expression following immunocytochemistry. a) WT H82 cells, b) transfected H82 cells, c) transfected H82 cells + cadmium, d) transfected H82 cells + 1,25D, e) HKC-8 control cells, and then after 24 h treatment with f) 1,25D, g) PMA and h) Fsk.

Results Summary

Table 1 summarises the effects of 1,25D, PMA and Fsk on the expression of VDR protein and 1∝- and 24-OHase mRNA's in WT and VDR transfected H82 cells and HKC-8 cells.

Treat-ment	H82 WT			H82 transfected			HKC-8		
	VDR	1αOH	24OH	VDR	1αOH	24OH	VDR	1αOH	24OH
control	-	+	-	++	+	±	±	+	+
CdCl₂	-	+	-	+++	±	±	not determined		
1,25D	-	+	-	++	±	+	++	±	+++
PMA	-	++	-	not determined			++	+	+
Fsk	-	+	-	not determined			+	++	±

Table 1. VDR protein, 1α– & 24-OHase mRNA expression in WT H82 and HKC-8 cells following 24 h treatment with forskolin (Fsk, 25µM), phorbol ester (PMA, 10^{-7}M) and 1,25D (10^{-7}M), and in VDR transfected H82 cells ± 2µM CdCl₂ (expression vector contains a cadmium inducible promoter). Scores ranged from negative (-) to highly positive (+++).

Conclusion

These results indicate that in VDR transfected H82 cells, reduced 1,25D synthesis results from down regulation of 1$\propto$-OHase and induction of 24-OHase mRNAs. In HKC-8 cells, up regulation of 1$\propto$-OHase expression occurs via the cAMP pathway, but in WT H82 cells by the PKC pathway. The results show that in both renal and non renal cells, the presence of functional VDR is required for the induction of 24-OHase activity. Stimulation of 1$\propto$-OHase expression can occur via different pathways, which appear to be independent of VDR regulation, and may be due to differences in cell specific regulation of the 1$\propto$-OHase gene promoter.

1. Mawer E.B., Hayes M.E., Heys S.E., Davies M., White M., Stewart M.F. and Smith G. (1994) Journal of Clinical Enocrinology and Metabolism 79, 554-560.

2. Mee A.P., Davenport L.K., Hoyland J.A., Davies M. and Mawer, E.B. (1996) Journal of Molecular Endocrinology 16, 183-195.

Funded by Innovation Grant No G9723869 from the Medical Research Council

In Vitro AND *In Vivo* TRANSFECTION OF SKIN WITH THE 25-HYDROXYVITAMIN D-1α-HYDROXYLASE cDNA PLASMID.

John N. Flanagan*, Lyman W. Whitlatch*, Tai C. Chen, Xue Hong Zhu, Michael T. Holick, Xiang Kong & Michael F. Holick*
Vitamin D, Skin and Bone Research Laboratory; Endocrinology, Nutrition, and Diabetes Section, Departments of Medicine and *Physiology, Boston University Medical Center, Boston, MA 02118, USA.

Introduction: Vitamin D is hydroxylated in the liver and kidney on carbons 25 and 1 respectively to become biologically active as 1,25-dihydroxyvitamin D_3 (1α,25(OH)$_2$D$_3$) (1) . 1α,25(OH)$_2$D$_3$ interacts with a nuclear vitamin D receptor (VDR) in the small intestine and osteoblasts to increase intestinal calcium transport and induce osteoclast maturation respectively. VDR exists in a wide variety of other tissues including the skin. 1α,25(OH)$_2$D$_3$ and its analogs exert antiproliferative and prodifferentiation effects on these cells both *in vitro* and *in vivo* (1). The renal cytochrome P_{450} 25-hydroxyvitamin D-1α-hydroxylase (1α-OHase), converts 25(OH)D$_3$ to 1α,25(OH)$_2$D$_3$, and is the major source of 1α,25(OH)$_2$D$_3$ in the circulation which is responsible for regulating calcium metabolism (1). The 1α-OHase is also present in several non-renal cells including keratinocytes. Recently, the cDNAs encoding the mouse, rat, and human 1α-OHase were cloned (2-5). The human renal and non-renal 1α-OHase cDNA sequences are 100% identical (4,5). The presence of 1α-OHase in the keratinocytes suggests an autocrine/paracrine role for 1α,25(OH)$_2$D$_3$ that maybe responsible for locally modulating cell proliferation and differentiation. The potent antiproliferative and prodifferentiation effects of 1α,25(OH)$_2$D$_3$ and its analogs on keratinocytes has led to the development of these compounds as potential new therapies for the hyperproliferative skin disease psoriasis.

During the past decade, advances in the introduction of genes to tissues and organs have greatly enhanced the prospect of gene therapy for humans (6). The topical application of the 1α-OHase gene to the skin to increase local 1α-OHase activity may be a unique and effective therapeutic approach for hyperproliferative disorders of the skin such as psoriasis. We report on the feasibility of introducing the 1α-OHase gene into cultured human keratinocytes which increased the 1α-OHase activity and sensitivity to the antiproliferative potential of 25(OH)D$_3$ *in vitro*. We also show that the topical application of the 1α-OHase cDNA plasmid on mice enhanced the cutaneous expression of the 1α-OHase *in vivo*.

Methods:

1α-OHase-GFP plasmid construction: PCR mutagenesis was used to generate the 1α-OHase-GFP fusion construct from 1α-OHase cDNA as described (4). First, 1α-OHase(-stop) fragment was generated, and ligated into pCR3.1 T/A cloning vector, followed by ligating 1α-OHase(-stop).pCR3.1 to pEGFP vector (Invitrogen, San Diego, CA, USA).

Cell culture and Transfection: Normal human keratinocytes were obtained from neonatal foreskin as previously described and grown in serum-free defined medium (7). Cells were grown to about 60% confluency in the absence of antibiotics, at which time the cells were exposed to fresh medium and added with freshly prepared 1α-OHase-GFP cDNA-LipofectAmine Reagent complexes (0.05 ml) as described in the protocol supplied by the company.

1α-OHase enzyme activity: The 1α-OHase enzyme activity was determined 24 hours after transfection in the presence of 0.1μCi of [³H]-25(OH)D₃ (New England Nuclear, Boston, MA, USA) and 10 μM 1,2-dianilinoethane (DPPD) by high performance liquid chromatography using methylene chloride/isopropanol (19:1) as mobile phase as described (8). The retention volumes for [³H]-25(OH)D₃ and [³H]-1α,25(OH)₂D₃ were confirmed with standard non-radioactive 25(OH)D₃ and 1α,25(OH)₂D₃. The enzyme activity was expressed as pmol of 1α,25(OH)₂D₃/mg protein/hour.

Cell proliferation assay: ³H-Thymidine incorporation was performed in the presence of 1α,25(OH)₂D₃ or 25(OH)D₃ as described (8).

Topical application and Immunohistochemistry: Topical Application of 1α-OHase-GFP plasmid and immunohistochemistry of the C57/BL6 mice skin was previously described (9,10). Twenty-four hours after topically applying naked cDNA to abraded mouse skin, biopsies were obtained, frozen embedded, sectioned and incubated with a rabbit anti-GFP antibody (Invitrogen, San Diego, CA, USA). Sections were examined for fluorescence using a Nikon fluorescence microscope (Melville, NY, USA) with a rhodamine filter system and standard compound light microscope.

Results and Discussion: The expression vector encoding the 1α-OHase-GFP fusion protein driven by the cytomegalovirus (CMV) promoter was transfected into normal human cultured keratinocytes to examine the expression and the appearance of cellular distribution of the 1α-OHase-GFP fusion protein using scanning laser confocal microscopy. The fluorescence of the GFP protein alone showed a diffused distribution (Fig. 1A), whereas the fluorescence of the 1α-OHase-GFP protein in transfected keratinocytes showed a mitochondrial distribution, consistent with the location of the cytochrome P₄₅₀-1α-OHase (Fig. 1B). The same transfected keratinocytes were also stained with a mitochondrial specific dye. When both images were superimposed the resulting image showed co-localization with in the keratinocytes confirming that the 1α-OHase-GFP protein was expressed in the mitochondria (data not shown).

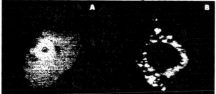

Figure 1. 1α-OHase-GFP or GFP expression in transfected normal human keratinocytes

To determine whether the expressed 1α-OHase-GFP was functional we examined the efficiency in the conversion of [³H]-25(OH)D₃ to [³H]-1α,25(OH)D₃ in keratinocytes transfected with 1α-OHase-GFP. High performance liquid chromatography analysis revealed an 85 ± 4.7% increase (from 25 ± 1.1% to 54 ± 2%) in the conversion of 25(OH)D₃ to 1α,25(OH)₂D₃ in keratinocytes transfected with 1α-OHase-GFP above basal activity (mock transfected with GFP vector alone) (Table 1). The 1α-OHase gene alone without the GFP tag was also tested in transfected keratinocytes which showed a $111\pm5.7\%$ increase (from $27\pm5\%$ to $60\pm2.1\%$) in the conversion of $[^3H]$-25(OH)D$_3$ to $[^3H]$-1α,25(OH)D$_3$.

After we established that keratinocytes transfected with 1α-OHase and 1α-OHase-GFP had enhanced 1α-OHase activity we evaluated whether the enhanced conversion of 25(OH)D$_3$ to 1α,25(OH)$_2$D$_3$ would result in an increased sensitivity to the antiproliferative effects of 25(OH)D$_3$. The antiproliferative activity of 25(OH)D$_3$ was determined in the transfected keratinocytes using the thymidine incorporation assay (7). In figure 2b, keratinocytes transfected with 1α-OHase showed significant decrease in ^3H-thymidine incorporation of $60\pm2\%$ at $10^{-7}M$ of 25(OH)D$_3$, compared to control.

Table 1. Effect of transfection of 1α-OHase cDNA in cultured normal human keratinocytes on the conversion of ^3H-25(OH)D$_3$ to ^3H-1α,25(OH)$_2$D$_3$ and ^3H-thymidine incorporation into DNA in the presence of 25(OH)D$_3$. *Means$\pm$SE of 5 determinations, ** Means$\pm$SE of 8-24 determinations.

Treatment	% Conversion ^3H-25(OH)D$_3$ to ^3H-1α,25(OH)$_2$D$_3$*	^3H-Thymidine Incorporation** (% of control in the absence 10^{-8} M of 25(OH)D$_3$)
NonTransfected Control	$27\pm5\%$	$100\pm2\%$
GFP Vector	$25\pm1.1\%$	
1α-OHase-GFP cDNA	$54\pm2\%$	
1α-OHase cDNA	$60\pm2.1\%$	$60\pm2\%$

Naked 1α-OHase-GFP plasmid DNA in water was topically applied to mouse skin to see whether the gene could be expressed *in vivo* in epidermis. No cross-reactivity of the GFP antibody was detected in either the epidermis or dermis of the skin treated with water alone (Figure 2A). However, there was marked expression of the 1α-OHase-GFP in the epidermis of the mice that received a single topical application of the 1α-OHase-GFP plasmid DNA 24 hours previously [indicated by the dark fluorescence of the fluorophore secondary antibody, Vector Bioscience, Eugene, OR (Figure 2B)]. These results were confirmed using compound light microscopy with expression located in the epidermis and epidermis appendages (data not shown).

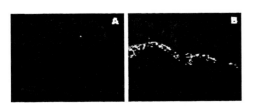

Figure 2. Immunofluorescent staining of the 1α-OHase-GFP protein in mouse skin.

Results from this study demonstrates the feasibility of using the 25-hydroxyvitamin D-1α-hydroxylase for gene therapy to treat hyperproliferative disorders of the skin such as psoriasis and skin cancer. *In vitro* the increase in expression of 1α-OHase led to increased conversion of 25(OH)D$_3$ to 1α,25(OH)$_2$D$_3$ and increased sensitivity to the antiproliferative potential 25(OH)D$_3$. Thus, it may be possible to selectively enhance the cutaneous expression of the 1α-OHase in psoriatic keratinocytes that could lead to an enhanced conversion of cellular 25(OH)D$_3$ to 1α,25(OH)$_2$D$_3$. The increased cellular levels of 1α,25(OH)$_2$D$_3$ could be an effective method to down-regulate the hyperproliferative activity of psoriatic keratinocytes (1, 7). This maybe a preferred method of treatment. Increasing 1α,25(OH)$_2$D$_3$ locally in psoriatic keratinocytes has the advantage of attaining high intracellular concentrations of 1α,25(OH)$_2$D$_3$ for at least several days and not having any systemic effects such as hypercalcemia.

References:
1. Holick, M.F. Vitamin D: photobiology, metabolism, mechanism of action, and clinical applications. In: M.J. Favus (ed.) *Primer on the Metabolic Bone Diseases and Disorders of Mineral Metabolism*, Fourth Edition, pp. 92-98, Lippincott-Raven:Philadelphia (1999).
2. Takeyama, K.I., Kitanaka, S., Sato, T., Kobori, M., Yanagisawa, J. & Kato, S.. *Science* 277, 1827-1830 (1997).
3. Kitanaka, S., Takeyama, K.I., Murayama, A., Sato, T., Okumura, K., Nogami, M., Hasegawa, Y., Nimi, H., Yanagisawa, J., Tanaka, T. & Kato, S.. *N. Engl. J. Med.* 338, 653-661 (1998).
4. Kong, X.F., Zhu, X.H., Pei, Y.L., Jackson, D.M. & Holick, M.F.. *Proc. Natl. Acad. Sci.* 96, 6988-6993 (1999).
5. Fu, G.K., Lin, D., Zhang, M.Y.H., Bikle, D.D., Shackleton, C.H.L., Miller, W.L. & Portale, A.A.. *Molecul. Endocrinol.* 11, 1961-1970 (1997).
6. Katz, S.I. Thematic Review Series VI: Skin Gene Therapy. *Proceedings of Association of American Physicians* 111, 183-219 (1999).
7. Chen,T.C., Persons, K, Liu, W-W, Chen, M.L. & Holick M.F. *J. Invest. Dermatol.* 104, 113-117 (1995).
8. Schwartz G.G., Whitlatch L.W., Chen T.C., Lokeshwar B.L. & Holick M.F.. *Cancer Epidemiol, Biomark & Prev.* 7, 391-395, (1998).
9. Yu, W.H., Kashani-Sabet, M., Liggitt, D., Moore, D., Heath, T.D. & Debs, R.J.. *J. Invest. Dermatol.* 112, 370-375 (1999).
10. Fan, H., Lin, Q., Morrissey, G.R. & Khavari P.A.. *Nat. Biotechnol.* 17, 870-872 (1999).

Acknowledgements
We appreciate the generous gift of the confocal microscope from Mr. Donald Christal and the California Sun Care Inc. Los Angeles, CA and the 25(OH)D$_3$-1α-hydroxylase antibody from A&D Bioscience Inc. Boston, MA. This work was supported in part by NIH Grants AR36963 and MO1RR00533.

1α,25(OH)$_2$D$_3$
NUCLEAR RECEPTOR

LIGAND BINDING TO THE NUCLEAR RECEPTOR FOR VITAMIN D.

G.D. Tocchini-Valentini, N. Rochel, J.M. Wurtz, A. Mitschler, D. Moras

Laboratoire de Biologie et Génomique structurale, Institut de Génétique et de Biologie Moléculaire et Cellulaire, CNRS/INSERM/ULP, BP 163, 67404 Illkirch Cedex, France.

Introduction:

The superfamily of the nuclear receptor (NR) includes receptors for the steroid, retinoid, thyroid hormones and receptors that mediate the peroximal proliferation in response to fatty acids (1,2). The NRs are ligand-activated transcription factors that control cell growth and differentiation, homeostasis, development and several physiological processes. They share the same modular structure in 6 domains with a N-terminal A/B domain highly variable, a DNA binding domain (DBD) highly conserved and a moderately conserved ligand binding domain (LBD). The LBD presents a dimerization interface and a ligand-dependent transcription activation domain, AF-2. Several crystal structures of apo or ligand-bound LBDs have been published (3-11). They all show a common fold of 11-13 α-helices sandwiched in three layers. All the agonist-bound LBD structures have the same unique conformation with the AF-2 helix in the same position (Figure 1b) which is determinant for coactivator interactions (12-13). In the apo structures (Figure 1a for the retinoid X nuclear receptor, RXR (3)), the AF-2 helix protrudes from the protein core or is packed against the body of the receptor as for PPAR α or γ (8,10). Comparison of the apo and holo structures allowed to propose a "mouse trap" mechanism in which the AF-2 domain undergoes a conformational change upon ligand binding (14). In the antagonist bound LBDs (Figure 1c for the estrogen nuclear receptor bound to OHT (13)), the ligand binds at the same site but prevents the position of the AF-2 helix over the ligand pocket.

The vitamin D nuclear receptor (VDR) mediates the genomic action of the active form of vitamin D, $1\alpha,25(OH)_2$dihydroxyvitamin D_3 ($1,25(OH)_2D_3$) (Figure 2) which regulates calcium and phosphate metabolism, induces potent cell differentiation and has immunosuppressive effects (15-16). Therapeutic applications of vitamin D analogs are treatments for renal osteodystrophy, osteoporosis, psoriasis, cancer and autoimmune diseases. These applications are limited by the calcemic side effects of the natural ligand. Hundreds of vitamin D analogs have been synthesized (15). Some of them exhibit efficient antiproliferative and prodifferentiation with less side effects. Figure 2 shows 4 different synthetic analogs that are all potent antiproliferative drugs. In this study we present the crystal structures of the VDR LBD bound to $1,25(OH)_2D_3$ and to several agonists.

208

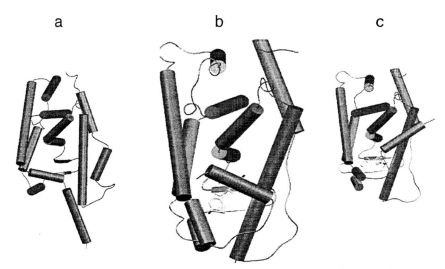

Figure 1: Different conformations adopted by the LBD in the apo form (a) for the RXRα (3), the agonist LBD complex (b) for the ER bound to DES (DiethylStyllbestrol) (13) and the antagonist bound LBD (c) for the ER bound to OHT (4-hydroxyTamoxifen) (13).

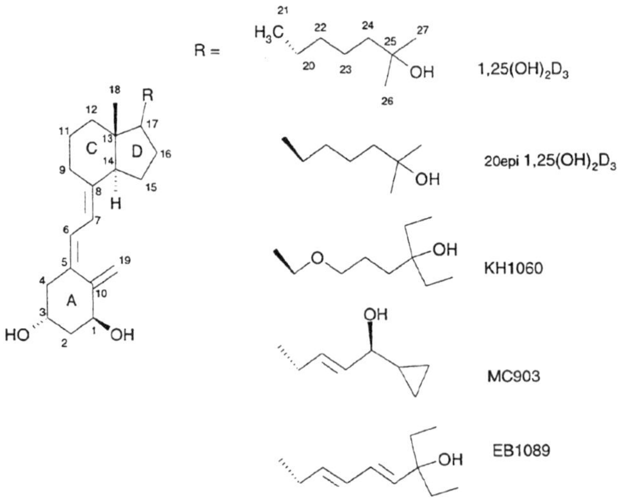

Figure 2: Chemical structure of 1,25(OH)$_2$D$_3$ analogs.

Engineering of the VDR construct and Characterization: VDR contrary to other NR presents an insertion domain in the peptide connecting helices H1 and H3 (Figure 3a). This insertion domain varies in length between 72 and 81 residues in the VDR family and shows low sequence homology (9% of identity between amino acids 157 and 215 of hVDR in the VDR family). This region is accessible to proteases with a cleavage site after ARG174 of hVDR and is poorly structured as seen by secondary structure prediction. We engineered a VDR LBD mutant without this insertion domain (118-425Δ165-215). The absence of this region doesn't affect the ligand binding or transactivation which remain the same for the VDR mutant and the VDR wild-type. Figure 3b shows the relative binding affinity of 1,25(OH)$_2$D$_3$ and of the synthetic analogs MC903, KH1060 and EB1089 for the VDR mutant compared to the VDR wild-type. The VDR mutant binds these analogs with similar affinity compared to the wild-type. The removal of the insertion domain results in a more stable protein that could be crystallized as a complex with agonists.

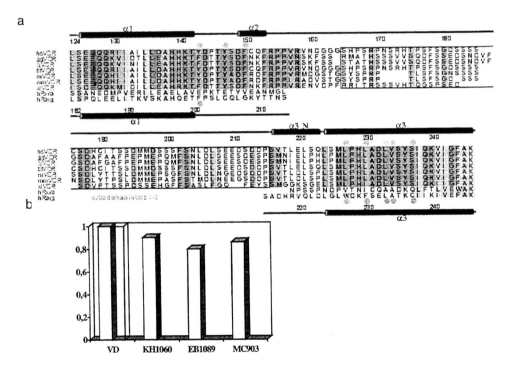

together with the hRXRα and hRARγ. h: *Homo sapiens*, j: *Coturnix japonica*, m: *Mus Musculus*, r: *Rattus norvegicus*, t: *Bos taurus*. The sequence numbering above and below are for hVDR and hRARγ sequences respectively. The secondary structures above and below the alignment corresponds to hVDR and hRARγ respectively. Identical residues are highlighted in dark grey. b: Relative binding affinity of 1,25(OH)$_2$D$_3$ and analogs to VDR wild-type (white) and mutant (grey).

High resolution crystal structure of VDR LBD complexed to 1,25(OH)$_2$D$_3$: The overall topology of the VDR LBD (11) is similar to that of the other NRS with 13 α-helices and a three-stranded β sheet (Figure 4). Helices H1 and H3 are connected by two small helices H2 and H3n. The truncation is distant from the ligand and therefore unlikely to affect the ligand binding. The relative position of helix H1 is conserved in all NRs and stabilizes the overall LBD architecture.

Helix H12, the activation helix which is critical for coactivator binding and transactivation is in the unique agonist position. Two residues Val418 and Phe422 of helix H12 are in Van der Waals contacts with the methyl group of 1,25(OH)$_2$D$_3$. The helix position is stabilized by several hydrophobic contacts and two polar interactions, which involve the conserved salt bridge Lys264(H4)-Glu420(H12) and a hydrogen bond between Ser235(H3) and Thr415(11-12). Some of the residues that stabilize H12 are directly interacting with the ligand suggesting that the ligand controls indirectly the position of helix H12.

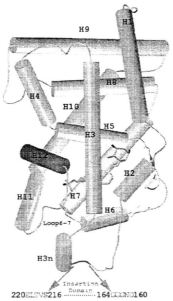

Figure 4: Overall topology of the VDR LBD bound to 1,25(OH)$_2$D$_3$.(11).

The hereditary vitamin D-resistant rickets, HVDRR, is a rare genetic disease caused by generalized resistance to 1,25(OH)$_2$D$_3$ action. The causes have been ascertained to several mutations, some of them in the VDR LBD: Cys190Trp (18), Gln259Pro (19), Arg274Leu (20), Trp286Arg (21), His305Gln (22), Ile314Ser (23), Arg391Cys (23) (Figure 5b). These mutations result in a VDR activity either resistant to the hormone or drastically reduced. All these residues except Cys190 are conserved in the VDR family. The mutation Cys190Trp is found in the insertion domain with no effect on ligand binding (17). Gln259 (H4) interacts with the loop 8-

heterodimerize, thus explaining the impaired VDR-RXR-VDRE formation (19). Arg274 (H5) is hydrogen-bonded to the 1-OH group of 1,25(OH)$_2$D$_3$ and its mutation affects the affinity of VDR for 1,25(OH)$_2$D$_3$. Trp286Arg (β1) results into a loss of ligand binding ablity because this critical residue contacts the ligand near the Cdrings and is part of a hydrogen bond network involving Ser275. His 305 (loop H6-H7) is hydrogen bonded to 25-OH of 1,25(OH)$_2$D$_3$ and its mutation decreases the hormone affinity. The mutation Ile314Ser (H7) closed to Leu313 that is in hydrophobic contact with the ligand, affects also the binding of the ligand. The last mutation Arg391Cys located in helix H10 is in the dimerization interface observed in the heterodimer RAR/RXR structure (24), thus affecting the heterodimerization. Premature stop codon found in HVDRR patients, occurs at Gln152 (H2) (20) and at Tyr295 (β2) (17). These modifications delete a large part of the LBD.

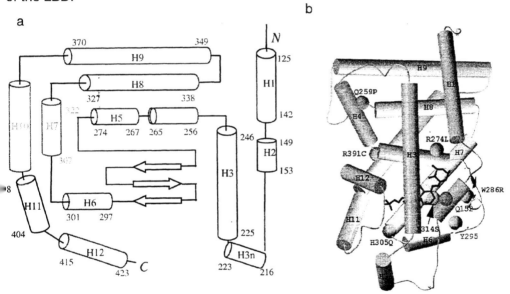

Figure 5 a: Topology of the VDR LBD.

       b : Natural mutants found in the VDR LBD are shown as spheres.

The active conformation of the vitamin D in the VDR complex is shown in Figure 6a. The ligand binding pocket is essentially hydrophobic. The elongated ligand embraces H3 with the A ring is oriented toward the C-termini of H5 and the 25-OH is near helices H7 and H11. The A ring adopts a chair B conformation with the 1-OH and 3-OH groups in equatorial and axial orientations. The conjuguated triene is tightly fitted in a hydrophobic channel between Ser275 (loop H5-β) and Trp286 (β2) on one side and Leu233 (H3) on the other side. The C6-C7 bond deviates by 30° from the planar geometry. The 1-OH makes two hydrogen bonds with Ser237 (H3) and Arg274 (H5) and the 3-OH with Ser278 (H5) and Tyr143. The 25-OH group is hydrogen bonded to His305 (loop6-7) and His397 (H11).

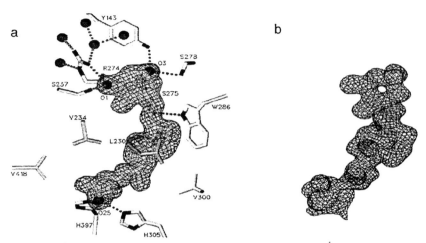

Figure 6: Experimental electron density omit maps of the (a) 1,25(OH)$_2$D$_3$ in the hVDR LBD pocket at 1.8 Å contoured at 1.0 σ and of (b) KH1060 VDR complex at 1.4 Å and contoured at 2.0 σ.

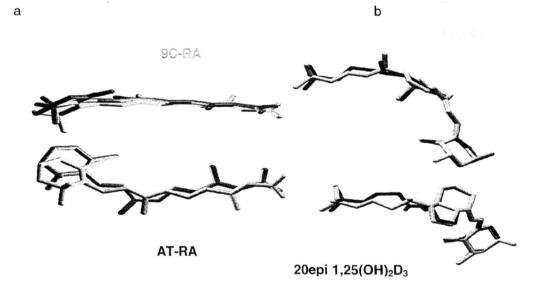

Figure 7 a: Superposition of 9cis retinoic acid and of all-trans retinoic acid in the superimposed RARγ complexes (7).

b : Superposition of 1,25(OH)$_2$D$_3$ and the 20epi 1,25(OH)$_2$D$_3$ in the superimposed VDR complexes.

We have now solved the structures at high resolution of the VDR LBD bound to several agonists. Figure 6b shows the experimental electron density omit map of the VDR LBD complexed to KH1060. The VDR in complex with the different synthetic agonists adopts the same unique conformation of the complex with the natural ligand shown on figure 4. The rmsd on the backbone between the VDR-1,25(OH)$_2$D$_3$ complex and the VDR-KH1060 complex is only 0.12 Å. The agonist dependent conformation of helix H12 is strictly maintained thereby allowing the same crystal packing. The vitamin D analogs are anchored in the pocket by the same residues making hydrogen bonds with the hydroxyl groups of the ligands. A similar observation has been seen for RAR complexed to several agonists (7). Only the anchoring points are conserved and the ligands adapt to the pocket. Figure 7b shows the superposition of the 1,25(OH)$_2$D$_3$ and the 20epi in the superimposed proteins together with on figure 7a the superposition of 9cis retinoic acid and all-trans retinoic acid in the RAR complexes. In the two cases the ligands adapts to a unique pocket in order to generate the unique agonist conformation of the LBD in order to interact with coactivators.

References:

1. Mangelsdorf, D.J., Thummel, C., Beato, M., Herrlich, P., Schütz, G., Umesono, K., Blumberg, B., Kastner, P., Mark, M. and Chambon, P (1995) Cell 83, 835-839.
2. Moras, D. and Gronemeyer, H. (1998) Curr. Opin. Cell Biol. 10, 384-391.
3. Bourguet , W., Ruff, M., Chambon, P., Gronemeyer H. and Moras, D. (1995) Nature 375, 377-382.
4. Renaud, J.P., Rochel, N., Ruff, M., Vivat, V., Chambon, P., Gronemeyer H. and Moras, D. (1995) Nature 378, 681-689.
5. Wagner, R.L., Apriletti, J.W., McGrath, M.E., West, B.L., Baxter, J.D. and Fletterick, R.J. (1995) Nature 378, 690-697.
6. Brzozowski, A.M., Pike, A.C.W., Dauter, Z., Hubbard, R.E., Bonn, T., Engström, L., Greene, G.L., Gustafsson, J.A. and Carlquist, M. (1997) Nature 389, 753-758.
7. Klaholz, B.P., Renaud, J.P., Mitschler, A., Zusi, C., Chambon, P., Gronemeyer, H. and Moras, D. (1998) Nat. Struct. Biol. 5, 199-202.
8. Nolte, R.T., Wisely, G.B., Westin, S., Cobb, J.E., Lambert, M.H., Kurokawa, R., Rosenfeld, M.G., Willson, T.M., Glass, C.K. and Milburn, M.V. (1998) Nature 395, 137-143.
9. Williams , S.P. and Sigler, P.B. (1998) Nature 393, 392-396.
10. Xu, H.E., Lambert, M.H., Montana, V.G., Parks, D.J., Blanchard, S.G., Brown, P.J., Sternbach, D.D., Lehmann, J.M., Wisely, G.B., Willson, T.M., et al. (1999) Mol. Cell 3, 397-403.
11. Rochel , N., Wurtz, J.M., Mitschler, A., Klaholz, B. and Moras, D. (2000) Mol. Cell 5, 173-179.
12. Darimont , B.D., Wagner, R.L., Apriletti, J.W., Stallcup, M.R., Kushner, P.J., Baxter, J.D., Fletterick, R.J. and Yamamoto, K.R. (1998) Genes Dev. 12, 3343-3356.

214

13. Shiau, A.K., Bastard, D., Loria, P.M. Cheng, L., Kushner, P.J., Agard, D.A. and Greene, G.L. (1998) Cell 95, 927-937.
14. Wurtz, J.M., Bourguet, W., Renaud, J.P., Vivat, V., Chambon, P., Moras, D. and Gronemeyer, H. (1996) Nat. Struct. Biol. 3, 87-94.
15. Bouillon, R., Okamura, W.H. and Norman, A.W. (1995) Endocr. Rev. 16, 200-257.
16. DeLuca, H.F. and Zierold, C (1998) Nutr. Rev. 56, 54-75.
17. Malloy, P.J., Pike, J.W. and Feldman, D. (1999) Endo. Rev. 20(2), 156-188.
18. Thompson, E., Kristjansson, K. and Hughes, M. (1991) In: Vitamin D: gene regulation, structure-function analysis and clinical application, Norman, A.W., Bouillon, R., Thomasset, M., eds. Eighth Workshop on Vitamin D. W. de Gruyter, New-York, Abstract p. 6.
19. Cockerill, F.J., Hawa, N.S., Yousaf, N., Hewison, M., O'Riordan, J.L. and Farrow, S.M. (1997) J. Clin. Endocrinol. Metab. 82, 3156-3160.
20. Kristjansson, K., Rut, A.R., Hewison, M., O'Riordan, J.L. and Hughes, M.R. (1993) J. Clin. Invest. 92, 12-16.
21. Nguyen, T.M., Petrovic, M., Guillozo, H., Alvarez, M.L., Kottler, M.L., Walrant-Debray, O., Rizk-Rabin, M. and Garabédian, M. (2000). In: Eleven Workshop on Vitamin D. Abstract 44, p. 188.
22. Malloy. P.J., Eccleshall, T.R., Gross, C., Van Maldergem, L., Bouillon, R. and Feldman, .D (1997) J. Clin. Invest. 99, 297-304.
23. Whitfield, G.K., Selznick, S.H., Haussler, C.A., Hsieh, J.C., Galligan, M.A., Jurutka, P.W., Thompson, P.D., Lee, S.M., Zerwekh, J.E. and Haussler, M.R. (1996) Mol. Endocr. 10, 1617-1631
24. Bourguet, W., Vivat, V., Wurtz, J.M., Chambon, P., Gronemeyer, H. and Moras, D. (2000) Mol. Cell 5, 289-298.

MECHANISM OF ACTION OF 20-EPI ANALOGS OF $1\alpha,25(OH)_2D_3$ WITH RESPECT TO ACTIVATION OF GENE TRANSCRIPTION

Pekka H. Mäenpää, Sami Väisänen, Tiina Jääskeläinen, and Sanna Ryhänen, Department of Biochemistry, University of Kuopio, 70210 Kuopio, Finland

Introduction A number of synthetic 20-epi analogs of $1\alpha,25(OH)_2D_3$ (calcitriol) are biologically powerful superagonists of calcitriol (1-3). We have been interested in studying, whether the 20-epi configuration as such is a determinant allowing more efficient activation of gene transcription as compared with the corresponding 20-natural analogs. A series of synthetic 20-natural and 20-epi analogs have been kindly made available for us by Drs. Lise Binderup and Fredrik Björkling from the Leo Pharmaceutical Products, Ltd, Ballerup, Denmark for these studies.

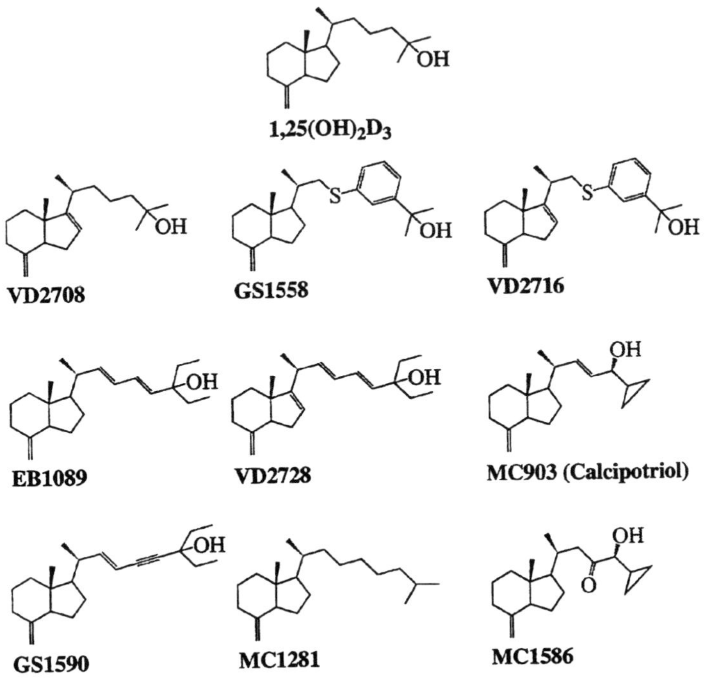

Figure 1: Side-chain structures of the 20-natural calcitriol analogs used in this study.

Materials and Methods Cell culture experiments using MG-63 human osteoblast-like osteosarcoma cells were performed as described previously (4). Limited trypsin digestion of in vitro-produced hVDR protein followed by SDS-PAGE and autoradiography was used to study the conformational change of the hVDR ligand-binding domain (LBD) caused by the different ligands (4-5).

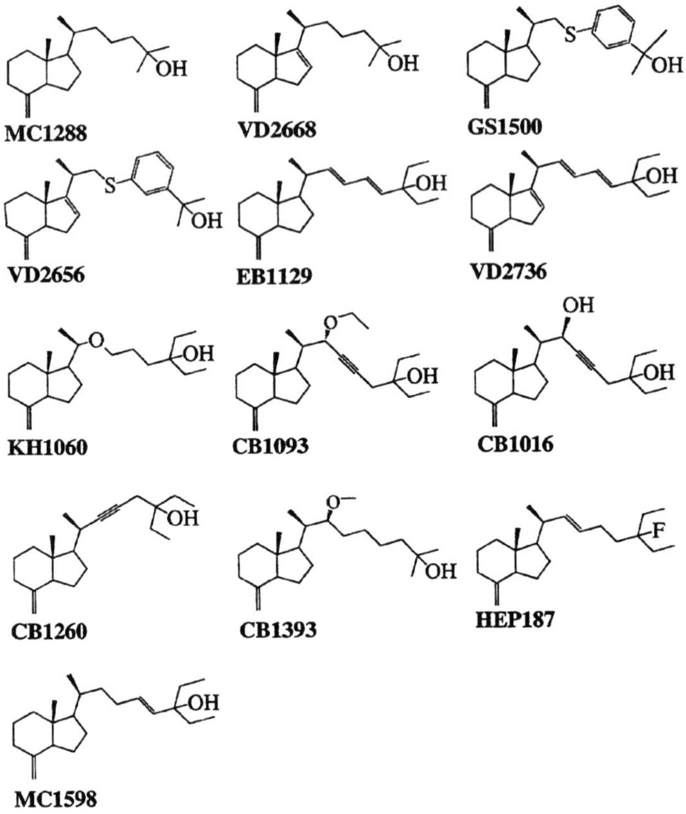

Figure 2: Side-chain structures of the 20-epi calcitriol analogs used in this study.

Results Based on our previous findings (5) that the 20-epi analog of calcitriol, MC1288, apparently does not form 1-OH hydrogen bond to Ser-237 as calcitriol does, we performed a series of experiments with point-mutated hVDRs and the various analogs to determine the destabilizing effect caused by the different vitamin D_3 compounds on hVDR conformation. In addition to Ser-237 (helix 3), Arg-274 (helix 5), which also forms a hydrogen bond to 1-OH with calcitriol, and Tyr-143 as well as Ser-278 (helix 5), which both form hydrogen bonds to 3-OH, were separately mutated for these studies.

Hydrogen bonding of the 1-OH to Ser-237 is apparently not important for all the analogs, since its substitution to Ala had no major effect on the stability of the LBD after treatment with analogs VD2708, VD2728, MC1288, KH1060, MC1598, or CB1093 (Table 1). However, there was no specificity in this effect with respect to the C-21 methyl group orientation. In contrast, Arg-274 is essential for ligand binding, since calcitriol and all the analogs studied altered the LBD conformation and caused a rapid breakdown of the receptor during trypsin digestion, when Arg-274 was changed to Ala.

Table 1: Effects of point mutations of selected natural amino acid residues to Ala. With calcitriol, 1-OH forms hydrogen bonds to Ser-237 and Arg-274, while 3-OH forms hydrogen bonds to Tyr-143 and Ser-278 (6). Protease digestion was for 10 min at 22°C with 25 μg/ml trypsin. Symbols: (-) conformation of the LBD is changed, (+) conformation is unaltered.

		Wild type hVDR	1α-OH		3β-OH	
			S237A	R274A	Y143A	S278A
20-normal analogs	1,25(OH)₂D₃	+	-	-	-	+
	VD2708	+	+	-	+	+
	VD2728	+	+	-	+	+
	MC903	+	-	-	-	-
	EB1089	+	-	-	-	+
20-epi analogs	MC1288	+	+	-	+	+
	VD2668	+	-	-	-	-
	GS1500	+	-	-	-	+
	VD2656	+	-	-	-	-
	KH1060	+	+	-	+	-
	CB1260	+	-	-	-	-
	CB1393	+	-	-	+	+
	MC1598	+	+	-	-	+
	CB1093	+	+	-	+	+
	HEP187	+	-	-	-	-
	CB1016	+	-	-	-	+

With respect to hydrogen bonding to 3-OH, replacement of Tyr-143 with Ala caused a conformational change with calcitriol but not with VD2708, VD2728, MC1288, KH1060, CB1393, and CB1093 whereas, with the other analogs, the conformation was changed. With respect to Ser-278, calcitriol protects the receptor also well, when it is changed to Ala. The analogs VD2708, VD2728, EB1089, MC1288, GS1500, CB1393, MC1598, CB1093, and CB1016 allow stable conformation, when Ser-278 is replaced by Ala. Again, when comparing the 20-normal and 20-epi analogs in this respect, there seems to be no specific effect caused by the C-21 methyl group orientation.

Next, we compared the biological properties of the various analogs, when the indicators were trypsin sensitivity of the LBD and induction of osteocalcin mRNA (Fig. 3) or secretion of osteocalcin protein into the medium (Fig. 4).The results from these experiments indicated that the orientation of the C-21 methyl group does not have any specific effect on the biological indicators of these compounds.

218

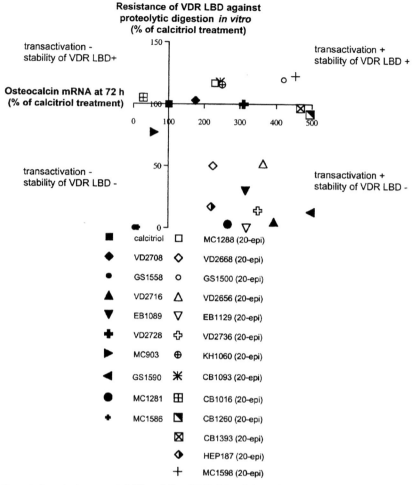

Figure 3: Correlation between stability of the LBD (Y-axis) and transcriptional activity (X-axis) after treatment with the different analogs. The hVDR protein was preincubated with 1 µM calcitriol or the analogs before partial proteolytic digestion with 100 µg/ml trypsin. The digestion products were analyzed by SDS/PAGE and autoradiography. Transcriptional activities of the vitamin D_3 compounds were measured by determining induced osteocalcin mRNA levels using Northern analysis. MG-63 cells were treated with calcitriol or the analogs for 6 h, the medium was replaced, and the osteocalcin mRNA levels were determined after a 72-h incubation without the vitamin D_3 compounds. Stability of the LBD against trypsin digestion *in vitro* and transcriptional activity in the presence of calcitriol were set to 100%.

Similarly, we compared biological effects of the 20-normal and 20-epi analogs after ligand binding in MG-63 cells by determining hVDR half-life (7) and osteocalcin mRNA levels (4). As can be seen from Fig. 5, most analogs behaved as superagonists, when compared with calcitriol, but no specific differences were observed with respect to the orientation of the C-21 methyl group.

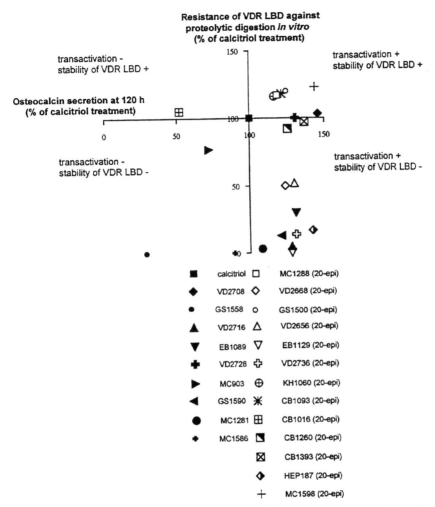

Figure 4: Correlation between stability of the VDR LBD (Y-axis) and transcriptional activity (X-axis) after treatment with the different analogs. Trypsin sensitivity of the hVDR protein was determined as in Fig. 3. Transcriptional activities of the vitamin D_3 compounds were measured as osteocalcin production into the medium by radioimmunoassay. MG-63 cells were treated with calcitriol or the different analogs as in Fig. 3. Stability of the LBD against trypsin digestion in vitro and transcriptional activity in the presence of calcitriol were set to 100%.

Discussion Structural requirements for VDR activation depend primarily on three structural features of the VDR; the A-ring, the side chain, and the D-ring (3). High affinity of the vitamin D_3 compounds for VDR depend on the hydroxyl groups in the A-ring, particularly the presence of the 1α-hydroxyl group, since precursors of calcitriol, which lack this hydroxyl group, bind in general poorly to VDR. It was therefore somewhat surprising that some vitamin D_3 analogs protected the tight LBD conformation of the VDR even when one of the hydrogen pairing amino acid residues (Ser-237) was changed to Ala. However, the presence of Arg-274 was essential with all the studied analogs for the native conformation. The hydrogen bonding of 3-OH to Tyr-143 and Ser-278 allowed more variation between the different analogs but, collectively, the VDR stability experiments did not reveal any specific effects between the 20-normal and 20-epi analogs.

Some biologically potent vitamin D_3 analogs contain 20-epi configuration in the side chain. It was therefore interesting to examine, whether the high biological potency is a general phenomenon of the 20-epi analogs compared with the corresponding 20-normal analogs. The osteocalcin mRNA and protein induction data as well as the determination of VDR half-lives with selected analogs did not, however, reveal any specific differences between the 20-normal and 20-epi analogs.

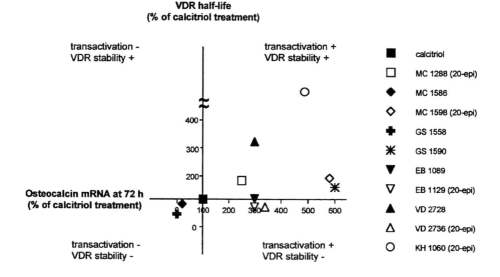

Figure 5: Correlation between VDR half-life (Y-axis) and transcriptional activity (X-axis) as influenced by the different analogs. The half-life was determined by Western-immunoblotting from nuclear extracts of MG-63 cells treated with cycloheximide (20 µg/ml) and the vitamin D_3 compounds (0.1 nM) for different periods of time (6 to 48 h). Transcriptional activities of the vitamin D_3 compounds were measured by determining induced osteocalcin mRNA levels using Northern analysis. MG-63 cells were treated with calcitriol or the analogs as in Fig. 3. The VDR half-life and the transcriptional activity in the presence of calcitriol were set to 100%.

Molecular modeling with vitamin D_3 analog docking into the binding pocket of modified LBD has suggested that the analogs with a rather rigid aliphatic side chain, such as MC903 and EB1089, can be accommodated with only minor adjustments of the geometry of calcitriol, while the 20-epi analogs, MC1288 and KH1060, could be docked only as low-energy conformers. With such geometry, the C-21 methyl group points in the same cavity as the natural ligand, while the rest of the chain is lining the opposite side of the binding cavity (6). This modeling result may also explain the present findings on the absence of specific biological effects between the 20-natural and 20-epi analogs. Apparently, the structure of the remaining side chain of the analogs, its contacts with the binding cavity and, consequently, the modified final conformation of the ligand binding pocket are more important for additional contacts with coactivators, corepressors, dimerization partners, and degradation specific factors (2,7,8,9).

References
1. Peleg, S., Sastry, M., Collins, E.D., Bishop, J.E., and Norman, A.W. (1995) J. Biol. Chem. 18: 10551-10558.
2. Rachez, C., Suldan, Z., Ward, J., Chang, C.P.B., Burakov, D., Erdjument-Bromage, H., Tempst, P., and Freedman, L.P. (1998) Genes Dev. 12: 1787-1800.
3. Peleg, S., in Vitamin D (Feldman D, Glorieux F.H. and Pike, J.W., eds, Academic Press, San Diego 1997), p. 1011-1025.
4. Väisänen, S., Ryhänen, S., Saarela, J.T.A., and Mäenpää, P.H. (1999) Eur. J. Biochem. 261: 706-713.
5. Väisänen, S., Rouvinen, J., and Mäenpää, P.H. (1998) FEBS Lett. 440: 203-207.
6. Rochel, N., Wurtz, J.M., Mitschler, A., Klaholz, B., and Moras, D. (2000) Mol. Cell: 5: 173-179.
7. Jääskeläinen, T., Ryhänen, S., Mahonen, A., DeLuca, H.F., and Mäenpää, P.H. (2000) J. Cell. Biochem. 76: 548-558.
8. Masuyama, H. and MacDonald, P.N. (1998) J. Cell. Biochem. 71: 429-440.
9. Yang, W. and Freedman, L.P. (1999) J. Biol. Chem. 274: 16838-16845.

CONFORMATIONS OF VDR-RXR HETERODIMERS AS THE MOLECULAR SWITCHES OF 1α,25(OH)₂D₃ SIGNALING

Carsten Carlberg

Institut für Physiologische Chemie I, Heinrich-Heine-Universität, D-40001 Düsseldorf, Germany

Summary: The vitamin D_3 receptor (VDR) acts primarily as a heterodimer with the retinoid X receptor (RXR) on different types of 1α,25-dihydroxyvitamin D_3 (1α,25(OH)$_2$D$_3$) response elements (VDREs). Therefore, DNA-bound VDR-RXR heterodimers can be considered as the molecular switches of 1α,25(OH)$_2$D$_3$ signaling. Functional conformations of these molecular switches are of central importance for describing the biological actions of 1α,25(OH)$_2$D$_3$ and its analogues. Moreover, VDR conformations provide a molecular basis for understanding the potential selective profile of VDR agonists and antagonists, which is critical for a therapeutic application. This review discusses VDR conformations and their selective stabilization by 1α,25(OH)$_2$D$_3$ and its analogue, when VDR is in solution, i.e. acting DNA-independent, or is complexed with RXR on different VDREs in the presence of coactivator or corepressor proteins.

Introduction: The transcription factor, VDR is the nuclear receptor for 1α,25(OH)$_2$D$_3$, and the mediator of all genomic actions of 1α,25(OH)$_2$D$_3$ and its analogues (1). The VDR is a member of a superfamily of structurally related nuclear receptors (2) that contain two zinc finger structures forming a characteristic DNA-binding domain (DBD) of 66 amino acids (3) and a carboxy-terminal ligand-binding domain (LBD) of approximately 300 amino acids (Fig. 1) (4).

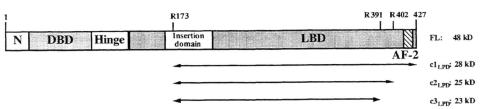

Figure 1: Primary structure of the VDR. Schematic overview on the primary structure of the VDR containing an amino-terminal region (N), DBD, hinge region and LBD. Furthermore, the LBD contains the insertion domain and the AF-2 domain. The trypsin restriction sites (after arginines at position 173, 391 and 402), that are critical for the generation of VDR fragments 1, 2 and 3 in the LPD assay, are indicated.

The LBD is formed by 12 α-helices (5) and has diverse functions in addition to ligand binding (6). These include interaction with other nuclear receptors for the formation of dimeric complexes and contact with cofactors, such as coactivators and corepressors, for modulation of transcriptional activities. Ligand binding causes a conformational change in the LBD whereby the ligand-binding pocket is closed by α-helix 12 via a "mouse-trap like" intramolecular folding (7). This α-helix contains a relatively conserved, seven amino acid region (the so-called activation function (AF)-2 domain) that serves as an interface for interaction with coactivator proteins (Fig. 2) (6).

224

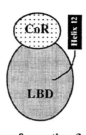 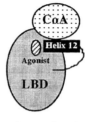 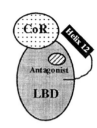

Figure 2: Three-conformation-model. In the absence of ligand, helix 12 of the LBD is displaced and an interaction with corepressor (CoR) proteins is possible ($c3_{LPD}$). In the presence of an agonist, helix 12 closes the ligand-binding pocket and enables an interaction with coactivator (CoA) proteins ($c1_{LPD}$). In the presence of an antagonist, helix 12 is shifted and not able to interact with coactivators ($c2_{LPD}$).

conformation 3
non-agonistic

conformation 1
agonistic

conformation 2
antagonistic

An essential prerequisite for a direct modulation of transcription by $1\alpha,25(OH)_2D_3$ is for ligand-activated VDR to be located in close proximity to the basal transcriptional machinery. This is initially achieved through the specific binding of the VDR to a VDRE in the regulatory region of a primary $1\alpha,25(OH)_2D_3$ responding gene. The DBD of VDR contacts the major grove of a hexameric sequence, referred to as core binding motif, with the consensus sequence RGKTCA (R = A or G, K = G or T) (8). The VDR requires formation of homo- and/or heterodimeric complexes with a second partner receptor in order to allow efficient DNA binding (8). Most nuclear $1\alpha,25(OH)_2D_3$ signaling models assume that VDR can only act as a heterodimer with RXR on a directly repeated arrangement of two hexameric core binding motifs spaced by 3 nucleotides, so-called DR3-type VDREs (9) (for more details see Toell & Carlberg in these proceedings). Several examples of simple VDREs fit into this rule, but other VDRE structures have also been identified (for more details see Quack & Carlberg in these proceedings) (10). On DR3- and DR4-type VDREs, the DBDs of VDR and RXR bind to the same side of the DNA, but on DR6- and IP9-type VDREs, the distance of the VDR-DBD relative to the RXR-DBD is too wide to allow direct contact of both DBDs (Fig. 3) (11). This suggests that alternative dimerization interfaces between VDR and RXR are used and that VDR-RXR heterodimers are taking different conformations on the different VDRE types.

Figure 3: VDR-RXR complexes on DR3- and IP9-type VDREs. Schematic representation of VDR-RXR heterodimers that have been modelled on DR3- and IP9-type VDREs based on the crystal structure of T_3R-RXR heterodimers bound to a DR4-type response element. On a DR3-type VDRE, both DBDs are located on the same side of the DNA and contact each other. In contrast, on an IP9-type VDRE the DBDs theoretically contact different sides of the DNA as they are too distant for a direct contact. Thus, the model postulates an alternative dimerization interface within the hinge region of both receptors.

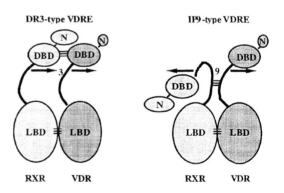

In vitro evaluation of VDR conformations: The activation of VDR-RXR heterodimers by ligand is the key reaction in nuclear $1\alpha,25(OH)_2D_3$ signaling (12) and allows for DNA-bound VDR-RXR heterodimers as the molecular switches in the vitamin D_3 endocrine system to be considered. Novel *in vitro* assay systems, such as limited protease digestion (LPD) (13,14) and gel shift clipping (GSC) (11,15-17) (Fig. 4), were developed to get a more detailed understanding of these molecular switches. In DNA-independent LPD assays, ligand-bound monomeric VDR is incubated with an endoprotease such as trypsin, which allows for the detection of up to three different protease-resistant VDR fragments (14,18,19) (Fig. 1). These VDR fragments are interpreted as representatives of the ligand-stabilized VDR conformations $c1_{LPD}$, $c2_{LPD}$ and $c3_{LPD}$ (13,20,21) (Fig. 2). However, with most VDR agonists, only conformations $c1_{LPD}$ and $c3_{LPD}$ are observed (21) (Fig. 4). In the GSC assay, VDR-RXR heterodimers are formed on a VDRE and consequently incubated with trypsin, which provides two truncated DNA-bound VDR-RXR complexes that are interpreted as conformations of ligand-stabilized VDR-RXR heterodimers ($c1_{GSC}$ and $c2_{GSC}$) (Fig. 4). Both assay systems promise a fast and accurate *in vitro* evaluation of $1\alpha,25(OH)_2D_3$ analogues, but differ in their perspectives on ligand-induced VDR conformations: in its "classical", DNA-independent form, the LPD assay studies monomeric VDR in solution, whereas the GSC assay analyses DNA-bound VDR-RXR heterodimers.

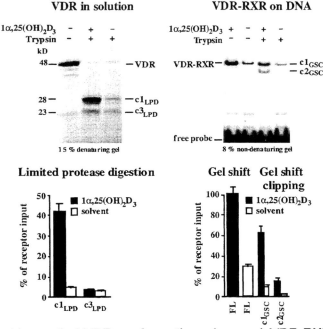

Figure 4: Analysis of VDR conformations by LPD and GSC assays. *In vitro* translated VDR in solution or *in vitro* translated VDR-RXR heterodimers bound to DNA in the presence of 10 µM $1\alpha,25(OH)_2D_3$ or solvent was analyzed by LPD and GSC assays. Representative experiments are shown. The molecular mass of full-length VDR and VDR fragments 1 and 3 ($c1_{LPD}$ and $c3_{LPD}$) is indicated. Phosphorimaging quantified the amount of $c1_{LPD}$ and $c3_{LPD}$ in relation to VDR input and of digested VDR-RXR heterodimer-DNA complexes 1 and 2 ($c1_{GSC}$ and $c2_{GSC}$) in relation to ligand-induced, non-digested VDR-RXR heterodimers. For experimental details see (16).

There are several lines of evidence that VDR conformation $c1_{LPD}$ and VDR-RXR conformations $c1_{GSC}$ and $c2_{GSC}$ represent activated VDR-RXR heterodimers (Fig. 2). The size difference between VDR-RXR heterodimer-VDRE complexes that represent conformations $c1_{GSC}$ and $c2_{GSC}$ (Fig. 4) appears to be based on the truncation of the amino-terminal region of RXR, i.e. the VDR component of both conformations is identical and comparable to VDR conformation $c1_{LPD}$ (16). In contrast, VDR conformation $c3_{LPD}$ does not appear to be of relevance for the characterization of an agonistic behaviour of a VDR ligand and is therefore referred to as a non-agonistic conformation (Fig. 2). This is supported by the observation that truncation of the 14 most carboxy-terminal amino acids of the VDR, i.e. of helix 12 containing the AF-2 domain (Figs. 1), resulted in a clear loss in ligand sensitivity, of the whole VDR, by affecting $c1_{LPD}$ (16). The size of the VDR fragment 1 that represents $c1_{LPD}$ decreased in relation to the constant size of VDR fragment 3 (representing $c3_{LPD}$), when an increasing number of amino acids were truncated from the carboxy-terminus. This suggests that the major difference between $c1_{LPD}$ and $c3_{LPD}$ are the 40 most carboxy-terminal amino acids, which would perfectly explain the size difference between VDR fragments 1 and 3 (Figs. 1 and 2). Further analysis of amino- and carboxy-terminal truncations of the VDR defined the position of the high-affinity LBD between amino acids 128 and 427 (carboxy-terminus, see Fig. 1). Interestingly, the VDR fragments that represent $c1_{LPD}$ (28 kD) and $c3_{LPD}$ (23 kD) do not contain all of these 300 amino acids. Microsequencing has indicated that the VDR fragments are generated by digestion after arginine 173 (24) (Fig. 1). This cutting site is located within a subdomain of the LBD, referred to as insertion domain (Fig. 1), as it does not show homology to any other member of the nuclear receptor superfamily (4). Thus, it is likely that this subdomain is not involved in complexing the ligand in the ligand-binding pocket and may therefore be exposed enough for accessing the protease.

Carboxylic ester VDR antagonists function via selective stabilization of an antagonistic conformation ($c2_{LPD}$) of the VDR-LBD, which is not observed with VDR agonists (25) (for more details see Herdick *et al.* in these proceedings). The observation that these antagonists cannot induce supershifts with the coactivator protein TIF2 suggests that, in this antagonistic conformation, helix 12 of the LBD does not appear to be positioned correctly, so that the AF-2 domain on this helix is not able to interact with the LXXLL (L = leucine, X = any amino acid) core nuclear receptor interaction motifs of coactivator proteins (26,27) (Fig. 2). Moreover, GSC assays with the endoprotease chymotrypsin allowed for a visualization of different conformations representing antagonist-complexed VDR-RXR heterodimers and agonist-complexed VDR-RXR heterodimers. Interestingly, these different heterodimer conformations cannot only be observed with receptors that were translated *in vitro*, but also with receptor complexes within nuclear extracts from different agonist- and antagonist-treated cells (M. Herdick, A. Steinmeyer, C. Carlberg, unpublished results). This confirms that antagonist-specific conformations also exist in living cells, i.e. that an *in vitro* evaluation of antagonistic receptor conformations represents the *in vivo* situation.

Molecular basis of promoter selectivity: The $1\alpha,25(OH)_2D_3$ analogue, EB1089, shows potent anti-proliferative effects in breast cancer cells both *in vitro* and *in vivo* with a potency that is 10-100 times higher than that of the natural hormone (28). This sharp biological profile was associated with the higher selectivity (approximately 15-times) of EB1089 to activate IP9-type VDREs rather than DR3-type VDREs in MCF-7 human breast cancer cells (18). It was hypothesized that primary $1\alpha,25(OH)_2D_3$ responding genes, that are involved in mediating growth arrest, should preferentially contain IP9-type VDREs in their promoter region (8,29). Due to the relatively low number of known primary $1\alpha,25(OH)_2D_3$ responding genes with characterized VDREs, this idea has not yet statistically been proven, but, for e.g., the genes for mouse *c-fos* and human and mouse

$p21^{WAF1/CIP1}$ each contain an IP9-type VDRE in their regulatory regions (10). This suggests that these genes should selectively be activated by EB1089, which is the analogue with the highest preference for the activation of IP9-type VDREs within a group of approximately 30 analogues that have presently been analyzed for promoter selectivity (18,19,22,30,31). Moreover, promoter selectivity appears to be closely linked to the exact structure of EB1089, as metabolites and close structural relatives of the analogue have lost this property almost entirely (30,31).

The molecular basis of this promoter selectivity was found to be a VDRE-selective stabilization of VDR-RXR heterodimers (15). Ligand-dependent gel shift assays demonstrated that EB1089 mediated the stabilization of VDR-RXR heterodimers on IP9-VDREs at approximately 8-fold lower concentrations than on DR3-type VDREs (15). As a reference, the natural hormone $1\alpha,25(OH)_2D_3$ did not show a significant selectivity. GSC assays demonstrated similar results and in addition allowed for the two VDR-RXR heterodimers conformations $c1_{GSC}$ and $c2_{GSC}$, to be differentiated. On an IP9-type VDRE, $c1_{GSC}$ was found to be stabilized by EB1089 at approximately 9-fold lower concentrations than on a DR3-type VDRE. This selectivity could not be observed with $c2_{GSC}$ or with $1\alpha,25(OH)_2D_3$ as a ligand (15).

Taken together, two functional conformations of the VDR can be differentiated on each VDRE, therefore allowing a more detailed view on DNA-complexed VDR-RXR heterodimers. VDR-RXR heterodimers in $c1_{GSC}$ clearly gain a higher affinity for DNA, through EB1089 and are activated more sensitively on an IP9-type VDRE than on a DR3-type VDRE, whereas VDRE-type preference is not observed with the natural hormone, $1\alpha,25(OH)_2D_3$. This indicates that a promoter selectivity of VDR agonists is based on their property to selectively increase affinity for VDREs and to quite sensitively stabilize VDR conformations in VDR-RXR-VDRE complexes.

Modulation of functional VDR conformations by DNA: In DNA-independent, LPD assays, most of the potent VDR agonists such as $1\alpha,25(OH)_2D_3$, its 20-epi and 20-methyl analogues (MC1288 and ZK161422) and EB1089, preferentially stabilize the VDR in conformation $c1_{LPD}$, but other agonists, such as Gemini (also called Ro27-2310, having two side chains at carbon 20) and EB1436 (an EB1089 metabolite (32)) stabilize the receptor exclusively or in majority in conformation $c3_{LPD}$ (16,33). According to the three-conformation-model (Fig. 2), this is interpreted as a sign for a weak agonist, as the stabilization of $c3_{LPD}$ requires rather high ligand concentrations (30,31). Interestingly, heterodimerization of VDR with RXR in the absence of DNA did not result in a significant effect on the ligand affinity and the ratio of VDR conformations. However, complex formation of VDR-RXR heterodimers on VDREs was very effective in increasing the ligand sensitivity of the VDR (16,33). DNA-dependent, LPD assays demonstrated that the sensitivity of $c1_{LPD}$ for $1\alpha,25(OH)_2D_3$ increased by a factor of approximately 30 to a value of 0.1 nM. Supershift and GSC assays confirmed that the affinity of VDR-RXR heterodimer conformations for $1\alpha,25(OH)_2D_3$ was in the order of 0.1 nM (33). The complex formation of the VDR with DNA increased the affinity of $c3_{LPD}$ for Gemini by a factor of 60 and allowed the stabilization of $c1_{LPD}$ by the analogue (33) (for more details see Bury et al. in these proceedings). GSC assays confirmed this drastic increase in affinity of VDR-RXR heterodimer conformations for Gemini. Moreover, complex formation of the VDR on DNA also results in a shift from VDR conformation 3 to 1, i.e. the relative amount of VDR molecules that are stabilized in $c3_{LPD}$ are decreased in favour for those that occupy $c1_{LPD}$ (16). This suggests that a VDR agonist, which appears to be weak in DNA-independent assays, may show unexpected potency in DNA-dependent assays. In summary, an apparent discrepancy between *in vitro* and *in vivo* assays that is observed with some VDR agonists could be solved by using *in vitro* assays that take advantage of the fact that VDR-RXR complex formation on VDREs clearly enhances agonist affinity and can facilitate conformational changes of the VDR.

Modulation of functional VDR conformations by coactivators: Coactivators mediate ligand-activated transcription by enhancing nuclear receptor transactivation through contacts with the basal transcriptional machinery and initiation of chromatin opening by histone acetylase activity (34). In the past years, several coactivators have been cloned and characterized, of which the three members of the SRC-family, SRC-1, TIF2 and RAC3 (reviewed in (35)) appear to be the most prominent. The binding of $1\alpha,25(OH)_2D_3$ or its analogues induces the above discussed conformational changes in the VDR-LBD, which then facilitate the interaction with coactivator proteins (Fig. 2). VDR has been shown to interact with all three members of the SRC-family and their contact points have been mapped in helix 12 (AF-2 domain) and helix 3 of the LBD. A direct comparison of the affinity of the interaction of SRC-1, TIF2 and RAC3 with the VDR for a selection of VDR agonists did not provide significant evidence for a coactivator-analogue selectivity (33). In contrast to the recently suggested coactivator selectivity of the $1\alpha,25(OH)_2D_3$ analogue OCT (36), the three members of the SRC-coactivator family appear to act similarly with most VDR agonists (33) and may therefore replace each other in the *in vivo* situation (37). The VDR-coactivator interaction further facilitates recruitment of other factors to form a larger complex that modulates chromatin structure and initiates transcription (38). This also involves the recently described DRIP/ARC cofactor complexes (39,40), which appear to contact the VDR and other nuclear receptors as a second step after their interaction with SRC-family coactivator proteins (34).

When comparing the *in vitro* profile of $1\alpha,25(OH)_2D_3$ with the model analogues MC1288, ZK161422 and Gemini (33), the latter analogue showed interesting, coactivator-dependent effects. Since Gemini behaves in DNA-independent LPD assays as a weak VDR agonist, it is surprising that mammalian one-hybrid assays (in the presence of endogenous coactivators) indicated a higher potency for Gemini than for $1\alpha,25(OH)_2D_3$ (33). Moreover, Gemini appeared to be quite ineffective in mediating an *in vitro* interaction of VDR with any of the three SRC-family members in solution, but in reporter gene assays the overexpression of TIF2 (as a representative coactivator family member) resulted in a 36-fold increased sensitivity of Gemini for gene activation from DR3-type VDREs (33). In DNA-dependent LPD assays the addition of TIF2 shifted the majority of agonist-stabilized VDR molecules into $c1_{LPD}$ and as a consequence drastically increased the ligand sensitivity of this conformation (for more details see Bury *et al.* in these proceedings). These results suggest that with some VDR agonists, such as Gemini, the complex formation of VDR-RXR heterodimers on a VDRE (which shifts most of the VDR molecules into $c1_{LPD}$) is a prerequisite for an efficient interaction with coactivators. In contrast, with VDR agonists that readily stabilize most VDR molecules in solution in $c1_{LPD}$, such as the natural hormone $1\alpha,25(OH)_2D_3$ and its 20-epi and 20-methyl analogues, the DNA-dependent interaction with a coactivator does not result in significant effects on the stabilization of functional VDR conformations (33).

Modulations of functional VDR conformations by corepressors: Corepressors silence non-liganded nuclear receptors by recruitment of histone deacetylases, which maintain chromatin in a transcriptionally repressive state (Fig. 2) (6,41). The VDR was described as a nuclear receptor with intrinsic repression activity that, as being sensitive to histone deacetylase inhibitors, appears to act through the established Sin3-HDAC pathway (42). The nuclear receptor corepressor (NCoR) was demonstrated to directly contact the VDR with similar binding affinity of both of its nuclear receptor interaction domains (42,43). The VDR-NCoR complex dissociates with increasing $1\alpha,25(OH)_2D_3$ concentrations suggesting that VDR-NCoR interaction is valid (42) and can be compared to established T_3R- or RAR-NCoR interactions (44-46). In addition, a protein-protein interaction of VDR with the novel corepressor Alien was demonstrated, both in vivo and in vitro (42) (for more details see Polly et al. in these proceedings). The interaction of the VDR with NCoR results in a preferential stabilization of the VDR in the non-agonistic conformation $c3_{LPD}$, whereas within a complex with SRC-1 VDR takes the agonistic conformation $c1_{LPD}$. Again helix 12 was found to be a critical sensor for the differential stabilization of the activated and silent state of the receptor. VDR agonists that showed similar sensitivity in inducing VDR-RXR-VDRE complex formation were found to mediate a different dose-dependent release of NCoR from these complexes, which correlates with their ability to stabilize the silent state of the VDR in the presence of NCoR. Interestingly, a reasonable amount of VDR-NCoR complexes were found to be stable even in the presence of saturating agonist concentrations. This was confirmed by a quenching effect of overexpressed NCoR on agonist-induced gene activity mediated by VDR-RXR heterodimers (M. Herdick & C. Carlberg, unpublished results).

Conclusion: DNA-bound VDR-RXR heterodimers are the molecular switches in $1\alpha,25(OH)_2D_3$ signaling and their different conformations may explain the selectivity of VDR agonists and antagonists. The induction of response element- and coactivator-modulated VDR conformations is a key step for the gene regulatory function of a VDR agonist. Therefore, analyzing the interaction of $1\alpha,25(OH)_2D_3$ analogues with VDR and VDR-RXR conformations, presently appears to be the most informative way of an in vitro evaluation of $1\alpha,25(OH)_2D_3$ analogues.

References:
1. Carlberg, C., and Polly, P. (1998) Crit Rev Eukaryot Gene Expr 8, 19-42
2. Mangelsdorf, D. J., Thummel, C., Beato, M., Herrlich, P., Schütz, G., Umesono, K., Blumberg, B., Kastner, P., Mark, M., Chambon, P., and Evans, R. M. (1995) Cell 83, 835-839
3. Freedman, L. P. (1992) Endocrine Rev 13, 129-145
4. Wurtz, J.-M., Bourguet, W., Renaud, J.-P., Vivat, V., Chambon, P., Moras, D., and Gronemeyer, H. (1996) Nat Struc Biol 3, 87-94
5. Rochel, N., Wurtz, J. M., Mitschler, A., Klaholz, B., and Moras, D. (2000) Mol Cell 5, 173-179
6. Moras, D., and Gronemeyer, H. (1998) Curr Opin Cell Biol 10, 384-391

230

7. Renaud, J.-P., Rochel, N., Ruff, M., Vivat, V., Chambon, P., Gronemeyer, H., and Moras, D. (1995) *Nature* **378**, 681-689
8. Carlberg, C. (1995) *Eur J Biochem* **231**, 517-527
9. Umesono, K., Murakami, K. K., Thompson, C. C., and Evans, R. M. (1991) *Cell* **65**, 1255-1266
10. Carlberg, C. (1997) *Proc 10th Int Vitamin D Workshop*, 268-275
11. Quack, M., Szafranski, K., Rouvinen, J., and Carlberg, C. (1998) *Nucleic Acids Res* **26**, 5372-5378
12. Carlberg, C. (1996) *Endocrine* **4**, 91-105
13. Nayeri, S., and Carlberg, C. (1997) *Biochem J* **327**, 561-568
14. Peleg, S., Sastry, M., Collins, E. D., Bishop, J. E., and Norman, A. W. (1995) *J Biol Chem* **270**, 10551-10558
15. Quack, M., and Carlberg, C. (1999) *Mol Pharmacol* **55**, 1077-1087
16. Quack, M., and Carlberg, C. (2000) *Mol Pharmacol* **57**, 375-384
17. Quack, M., and Carlberg, C. (2000) *J Mol Biol* **296**, 743-756
18. Nayeri, S., Danielsson, C., Kahlen, J. P., Schräder, M., Mathiasen, I. S., Binderup, L., and Carlberg, C. (1995) *Oncogene* **11**, 1853-1858
19. Nayeri, S., Mathiasen, I. S., Binderup, L., and Carlberg, C. (1996) *J Cell Biochem* **62**, 325-333
20. Liu, Y.-Y., Collins, E. D., Norman, A. W., and Peleg, S. (1997) *J Biol Chem* **272**, 3336-3345
21. Nayeri, S., Kahlen, J. P., and Carlberg, C. (1996) *Nucleic Acids Res* **24**, 4513-4518
22. Danielsson, C., Mathiasen, I. S., James, S. Y., Nayeri, S., Bretting, C., Hansen, C. M., Colston, K. W., and Carlberg, C. (1997) *J Cell Biochem* **66**, 552-562
23. Danielsson, C., Nayeri, S., Wiesinger, H., Thieroff-Ekerdt, R., and Carlberg, C. (1996) *J Cell Biochem* **63**, 199-206
24. Väisänen, S., Juntunen, K., Itkonen, A., Vihko, P., and Mäenpää, P. H. (1997) *Eur J Biochem* **248**, 156-162
25. Herdick, M., Steinmeyer, A., and Carlberg, C. (2000) *J Biol Chem* **275**, in press
26. Brzozowski, A. M., Pike, A. C. W., Dauter, Z., Hubbard, R. E., Bonn, T., Engström, O., Öhman, L., Greene, G. L., Gustafsson, J.-A., and Carlquist, M. (1997) *Nature* **389**, 753-758
27. Shiau, A. K., Barstad, D., Loria, P. M., Cheng, L., Kushner, P. J., Agard, D. A., and Greene, G. L. (1998) *Cell* **95**, 927-937
28. Mørk Hansen, C., and Mäenpää, P. H. (1997) *Biochem Pharmacol* **54**, 1173-1179
29. Carlberg, C. (1996) *J Invest Dermatol Symp Proc* **1**, 10-14
30. Quack, M., Clarin, A., Binderup, E., Björkling, F., Hansen, C. M., and Carlberg, C. (1998) *J Cell Biochem* **71**, 340-350
31. Quack, M., Mork Hansen, C., Binderup, E., Kissmeyer, A. M., and Carlberg, C. (1998) *Br J Pharmacol* **125**, 607-614
32. Kissmeyer, A.-M., Binderup, E., Binderup, L., Mørk Hansen, C., Rastrup Andersen, N., Makin, H. L. J., Schroeder, N. J., Shankar, V. N., and Jones, G. (1997) *Biochem Pharmacol* **53**, 1087-1097
33. Herdick, M., Bury, Y., Quack, M., Uskokovic, M., Polly, P., and Carlberg, C. (2000) *Mol Pharmacol* **57**, 1206-1217
34. Freedman, L. P. (1999) *Cell* **97**, 5-8
35. Chen, J. D., and Li, H. (1998) *Crit Rev Eukaryot Gene Expr* **8**, 169-190
36. Takeyama, K.-I., Masuhiro, Y., Fuse, H., Endoh, H., Murayama, A., Kitanaka, S., Suzawa, M., Yanagisawa, J., and Kato, S. (1999) *Mol Cell Biol* **19**, 1049-1055
37. Xu, J., Qiu, Y., DeMayo, F. J., Tsai, S. Y., Tsai, M.-J., and O'Malley, B. W. (1998) *Science* **279**, 1922-1925
38. Spencer, T. E., Jenster, G., Burcin, M. M., Allis, C. D., Zhou, J., Mizzen, C. A., McKenna, N. J., Onate, S. A., Tsai, S. Y., Tsai, M.-J., and O'Malley, B. W. (1997) *Nature* **389**, 194-198
39. Rachez, C., Lemon, B. D., Suldan, Z., Bromleigh, V., Gamble, M., Näär, A. M., Erdjument-Bromage, H., Tempst, P., and Freedman, L. P. (1999) *Nature* **398**, 824-828
40. Näär, A. M., Beaurang, P. A., Zhou, S., Abraham, S., Solomon, W., and Tjian, R. (1999) *Nature* **398**, 828-832
41. Torchia, J., Glass, C., and Rosenfeld, M. G. (1998) *Curr Opin Cell Biol* **10**, 373-383
42. Polly, P., Herdick, M., Moehren, U., Baniahmad, A., Heinzel, T., and Carlberg, C. (2000) *FASEB J* **13**, in press
43. Dwivedi, P. P., Muscat, G. E. O., Bailey, P. J., Omdahl, J. L., and May, B. K. (1998) *J Mol Endocrinol* **20**, 327-335
44. Hörlein, A. J., Näär, A. M., Heinzel, T., Torchia, J., Gloss, B., Kurokawa, R., Ryan, A., Kamei, Y., Söderström, M., Glass, C. K., and Rosenfeld, M. G. (1995) *Nature* **377**, 397-404
45. Chen, J. D., and Evans, R. M. (1995) *Nature* **377**, 454-457
46. Dressel, U., Thormeyer, D., Altincicek, B., Paululat, A., Eggert, M., Schneider, S., Tenbaum, S. P., Renkawitz, R., and Baniahmad, A. (1999) *Mol Cell Biol* **19**, 3383-3394

VITAMIN D RECEPTOR KNOCKOUT MOUSE AND REPRODUCTION

KEIKO KINUTA, HIROYUKI TANAKA, SHIGEAKI KATO and YOSHIKI SEINO
Department of Pediatrics, Okayama University Medical School, Okayama, 700-8558, Japan and Institute of Molecular and Cellular Biosciences, The University of Tokyo, Tokyo, 113-0032, Japan.

Introduction The vitamin D receptor (VDR) is expressed in calcium regulating tissues such as the intestine, the skeleton, and the parathyroid gland, as well as in the ovary and the testis (1), however the VDR function in gonads remains unclear. VDR knockout mouse (VDRKO) was established as a model for VDR itself and vitamin D function (2). In addition to the hypocalcemic rickets, uterine hypoplasia and impaired folliculogenesis were found in most of the female VDR KO, and estrogen supplementation increased the uterine weight of the mice (2). These results indicated that the uteri of the mice were in an estrogen-deficient state and suggested that VDR plays a role in estrogen production in the ovary. In male gonads, certain abnormalities may exist, although macroscopically the testis of the male VDRKO appeared normal. To clarify the pathophysiology of the disorder of gonads in the VDRKO, the activity of aromatase cytochrome P450 (P450arom), a key enzyme in estrogen biosynthesis, and the expression of CYP19 gene encoding P450arom were investigated.

Methods VDRKO were generated by gene targeting as described previously (2). Mice were weaned at 3 weeks of age, and were then fed a chow diet, MF (Ca, 11.1 mg/g; P, 8.3 mg/g; vitamin D_3, 1.08 IU/g) or high calcium diet (3) (Ca, 20.0 mg/g; P, 12.5 mg/g; vitamin D_3, 1.08 IU/g; lactose, 200mg/g). Activities of P450arom in ovaries were determined from the liberation of $[^3H]H_2O$ from $[1\beta-^3H]$ androstenedione essentially according to previously reported methods (4). The P450arom activities were determined in terms of picomoles of $[^3H]H_2O$ liberated per min per mg of protein. The expression level of the CYP19 gene after the calcium supplementation was analyzed by competitive PCR.

Results The activities of P450arom in the ovaries, testes and epididymis were measured. The P450arom activity in the 7-week-old VDR-/- mice was 0.087±0.011 (n=4). This value was 24.4% of that in the 7-week-old VDR+/+ mice and was similar to that in the 4-week-old VDR+/+ mice (just after weaning). The P450arom activity in the testes of the 10-week-old VDR+/+ mice was 0.354±0.020 picomoles of $[^3H]H_2O$ liberated per hour per mg of protein (mean ± SEM; n=4), which is approximately one sixtieth the value in the ovaries of 7-week-old VDR+/+ female mice. The P450arom activity in the testes of the 10-

week-old VDR-/- mice was 0.207±0.028 (n=5) picomoles of [^{3}H]H$_2$O liberated per hour per mg of protein. This level was 58.5% of that in the 10-week-old VDR+/+ mice ($p<0.005$). In the epididymis, the level of P450arom activity of the 10-week-old VDR-/- mice was 0.225±0.049, which was 34.6 % of that in the VDR+/+ mice (0.650±0.118;n=4,$p<0.01$). To evaluate the level of CYP19 gene expression, we applied a RT-PCR procedure. The ovary and the testis of VDR-/- mice expressed the mRNA of the CYP19 gene, but the expression levels of the CYP19 gene were markedly decreased. The results of competitive PCR were consistent with those of this RT-PCR.

Sperm functions: After incubation in capacitation medium for 15 min, 50-60% of the sperm from the cauda epididymides of the male VDR+/- mice were motile, whereas the percentage of sperm motile in the VDR-/- males declined from 15 % to less than 1% at 10-weeks of age. As shown in Table 1, the sperm counts of the VDRKO were half those of the VDR+/- mice. These results revealed that the functional sperm were markedly decreased in VDRKO as compared to VDR+/- mice. Testicular weight: Testicular weights were evaluated as the ratio of testis weight to body weight (mg/g). A transient increase in testicular weight in VDR-/- males was observed at 10 weeks of age ($p<0.01$ compared with VDR +/- mice), although the weight had decreased to the normal level by 15 weeks, as was reported in ERα gene knockout mice (5). Histology of the testes: As shown in Figure 1-B, the testes of 10-week-old VDRKO showed dilated lumen of seminiferous tubules, a thinner layer of epithelial cells and decreased spermatogenesis. The testes of 15-week-old VDRKO revealed rare spermatogenesis. A more widely dilated lumen of seminiferous tubules and atrophy of the seminiferous epithelium cells were observed (Figure 1-C).

The serum levels of estradiol in the female VDRKO are 3.3±1.3pg/ml (VDR+/-; 19.4±1.8pg/ml). The circulating estradiol level in the female VDRKO was significantly lower than that of in the heterozygous mice. The serum levels of LH and FSH in the VDRKO are shown in Table 1. The LH level was elevated 5-10 fold in both female and male VDR-/- mice as compared with VDR+/+ mice at 8 weeks-of-age. And the FSH level in VDR-/- mice was twice that in VDR+/+ mice at 8 weeks-of-age.

After the supplementation of estrogen to the male VDRKO, the histology of the testes revealed no apparent abnormality of the lumen of the seminiferous tubules or epithelial cells at age 10-weeks as shown in Figure 1-D. The sperm count and motility in the estrogen treated mice (n=3) was increased to the same level of the heterozygous mice (count: 47.7±5.0 x10^6/ml vs. 26.3 ± 7.3 x10^6/ml in VDR-/- without treatment, p<0.05, motility: 47.0±3.6 % vs. 6.0 ± 4.6 % in VDR-/- without treatment, *p*=0.0001). The serum calcium level was not increased (6.4± 0.1 mg/dl vs. 8.30±0.26 mg/dl in the VDR+/+ mice, *p*=0.0008).

The serum calcium level of the VDR null mutant mice given a normal diet (MF) was 5.36±0.25 mg/dl (mean±SEM; n=9) at the age of 7 weeks. The serum calcium level of VDR+/+ mice was 8.30±0.26 mg/dl (n=10) at this age. To correct the hypocalcemia, the VDR null mutant mice (n=10) were fed a high calcium diet from the time of weaning (3 week of age). The serum calcium increased to 8.65± 0.25 mg/dl (n=8). The serum level of calcium in the VDRKO was completely normalized after calcium supplementation. The P450arom activity in the ovary at the age of 7 weeks was 0.223±0.015 picomoles of [^{3}H]H$_2$O per min per mg of protein after the calcium supplementatin. The P450arom activity was increased to 60% of that in the wild type mice (*p*=0.005). The P450arom activity in the testis at the age of 10 weeks was 0.272±0.013 picomoles of [^{3}H]H$_2$O per hour per mg of protein after the calcium supplementation. The P450arom activity was increased to 77% of that in the wild type mice (*p*=0.024). The competitive PCR analysis of CYP19 is shown in Figure2. These results indicated that the expression of CYP19 gene was increased by calcium supplementation both in ovary and testis. However, the same as aromatase activity, the expression level of the aromatase gene was not completely recovered after normalization of serum calcium, being one fifth of that of the wild type in the ovary, (*P*=0.004) and one fourth of that of the wild type in the testis (*p*=0.02). The circulating estradiol level did not increased after calcium supplementation. In the female the estradiol level was 5.6±2.6 pg/ml (n=4) (*p*=0.03 compared with VDR+/- female mice at 8-weeks-of-age). The serum levels of LH and FSH were not corrected and remained high despite that the serum calcium level was normal after calcium supplementation. In the male VDRKO given calcium supplements, dilated lumens were observed in certain seminiferous tubules (Figure 1-E). The sperm count was increased to 44.0±5.3 x10^6/ml, but not significantly different compared to VDR-/- without treatment (*p*=0.09). The sperm motility was significantly increased to 39.3% compared to VDR-/- without treatment (*p*=0.0015).

Discussion The VDR is expressed in the ovary and the testis (1), suggesting that vitamin D has a role in these organs. Vitamin D-deficiency caused gonadal insufficiency in rats. The overall fertility of the female vitamin D-deficient rats was reduced to 75% and the litter size to 30% of the values for the vitamin D-replete females (6). The presence of sperm in the vaginal tract of females mated by vitamin D-deficient males was reduced to 45% compared to the matings by the vitamin D-replete males (7).

In the female VDRKO, uterine hypoplasia with impaired folliculogenesis was observed, and estrogen supplementation increased the uterine weight (2). These results indicated that estrogen deficiency caused impaired folliculogenesis and uterine hypoplasia in the female VDRKO. In the male VDRKO in this study, a transient increase in testicular weight was observed and decreased sperm counts and motility with histological abnormality in the testis was found. These findings in the VDRKO were similar to those in ERα knockout mice (5,8). In the male gonads of ERα knockout mice, the fluid reabsorption in efferent ductules of the testis was abnormal (8). In our study of the VDRKO, estrogen deficiency appeared to cause gonadal insufficiencies by a mechanism similar to that observed in ERα knockout mice. In addition, aromatase gene deficient mice (ArKO) showed gonadal insufficiencies, such as underdeveloped uteri and ovaries (9), and impaired spermatogenesis (10). The phenotype of gonads of ERα and ArKO paralleled those of the VDRKO.

No histological abnormality was observed in the testes of the male VDRKO supplemented with estrogen. The estrogen supplementation protected the testis of the VDRKO from histological changes. These results strongly suggested that estrogen deficiency induced by VDR ablation is the cause of the abnormal spermatogenesis in VDRKO.

Decreases in the activity of P450arom and the suppression of CYP19 gene expression in both female and male gonads of the VDRKO were demonstrated. The CYP19 gene encodes P450arom, the key enzyme for estrogen biosynthesis, which dominantly influences the estrogen level. These results indicated that the estrogen deficient state in the VDRKO caused by decreased P450arom activity depended on suppressed CYP19 gene expression.

It was reported that normalization of the serum calcium level restored fertility in vitamin D-deficient female and male rats (11,12), and also prevented some phenotypic abnormalities in the VDRKO(9). To clarify the influences of severe hypocalcemia, calcium supplementation was performed in the VDRKO. A high calcium diet increased the serum calcium level to near that of the wild type mice. The normalization of the serum calcium level increased the aromatase activity in the ovary to 60% of that in the wild type. Furthermore, the expression level of CYP19 gene was increased to ten-fold of that in the VDRKO without calcium supplementation. The high levels of LH and FSH after the normalization of serum calcium meant that the endocrinological state remained abnormal.

Despite the abnormal endocrinologocal state, some VDRKO with a normal serum calcium level were fertile. This may explain why other VDR ablated mice (13) did not show infertility, although the details of the gonadal functions were not reported. The serum calcium levels of these mice were much higher than those of our VDRKO (1.00 - 1.09 mM, 82% of wild type mice vs. 5.36 ± 0.25 mg/dl, 65% of wild type mice). In human cases of vitamin D dependent rickets type II, no gonadal insufficiencies were detected (14,15). Calcium had been administered to these patients from an early phase. Normalization of the serum calcium level might therefore restore the infertility.

It was recently reported that the P450arom activity of human choriocarcinoma cell lines was stimulated by $1,25\text{-}(OH)_2D_3$ and that the VDR response element was identified in the CYP19 gene (17). This would suggest that vitamin D regulates the CYP19 gene directly. Using VDRKO not vitamin D-deficient mice, we demonstrated that vitamin D acted to regulate estrogen biosynthesis: this regulation could not be explained by the calcitropic activities alone. These results indicated that vitamin D plays a role in estrogen biosynthesis partially by maintaining extracellular calcium homeostasis. However, the direct regulation of the expression of aromatase gene was also considered.

References

1. Stumpf, W.E (1995) *Histochemistry and Cell Biology.* 104:417-427.
2. Yoshizawa, T., Handa, Y., Uematsu, Y., Takeda, S., Sekine, K., Yoshihara, Y., Kawakami ,T., Arioka, K., Soto, H., Uchiyama, Y., Masushige, S., Fukamizu, A., Matsumoto, T., Kato, S (1997) *Nature genetics.* 16:391-396.
3. Nelson, D.R., Kamataki,T., Waxman, D.J., Guengerich, F.P., Estabrook, R.W., Feyereisen, R., Gonzalez, F.J., Coon, M.J., Gunsalus, I.C., Gotoh, O., Okuda, K., Nebert, D.W (1993) *DNA Cell Biol.* 12:1- 51.
4. Li, Y.C., Amling, M., Pirro, A.E., Priemel, M., Meuse, J., Baron, R., Delling, G. and Demay M.B (1998) *Endocrinology.* 139:4391-4396.
5. Roselli, C.E., Ellnwood, W.E. and Resko, J.A (1984) *Endocrinology.* 114:192-200.

236

6. Eddy, E.M., Washburn, T.F., Bunch, D.O., Goulding, E.H., Gladen, B.C., Lubahn, D.B., and Korach, K.S (1996) *Endocrinology.* 137:4796-4805.

7. Halloran, B.P. and Deruca H.F (1980) *J. Nutr..* 110:1573-1580.

8. Kwiecinski, G.G., Petrie, G.I. and DeLuca H.F (1989) *J. Nutr..* 119:741-744.

9. Hess, R.A., Bunick, D., Lee, K.H., Bahr, J., Taylor, J.A., Korach, K.S. and Lubahn, D.B (1997) *Nature.* 390:509-512.

10. Fisher, C.R., Graves K.H., Parlow, A.F. and Simpson, E.R (1998) *Proc. Natl. Acad. Sci. USA.* 95:6965-6970.

11. Robertson, K.M., O'Donnell, L., Jones, M.E.E., Meachem, S.J., Boon, W.C., Fisher, C.R., Graves K.H., McLachlan, R.I. and Simpson, E.R (1999) *Proc. Natl. Acad. Sci. USA.* 96:7986-7991.

12. Kwiecinski, G.G.,Petrie, G.I.and DeLuca H.F(1989)*Am.J.Physiol.*256:E483-487.

13. Uhland, A.M., Kwiecinski, G.G.and DeLuca H.F(1992)*J.Nutr..*122:1338-1344.

14. Li, Y.C., Pirro, A.E., Amling, M., Delling, G., Baron, R., Bronson, R. and Demay, M.B (1997) *Proc. Natl. Acad. Sci. USA.* 94:9831-9835.

15. Malloy, P.J,, Hochberg, Z., Tiosano, D., Pike, J.W., Hughes, M.R., Feldman, D (1990) *J. Clin. Invest.* 86:2071-2079.

16. Hawa, N.S., Cockerill, F.J. Vadher, S., Hewison, M., Rut, A.R., Pike, J.W., O'Riordan, J.L., Farrow, S.M (1996) *Clinical Endocrinology.* 45(1):85-92.

17. Sun, T., Zhao, Y., Mangelsdorf, D.J. and Simpson, E.R (1997) *Endocrinology.* 139:1684-1691.

Table 1.   Serum LH and FSH values (ng/ml).

			3w	8w	12w
VDR+/+	female	LH	0.7± 0.1 (n=4)	1.2 ± 0.3 (n=4)	ND (not determined)
		FSH	165.0± 18.0 (n=4)	262.8± 6.1 (n=4)	ND
	male	LH	ND	0.97± 0.04 (n=4)	ND
		FSH	ND	208.5 ± 12.8 (n=4)	ND
VDR-/-	female	LH	0.98±0.04 (n=3)	5.8 ± 0.4 * (n=4)	8.4 ± 1.0 (n=4)
		FSH	204.0±24.0 (n=3)	409.8± 43.6 * (n=4)	473.0± 25.0 (n=4)
	male	LH	ND	8.5 ± 0.8 *(n=4)	7.1± 0.5 (n=3)
		FSH	ND	426.3± 23.5 * (n=4)	445.5± 5.5 (n=3)
VDR-/- with calcium supplementation (8w)			female LH 5.9 ± 0.2 * (n=3) FSH 385.0 ± 32.0 * (n=3)		
			male LH 8.1 ± 0.3* (n=3) FSH 310.0 ± 16.0 * (n=3)		

*;$p \leq 0.01$ compared with VDR+/+ mice at 8-weeks-of-age. *;$p < 0.001$ compared with VDR-/- mice at 8-weeks-of-age.

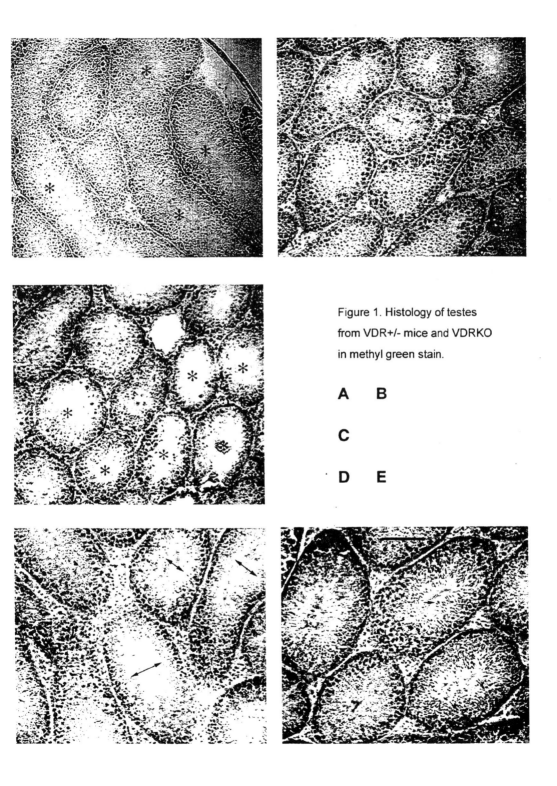

Figure 1. Histology of testes
from VDR+/- mice and VDRKO
in methyl green stain.

A   B

C

D   E

Figure 1. A, The testis of a 10-week-old VDR+/- mouse. The seminiferous tubules were at different stages of spermatogenesis, and the diameter of the lumen and the thickness of the seminiferous epithelium vary with the stage of spermatogenesis (arrow); B, the testis of a 10-week-old VDR-/- mouse. The lumen of the seminiferous tubules was often dilated (arrows). The thickness of the seminiferous epithelium is less than in 10-week-old control mice; C, The testis of a 15-week-old VDR-/- mouse. The lumen was more widely dilated (asterisks), the seminiferous epithelium is atrophic in many tubules, and spermatogenesis is rare; D, The testis of a 10 week-old VDR-/- mouse with estrogen treatment revealed no change. The seminiferous tubules were at different stages of spermatogenesis (arrow), and the diameter of the lumen and the thickness of the seminiferous epithelium vary with the stage of spermatogenesis; E, The testis of a 10 week-old VDR-/- mouse with calcium supplementation revealed dilated lumen in some seminiferous tubules (asterisks). *bar* = 100 µm.

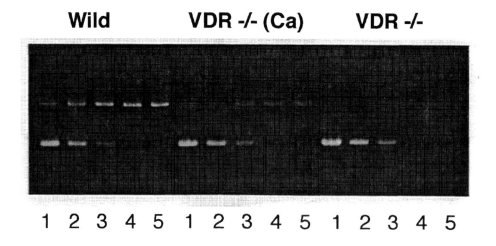

Figure 2. The effect of calcium supplementation. The competitive RT-PCR amplification of mRNA of the CYP19 gene in ovary at 7 weeks of age of wild (VDR+/+) and VDR-/- with calcium supplementation and VDR-/- without treatment. The size of the CYP19 gene product was 526 bp and competitor product was 350 bp. The competitive template used was 4fM, 4×10^{-1}fM, 4×10^{-2}fM, 4×10^{-3}fM, and 4×10^{-4}fM from lane 1 to lane 5 respectively. The expression of the CYP19 gene in the ovary of VDR-/- mice given calcium supplements was increased.

FIRST IDENTIFICATION OF A NATURAL POINT MUTATION IN THE VDR GENE CAUSING TOTAL FAILURE OF LIGAND-BINDING AND SEVERE CLINICAL RESISTANCE TO 1,25-(OH)$_2$D$_3$.

T.M.Nguyen, M.Petrovic, H.Guillozo, M.L.Alvarez, M.L.Kottler*, O.Walrant-Debray, M.Rizk-Rabin, M.Garabédian.
CNRS-UPR 1524, Hôpital St Vincent de Paul, Paris 14; * Unité de Génétique Moléculaire, CHU Pitié-Salpétrière, Paris 13, France.

Introduction: Mutations in the vitamin D receptor (VDR) gene have been shown to cause hereditary vitamin D-resistant rickets (HVDRR) (1). In this study, two Algerian patients, a boy and a girl with known consanguinity in their family, exhibited the clinical characteristics of severe HVDRR with early onset rickets, hypocalcemia and elevated 1,25-dihydroxyvitamin D levels as well as total alopecia. Fibroblasts were cultured from a skin biopsy of patients and used to assess the VDR, to investigate the VDR functional defect and to sequence the VDR cDNA.

Materials and methods:

- Patients fibroblasts culture
Fibroblasts from the two affected subjects and from one age-matched control child were started from skin biopsies and grown in Dulbecco's modified Eagle's medium (DMEM) (Gibco BRL, Gaithersburg, MD) supplemented with 10% fetal bovine serum, penicillin, streptomycin and fungizone. Cells were incubated at 37°C under a 5% CO$_2$ atmosphere.

- Preparation of cytosol and ligand binding
Cultured fibroblasts were incubated for 16h in bovine serum free DMEM with either solvent (ethanol) or 1,25-(OH)$_2$D$_3$ at different concentrations (10^{-12} to 10^{-6} M). At the end of incubation, cells were harvested and washed twice with PBS by centrifugation at 2,000g for 5 min. Cell pellets were resuspended in 2 vol of high salt buffer (0.3 M KCl, 1.5 mM EGTA, 0.01 M Na$_2$MoO$_4$, 1 mM DTT). Cells were disrupted by sonication on ice and their cytosols prepared by ultracentrifugation at 100,000 g for 1h. For ligand binding, cytosols were diluted to a protein concentration of 1 mg/ml with the high salt buffer supplemented with Aprotinin (Sigma) (0.4 Trypsin inhibitor unit per ml of buffer). They were incubated with 2nM ^{3}H1,25-(OH)$_2$D$_3$ (specific activity:160 Ci/mmol) (Amersham, Buckinghamshire, UK) in the presence or absence of a 50-fold excess of radioinert hormone. After 1h on ice, bound and free steroid were separated by hydroxylapatite (Biorad) (2) .

- cDNA synthesis and sequencing
Total RNA was extracted from fibroblasts of the two affected patients. After reverse transcription by using Superscript II-RNase H Reverse Transcriptase (Gibco), each half of the coding region of patient VDR was amplified by a nested PCR reaction, using the following primers: 1a (5'-ACC AGA AGC CTT TGG GTC TG) and 1b (5'-TAA CTG ACC AGG TCA GCC AG) for the 5' half; 2a (5'-TGA TGG ACT CGT CCA GCT TC) and 2b (5'-ACA GGA GAG AGA ATG GGC TG) for the 3' half. PCR was performed using Taq polymerase (Appligene) with 0.16 μM of each primer in buffer containing 2mM MgCl$_2$, 2.5% DMSO for 35 cycles.

Each cycle consisted of denaturation at 95°C for 1 min, annealing at 58°C for 1 min, primer extension at 72°C for 2 min with a final elongation step at 72°C for 10 min. Following amplification, PCR products were purified with a High pure PCR product purification Kit (Boehringer). Sequencing was carried out using the Taq Dye-Deoxy Terminator cycle sequencing Kit and a ABI PRISM 377 DNA sequencer (Perkin-Elmer, Biosystem, France).

-VDR immunocytochemical expression and response to 1,25-(OH)$_2$D$_3$

VDR was detected by immunocytochemistry using a modification of the method of Clemens et al.. Before immunostaining, fibroblasts (control and patient 2) were first cultured in Lab-Tek chambers in DMEM +10% FCS, at a density of 12x10^3 cells per well for 4 days at 37°C under a 5% CO$_2$ atmosphere, then in DMEM without FCS for another 16h. Ethanol or 1,25-(OH)$_2$D$_3$ (10^{-9} M) was added to the cultures for the last 24h of the incubations. Fibroblasts were then washed with phosphate-buffered saline (PBS), fixed in paraformaldehyde (4%) for 15 min at ambient temperature and washed twice in PBS. Endogenous peroxidase was blocked with 1%H$_2$O$_2$ for 10 min, and cells were incubated overnight at 4°C with 9A7 gamma, a monoclonal antibody against VDR (a gift from Dr Pike), or with rat serum as negative control (diluted 1:200 in PBS plus 0.005% bovine serum albumin). They were washed and treated with biotinylated rabbit anti-rat immunoglobulin G (1:100, Pharmacia) for 2h at room temperature. Cells were then treated with biotinylated protein A (1:100 for 1h), followed by streptavidin biotin horseradish peroxidase (1:200 for 45min) at room temperature. Receptors were visualized with the use of diaminobenzidine tetrahydrochloride (0.5%)-H$_2$O$_2$ (0.3%) in Tris-HCl 0.1M, pH 7.4.

-25-(OH)D$_3$ 24-hydroxylase activity determination

Fibroblasts (control and patient 2) were incubated in 24-well culture plates (5x10^5 cells/well) in 1 ml serum free DMEM in presence of non radioactive 1,25-(OH)$_2$D$_3$ (1pM-1µM) or its solvent (ethanol) for 16h. After rinsing with fresh serum free medium, 2.5nM ^{3}H25-(OH)D$_3$ (0.05µCi) (S.A.:23 Ci/mmol) (Amersham, UK) were added and the cultures were incubated for an additional 120min. The medium was removed and the ^{3}H vitamin D$_3$ derivatives present in the medium were extracted by adding 2ml methanol plus 2ml chloroform. The chloroform extract was cochromatographed with 100ng unlabeled 24,25-(OH)$_2$D$_3$ using a straight phase HPLC system (Beckman, Berkeley, CA,USA) equipped with a 4.6x250 mm Ultrasphere Si column (Altex, Berkeley, CA) and equilibrated with n-hexane-isopropanol (95:5) (flow rate 1.5 ml/min). Absorbance at 254nm was monitored continously and effluent fractions were collected every minute. After evaporation to dryness, fractions were dissolved in scintillation fluid (Ultimagold MV, Packard) and their radioactivity was measured.

Results:

-VDR binding studies

Control fibroblasts had detectable 1,25-(OH)$_2$D$_3$ binding capacity (12±0.2 fmoles/mg protein). Incubation of these cells with 10^{-10} M 1,25-(OH)$_2$D$_3$ led to the doubling of the cytosol ability to bind 1,25-(OH)$_2$D$_3$ (26±1 fmoles/mg protein) (p<0.001). In contrast, fibroblasts from both affected children completely failed to bind $1,25\text{-}(OH)_2D_3$, even after preincubation of the cells with $1,25\text{-}(OH)_2D_3$ concentrations ranging from 10^{-12} to 10^{-6} M.

-Amplification of cDNA and nucleotides sequence analysis
Sequencing of the total cDNA from both patients revealed a unique T to C point mutation at nucleotide 971, which resulted in the substitution of Tryptophan (TGG) by Arginin (CGG), at amino acid position 286 (W286R) in the ligand-binding domain (exon7). Both patients cDNAs were found to be homozygous for the mutation.

-Immunocytochemical VDR expression and response to $1,25\text{-}(OH)_2D_3$
VDR expression, visualized after treatment of the cultured skin fibroblasts with a monoclonal antibody to purified avian VDR, was easily detectable in control as well as in patient cells. It was mainly localized in the nucleus. Cells incubated with adult rat serum and no 9A7 gamma were not immunostained. As expected, preincubation of the control cells, with 10^{-9} M $1,25\text{-}(OH)_2D_3$ for 16h, significantly increased the number of stained cells (9.7 ± 0.9 versus 6.4 ± 0.9 percent) ($p<0.01$) as well as the intensity of staining, suggesting an up-regulation of VDR expression by $1,25\text{-}(OH)_2D_3$.In basal conditions, the percentage of immunostained cells in the patient fibroblast cultures was similar to that found in controls (6.8 ± 1.9 versus 6.4 ± 0.9 percent). By contrast, preincubation of the patient fibroblasts with $1,25\text{-}(OH)_2D_3$ (10^{-9} M) had no effect on the number of stained cells and on the intensity of staining.

-24-hydroxylase activity and response to $1,25\text{-}(OH)_2D_3$
An in vitro conversion of $25\text{-}(OH)D_3$ into $24,25\text{-}(OH)_2D_3$ was found in both the control and patient fibroblasts cultured in basal conditions (35.0 ± 4.4; 20.0 ± 4.4 fmoles/10^5 cells/120 min respectively).Treatment with 10^{-12} to 10^{-8}M $1,25\text{-}(OH)_2D_3$ for 16h significantly stimulated the $25\text{-}(OH)D_3$-24-hydroxylase activity of control fibroblasts. The stimulation was dose-dependent and a maximal 6-fold increase was observed after cell incubation with 10^{-8}M $1,25\text{-}(OH)_2D_3$. A similar dose-dependent response was found with the patient fibroblasts, a maximal effect being obtained with $1,25\text{-}(OH)_2D_3$ concentrations of 10^{-12}-10^{-10}M. But the magnitude of the response, 3-fold, and the maximal 24-hydroxylase activity reached in the presence of $1,25\text{-}(OH)_2D_3$ were lower in patients fibroblasts than in controls (65 ± 17 versus 191 ± 20 fmoles/10^5 cells/120 min, $p<0.001$).

In conclusion: a new point mutation was identified in exon 7 concerning the unique Tryptophan residue of the VDR gene. This natural mutation caused severe clinical resistance to $1,25\text{-}(OH)_2D_3$ and the total inability of patients fibroblasts to bind $^3H1,25\text{-}(OH)_2D_3$. In spite of this alteration, a partial response to $1,25\text{-}(OH)_2D_3$ was observed in cultured skin fibroblasts. These results emphasize the critical role played by the unique Tryptophan residue of the VDR and suggest that some VDR-mediated transcriptional activation does not require ligand binding.

References:
1-Malloy P.J, Pike J.W, Feldman D. (1999) Endocr Rev 20 (2):156-188
2-Wecksler W.R., Norman A.W. (1979) Anal Biochem 92:314-323

3D STRUCTURE OF VDR LIGAND BINDING DOMAIN AND STRUCTURE-FUNCTION RELATIONSHIP OF VITAMIN D (1): ALANINE SCANNING MUTATION ANALYSIS OF AMINO-ACID RESIDUES LINING LIGAND BINDING POCKET AND ASSIGNMENT OF THE ROLE OF EACH AMINO ACID.

M. Choi,[1] K. Yamamoto,[1] H. Masuno,[1] K. Nakashima,[2] T. Taga[2] and S. Yamada.[1]
[1]Institute of Biomaterials and Bioengineering, [2]Medical Research Institute, Tokyo Medical and Dental University, Kanda-Surugadai, Chiyoda-ku, Tokyo 101, Japan

Introduction   In the studies of structure-function relationship of vitamin D, we firstly focused our attention on the side chain of vitamin D, since most of potent vitamin D analogs are found in the side-chain modified derivatives. We used systematic conformational analysis technique of molecular mechanics as a basic tool and suggested the active space group concept (1,2). We grouped mobile regions of vitamin D side chain, termed them A, G, F, EA and EG and showed the potency (the cell differentiating activity) to increase in the order G<EG<A<F<EA (3,4) (see the part 2). To develop this theory to that including vitamin D receptor (VDR), we modeled ligand-binding domain (LBD) of VDR by homology modeling technique (5). Nearly the same time, the x-ray crystal structure of a deletion mutant (Δ165-215) of VDR was reported by Moras' group (6).   Fortunately our model was essentially the same as the crystal structures except for some detailed parts.   Although it is believed that crystal structures are absolutely reliable, this VDR case left some ambiguity because in the mutVDR-LBD 51 residues are deleted from the long loop between helices 1 and 3 for crystallization engineering.   To study the interaction between the VDR and its natural as well as synthetic ligands in more detail, we prepared twelve one-point mutants of amino acid residues facing the ligand binding pocket (LBP), evaluated their transcriptional potency when activated by natural and synthetic ligands, and assigned the role of each amino acid residue (part 1).   In the 2nd part of these papers, we will examine the docking of typical vitamin D synthetic ligands having high potency and discuss its relationship with biological activity.

Materials and method   Vitamin D analogs, OCT (Chugai Pharmaceutical Co. Ltd.), 20-epi-1,25-(OH)2D3 and KH1060 (Leo Pharmaceutical Products) were kindly donated by these companies.

The human VDR expression vector pCMX-hVDR was constructed as described previously (5) and was used as a template for site-directed mutagenesis. Twelve clones of mutated hVDRs (L233A, V234A, S237A, R274A, S275A, S278A, W286A, C288A, H305A, H397A, Q400A and Y401A) were produced by changing the corresponding amino acid residue into alanine by using commercial site-directed mutagenesis kit (Stratagene, CA, USA). E. coli DH5α competent cells were transformed with the vectors incorporating the desired mutations. The cDNAs of the clones were purified and sequenced completely to ensure that no other base changes were produced. The level and stability of wild-type and twelve mutant hVDRs were assessed by Western blot using VDR antibody.

Dual luciferase assay was performed as described previously (5). All experiments were done in triplicates.

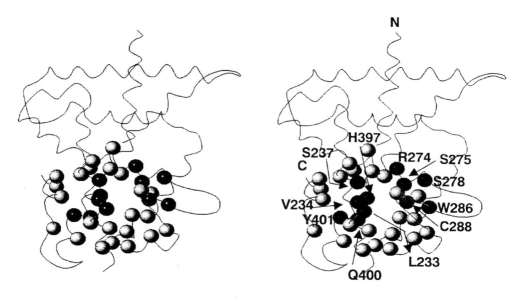

1   2   3   4

Results and discussion   Twelve one-point mutants [L233A, V234A, S237A (H3); R274A, S275A, S278A (H4/5); W286A, C288A (β-sheet); H305A (loop 6-7); H397A, Q400A, Y401A (H10/11)] of amino acids lining LBP (Fig. 1) were prepared and used to analyze the effect of one-point mutation in the transactivation induced by various ligands.

N

H397
S237   R274 S275
C   S278
V234   W286
Y401   C288
              L233
Q400

Fig. 1. Amino acid residues (balls) lining ligand binding pocket of VDR. The VDR-LBD was shown with single ribbon presentation and the residues mutated in this study are shown with black balls.

The results of the transactivation induced by 1,25-$(OH)_2D_3$ (**1**) and synthetic ligands, 22-oxa-1,25-$(OH)_2D_3$ (OCT, **2**), 20-epi-1,25-$(OH)_2D_3$ (**3**)   and 22-oxa-24,26,27-trihomo-1,25-$(OH)_2D_3$ (KH1060, **4**) are shown in Fig. 2.

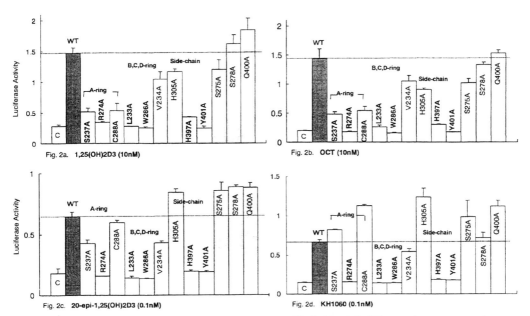

Fig. 2a. 1,25(OH)2D3 (10nM)

Fig. 2b. OCT (10nM)

Fig. 2c. 20-epi-1,25(OH)2D3 (0.1nM)

Fig. 2d. KH1060 (0.1nM)

The transactivation induced by 1,25-$(OH)_2D_3$ (1) (Fig. 2a) was significantly reduced by the mutations L233A, R274A, W286A, H397A and Y401 A, moderately reduced by V234A, S237A, S275A, C288A, and little affected by S278A and Q400A. We assigned the role of the important amino acids as follows (Table 1): Around the A-ring, R274 and S237 together form pincer-type hydrogen bond with the 1α-hydroxyl group , with R274 playing major role and S237 assisting role. S278 or C288 forms weak hydrogen bond with the 3β- hydroxyl group . At the C- to seco-B-ring part, W286 and L233 together hold this hydrophobic core part of the ligand from both bottom and top sides by hydrophobic interaction. At the side chain part, H397 strongly anchors the 25-hydroxyl group with H305 supporting this. Y401 at the tail of H11 is likely to be important in holding H12 in the active form by hydrophobic interaction with a lipophilic residue at H12.

Table 1

1,25$(OH)_2D_3$	Residues	Location	Natural Mutant	Assumed Function
A-ring	S237	H3		Assist 1-OH Hydrogen Bonding
	R274	H5	R274L	1-OH Hydrogen Bonding
	S278	H5		3-OH Hydrogen Bonding (mutant VDR)
	C288	β-sheet		3-OH Hydrogen Bonding (our model)
B,C,D-ring	L233	H3	L233fs	Hydrophobic Interaction
	W286	β-sheet		Hydrophobic Interaction
	V234	H3		Hydrophobic Interaction
Side Chain	H305	loop 6-7	H305Q	Assist 25-OH Hydrogen Bonding
	H397	H11		25-OH Hydrogen Bonding
	Y401	H11		Interaction with H12

The transactivation spectrum induced by OCT (2) (Fig 2b) is similar to that induced by the natural hormone (1). This result indicates that OCT binds to the VDR in the same manner as 1,25-$(OH)_2D_3$ does. It should be noted that OCT can be harbored in the VDR with stable conformation (gauche(-)), in contrast to the natural hormone that is docked in the LBP with its unstable conformation (see the part 2). This explain why vitamin D analogs in the F region including OCT and 16-ene-vitamin D derivatives have high potency.

The transactivation of the series of one point mutants by 20-epi-1,25-$(OH)_2D_3$ (3) shows different pattern (Fig. 2c). Although the residues which anchor 1,25-$(OH)_2D_3$ (1) strongly were also important in anchoring the 20-epi analog (3), the residues that moderately hold 1,25-$(OH)_2D_3$ were no more important to anchor the epi compound (3). H305A showed higher potency than the wild-type VDR in activating the transcription, suggesting that no hydrogen bond would be formed between this residue and the 25-OH of the epi-analog (3). S275A is also more potent than the WT-VDR. Changing of Ser to Ala may somewhat reduces steric repulsion with the ligand and elevates the transactivation potency.

The transactivation spectrum of the mutants induced by KH1060 (4) is similar to that by 20-epi-1,25-$(OH)_2D_3$ (Fig. 2d). Here, however, C288A is more potent than WT-VDR in the transactivation. The potency of C288A is even higher than that of S278A. This indicates that S278 is more important than C288 in interacting with the 3β-OH (or the A-ring part). These results are in contrast with the results with 1,25-$(OH)_2D_3$. This may suggest that KH1060 adopt different A-ring conformation from that of the natural hormone.

In conclusion, we noticed that the key residues to anchor the natural ligand are likely to be essential to bind synthetic ligands regardless of their structure, while the moderately important residues varies their role depending on the structure of the ligand. Thus, among the twelve residues mutated in this study, L233, R274, W286 and H397 were found to play most important role in anchoring vitamin D ligands.

References

(1) Yamamoto, K., Ohta, M., DeLuca, H.F. and Yamada, S. (1995) *Bioorg. Med. Chem. Lett.* **5**, 979-984..

(2) Yamamoto, K., Sun, W. Y., Ohta, M., Hamada, K., DeLuca, H.F. and Yamada, S. (1996) *J. Med. Chem.* **39**, 2727-2737.

(3) Yamada, S., Yamamoto, K., Masuno, H. and Ohta M. (1998) *J. Med. Chem.* **41**, 1467-1475.

(4) Yamamoto, K., Ooizumi, H., Umesono, K., Verstuyf, A., Bouillon, R., DeLuca, H.F., Shinki, T., Suda, T. and Yamada, S. (1999) *Bioorg. Med. Chem. Lett.* **9**, 1041-1046.

(5) Yamamoto, K., Masuno, H., Choi, M., Nakashima, K., Taga, T., Ooizumi, H., Umesono, K., Sicinska, W., VanHooke, J., DeLuca, H.F. and Yamada, S. (2000) *Proc. Natl. Acad. Sci. USA*, **97**, 1467-1472.

(6) Rochel, N., Wurtz, J.M., Mitschler, A., Klaholz, B. and Moras, D. (2000) *Molecular Cell.* **5**, 173-179.

3D STRUCTURE OF VDR LIGAND BINDING DOMAIN AND STRUCTURE-FUNCTION RELATIONSHIP OF VITAMIN D (2): VDR-DOCKING BEHAVIOR AND ACTIVITY RELATIONSHIP OF TYPICAL VITAMIN D ANALOGS

K. Yamamoto,[1] H. Masuno,[1] M. Choi,[1] K. Nakashima,[2] T. Taga[2] and S. Yamada.[1]
[1]Institute of Biomaterials and Bioengineering, [2]Medical Research Institute, Tokyo Medical and Dental University, Kanda-Surugadai, Chiyoda-ku, Tokyo 101, Japan

Introduction. In the course of systematic structure-function studies using conformational analysis and conformationally restricted vitamin D analogs as tools, we proposed active space group concept (1-3). We grouped mobile regions of vitamin D side chain, termed them A, G, F, EA and EG and proposed relationships between the space group and activities as shown in Fig. 1. To develop this theory to that including vitamin D receptor (VDR), we modeled ligand-binding domain (LBD) of VDR (4). In this paper, we examined docking manner of typical vitamin D synthetic ligands in the ligand-binding pocket (LBP) of VDR based on the alanine scanning mutation analysis described in part 1 of these papers. These reveal that the space group concept is well correlated to the docking manner of each vitamin D compound.

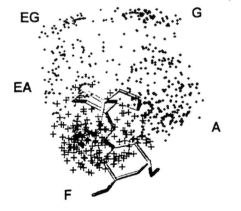

VDR:
   EA>A>F>G>EG
Cell differentiating:
   EA>F>A>EG,G
Calcemic:
   EA>A,G>>F

Fig. 1 Active space group concept of vitamin D side-chain

3D structure of VDR-LBD: The overall fold of VDR-LBD (Fig. 2) is quite similar to those of the same nuclear receptor (NR) subfamily (group 1) members as VDR except for insertion of a long loop between the helices 1 and 3 in VDR. Our model was constructed eliminating this loop (4), and in the crystal structure of engineered VDR (5), 51 residues are deleted from this long loop. The structure of the ligand VDR-LBP is spacious at the site 2 (helix 11 site) and narrow at the site 1 (β-sheet site).

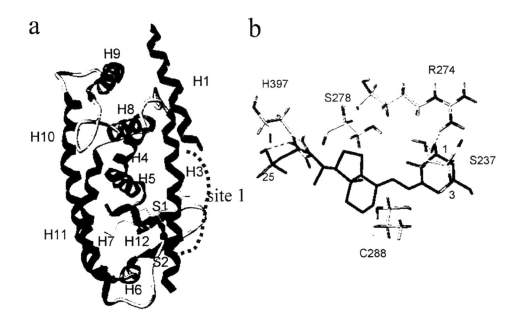

a

H9
H1
H8
H10
H4
H3
H5
Site 1
S1
H11
H7 H12
S2
H6

b

R274
H397
S278
25
1
S237
3
C288

Fig. 2 3 D model of VDR-LBD (a) and residues interacting with 1,25-(OH)$_2$D$_3$ (b)

Docking of 1,25-(OH)$_2$D$_3$. 1,25-(OH)$_2$D$_3$ is harbored in the VDR-LBP with the side chain heading the site 2 and the A-ring site 1 (Fig. 2a). Orientation of the short axis is the same as other steroid NR ligands harbored in their cognate receptor (estradiol in ER and progesterone in PR). We assumed the A-ring to adopt the α-form but in the crystal structure of deletion mutant VDR the A-ring was the β-form. The 1α-OH group forms pincer type hydrogen bonds (H-bond) with S237 and R274 (Fig. 2b) of which R274 plays the major role in anchoring the ligand as the results of the mutation analysis show (see part 1). The 3β-OH group form a H-bond with S278 in the crystal structure. We assume that 3β-hydroxyl group forms a H-bond with C288 on the basis of the mutation analysis (see part 1). It is also anticipated that the α-form is favorable to form H-bond with C288. The 25-OH group forms a H-bond with H397 (helix 11). In the crystal structure H305 is also a partner of the H-bond with 25-OH. Unexpectedly, the side chain of 1,25-(OH)$_2$D$_3$ adopts less stable conformation in the LBP. The side chain is directed toward the direction of the angular C(18)-methyl group. In the dot map, this conformation is found at the far end of the A region.

Docking of typical vitamin D analogs. 22-Oxa-1,25-(OH)$_2$D$_3$ (OCT, 2): As described in part 1 of these papers, transactivation pattern of the series of one-point mutants initiated by OCT was quite similar to that induced by the natural hormone. This suggests that OCT is harbored in the LBP in a similar manner to 1,25-(OH)$_2$D$_3$. Furthermore OCT can adopt the stable side-chain conformation, gauche(-) at C(16-17-20-22), in the LBP. This fact explains why vitamin D analogs categorized

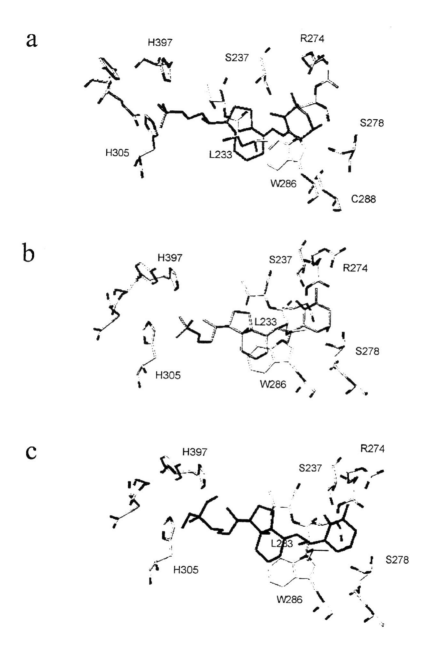

Fig. 3 Docking models of OCT/VDR-LBD (a), 20-epi-1,25-(OH)$_2$D$_3$/VDR-LBD (b), and KH1060/VDR-LBD (c)

in the F region, such as OCT, 16-ene-1,25-(OH)$_2$D$_3$ derivatives and 18-nor-1,25-(OH)$_2$D$_3$ have high potency. The reason is that these F oriented analogs can be harbored in the LBP with their stable conformation.

20-Epi-1,25-(OH)$_2$D$_3$ (**3**): 20-Epimerization of the natural hormone yields 20-epi-1,25-(OH)$_2$D$_3$ which has significantly higher biological activity than the natural hormone. Most of vitamin D chemists have been curious why the 20-epi analogs have such high potency. The 3D structure of VDR-LBP answered the question. The 20-epi analog **3** can be harbored in the LBP with its stable side-chain conformation, anti at C(16-17-20-22). Furthermore in that stable conformation the side chain directed to the H12. So the side chain terminal can have favorable hydrophobic interaction with the residues of H12 facing LBP. As described in part 1, transactivation spectrum induced by **3** is considerably different. S275A, S278A and H305A are more potent than the WT-VDR in the transactivation. H305 is likely not to form a H-bond with the 25-OH of **3**.

24,26,27-Trihomo-22-oxa-20-epi-1,25-(OH)$_2$D$_3$ (KH1060, **4**): This analog with 20-epi configuration has been known as the most potent vitamin D analog. The high potency of this compound can be similarly explained. The elongation of the side chain and addition of the two terminal methyl groups probably increase the hydrophobic interaction with H12 making the active VDR conformation more stable. As described in part 1, transactivation spectra induced by **3** and **4** are similar to each other but considerably different from that induced by 1,25-(OH)$_2$D$_3$ and OCT. Especially C288 which is supposed to be contributing in the H-bond with 3β-OH seems to have no significant role, since the mutation to Ala rather elevated the potency.

Conclusion. It is concluded that in terms of the ligand conformation adopted in the VDR-LBP, the compounds which can be harbored with their stable conformation in the LBP have high biological potency. The importance of hydrophobic interaction was highly recognized in these studies. We also noticed that the conformations of ligands adopted in the VDR were all found at the border of the three active regions A, F and EA. Thus the structure-activity relationship derived from the studies of the ligand side (active space group concept) and that from the receptor side (the docking studies) were compatible each other.

References
(1) Yamamoto, K., Sun, W. Y., Ohta, M., Hamada, K., DeLuca, H.F. and Yamada, S. (1996) *J. Med. Chem.* **39**, 2727-2737.
(2) Yamada, S., Yamamoto, K., Masuno, H. and Ohta M. (1998) *J. Med. Chem.* **41**, 1467-1475.
(3) Yamamoto, K,. Ooizumi, H,. Umesono, K,. Verstuyf, A,. Bouillon, R,. DeLuca, H.F., Shinki, T., Suda, T. and Yamada, S. (1999) *Bioorg. Med. Chem. Lett.* **9**, 1041-1046.
(4) Yamamoto, K., Masuno, M., Choi, M., Nakashima, K., Taga, T., Ooizumi, H., Umesono, K., Sicinska, W., VanHooke, J., DeLuca, H.F. and Yamada, S. (2000) *Proc. Natl. Acad. Sci. USA*, **97**, 1467-1472.
(5) Rochel, N., Wurtz, J.M., Mitschler, A., Klaholz, B. and Moras, D. (2000) Molecular Cell. **5**, 173-179.

STUDIES IDENTIFYING KEY INTERACTION POINTS BETWEEN 1,25-DIHYDROXYVITAMIN D3 AND THE LIGAND BINDING DOMAIN OF THE VITAMIN D NUCLEAR RECEPTOR USING MOLECULAR MODELING AND SITE-DIRECTED MUTAGENESIS

Elaine D. Collins[*] and Anthony W. Norman[+], [*]Department of Chemistry, San Jose State University, San Jose, CA 95192 and [+]Department of Biochemistry, University of California, Riverside, CA 92521.

Introduction   Most of the biological effects of the steroid hormone $1,25(OH)_2$-vitamin D_3 are mediated through its interaction with the nuclear vitamin D receptor (VDR). VDR is a member of a superfamily of nuclear receptors which are ligand-dependent transcription factors. Other members of the family include receptors for steroid hormones, retinoids, thyroid hormone and several orphan receptors. Ligand binding induces conformational changes in the VDR that enable the receptor to form heterodimers with RXR, interact with other coactivators, and modulate gene transcription. The first steps in $1,25(OH)_2D_3$ modulation of gene transcription involve binding of the $1,25(OH)_2D_3$ ligand to VDR which results in conformational changes in the ligand binding domain (LBD) of VDR. We have previously generated a 3-dimensional model of the LBD of the human VDR based on its alignment with the rat $\alpha 1$ isoform of the nuclear thyroid receptor (TR) and applied the atomic coordinates of TR obtained from its 2.0 A x-ray crystallographic structure. Next we docked a 6-s-cis-conformation of $1,25(OH)_2D_3$ and identified candidate amino acids which might interact with the three critical hydroxyl groups of the ligand.   We then constructed a series of mutant VDRs to assess the requirement of specific amino acid residues for ligand binding and receptor function. We are in the process of analyzing these mutant VDRs by: (a) saturation binding analysis with $1,25(OH)_2D_3$; (b) limited proteolysis of the receptor-ligand complex to examine conformational changes induced by ligand binding; (c) ability of VDR mutant to activate gene transcription from an osteocalcin VDRE.

Results Using site-directed mutagenesis we have constructed several mutants of VDR LBD and have begun to characterize these variants.   Figure 1 shows representative saturation analysis data of wild-type VDR and four variants. The data are summarized in Table 1. The binding studies revealed that changing the amino acid residues S237A, H397F, Y401F, T415V, did not result in large differences in affinity for radiolabeled $1,25(OH)_2D_3$. There was a two-fold decrease in affinity for variant S237A and a five-fold decrease in affinity for variant H397F.

Although all four variants were able to bind radiolabeled $1,25(OH)_2D_3$ with about the same affinity as wild-type VDR, $1,25(OH)_2D_3$ was not able to induce the same conformational changes in the variant VDRs as shown by protection from trypsin digestion. Figure 2 shows representative protease sensitivity data of wild-type VDR and three variants. The data are summarized in Table 1. The dose response curves yield an ED_{50} which is the concentration of $1,25(OH)_2D_3$ needed to protect the 35-kDa band from being half-digested. The ED50 for wild-type VDR

252

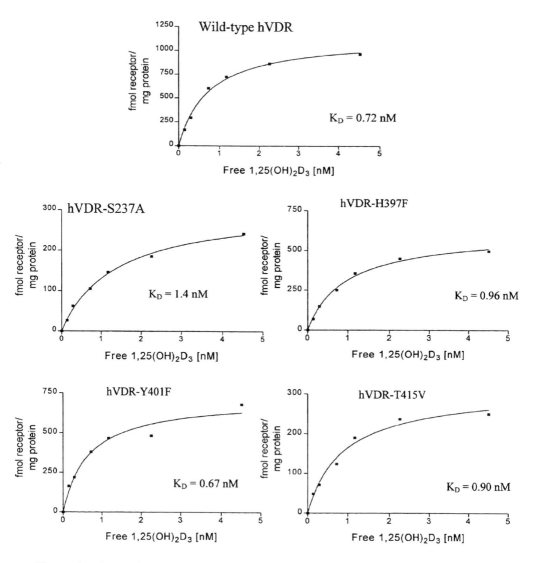

Figure 1. Increasing concentrations of radiolabeled $1,25(OH)_2D_3$ (specific activity 98 Ci/mmol) were added to aliquots of cell homogenates transfected with wild-type or mutant VDR cDNA in the presence or absence of 200-fold excess nonradioactive $1,25(OH)_2D_3$. Hormone bound to receptor was separated from free ligand using hydroxylapatite batch assay. Specific binding was calculated by subtracting nonspecific binding from total binding. The data for total binding are the mean of triplicate points and for nonspecific binding are the mean of duplicate points.

was about the same as that for variant H397F but was ten to 100-fold less than that for variants S237A and T415V. Although variants S237A and T415V can bind

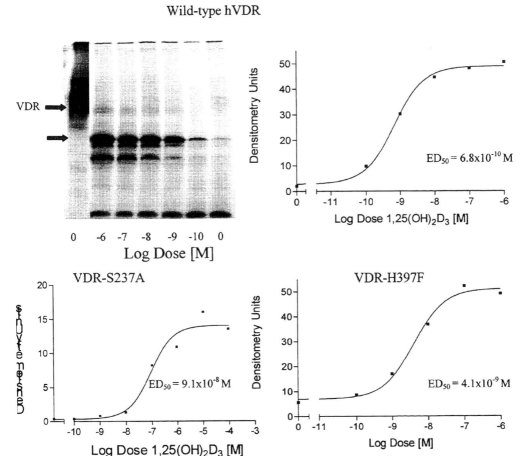

Figure 2. Wild-type or mutant VDR was transcribed and translated *in vitro* in the presence of [^{35}S]-methionine. Receptor was incubated with increasing doses of 1,25(OH)$_2$D$_3$ or ethanol for 2- min at room temperature then incubated with 15 mg/ml trypsin for 20 min at room temperature. Reaction was stopped by heating at 70° C for 5 min then resolved on 14% polyacrylamide gel electrophoresis. The gel was dried and autoradiographed. The 35 kDa protected band (lower arrow) was quantitated using Stratgene's Eagle Eye II gel documentation system.

1,25(OH)$_2$D$_3$ with the same affinity as wild-type VDR, binding did not result in conformational changes seen with wild-type VDR.

Conformational changes in LBD induced by 1,25(OH)$_2$D$_3$ binding results in the formation of new surfaces on the LBD that can interact with coactivators leading to activation of gene transcription. The ability of 1,25(OH)$_2$D$_3$ to activate gene transcription of wild-type and four variant VDRs is shown in Figure 3 and summarized in Table 1. Variants H397F and T415V were able to activate gene transcription at slightly higher doses than wild-type VDR, although H397F was not

254

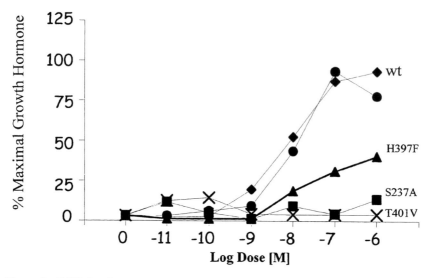

Figure 3. COS-1 cells were co-transfected with a thymidine kinase-growth hormone fusion gene containing the osteocalcin VDRE and a cDNA for VDR (wild-type or mutant) using DEAE-dextran. After 24 h. cells were treated with increasing doses of $1,25(OH)_2D_3$ or ethanol. Forty-eight h. after transfection, culture medium was collected and growth hormone levels were determined by radioimmunoassay. Each point is the average of triplicate transfections.

able to reach the same levels of transcription as wild-type of T415V. Variants S237A and Y401F were both unable to activate gene transcription.

Conclusions Mutant VDRs will be useful in studying ligand binding and receptor function.

Table 1. SUMMARY OF PRELIMINARY RESULTS

VDR Construct	Saturation Analysis* K_D [nM]	Protease Sensitivity* ED_{50} [nM]	Transcriptional Activation ED_{50} [nM]
Wild-type	0.67 ± 0.18	5.9 ± 0.62	1.4 4.1
S237A	1.5 ± 0.34	72 ± 36	No Induction
H397F	3.7 ± 2.0	6.6 ± 4.1	28 13
Y401F	0.84 ± 0.54	ND	No Induction
T415V	1.0 ± 0.36	820 ± 470	10

* n = 3

AMINO ACID RESIDUES OF HUMAN VITAMIN D RECEPTOR IMPORTANT FOR CONFORMATION VARY BETWEEN CALCITRIOL AND ITS SYNTHETIC ANALOGS

Sami Väisänen, Sanna Ryhänen, Teemu Andersin, and Pekka H. Mäenpää, Department of Biochemistry, University of Kuopio, P. O. Box 1627, FIN-70211 Kuopio, Finland

Introduction   Recently the crystal structure of the modified ligand binding domain (LBD) of human vitamin D receptor (hVDR) was published (1). The structure revealed the exact contact sites of $1\alpha,25$-dihydroxyvitamin D_3 (calcitriol) within hVDR as well as the location of several amino acid residues important for stable structure of the ligand binding pocket. In this study we have clarified the role of a number of amino acid residues for ligand binding and conformation of hVDR with several vitamin D analogs by site-directed point mutagenesis, limited proteolytic digestion and ligand binding assays. All studied analogs stabilized the LBD of wild type hVDR against limited proteolytic digestion by trypsin. All but one of the studied analogs were biologically more active than calcitriol as detected in MG-63 cells by analysis of the levels of osteocalcin mRNA and the translated osteocalcin protein (Fig. 1).

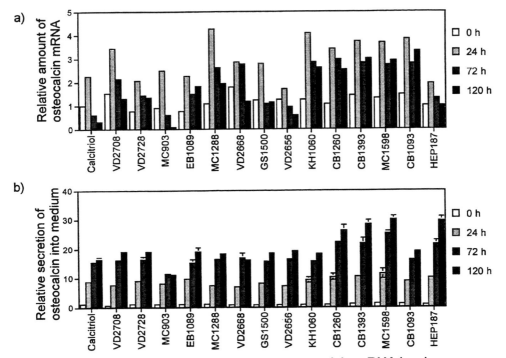

Figure 1: Biological activity of the analogs. a) osteocalcin mRNA levels, b) relative osteocalcin secretion into the culture medium.

<u>Materials and Methods</u>   The amino acid residues for site-directed mutagenesis were chosen based on the crystal structure of modified hVDR (pdb entry 1DB1)(1) and selecting amino acid residues that could possibly interact with differently positioned ligands. The cDNA of hVDR was subcloned into expression vector pSP65 and used as a template for site-directed mutagenesis using QuickChange™ Site-Directed Mutagenesis Kit (Stratagene, Cambridge, England). Nineteen substitutions and one deletion were produced by changing the chosen amino acid residues separately into alanines as described by the manufacturer. The wild type and mutated hVDRs were prepared *in vitro* by the coupled wheat germ extract system with either wild type or modified hVDR cDNA inserted into plasmid pSP65 as described by the manufacturer (Promega, Madison, WI). Binding of calcitriol to wild type and mutated, *in vitro* translated, hVDRs was assessed by one point analysis. Statistical analysis was performed by the SPSS (6.1.1.) program. For conformational analysis, the L-[^{35}S]methionine (>1000 Ci/mmol, Amersham International plc, Buckinghamshire, England) labeled hVDRs were pre-incubated for 30 min at 22 °C with 1 µM of nonradioactive calcitriol or its analogs (a generous gift from Leo Pharmaceutical Products Ltd, Ballerup, Denmark) before exposing them to partial proteolytic digestion by 25 µg/ml trypsin for 10 min at 22 °C. The digestion products were separated by 15% SDS-polyacrylamide gel electrophoresis and the gels were dried and autoradiographed. The biological activity of the analogs was assessed by using human osteocalcin gene activity as an indicator of both transcriptional and translational effects of calcitriol and its analogs in MG-63 human osteosarcoma cells. MG-63 cells were treated 24 h after seeding with calcitriol or the analogs (10 nM) for 6 h. The medium was replaced with a medium containing 2% charcoal-treated FCS and the cells were cultured without hormones for the next 120 h. Osteocalcin protein levels were detected from the media and mRNA levels were detected from the collected cells.

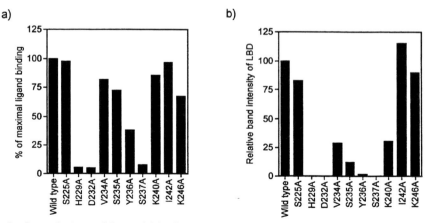

Figure 2: Correlation of ligand binding with stability of the mutated hVDR LBDs. a) effect of point mutations within helix 3 to the maximal ligand binding, b) effect of point mutations within helix 3 to the stability of LBD against limited proteolytic digestion by trypsin.

Results and Discussion   The ligand binding studies and the limited proteolytic digestion by trypsin suggest a correlation between ligand binding and stability of the LBD (Fig. 2)(2-3). This observation made it possible for us to use site-directed point mutagenesis and limited proteolytic digestion as tools to get an insight into those amino acid residues that are important for ligand binding and correct conformation of hVDR with the different analogs. Limited proteolytic digestion revealed that the analogs stabilize the mutated hVDR LBDs differently suggesting that different amino acid residues are important for the mechanism of action of the different ligands (Table 1).

Table 1: Stability of the mutated hVDR LBDs treated with calcitriol or its synthetic analogs.

		20-normal analogs					20-epi analogs									
		Calcitriol	VD2708	VD2728	MC903	EB1089	MC1288	VD2668	GS1500	VD2656	KH1060	CB1260	CB1393	MC1598	CB1093	HEP187
Coil	Y143A	-	+	+	-	-	+	-	-	-	+	-	+	-	+	-
	Y147A	+	+	+	+	+	+	+	+	+	+	+	+	+	+	+
	R158A	+	+	+	+	+	+	+	+	-	+	-	+	+	+	-
Helix 3	H229A	-	-	-	-	-	-	-	-	-	-	-	-	-	-	-
	D232A	-	-	-	-	-	-	-	-	-	-	-	-	-	-	-
	V234A	+	+	+	+	-	+	+	+	-	+	+	+	+	+	-
	S235A	+	+	+	+	+	+	+	+	+	+	-	-	-	+	+
	Y236A	+	+	+	-	-	+	-	-	-	+	-	-	+	+	-
	S237A	-	+	+	-	-	+	-	-	-	+	-	-	+	+	-
	K240A	+	+	+	+	+	+	+	+	-	+	-	+	+	+	+
Helix 5	S266A	+	+	+	+	+	+	+	+	+	+	+	+	+	+	+
	E269A	-	-	-	-	-	-	-	-	-	-	-	-	-	-	-
	R274A	-	-	-	-	-	-	-	-	-	-	-	-	-	-	-
	S275A	+	+	+	-	+	+	-	+	-	+	-	-	+	+	+
	E277A	+	+	+	+	+	+	+	+	+	+	+	+	+	+	+
	S278A	+	+	+	-	+	+	-	+	-	-	-	+	+	+	-
β-sheet	C288A	+	+	+	+	+	+	+	+	+	+	-	+	+	+	-
	Y293A	+	+	+	+	+	+	+	+	+	+	+	+	+	+	+
Coil	H305A	-	-	+	+	+	-	-	+	+	+	-	+	-	-	-
Helix 12	Deletion of P416-S428	-	+	-	+	-	+	-	-	+	+	-	+	+	-	-

This suggests that the ligand binding pocket slightly changes its conformation depending on the side chain structure of the ligand. In this case, binding of different ligands may induce different overall receptor conformations, which in turn may either stabilize or destabilize binding of transcription coactivators such as DRIPs, resulting in higher or lower transactivation efficiencies (Fig. 1). Another possibility is that the different conformations of hVDR may stabilize or destabilize binding of degradative factors, such as SUG-1, resulting in altered degradation rates of the hVDR complex, which in turn is reflected in the transcription efficiency. When our results are compared with the known natural point mutations causing decreased ligand binding and vitamin D-dependent rickets, type II (Table 2), it can be observed that many analogs can stabilize the LBDs of the mutated hVDRs. This suggests that these analogs have not lost their ability to bind to hVDR, while calcitriol itself has, indicating that these analogs have different contact amino acid residues within hVDR when compared to calcitriol. Interestingly, the studied analogs can stabilize the mutated hVDRs very differently. Some analogs are very sensitive to hVDR modifications (VD2656, CB1260, HEP187) while some analogs ignore most of the substitutions (VD2728, MC1288, KH1060, CB1093). In addition, there are analogs (MC903, EB1089, VD2668) that act very similarly with calcitriol. This suggests that different areas of hVDR ligand binding pocket are important for different analogs.

Table 2: Natural point mutations of hVDR resulting in decreased ligand binding.

Mutation	Consequence	Reference
Arg274Leu	Impaired ligand binding; VDRR-II syndrome	Kristjansson et al., 1993
Cys288Gly	Impaired ligand binding; VDRR-II syndrome	Nakajima et al., 1996
His305Gln	Ligand binding decreased by 80%; decreased transactivation	Malloy et al., 1997

References

1. Rochel, N., Wurtz, J.M., Mitschler, A., Klaholz, B.,and Moras, D. (2000) Mol. Cell 5:173-179.
2. Väisänen, S., Rouvinen, J. and Mäenpää, P.H. (1998) FEBS Lett. 440, 203-207.
3. Väisänen, S., Duchier, C., Rouvinen, J., and Mäenpää, P.H. (1999) Biochem. Biophys. Res. Comm. 264, 478-482.
4. Kristjansson, K., Rut, A.R., Hewison, M., O'Riordan, J.L., and Hughes, M.R. (1993) J. Clin. Invest. 92, 12-16.
5. Nakajima, S., Hsieh, J.C., Jurutka, P.W., Galligan, M.A., Haussler, C.A., Whitfield, G.K., and Haussler, M.R. (1996) J. Biol. Chem. 271, 5143-5149.
6. Malloy, P.J., Eccleshall, T.R., Gross, C., Van Maldergem, L., Bouillon, R., and Feldman, D. (1997) J. Clin. Invest. 99, 297-304.

MECHANISM OF THE ANTAGONISTIC ACTION OF A 25-CARBOXYLIC ESTER ANALOGUE OF 1α,25-DIHYDROXYVITAMIN D3

Michaela Herdick[1], Andreas Steinmeyer[2] and Carsten Carlberg[1],

[1]Institut für Physiologische Chemie I, Heinrich-Heine-Universität, D-40001 Düsseldorf, Germany, [2]Institut für Arzneimittelchemie, Schering AG, D-13342 Berlin, Germany

Summary: ZK159222, a 25-carboxylic ester analogue of 1α,25-dihydroxyvitamin D_3 (1α,25(OH)$_2$D$_3$), was described as a novel type of antagonist of 1α,25(OH)$_2$D$_3$ signalling. ZK159222 was not able to promote a ligand-dependent interaction of the VDR with the coactivator proteins SRC-1, TIF2 and RAC3. Functional analysis in HeLa and Cos-7 cells demonstrated a 10- to 100-fold lower ligand sensitivity for ZK159222 and most interestingly, a potency that was drastically reduced. A cotreatment of 1α,25(OH)$_2$D$_3$ with a 100-fold higher concentration of ZK159222 resulted in a prominent antagonistic effect. These data suggest that the antagonistic action of ZK159222 is due to a lack of ligand-induced interaction of the VDR with coactivators.

Introduction: A critical step in 1α,25(OH)$_2$D$_3$ signalling is the specific ligand-triggered induction of a conformational change within the ligand binding domain (LBD) of the VDR (1,2). This conformational change facilitates the interaction with coactivator proteins with members of the p160-family, such as SRC-1, TIF2 and RAC3 (3). This VDR-coactivator interaction then further facilitates recruitment of other factors to form a larger complex that modulates chromatin structure and initiates transcription (4). Antagonists have been known for some time, for some members of the nuclear hormone receptor superfamily (5). In this study, a 25-carboxylic ester analogue of 1α,25(OH)$_2$D$_3$, ZK159222 was characterized as a novel type of 1α,25(OH)$_2$D$_3$ antagonist (6).

Results: Conformations of the VDR, bound by saturating concentrations (10 µM) of 1α,25(OH)$_2$D$_3$ or the 25-carboxylic ester analogue ZK159222 (for structures see Fig. 1), were analyzed by limited protease digestion assays (7,8), which provided two digestion products, c1$_{LPD}$ and c3$_{LPD}$ for 1α,25(OH)$_2$D$_3$ and an additional digestion product, c2$_{LPD}$ for ZK159222 (data not shown).

Gel shift assays were performed with in vitro translated VDR-RXR heterodimers bound to the rat ANF DR3-type 1α,25(OH)$_2$D$_3$ response element (VDRE) (9) in the presence of GST-fusion proteins of the SRC-1 family proteins and saturating concentrations (10 µM) of 1α,25(OH)$_2$D$_3$ and ZK159222 (data not shown). In the presence of 1α,25(OH)$_2$D$_3$, VDR-RXR-VDRE-coactivator complexes were observed with all three p160-family members, whereas in the presence of ZK159222, a supershift could not be detected with any of the tested coactivators. Quantification of the relative intensities of these VDR-RXR and VDR-

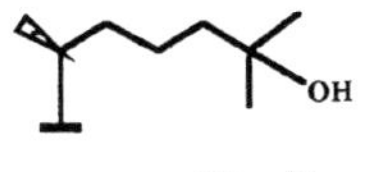

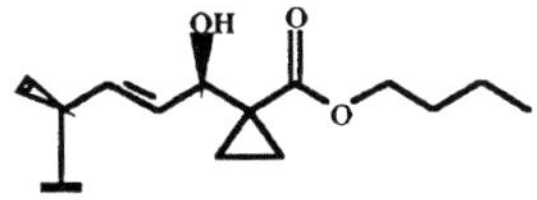

Figure 1: Structure of 1α,25(OH)$_2$D$_3$ and ZK159222. ZK159222 is a 25-carboxylic ester of 1α,25(OH)$_2$D$_3$, the structure of the side chain of both compounds is given.

RXR-coactivator complexes indicated that ZK159222 stabilized the same amount of VDR-RXR heterodimers compared to $1\alpha,25(OH)_2D_3$ and that both compounds provided EC_{50}-values of 0.14 and 1.0 nM for $1\alpha,25(OH)_2D_3$ and ZK159222, respectively. However, in the case of ZK159222 these heterodimers did not demonstrate interaction with coactivator proteins (data not shown).

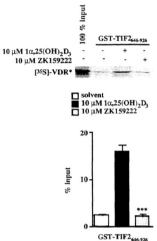

GST pull down assays were performed with bacterially produced GST-TIF2$_{646-926}$ fusion protein (containing the nuclear receptor interaction domains) and *in vitro* translated [^{35}S]-labelled VDR protein at a saturating concentration (10 μM) of $1\alpha,25(OH)_2D_3$ and ZK159222 (Fig. 2). $1\alpha,25(OH)_2D_3$ mediated a precipitation of up to 18 % of VDR input, whereas in the presence of ZK159222, the precipitation of VDR protein was not significantly higher than that of solvent control.

Mammalian one-hybrid assays were performed in HeLa cells that were transiently transfected with an expression vector for a fusion protein containing the DNA binding domain (DBD) of the yeast transcription factor GAL4 and the LBD of the VDR together with a reporter gene construct containing a GAL4 binding site-driven luciferase gene in the presence of graded concentrations of $1\alpha,25(OH)_2D_3$ and ZK159222 (Fig. 3). In this assay system, $1\alpha,25(OH)_2D_3$ induced reporter gene activity in a typical dose response (potency of 14-fold induction and ligand sensitivity, i.e. EC_{50}-value, of 1.0 nM), whereas ZK159222 showed very weak potency (2-fold induction at saturating concentrations) and low ligand sensitivity (EC_{50}-value of 120 nM).

Figure 2: ZK159222 does not stimulate VDR-coactivator interactions. GST pull-down assays (A) were performed with *in vitro* translated [^{35}S]-labelled VDR and bacterially expressed GST-TIF2$_{646-926}$. The VDR was preincubated with saturating (10 μM) concentrations of $1\alpha,25(OH)_2D_3$ or ZK159222. *** represent p < 0.0001 compared with the activity of $1\alpha,25(OH)_2D_3$.

Antagonistic effects of ZK159222 on $1\alpha,25(OH)_2D_3$ signalling were tested *in vivo* and *in vitro* by applying a saturating concentration of $1\alpha,25(OH)_2D_3$ with a concentration of ZK159222 which was up to 1000-fold higher. Luciferase assays in Cos-7 cells (Fig.4), in which ZK159222 was titrated at constant concentrations of $1\alpha,25(OH)_2D_3$ (10 nM), indicated a half-maximal antagonistic effect of 20-30 nM ZK159222, i.e. at concentrations 2- to 3-times higher than that of $1\alpha,25(OH)_2D_3$.

Supershift experiments with GST-TIF2$_{646-926}$ (Fig.5) were performed at different doses of ZK159222 and indicated the dose-dependent, antagonistic action of ZK159222. The combination of 10 nM $1\alpha,25(OH)_2D_3$ with 10 μM ZK159222 resulted in

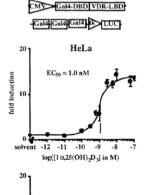

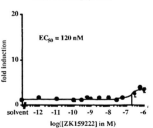

Figure 3: ZK159222 shows reduced potency *in vivo*. Mammalian-one-hybrid assays were performed with extracts from HeLa cells that were transiently transfected with a reporter gene construct-driven by three copies of the GAL4 binding site and an expression vector for a GAL4$_{DBD}$VDR$_{LBD}$ fusion protein as schematically depicted above.

an equal amount of VDR-RXR-VDRE and VDR-RXR-VDRE-TIF2 complexes.

Discussion: The antagonistic mechanism described here for ZK159222 is also likely to apply to other VDR ligands. If a compound, which does not necessarily have to be a classical $1\alpha,25(OH)_2D_3$ analogue, binds with an affinity to the ligand binding cleft of the VDR that is in the order of the EC_{50}-value for VDR-$1\alpha,25(OH)_2D_3$ interaction, i.e. 0.1 nM, but in parallel does not enable the receptor to interact with coactivators, it may act as an antagonist of $1\alpha,25(OH)_2D_3$ signalling. This suggests that the

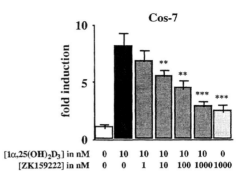

Figure 4: Antagonistic effects of ZK159222 in vivo. Luciferase reporter gene assays were performed with extracts from Cos-7 cells that were transiently transfected with a luciferase reporter gene construct driven by four copies of the DR3-type VDRE from the rat ANF gene promoter together with the expression vectors for VDR and RXR. *** and ** represent p < 0.001 and p < 0.01, respectively, compared with the activity of $1\alpha,25(OH)_2D_3$ alone.

transactivation potency of a VDR-binding ligand, i.e. its fold induction, should be taken in relation to its interaction sensitivity with the VDR, i.e. its EC_{50}-value. Tissue-specific differences in coactivator expression as well as in analogue metabolism may in turn cause tissue-specific differences in the extent of VDR ligand antagonistic effects. However, there may also be other mechanisms of antagonism in $1\alpha,25(OH)_2D_3$ signalling, e.g., a prevention of VDR-RXR complex formation on DNA, as suggested for the 26,23-lactone $1\alpha,25(OH)_2D_3$ analogue TEI-9647 (10). The AF-2 domain in helix 12 was described to be repositioned after ligand binding to the LBD and provides an interface for nuclear receptors together with amino acids of helices 3 and 5 for the binding of coactivators (Fig.6). A comparison of the crystal structure of agonist- and antagonist-bound estrogen receptor (ER) (11) suggests that antagonists block AF-2 function by disrupting the topography of the AF-2 surface. In analogy to this, one would expect that ZK159222 also stabilizes a VDR conformation that

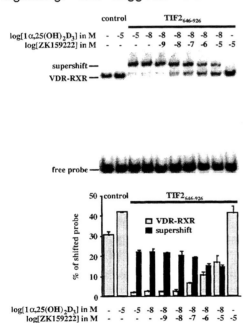

Figure 5: Antagonistic effects of ZK159222 in vitro. Gel shift experiments were performed with in vitro translated VDR-RXR heterodimers that were preincubated with approximately 3 μg of bacterially expressed GST-TIF2$_{646-926}$, the indicated concentrations of $1\alpha,25(OH)_2D_3$ and ZK159222 and the [^{32}P]-labelled DR3-type VDRE from the rat ANF gene promoter.

differs from the agonistic conformation $c1_{LPD}$ and in which the AF-2 is functionally blocked. This could be $c2_{LPD}$, which is only stabilized by ZK159222 and its antagonistic relatives and not by agonists, if physiological ionic strength conditions are used (data not shown). One could speculate that the rather long side chain of ZK159222 results in an alternative packing arrangement of ligand binding pocket residues. This may then result in a conformation of the LBD, where helix 12 reaches the static region of the AF-2 surface, which was shown in the case of ER to mimic bound coactivator (11).

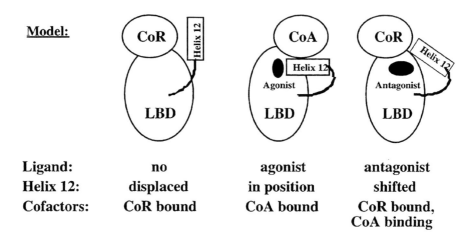

Ligand:	**no**	**agonist**	**antagonist**
Helix 12:	**displaced**	**in position**	**shifted**
Cofactors:	**CoR bound**	**CoA bound**	**CoR bound, CoA binding**

<u>Figure 6:</u> The model shows the conformational change of the LBD induced by agonists or antagonists. CoR = corepressor, CoA = coactivator.

References:
1. Carlberg, C., and Polly, P. (1998) *Crit Rev Eukaryot Gene Expr* **8,** 19-42
2. Moras, D., and Gronemeyer, H. (1998) *Curr Opin Cell Biol* **10,** 384-391
3. Chen, J. D., and Li, H. (1998) *Crit Rev Eukaryot Gene Expr* **8,** 169-190
4. Freedman, L. P. (1999) *Cell* **97,** 5-8
5. Fuhrmann, U., Parczyk, K., Klotzbücher, M., Klocker, H., and Cato, A. C. B. (1998) *J Mol Med* **76,** 512-524
6. Herdick, M., Steinmeyer, A., and Carlberg, C. (2000) *J Biol Chem*, in press
7. Nayeri, S., and Carlberg, C. (1997) *Biochem J* **327,** 561-8
8. Quack, M., and Carlberg, C. (2000) *Mol Pharmacol* **57,** 375-84
9. Kahlen, J. P., and Carlberg, C. (1996) *Biochem Biophys Res Commun* **218,** 882-6
10. Ozono, K., Saiti, M., Miura, D., Michigami, T., Nakajima, S., and Ishizuka, S. (1999) *J Biol Chem* **274,** 32376-32381
11. Shiau, A. K., Barstad, D., Loria, P. M., Cheng, L., Kushner, P. J., Agard, D. A., and Greene, G. L. (1998) *Cell* **95,** 927-937

ANTAGONISTIC ACTION OF 25-DEHYDRO-1α-DIHYDROXYVITAMIN D$_3$-26,23S-LACTONE DEPENDS ON THE AGONIST AND RESULTS IN A UNIQUE PROTEIN CONFORMATIONAL CHANGE IN THE NUCLEAR VITAMIN D RECEPTOR.

C. M. Bula, J. E. Bishop, S. Ishizuka* and A. W. Norman. Department of Biochemistry, University of California-Riverside, Riverside, CA USA 92521; and *Department of Bone and Calcium Metabolism, Teijin Institute for Bio-Medical Research, Tokyo 191-8512, Japan

Introduction.   Recently, an analog of the natural metabolite 1α,25(OH)$_2$D$_3$-26,23S-lactone has been discovered to function as an antagonist of the 1α,25(OH)$_2$D$_3$ mediated nuclear receptor VDR. This antagonistic analog, 25-dehydro-1α-OH-D$_3$-26,23S-lactone [TEI-9647 or MK], has been shown to block 1α,25(OH)$_2$D$_3$ induced cellular differentiation in HL-60 but not in NB4 cells (1). In cells over-expressing a transiently transfected VDR, a 10-fold excess of analog MK in combination with 1α,25(OH)$_2$D$_3$ results in a 50% reduction in transactivation of a reporter plasmid driven by the 24-hydroxylase promoter. The same concentration ratio also was shown to reduce 1α,25(OH)$_2$D$_3$ induced p21[WAF1,CIP1] expression (2) and modulate the protein-protein interaction between VDR and SRC-1 without modifying the nuclear localization or DNA binding properties of the VDR (3).

Presently, the molecular basis of antagonistic action of the 25-dehydro-1α-OH-D$_3$-26,23S-lactone is not known. One possibility is that the reactive C-25/C-26 primary alkene may bind covalently within the hydrophobic pocket of the ligand-binding domain of the VDR to block the transcriptional action of the receptor. In this communication we extend the action of the antagonistic analog to the osteocalcin VDRE and indicate that it functions not by the covalent modification of the VDR but rather by displacing the far more active agonist 1α,25(OH)$_2$D$_3$ in a concentration-dependant manner. The antagonistic action occurs only over a limited concentration range, however, that is dependent on the activity of the agonist. Furthermore, evidence for a unique conformational change in the ligand-binding domain of the VDR upon antagonist binding is also shown. Together, these results support a mechanism by which MK when, in appropriate excess, acts as a potent partial antagonist for 1α,25(OH)$_2$D$_3$ and its analogs.

Materials and Methods. For transfection, Cos-1 cells were seeded at 3×10^5 cells per well on 6-well plates. After 30 hours incubation at approximately 50% confluence, cells were washed in PBS and transfected using a 9-minute pre-treatment with 1 mg/ml DEAE-dextran in PBS. After washing twice more in PBS, pre-treated cells were incubated for 24 minutes with 0.5 µg/well pGEM-4 VDR plasmid(4) and 1.5 µg/well pTKGH plasmid, containing the osteocalcin VDRE (4).   Transfected cells were incubated in 80 µM chloroquine in Dulbecco's Modified Eagle's Medium Nutrient Mixture-F12 Ham with 4.5% charcoal-stripped fetal bovine serum for 3.5 hours followed by the same culture medium without chloroquine for 27 hours. Thirty hours after transfection, the cell medium was replaced with the same medium containing analogs with a final ethanol concentration of 0.1%. At 30 hours after analog treatment, the cell medium was harvested to measure the growth hormone reporter as an indicator of transcriptional activity by radioimmunoassay (Nichols Institute, San Juan Capistrano, CA). The data is presented as fold activation relative to ethanol control. All experiments were carried out on triplicate samples and the data is expressed as the mean ± SEM.

For exchange assays, duodenal mucosa from three week-old vitamin D-deficient White Leghorn cockerels fed from hatch on a standard rachitogenic diet (5), was homogenized in 10 mM Tris, 1.5 mM EDTA, 1 mM dithiothreitol, pH 7.4 to make a 10% homogenate.

The crude chromatin fraction was prepared by our standard procedure (6). The proportion of occupied receptor in each sample was measured using our exchange assay (7).

Protease sensitivity assays were performed as previously described (4).

Results and Discussion. One possible mechanism for the antagonistic action of MK suggests that the C-25, C-26 primary alkene adjacent to a carbonyl group of the lactone could serve as a nucleophile that can form a 1,4-nucleophilic addition to either histidine 305 or histidine 397 of the VDR. To test this hypothesis we pre-incubated analog MK or $1\alpha,25(OH)_2D_3$ as a control with VDR present in vitamin D-deficient chick duodenal mucosal chromatin. After a 4-hour incubation at 0°C, TPCK (L-1-tosylamido-2-phenylalanine-chloromethyl-ketone) was added to covalently bind in the ligand-binding site of any unoccupied VDR (8). After washing away any unreacted TPCK, the VDR was incubated at 37°C in the presence of excess $[^3H]-1\alpha,25(OH)_2D_3$. The radioactive ligand can then be exchanged with ligand in the sites previously protected by a non-covalently bound ligand. Exchanged ligand, as determined by liquid scintillation, was reported as percent re-occupancy. High concentrations of $1\alpha,25(OH)_2D_3$ (2 nM) or MK (200nM) were able to bind nearly all of the VDR (better than 96% and 89%, respectively; data not shown) which would indicate the VDR is nearly saturated and both $1\alpha,25(OH)_2D_3$ and MK are fully exchangeable with the tritium labeled ligand. This then would indicate that analog MK does not bind irreversibly to the VDR.

Another mechanism for MK antagonism suggests that MK acts in a similar manner as raloxifene to the estrogen receptor or RU-486 to the progesterone receptor by binding to the receptor without generating a transcriptionally competent protein. If this is true then MK should be able to antagonize other VDR agonists in a manner that is proportional to their agonistic activities. To test this theory, four ligands with similar RCI and cell differentiation ratio values were randomly chosen. Each of these analogs was added both in the presence and absence of 20 nM analog MK to transiently transfected Cos-1 cells over-expressing the VDR and a plasmid vector containing the osteocalcin VDRE reporter construct (4). The transcriptional activity of each of these analogs with and without MK as compared to $1\alpha,25(OH)_2D_3$ is shown in figure 2. Antagonism ranges from 44% for analog AW to 30% for both analogs Q and HQ. Therefore, agonists of lesser transcriptional activity exhibit proportionally less antagonism by MK on the VDR.

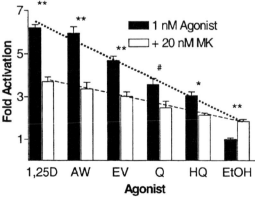

Figure 1. MK antagonizes agonists of VDR in proportion to their transcriptional activity. 1 nM agonists with and without 20 nM MK in 0.1% ethanol were used to treat Cos-1 cells transfected with an osteocalcin VDRE driven reporter. Data shown is average of 2 triplicate experiments. Symbols **, * and # indicate an antagonistic difference for p < 0.99, 0.95 and 0.90- respectively. Broken lines illustrate that antagonism is a constant proportion of transactivation by agonist alone.

A corollary to the stronger agonist displacement theory is that an analog with significantly higher affinity will require an increased molar excess of antagonist to displace the agonist thus inducing antagonism. To test this hypothesis analog IE, 20-epi-1α,25(OH)$_2$D$_3$ (9), and analog V, 16-ene,23-yne-1α,25(OH)$_2$D$_3$ (10), which have an increased transactivational activity for the VDR relative to 1α,25(OH)$_2$D$_3$, were used. A dose response curve of both analogs IE and V from 0.001 to 10 nM show that analog IE is antagonized 70% after the addition of 20 nM MK at 0.01 and analog V is antagonized 42% by 20 nM MK at 0.1 nM. When the ligand being antagonized is comparatively much more active than MK, as is the case of V and IE the equilibrium of interaction with the VDR is shifted away from MK because of its poorer affinity so that the antagonistic activity of MK is again reduced. These analogs require a 200- to 2000-fold excess of MK respectively as compared to only a 20-fold excess shown for 1α,25(OH)$_2$D$_3$. This would imply that, using this system, the effective range of MK antagonism is only useful for agonists with a level of transactivation in the range of 1α,25(OH)$_2$D$_3$.

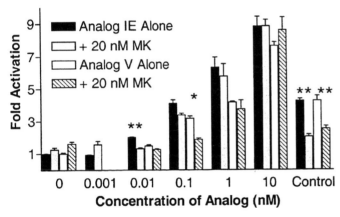

Figure 2. MK antagonism acts over a concentration range dependant on the activity of the agonist. Dose response curves of both analog IE and V either alone or with 20 nM MK are presented. Data is a representative of 3 independent triplicate experiments. Symbols ** and * indicate a difference for p < 0.99 and 0.95 respectively. Analog IE and V are antagonized only at a molar excess of 2000 and 200 fold, respectively. As a control, 1 nM 1α,25(OH)$_2$D$_3$ is included.

For MK to function as an antagonist, the conformation of the VDR with MK bound should be different than with 1α,25(OH)$_2$D$_3$. To address this hypothesis, the VDR was subjected to limited proteolysis by trypsin in the presence of a saturating concentration of ligand. Alterations in protein conformation are reflected by fragmentation pattern changes as shown by SDS-PAGE. This occurs by exposing or shielding trypsin sites. In the case of the VDR, the binding of 1α,25(OH)$_2$D$_3$ produces protease resistant fragments at 34 kDa and 30 kDa (4). Similar fragments have been shown by N-terminal sequencing to be cleaved at the C-terminus of arginine 173 (11). The 30 kDa band, which is very minor in the 1α,25(OH)$_2$D$_3$ fragmentation pattern, is seen as the predominant band for the natural metabolite lactone BS, 1α,25R(OH)$_2$-D$_3$-26,23S-lactone, and is possibly derived from the apo-VDR conformation. Using this method we have observed the MK antagonist forms a unique conformation with the VDR. A doublet of bands at 34 kDa (specifically 34.6 kDa and 33.3 kDa mass apparent) and a fragment at 30 kDa characterizes this fragment pattern. The nearest trypsin site C-terminal to the end of the VDR is at Lys413, which is also 1.5 kDa, as determined from the primary sequence (12). This value is almost the difference in molecular weight between the two fragments reported here. The example of an altered positioning of helix 12 resulting from antagonist binding into the estrogen receptor has been previously reported (13;14). This further supports the idea that the

266

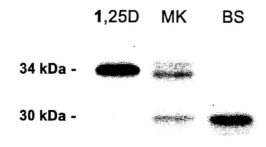

1,25D   MK   BS

34 kDa -

30 kDa -

Figure 3. MK induces a unique conformational change in the VDR-LBD. Limited proteolysis of VDR labeled by [^{35}S]-methionine with saturating concentrations of indicated ligand are shown on SDS-PAGE. BS, 1α,25(OH)$_2$D$_3$-26, 23S-lactone, and MK are added at 10 μM and 1α,25(OH)$_2$D$_3$ at 1 μM. Apparent molecular weight of bands are shown on the left.

doublet of fragments centered at 34 kDa upon MK binding results from proteolysis of a differentially exposed trypsin site near helix 12 of the VDR.

In conclusion, we have shown that the antagonism of MK toward the nuclear receptor for 1α,25(OH)$_2$D$_3$ is not due to a covalent binding to the VDR but, rather, the freely reversible interaction with a poorly agonistic ligand. For the osteocalcin VDRE in Cos-1 cells, this antagonism has been shown to occur against all ligands tested but the useful range of antagonism is dependant on the transactivation activity of the agonist relative to MK. Agonists that are significantly more active than 1α,25(OH)$_2$D$_3$ require too large an excess of MK to prove useful and significantly weaker agonists have little different agonist activity than MK. For this reason MK may be described as a partial antagonist especially since variable results have been shown using other cell systems. Future studies will expand upon the differential effects of this ligand on VDR as both an agonist and antagonist. These differential actions may serve useful in modulating the activity of the vitamin D endocrine system.

References

1. Miura,D., Manabe,K., Gao,Q., Norman,A.W., and Ishizuka,S. (1999) *FEBS Lett.* **460**, 297-302.
2. Miura,D., Manabe,K., Ozono,K., Saito,M., Gao,Q., Norman,A.W., and Ishizuka,S. (1999) *J.Biol.Chem.* **274**, 16392-16399.
3. Ozono,K., Saito,M., Miura,D., Michigami,T., Nakajima,S., and Ishizuka,S. (1999) *J Biol.Chem.* **274**, 32376-32381.
4. Liu,Y.Y., Collins,E.D., Norman,A.W., and Peleg,S. (1997) *J.Biol.Chem.* **272**, 3336-3345.
5. Norman,A.W. and Wong,R.G. (1972) *J.Nutr.* **102**, 1709-1718.
6. Walters,M.R., Hunziker,W., and Norman,A.W. (1980) *J.Recept.Res.* **1(2)**, 313-327.
7. Hunziker,W., Walters,M.R., and Norman,A.W. (1980) *J.Biol.Chem.* **255**, 9534-9537.
8. Norman,A.W., Hunziker,W., Walters,M.R., and Bishop,J.E. (1983) *J.Biol.Chem.* **258**, 12876-12880.
9. Peleg,S., Sastry,M., Collins,E.D., Bishop,J.E., and Norman,A.W. (1995) *J.Biol.Chem.* **270**, 10551-10558.
10. Zhou,J.Y., Norman,A.W., Chen,D., Sun,G., Uskokovic,M.R., and Koeffler,H.P. (1990) *Proc.Natl.Acad.Sci.USA* **87**, 3929-3932.
11. Vaisanen,S., Juntunen,K., Itkonen,A., Vihko,P., and Maenpaa,P.H. (1997) *Eur.J.Biochem.* **248**, 156-162.
12. Baker,A.R., McDonnell,D.P., Hughes,M., Crisp,T.M., Mangelsdorf,D.J., Haussler,M.R., Pike,J.W., Shine,J., and O'Malley,B.W. (1988) *Proc.Natl.Acad.Sci.USA* **85**, 3294-3298.
13. Nichols,M., Rientjes,J.M., and Stewart,A.F. (1998) *EMBO J.* **17**, 765-773.
14. Lazennec,G., Ediger,T.R., Petz,L.N., Nardulli,A.M., and Katzenellenbogen,B.S. (1997) *Molecular Endocrinology* **11**, 1375-1386.

IN VITRO EVALUATION OF THE FUNCTIONALITY OF NATURAL DR3-TYPE VITAMIN D RESPONSE ELEMENTS

Andrea Toell and Carsten Carlberg
Institut für Physiologische Chemie I, Heinrich-Heine-Universität, D-40001 Düsseldorf, Germany

Summary: All presently known natural DR3-type (direct repeat of two hexameric binding sites with three spacing nucleotides) vitamin D_3 response elements (VDREs) have been compared and classified for their in vitro functionality, i.e. for their complex formation with VDR-RXR heterodimers, their ability to stabilize VDR-RXR heterodimer conformations and the interaction VDRE-bound VDR-RXR heterodimers with coactivators and corepressors. The affinity of VDR-RXR heterodimers for each VDRE appears to be the major discriminative parameter between the DR3-type VDREs. Based on this aspect, DR3-type VDREs were divided into three classes. A significant difference was not found for ligand sensitivity of complex formation and conformation stabilization (EC_{50} = 0.1 nM) and for the $1\alpha,25$-dihydroxyvitamin D_3-($1\alpha,25(OH)_2D_3$-)modulated interaction of the VDR-RXR-VDRE complex with cofactors. Taken together, this will not only facilitate further investigation of the principles of DR3-type VDRE-mediated gene regulation, but also strongly suggests that DR3-type VDREs alone can not explain the pleiotropic genomic action of $1\alpha,25(OH)_2D_3$.

Introduction: The most important step in $1\alpha,25(OH)_2D_3$ signalling is probably the complex formation of VDR-RXR heterodimers with VDREs in the promoter of primary $1\alpha,25(OH)_2D_3$ regulated genes. The majority of the presently known VDREs show a DR3-type structure (1). However, other VDRE structures (DR4, DR6, IP9) have also been described (2). Binding of ligand results in a conformational change of VDRE-bound VDR-RXR heterodimers followed by the dissociation of corepressors and subsequent interaction with coactivators (3). VDR-coactivator interaction then further facilitates recruitment of other factors to form a larger complex that modulates chromatin structure and initiates transcription (4). The central question of this study is whether each DR3-type VDRE has an individual functionality that may explain specific effects of $1\alpha,25(OH)_2D_3$ or whether all DR3-type VDREs function in the same way.

Results and discussion: Ligand-dependent gel shift assays were performed using in vitro translated VDR and RXR proteins and all presently known natural DR3-type VDREs (for their core sequences see Tab. 1) in the absence and presence of a saturating concentration of $1\alpha,25(OH)_2D_3$ (Fig. 1). The rPit-1 DR4-type VDRE was included as a reference in all experimental series. The affinity of VDR-RXR heterodimers for the tested VDREs (at a fixed protein-DNA ratio) was found to be different, which allowed a grouping of the VDREs into three classes. The DR3-type VDREs from the rANF, the mouse and pig OPN and the cCAII promoter showed the strongest VDR-RXR heterodimer binding and were categorized into class I (Tab. 1), but the binding affinity of VDR-RXR heterodimers for each of them was found to be lower (10-30 %) than of the rPit-1 DR4-type VDRE. The affinity of VDR-RXR heterodimers for the six VDREs that form class II (from the human genes CYP24, NaP_i and PTH and the rat genes CYP24, OC and PTHrP) is reduced (2-10 %), but they are also ligand sensitive. The binding of VDR-RXR heterodimers to the ten DR3-type VDREs of class I and II as well as to the Pit-1

abbrev.	sequence	pos.	species	gene	ref.
reference DR4-type VDRE					
rPit-1	GAAGTTCATGAGAGTTCA	-683	rat	Pit-1	(9)
Class I DR3-type VDREs					
rANF	AGAGGTCATGAAGGACA	-907	rat	atrial natriuretic factor	(10)
mOPN	AAGGTTCACGAGGTTCA	-759	mouse	osteopontin	(11)
pOPN	ATGGGTCATATGGTTCA	-2261	pig	osteopontin	(12)
cCAII	GAAGGGCATGGAGTTCG	-62	chicken	carbonic anhydrase II	(13)
Class II DR3-type VDREs					
hCYP24	GGAGTTCACCGGGTGTG	-291	human	24-hydroxylase	(14)
hNaPi	CAGGGGCAGCAAGGGCA	-1977	human	Na+-dependent inorganic phosphate transporter type II	(15)
rOC	CTGGGTGAATGAGGACA	-457	rat	osteocalcin	(16,17)
rCYP24	AGGGTTCAGCGGGTGCG	-259	rat	24-hydroxylase	(18)
hPTH	ATGGTTCAAAGCAGACA	-122	human	parathyroid hormone	(19)
rPTHrP1	TAAGGTTACTCAGTGAA	-805	rat	PTH related peptide	(20)
Class III DR3-type VDREs					
rPTHrP2	AGGGTGGAGAGGGGTGA	-1107	rat	PTH related peptide	(21)
rD9k	GAGGGTGTCGGAAGCCC	-490	rat	calbindin D9k	(22)
aMyHC	GAAGGACAAAGAGGGGA	-801	quail	slow myosin heavy chain	(23)
hGH	TGGGGTCAACAGTGGGA	-59	human	growth hormone	(24)
cIntβ	GCGAGGCAGAAGGGAGA	-772	chicken	integrin β3	(25)
cPTH	GAGGGTCAGGAGGGTGT	-76	chicken	parathyroid hormone	(26)
hp21	GTAGGGAGATTGGTTCA	-779	human	p21	(27)

Table 1: Natural DR3-type VDREs. The core sequence of the 17 examined DR3-type VDREs and the reference rat Pit-1 DR4-type VDRE in relation to the transcription start site are indicated. Hexameric core binding motifs are in bold and deviations from the consensus sequence RGKTSA are underlined.

element was found to be enhanced by $1\alpha,25(OH)_2D_3$ by a factor of 2 to 5. In contrast, the seven VDREs grouped into class III show a very weak binding of VDR-RXR heterodimers (less than 2 %) and no significant ligand inducibility. According to the stringent *in vitro* criteria, the core sequences of the class III members cannot be considered as functional VDREs. However, these findings do not exclude the possibility that class III VDREs may gain responsiveness to $1\alpha,25(OH)_2D_3$ in their natural promoter context through the help of flanking partner proteins or a potential cooperative action with additional VDREs, such as in the case of the CYP24 gene (5).

For the analysis of ligand-stabilized VDR-RXR conformations, gel shift clipping assays were performed with all VDREs of classes I and II (reference: rPit-1 element; data not shown). The digestion of VDR-RXR-VDRE complexes in the absence or presence of saturating concentrations of $1\alpha,25(OH)_2D_3$ with a limited concentration of the endoprotease trypsin resulted in the same two protein-DNA complexes ($c1_{GSC}$ and $c2_{GSC}$) representing different conformations of DNA-bound VDR-RXR heterodimers (6). The conformations $c1_{GSC}$ and $c2_{GSC}$ were quantified in relation to the respective ligand-induced, non-digested VDR-RXR and provided a very similar pattern for all VDREs, although the absolute amount of ligand-triggered VDR-RXR complex formation differed between the tested VDREs. In the presence of $1\alpha,25(OH)_2D_3$, 37-72 % of DNA-bound VDR-RXR heterodimers were found to be stabilized in $c1_{GSC}$, whereas 17-32 % was stabilized in $c2_{GSC}$. This suggests, that VDR-RXR heterodimers form identical complexes on the ten VDREs of classes I and II.

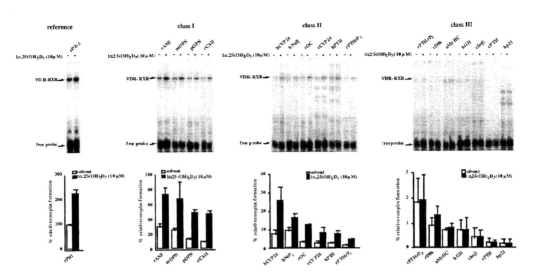

Figure 1: Classification of DR3-type VDREs. Ligand-dependent gel shift assays were performed using *in vitro* translated VDR-RXR heterodimers, 10 µM 1α,25(OH)$_2$D$_3$ (or solvent as control) and 17 different [^{32}P]-labelled DR3-type VDREs. Protein-DNA complexes were separated from free probe through 8 % non-denaturing polyacrylamide gels. Representative experiments are shown. The amount of VDR-RXR-VDRE complexes was quantified in relation to the free probe by phosphorimaging. Relative complex formation is presented in reference to the VDR-RXR heterodimer complex on the rat Pit-1 DR4-type VDRE in absence of 1α,25(OH)$_2$D$_3$.

The ligand sensitivity of VDR-RXR heterodimers bound to representative DR3-type VDREs from class I (rANF, mOPN) and class II (hCYP24, hPTH) did not demonstrate a significant deviation from an average EC$_{50}$-value of 0.1 nM, as confirmed independently on the level of VDR-RXR-VDRE complex formation and of stabilization of VDR-RXR heterodimer conformations c1$_{GSC}$ and c2$_{GSC}$ (data not shown). Moreover, a potentially differential effect of the RXR-selective ligand CD2425 on conformations of VDR-RXR bound to those DR3-type VDREs assessed by gel shift clipping assays using the endoprotease chymotrypsin was not observed (data not shown).

Finally, the interaction of DR3-type VDRE-bound VDR-RXR heterodimers with cofactors was examined in supershift experiments with bacterially expressed GST-fusions of the representative coactivator SRC-1 (GST-SRC-1$_{596-790}$) and the representative corepressor NCoR (GST-NCoR$_{1679-2453}$) with the same set of representative VDREs at saturating concentrations of 1α,25(OH)$_2$D$_3$ (data not shown). Interestingly, despite the different individual affinity of VDR-RXR heterodimers for the five selected VDREs, in the presence of 1α,25(OH)$_2$D$_3$, 46-82 % of all VDRE-bound VDR-RXR heterodimers formed complexes with SRC-1. Complex formation with NCoR was also observed on all five representative VDREs, but the analysis of the ligand-dependent dissociation of VDR-RXR-VDRE-NCoR complexes is complicated by the fact that ligand enhances VDR-RXR-VDRE complex formation in parallel. Therefore, the individual ratio of VDR-RXR-VDRE-NCoR complexes to VDR-RXR-VDRE complexes was calculated for each VDRE. This ratio decreased from a value of 0.34-0.76 to a level of 0.23-0.39 after addition of 1α,25(OH)$_2$D$_3$. Thus, these cofactor-dependent assays did not demonstrate a significant difference in the *in vitro* functionality of VDR-RXR heterodimers that are bound to DR3-type VDREs. Interestingly, VDREs from genes that are negatively regulated by $1\alpha,25(OH)_2D_3$, e.g. from the rANF and the hPTH gene, show the same interaction with cofactors than VDREs from positively regulated genes. This suggests that positive and negative regulation by $1\alpha,25(OH)_2D_3$ is not related to the VDRE sequence.

In conclusion, natural DR3-type VDREs were found to differentiate in the affinity of VDR-RXR heterodimers for each VDRE, but the heterodimers appear to take identical conformations on all of them and show also similar interaction with cofactors. This facilitates further investigation of the principles of DR3-type VDRE-mediated gene regulation, but also strongly suggests that DR3-type VDREs alone can not explain the pleiotropic genomic action of $1\alpha,25(OH)_2D_3$.

References:

1. Carlberg C. (1995) *Eur J Biochem* **231**, 517-27
2. Carlberg C. (1997) *Proc. 10th Int. Vit. D Workshop*, 268-275
3. Torchia J, Glass C and Rosenfeld MG. (1998) *Curr. Opin. Cell Biol.* **10**, 373-383
4. Spencer TE, Jenster G, Burcin MM, Allis CD, Zhou J, Mizzen CA, McKenna NJ, Onate SA, Tsai SY, Tsai M-J and O'Malley BW. (1997) *Nature* **389**, 194-198
5. Kerry DM, Dwivedi PP, Hahn CN, Morris HA, Omdahl JL and May BK. (1996) *J. Biol. Chem.* **271**, 29715-29721
6. Quack M and Carlberg C. (2000) *Mol Pharmacol* **57**(2), 375-84
7. Herdick M, Steinmeyer A and Carlberg C. (2000) *J Biol Chem*, in press
8. Polly P, Herdick M, Moehren U, Baniahmad A, Heinzel T and Carlberg C. (2000) *FASEB J.* **13**, in press
9. Rhodes SJ, Chen R, DiMattia GE, Scully KM, Kalla KA, Lin S-C, Yu VC and Rosenfeld MG. (1993) *Genes & Dev.* **7**, 913-932
10. Kahlen JP and Carlberg C. (1996) *Biochem Biophys Res Commun* **218**, 882-6
11. Noda M, Vogel RL, Craig AM, Prahl J, DeLuca HF and Denhardt DT. (1990) *Proc. Natl. Acad. Sci. USA* **87**, 9995-9999
12. Zhang Q, Wrana JL and Sodek J. (1992) *Eur. J. Biochem.* **207**, 649-659
13. Quélo I, Machuca I and Jurdic P. (1998) *J. Biol. Chem.* **273**, 10638-10646
14. Chen K-S and DeLuca HF. (1995) *Biochim. Biophys. Acta* **1263**, 1-9
15. Taketani Y, Segawa H, Chikamori M, Morita K, Tanaka K, Kido S, Yamamoto H, Iemori Y, Tatsumi S, Tsugawa N, Okano T, Kobayashi T, Miyamoto K and Takeda E. (1998) *J. Biol. Chem.* **273**, 14575-14581
16. Lian JB, Steward C, Puchacz E, Mackowiak S, Shalhoub V, Collart D, Zambetti G and Stein G. (1989) *Proc. Natl. Acad. Sci. USA* **86**, 1143-47
17. Demay MB, Gerardi JM, DeLuca HF and Kronenberg HM. (1990) *Proc. Natl. Acad. Sci. USA* **87**, 369-373
18. Zierold C, Darwish HM and DeLuca HF. (1994) *Proc. Natl. Acad. Sci. USA* **91**, 900-902
19. Demay MB, Kieran MS, DeLuca HF and Kronenberg HM. (1992) *Proc. Natl. Acad. Sci. USA* **89**, 8097-8101
20. Falzon M. (1996) *Mol. Endocrinol.* **10**, 672-681
21. Kremer R, Sebag M, Champigny C, Meerovitch K, Hendy GN, White J and Goltzman D. (1996) *J. Biol. Chem.* **271**, 16310-16316
22. Darwish HM and DeLuca HF. (1992) *Proc. Natl. Acad. Sci. USA* **89**, 603-607
23. Wang GF, Nikovits W, Schleinitz M and Stockdale FE. (1998) *Mol. Cell. Biol.* **18**, 6023-6034
24. Alonso M, Segura C, Dieguez C and Perez-Fernandez R. (1998) *Biochem. Biophys. Res. Commun.* **247**, 882-887
25. Cao X, Ross FP, Zhang L, MacDonald PN, Chappel J and Teitelbaum SL. (1993) *J. Biol. Chem.* **268**, 27371-27380
26. Liu SM, Koszewski N, Lupez M, Malluche HH, Olivera A and Russell J. (1996) *Mol. Endocrinol.* **10**, 206-215
27. Liu M, Lee M-H, Cohen M, Bommakanti M and Freedman LP. (1996) *Genes & Dev.* **10**, 142-153

The Mouse Vitamin D Receptor is Expressed Through an Sp1-Driven Promoter.

Frederic Jehan[1] and Hector F. DeLuca
Department of Biochemistry, University of Wisconsin-Madison, Madison, WI 53706
[1]Present Address: CNRS UPR 1524, Hopital Saint Vincent de Paul, 82 Avenue Denfert-Rochereau, 75014, Paris, France

INTRODUCTION

Vitamin D exerts a number of biological functions in the body, the main one being the regulation of calcium and phosphorus homeostasis (1-3). The active form of vitamin D, 1,25-dihydroxyvitamin D_3 (1,25-$(OH)_2D_3$), acts through binding to its receptor, the VDR, a ligand-inducible transcription factor member of the steroid hormone superfamily. The VDR forms heterodimers with the retinoid X receptor and the complex binds to specific response elements found in the promoter of vitamin D target genes (1-3). The availability of the mouse VDR (mVDR) gene has allowed a characterization of a TATA-less promoter containing a cluster of 4 Sp1 sites named Sp1-1, Sp1-2, Sp1-3 and Sp1-4 (4). Similarly, the human VDR promoter (5) and the chicken VDR promoter (6) reveal TATA-less, multiple Sp1 site promoters. In order to understand the transcriptional regulation of the mouse VDR gene, we have investigated the functional role of the 4 clustered Sp1 binding sites in promoter activity of the mVDR gene.

A

Figure 1. Gel shift analysis of the putative Sp1 sites present in the mVDR promoter.

A. Characterization of the Sp1 complexes bound to the Sp1 sites of the mVDR promoter. Binding reactions were performed using 10 µl of porcine intestinal nuclear extract (PNE) and 0.1 ng of each labeled probe as indicated, in the presence (+) or absence (-) of 400-fold unlabeled Sp1-DHFR oligonucleotide as competitor. The complexes formed were resolved by electrophoresis on a 4% nondenaturing polyacrylamide gel.

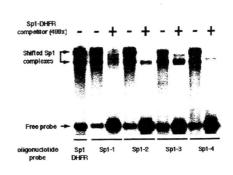

B. Ability of the mVDR promoter Sp1 sites to compete for the binding of Sp1 complexes to the canonical Sp1-DHFR site. Binding reactions have been performed with 10 µl PNE and 0.1 ng of radiolabeled Sp1-DHFR oligonucleotide in the absence (lane 1) or presence of 400 fold excess of unlabeled Sp1-DHFR (lane 2), Sp1-1 (lane 3), Sp1-2 (lane 4), Sp1-3 (lane 5) or Sp1-4 (lane 6) oligonucleotides.

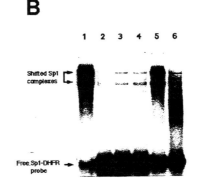

RESULTS

Binding affinity analysis of the putative sp1 sites for the transcription factor Sp1

To characterize the Sp1 sites found in the mVDR promoter, gel shift experiments have been performed using the canonical Sp1 site GGGGCGGGGC found in the Dihydrofolate reductase (DHFR) gene (7). Labeled Sp1-DHFR or mVDR Sp1 oligonucleotides have been incubated with Pig intestinal nuclear extract (PNE) (Fig. 1) or ROS 17/2.8 nuclear extract (data not shown). Similar results have been obtained with both nuclear extracts. After resolution on a 4 % polyacrylamide gel electrophoresis, two complexes w ere formed with the Sp1-DHFR probe that shifted in the presence of any of the four mVDR Sp1 oligonucleotides. Unlabeled Sp1-DHFR oligonucleotide used as competitor (400-fold excess) eliminated the two complexes bound to Sp1-1, Sp1-2 and Sp1-4 probes (Fig. 1A). However, the lower complex bound to the Sp1-3 probes remained (Fig. 1A), suggesting that this complex is not related to a Sp1 site complex while having the same migration properties. To confirm the nature of the complexes bound to the four mVDR Sp1 sites, mVDR Sp1 oligonucleotides were used in competition experiments to determine their ability to eliminate the binding on the canonical Sp1-DHFR. In the same manner, the two Sp1 (or Sp1-related) complexes bound to the canonical Sp1-DHFR site were eliminated by competition with a 400-fold excess of unlabeled Sp1-1, Sp1-2 or Sp1-4 oligonucleotides but not by a 400-fold excess of Sp1-3 oligonucleotide (Fig. 1B). This indicates that the mVDR Sp1-3 is not a Sp1 site. A one base difference from the consensus Sp1 sequence is obviously responsible.

The relative affinity of the mVDR Sp1 sites for the Sp1 complexes, competition experiments has been determined with increasing amounts of unlabeled competitor (12-fold to 200-fold) in the presence of PNE. The results have shown that the most efficient competitor for the strong canonical Sp1-DHFR site is itself. However, Sp1-1 and Sp1-2 are only two times less efficient, and Sp1-4 is only 4 times less efficient, than Sp1-DHFR itself data not shown.

Role of Sp1 sites in the mVDR promoter activity

The role of the Sp1 sites in the mVDR promoter activity has been further investigated by mutation analysis. For that purpose, one or several Sp1 sites have been mutated in the 0.842 kb promoter construct (corresponding to the 0.8 kb promoter construct in ref. 4). Mutations of Sp1 sites have been done by replacing the central GCG core in the consensus sequence GGGGCGGGGC by AAA, as described by Gidoni et al. (8). To produce 0.842 kb constructs with precise mutation, an Sp1-less construct has been generated by fusion of the PCR products generated by amplification of the 5' and 3' flanking regions of the two half sites of MscI, conveniently located on both side of the Sp1 cluster. This has generated a construct with an unique MscI site. Each mutated Sp1 oligonucleotide was inserted in this unique MscI cloning site where the four Sp-1 sites have been deleted. Sequences of the plasmid constructs were checked and are identical to the 0.842 kb construct except for the Sp1 mutation. The activity of the mutated constructs has been tested using transfection/transactivation experiments in ROS17/2.8 cells (Fig. 2).

As expected, removal of the Sp1 site region, by deletion of 107 bases at the 3' end of this 0.842 kb construct or the 51 bp between the two MscI half-sites (M1 and M2), dramatically decreased the promoter activity. To further identify their role in the promoter activity, each Sp1 site has been mutated separately in different constructs. Individual mutation of the mVDRp Sp1 sites did not significantly decrease the luciferase activity, suggesting that at least several Sp1 sites are involved in the basal activity of the mVDR gene. We have seen previously that Sp1-3 element barely competes with Sp1 (or Sp1-related) complexes bound to the DHFR Sp1 site (Fig. 1B). Interestingly, mutation of the Sp1-3 site has induced a 3- to 5-fold increase in promoter activity. When Sp1-1 and Sp1-2 elements, believed to be important in the promoter activity, are mutated together, a decrease of only 50% of the promoter activity was observed. Mutation of all four Sp1 sites was necessary to eliminate all promoter activity (Fig. 2). _

DISCUSSION

TATA-less Sp1-controlled promoters are common among housekeeping genes and these promoters are not subject to environmental control (7). However, such promoters are also found in genes that have paradoxically a restricted pattern of expression in the body. Such characteristics exemplified in the nerve growth factor receptor gene (9), or the malic enzyme gene (10), has been found in the gene of most members of the steroid/thyroid receptor superfamily (11).

The two Sp1 or Sp1-related complexes we have seen in gel shift experiment have been commonly observed on Sp1 sites (e.g. references 12,13). Furthermore, competition experiments have evidenced that the complexes formed contain Sp1 or Sp1-related proteins. The Sp1-3 site bound an unknown factor with similar migration properties to the lower band of the Sp1 complexes (Fig. 1B). The presence of this unknown complex was demonstrated by eliminating any Sp1 related complexes with 400-fold excess of Sp1-DHFR oligonucleotide. This suggests that this unknown complex is not related to Sp1 factor. This unknown factor has been found in both porcine intestine and osteoblast-like Ros 17/2.8 cell nuclear extracts, two cell types that express VDR. This factor may play an important role in repression of the mVDR promoter activity since mutation of the binding site has produced a 3- to 5-fold increase in transactivation (Fig. 2).

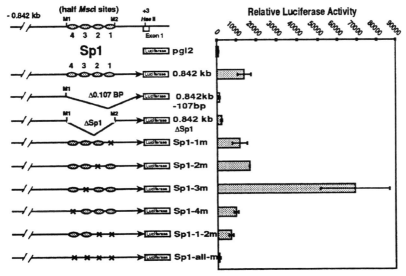

Figure 2. Functional analysis of the m VDR Sp1 sites in ROS17/2.8 cells.
ROS 17/2.8 cells were maintained in F-12 medium supplemented with 10% fetal calf serum. Twenty hours before transfection, cells were plated at a density of 150,000 cells per square cm in a six-well plate. ROS17/2.8 cells were transfected with constructs containing the 0.8 kb fragment of the mVDR promoter inserted in the pGL2b reporter vector and mutated or deleted in various positions. These constructs are shown schematically on the left side. Oval symbols represent Sp1 sites. Mutation of one Sp1 sit is symbolized by (**X**). Restriction sites used to generate these constructs are indicated on the top left panel. ROS cells were grown for 24 h before transfection. They were cotransfected with 1 µg of the mVDR promoter reporter constructs and 30 ng of the pCMVβ vector using 5 ul of lipofectin reagent. Cells were harvested 48 h after transfection. Luciferase activity was corrected for β-galactosidase activity. Data are mean of three transfections +/- SD.

The involvement of the four Sp1 elements in the activation of basal transcription of the mVDR was demonstrated in transfection experiments using the luciferase gene of the pGL2 basic vector as reporter. ROS 17/2.8 cells have been used for transfection because they naturally express high level of VDR protein and mRNA. Deletion experiments have shown that sequence -177 to −54 containing the four Sp-1 sites is responsible for most if not all activity of the mVDR promoter. This has been further shown by deletion of the -177 to +3 sequence of the promoter in the 1.494 kb promoter construct (corresponding to the -1.5 kb construct in ref. 4). Interestingly, doing the same type of deletion experiment in Hepa1c1c7, a mouse liver cell line that does not express VDR (data not shown), has given a similar pattern of expression. Transfection experiments in this liver cell line have shown a 20-fold decrease in luciferase activity when -177 to +3 sequence of the promoter was eliminated in the 1.494 kb construct (data not shown). The fact that the mVDR promoter is active in cells that do not express the VDR suggests the binding of activating or inhibiting factors upstream of the 1.494 kb promoter region. Supporting this point, the binding of an intestine-specific activating factor, Cdx-2, has been evidenced 3.7 kb upstream of the transcriptional start site in the human VDR gene (14). Therefore, the Sp1 region may not be involved in the difference in VDR expression seen in liver and osteoblasts.

The mutation of every Sp1 site of the 0.842 kb construct has eliminated all promoter activity, giving the most convincing evidence of the role of the 4 Sp1 sites in promoter activity. However, mutation of individual Sp1 sites produced no dramatic decrease in the promoter activity. Such a result is not surprising since, in other promoters controlled by a cluster of Sp1 sites, it has been shown that elimination of one Sp1 site had little consequence in promoter activity (8, 12). Since the Sp1-1 is the downstream Sp1 site in the mVDR promoter, its mutation was likely to change the main start location, controlled then by the next upstream Sp1 site, Sp1-2 (8, 15). Mutation of the two strong Sp1 sites, Sp1-1 and Sp1-2, have produced no more than about 50% decrease in promoter activity, suggesting that either the remaining Sp1 site (Sp1-4) has supported the promoter activity or that the complexes bound to Sp1-3 have played a role in generating promoter activity. The increase in activity due to mutation of the Sp1-3 site does not support the latter hypothesis, meaning that one Sp1 site with a medium affinity for Sp1 complexes (Sp1-4) is sufficient to drive half of the mVDR promoter activity. This is supported by the fact that Sp1-4, which differs by a T in position 7 of the consensus Sp1 sequence, has been shown to be a good competitor for Sp1-DHFR.

In conclusion, our results show that this TATA-less mVDR promoter is the main VDR promoter in normal mouse intestine and kidney and is effectively driven by 3 Sp1 sites.

ACKNOWLEDGMENTS

This work was supported in part by a program project grant, no. DK14881, from the National Institutes of Health and a fund from the Wisconsin Alumni Research Foundation.

REFERENCES

1. Darwish, H.M. & DeLuca, H.F. (1993) *Crit. Rev. Eucaryotic Gene Exp.* **3**, 89-116.
2. Haussler, M.R., Whitfield, G.K., Haussler, C.A., Hsieh, J.-C., Thompson, P.D., Selznick, S.H., Dominguez,C.E. & Jurukta, P. (1998). *J. Bone Min. Res.* **13**, 325-349.
3. Jones, G., Strugnell, S.A. & DeLuca,H.F. (1998) *Physiological reviews* **78**, 193-1231.
4. Jehan, F. & DeLuca, H.F (1997). *Proc. Natl. Acad. Sci. USA* **94**, 10138-10143.
5. Miyamoto,K.-I., Kesterson, R.A., Yamamoto, H., Taketani, Y., Nishiwaki, E., Tatsumi, S., Inoue, Y., Morita, K., Tadeka, E. & Pike,J.W. (1997) *Mol. Endoc.* **11**. 1165-79.
6. Lu, Z., Jehan, F., Zierold, C. & DeLuca H.F. (1999) J. Cell. Biochem, in press.
7. Dynan, W.S., Sazer, S., Tjian, R. & Schimke, R.T. (1986) *Nature.* **319**, 246-248.
8. Gidoni, D., Kadonaga, J.T., Barrera-Saldana, H., Takahashi, K., Chambon,P. & Tjian, R. (1985) *Science* **230**, 511-517.
9. Seghal, A., Patil,N. & Chao, M. (1988), V.M. (1988) *Mol. Cell. Biol.* **8**, 3542-3545.
10. Morioka,H., Tennyson, G.E. & Nikodem,V.M. (1988). *Mol. Cell. Biol.* **8**, 3542-3545.
11. Gronemeyer, H. & Laudet, V. (1995) *Nuclear Receptors Prot. Profile* **2**, 1173-1235.
12. Boisclair, Y.R., Brown, A.L., Casola, S. & Rechler, M.M. (1993) *J. Biol. Chem.* **268**, 24892-24901.
13. Li, J., Qu, X. & Schmidt, A.M. (1998) *J. Biol. Chem.* **273**, 30870-30878.
14. Yamamoto,H., Miyamoto,K.-I., Li, B., Taketani, Y., Kitano, M., Inoue, Y., Morita, K., Pike, J.W. & Takeda,E. (1999) *J. Bone Miner. Res.* **14**, 240-247.
15. Kadonaga, J.T., Jones, K. A. & Tjian, R. (1986) *Trends Biochem. Sci.* **11**, 20-23.

HORMONE REGULATION OF THE HUMAN VITAMIN D RECEPTOR GENE

Ian Byrne, Saara Romu, Sarah Smyzcek, Martin Tenniswood and JoEllen Welsh, University of Notre Dame, Notre Dame, IN 46556

Introduction Vitamin D receptor (VDR) abundance is an important determinant of cellular sensitivity to $1,25(OH)_2D_3$ and is affected by many physiological factors through a variety of mechanisms. Specific regulators of the VDR include $1,25(OH)_2D_3$ itself and other steroids such as 17β-estradiol, dexamethasone and retinoic acid, all of which have been shown to up-regulate the VDR protein and/or mRNA in vitro. Characterization of the transcriptional regulation of the human VDR (hVDR) gene has primarily been hampered by the complexity of its promoter region. The untranslated exon 1 is present in multiple copies and is associated with at least two and probably three differentially utilized promoters (1,2). Attempts to demonstrate regulation of these promoter regions, using reporter gene assays in numerous cell lines, have been largely unsuccessful, with one exception - the demonstration of a retinoic acid responsive region in the intronic region located between exon 1c and exon 2 (1). In these studies we have cloned and characterized the 5' flanking region of exon 1c of the hVDR and provide evidence that this region represents a hormone regulated promoter in breast cancer cells.

Materials and Methods The region upstream of exon 1c of the hVDR gene was amplified by PCR and products of 1300bp and 800 bp were cloned into TA cloning vectors and sequenced. The 800 and 1300bp products were subcloned into the promoterless pRL null vector which contains the renilla luciferase reporter gene. For transient transfections, MCF-7 and SUM-159PT human breast cancer cell lines (3) cultured in phenol red-free media were co-transfected with 0.75 µg of the designated pRL construct and 0.25 µg of pGL-3 SV40. After 1h, media containing 5% charcoal stripped serum (CSS), supplemented with the appropriate treatment, or an equal volume of ethanol vehicle, was added to each well. After 18 h, cells were lysed and luciferase activity was determined with the Dual Luciferase Assay Kit. Transfection efficiency was normalized using the pGL-3 SV40 construct and data are expressed as relative luciferase units (RLUs).

Results The sequence of the 5' flanking region of exon 1c displays an organization reminiscent of a typical TATA containing promoter. A consensus TATA sequence (GATAAAA) is present 29 bp upstream from the transcription start site. A number of putative regulatory regions are present in this region, including several Sp1 and AP-2 sites upstream of the TATA box in addition to consensus sequences corresponding to AP-1 and glucocorticoid receptor response element half sites. Notably, no sequences corresponding to consensus direct repeat vitamin D_3 response elements (VDRE) or estrogen response elements (ERE) are present in this region.

Primer extension analysis was used to identify transcripts initiated immediately upstream of the predicted start site of exon 1c (not shown). These studies identified a 79bp extension product in MCF-7 cells, consistent with a VDR transcript containing only exon 1c. Several larger primer extension products were also present which likely represent splice variants containing exon 1c and several of the alternative exons identified further upstream. While

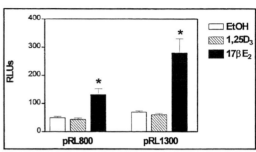

Figure 1. Effects of $1,25D_3$ and 17β-estradiol on pRL800 and pRL1300 luciferase reporter constructs in MCF-7 cells.

confirmation of these assignments will require cloning and sequencing of these products, the primer extension analysis indicates that the putative promoter upstream of exon 1c of the hVDR gene is active in MCF-7 human breast cancer cells. This was confirmed using the pRL800 and pRL1300 luciferase reporter constructs. Both of these constructs are constitutively active in untreated MCF-7 cells and are induced by 10 nM 17β-estradiol but not 100nM $1,25(OH)_2D_3$ (Fig. 1). This data suggests that the up regulation of the VDR that is seen in MCF-7 cells (4) is not mediated by transcriptional regulation of the VDR through exon 1c.

To determine whether the effects of 17β-estradiol on the hVDR constructs are mediated by the estrogen receptor, pRL800 activity was measured in MCF-7 cells treated with 4-hydroxytamoxifen, the biologically active form of the anti-estrogen tamoxifen. Treatment of MCF-7 cells with 1μM 4-hydroxytamoxifen does not alter reporter gene activity, but when administered simultaneously, 4-hydroxytamoxifen completely blocks the stimulation of the pRL800 reporter construct by 1nM 17β-estradiol (Fig. 2). Similar results are observed with the pRL1300 construct. We have also

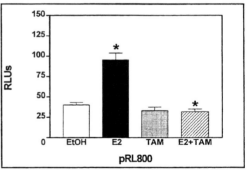

Figure 2. Effects of tamoxifen on basal and estradiol stimulated pRL800 activity in MCF-7 cells.

found that 17β-estradiol does not induce either reporter gene construct in an estrogen receptor negative cell line, SUM159PT (not shown). Thus, the effect of 17β-estradiol on transcription initiated in the promoter region upstream of exon 1c is directly mediated via the estrogen receptor.

As shown in Fig. 3, 1nM ATRA or 1μM forskolin upregulate the promoter activity of both the pRL800 and pRL1300 constructs in MCF-7 cells, while neither 1nM TPA or 10nM dexamethasone induce transcription above the basal levels seen in vehicle treated control cells. Forskolin induces the promoter activity by approximately 5 fold with both the pRL1300 and pRL800 constructs, suggesting that the sequences responsible for this regulation are localized in the first 800bp upstream of the promoter. On the other hand, the induction by ATRA is greater when the longer construct is utilized, suggesting that the retinoid mediated regulation of the promoter lies, at least in part, in the more distal region of the pRL1300 construct.

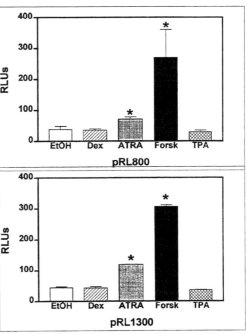

Figure 3. Effects of dexamethasone, all trans retinoic acid, forskolin and TPA on pRL800 and pRL1300 activity in MCF-7 cells.

Discussion

We describe a TATA containing promoter immediately upstream of exon 1c of the hVDR, and demonstrate that this region represents a hormonally regulated hVDR promoter active in breast cancer cells. Exon 1 of the hVDR gene is present in multiple copies (exons 1a through 1f), and the existence of at least three differentially utilized promoters (exons 1a, 1d, and 1f) has been demonstrated (1, 2). In the studies reported here, primer extension using RNA isolated from untreated MCF-7 cells identifies transcripts containing only exon 1c, as well as additional transcripts initiated from other promoters further upstream which contain exon 1c. These data are consistent with earlier studies which demonstrated numerous transcripts containing exon 1c (1, 2). Miyamoto et al (1) identified transcripts originating upstream of exon 1a which contained exon 1c using human kidney RNA as a template. Crofts et al (2) identified transcripts initiated upstream of exons 1a, 1d and 1f which contained exon 1c in a panel of 15 cell lines, but did not utilize primers which would identify transcripts initiated immediately upstream of exon 1c. Notably, transcripts originating upstream of exon 1f were restricted to kidney, parathyroid and intestinal cell lines, while transcripts originating upstream of exons 1a and 1d were equally expressed in all 15 cell lines examined, including the estrogen responsive breast cancer cell line T47D (2). The data presented here suggest that in unstimulated MCF-7 cells transcription of the VDR gene is initiated primarily from exon 1f promoter, but alteration of promoter usage occurs after stimulation with estradiol, forskolin or ATRA, and transcription from the exon 1c promoter is induced (Fig. 4). Interestingly, even though these agents induce transcription through this promoter, the effects appear to be mediated by AP-2 and Sp-1 sites rather than the more classical motifs.

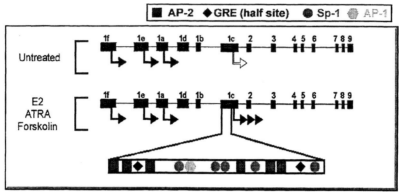

Figure 4. Proposed promoter usage in MCF-7 cells before and after stimulation.

REFERENCES

1. Miyamoto K, Kesterson R, Yamamoto H, Taketani Y, Nishiwaki E, Tatsumi S, Inoue Y, Morita K, Takeda E and Pike, JW (1997) *Mol. Endocrinol.* 11,1165-1179

2. Crofts L, Hancock M, Morrison N and Eisman J (1998) *Proc. Natl Acad. Sci. USA* 95, 10529-10534

3. Flanagan, L, VanWeelden K, Ammerman C, Ethier S and Welsh JE (1999) *Breast Cancer Res. Treat* 58,193-204

4 Narvaez CJ, VanWeelden K, Byrne I and Welsh JE. (1996) *Endocrinology* 137, 400-409

LIGAND-TRIGGERED STABILIZATION OF VITAMIN D RECEPTOR-RETINOID X RECEPTOR HETERODIMER CONFORMATIONS ON DR4-TYPE RESPONSE ELEMENTS

Marcus Quack and Carsten Carlberg
Institut für Physiologische Chemie I, Heinrich-Heine-Universität, D-40001 Düsseldorf, Germany

Summary: The vitamin D_3 receptor (VDR) is the nuclear receptor for $1\alpha,25$-dihydroxyvitamin D_3 ($1\alpha,25(OH)_2D_3$) and is known to function as a heterodimer with the retinoid X receptor (RXR) on DR3-type $1\alpha,25(OH)_2D_3$ response elements (VDREs). It was demonstrated, in this study, that DR4-type response elements (REs) are, at least, as effective as DR3-type VDREs. Gel shift clipping analysis showed that VDR-RXR heterodimers form, in response to $1\alpha,25(OH)_2D_3$ and RXR ligands, 9-*cis* retinoic acid (9cRA) and CD2425, different conformations on the DR4-type element of the rat Pit-1 gene and showed a synergistic interaction of both ligands. Complexes of RXR with the thyroid hormone receptor (T_3R), the retinoic acid receptor (RAR) and the benzoate ester receptor (ONR) also displayed characteristic individual ligand-dependent complex formation on this RE. Taken together, this study establishes DR4-type REs as multi-functional DNA binding sites with a potential to integrate various hormone signalling pathways.

Introduction: VDR and the receptors for thyroid hormone 3,5,3'-triiodo-thyro-nine (T_3), T_3R, the vitamin A derivative all-*trans* retinoic acid (atRA), RAR and benzoate esters (4-amino-butyl-benzoate (4-ABB)) ONR (1) form heterodimeric complexes with the RXR. These heterodimers bind to DNA via response elements (REs). According to the 3-4-5 rule (2) simple REs are formed by two AGGTCA motifs in a directly repeated (DR) arrangement and the number of spacing nucleotides is the major discriminating parameter for a specific DNA recognition. Stabilization of a functional nuclear receptor ligand binding domain (LBD) conformation is the second important factor in nuclear hormone signalling (3). The multiple $1\alpha,25(OH)_2D_3$ signalling model (4) suggests that the different physiological functions of the hormone may be represented by different types of VDR-VDRE complexes. This may include different RE structures (5), but also different conformations of the same heterodimer complex type. Non-DR3-type VDREs, such as inverted palindromic arrangements of the core binding sites with 9 intervening nucleotides (IP9) (6) have been demonstrated to mediate some aspects of the selective functional profile of $1\alpha,25(OH)_2D_3$ analogues (7,8). VDRE types that have not been intensively investigated thus far are DR4-type elements, i.e. direct repeats with 4 intervening nucleotides. This study shows that DR4-type REs are recognized by variety of heterodimeric complexes.

Results: The DNA binding profile of VDR-RXR, T_3R-RXR, RAR-RXR and ONR-RXR heterodimers was analyzed by gel shift experiments on REs that consist of two copies of the core binding motifs AGTTCA (DRX_T, Fig. 1A-D) or AGGTCA (DRX_G, Fig. 1E-H) in a directly repeated orientation with 2 to 6 intervening nucleotides ($DR2_T$ to $DR6_T$ or $DR2_G$ to $DR6_G$). The amount of protein-complexed REs was quantified in relation to that on the DR4-type RE of the rat Pit-1 gene ($DR4_T$). VDR-RXR heterodimers demonstrated strong binding to DR3- and DR4-type REs, with higher preference for elements with AGTTCA motifs (Figs. 1A+E). In addition, VDR-RXR heterodimers showed binding on DR2-, DR5- and DR6-type

REs. RAR-RXR heterodimers (Figs. 1C+G) bind to DR5- and DR2-type REs and to the $DR4_T$ element. T_3R-RXR (Figs. 1B+F) and ONR-RXR heterodimers (Figs. 1D+H) displayed a sharp binding profile with a maximum at DR4-type REs.

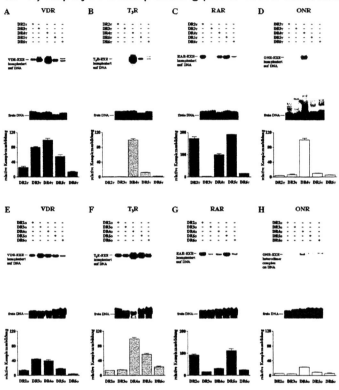

Figure 1: Binding pattern of RXR heterodimers to DR-type response elements with AGT(G)TCA motifs. Gel shift experiments were performed with heterodimers formed by *in vitro* translated RXR and VDR (A, E), T_3R (B, F), RAR (C, G) or ONR (D, H) on a series of [^{32}P]-labelled DR-type response elements that consists of two AGTTCA motifs (A-D) or two AGGTCA motifs (E-H) with 2 to 6 intervening nucleotides. The respective heterodimer-DNA complexes were separated from free probe on 10 % non-denaturing polyacrylamide gels. The amount of protein-complexed response elements was quantified on a Bioimager in relation to non-complexed response elements. For each heterodimer type, relative complex formation is expressed in relation to that of the DR4-type response element of the rat Pit-1 gene ($DR4_T$).

The influence of ligands for the RXR partner receptors, was analyzed by gel shift clipping assays performed on the $DR4_T$ element (Fig. 2). Separation of the reaction products provided protein-DNA complexes ($c1_{GSC}+c2_{GSC}$) that migrated faster than non-digested heterodimers and therefore represent a sub-population of all DNA–binding receptor complexes. The digested complexes may be interpreted as individual heterodimer conformations. With VDR-RXR heterodimers (Fig. 2A) two complexes with a migration difference could be discriminated. In presence of solvent (or RXR ligands), the faster migrating $c2_{GSC}$ was observed. The addition of $1\alpha,25(OH)_2D_3$ provided a complete shift from $c2_{GSC}$ to $c1_{GSC}$ and resulted in a 3.5-fold protection against protease digestion. This induction could be synergistically enhanced by additional treatment with 9cRA (2.6-fold) or CD2425 (4.5-fold). Two complexes with a faint migration difference were observed with T_3R-RXR heterodimers (Fig. 2B). A treatment with solvent (or RXR ligands) resulted in $c1_{GSC}$. The addition of T_3 resulted in a complete shift from $c1_{GSC}$ to $c2_{GSC}$. However, the additional treatment with 9cRA and CD2425 synergistically enhanced the protection against protease digestion by a factor of 2.8 and 3.2.

Two different complexes were observed with RAR-RXR heterodimers (Fig. 2C). The $c1_{GSC}$ complex was induced 2.0-fold by atRA compared with the solvent-treated control. A combined treatment with RAR and RXR ligands was found to be neutral. The smaller $c2_{GSC}$ probably only represents the DNA-binding domains.

ONR-RXR heterodimers (Fig. 2D) provided one complex ($c1_{GSC}$) that was stabilized by addition of 4-ABB (factor 3.0). The combination of 4-ABB with 9cRA or CD2425 resulted in a significant reduction (2-fold) of protease protection.

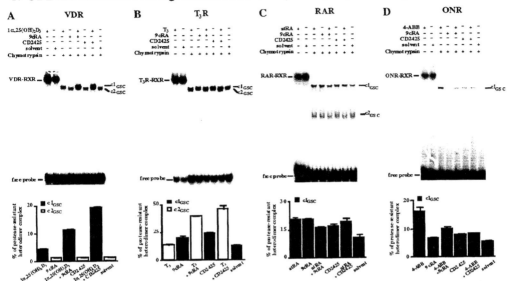

Figure 2: **Ligand-stabilized conformations of RXR heterodimers.** Gel shift clipping experiments were performed with heterodimers formed by *in vitro* translated RXR and VDR (A), T_3R (B), RAR (C) or ONR (D) on the [^{32}P]-labelled DR4-type response elements of the rat Pit-1 gene. Heterodimers were formed in the presence of 1 µM of the RXR-ligands 9cRA or CD2425 alone or in combination with 1 µM of VD, T_3, atRA or 100 µM 4-ABB. Protein-DNA complexes were incubated for 45 min with 33 ng/µl chymotrypsin in the case of VDR-RXR and T_3R-RXR heterodimers, for 10 min with 4.1 ng/µl chymotrypsin in the case of RAR-RXR heterodimers and for 10 min with 8.3 ng/µl chymotrypsin in the case of ONR-RXR heterodimers. The resulting protein-DNA complexes were separated from free probe through 13 % non-denaturing polyacrylamide gels. Representative experiments are shown. The amount of digested receptor-DNA complexes were quantified on a Bioimager in relation to the respective ligand-induced, non-digested receptor-DNA complexes.

Finally, the synergistic interaction of $1\alpha,25(OH)_2D_3$ with RXR was analyzed by gel shift clipping assays on structurally different natural VDREs, such as the DR3-type element of the rat ANF gene (Fig. 3A) and the IP9-type element of the mouse c-*fos* gene promoter (Fig. 3B). In the absence of ligand, $c2_{GSC}$ was stabilized on the two VDRE types. Moreover, a treatment with $1\alpha,25(OH)_2D_3$ resulted in a shift from $c2_{GSC}$ to $c1_{GSC}$ and an additional treatment with 9cRA or CD2425 resulted in a further increase of protease resistant receptors.

Discussion: According to the 3-4-5 rule (2), complexes of VDR, T_3R and RAR with RXR should bind to DR3-, DR4- and DR5-type REs (9). These predictions could be confirmed in this study, but it was also found that their DNA binding profile is broader than initially assumed. VDR-RXR, T_3R-RXR and ONR-RXR heterodimers showed most effective binding to the DR4-type RE of the rat Pit-1 gene ($DR4_T$) and also RAR-RXR heterodimers bind to this element with reasonable affinity. On DR4-type REs the heterodimeric partners bind to the same side of the DNA and therefore have ideal prerequisites for a dimeric interaction. Since the recognition of DR4-type REs appears to be competitive between most RXR heterodimers,

282

further individual properties of a nuclear receptor are important for a specific transactivation from these types of REs. This study demonstrates that ligand-induced conformations of heterodimeric complexes may represent the required additional level of complexity in nuclear hormone signalling. Gel shift clipping assays allow heterodimer subpopulations, that have taken ligand-stabilized conformations and the remaining heterodimers, which bind to DNA independent of ligand and are therefore eliminated through protease digestion to be distinguished. RXR appears to have a central role in a variety of nuclear signalling processes (10). When the RXR partner receptor is already activated by its specific ligand, gel shift clipping analysis suggested a discrimination between three different type of responses to RXR ligands to be made: a synergistic reaction (VDR-RXR and T_3R-RXR), a neutral result (RAR-RXR) and a destabilizing reaction (ONR-RXR). The role of RXR ligands for the VDR still remains unclear (11,12). However, the potential of a synergistic interaction of $1\alpha,25(OH)_2D_3$ and RXR ligands was demonstrated by gel shift DNA-competition assays (13) and is not limited to DR4-type VDRE, but is also observed on DR3- and IP9-type VDREs. In conclusion the VDR recognizes a broad variety of REs and VDR and RXR ligands show a synergistic interaction.

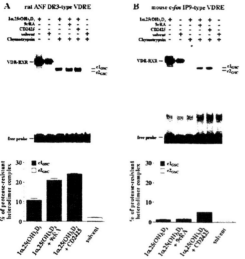

Figure 3: Synergistic ligand effects on VDR-RXR heterodimers on different natural VDREs. Gel shift clipping experiments were performed with in vitro translated RXR-VDR heterodimers on the [^{32}P]-labelled DR3-type VDRE of the rat ANF gene (A) or the IP9-type VDRE of the mouse c-fos gene (B). Heterodimers were formed in the presence of 1 µM $1\alpha,25(OH)_2D_3$ alone or in combination with the RXR-ligands 9cRA or CD2425. Chymotrypsin was then added to a final concentration of 66 ng/µl and the incubation was continued for 45 min. Protein-DNA complexes were separated from free probe on 10 % non-denaturing polyacrylamide gels. The amount of digested receptor-DNA complexes were quantified on a Bioimager in relation to the ligand-induced, non-digested VDR-RXR heterodimers.

References:

1. Blumberg, B., Kang, H., Bolado, J., Chen, H., Craig, G., Moreno, T. A., Umesono, K., Perlmann, T., De Robertis, E. M., and Evans, R. M. (1998) Genes & Dev 12, 1269-1277

2. Umesono, K., Murakami, K. K., Thompson, C. C., and Evans, R. M. (1991) Cell 65, 1255-1266

3 Nayeri, S., and Carlberg, C. (1997) Biochem J 327, 561-568

4. Carlberg, C. (1996) J Invest Dermatol Symp Proc 1, 10-14

5. Carlberg, C. (1995) Eur J Biochem 231, 517-527

6. Schräder, M., Kahlen, J. P., and Carlberg, C. (1997) Biochem Biophys Res Commun 230, 646-651

7. Nayeri, S., Danielsson, C., Kahlen, J. P., Schräder, M., Mathiasen, I. S., Binderup, L., and Carlberg, C. (1995) Oncogene 11, 1853-1858

8. Quack, M., and Carlberg, C. (1999) Mol Pharmacol 55, 1077-1087

9. Smith, W. C., Nakshatri, H., Leroy, P., Rees, J., and Chambon, P. (1991) EMBO J 10, 2223-2230

10. Mangelsdorf, D. J., and Evans, R. M. (1995) Cell 83, 841-850

11. Allegretto, E. A., Shevde, N., Zou, A., Howell, S. R., Boehm, M. F., Hollis, B. W., and Pike, J. W. (1995) J Biol Chem 270, 23906-23909

12. Cheskis, B., and Freedman, L. P. (1994) Mol Cell Biol 14, 3329-3338

13. Quack, M., and Carlberg, C. (2000) J Mol Biol 296, 743-756

REGULATION OF VITAMIN D RECEPTOR PROTEIN LEVELS AND TRANSACTIVATION BY 9-CIS RETINOIC ACID

Tiina Jääskeläinen, Sanna Ryhänen, and Pekka H. Mäenpää, Department of Biochemistry, University of Kuopio, 70210 Kuopio, Finland.

Introduction Vitamins A and D have diverse effects on cellular growth and differentiation. They both act via nuclear hormone receptors by a classical steroid hormone mechanism. The existence of different retinoic acid (RARα, β, γ) and retinoid X (RXRα, β, γ) receptors, which all bind the metabolites of vitamin A, can in part explain the various biological effects of retinoids. RXRs form homodimers or heterodimers with RARs and bind to hormone response elements (HREs) of the DR1 and DR5 type, respectively. The RXRs can also heterodimerize with several other nuclear receptors, such as vitamin D receptor (VDR) and thyroid hormone receptor (TR). These heterodimers bind to their specific HREs at promoter regions of the hormone-regulated genes and mediate the actions of vitamin D and thyroid hormone, respectively. Thus, the availability of RXR for heterodimerization is a key step regulating the effects of these ligands. The role of RXR in these heterodimers was originally believed to be a "silent" partner, a structural element needed for proper DNA binding and conformation of the heterodimer. Only recently it has been shown that RXR in a heterodimer can bind its ligand 9-cis retinoic acid (9-cisRA) and that this can modulate the transcriptional activity of the heterodimer, further expanding the actions of retinoids. In this study, we show that 9-cisRA inhibits proliferation and promotes differentiation of osteoblastic cells during the proliferative period of cell growth alone or in combination with different vitamin D_3 compounds. We also show that 9-cisRA promotes degradation of its own receptor and also VDR, thus providing a delicate mechanism to control the differentiation promoting effects of calcitriol in these cells.

Results MG-63 human osteoblastic sarcoma cells were treated with 1 nM concentration of calcitriol or its analogs GS1558 and KH1060 either alone or in combination with 0.1 µM 9-cisRA. Effects on cell numbers were measured after 24-h, 72-h and 120-h incubation (Fig. 1). In vehicle-treated cells, the cell numbers were 5.5 fold higher after the 120-h incubation than they were at the starting point (Fig. 1). In calcitriol-treated cells, the respective fold induction was 5.1, whereas the analog KH1060 very efficiently inhibited cell growth at 1 nM concentration and the cell numbers after the 120-h incubation were only 3.5-fold. GS1558 had no effect on cell numbers. 9-cis RA (0.1 µM) was even more potent than KH1060 during the first 72 h, but thereafter cell numbers started to rise again and the fold induction after 120 h was 3.8. With combination treatments, 9-cisRA potentiated the effects of the different vitamin D_3 compounds. The most potent inhibitor of cell growth was the combination of KH1060 and 9-cis RA, since the cell numbers after the 120-h incubation were only 1.4-fold higher than in the beginning.

The effect of 9-cisRA on transactivation through RXR-VDR was measured as osteocalcin mRNA induction and osteocalcin protein secretion in the MG-63 cells. During the proliferative period, osteocalcin mRNA levels were 1.7-fold higher in the

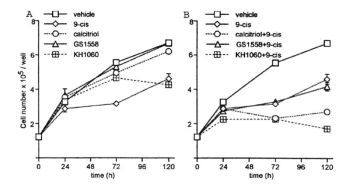

Figure 1: Inhibition of cell growth by calcitriol, GS1558 and KH1060 (1 nM) and 9-cisRA (9-cis, 0.1 µM) either alone (A) or in combination (B).

cells treated with 0.1 µM calcitriol and 9-cisRA than obtained with calcitriol alone and, at protein level, the respective fold induction was 1.5 (Fig. 2). 9-cisRA alone also induced osteocalcin production in these cells as determined by radioimmunoassay (Fig. 2B). Induction was also seen at mRNA level after longer exposure of the Northern blots or by RT-PCR (not shown). When calcitriol or its analogs GS1558, GS1500, EB1089 or KH1060 were used at 1 nM concentration, 9-cisRA (0.1 µM) similarly increased osteocalcin production during the proliferative cell growth (not shown).

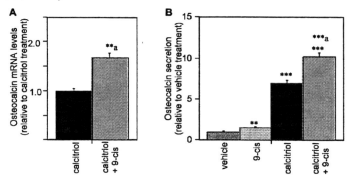

Figure 2: The effects of 9-cisRA (9-cis, 0.1 µM) on osteocalcin mRNA (A) and protein (B) levels. Statistical significance between vehicle treatment vs. treatment with the different compounds and (a) between calcitriol vs. combination treatment, **$p \leq 0.01$ and ***$p \leq 0.001$.

Next, we measured the effects of 9-cisRA on the levels of both VDR and RXRβ to examine, whether the stimulation of transactivation through VDR was related to increased receptor levels. After a 16-h incubation of the cells with protein synthesis inhibitor cycloheximide (20 µg/ml), 58% of the initial RXRβ was left and 9-cisRA (0.1 µM) promoted receptor degradation (only 28% remained, Fig. 3A). 9-cisRA also promoted the degradation of VDR. In vehicle-treated cells, VDR half-life was about 4 h 30 min and, in the presence of 0.1 µM 9-cisRA, it was 3 h 20 min (Fig. 3B). Calcitriol (1 nM) prolonged the half-life to about 13 h 30 min but, when it was used in combination with 0.1 µM 9-cis RA, the half-life was reduced to 4 h 30 min, i.e., to the level obtained with vehicle-treated cells.

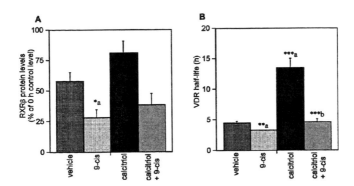

Figure 3: Degradation of RXRβ and VDR in the presence of 9-cisRA (9-cis, 0.1 µM) and calcitriol (1 nM). MG-63 cells were treated with cycloheximide (20 µg/ml), 9-cisRA (0.1 µM) and calcitriol (1 nM) for 16 h (A) and 4 to 30 h (B). RXRβ and VDR protein levels were measured by Western immunoblotting. Statistical significance between vehicle treatment vs. treatment with the different compounds (A) and between calcitriol treatment vs. combination treatment (B).

Discussion Both calcitriol and 9-cisRA have antiproliferative and differentiation inducing effects on different cell lines and different tissues (1-4). In this study, 9-cisRA inhibited the growth and also induced differentiation of the osteoblastic MG-63 cells. When it was used in combination with calcitriol or the different calcitriol analogs, it further potentiated the effects of these vitamin D_3 compounds on the inhibition of proliferation and induction of differentiation of these cells. In the presence of 1 nM calcitriol or GS1558, cell numbers increased throughout the 120-h incubation, whereas in KH1060-treated cells, cell numbers were decreased after the 72-h incubation. 9-cisRA was even more potent than KH1060 at 0.1 µM concentration during the first 72 h, but after that cell numbers rapidly increased, possibly due to catabolism of the compound. Calcitriol and KH1060 potentiated the effects of 9-cisRA and cell numbers were decreased already between 24 and 72 h of incubation. In the presence of calcitriol and 9-cisRA, however, cell numbers again increased after the 72-h incubation, possibly due to catabolism of both compounds. In KH1060-treated cells, in turn, the biologically active metabolites (5) may have inhibited cell proliferation throughout the experiment and the fold induction in cell numbers after the 120-h incubation with 9-cisRA was only 1.4.

Even though both calcitriol and 9-cis RA have been widely studied both alone and in combination, the combinatorial effects on transcriptional regulation through RXR-VDR acting via different DR3-type elements are controversial (6-10). Here we describe for the first time the regulation of VDR protein levels by 9-cisRA, whereas the down-regulatory effects of 9-cisRA on its own receptor levels have been previously described for RXRα (11). The effects of 9-cisRA on VDR protein levels seem to be a unique feature among nuclear receptors since, in our hands, 9-cisRA had no effects on the levels of other dimerization partners of RXR, such as TR and RAR (data not shown). The discrepancy in the results on transcriptional regulation through RXR-VDR by 9-cisRA may derive from different growth states of the cells used and, accordingly, from different amounts of the receptors present. When considering the effects described here for the down-regulation of VDR protein levels by 9-cisRA, it seems that 9-cisRA influences interactions between RXR-VDR and co-activators thus resulting in enhanced transcriptional activation by the heterodimer even with reduced receptor levels. This has previously been shown for RXR-RAR, where binding of the RXR-specific ligand LG268 to the heterodimer exposes the AF-2 domain of RXR for proper binding of Src-1, a member of the p160 family of co-activators (12). The finding that overexpression of RXR mutated in its AF-2 domain inhibits the activity of endogenous RXR-VDR on DR3 elements in keratinocytes further supports this idea (10).

Collectively, the present results and the results published previously by others suggest that, during the proliferative cell growth, 9-cisRA alone promotes differentiation of osteoblasts and further stimulates differentiation induced by calcitriol, possibly by facilitating interactions between RXR-VDR and the co-activators. Further, the reduction of both RXR and VDR protein levels by 9-cisRA suggests that reduction of the VDR protein levels by 9-cisRA treatment may result in controversial effects on calcitriol-induced transactivation.

References
1. Blutt, S.E., Allegretto, E.A., Pike, J.W. and Weigel, N.L. (1997) Endocrinology 138, 1491-1497.
2. Elstner E, Campbell, M.J., Munker, R., Shintaku, P., Binderup, L., Heber, D., Said, J., Koeffler, H.P. (1999) Prostate 40, 141-149.
3. Güzey, M., Sattler, C. and DeLuca, H.F. (1998) Biochem. Biophys. Res. Commun. 249, 735-744.
4. Verstuyf, A., Methieu, C., Verlinden, L., Waer, M., Tan, B.K. and Bouillon, R. (1995) J. Steroid Biochem. Molec. Biol. 53, 431-441.
5. Dilworth, F.J., Williams, G.R., Kissmeyer, A.M., Nielsen, J.L., Binderup, E., Calverley, M.J., Makin, H.L. and Jones, G. (1997) Endocrinology 138, 5485-5496.
6. MacDonald, P.N., Dowd, D.R., Nakajima, S., Galligan, M.A., Reeder, M.C., Haussler, C.A., Ozato, K. and Haussler, M.R. (1993) Mol. Cell. Biol. 13, 5907-5917.
7. Carlberg, C., Bendik, I., Wyss, A., Meier, E., Sturzenbecker, L.J., Grippo, J.F. and Hunziker, W. (1993) Nature 361, 657-660.
8. Kato, S., Sasaki, H., Suzawa, M., Masushige, S., Tora, L., Chambon, P. and Gronemeyer, H. (1995) Mol. Cell. Biol. 15, 5858-5867.
9. Ferrara, J., McCuaig, K., Hendy, G.N., Uskokovic, M. and White, J.H. (1994) J. Biol. Chem. 269, 2971-2981.
10. Li, X.Y., Xiao, J.H., Feng, X., Qin, L. and Voorhees, J.J. (1997) J. Invest. Dermatol. 108, 506-512.
11. Nomura, Y., Nagaya, T., Hayashi, Y., Kambe, F. and Seo, H. (1999) Biochem. Biophys. Res. Commun. 260, 729-733.
12. Westin, S., Kurokawa, R., Nolte, R.T., Wisely, G.B., McInerney, E.M., Rose, D.W., Milburn, M.V., Rosenfeld, M.G. and Glass, C.K. (1998) Nature 395, 199-202.

DIFFERENT RETINOID X RECEPTOR ACTIVATION FUNCTION-2 RESIDUES DETERMINE TRANSCRIPTION IN HOMODIMERIC AND VITAMIN D RECEPTOR HETERODIMERIC CONTEXTS

Paul D. Thompson, Lenore S. Remus, Jui-Cheng Hsieh, Peter W. Jurutka, G. Kerr Whitfield, Michael A. Galligan, Carlos Encinas Dominguez, Carol A. Haussler and Mark R. Haussler, Department of Biochemistry, University of Arizona College of Medicine, Tucson, AZ 85724 U.S.A.

Introduction: Upon binding to 1,25-dihydroxyvitamin D_3 (1,25(OH)$_2$D$_3$), the vitamin D receptor (VDR) activates transcription of vitamin D responsive genes as a heterodimer with retinoid X receptor (RXR) (1). RXR itself can regulate the transcription of genes responsive to its cognate ligand, 9-*cis* retinoic acid (9-*cis* RA), as an RXR-RXR homodimer (2,3). A C-terminal hormone-dependent activation function-2 (AF-2) domain (Fig. 1) has been shown to play a crucial role in the transcriptional response of both receptors (4-9) to their respective cognate ligands. Studies of different members of the nuclear receptor superfamily have confirmed the function of this region as mediating ligand-dependent interactions with members of the p160 class of coactivator such as GRIP 1 (10) and ACTR (11), that ultimately lead to the activation of target genes. With respect to hVDR, it has been shown that residues L417 and E420 represent vital sites of interaction between the receptor and coactivator (4,5,12), however, the role of the AF-2 that resides in RXR, when in the context of a VDR containing heterodimer, has not been clearly defined. The present study was undertaken in order to decipher the comparative functional importance of the AF-2 of RXR in mediating both 1,25(OH)$_2$D$_3$ and 9-*cis* RA transcriptional responses, via RXR-VDR and RXR-RXR dimeric complexes, respectively.

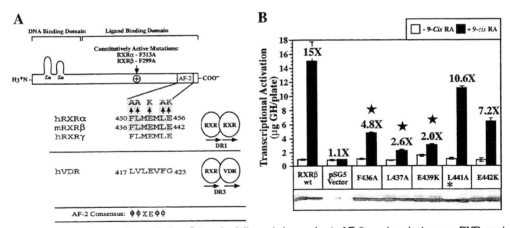

Fig. 1. (A) Comparison of the C-terminal ligand-dependent AF-2 region between RXR and VDR, and amino acid alterations made in RXRs in the present study. (B) Effect of mutational changes within the AF-2 region of mRXRβ on RXRE-driven transcriptional response to 9-*cis* RA, as mediated by the RXR homodimer.

Results: The sequence of the AF-2 regions of human RXRα (hRXRα), mouse RXRβ (mRXRβ) and human RXRγ (hRXRγ) (top alignment) are shown in Fig. 1A in relation to that present in the homologous region of hVDR (lower alignment). The AF-2 consensus (a Glu residue flanked by hydrophobic (φ) amino acids) is shown below the AF-2 sequence alignment for hVDR. We generated a series of single point mutations within the AF-2 domains of both hRXRα and mRXRβ as indicated by the gray vertical bars. Also depicted (⊕) is a mutation that we generated within the ligand binding domain of mRXRβ, F299A, that is homologous to the point mutation that creates a constitutively active form of mRXRα, namely F318A (13). The ability of the series of mRXRβ AF-2 mutants, when cotransfected into COS-7 cells in combination with an RXR responsive element (RXRE)-containing reporter plasmid, to mediate a transcriptional response to 9-*cis*

288

RA (10^{-6} M), is shown in Fig. 1B. As is indicated (★), mRXRβ AF-2 mutants F436A, L437A and E439K in the N-terminal region of the AF-2 exhibit a marked decrease in their transcriptional responsiveness to retinoid ligand. Conversely, the L441A mutation, located in the C-terminal portion of the AF-2, displays a transcriptional response closer to that of wild type mRXRβ. A similar profile of transactivation is observed employing the homologous set of hRXRα mutations (data not shown). Note that the L441A mRXRβ and its hRXRα equivalent, L455A, are designated in Figs. 1B, 2A, B and 3 by an asterisk (✳) to distinguish this residue from the more N-terminal L437/L451 residues. Western blot analysis verifies that the protein expression levels for both the mRXRβ (lower panel of Fig. 1B) and hRXRα (data not shown) set of AF-2 mutations are essentially equivalent to that of the wild type isoform. The conclusion at this point is that the N-terminal region of the RXR AF-2 is crucial in facilitating an RXR homodimer-mediated response to 9-*cis* RA.

Fig. 2A describes an RXR "rescue" experiment to define the effect of RXR AF-2 mutations on RXR-VDR mediated transcription. Our approach utilizes the R391C mutant hVDR, which is a naturally occurring mutation exhibiting impaired ability to heterodimerize with its RXR partner (14). In cotransfection studies employing COS-7 cells, the transcriptional activity of R391C hVDR can be restored to levels comparable to wild type hVDR by the cotransfection of exogenous RXR. As is illustrated in Fig. 2A, the impaired transcriptional response of hVDR R391C (panel 3 from the left) is significantly boosted by the addition of exogenous mRXRβ (panel 4) to levels approaching that of wild type hVDR (panels 1 and 2). The transactivation profile indicates that an impaired rescue was exhibited only by the mRXRβ L441A mutant (as denoted by ★), with the remaining AF-2 mutants demonstrating rescue properties similar to wild type mRXRβ.

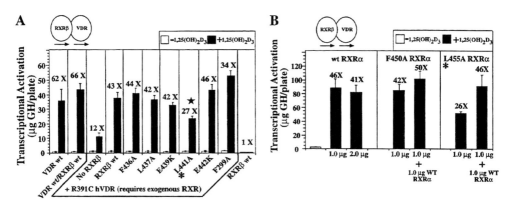

Fig. 2. (A) Effect of mRXRβ AF-2 mutations on VDRE-mediated transcription by the RXR-VDR heterodimer in response to 1,25(OH)₂D₃. (B) L455A hRXRα exerts a dominant negative effect on RXR-VDR mediated transcription that can be reversed by the addition of wild type hRXRα.

A similar rescue profile was obtained using the series of hRXRα mutants, with the L455A hRXRα mutant, equivalent to L441 mRXRβ, also displaying a significant reduction in its ability to restore the transcriptional competency of R391C hVDR (data not shown). As each of the RXR AF-2 mutants are observed to heterodimerize normally with hVDR in a 1,25(OH)₂D₃-dependent manner (data not shown), the blunted transcriptional rescue observed using L441A mRXRβ and L455A hRXRα is not likely to be due to an impaired ability of these mutants to heterodimerize with VDR. Panel 10 of Fig. 2A illustrates that an RXR mutant (F299A mRXRβ) which exhibits constitutive activity when driving an RXRE-containing reporter (13), can neither confer transcriptional potency on an unliganded RXR-VDR heterodimer nor induce synergistic activity in the presence of the 1,25(OH)₂D₃ ligand. The conclusion from these experiments is while RXR plays a subordinate role in RXR-VDR mediated transcription, an intact AF-2 of the RXR heteropartner is nonetheless required for full transcriptional potency of RXR-VDR.

In order to evaluate further the importance of L441 in mRXRβ, and its hRXRα equivalent, residue L455, in the full transcriptional competency of the RXR-VDR response to 1,25(OH)$_2$D$_3$, we determined whether mutation of this residue could confer a dominant negative phenotype in 1,25(OH)$_2$D$_3$-dependent transcription assays. Fig. 2B indicates that cotransfection of the L455A hRXRα and hVDR expression vectors into COS-7 cells results in a significant reduction in the transcriptional response to 1,25(OH)$_2$D$_3$ from a VDRE-driven reporter plasmid (panel 3). This inhibition can be overcome by the addition of wild type hRXRα. In contrast, the F450A hRXRα mutant did not exert dominant negative activity (panel 2), because its effect on the 1,25(OH)$_2$D$_3$ transcriptional response was not different from that of wild type hRXRα (panel 1). Thus, leucine 455 and 441 in hRXRα and mRXRβ, respectively, are both essential in 1,25(OH)$_2$D$_3$-triggered RXR-VDR transcriptional signaling, and exert a dominant negative effect when mutated to alanine.

Conclusions and Discussion: Data using the F299A mRXRβ constitutive mutant, (Fig. 2A, panel 10) imply that, although RXR is an essential component in the binding of VDR to its responsive element in DNA, it plays a subordinate role in RXR-VDR-mediated transcription. It is clear, however, from the rescue assay that an intact RXR AF-2 is required for a full transcriptional response to 1,25(OH)$_2$D$_3$ via the VDR heterodimer; therefore the RXR partner is active rather than silent in vitamin D control of gene expression. In addition, we describe here a functional switch in the AF-2 residues that mediate transactivation when RXR is transformed from the context of an RXR homodimer to that of a RXR-VDR heterodimer. Residue L441 of mRXRβ (or its hRXRα equivalent L455) that is located toward the C-terminal end of the AF-2, is seemingly less involved in the transcriptional response of the RXR homodimer to 9-cis RA (Fig. 1B). The same residue, however, is vital for ensuring the full transcriptional competency of the RXR-VDR heterodimer (Fig. 2). Conversely, those same residues observed in Fig. 1B to be crucial for the transcriptional competency of the RXR homodimer appear to be relatively uninvolved on a transcriptional level in the context of the RXR-VDR heterodimer.

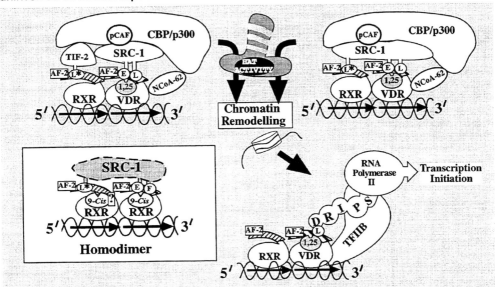

Fig. 3. Model for the potential roles of the RXR AF-2 in the context of an RXR-RXR homodimer vs. that of an RXR-VDR heterodimer.

As depicted in the model presented in Fig. 3, the L417 and E420 AF-2 residues of the VDR "primary" partner are postulated to interact with a coactivator such as SRC-1. A potential role for the AF-2 of the "secondary" RXR partner may be in contacting a less dominant, but still important coactivator, in this case represented by TIF-2, via a leucine located toward the C-terminal end of the AF-2 region (L441 and L455 of mRXRβ and hRXRα, respectively). An alternative mechanism involving the RXR AF-2 may consist of its contacting a second, less critical region of the same coactivator associated with the primary receptor, again through interactions involving the same leucine residue. In the case of the AF-2 homodimer, in the model we speculate that the RXR monomer that resides on the 3' half-site of the DR-1 RXRE functions as the "primary" partner and mediates coactivator interactions via a phenylalanine and glutamic acid, homologous to L417 and E420 of VDR. The AF-2 of the RXR positioned on the 5' half-site is proposed to have a secondary role, analogous to its role in the context of the RXR-VDR. As depicted in Fig. 3, the combined action of these interactions leads to chromatin remodeling through coactivator-mediated HAT activity, and to the eventual recruitment of a transcriptional multicomplex comprised of the DRIP/TRAP coactivators, basal transcription factors and RNA polymerase II to result in transcriptional initiation (reviewed in (15)).

Acknowledgements: Supported by N.I.H. grants to Mark R. Haussler.

References:
1. MacDonald, P. N., Dowd, D. R., Nakajima, S., Galligan, M. A., Reeder, M. C., Haussler, C. A., Ozato, K., and Haussler, M. R. (1993) *Mol. Cell. Biol.* **13**, 5907-5917
2. Mangelsdorf, D. J., Ong, E. S., Dyck, J. A., and Evans, R. M. (1990) *Nature* **345**, 224-229
3. Heyman, R. A., Mangelsdorf, D. J., Dyck, J. A., Stein, R. B., Eichele, G., Evans, R. M., and Thaller, C. (1992) *Cell* **68**, 397-406
4. Masuyama, H., Brownfield, C. M., St-Arnaud, R., and MacDonald, P. N. (1997) *Mol. Endocrinol.* **11**, 1507-1517
5. Jurutka, P. W., Hsieh, J.-C., Remus, L. S., Whitfield, G. K., Thompson, P. D., Haussler, C. A., Blanco, J. C. G., Ozato, K., and Haussler, M. R. (1997) *J. Biol. Chem.* **272**, 14592-14599
6. Schulman, I. G., Chakravarti, D., Juguilon, H., Romo, A., and Evans, R. M. (1995) *Proc. Natl. Acad. Sci. USA* **92**, 8288-8292
7. Le Douarin, B., Zechel, C., Garnier, J.-M., Lutz, Y., Tora, L., Pierrat, B., Heery, D., Gronemeyer, H., Chambon, P., and Losson, R. (1995) *EMBO J.* **14**, 2020-2033
8. vom Baur, E., Zechel, C., Heery, D., Heine, M. J. S., Garnier, J. M., Vivat, V., Chambon, P., and Losson, R. (1996) *EMBO J.* **15**, 110-124
9. Voegel, J. J., Heine, M. J., Zechel, C., Chambon, P., and Gronemeyer, H. (1996) *EMBO J.* **15**, 3667-3675
10. Hong, H., Kohli, K., Garabedian, M. J., and Stallcup, M. R. (1997) *Mol. Cell. Biol.* **17**, 2735-2744
11. Chen, H., Lin, R. J., Schiltz, R. L., Chakravarti, D., Nash, A., Nagy, L., Privalsky, M. L., Nakatani, Y., and Evans, R. M. (1997) *Cell* **90**, 569-580
12. Oñate, S. A., Tsai, S. Y., Tsai, M.-J., and O'Malley, B. W. (1995) *Science* **270**, 1354-1357
13. Vivat, V., Zechel, C., Wurtz, J.-M., Bourguet, W., Kagechika, H., Umemiya, H., Shudo, K., Moras, D., Gronemeyer, H., and Chambon, P. (1997) *EMBO J.* **16**, 5697-5709
14. Whitfield, G. K., Selznick, S. H., Haussler, C. A., Hsieh, J.-C., Galligan, M. A., Jurutka, P. W., Thompson, P. D., Lee, S. M., Zerwekh, J. E., and Haussler, M. R. (1996) *Mol. Endocrinol.* **10**, 1617-1631
15. Freedman, L. P. (1999) *Cell* **97**, 5-8

DIFFERENTIAL REGULATION OF HETERODIMERIZATION AND COACTIVATOR INTERACTION BY THE ACTIVATION FUNCTION 2 DOMAIN OF THE VITAMIN D RECEPTOR

Sara Peleg and Yan-Yun Liu. Department of Medical Specialties,. The University of Texas, M. D. Anderson Cancer Center, Houston, TX 77030.

INTRODUCTION

The transcriptional activity of the vitamin D receptor (VDR) depends on binding of VDR/retinoid X receptor (RXR) heterodimers to specific DNA sequences called vitamin D-responsive elements (VDREs) and on the interaction of VDR with transcription coactivators and bridging factors of the basal transcriptional machinery (1-3). Heterodimerization of VDR with RXR is a ligand-modulated process that depends on availability of dimerization interfaces in the DNA- and ligand-binding domains (1,4,5). Interaction of VDR with coactivators of transcription and with the basal transcription apparatus is also a ligand-modulated process, but is dependent on amino acid residues in the ligand binding domain (LBD), especially C-terminal residues called activation function-2 domain (AF-2) (3,6). The 20-epi analogs are a group of deltanoids that attracted significant research interest because they have up to a 1000 times greater transcriptional potency than the natural hormone does. The exceptional transcriptional potency of these superagonists has been proposed to be mediated, in part, through differential modulation of the VDR (7,8). The 20-epi analogs enhance dimerization and DNA binding potency of VDR-RXR heterodimers more effectively than $1,25D_3$ does, and occupy the ligand-binding pocket of VDR without contacting its AF-2 residues (8). The mechanism that leads to the enhanced dimerization by the 20-epi analogs and the consequences of the differential interaction with the AF-2 on their transcriptional potency are not known. Therefore, two questions that are raised with respect to the mechanism of 20-epi analogs action are: does differential interaction of $1,25D_3$ and its 20-epi analogs with the AF-2 residues affect the ability of VDR to recruit coactivators, and alternately, do AF-2 residues have any role in regulating the dimerization ability of VDR? In the study presented here we investigated the role of AF-2 residues in regulating $1,25D_3$- and 20-epi analog-mediated dimerization and interaction with coactivators of transcription.

RESULTS

Quantification of heterodimerization and coactivator recruitment potency of VDR-ligand complexes. To study the ligand-dependent interaction of VDR with RXR and with SRC-1 we used constructs expressing the following fusion proteins: GST-RXR, which contained the ligand-binding domain of RXRα fused to GST, and GST-SRC-1 which contained the SRC-1 peptide (nuclear receptor interacting motifs 1 and 2, amino acid residues 635-734). These fusion proteins were incubated with ^{35}S-labeled VDR in the absence or presence of ligands and the VDR-RXR complexes or VDR-SRC complexes were isolated by binding to glutathione-sepharose beads. Using these assays, we found that in the absence of $1,25D_3$ there was little dimerization of VDR with RXRα, but in the presence of the hormone, significant heterodimerization was induced. The level of dimerization depended on the ligand concentration and appeared to reach a maximum at 10 nM. Likewise, we found that the interaction of VDR and SRC-1 peptide was completely ligand dependent. We proceeded to use these assays to compare $1,25D_3$- and 20-epi analog-mediated interaction of VDR with RXR or with SRC-1. By performing a ligand dose response we found that the effective dose required to reach 50% of maximal interaction (ED_{50}) for $1,25D_3$-mediated dimerization was 1.8 nM, whereas the potency of the 20-epi analog to induce dimerization had an ED_{50} of 0.05 nM. In contrast, when we compared the potencies of the two compounds to induce interaction with SRC we found it to be similar (an ED_{50} of 0.7-1 nM). These assays suggest that the mechanism by which the 20-epi analog enhances transcription involves enhanced dimerization rather than enhanced recruitment of coactivators of the p160 family.

Regulation of ligand-mediated dimerization through residues in heptad 4, heptad 9 and the E-1 domain

The dimerization of nuclear receptors is regulated by regions in the DNA binding domain and the ligand binding domain (1,4,5). The ligand-mediated dimerization we measured in the assays described above was completely dependent on amino acid sequences in the LBD. We hypothesized that the difference in dimerization potency induced by $1.25D_3$ and the 20-epi analog may be due to differences in the nature of the dimerization interface(s) exposed after binding of these ligands to the VDR. Studies by others have mapped three regions within the LBD that regulate this function: heptad 9 (residues 383-390), heptad 4 (residues 325-332) and the E1 domain (residues 244-263) (4,5). By using site-directed mutagenesis we attempted to define if these regions regulate differently dimerization induced by $1,25D_3$ and the 20-epi analog. Our results (Figure 1) showed that mutations in these regions abolished either dimerization induced by $1,25D_3$ or by the analog, thus suggesting the mechanism by which the 20-epi analog enhances dimerization is not by changing the amino acid composition of the dimerization interface.

Regulation of heterodimerization by the AF-2 domain. The X-ray crystallography studies of nuclear receptors demonstrate that the most significant structural difference between unoccupied LBD and ligand-bound LBD is the position of the AF-2 core residues/helix 12 (9,10). Furthermore, agonist-bound and antagonist-bound LBDs are also distinguishable primarily by the position of their AF-2 core with respect to other residues that form coactivator binding site: in the antagonist-bound receptor, the AF-2 residues are presumably masking the coactivator binding site (11,12). Because of this flexibility of the AF-2 core, it is reasonable to hypothesize that its position in the ligand-occupied VDR may also contribute to the availability of the dimerization interface, and that $1,25D_3$ and its analogs may have different effects on AF-2 position with respect to the dimerization interface. To examine the role of the AF-2 core in dimerization, we used WT or AF-2-mutated VDRs and compared their potency to dimerize with GST-RXR in the presence of $1,25D_3$ or its 20-epi analog. The substituted AF-2 residues were 419 (L419S), 420 (E420A), 421 and 422 (V421M/F422A). Our results clearly indicate that three of these four AF-2 residues (L419, V421 and F422 but not residue E420) were necessary for 1,25D$_3$-mediated dimerization. In contrast, none of these AF-2 residues were necessary for the 20-epi analog-mediated dimerization (Figure 1).

To determine the reason for these differences we considered the possibility that the AF-2 residues were differently used to stabilize VDR conformation that expose the dimerization interface in VDR-hormone and VDR-analog complexes. Indeed, when we compared the ability of the two ligands to stabilize a VDR conformation we found significant differences: residues L419, V421 and F422 were essential for stabilization of VDR-1,25D$_3$ complexes, but not for VDR-20-epi analog complexes.

Dimerization interfaces in the ligand binding domain of VDR

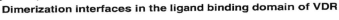

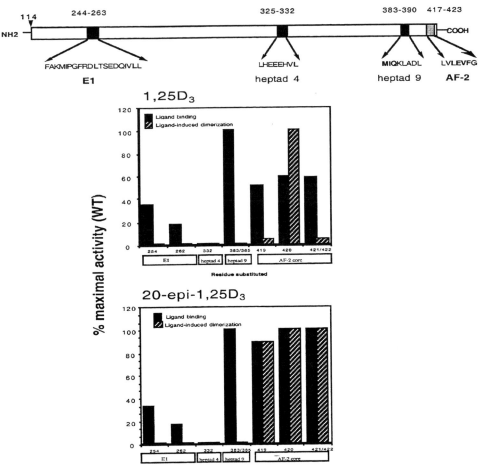

Figure 1: Examination of putative dimerization interfaces in the VDR's LBD. Regulation of dimerization and ligand binding by the 4 regions indicated at the top was examined by substituting the amino acid residues indicated at the bottom of each panel and performing competition assays or pull-down assays in the presence of either 1,25D$_3$ or its analog.

Regulation of coactivator recruitment by the AF-2 domain of VDR. The AF-2 core is defined by conserved C-terminal residues of ligand-binding nuclear receptors (6). These residues have been shown to contribute direct contact points for coactivator interaction, as well as to form ligand-mediated intramolecular interactions that distinguish agonist and antagonist conformations of the ligand-bound receptor. The agonist-mediated position of the AF-2 core contributes to a hydrophobic cleft that comprises the coactivator binding site on the surface of the LBD, and includes residues from helix 3 and helix 5 in addition to the AF-2 core residues. To determine if the AF-2 core is differently used for recruitment of coactivators by $1,25D_3$ or by the 20-epi analog, we performed pull-down experiments, as describe above, using the GST-SRC-1 fusion protein and ^{35}S-VDR, in the presence of $1,25D_3$ or its 20-epi analog. The experiments were performed with WT VDR and the three AF-2 mutants, L419S, E420A, and V421M/F422A. We found that all of these mutations diminished the binding of VDR to GST-SRC, either in the presence of $1,25D_3$ or in the presence of the 20-epi analog. These results suggest that the requirement for AF-2 residues with respect to recruitment of coactivators of the p160 family is indistinguishable for $1,25D_3$-VDR complexes and 20-epi-$1,25D_3$-VDR complexes.

DISCUSSION

This study is an extension of our efforts to explain the mechanism of action of superagonists with 20-epi side-chain stereochemistry (7, 8). Here, we used a cell-free system to investigate directly whether the 20-epi analogs enhanced the dimerization potency of VDR or its potency to interact with transcriptional coactivators. We also used this system to examine the nature of the biophysical changes in VDR that lead to that enhancement. We found that the potency of the analog to induce interaction of the ligand-binding domains of VDR and RXR was 100 times greater than that induced by $1,25D_3$. In contrast, the analog did not enhance the potency of the VDR to recruit transcriptional coactivators. In pursuit of an explanation for the mechanism by which the 20-epi analog enhanced dimerization potency of VDR we considered the possibility that the binding of the analog to the VDR induces a conformation that changes the structure of the dimerization interface. If this was correct, than the residues that contribute to the interaction of VDR-20-epi analog complexes with RXR should have been different from the residues that regulate heterodimerization of VDR-$1,25D_3$. Three regions in the ligand binding domain have been shown to regulate heterodimerization of VDR, including the E1 domain, heptad 4 and heptad 9. Because it is not known which of these regions provide actual contact points with RXR, we have examined each of these regions for their regulation of hormone- and analog-mediated dimerization. By substituting amino acid residues in each of these three regions and testing the effects of these substitutions on dimerization of VDR with RXR, we found that all three regions were equally necessary for the hormone- or the analog-mediated heterodimerization.

A second explanation for enhanced dimerization could be that the 20-epi analog is more potent than $1,25D_3$ to induce a conformation that exposes the dimerization interface of VDR. We rationalized that the AF-2 core, a region that functions to either expose or mask residues that function in protein-protein contact of nuclear receptors, may also regulate dimerization-competent conformations of VDR. Indeed, our experiments showed that the AF-2 residues were necessary for $1,25D_3$, but not for the 20-epi analog, to form a dimerization-competent conformation. In contrast, these residue were equally important to form a coactivator-competent conformation of the VDR-hormone and the VDR-analog complexes. Our interpretations of these results are that the AF-2 residues regulate coacitvators binding directly, by providing contact points for their interaction, whereas the AF-2 core probably regulates dimerization interface indirectly, by exposing residues that are essential for VDR interaction with RXR.

The implications of these findings for the ligand-mediated transcriptional activities of VDR is that the stability of the heterodimerized and DNA-bound VDR-$1,25D_3$ complexes may be susceptible to AF-2-mediated intermolecular and intramolecular interactions, whereas AF-2's interactions of VDR-20-epi analog complexes have little or no effect on the stability of the heterodimers and DNA binding. Overall, these experiments confirmed our initial hypothesis that the incredible potency of the 20-epi analogs is due primarily to their ability to form a stable complexes with the VDR monomer and even more so with the heterodimerized VDR.

References
1. Haussler, M. R., Jurutka, P. W., Hsieh, J-C., Thompson, P.D., Haussler, C. A., Selznick, S. H., Remus, L. S., and Whitfield., G. K. (1997) In: Vitamin D, Feldman D., Glorieux FH, and Pike J. W. (eds). Academic Press, San Diego CA. pp. 149-177
2. Gill, R. K., Atkins, L. M., Hollis, B. W., Bell, N. H. (1998) Mol Endocrinol 12, 57-65
3. Hong, H., Kohli, K., Garabedian, M. J., Stallcup, M. R. (1997) Mol Cell Biol 17, 2735-2744
4. Nakajima, S., Hsieh, J-C, MacDonald, P. N., Galligan, M. A., Haussler, C. A., Whitfield, G. K., Haussler, M. R. (1994) Mol Endocrinol 8, 159-172
5. Rosen, E. D., Beninghof, E. G., Koenig, R. J. (1993) J Biol Chem 268, 11534-11541
6. Danielian, P. S., White, R., Lees, J. A., Parker, M. G. (1992) EMBO J 11, 1025-1033
7. Peleg, S., Sastry, M., Collins, E. D., Bishop, J. E., and Norman, A. W. (1995) J Biol Chem 270, 10551-10558
8. Liu, Y. Y., Collins, E. D., Norman, A. W., and Peleg, S. (1997) J. Biol. Chem, 272, 3336-3345
9. Bourguet, W., Ruff, M., Chambon, P., Gronemeyer, H., and Moras, D. (1995) Nature 375, 377-382
10. Renaud, J. P., Rochel, N., Ruff, M., Vivat, V., Chambon, P., Gronemeyer, H., Moras, D. (1995) Nature 378, 681-689
11. Brozozowski, A. M., Pike, A. C. W., Dauter, Z., Hubbard, R. E., Bonn, T., Engstrom, O., Ohman, L., Greene, G. L., Gustafsson, J-A., Carlquist, M. (1997)

Nature 389, 753-758.
12. Shiau, A. K., Barstad, D., Loria, P.M., Cheng, L., Kushner, P. J., Agard, D.A., Greene, G. L. (1998) Cell 95, 927-937

BIOCHEMICAL EVIDENCE FOR A 170 KILODALTON, AF-2-DEPENDENT VITAMIN D RECEPTOR/RETINOID X RECEPTOR COACTIVATOR THAT IS HIGHLY EXPRESSED IN OSTEOBLASTS

Peter W. Jurutka, Lenore S. Remus, G. Kerr Whitfield, Michael A. Galligan, Carol A. Haussler, and Mark R. Haussler, Department of Biochemistry, University of Arizona College of Medicine, Tucson, AZ, 85724, U.S.A.

Introduction The actions of 1,25-dihydroxyvitamin D_3 (1,25(OH)$_2$D$_3$) are mediated by the vitamin D receptor (VDR), a nuclear protein that belongs to a superfamily including receptors for steroids, retinoids, and thyroid hormone (1). The binding of 1,25(OH)$_2$D$_3$ results in a presumed conformational change in VDR, enhancing its interaction with any one of several isoforms of retinoid X receptor (RXR) to generate a heterodimer (2), the biologically active species in recognizing high affinity vitamin D responsive elements (VDREs) located in the upstream promoter region of target genes (2,3). Both ligand binding and heterodimerization are mediated by the C-terminal ligand binding domain of VDR, which also contains an activation function-2 (AF-2) located in a helix-12 region near the C-terminus (4). Upon association with 1,25(OH)$_2$D$_3$, the resulting VDR-RXR heterodimer not only interacts with the VDRE, but also stimulates the transcription of downstream target genes, with apparent participation by the AF-2 domains in both VDR (5) and RXR (4,6). Other members of the nuclear receptor superfamily also possess AF-2 regions that are thought to facilitate interactions with several recently described coactivators (7), including steroid receptor coactivator-1 (SRC-1) (8), glucocorticoid receptor (GR) interacting protein (GRIP1) (9), and the activator of thyroid and retinoid receptors (ACTR) (10). Also, a large complex of multiple vitamin D receptor interacting proteins (DRIPs) (11) may be involved in transcriptional control by VDR through its AF-2. One proposed mechanism for transactivation is that these coactivators act as a bridge to RNA polymerase II and stabilize the transcriptional pre-initiation complex (11,12). An alternative or concomitant function of a subset of coactivators may be an ability to remodel chromatin nucleosome structure within the promoter region of the target gene via the histone acetyl transferase (HAT) activity possessed by some SRC-1/p160 proteins (12).

Results In order to study the role of the VDR AF-2 domain in mediating coactivator interactions, we developed a transcriptional interference assay with a glucocorticoid responsive element (GRE)-linked reporter gene and an expression vector for GR (Fig. 1A). Treatment of cotransfected cells with dexamethasone results in a 25- to 30-fold increase in the transcription of the GH reporter gene (first two bars of each panel). When increasing amounts of a pSG5 vector expressing hVDR (pSG5-WT hVDR) are cotransfected into the cells along with GR/GRE constructs, the induction of GH transcription (gray bars) is significantly reduced (to approximately 15-fold; black bars) when the cells are simultaneously treated with 1,25(OH)$_2$D$_3$. As a control for non-specific squelching, 2.5 μg of pSG5 vector lacking insert were transfected with the GR/GRE, yielding only a slight reduction in overall transcription, but no squelching in the presence of 1,25(OH)$_2$D$_3$. Importantly, when an AF-2 mutant hVDR (E420A) that is transcriptionally inactive (5) was utilized, squelching was not observed under any conditions tested (Fig. 1A, right panel). These results demonstrate that VDR can interact with at least one transcriptional coactivator that also functions in GR-mediated signaling, and that this association is dependent upon both the 1,25(OH)$_2$D$_3$ ligand and the integrity of the VDR AF-2 domain. In order to identify such VDR-interacting proteins (VIPs), WT and E420A hVDRs were cloned into a pGEX vector to create in-frame GST-hVDR fusion proteins that were then linked to glutathione-Sepharose. Employing the GST-hVDR-Sepharose beads, we then precipitated a major VIP from cellular extracts of rat osteoblast-like ROS 17/2.8 cells. The cells had been metabolically labeled with ^{35}S-methionine followed by incubation of lysates with either GST-WT-hVDR (Fig. 1B, lanes 1 and 2) or GST-E420A-hVDR (lanes 3 and 4) in the absence (lanes 1 and 3) or presence (lanes 2 and 4) of 10^{-7} M 1,25(OH)$_2$D$_3$. The VIP (lane 2) appears as a doublet with a molecular mass of approximately 170 kDa, and is not

298

bound in the absence of $1,25(OH)_2D_3$ (lane 1) or by an hVDR with a mutated AF-2 (E420A; lanes 3 and 4), implying that VIP_{170} represents a coactivator that may be required for VDR-mediated transcriptional activation.

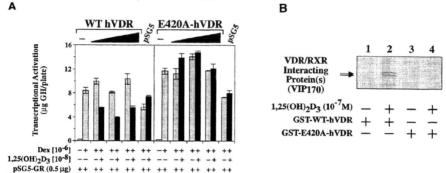

Figure 1: hVDR can squelch GR-mediated transcription in transfected COS-7 cells and can interact with VIP_{170} from ROS 17/2.8 cells in a $1,25(OH)_2D_3$- and AF-2-dependent manner.

Next, we performed similar coprecipitations using lysates from monkey kidney (COS-7) cells cotransfected with hRXRα (Fig. 2A). Again, a VIP_{170} doublet was coprecipitated in a $1,25(OH)_2D_3$- and AF-2-dependent fashion (Fig. 2A, lanes 2 and 6); however, in both COS-7 and human cervical carcinoma cells (HeLa, data not shown), VIP_{170} appeared less abundant than in ROS 17/2.8 cells. Interestingly, overexpression of RXR in COS-7 cells led to an enhanced level of association between VDR and VIP_{170} (compare lanes 2 and 6). Excess RXR did not, however, induce VIP_{170} binding to E420A. Interestingly, this AF-2 mutation also appears to attenuate the interaction of E420A hVDR with RXR (compare lanes 2 and 4; 6 and 8). Finally, we tested a pure RXR heterodimerization mutant with an intact AF-2, namely L254G-hVDR (13), in the transcriptional interference assay (Fig. 2B). Similar to results in Fig. 1A, WT hVDR can squelch GR/GRE-mediated transcription in the presence of $1,25(OH)_2D_3$ (Fig. 2B, left panel), but the L254G mutant caused only slight squelching similar to the pSG5 control (Fig. 2B, right panel). Taken together, these results argue that the VDR/RXR heterodimer is the biologically functional species, especially since ablation of heterodimerization also abrogates coactivator association as demonstrated by the lack of L254G-mediated squelching. Conversely, because a mutation in the VDR AF-2 region not only abolishes receptor mediated transactivation and VIP_{170} binding, but also attenuates interaction with RXR, VDR association with the VIP_{170} putative coactivator likely also stabilizes the interaction of the receptor with RXR and facilitates the formation of a functionally relevant multimeric VDR complex.

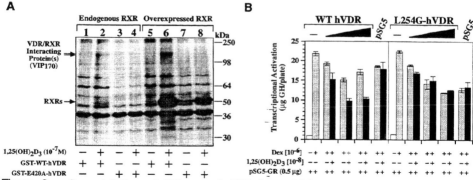

Figure 2: Coprecipitation of VIP_{170} and RXR from COS-7: evaluation of the role of heterodimerization in the formation of the VDR/VIP_{170} complex.

Discussion A goal of the present study was to screen cellular proteins from osteoblast-like cells (ROS 17/2.8), a major target of $1,25(OH)_2D_3$ action, for an ability to interact with VDR. A 170 kDa protein, termed VIP_{170}, was demonstrated to associate with VDR in a $1,25(OH)_2D_3$ ligand- and AF-2-dependent manner, suggesting that this protein may function as a VDR coactivator. The apparent molecular mass of VIP_{170} (approximately 170 kDa) suggests a relationship to other known "p160" coactivators such as SRC-1, GRIP-1 or ACTR. However, the abundance of VIP_{170} specifically in osteoblasts makes it a candidate for a novel bone-cell coactivator. In a similar study, Nakajima *et al.* (14) have reported the isolation of an AF-2-dependent, 65 kDa protein from human osteoblastic cells (MG-63) employing histidine-tagged, bacterially expressed hVDR bound to the VDRE and $1,25(OH)_2D_3$, again suggesting, as have other investigators, the existence of tissue- and/or receptor-specific coactivator subclasses (15,16) or splicing variants (17). The observation that the E420A hVDR mutant exhibits concomitant loss of transactivation ability, VIP_{170} association, and ability to squelch GR signaling intimates that VIP_{170} may also serve in GR signaling. While it is possible that VIP_{170} has a broad activity spectrum for nuclear receptor superfamily members, it is still conceivable that VIP_{170} may be VDR-specific. Thus, GR/GRE squelching by VDR-VIP_{170} could be explained by the ability of this complex to recruit additional limiting factors that are required for GR signaling.

The current data demonstrate that hVDR interacts in solution with RXR, the heterodimeric partner for hVDR that participates in high affinity VDRE binding (4,18). The association of hVDR with RXR is evident with endogenous as well as with overexpressed RXR (Fig. 2A) and, in all cases, the binding is strictly dependent on the presence of $1,25(OH)_2D_3$. Interestingly, overexpression of RXR enhances recruitment of VIP_{170} by hVDR in the presence of ligand, suggesting that heterodimerization with RXR influences VIP_{170} binding to VDR, as would be expected for a transcriptionally relevant interaction. Figure 3 depicts a schematic model of a hVDR/RXR heterocomplex forming upon $1,25(OH)_2D_3$ binding, then interacting with VDR coactivator/VIP_{170} as well as an RXR coactivator; intermolecular associations between each member of the quaternary complex are hypothesized to reinforce and stabilize this multimeric species. The model predicts that an hVDR heterodimerization mutant unable to bind RXR also would be impaired in its ability to recruit a coactivator, and the present data (Fig. 2B) support this hypothesis, in that the L254G heterodimerization mutant is unable to squelch GR/GRE-mediated transcription. Also consistent with the model are observations that interaction of the hVDR AF-2 mutant (E420A) with either endogenous or overexpressed RXR is significantly reduced in an *in vitro*, protein-protein binding assay system (Fig. 2A). We would also argue that, because mutational studies with VDR (5,19), and several closely related nuclear receptors (20-22), do not support a direct role for the AF-2/helix-12 region in heterodimerization, the effect of the hVDR E420A mutation on heterodimerization with RXR is likely mediated by the loss of cooperative interactions within the VDR/RXR multimeric complex (Fig. 3).

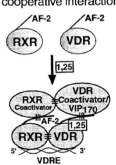

Figure 3: Model for cooperative interactions between VDR, RXR and coactivators. Wild type RXR and VDR exist in an inactive conformation with the AF-2 of each receptor extended in a conformation incompatible with coactivator association. Upon binding the $1,25(OH)_2D_3$ ligand, VDR assumes an active configuration that allows for heterodimerization with RXR and the concomitant repositioning of both the VDR and RXR AF-2 helices such that they are able to interact with coactivators. VIP_{170} is postulated to bind to VDR, while a different coactivator associates with the RXR AF-2 (strong protein-protein interactions are depicted as three solid lines). Alternatively (not shown), the RXR and VDR AF-2s may bind to two separate domains of the same coactivator.

The participation of an integrated network of protein-protein interactions that facilitate the formation of a multimeric complex in signal transduction has also been reported for the RXR/RAR heterodimer (23). When the endogenous retinoic acid receptor β (RARβ) gene promoter was examined in P19 EC cells by *in vivo* footprinting, retinoic acid treatment resulted in promoter occupancy by the RXR/RAR heterodimer but not in the presence of a mutant RXR that lacked the AF-2 domain (23). These results imply that the AF-2 region of RXR is required for full retinoic acid responsive element (RARE) occupancy *in vivo,* and that retinoic acid treatment leads to the recruitment of multiple factors to the promoter that are ultimately required for sustained RARE binding and transactivation. The model in Figure 3 proposes the existence of two separate coactivators, one directly binding to RXR and the other associating with VDR. This concept is suggested by the observation that VIP_{170} is reproducibly coprecipitated by the VDR/RXR heterodimer as a doublet of two equal intensity bands (Fig. 1B), and is also consistent with the observation that additional RXR overexpression enhances the precipitation of the VIP_{170} doublet (Fig. 2A). However, it is possible that the doublet represents a degradation product of a single VIP protein or, alternatively, a post-translationally modified (e.g., phosphorylated) VIP, and that only one coactivator interacts with the VDR/RXR heterocomplex. If so, then it appears that the VDR AF-2 domain associates with one region of this coactivator while the RXR AF-2 region interacts with a different domain. The notion that RXR associates with a coactivator is further supported by: i) the fact that RXR AF-2 mutants act as dominant negative effectors of VDR-mediated transcription (23), ii) the present data indicating that a heterodimerization mutant in VDR is also compromised in coactivator association (Fig. 2B), and iii) the present finding that an AF-2 mutation in VDR attenuates heterodimerization with RXR (Fig. 2A). Ultimately, it will be necessary to clone and sequence the VIP_{170} protein(s) to determine if it truly represents a novel, perhaps VDR-specific, coactivator in osteoblasts. The availability of a cloned VIP_{170} would also allow for direct functional testing of this AF-2 associated protein.

References

1. Whitfield, G. K., Jurutka, P. W., Haussler, C. A., and Haussler, M. R. (1999) *J. Cell. Biochem.* **32/33,** (Suppl.) 110-122
2. MacDonald, P. N., Dowd, D. R., Nakajima, S., Galligan, M. A., Reeder, M. C., Haussler, C. A., Ozato, K., and Haussler, M. R. (1993) *Mol. Cell. Biol.* **13**(9), 5907-5917
3. Sone, T., Kerner, S., and Pike, J. W. (1991) *J. Biol. Chem.* **266**(34), 23296-23305
4. Haussler, M. R., Whitfield, G. K., Haussler, C. A., Hsieh, J.-C., Thompson, P. D., Selznick, S. H., Encinas Dominguez, C., and Jurutka, P. W. (1998) *J. Bone Miner. Res.* **13**(3), 325-349
5. Jurutka, P. W., Hsieh, J.-C., Remus, L. S., Whitfield, G. K., Thompson, P. D., Haussler, C. A., Blanco, J. C. G., Ozato, K., and Haussler, M. R. (1997) *J. Biol. Chem.* **272,** 14592-14599
6. Haussler, M. R., Jurutka, P. W., Hsieh, J.-C., Thompson, P. D., Selznick, S. H., Haussler, C. A., and Whitfield, G. K. (1995) *Bone* **17,** (Suppl.) 33S-38S
7. Perlmann, T., and Evans, R. M. (1997) *Cell* **90,** 391-397
8. Oñate, S. A., Tsai, S. Y., Tsai, M.-J., and O'Malley, B. W. (1995) *Science* **270,** 1354-1357
9. Hong, H., Kohli, K., Garabedian, M. J., and Stallcup, M. R. (1997) *Mol. Cell. Biol.* **17**(5), 2735-2744
10. Chen, H., Lin, R. J., Schiltz, R. L., Chakravarti, D., Nash, A., Nagy, L., Privalsky, M. L., Nakatani, Y., and Evans, R. M. (1997) *Cell* **90**(3), 569-580
11. Rachez, C., Lemon, B. D., Suldan, Z., Bromleigh, V., Gamble, M., Naar, A. M., Erdjument-Bromage, H., Tempst, P., and Freedman, L. P. (1999) *Nature* **398**(6730), 824-828
12. McKenna, N. J., Lanz, R. B., and O'Malley, B. W. (1999) *Endocr. Rev.* **20**(3), 321-344
13. Whitfield, G. K., Hsieh, J.-C., Nakajima, S., MacDonald, P. N., Thompson, P. D., Jurutka, P. W., Haussler, C. A., and Haussler, M. R. (1995) *Mol. Endocrinol.* **9,** 1166-1179
14. Nakajima, S., Yanagihara, I., and Ozono, K. (1997) *Biochem. Biophys. Res. Commun.* **232**(3), 806-809
15. Li, H., Gomes, P. J., and Chen, J. D. (1997) *Proc. Natl. Acad. Sci. USA* **94**(16), 8479-84
16. Takeshita, A., Cardona, G. R., Koibuchi, N., Suen, C. S., and Chin, W. W. (1997) *J. Biol. Chem.* **272**(44), 27629-27634
17. Kamei, Y., Xu, L., Heinzel, T., Torchia, J., Kurokawa, R., Gloss, B., Lin, S.-C., Heyman, R. A., Rose, D. W., Glass, C. K., and Rosenfeld, M. G. (1996) *Cell* **85,** 403-414
18. MacDonald, P. N., Haussler, C. A., Terpening, C. M., Galligan, M. A., Reeder, M. C., Whitfield, G. K., and Haussler, M. R. (1991) *J. Biol. Chem.* **266**(28), 18808-18813
19. Nakajima, S., Hsieh, J.-C., MacDonald, P. N., Galligan, M. A., Haussler, C. A., Whitfield, G. K., and Haussler, M. R. (1994) *Mol. Endocrinol.* **8**(3), 159-172
20. Forman, B. M., and Samuels, H. H. (1990) *Mol. Endocrinol.* **4,** 1293-1301
21. Zhang, X.-k., Hoffman, B., Tran, P. B.-V., Graupner, G., and Pfahl, M. (1992) *Nature* **355,** 441-446
22. Tone, Y., Collingwood, T. N., Adams, M., and Chatterjee, V. K. (1994) *J. Biol. Chem.* **269,** 31157-31161
23. Blanco, J. C. G., Dey, A., Leid, M., Minucci, S., Park, B.-K., Jurutka, P. W., Haussler, M. R., and Ozato, K. (1996) *Genes Cells* **1,** 209-221

VITAMIN D AND PEROXISOMAL PROLIFERATOR ACTIVATED RECEPTORS COOPERATE TO INHIBIT LEUKEMIC CELL PROLIFERATION

Mark English, Sarah Fenton, Susan Hughes, Rosemary Bland, Christopher Bunce and Martin Hewison.
Division of Medical Sciences, The University of Birmingham, Birmingham B15 2TH, UK.

Introduction

The antiproliferative/differentiative properties of agents such as 1,25-dihydroxyvitamin D_3 ($1,25D_3$) and retinoic acids (RAs) has led to their potential use in the treatment of haempoietic malignancies. However, with the single exception of *all trans* retinoic acid (ATRA) in acute promyelocytic leukemia these trials have been disappointing. In part the inability to recapitulate the *in vitro* capacity of RAs and $1,25D_3$ to induce differentiation *in vivo* has been due to unacceptable side effects of the treatment. One approach to this problem has been the development of vitamin D analogs, that have potent antiproliferative/differentiative effects but exert tolerable effects on serum calcium levels. Another potential solution is the use of $1,25D_3$ or RAs in combination with other therapeutic agents including cytotoxic compounds. In recent studies we have sought to determine the mechanism whereby non-toxic agents are able to potentiate the antiproliferative effects of $1,25D_3$. Nilsson *et al* 1995 demonstrated that clofibric acid (CA) the ligand for $PPAR\alpha$ in combination with ATRA enhanced HL60 neutrophil differentiation [1]. The potentiation of HL60 responses to ATRA has been shown to be mediated by a suppression of cell proliferation [2]. Antiproliferative effects of troglitazone, the ligand for $PPAR\gamma$ was also demonstrated in a panel of myeloid leukemic cell lines [3]. More recently we demonstrated that potentiation of differentiation also occurred with $1,25D_3$. Clearly elucidation of the mechanism through which CA mediates this effect could provide novel molecular targets for 'differentiation' therapy. In this report we have investigated various mechanisms whereby CA modulates $1,25D_3$ action in leukemic cells *in vitro*.

Materials and Methods

Exponentially growing HL60 cultures were maintained in RPMI 1640 medium supplemented with 10% fetal bovine serum (Gibco). Cells were treated with either 100nM or 5nM $1,25D_3$, 0.5mM CA and 0.5mM CA combined with 5nM $1,25D_3$. At various time points, cells were analyzed for viability and differentiation towards monocytes. Differentiation was confirmed by staining cytospins for α-naphthylacetate esterase (ANAE), Jenner Giemsa and reduction of nitrotetrazolium blue (NBT). Cell proliferation was assessed using total cell counts and ^{3}H-thymidine incorporation (1μCi/ml). RT-PCR analysis with primers specific for $PPAR\alpha$, β and γ were used to examine PPAR isoform expression. Quantitative thin layer chromatography (TLC) analysis was used to assess 24-hydroxylase activity (conversion of ^{3}H-$1,25D_3$ to ^{3}H-$24,25D_3$) and 17β-hydroxysteroid dehydrogenase (HSD) activity (conversion of ^{3}H-estradiol (E_2) to ^{3}H-estrone (E_1), the latter being a recently identified rapid marker of HL60 differentiation. Vitamin D receptor (VDR) expression was determined using

Western blot analysis (monoclonal antibody 9A7γ) and by nuclear association assays. The latter were carried out by determining the nuclear binding of ^{3}H-1,25D$_3$ (0.03 - 1nM) in the presence of a 200-fold excess of unlabelled 1,25D$_3$, followed by Scatchard analysis. Gel-shift mobility assays were performed using HL60 nuclear protein in the presence of 150mM KCl binding buffer (10mM Tris-HCl, pH 7.6, 150mM KCl, 1.0mM dithiothreitol, 15% glycerol, 1mg/ml acetylated bovine serum albumin and 5μg/ml of poly(dl-dC). Nuclear proteins were incubated with double-stranded ^{32}P-dTTP labeled idealized vitamin D response element (VDRE) and p21 VDRE.

Results

RT-PCR analysis demonstrated the presence of PPARα, and β in HL60 cells (data not shown). Having demonstrated the presence of the receptor for clofibric acid (PPARα), further studies were then carried out to investigate the effect of CA on 1,25D$_3$-induced differentiation of HL60 cells.

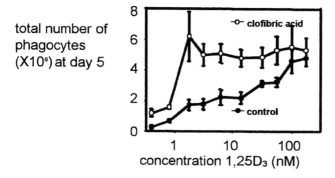

Figure 1. Effect of clofibric acid on 1,25D$_3$ induced differentiation in HL60 cells. Clofibric acid increased the sensitivity of HL60 cells to 1,25D$_3$. Similar studies were then carried out on HL60 cell proliferation (figure 2).

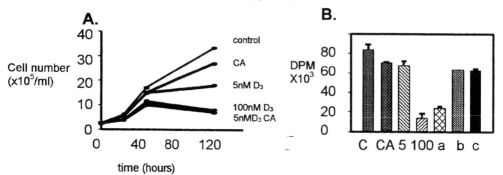

Figure 2. Inhibition of HL60 proliferation by 1,25D$_3$ and clofibric acid.
(A) Cell number and (B) Cell proliferation (^{3}H-thymidine incorporation) at 48 hours. Treatments (48hrs): control cells (C), 0.5mM clofibric acid (CA), 5nM 1,25D$_3$ (5), 100nM 1,25D$_3$ (100), 0.5mM clofibric acid and 5nM 1,25D$_3$ (a), CA plus 5nM 1,25D$_3$ included for final 24 hrs (b), 5nM 1,25D$_3$ plus CA included for final 24 hrs (c).

Data in figure 2 indicated that CA in combination with 5nM 1,25D₃ potentiated the anti-proliferative effects of 1,25D₃. Additionally, co-administration of CA and 1,25D₃ is required for this response. We then investigated other responses to 1,25D₃, as shown in figure 3.

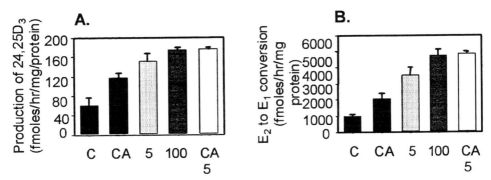

A.

B.

Figure 3. Effect of clofibric acid on functional responses to 1,25D₃ after 48 hours treatment. (A) 24-hydroxylase activity and (B) 17β-HSD activity. E_2; estradiol; E_1: estrone.

HL60 cells have basal 24-hydroxylase activity, which is increased with CA alone , 5nM and 100nM 1,25D₃ and CA in combination with 5nM 1,25D₃. 17β-HSD4 is a peroxisomal enzyme, which catalyses the conversion of E_2 to E_1 and has recently been identified as an early marker of HL60 differentiation [4]. A similar pattern of activity is seen as with 24-hydroxylase activity. Therefore we concluded that cooperativity between 1,25D₃ and CA was not mediated by increased catabolism of 1,25D₃ and that CA alone was able to regulate 1,25D₃ target gene expression. Therefore we investigated this further by examining the effect of CA on VDR expression in HL60 cells.

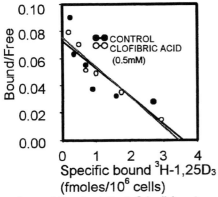

Figure 4. Clofibric acid has no effect on 1,25D₃ nuclear binding
CA did not alter VDR number (B_{MAX}) or binding affinity (k_d). Also there was no significant change in VDR expression as demonstrated by Western analysis (data not shown).

In view of the fact that CA did not appear to inhibit catabolism of 1,25D₃ or increase VDR expression, we then investigated the ability of CA to modulate the association of nuclear proteins to bind to an idealized VDRE, as shown in figure 5.

304

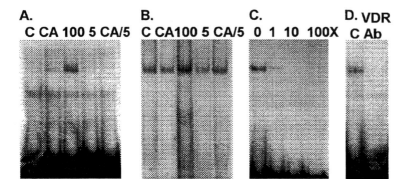

A.
C CA 100 5 CA/5

B.
C CA100 5 CA/5

C.
0 1 10 100X

D. VDR
C Ab

Figure 5 Effect of clofibric acid on VDR/VDRE binding specificity. (A) *In vitro* (B) *in vivo*, (C) Increasing amounts of unlabeled VDRE, (D) Gel Shift inhibition of complex formation with a VDR antibody.

100nM 1,25D$_3$ induced VDR/VDRE complex formation on an idealized VDRE (AGGTCAxxxAGGTCA) when treatments were added to the binding reaction (figure. 5A). and when cells were treated for 4 hours and subsequently nuclear proteins isolated and used for gel shift assays (figure 5B). CA alone or in combination with 5nM 1,25D3 had not significant effect on induction of complex formation. Specificity of this interaction was demonstrated by competition with increasing amounts of cold VDRE (figure 5C) and by super-shift studies using a monoclonal VDR antibody (figure. 5D).

Discussion
In data presented here we have demonstrated that CA sensitizes HL60 cells to 1,25D$_3$-induced differentiation. The mechanism whereby CA potentiates this 1,25D$_3$ effect does not appear to occur via modulation of 1,25D$_3$ catabolism, changes in VDR expression or 1,25D$_3$ induced VDR/VDRE binding. Although CA does not appear to modulate VDR/VDRE binding directly, PPARα may interact with vitamin D signaling pathways through novel VDR-VDRE complexes. Putative mechanisms may also include altered VDR translocation to the nucleus, increased cellular uptake or indirect activation of late CA responsive genes. However, irrespective of the mechanism involved, these studies indicate a potential role for CA as a potentiator of the effects of 1,25D$_3$. Future studies will be carried out to determine the specificity of this combination therapy for differentiative versus calciotropic response. This may lead to an exciting novel approach to vitamin D therapy *in vivo*.

References
[1] Nillson A, Farants AK, Nesland JM, Finstad HS, and Pederson JL. (1995) Eur J Cell Biol. 67, 379-85.
[2] Fenton SL, Drayson MT, Hewison M, Vickers E, Brown G and Bunce CM. (1999) B J Haematol. 105, 448-51.
[3] Asou H, Verbeek W, Williamson E, Elstner E, Kubota T, Kamada K, Koeffler HP. (1999) Int J Oncol. 15, 1027-31.
[4] Mountford J, Bunce CM, Hughes SV, Drayson MT, Webb D, Hewison M. (1999) Exp Haematol. 27, 451-60.

IDENTIFICATION OF A PHOSPHORYLATED REGION WITHIN THE HIGHLY CONSERVED SNW DOMAIN OF THE VITAMIN D RECEPTOR COACTIVATOR PROTEIN NCOA-62.

Hisashi Tokumaru and Paul N. MacDonald Department of Pharmacology, Case Western Reserve University, Cleveland, OH 44106

Introduction Vitamin D receptor (VDR) and retinoid X receptor (RXR) heterodimers bind to vitamin D responsive elements (VDREs) and form complexes with a variety of nuclear receptor coactivator proteins that are necessary to drive transcription by the preinitiation complex. NCoA-62 is one important nuclear receptor coactivator protein that interacts with VDR and augments 1,25-dihydroxyvitamin D3-dependent transcription. It may function as a bridging factor between the nuclear receptor and the transcription machinery. NCoA-62 also augments ligand-activated transcription mediated by other nuclear receptors including gucocorticoid receptor (GR) , retinoic acid receptor (RAR) and estrogen receptor (ER) (1). The precise role of NCoA-62 in this complex process in unknown. Phosphorylation is an important aspect of the mechanism of many transcriptional regulatory proteins including nuclear receptors. Therefore, in the present study, we examined whether NCoA-62 was phosphorylated and the potential role of phosphorylation in the coactivator function of NCoA-62 .

Materials and Methods COS-7 cells seeded at 2×10^5 per 6 cm diameter culture dish were transiently transfected with 1µg of FLAG-CMV2 NCoA-62 expression vector and 9 µg of BlueScript II KS$^+$ as a carrier DNA using standard calcium phosphate precipitation procedures. Forty eight hours later, the cells were metabolically labeled with 1mCi [^{32}P]orthophosphate in phosphate-free DMEM media containing 2% dialyzed Calf Bovine Serum). Four hours later, the cells were harvested with 500 µl of ice-cold lysis buffer(25mM Tris-HCl,pH 7.4, 150mM NaCl, 1mM EDTA, 0.1mM NaVO$_3$, 50mM NaF, 1% NP-40). The lysate was centrifuged at 14000 rpm for 10 min, cell extract was added to 30 µl of a 50 % slurry FLAG-M2 affinity beads(SIGMA). Following an overnight incubation at 4 °C, the beads were washed five times with 1 ml of lysis buffer lacking NP-40, mixed with 100µl of final sample buffer and boiled for 5 min. The samples were subjected to SDS-PAGE analysis, stained by Coomasie Blue, dried on 3M filter paper and exposed to X-ray film. For phospho-amino analysis, the radiolabeled protein was cut out of the gel, acid hydrolyzed and analyzed by thin-layer chromatography. Reporter gene assays used 2 µg of (VDRE)^4-TATA GH, 10 ng of SG5 VDR or SG5 GR, 250ng of SG5 NcoA-62 or SG5 NCoA-62 triple mutant and 12µg of Blue Script II. The DNA were transfected into COS7 cells as described above. The cells were treated with ligand or vehicle for 24 hours, and the amount of secreted growth hormone was determined with an immunoassay kit (Nichols Institute).

Results Immunoprecipitation of metabolically-labeled cellular extracts with FLAG M2 antibody demonstrated that NCoA-62 is a phosphoprotein. Phospho-amino acid analysis revealed that NCoA-62 is phosphorylated exclusively on serine residues. To identify the site(s) of phosphorylation, several amino terminal and carboxyl terminal deletion constructs of NCoA-62 were expressed and examined for relative phosphorylation in the COS-7 system. Each FLAG tagged deletion mutant was radiolabeled with [^{32}P]orthophoshate and immunoprecipitated by FLAG-M2 antibody. Deletion from both the amino-terminus and carboxy-terminus identified a major phosphorylated region within a 17 residue segment between P223 and K240 in the highly conserved SNW domain of NCoA-62 (fig 1).

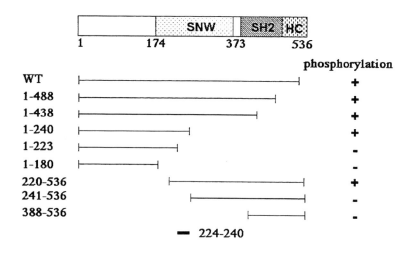

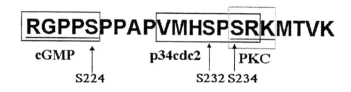

Figure 1 Deletion mutant constructs of FLAG NCoA-62 and protein kinase phosphorylation sites sequence in R220 to K240

Three serine residues are located in this 17 amino acid segment, S224, S232, and S234. All three exist within known consensus phosphorylation sites for cGMP-dependent protein kinase, p34cdc2 protein kinase and protein kinase C, respectively (fig 1). Point mutations were introduced alone or in combination into each of these three codons and these serine to alanine mutants were examined for relative phosphorylation. While the NCoA-62(S234A) mutant was phosphorylated to a similar extent as wild-type NCoA-62, the S224A, the S232A, and the S232,234A double mutant exhibited 50 % reduced levels of phosphorylation. Importantly, phosphorylation was nearly abolished (> 95 %) in the NCoA-62(S224,232,234A) triple mutant suggesting that S224 and S232 account for the vast majority of the phosphorylation observed in these studies. Coomasie staining of the immunoprecipitated proteins showed that differences in phosphorylation were not due to differences in the level of NCoA-62 derivatives isolated in these experiments (fig 2). We conclude that NCoA-62 is phosphorylated on multiple serine residues within the central SNW domain.

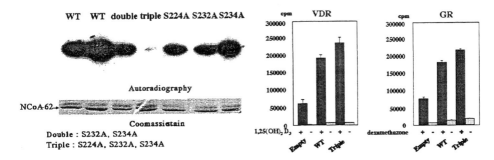

Figure 2 [^{32}P]Orthophosphate labeled point mutants, double and triple mutant

Figure 3 Nuclear receptor mediated reporter gene assay with NcoA-62 wild type or triple mutant

To examine whether phosphorylation of NCoA-62 affects vitamin D-mediated transcription, a VDR-responsive reporter gene expression vector [(VDRE)^4-Osteocaiclin TATA-GH] was co-transfected with 250ng of wild type SG5 NCoA-62 or SG5 NCoA-62 (triple mutant) into COS-7 cells. Following treatment with 10^{-8}M 1,25(OH)$_2$D$_3$, we observed a 3-fold increase in VDR-activated transcription by WT NCoA-62 expression. Little or no difference in this coactivator activity was noted in the NCoA-62 triple mutant Similar results were observed using a glucocorticoid responsive reporter system. Thus, eliminating phosphorylation of NCoA-62 in the triple mutant did not have a significant impact in nuclear receptor activated transcription (fig 3).

308

Discussion By deletion mutant analysis, phoshorylation sites of NCoA-62 were revealed within a 17 residue segment between P223 and K240 in the highly conserved SNW domain of NCoA-62. The SNW domain was designated from the SNW1 gene previously cloned as a homolog of BX42, a hormonally regulated chromatin binding protein from *Drosophila melanogaster.* The functional role of the SNW1 gene is not well understood. Coactivators such as CBP/p300 and SRC-1 have histones acetyltransferase activity (HAT) which loosens chromatin structure to expose DNA from core histones and facilitate transcription. The SNW domain of NCoA-62 may take part in this nucleosome remodelling process. Eliminating phosphoryation in the triple mutant had little or no impact on nuclear receptor coactivator function. One possible explanation is that phosphorylation of NCoA-is not required for nuclear receptor mediated transcription. Alternatively, the role of phosphorylated NCoA-62 may be cell selective and does not occur in the COS7 cell system examined here. Furthermore, we have thus far tested only VDR and GR. Using different cell lines and other nuclear receptors may reveal roles for thus phosphorylation event. NCoA-62 was also cloned by another group as Ski oncoptotein interacting protein(SKIP). Ski oncoptotein is involved in muscle cell differentiation and proliferation (2). Most recently, the other group found NCoA-62/SKIP is a repressor forming a complex with CBF-1 and SMRT of Notch receptor pathway which influence a broad spectrum of developmental processes (3). Phosphorylated NCo-A-62 might be important to interact with these pathway rather than nuclear receptors, otherwise unknown factors which have not been detected yet (fig 4). Further studies are required to test these possibilities.

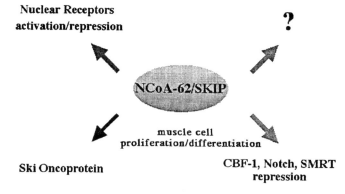

Figure 4 multi functional role of NCoA-62/SKIP

Reference

1. Baudino T.A., Kraichely D.M. and MacDonald P.N. (1998) J. Biol. Chem. 273 16434-16441
2. Dahl R, Wani B, Hayman M.J. (1998) Oncogene. 16, 1579-1586.
3. Zhou S., Fujimuro M. And Hayward S.D. (2000) Mol . cell. Biol. 20, 2400-2410

VDR-ALIEN: A NOVEL, DNA-SELECTIVE, VITAMIN D3 RECEPTOR-COREPRESSOR PARTNERSHIP.

Patsie Polly[§], Michaela Herdick and Carsten Carlberg.
Institut für Physiologische Chemie I, Heinrich-Heine-Universität, D-40001 Düsseldorf, Germany.

Summary: The vitamin D receptor (VDR) is a transcription factor that transmits incoming 1,25-dihydroxyvitamin D3 (1,25-D_3) signalling via combined contact with coactivator proteins and specific DNA binding sites (VDREs), which ultimately results in activation of transcription. This study documents direct, ligand-sensitive protein-protein interaction of the VDR with the nuclear receptor corepressor (NCoR) and a novel corepressor, called Alien. Functional assays indicated that Alien, but not NCoR, displays selectivity for different VDRE structures for transferring these repressive effects into gene regulatory activities. Taken together, association of the VDR with corepressor proteins provides a further level of transcriptional regulation, which is emerging as a complex network of protein-protein interaction mediated control.

Introduction: Many coactivators and corepressors, generally grouped as families, have been identified, characterized and studied in the context of transcriptional activation or repression. NCoR (2) and silencing mediator for retinoid and thyroid hormone receptors (SMRT) (3) were the 'founding' members of the corepressor family, which has grown to include a recent member, Alien (4). Interaction of corepressors with nuclear receptors has been described, especially for T_3R and RAR, but also for orphan members of the nuclear receptor superfamily, such as RevErbα. Several mechanisms are postulated to be operating to mediate repression. Identification of several histone deacetylases (HDACs) has provided a molecular link between histone deacetylation, corepressor activity and transcriptional regulation. In addition, corepressor interaction with components of the basal transcriptional machinery, which represent alternative pathways to HDAC-nuclear receptor interaction, has also been suggested. In this report, VDR-mediated repression and corepressor-mediated superrepression was studied in solution and on VDREs. VDR was confirmed to interact effectively with NCoR and was demonstrated, for the first time, to interact with the novel corepressor Alien. VDR-Alien interaction was found to be comparable to T_3R-Alien interaction. VDR-Alien complexes showed DNA selectivity by mediating repression only through DR3-type VDREs and not through IP9-type VDREs.

Results: In order to test whether VDR contains intrinsic repressive activity, fusion proteins each containing the GAL4DBD and either the LBD of VDR, the LBD of T_3R or the first repression domain of NCoR, respectively, were overexpressed in HeLa cells. GAL4 binding site driven luciferase reporter gene activity was then determined. In this mammalian-one-hybrid assay the VDR-LBD showed 28.6-fold repression, the T_3R-LBD mediated 9.7-fold repression and the repression domain I of NCoR displayed 45.1-fold repression (Fig. 1).

310

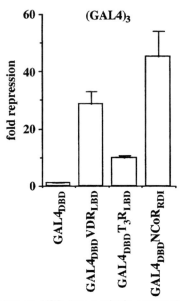

Figure 1: VDR has intrinsic repression activity. Transient transfections of HeLa cells were performed with luciferase reporter constructs driven by three copies of the GAL4 binding site and the indicated expression vectors for the indicated GAL4 fusion proteins. Cells were transfected for 16 hours then β-galactosidase-normalized luciferase activities were determined. GAL4-fusion protein-mediated repression of basal transcriptional activity was expressed as fold repression of basal transcriptional activity.

VDR-corepressor interactions were assessed, *in vitro*, with the use of bacterially overexpressed GST fusion proteins. GST pull-down assays demonstrated that VDR can interact with the corepressor Alien in a ligand-dependent manner (Fig. 2A). The intensity of VDR-Alien interaction appeared to be similar to the T_3R-Alien interaction. A ligand-mediated dissociation of the VDR-Alien complex was seen upon treatment with 1,25-D_3 (10 µM), where VDR-Alien interaction appeared to be reduced by 50-60 % in the presence of 1,25-D_3, which was slightly weaker than T_3-mediated dissociation of T_3R-Alien interaction. As a control, VDR and T_3R interaction with the two established nuclear receptor

interaction domains of NCoR, i.e. NCoR$_{1954-2215}$ and NCoR$_{2218-2453}$, was also tested in GST pull-down assays. VDR showed comparable, ligand-dependent interaction with both NCoR interaction domains (data not shown). The role of the VDR activation function 2 (AF-2) domain for an interaction with corepressors was investigated using VDR$_{413Stop}$, an AF-2 deletion mutant of the VDR deleting the entire VDR AF-2 domain from aa 417 to 427, in ligand-dependent GST pull-down assays. When assessing VDR$_{413Stop}$, the effect of ligand-dependent dissociation of Alien or NCoR was still present. Taken together, this suggested that VDR-Alien and VDR-NCoR interaction was independent of the AF-2 domain (data not shown). Finally, yeast two-hybrid assays were performed in order to assess VDR-corepressor association *in vivo* (Fig. 2B). Yeast cells were transformed with expression vectors for LexA$_{DBD}$-VDR$_{80-427}$ fusion protein as the bait and activation domain fusion proteins containing Alien or NCoR$_{2240-2453}$ as activators. β-galactosidase reporter gene assays demonstrated VDR-Alien and VDR-NCoR interaction and an ligand-dependent dissociation of these complexes.

Luciferase reporter gene assays were performed to assess the functional consequences of DNA-dependent effects of corepressor-VDR interaction. Cos-7 cells were transfected with expression vectors for VDR, RXR, Alien or NCoR$_{1-2453}$ together with luciferase reporter gene constructs driven by the DR3-type VDRE of the rat ANF gene promoter or IP9-type VDRE of the mouse c-*fos* gene promoter (1). Cells were then stimulated for 16 hours, graded 1,25-D_3, and β-galactosidase normalized luciferase reporter gene activities were expressed as fold-induction.

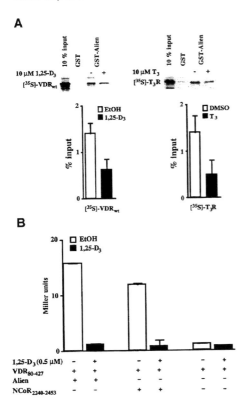

A

B

Figure 2: VDR-corepressor interaction *in vitro* and *in vivo*. GST pull-down assays (A) were performed with *in vitro* translated [^{35}S]-labelled VDR$_{wt}$, [^{35}S]-labelled T$_3$R and bacterially overexpressed GST-Alien (A). Nuclear receptors were pre-incubated for 20 min at room temperature with solvent (ethanol or DMSO) or the indicated ligands (10 µM). Yeast two-hybrid assays (B) were performed by transforming yeast cells with expression vectors for LexA$_{DBD}$-VDR$_{80-427}$ fusion protein and Alien or NCoR$_{2240-2453}$ activation domain fusion proteins together with a LexA binding site driven β-galactosidase reporter gene construct. Cells were then treated with either ethanol (0.1 %) or 1,25-D$_3$ (500 nM) and 16 hours after onset of stimulation, β-galactosidase assays were performed. The intensity of solvent-treated or ligand-treated VDR-corepressor interaction was expressed as Miller units.

Overexpressed Alien and NCoR in direct comparison on DR3- and IP9-type VDREs could confirm the selectivity of Alien to mediate 'superrepression' of VDR-RXR heterodimer activity only via DR3-type VDREs (Fig. 3). Moreover, in this experimental series, the effect of TSA was demonstrated to partially relieve the NCoR-mediated superrepression. In contrast, the incomplete reduction of the repressive effect of VDR-Alien on DR3-type VDREs suggested that Alien is relatively TSA insensitive and is using, at least in part, alternate molecular pathways.

Discussion: This report describes VDR as a nuclear receptor with intrinsic repression activity that, as being sensitive to TSA treatment, appears to act through the established Sin3-HDAC pathway. In the mammalian-one-hybrid system the VDR-LBD demonstrated a potent repressive activity. The most significant finding of this report is the demonstration of a protein-protein interaction of VDR with the novel corepressor Alien, both *in vivo* and *in vitro*. Compared to NCoR (2453 aa and a molecular mass of 270 kD), Alien is much smaller (305 aa and a molecular mass of 34 kD) and shows no obvious sequence homology to known corepressor molecules (4). Alien is known to interact with T$_3$R and ecdysone receptor but not with RAR (4). This study shows that in its functionality as a corepressor of VDR, Alien appears to be, at least, as potent as NCoR. Alien even appears to interact more effectively with VDR than NCoR does with VDR, as higher 1,25-D$_3$ concentrations are needed to dissociate the VDR-Alien complex than VDR-NCoR complexes both *in vitro* and *in vivo* (data not shown).

312

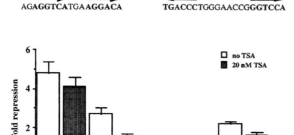

rat ANF DR3-type VDRE

AGAGGTCATGAAGGACA

mouse c-*fos* IP9-type VDRE

TGACCCTGGGAACCGGGTCCA

□ no TSA
■ 20 nM TSA

fold repression

Alien   NCoR
DR3-type VDRE

Alien   NCoR
IP9-type VDRE

Figure 3: Alien and NCoR display differences in VDRE selectivity and ligand sensitivity. Transient transfections of Cos-7 cells were performed with the DR3-VDRE and IP9-type VDRE driven luciferase reporter constructs (for details see Fig. 3), together with the expression vectors for VDR and RXR (in all cases) and Alien or NCoR (as indicated). Cells were treated for 16 hours with ethanol (0.1 %) or TSA (20 nM), then β-galactosidase-normalized luciferase activities were determined in relation to solvent-treated activity. Corepressor-mediated superrepression was expressed as fold repression of VDR activity.

However, the most interesting characteristic of Alien is that it mediates repression only from VDR-RXR complexes that are bound to DR3-type VDREs and not from those bound to IP9-type VDREs. The protein-DNA complexes that are formed on these two types of response elements are clearly distinct. On DR3-type elements, the DBDs of VDR and RXR bind to the same side of the DNA, they contact each other and show a head-to-tail orientation, whereas on IP9-type elements the two DBDs bind to opposite sides of the DNA at a distance that is too wide for a direct contact of the core DBDs (1). Since the LBDs of VDR and RXR in both types of protein-DNA complexes are assumed to interact in a similar fashion, it is more likely that a differential effect of Alien is due to its interaction with the hinge region rather than with the LBD of VDR. The conformation of VDR-RXR heterodimers on IP9-type VDREs suggests that the interaction interface of VDR with Alien may not be accessible due to steric hindrance. For interaction with nuclear receptors, NCoR requires the so-called CoR-box, a conserved aa sequence within helix 1 of the LBD, within nuclear receptors such as T_3R and RAR (3). This suggests that Alien and NCoR are using different interaction interfaces within the VDR. In summary, an alternate pathway for repression involving the VDR has been presented. The novel interaction between the VDR and Alien, which is representative of a new class of corepressor, presents a mechanism for repression which appears to be VDRE selective.

§Acknowledgments: P. Polly was the recipient of a fellowship from the Alexander von Humboldt Foundation for the duration of these studies and is presently at the Children's Medical Research Institute, Sydney, NSW 2145, Australia.

References:
1.   Carlberg C., and Polly P. (1998). *Crit. Rev. Eukaryot. Gene Expr.* **8**, 19-42
2.   Hörlein A. J., Näär A. M., Heinzel T., Torchia J., Gloss B., Kurokawa R., Ryan A., Kamei Y., Söderström M., Glass C. K., and Rosenfeld M.-G. (1995. *Nature* **377**, 397-404
3.   Chen J. D., and Evans R. M. (1995. *Nature* **377**, 454-457
4.   Dressel U., Thormeyer D., Altincicek B., Paululat A., Eggert M., Schneider S., Tenbaum S. P., Renkawitz R., and Baniahmad A. (1999). *Mol. Cell. Biol.* **19**, 3383-3394

ENHANCEMENT OF VITAMIN D RECEPTOR MEDIATED TRANSCRIPTION BY PHOSPHORYLATION INVOLVES INCREASED INTERACTION BETWEEN THE VITAMIN D RECEPTOR AND DRIP205, A SUBUNIT OF THE DRIP COACTIVATOR COMPLEX.

Frank Barletta[*], Leonard P. Freedman[+], Mihali Raval-Pandya[*] and Sylvia Christakos[*], [*]Department of Biochemistry and Molecular Biology, UMNDJ-New Jersey Medical School, Newark, NJ and [+]Cell Biology Program, Memorial Sloan-Kettering Cancer Center, New York, NY

Introduction: The action of 1,25 dihydroxyvitamin D_3 [1,25$(OH)_2D_3$] is mediated through the vitamin D receptor (VDR), a member of the superfamily of nuclear receptors, that function as ligand activated transcription factors. VDR, like the progesterone receptor (PR) (1,2), glucocorticoid receptor (GR) (3,4), androgen receptor (AR) (5,6), estrogen receptor (ER) (7,8), and the retinoic acid receptor β (RAR β) (9,10), is a phosphoprotein. It has been determined that VDR is hyperphosphorylated upon 1,25$(OH)_2D_3$ treatment (11-13). VDR has been shown to be phosphorylated by PKA(14), PKC(15), and casein kinase II(16). It has been suggested that the phosphorylation of nuclear hormone receptors may play a role in nuclear localization, hormone binding, DNA binding, cofactor recruitment, and has been implicated in transcriptional activation as well as transcriptional repression (17). The role that phosphorylation plays in vitamin D mediated gene expression is not well understood. The objective of this study was to further characterize VDR mediated transcriptional activation by phosphorylation. The results of this investigation show that okadaic acid (OA), an inhibitor of protein phosphatase-1 and 2A, enhances 1,25$(OH)_2D_3$ dependent transcription and this enhancement may be due to an increased interaction between the VDR and specific coactivator proteins.

Results: When LLCPK1 kidney cells, UMR 106-01 osteoblastic cells and COS cells were transfected with the rat 24-hydroxylase [24(OH)ase] promoter (-1367/+74) (Figure 1) or the osteopontin (OPN) promoter (-777/+79) we found that the response to 1,25dihydroxvitamin D_3 [1,25$(OH)_2D_3$] could be significantly enhanced 3-4 fold by okadaic acid (OA;50nM). OA was also observed to enhance levels of 24(OH)ase and OPN mRNA in UMR osteoblastic cells as determined by Northern blot analysis. Transfection of a synthetic proximal rat 24(OH)ase vitamin D response element (VDRE) thymidine kinase (tk) chloramphenicol acetyl transferase (CAT) reporter gene or an OPN VDRE tk CAT construct still resulted in a 3-4 fold enhancement of 1,25$(OH)_2D_3$ induced transcription by OA, suggesting that other promoter regulatory regions are not involved in the effect of the inhibitor. The effect of OA is not due to a general increase in transcription since OA did not affect transcription of the pSV2 minimal promoter CAT reporter construct. The stimulatory effect of OA on VDR mediated transcription was also not due to an upregulation of VDR levels (assessed by Western and Northern blot analysis) or to an increase in VDR-RXR interaction with the VDRE (assessed by electromobility shift assay).

314

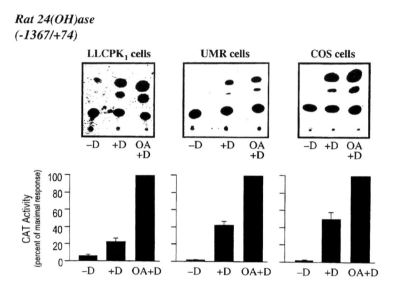

Rat 24(OH)ase
(-1367/+74)

<u>Figure 1:</u> *Enhancement of 1,25(OH)$_2$D$_3$ Induced 24(OH)ase Transcription by Inhibition of Protein Phosphatase 1 and 2A.* LLCPK1 (left panel), UMR (center panel) and COS cells (right panel) were transfected with 4ug of CAT reporter construct containing the rat 24(OH)ase promoter region from −1367/+74. COS cell were also transfected with 0.5ug of the VDR expression vector pAVhVDR. Transfected cells were treated with vehicle, 1,25(OH)$_2$D$_3$ (10^{-8}M) or 1,25(OH)$_2$D$_3$ +OA (50nM). After a 24h treatment cells were harvested, lysed, and CAT activities were measured at constant β-galactosidase activity. A typical autoradiogram and a graphical representation of three or more separate experiments are shown for each cell line.

Enhancement of cellular phosphorylation was found not only to increase 1,25(OH)$_2$D$_3$ induced transcription but also to reverse inhibition of 24(OH)ase transcription mediated by the transcription factor YY1. To investigate whether phosphorylation regulates VDR mediated transcription by modulating interactions with protein partners we examined the effect of phosphorylation on the protein-protein interaction between VDR and DRIP205 using GST pull down assays. COS cells transfected with VDR were treated with vehicle, 1,25(OH)$_2$D$_3$ (10^{-8}M) or 1,25(OH)$_2$D$_3$ +OA (50nM) for 24h. Nuclear extracts containing equal amounts of VDR were incubated with immobilized GST-DRIP205 and bound VDR was subsequently visualized by Western analysis (<u>Figure 2</u>).
Binding to DRIP was 1,25(OH)$_2$D$_3$ dependent. Similar to the functional studies, OA was consistently found to enhance the interaction of VDR with DRIP205 3-4 fold above the interaction observed in the presence of 1,25(OH)$_2$D$_3$ alone.

These findings suggest for the first time that a major mechanism of the effect of phosphorylation on VDR mediated transcription may be by the modulation of protein-protein interactions.

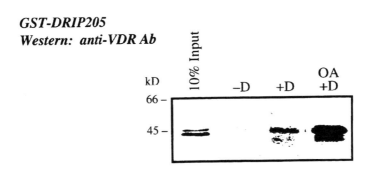

GST-DRIP205
Western: anti-VDR Ab

Figure 2: *Enhancement of VDR Mediated Transcription by Phosphorylation Involves Increased Interaction Between VDR and DRIP205.* COS cells were transfected with 2ug of the VDR expression vector pAVhVDR. Transfected cells were treated with vehicle, 1,25(OH)$_2$D$_3$ (10^{-8}M) or 1,25(OH)$_2$D$_3$ +OA (50nM) for 24h. Nuclear extracts were prepared and equal amounts of VDR protein were incubated with immobilized GST-DRIP205 for 16h. Pellets were washed and bound VDR was visualized by Western analysis using a VDR monoclonal antibody.

References:
1.   Denner, L. A., Schrader, W. T., O'Malley, B. W., and Weigel, N. L. (1990) *J. Biol. Chem.* **265**(27), 16548-55
2.   Sheridan, P. L., Evans, R. M., and Horwitz, K. B. (1989) *J. Biol. Chem.* **264**(11), 6520-8
3.   Hoeck, W., and Groner, B. (1990) *J. Biol. Chem.* **265**(10), 5403-8
4.   Bodwell, J. E., Orti, E., Coull, J. M., Pappin, D. J., Smith, L. I., and Swift, F. (1991) *J. Biol. Chem.* **266**(12), 7549-55
5.   Zhou, Z. X., Kemppainen, J. A., and Wilson, E. M. (1995) *Mol. Endocrinol.* **9**(5), 605-15
6.   van Laar, J. H., Berrevoets, C. A., Trapman, J., Zegers, N. D., and Brinkmann, A. O. (1991) *J. Biol. Chem.* **266**(6), 3734-8
7.   Migliaccio, A., Di Domenico, M., Green, S., de Falco, A., Kajtaniak, E. L., Blasi, F., Chambon, P., and Auricchio, F. (1989) *Mol. Endocrinol.* **3**(7), 1061-9
8.   Washburn, T., Hocutt, A., Brautigan, D. L., and Korach, K. S. (1991) *Mol. Endocrinol.* **5**(2), 235-42
9.   Rochette-Egly, C., Oulad-Abdelghani, M., Staub, A., Pfister, V., Scheuer, I., Chambon, P., and Gaub, M. P. (1995) *Mol. Endocrinol.* **9**(7), 860-71

10. Rochette-Egly, C., Gaub, M. P., Lutz, Y., Ali, S., Scheuer, I., and Chambon, P. (1992) *Mol. Endocrinol.* **6**(12), 2197-209

11. Pike, J. W., and Sleator, N. M. (1985) *Biochem. Biophys. Res. Commun.* **131**(1), 378-85

12. Brown, T. A., and DeLuca, H. F. (1990) *J. Biol. Chem.* **265**(17), 10025-9

13. Brown, T. A., and DeLuca, H. F. (1991) *Biochim. Biophys. Acta.* **1073**(2), 324-8

14. Jurutka, P. W., Hsieh, J. C., and Haussler, M. R. (1993) *Biochem. Biophys. Res. Commun.* **191**(3), 1089-96

15. Hsieh, J. C., Jurutka, P. W., Galligan, M. A., Terpening, C. M., Haussler, C. A., Samuels, D. S., Shimizu, Y., Shimizu, N., and Haussler, M. R. (1991) *Proc. Natl. Acad. Sci. U S A* **88**(20), 9315-9

16. Jurutka, P. W., Hsieh, J. C., MacDonald, P. N., Terpening, C. M., Haussler, C. A., Haussler, M. R., and Whitfield, G. K. (1993) *J. Biol. Chem.* **268**(9), 6791-9

17. Weigel, N. L. (1996) *Biochem. J.* **319**(Pt 3), 657-67

GENE REGULATION

MOLECULAR MECHANISMS OF TRANSCRIPTIONAL ACTIVATION BY THE VITAMIN D3 RECEPTOR

Christophe Rachez and Leonard P. Freedman

Cell Biology Program, Memorial Sloan-Kettering Cancer Center,1275 York Avenue
New York, NY 10021 USA

Introduction

Vitamin D3 receptor (VDR) regulates transcription in direct response to its hormonal ligand, 1,25(OH)$_2$D3. Ligand-binding leads to the recruitment of coactivators which can be defined as proteins that potentiate the activity of specific transcription factors. Many of these coactivators, present in large complexes, act, in part, by chromatin remodeling through intrinsic histone modifying activities. In addition, other ligand-recruited complexes appear to act more directly on the transcriptional appartus. This suggests that transcriptional regulation by VDR and other nuclear receptors may involve a process of both chromatin alterations and direct recruitment of key initiation components at regulated promoters.

Nuclear receptors and the basal machinery of transcription

Transcriptional activation of genes regulated by nuclear receptors and other transcription factors is currently understood as a multi-step process that is initiated at the promoter region of expressed genes. It is catalyzed by RNA polymerase II (RNA Pol II) and requires the assembly of general transcription factors (GTFs) including TFIIA, -B, -D, -E, -F, -H, at the promoter (illustrated in Fig 1; for review see refs 1,2). This process is regulated by a combination of transcription factors recruited on a given promoter by direct DNA binding to their specific response elements. DNA-bound factors mediate protein-protein interactions with components of the transcription machinery, ultimately targeting the recruitment and/or control of RNA Pol II.

Several direct contacts have been identified between VDR or other nuclear receptors and the basal transcription apparatus. TFIIB has been reported to interact directly with VDR-LBD. Interestingly, this interaction does not include the transactivation motif (AF-2) of VDR (3) (4). Moreover, the ligand may have distinct effect on this interaction depending on the cell type (5) (3) (6). These data taken together may suggest the requirement of additional targets for VDR transcription activity. For example, another basal factor, TFIIA, has also been shown to bind VDR. This effect is strongly stimulated by ligand and occurs in the context of VDR bound to a promoter DNA template (7). VDR has also been found to bind several TBP-associated factors TAFs [TATA box-binding protein (TBP) associated factors] that comprise the basal factor TFIID. TAF$_{II}$135 and TAF$_{II}$55 bind to VDR, RAR and TR and enhance their activity (8) (9). TAF$_{II}$28 has a potentiating or repressive effect on VDR and ER activity, depending on the cell type (Cos versus HeLa cells, respectively, (10). Finally, VDR binds a number of newly discovered factors that appear to bridge or recruit other activities important for the activation process, as described at length below.

The SRC/p160 family of coactivators

Over the last few years, a growing number of proteins have been identified as coactivators for various nuclear receptors (for review: 11-13). Many of these putative coactivators have been cloned by yeast two-hybrid or GST pull down assays by virtue of their interaction with members of the nuclear receptor family, and their ability to potentiate transcriptional activity. Among the many nuclear receptor coactivators characterized so far, a homologous family of proteins has emerged. It has been alternatively named SRC, NCoA, or more generically, p160, based on one of its first identified members, the 160 kDa protein steroid receptor coactivator-1 (SRC-1) (14). The SRC/p160 family comprises three types of factors, on the basis of their homologies, including SRC-1/NCoA-1, GRIP1/TIF2/NCoA-2, and pCIP /RAC3/ACTR/AIB1/TRAM-1 (for review: (15,16). The original enzymatic activity found to be common to these factors is histone acetyl-transferase (HAT) activity, which catalyzes the acetylation of lysine residues at the N-terminal tails of histones (17,18). Acetylation is thought to destabilize the interactions between DNA and the histone cores that form its nucleosomal structure in the nucleus. The SRC/p160 family members would thereby act as coactivators by loosening the repressive effect of chromatin on gene expression. In the original publications describing these proteins, ligand-dependent binding to VDR was only documented with the coactivator ACTR, but subsequent analyses has shown that VDR is also the target of GRIP1/TIF-2 and SRC-1 (19,20; our observations).

Specific inactivation of SRC-1 by gene targeting shows that there may be at least partial functional redundancy between the different SRC/p160 family members, since only a partial resistance to hormonal response is observed in SRC-1(-/-) mice. This phenomenon is concommitant to increased mRNA levels of other coactivators like TIF2, perhaps compensating for the loss of SRC-1 (21). The coactivator effects of SRC-1 on nuclear receptors has also been demonstrated in vitro in the presence of chromatin assembled templates (22). Under these conditions, SRC-1 strongly potentiates the ligand-dependent activity of the progesterone receptor (PR-B). Interestingly, this potentiation also occurs to a certain extent on naked DNA, in the absence of chromatin. These results may suggest a dual effect of SRC-1, both on chromatin remodelling and on other activities or interactions yet to be identified.

Beyond this homogeneous family, several proteins that have been found to act as coregulators of VDR cannot be classified in any of the previous categories. NCoA-62, identified by yeast two-hybrid, coactivates VDR in a ligand-dependent fashion, but no function has been assigned to this protein (23). TIF1 was found to interact with VDR and other nuclear receptors (24). TIF1 also interacts with heterochromatin-associated proteins and has a kinase activity that can phosphorylate several general transcription factors (TFIIEa, TAFII28 and TAFII55), suggesting a novel mechanism of transcription regulation for nuclear receptors (25).

Large coactivator assemblies provide multifunctional HAT activity
The SRC/p160 family of coactivators form complexes with CBP/p300 (18). The co-integrators CBP and p300 bind a large panel of transcription factors (26). They also bind nuclear receptors, but much more weakly than do SRC/p160. They also have HAT activity (27,28), and they appear to interact with nuclear receptors cooperatively with SRC/p160 and other components like p/CIP and PCAF, together forming a larger co-activator complex (11,29). Alternatively, CBP and SRC-1 may be stabilized by a specific RNA coactivator, SRA (Steroid receptor RNA Activator). Interestingly, SRA has been found to be part of a 600-700 kD ribonucleoprotein structure that includes SRC-1 (30). The fact that different components of the complex possess HAT activity suggests that they have a cooperative effect or/and an increased array of specificities. Recent reports present additional functions for CBP's HAT activity besides chromatin remodelling. CBP/p300 is able to acetylate non-histone proteins, such as the transcription factor p53, whose acetylation promotes its DNA binding activity (31). Components of the basal-machinery (TFIIEa, TFIIF) are also acetylated by p300, PCAF and TAFII250, but the effects of this modification are not yet understood (32). Intriguingly, CBP/p300 can regulate the association between ACTR and the estrogen receptor by directly acetylating ACTR at two lysines close to one of its NR boxes, thereby disrupting its association with ER (33). Currently, our view of how SRC/p160 functions is primarily to act as means of recruiting CBP/p300 to a nuclear

receptor. It is CBP/p300 rather than SRC/p160 that appears to be the primary source of HAT activity.

Identification of a new cofactor complex for transcription regulation--DRIP

Besides the SRC/p160 coactivators, several laboratories, including our own, have recently identified a novel type of nuclear receptor coactivator complex, alternatively called DRIP, TRAP, ARC, NAT, or mammalian Mediator (Table 1), depending on the purification process, and the activators tested as targets. These complexes are required for activation of transcription in vitro, in different transcription assays involving purified components of the transcription machinery. At the time of their respective discoveries, each one of these complexes was thought to be specific for a distinct transcription factor. DRIP (vitamin D Receptor Interacting Proteins;(34,35) and ARC (Activator Recruited Cofactor; (36,37) complexes were purified out of nuclear extracts by in vitro pull-down assays using GST fusions with VDR-LBD, or with the activation motifs of several transcription factors (SREBP-1a, NF-kB and VP16), respectively. The TRAP complex (TR Associated Proteins; (38,39) was isolated by co-immunoprecipitation of epitope-tagged TR stably expressed in HeLa cells. TRAP has later been identified as identical to the SMCC complex (Srb/Med-containing cofactor complex; (40), a complex purified by co-immunoprecipitation with antibodies directed against epitope-tagged Srb10. The cloning of these component subunits by independent groups revealed the near-identity of their sequences for many of them, which now suggests that these different complexes might actually constitute a single, universal one. Importantly, some subunits do differ from complex to complex. For example, TRAP150 has no homology with any of its candidate conterparts. In addition, DRIP/ARC/CRSP130, also identified as hSur2 (41), has not been identified in the TRAP complex. The various subunit compositions are summarized in Table 1.

Other complexes have close identities with the DRIP, ARC and TRAP complexes. CRSP (Cofactor Required for Sp1 Activation; (42), purified by multiple chromatographic steps, appears to be a subset of nine subunits of the DRIP/ARC complex and might represent a stable core of subunits or a conserved subcomplex among various functionally related complexes. The CRSP complex differs, however, by its two unrelated 34 and 70 kDa subunits (Table 1). The homology of CRSP70's N-terminus with the elongation factor TFIIS is a unique feature among all the complexes described so far. Despite its apparently limited number of subunits, CRSP potentiates the activity of the transcription factor Sp1 in vitro. The NAT complex (Negative regulator of Activated Transcription) was identified by co-immunoprecipitation out of HeLa nuclear extracts with an antibody against hSrb10/CDK8 (43). It shares many common subunits with DRIP, ARC and TRAP. However, when the NAT complex was tested in vitro in a purified transcription assay in the presence of RNA pol II, general transcription factors (TFIIA, to -H), and a cofactor activity PC4 (see below), it exhibited a repressing effect on transcription driven by various activators, without any influence on basal transcription. This unexpected result suggests that these complexes may not only have an activation potential, but also repressive activities on transcription in vitro, as will be discussed later. The mammalian Mediator complex was identified (44) through biochemical purification out of nuclear extracts of murine cells. Its name reflects its homologies with a yeast Mediator counterpart (Table 1; see below).

Functionality of the DRIP complex

The functional role of the DRIP and related complexes in human cells can be postulated on the basis of a series of studies in yeast (for review, (45,46). Genetic and biochemical analyses in yeast revealed the importance of several types of factors for transcription of target genes by RNA pol II in response to activators (46). They include the products of SRB genes, identified in a genetic screen as suppressors of the effect of truncations in the CTD of RNA pol II (47). Srb proteins point to the importance of CTD phosphorylation in

Table 1. Subunit composition of general coactivator complexes.

DRIP	ARC	SMCC /TRAP	CRSP	NAT	Mediator (mouse)	Mediator (Yeast S.c.)
	CBP/p300					
DRIP250	ARC250	TRAP240				
DRIP240	ARC240	TRAP230		p230	p160a	Nut1
DRIP205	ARC205	TRAP220	CRSP200		p160b	Gal11
DRIP150	ARC150	TRAP170	CRSP150	p150	Rgr1/p110	Rgr1
DRIP130	ARC130	TRAP150	CRSP130	p140/hSur2		
	ARC105/ TIG-1					
DRIP100	ARC100	TRAP100				Sin4
DRIP97		TRAP97		p95	Ring3/p96a	Srb4
DRIP92	ARC92	TRAP95		p90	p96b	Med1
		TRAP93				
DRIP77	ARC77	TRAP80	CRSP77		p78	
DRIP70-2	ARC70		CRSP70	p70		Med2
	ARC42				p55	Pgd1/Hrs1
		hSrb10		p56/Cdk8		Srb10
DRIP36	ARC36		CRSP34	p45	p34	Med4
DRIP34	ARC34	hMed7	CRSP33	p37	Med7/p36	Med7
				p36		Srb5
DRIP33	ARC33	hMed6		p33	Med6/p32	Med6
	ARC32	hTRF			TRF/p28a	Med8
		hSrb11		p31/Cycl.C		Srb11
	p28	hSoh1		p30	p28b	Rox3/Ssn7
				p23		Srb2
				p22		
				p21		Med9/Cse2
		hSrb7		p17	Srb7/p21	Srb7
		hNut2		p14		Med10/Nut2
						Med11
						Srb6

Subunits in Bold with highlight are equivalent in the different complexes, or homologs between mammalian and yeast complexes.
Subunits in the same lanes have similar molecular weights regardless of any homology.

the transition between transcription initiation at the promoter and elongation of the RNA transcript (48), and references therein). Biochemical fractionation resulted in the isolation of Mediator as a multi-subunit complex (49) that contained Srb proteins, and another set of components named Med proteins (50,51). Detailed functional studies in yeast revealed the importance of both Srb and Med components of the Mediator complex in either general transcription (Srb4, (52), or activation of transcription by specific factors both in vivo and in vitro, such as Gcn4, Gal4, or VP16 (observed for Med2, Med6, Pgd1/Hrs1, and Sin4; (50,51). This raised the definition of the yeast Mediator as a "global transcription coactivator" (53).

The existence of human homologs of a number of yeast Mediator proteins suggested that a corresponding complex would exists in higher organisms. Mammalian Mediator has been identified in mice by Kornberg's group (44). Its homology to the yeast Mediator is also suggested by some of its functional characteristics: the complex is able to bind the CTD of RNA pol II, and it stimulates in vitro CTD phosphorylation catalyzed by TFIIH. However, "mammalian Mediator", as isolated, has not yet been shown to function in transcription assays. Some of its subunits have yeast conterparts (Rgr1, Med6, Med7, Srb7), but several other subunits have not matched any yeast homologs. Some, but not all, of the mouse Mediator subunits are in fact also present within DRIP, ARC, TRAP/SMCC, and NAT (see Table 1). That DRIP, ARC and TRAP/SMCC complexes all contain Med components (35,37,40) may suggest that these complexes could be human homologs of the Mammalian Mediator. However, a side by side comparison of the respective subunits within human and mouse complexes favors a scenario where "mammalian Mediator" is distinct of DRIP, ARC and TRAP/SMCC complexes (Table 1). A larger diversity of complexes in higher eukaryotes relative to yeast, was previously suggested for the RNA Pol II holoenzyme on the basis of its different subunit compositions in mammalian preparations (i.e. variations in a subset of components) (45). The potential differences in composition of the DRIP, ARC, TRAP/SMCC, NAT and mammalian Mediator complexes may reflect this diversity. Whatever the case, the presence of Srb/Med subunits in DRIP, ARC, and TRAP/SMCC strongly suggests that at least part of how this complex functions is through recruitment of RNA pol II, and recent experiments demonstrate that DRIP bound to liganded VDR indeed can recruit RNA pol II and associated subunits.(54).

As mentioned previously, activities of all these complexes were tested in highly purified transcription assays in vitro, in response to specific activators. The DRIP complex strongly potentiated ligand-dependent VDR-RXR transcription on DNA templates assembled into chromatin, but interestingly had little or no effect on the same transcription in the absence of chromatin (naked templates). None of the previously identified SRC/p160 coactivators have been found to be part of the purified DRIP complex (35), and the absence of any HAT activity in the DRIP complex suggests that it may contain distinct chromatin remodelling activities, or may recruit them. The ARC complex tested on chromatin-assembled templates exhibits cooperativity between different activators, such as Sp1 and SREBP-1a, on the same template promoter, in conditions where ARC has no effect on the same activators tested individually (37). This is an interesting demonstration of the ability of these complexes to integrate multiple transcription pathways into a synergistic effect on gene activation. TRAP/SMCC, whose activity was tested only in the absence of chromatin, also enhances activator-dependent transcription in a purified in vitro system with RNA pol II, GTFs, and PC4, but only in the absence of TFIIH or at limiting concentrations of it (40). In a transcription system including both PC4 and TFIIH, the SMCC complex repressed transcription. This effect was specific for the presence of activators like Gal4-AH, since no strong effect was observed on basal transcription. By analogy with the effect of Mediator in yeast on phosphorylation of RNA pol II CTD, the kinase activity of SMCC was tested in vitro. Although the CTD was phosphorylated, the major substrate was the cofactor PC4, a single-stranded DNA binding protein which is required for activated transcription (55,56). PC4 has been shown to interact in vitro with TFIIA and VP16 (56). More importantly, PC4 binding and transcription activities are lost upon phosphorylation (55,56). The conservation of PC4 in yeast (as Tsp1) highlights its general requirement among eukaryotic systems (57). Interestingly, the repression effect by SMCC was also observed when a CTD-less form of RNA pol II was used. Based on this, the authors suggested that regulation of transcription by SMCC could be mediated in concert with PC4, but independently of modifications of the RNA pol II CTD (40).

More recently, Roeder's group demonstrated that TRAP/SMCC complex activity, at limiting amounts of TFIIH, can be synergistically stimulated by addition of PC4 and a distinct cofactor, PC2 (an unresolved positive cofactor activity (58). However, it appears that a further increase in the amounts of PC4 in this assay led to repression of the initial transcription effect. This might reflect the sensitivity of the highly purified assay to subtle variations in its individual components, like PC4. It could also explain why two highly similar complexes like SMCC and NAT have been independently characterized as an activator and repressor of activator-dependent transcription, depending on the equilibrium between constituents of the assays. These observations, however, could still reflect real and decisive variations in the subunit compositions of the two complexes that are biologially relevant.

Integration of signalling pathways

The SRC-1/p160 family and the DRIP complex represent two unrelated protein complexes, together carrying several distinct activities that have been shown to potentiate VDR (and other nuclear receptors) transcription activity. These activities may function together to provide a synergistic effect of $1,25(OH)_2D_3$-mediated activation, or to provide specificity of targeting to its regulation. VDR transcription regulation may require a combination of chromatin remodeling activities, as well as efficient recruitment of the RNA pol II machinery, via several of its basal factors. We have suggested a step-wise model that combines these distinct activities, where a CBP/p160 type coactivator complex might be required for chromatin remodelling, followed by the direct recruitment of the transcription machinery by the DRIP complex. Definitive experimental analysis has yet to confirm this view (12,59). In vitro, however, the SRC/p160 and DRIP coactivators appear to have no real intrinsic difference in their ability to interact with nuclear receptors. They both utilize the AF-2 of nuclear receptors and bind with similar affinities [TRAP220 vs TIF2 for TR (60); DRIP205 and GRIP1 for VDR (61). Thus we could envision a cooperative model where both CBP/p160 and DRIP complexes simulataneous occupy a promoter, and through their combined actions facilitate activation of transcription (Fig. 1). The observation that CBP can acetylate ACTR, leading to the latter's dissociation from liganded ER (33) suggests a mechanism for the sequential model, whereby the first complex functions to acetylate histones and disrupt chromatin structure, whereupon it itself dissociates from the receptor, allowing the DRIP complex to bind and act at the level of direct recruitment (Fig. 1).

Recent studies have revealed multiple binding motifs for coactivators within the DRIP and TRAP complexes. For example, GR interacts with the DRIP complex via both AF-1 and AF-2 motifs with DRIP150 and DRIP205 respectively (62). These results define the GR binding motif in the DRIP complex as a combination of two subunits, and might explain the presence of two unrelated activation functions in the same receptor. In the TRAP/SMCC complex, both p53 and VP16 interact via TRAP80, but binding of VP16 and TR (which binds TRAP220) to the TRAP complex are not mutually exclusive, suggesting that this complex may support activation by a combination of distinct transcription factors. The transactivation domain (conserved region 3, CR3) of E1A interacts directly with hSur-2, which corresponds to DRIP130 (41). This defines yet another novel and distinct target motif for an activator within the complexes.

Conclusions

Transcriptional regulation by $1,25(OH)_2D_3$ can be dissected into several functional activities that are mediated by VDR. Generally, transactivation requires that a repressed state of chromatin has to be disrupted in a given target gene's regulatory regions, together with the ability to promote productive elongation of RNA products by the RNA pol II machinery at the site of transcription initiation. Several candidates for such activities that are recruited

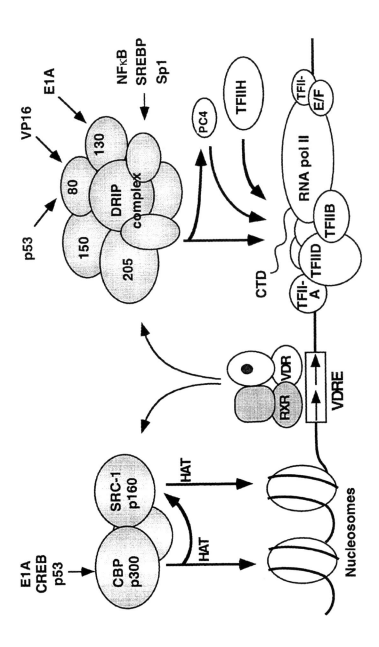

Figure 1 Interactions between VDR and its coactivators. SRC/p160 coactivators are specific for nuclear receptors, but the cointegrators CBP and p300 also bind a large number and classes of transcription factors (including E1A, CREB, p53,...). The DRIP complex and its analogous complexes ARC, TRAP/SMCC, NAT, CRSP, and Mediator are the target of nuclear receptors and multiple transcription factors that bind via specific subunits. The SRC/CBP complex appears to act, although perhaps not exclusively, by histone acetyltransferase activity (HAT) on histone and non-histone proteins. The DRIP and analogous complexes may provide RNA pol II with the ability to respond to activators through its direct recruitment to the basal machinery on the promoter, and may also regulate the initiation of transcription by phosphorylation of the RNA pol II C-terminal repeat domain (CTD) and one of its cofactors PC4.

by nuclear receptors in direct response to ligand binding have been recently identified, as has been described in this review. The HAT activity-containing coactivators (SRC/p160 family, CBP/p300, PCAF, etc.) at face-value appear to act primarily in the disruption of chromatin through histone modifications, although a series of additional, provocative targets corresponding to ATP-dependent chromatin remodellers have more recently been identified. The regulation of RNA pol II and its ability to respond to activators appears to be mediated by a distinct type of cofactor complex (DRIP/ARC/TRAP/SMCC/Mediator) whose functions are not yet completely elucidated. Given the fact that many classes of activators interact with DRIP beyond VDR and nuclear receptors, this complex must be considered as a regulatory panel for RNA pol II rather than an exclusive target for nuclear receptors. DRIP may be therefore viewed as a downstream target of multiple transcription activators, perhaps conferring to RNA pol II the ability to simultaneously integrate multiple signalling pathways onto a single promoter in vivo. This model may provide a key for an interpretation of some unresolved mechanisms involving the simultaneous cross-talk of several signalling systems.

Acknowledgements
This work was supported by grants from the NIH and Human Frontiers Science Program.

References

1. Zawel, L., and Reinberg, D. (1995) *Annu Rev Biochem* **64**, 533-61
2. Roeder, R. G. (1996) *Trends Biochem Sci* **21**, 327-35
3. Blanco, J. C., Wang, I. M., Tsai, S. Y., Tsai, M. J., O'Malley, B. W., Jurutka, P. W., Haussler, M. R., and Ozato, K. (1995) *Proc Natl Acad Sci U S A* **92**, 1535-9
4. Jurutka, P., Hsieh, J., Remus, L., Whitfield, G., Thompson, P., Haussler, C., Blanco, J., Ozato, K., and Haussler, M. (1997) *J Biol Chem* **272**(23), 14592-9
5. MacDonald, P., Sherman, D., Dowd, D., Jefcoat, S. J., and DeLisle, R. (1995) *J Biol Chem* **270**, 4748-4752
6. Masuyama, H., Jefcoat, S. C., Jr., and MacDonald, P. N. (1997) *Mol Endocrinol* **11**, 218-28
7. Lemon, B. D., Fondell, J. D., and Freedman, L. P. (1997) *Mol Cell Biol* **17**(4), 1923-37
8. Mengus, G., May, M., Carre, L., Chambon, P., and Davidson, I. (1997) *Genes Dev* **11**, 1381-95
9. Lavigne, A. C., Mengus, G., Gangloff, Y. G., Wurtz, J. M., and Davidson, I. (1999) *Mol Cell Biol* **19**(8), 5486-94
10. May, M., Mengus, G., Lavigne, A. C., Chambon, P., and Davidson, I. (1996) *EMBO J* **15**, 3093-104
11. Torchia, J., Glass, C., and Rosenfeld, M. G. (1998) *Curr Opin Cell Biol* **10**(3), 373-83
12. Freedman, L. P. (1999) *Cell* **97**, 5-8
13. Lemon, B. D., and Freedman, L. P. (1999) *Curr Opin Genet Dev* **9**(5), 499-504
14. Onate, S. A., Tsai, S. Y., Tsai, M. J., and O'Malley, B. W. (1995) *Science* **270**, 1354-1357
15. McKenna, N. J., Xu, J., Nawaz, Z., Tsai, S. Y., Tsai, M. J., and O'Malley, B. W. (1999) *J Steroid Biochem Mol Biol* **69**, 3-12
16. Xu, L., Glass, C. K., and Rosenfeld, M. G. (1999) *Curr Opin Genet Dev* **9**, 140-7
17. Spencer, T. E., Jenster, G., Burcin, M. M., Allis, C. D., Zhou, J. X., Mizzen, C. A., McKenna, N. J., Onate, S. A., Tsai, S. Y., Tsai, M. J., and Omalley, B. W. (1997) *Nature* **389**, 194-198
18. Chen, H. W., Lin, R. J., Schiltz, R. L., Chakravarti, D., Nash, A., Nagy, L., Privalsky, M. L., Nakatani, Y., and Evans, R. M. (1997) *Cell* **90**(3), 569-580

19. Hong, H., Kohli, K., Garabedian, M. J., and Stallcup, M. R. (1997) *Mol Cell Biol* **17,** 2735-44
20. Masuyama, H., Brownfield, C. M., StArnaud, R., and MacDonald, P. N. (1997b) *Mol Endocrinol* **11,** 1507-1517
21. Xu, J., Qiu, Y., DeMayo, F. J., Tsai, S. Y., Tsai, M. J., and O'Malley, B. W. (1998) *Science* **279,** 1922-5
22. Liu, Z., Wong, J., Tsai, S. Y., Tsai, M. J., and O'Malley, B. W. (1999) *Proc Natl Acad Sci U S A* **96,** 9485-90
23. Baudino, T. A., Kraichely, D. M., Jefcoat, S. C., Jr., Winchester, S. K., Partridge, N. C., and MacDonald, P. N. (1998) *J Biol Chem* **273**(26), 16434-41
24. Le Douarin, B., vom Baur, E., Zechel, C., Heery, D., Heine, M., Vivat, V., Gronemeyer, H., Losson, R., and Chambon, P. (1996) *Philos Trans R Soc Lond B Biol Sci* **351,** 569-78
25. Fraser, R. A., Heard, D. J., Adam, S., Lavigne, A. C., Le Douarin, B., Tora, L., Losson, R., Rochette-Egly, C., and Chambon, P. (1998) *J Biol Chem* **273,** 16199-204
26. Goldman, P. S., Tran, V. K., and Goodman, R. H. (1997) *Recent Prog Horm Res* **52,** 103-19
27. Bannister, A. J., and Kouzarides, T. (1996) *Nature* **384**(6610), 641-3
28. Ogryzko, V. V., Schiltz, R. L., Russanova, V., Howard, B. H., and Nakatani, Y. (1996) *Cell* **87,** 953-9
29. McKenna, N. J., Nawaz, Z., Tsai, S. Y., Tsai, M.-J., and O'Malley, B. W. (1998) *Proc. Natl. Acad. Sci. USA* **95,** 11697-11702
30. Lanz, R. B., McKenna, N. J., Onate, S. A., Albrecht, U., Wong, J., Tsai, S. Y., Tsai, M. J., and O'Malley, B. W. (1999) *Cell* **97**(1), 17-27
31. Gu, W., and Roeder, R. G. (1997) *Cell* **90**(4), 595-606
32. Imhof, A., Yang, X. J., Ogryzko, V. V., Nakatani, Y., Wolffe, A. P., and Ge, H. (1997) *Curr Biol* **7**(9), 689-92
33. Chen, H., Lin, R. J., Xie, W., Wilpitz, D., and Evans, R. M. (1999) *Cell* **98**(5), 675-86
34. Rachez, C., Suldan, Z., Ward, J., Chang, C. P., Burakov, D., Erdjument-Bromage, H., Tempst, P., and Freedman, L. P. (1998) *Genes Dev* **12**(12), 1787-800
35. Rachez, C., Lemon, B. D., Suldan, Z., Bromleigh, V., Gamble, M., Naar, A. M., Erdjument-Bromage, H., Tempst, P., and Freedman, L. P. (1999) *Nature* **398,** 824-8
36. Naar, A. M., Beaurang, P. A., Robinson, K. M., Oliner, J. D., Avizonis, D., Scheek, S., Zwicker, J., Kadonaga, J. T., and Tjian, R. (1998) *Genes Dev* **12,** 3020-31
37. Naar, A. M., Beaurang, P. A., Zhou, S., Abraham, S., Solomon, W., and Tjian, R. (1999) *Nature* **398,** 828-32
38. Fondell, J. D., Ge, H., and Roeder, R. G. (1996) *Proc. Natl. Acad. Sci. U.S.A.* **93,** 8329-8333
39. Ito, M., Yuan, C. X., Malik, S., Gu, W., Fondell, J. D., Yamamura, S., Fu, Z. Y., Zhang, X., Qin, J., and Roeder, R. G. (1999) *Mol Cell* **3,** 361-70
40. Gu, W., Malik, S., Ito, M., Yuan, C. X., Fondell, J. D., Zhang, X., Martinez, E., Qin, J., and Roeder, R. G. (1999) *Mol Cell* **3,** 97-108
41. Boyer, T. G., Martin, M. E., Lees, E., Ricciardi, R. P., and Berk, A. J. (1999) *Nature* **399,** 276-9
42. Ryu, S., Zhou, S., Ladurner, A. G., and Tjian, R. (1999) *Nature* **397,** 446-50
43. Sun, X., Zhang, Y., Cho, H., Rickert, P., Lees, E., Lane, W., and Reinberg, D. (1998) *Mol Cell* **2,** 213-22
44. Jiang, Y. W., Veschambre, P., Erdjument-Bromage, H., Tempst, P., Conaway, J. W., Conaway, R. C., and Kornberg, R. D. (1998) *Proc Natl Acad Sci U S A* **95,** 8538-43
45. Parvin, J. D., and Young, R. A. (1998) *Curr Opin Genet Dev* **8,** 565-70
46. Myer, V. E., and Young, R. A. (1998) *J Biol Chem* **273,** 27757-60
47. Koleske, A. J., and Young, R. A. (1994) *Nature* **368,** 466-9

48. Hengartner, C. J., Myer, V. E., Liao, S. M., Wilson, C. J., Koh, S. S., and Young, R. A. (1998) *Mol Cell* **2** 43-53
49. Kim, Y. J., Bjorklund, S., Li, Y., Sayre, M. H., and Kornberg, R. D. (1994) *Cell* **77**, 599-608
50. Lee, Y. C., Min, S., Gim, B. S., and Kim, Y. J. (1997) *Mol Cell Biol* **17**, 4622-32
51. Myers, L. C., Gustafsson, C. M., Bushnell, D. A., Lui, M., Erdjument-Bromage, H., Tempst, P., and Kornberg, R. D. (1998) *Genes Dev* **12**, 45-54
52. Thompson, C. M., and Young, R. A. (1995) *Proc Natl Acad Sci U S A* **92**(10), 4587-90
53. Myers, L. C., Gustafsson, C. M., Hayashibara, K. C., Brown, P. O., and Kornberg, R. D. (1999) *Proc Natl Acad Sci USA* **96**, 67-72
54. Chiba, N., Suldan, Z., Freedman, L. P., and Parvin, J. D. (2000) *J. Biol. Chem.* **275**, 10719-10722
55. Kretzschmar, M., Kaiser, K., Lottspeich, F., and Meisterernst, M. (1994) *Cell* **78**, 525-34
56. Ge, H., Zhao, Y., Chait, B. T., and Roeder, R. G. (1994) *Proc Natl Acad Sci USA* **91**, 2691-5
57. Henry, N. L., Bushnell, D. A., and Kornberg, R. D. (1996) *J Biol Chem* **271**, 21842-7
58. Kretzschmar, M., Stelzer, G., Roeder, R., and Meisterernst, M. (1994b) *Mol Cell Biol* **14**, 3927-37
59. Fondell, J. D., Guermah, M., Malik, S., and Roeder, R. G. (1999) *Proc Natl Acad Sci USA* **96**, 1959-64
60. Treuter, E., Johansson, L., Thomsen, J. S., A, W. r., Leers, J., Pelto-Huikko, M., Sjberg, M., Wright, A. P., Spyrou, G., and Gustafsson, J. (1999) *J Biol Chem* **274**, 6667-6677
61. Rachez, C., Gamble, M., Chang, C.-P. B., Atkins, G. B., Lazar, M. A., and Freedman, L. P. (2000) *Mol. Cell. Biol.* **20**, 2718-2726
62. Hittelman, A. B., Burakov, D., JA, I. i.-L., Freedman, L. P., and Garabedian, M. J. (1999) *EMBO J* **18**, 5380-5388

NUCLEAR RECEPTOR COACTIVATORS IN VITAMIN D-MEDIATED TRANSCRIPTION.

Paul N. MacDonald, Hisashi Tokumaru, Diane R. Dowd, and Chi Zhang. Department of Pharmacology, Case Western Reserve University, Cleveland, OH 44106.

Vitamin D-mediated transcription - The diverse effects of 1,25-dihydroxyvitamin D_3 [1,25-$(OH)_2D_3$] are mediated through the vitamin D receptor (VDR), a member of the superfamily of nuclear receptors for steroid hormones. VDR functions as ligand-activated transcription factor (1,2). Binding of the 1,25-$(OH)_2D_3$ hormonal ligand to VDR induces heterodimerization of VDR with RXR and high affinity binding of the VDR-RXR heterodimer to promoter sequences in vitamin D-responsive genes. These initial macromolecular interactions initiate a communication process that ultimately influences the rate of RNA polymerase II-directed transcription. A central aspect of this communication process involves protein-protein interactions between the VDR-RXR heterodimer and the transcription preinitiation complex. Nuclear receptor co-modulatory proteins (i.e. the coactivators and corepressors) may play key roles in this communication process (Fig. 1).

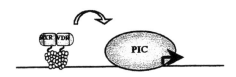

• Interact with nuclear receptors - ligand dependent or independent
• Required for efficient transcriptional regulation by the receptor
• Signal between receptor complex and transcription apparatus

Fig.1. General properties of putative nuclear receptor co-modulatory proteins in vitamin D-mediated transcription.

COACTIVATORS					COREPRESSORS	
SRC	Trip-1	NCoA-62	P/CIP	NSD-1	NCoR	SUNCoR
ERAP-160	E6-AP	Trip230	BRG-1	TRAPs/DRIPs	SMRT	NURD
RIP-140	TIF1	CBP	PCAF	SMADs	TRUP	
TIF2	ARA70	p300	HMG-1	ADA		

Nuclear receptor coactivator proteins have emerged as central players in the communication process connecting ligand-activated receptors to the preinitiation complex (3,4). The general functional properties of these transcriptional cofactors are their ability to interact with nuclear receptors and modulate their transcriptional responsiveness to the ligand. Thus far, the best characterized coactivators are the SRC family of nuclear receptor coactivators (4) which includes three members at present: SRC-1 (NCoA-1), SRC-2 (GRIP-1, TIF2, NCoA-2), and SRC-3 (pCIP, RAC3, ACTR, AIB-1, TRAM-1). The mechanisms through which coactivators function in VDR- and other nuclear receptor-mediated transcriptional pathways are largely unknown. Nuclear receptor coactivators may function as bridging proteins that link the receptor to RNA polymerase II and the basal transcription machinery and possibly recruit limiting components into preinitiation complex assembly. Indeed, SRC-1 interacts with general transcription factors, such as transcription factor IIB (TFIIB) and TATA-binding protein (TBP), as well as with other coactivators, such as CBP/p300. Coactivator proteins such as SRC-1 and CBP/p300 also possess intrinsic histone acetyltransferase activity. Thus, ligand-activated receptors may function to recruit coactivators that remodel chromatin structure and permit greater accessibility of the transcriptional machinery to DNA.

The SRC family of coactivators - The SRC family members interact in a ligand-dependent manner with the nuclear receptors (4). This interaction is mediated through three leucine-rich motifs located in the central region of SRC (5) which have the consensus sequence, LXXLL. These leucine-rich regions are termed nuclear receptor boxes or NR-boxes. Mutations of the NR-box abolish interaction with nuclear receptors and their coactivator activity. The key domain of the receptor that mediates interaction with the coactivator NR-box is the activation function-2 (AF-2) domain. The AF-2 domain is an amphipathic α-helical region at the carboxyl terminus of the LBD. Deletion of or mutations within the AF-2 domain selectively abolish ligand-activated transcription by disrupting receptor interaction with the SRC or other NR-box coactivators. The VDR AF-2 domain consists of a centrally conserved glutamic acid residue (E420 in the hVDR sequence) flanked on either side by hydrophobic residues. Mutation of residues in the hydrophobic or hydrophilic faces abolish $1,25$-$(OH)_2D_3$-activated transcription as well as SRC interaction with the VDR illustrating the importance of coactivator contacts with the AF-2 domain in the mechanism (6,7).

Structural studies of VDR and of related receptors provide insight into the mechanism of ligand-induced interaction of the VDR AF-2 domain with the NR-boxes of SRC coactivators. It is hypothesized that the $1,25$-$(OH)_2D_3$ ligand promotes coactivator interaction by inducing a repositioning of the AF-2 activation helix (helix H12). In the unliganded state, the AF-2 domain (helix H12) projects out away from the globular core of the LBD and in the liganded state the AF-2 domain is folded over onto the LBD globular core domain. One outcome of helix H12 folding is the creation of a platform or protein interaction surface through which nuclear receptor coactivator proteins effectively dock with the VDR. Scanning mutagenesis of the thyroid hormone receptor (TR) defined a coactivator interaction surface composed of helices H12, H3, H4, and H5 (8) and structural analysis of the estrogen, thyroid hormone, and PPARγ receptors complexed to NR-box peptides confirmed this model (9-11). We and others reported that a similar surface may exist on the VDR since select mutations within helices H12 and H3 disrupt SRC coactivator interaction and VDR-activated transcription (12,13). For example, a helix H3 mutant VDR [VDR(Y236A)] binds $1,25$-$(OH)_2D_3$ with high affinity and it heterodimerizes with RXR. However ,this H3 mutant did not interact with SRC-1 or GRIP1 and it did not activate $1,25$-$(OH)_2D_3$-mediated transcription. Based on our data and the structural data of others, it is likely that this region of the VDR (helix H3) together with the AF-2 domain (helix H12) forms a coactivator binding surface or platform through which proteins such as SRCs bind and mediate the transactivation properties of the VDR

NCoA-62/SKIP, a novel coactivator with distinct actions - P160 coactivator proteins, such as GRIP-1 and SRC-1 interact with nuclear receptors in a ligand-dependent manner through the AF-2 domain and this interaction is important in modulating the transcriptional response of the liganded receptor. However, a number of nuclear receptor coactivators are distinct from the p160 family and may function through alternate pathways. Other important coactivators that function in VDR-mediated transcription include the VDR-interacting protein complex or DRIP/TRAP complex, CBP/P300, SMAD3, and NCoA-62. The latter coactivator was cloned in our laboratory as a protein that interacted with the VDR (14). It was independently isolated by another group as a protein that interacts with the v-Ski oncogene and was termed SKIP, for Ski-interacting protein (15). This group suggested a role for NCoA-62/SKIP in cellular differentiation pathways including steroid hormone-mediated cellular differentiation. With regard to the nuclear receptor interaction, NCoA-62 interacts directly with VDR as well as other nuclear receptors tested including the retinoid X receptor (RXR), estrogen receptor (ER), and glucocorticoid receptor (GR) (Fig. 2).

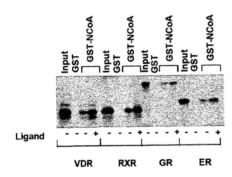

Ligand   - - - +   - - - +   - - - +   - - - +

VDR   RXR   GR   ER

Fig 2. NCoA-62 interacts with various nuclear receptors in an in vitro interaction assay. Purified GST-NCoA-62 was incubated with radiolabeled nuclear receptors and protein-protein complexes were visualized following SDS-PAGE analysis.

In addition to interacting directly with various nuclear receptors, NCoA-62 functions to modestly augment nuclear receptor-mediated transactivation as assessed in hormone responsive reporter gene assays. Coexpression of NCoA-62 in vitamin D, retinoic acid, estrogen, and glucocorticoid reporter gene expression assays augments ligand-activated transcription in each system by a factor of 2 or 3-fold (data not shown).

Based on its deduced amino acid sequence, NCoA-62 is a novel protein that is not related to p160 coactivators. None the less, it is classified as a nuclear receptor coactivator since it interacts directly with nuclear receptors to augment ligand-activated transcription. NCoA-62 is highly related to BX42, a Drosophila melanogaster nuclear protein putatively involved in ecdysone-stimulated transcription. Related proteins also exist in yeast and in C. elegans, but their function is unknown. Sequence comparisons between these related proteins identified three domains with varying degrees of conservation, the SNW domain, the SH2-like domain and the highly-charged (HC) carboxyl-terminal domain, but the function of these three domains is not well characterized (Fig. 3).

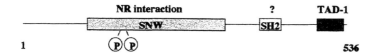

Fig. 3. Putative domains in the NCoA-62 protein

Deletion studies of NCoA-62 demonstrated that the highly charged COOH-terminal domain is essential for coactivator activity (12). Our more recent studies indicate that this region is a transactivation domain that we have designated TAD-1 for Transactivation Domain-1. Several lines of evidence support the definition of TAD-1 as a transactivation domain. First, deletion of the TAD-1 domain abolished coactivator function in VDR-, ER-, RAR-, and GR-mediated transcription without compromising NCoA-62 interaction with nuclear receptors (8 and data not shown). Second, removal of TAD-1 from the context of full-length NCoA-62 and fusing it to a heterologous DNA-binding domain [GAL4 (1-147)] was sufficient to confer transactivation activity to that fusion protein (Fig.4). Finally, an R449A mutant within the TAD-1 domain abrogated coactivator activity of full-length NCoA-62 in nuclear receptor-mediated transcription and similarly reduced the autonomous transactivation by the minimal TAD-1 domain. Thus, TAD-1 is a bona-fide transactivation domain that is both necessary and sufficient for transcriptional activation and for the coactivator activity of NCoA-62 in nuclear receptor-mediated transcription.

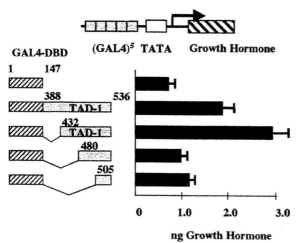

Fig. 4. The highly charged COOH-terminus of NCoA-62 contains a transactivation domain. Various lengths of the NCoA-62 C-terminus were fused to the Gal4 DNA-binding domain and the fusions were tested for the ability to transactivate a gal4-responsive growth hormone reporter gene.

The centrally conserved SNW domain of NCoA-62 seems to be essential for mediating interactions with the nuclear receptors including the VDR. Two-hybrid interaction studies showed that elimination of the SNW domain between residues 220 and 388 completely eliminated interaction with the VDR (12). Moreover, this domain alone was sufficient to form a specific protein-protein complex with VDR in GST-pulldown assays (Fig. 5). Thus, this highly conserved central domain is critical for mediating interactions with nuclear receptors. This region also contains two serine residues that are highly phosphorylated. The functional role of the phosphorylation in NCoA-62 action is still under investigation.

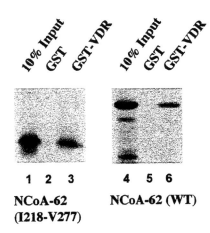

Fig. 5. The central SNW region of NCoA-62 is sufficient to mediate protein-protein interaction with the VDR. GST-VDR was incubated with radiolabeled gal4-NCoA62(218-277) and protein-protein complexes were analyzed by SDS-PAGE and autoradiography (lane 3). Gal4 DBD did not interact with GST-VDR in this system (data not shown). Radiolabeled full-length NCoA-62 was examined in lane 6.

1 2 3   4 5 6

NCoA-62   NCoA-62 (WT)
(I218-V277)

Distinct interactions of VDR with NCoA-62 and P160 coactivators - Importantly, NCoA-62 interaction with VDR does not require the AF-2 domain. Deletion of or mutations within the VDR AF-2 domain abolish ligand-dependent interaction with SRC coactivators. However, NCoA-62 retains interactions with these AF-2 mutants. This property is highlighted in Fig. 6, in which the VDR AF-2 deletion mutant [VDR(C403STOP)] abolishes ligand-dependent interaction with the SRC coactivator family, but it retains srong interaction with NCoA-62. Moreover, NCoA-62 does not contain canonical NR-box motifs (LXXLL) indicating that that this novel coactivator may contact other important domains within the VDR LBD. Thus, NCoA-62 belongs to a growing class of AF-2 independent coactivators. The likelihood exists that distinct classes of coactivator proteins may function through different mechanisms to cooperatively enhance VDR-activated transcription.

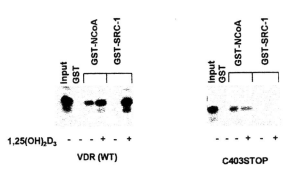

Fig. 6. NCoA-62 and SRC-1 interact with distinct domains on VDR. GST-NCoA-62 or GST-SRC-1 were incubated with radiolabeled wt VDR or with an AF-2 deletion mutant of VDR (C403STOP). Note that ligand-dependent interaction between VDR and SRC-1 is ablated in the VDR(C403STOP) mutant while NCoA-62 retains interaction with this mutant VDR.

1,25(OH)₂D₃   - - - + - +   - - - + - +

VDR (WT)   **C403STOP**

NCoA-62 interacts with unliganded receptors and ligand addition generally enhances formation of the complex by only two- or three-fold. Thus, an intriguing paradox arises. How is the modest effect of ligand on VDR/NCoA-62 interaction (2-fold) translated into the dramatic effect of ligand on VDR-activated transcription (generally over 20-fold). The answer likely resides in the cooperative interplay and requirement of multiple coactivator proteins in the nuclear receptor complex. To test this possibility, SRC-1 and GRIP-1, were examined in the vitamin D-responsive reporter gene assay in

COS-7 cells. GRIP-1 or SRC-1 expression augmented VDR-activated transcription by approximately 2-fold, a level of enhancement similar to that observed with NCoA-62 expression under these sub-optimal conditions (Fig. 7). However, coexpression of NCoA-62 and either GRIP-1 or SRC-1 resulted in a synergistic enhancement in 1,25-(OH)$_2$D$_3$-activated expression of the reporter gene construct (8-fold or 7-fold, respectively). As expected, coexpression of GRIP-1 and SRC-1, two related coactivators resulted in an additive effect of vitamin D-mediated transcription compared to each coactivator alone (Fig. 7).

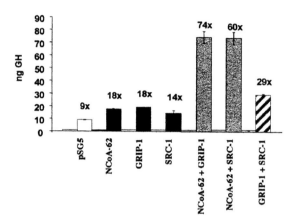

Fig. 7. Synergistic activation of vitamin D receptor-activated transccription by P160 coactivators and NCoA-62. COS-7 cells were transfected with a vitamin D responsive GH reproter gene construct and a VDR expression plasmid in the absence or presence of expression vectors for SRC-1 GRIP-1 or NCoA-62. GH values were determined 24 h following tretment with 10-8 M 1,25(OH)2D3

The synergism observed in these studies suggests that these two distinct coactivators function together to regulate nuclear receptor-mediated transcription. As discussed above, NCoA-62 interacts with the VDR through domains that are distinct from those involved in p160 coactivator interaction. If distinct domains of VDR mediate NCoA-62 interaction compared to P160 coactivator interaction, then the possibility exists that NCoA-62 and p160 coactivators may simultaneously contact the VDR to form a ternary complex. As illustrated in Fig. 8, in vitro GST pulldown studies demonstrated the formation of such a complex between NCoA-62, liganded VDR, and GRIP-1 or SRC-1 thus, providing strong support for this possibility.

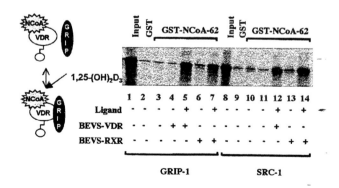

Fig. 8. P160 coactivators, NCoA-62, and liganded VDR form a ternary complex in an in vitro GST pulldown assay.

This ternary complex is completely dependent on the $1,25\text{-}(OH)_2D_3$ ligand in the binding assay indicating that a ligand-dependent interaction of SRC-1 or GRIP-1 with the VDR/NCoA-62 complex occurs. Thus, while the $1,25\text{-}(OH)_2D_3$ ligand may have only a modest effect on NCoA-62/VDR complex formation, it does have a profound effect on the formation of the NCoA-62/VDR/p160 ternary complex. It is likely that all three proteins within this complex are essential for the full transactivation potential of the system.

The mechanisms through which coactivators function are diverse. Some coactivators may function as macromolecular bridges between the nuclear receptor and the PIC. Their interaction with the PIC (either direct or indirect) may promote PIC assembly or enhance the stability of the PIC, thereby leading to activated transcription. An emerging property of several other coactivator proteins including CREB binding protein (CBP) and SRC-1 is that these coactivators possess intrinsic histone acetyltransferase (HAT). Histone acetylation may result in a disruption or loosening of the chromatin structure making promoters more accessible to the transcription machinery and ultimately leading to an increase in the rate of transcription. Thus, nuclear receptors may interact in a ligand-dependent manner to recruit enzymes that modify chromatin structure at a particular promoter. Thus, different classes of nuclear receptor coactivators may function through different mechanisms to augment ligand-activated transcription. This appears to be the case for NCoA-62 and the SRC coactivator family. Clearly, the effects are cooperative and coexpression in mammalian cells leads to synergistic effects on VDR-activated transcription. This is likely do to the fact that SRCs and NCoA-62 interact with distinct domains on the VDR. SRCs interact in a ligand-dependent manner with the H3, H4, H5, H12 coactivator interaction surface on VDR. Although the precise domain of VDR that mediates interactions with NCoA-62 is unknown, it is evident that this interaction is mediated exclusively through the VDR ligand binding domain and that it is independent of the AF-2 helix (helix H12). That the SRC and NCoA-62 interaction occurs via distinct domains on VDR is also evident in the observation of a ternary complex between NCoA-62, liganded VDR, and the SRC coactivator family members. We propose that this ternary complex exlains the cooperative, synergistic effects on NCoA-62 and SRC coactivators in VDR-activated transcription. Further studies are ongoing to test this model of coactivator action.

References

1. Haussler, M.R., Haussler, C.A., Jurutka, P.W., Thompson, P.D., Hsieh, J.C., Remus, L.S., Selznick, S.H., and Whitfield, G.K., (1997) J Endocrinol,. 154 Suppl: S57-73.
2. Kraichely, D.M. and MacDonald, P.N. (1998) Front Biosci,. 3: D821-33.
3. Horwitz, K.B., Jackson, T.A., Bain, D.L., Richer, J.K., Takimoto, G.S., and Tung, L. (1996) Mol. Endocrinol.,. 10: 1167-1177.
4. McKenna, N.J., Lanz, R.B., and O'Malley, B.W. (1999) Endocr Rev. 20(3): 321-44.
5. Heery, D.M., Kalkhoven, E., Hoare, S., and Parker, M.G. (1997) Nature 387: 733-6.

6. Masuyama, H., Brownfield, C.M., St.-Arnaud, R., and MacDonald, P.N. Mol. Endocrinol., 1997.

7. Jurutka, P.W., Hsieh, J.C., Remus, L.S., Whitfield, G.K., Thompson, P.D., Haussler, C.A., Blanco, J.C., Ozato, K., and Haussler, M.R. J Biol Chem, 1997. 272(23): 14592-9.

8. Feng, W., Ribeiro, R.C., Wagner, R.L., Nguyen, H., Apriletti, J.W., Fletterick, R.J., Baxter, J.D., Kushner, P.J., and West, B.L. (1998) Science 280: 1747-9.

9. Darimont, B.D., Wagner, R.L., Apriletti, J.W., Stallcup, M.R., Kushner, P.J., Baxter, J.D., Fletterick, R.J., and Yamamoto, K.R. Genes Dev, 1998. 12(21): 3343-56.

10. Nolte, R.T., Wisely, G.B., Westin, S., Cobb, J.E., Lambert, M.H., Kurokawa, R., Rosenfeld, M.G., Willson, T.M., Glass, C.K., and Milburn, M.V. Nature, 1998. 395(6698): 137-43.

11. Shiau, A.K., Barstad, D., Loria, P.M., Cheng, L., Kushner, P.J., Agard, D.A., and Greene, G.L. Cell, 1998. 95(7): 927-37.

12. Kraichely, D.M., Collins, J.J.r., DeLisle, R.K., and MacDonald, P.N. J Biol Chem, 1999. 274(20): 14352-8.

13. Jimenez-Lara, A.M. and Aranda, A. J Biol Chem, 1999. 274(19): 13503-10.

14. Baudino, T.A., Kraichely, D.M., Jefcoat, S.C., Jr., Winchester, S.K., Partridge, N.C., and MacDonald, P.N. J Biol Chem, 1998. 273(26): 16434-41.

15. Dahl, R., Wani, Bushra, and Hayman, M.J. Oncogene, 1998, 22: 1579-1586.

MECHANISM OF ACTION OF 1α,25-DIHYDROXYVITAMIN D3-26,23-LACTONE ANALOGUES WHICH FUNCTION AS ANTAGONISTS OF VDR GENOMIC ACTIVITIES MEDIATED BY 1α,25-DIHYDROXYVITAMIN D3.

Seiichi Ishizuka, Daishiro Miura, Keiichi Ozono[1], Mariko Saito[1], Hiroshi Eguchi, Manabu Chokki, Kenji Manabe, Qingzhi Gao, Ryo Sogawa, Kazuya Takenouchi, and Anthony W. Norman[2]

Teijin Institute for Bio-Medical Research, 4-3-2 Asahigaoka, Hino, Tokyo 191-8512, Japan, [1]Department of Environmental Medicine, Osaka Medical Center and Research Institute for Maternal and Child Health, 840 Murodo-Cho, Izumi, Osaka 594-1101, Japan, and [2]Department of Biochemistry and Division of Biomedical Sciences, University of California, Riverside, CA92521, U. S. A.

Introduction

It is widely accepted that the fundamental physiological functions of 1α,25-dihydroxyvitamin D3 (1α,25-(OH)2D3) are to stimulate intestinal calcium absorption and to increase bone calcium mobilization [1]. In recent years, however many new biological functions of 1α,25-(OH)2D3 different from those mentioned above have been reported [2]. 1α,25-(OH)2D3 is believed to mediate biological responses as a consequence of its interaction with both a nuclear receptor (VDRnuc) to regulate gene transcription [3,4] and with a putative cell membrane receptor (VDRmem) to generate rapid nongenomic actions [5], including opening of voltage-gated calcium and chloride channels [6], and activation of mitogen-activated protein kinase (MAP kinase) [7].

In order to better understand the interactions of the 1α,25-(OH)2D3-VDRnuc interacting with 9-cis-retinoic acid receptor (RXR) and then with a vitamin D responsive element (VDRE) located on the promoter of regulated genes, it would be helpful to identify analogues of 1α,25-(OH)2D3 that can antagonize these interactions. However, to date the only known antagonist of 1α,25-(OH)2D3 is 1β,25-(OH)2D3 that blocks rapid nongenomic actions, but which is without effect on the classical VDRnuc [8].

Discovery of antagonists to genomic actions of 1α,25-(OH)2D3

1. Synthesis of 1α,25-(OH)2D3-26,23-lactone analogues

(23S,25R)-1α,25-(OH)2D3-26,23-Lactone, a major metabolite of 1α,25-(OH)2D3, shows biological functions quite different from those of 1α,25-(OH)2D3 [9-11]. Recently, we have synthesized its analogues to investigate from the structural point of view where their unique biological actions are derived. The structures and biological characteristics of synthesized 1α,25-(OH)2D3-26,23-lactone analogues were shown in Fig. 1 and Table 1. (23S,25S)-1α-Hydroxyvitamin D3-

26,23-lactone (TEI-9616) is a 25-dehydroxylated version of the natural occurring (23S,25R)-1α,25-(OH)2D3-26,23-lactone. (23S)- and (23R)-25-dehydro-1α-hydroxyvitamin D3-26,23-lactone (TEI-9647 and TEI-9648) are also both 25-dehydrated versions of the (23S,25R)- and (23R,25R)-1α,25-(OH)2D3-26,23-lactone, respectively. Formally, TEI-9647 and TEI-9648 are 23-diastereoisomers of one another.

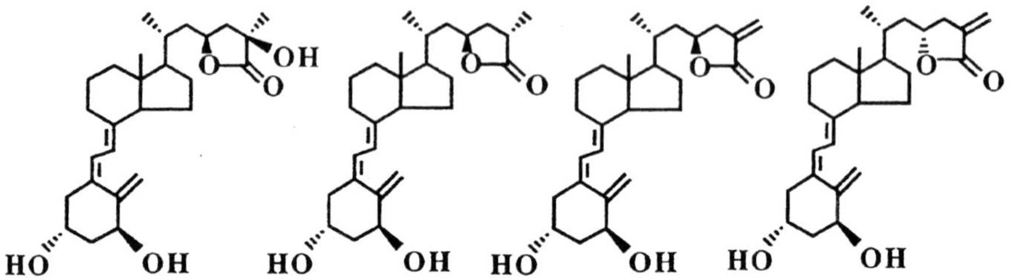

(23S,25R)-1α,25-(OH)₂D₃-26,23-lactone   (23S,25S)-1α-OH-D₃-26,23-lactone (TEI-9616)   (23S)-25-dehydro-1α-OH-D₃-26,23-lactone (TEI-9647)   (23R)-25-dehydro-1α-OH-D₃-26,23-lactone (TEI-9648)

Figure 1. Structures of 1α,25-(OH)2D3-26,23-lactone analogues.

Table 1. Biological characteristics of 1α,25-(OH)2D3-26,23-lactone analogues.

Assay	Relative Activity (%) [a]				
	1α,25-(OH)2D3	TEI-9616	TEI-9647	TEI-9648	1α,25-(OH)2D3-26,23- lactone
VDR BINDING AFFINITY					
HL-60 CELL VDR	100	0.42	10.0	8.3	0.07
CHICK INTESTINAL VDR	100	0.48	10.2	7.2	0.14
MG-63 CELL VDR	100	0.5	7.9	6.0	0.07
DBP BINDING AFFINITY	100	2.4	9.3	2.5	620
OSTEOCALCIN SYNTHESIS IN MG-63 CELL	100	15.9	< 1.0	< 1.0	11.8
HL-60 CELL DIFFERENTIATION	100	1.6	Not induced	Not induced	0.5

(a) The Relative Activity for each anlogue was calculated from their respective EC50 results and then normalized to the results obtained for 1α,25-(OH)2D3 which was set to 100%.

Among these lactone analogues, two novel 25-dehydro compounds, TEI-9647 and TEI-9648, neither stimulate osteocalcin synthesis in human osteosarcoma cells (MG-63 cells) nor induce HL-60 cell differentiation, even at high concentrations (10^{-6} M), although they have much stronger VDRnuc binding affinities than the natural (23S,25R)-1α,25-(OH)2D3-26,23-lactone (Table 1).

2. Effects of TEI-9647 and TEI-9648 on HL-60 cell differentiation

Through a VDRnuc/VDRE-mediated pathway occurs 1α,25-(OH)2D3 inducing HL-60 cell differentiation. Whose system is regarded as a good model for evaluateing its genomic actions. 10^{-8} M $1\alpha,25$-(OH)2D3 differentiated about 50% of the cells into nitro blue tetrazolium (NBT) reducing activity positive cells during 96 hr culture period. Neither TEI-9647 nor TEI-9648 induced HL-60 cell differentiation even after the treatment at 10^{-6} M. TEI-9647 dose dependently inhibited the cell differentiation induced by 10^{-8} M $1\alpha,25$-(OH)2D3; it caused 40% suppression at 10^{-9} M and almost complete inhibition was observed at 10^{-7} M. TEI-9648 showed a similar dose response curve, but its suppressive effect was consistently weaker than that of TEI-9647 as shown in Fig. 2 [12].

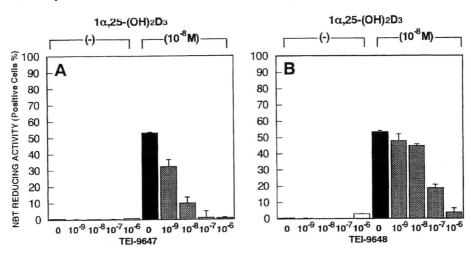

Figure 2. Effects of TEI-9647 and TEI-9648 on $1\alpha,25$-(OH)2D3 induced HL-60 cell differentiation as examined with NBT reducing activity. HL-60 cells were treated with TEI-9647 (A) or TEI-9648 (B) in the absence (-) or presence (+ 10^{-8} M) of $1\alpha,25$-(OH)2D3 for 96 hrs and NBT reducing activity was examined. Rectangles and bars show mean ± SD of triplicates, respectively.

However, TEI-9616 and (23S,25R)-$1\alpha,25$-(OH)2D3-26,23-lactone, so far from inhibiting, were found to stimulate HL-60 cell differentiation induced by $1\alpha,25$-(OH)2D3 [12,13]. In contrast, neither TEI-9647 nor TEI-9648 blocked the actions of retinoic acid and 12-O-tetradecanoylphorbol-13-acetate (TPA) on HL-60 cell differentiation, suggesting that their inhibitory actions might be $1\alpha,25$-(OH)2D3/VDRnuc specific ones [12,13]. Both TEI-9647 and TEI-9648 show considerable $1\alpha,25$-(OH)2D3 antagonistic activities on the cell differentiation of human monoblastic lymphoma cells (U-937 cells) [14], 25-hydroxyvitamin D3-24-hydroxylase (25-OH-D3-24-hydroxylase) gene expression and osteocalcin synthesis in human osteosarcoma cells (Saos-2 cells and MG-63 cells) [15,16], 25-OH-D3-24-hydroxylase gene expression in monkey kidney cells (COS-7 cells) [12], interleukin-2 and interferon-γ production in human peripheral mononuclear cells [Chokki, M. et al. in preparation] as well as HL-60 cell differentiation.

3. Effects of TEI-9647 and TEI-9648 on gene expression

The antagonistic activity of TEI-9647 and TEI-9648 has been confirmed in two other systems. p21[WAF1,CIP1] and 25-OH-D3-24-hydroxylase whose genes contain VDRE in their promoter region are known to have an important role in regulating cell proliferation, cell differentiation and metabolism of $1\alpha,25$-$(OH)2D3$ in HL-60 cells [17,18]. We examined 25-OH-D3-24-hydroxylase gene expression induced by $1\alpha,25$-$(OH)2D3$ in HL-60 cells using RT-PCR. The 25-OH-D3-24-hydroxylase mRNA was scarcely detectable 4 - 8 hrs after the treatment with 10^{-8} M $1\alpha,25$-$(OH)2D3$, but was significantly expressed after 24 hrs to 48 hrs. Even at high concentrations (10^{-6} M), neither TEI-9647 nor TEI-9648 caused the 25-OH-D3-24-hydroxylase gene expression, although both 10^{-6} M TEI-9616 or 10^{-6} M (23S,25R)-$1\alpha,25$-$(OH)2D3$-26,23-lactone remarkably did. However, 10^{-7} M TEI-9647 markedly suppressed 25-OH-D3-24-hydroxylase gene expression induced by 10^{-8} M $1\alpha,25$-$(OH)2D3$, and 10^{-6} M TEI-9647 blocked it by 86.2%. In the case of TEI-9648 the same is true, but its inhibitory action seemed much weaker than that of TEI-9647 [13]. Similarly, the gene expression of p21[WAF1,CIP1] was clearly invigorated by 10^{-8} M $1\alpha,25$-$(OH)2D3$; while it never emerged at 10^{-7} M TEI-9647. Impressively, 10^{-7} M TEI-9647 clearly suppressed p21[WAF1,CIP1] gene expression induced by 10^{-8} M $1\alpha,25$-$(OH)2D3$ 24 hrs after the treatment. Next, we examined the antagonistic actions of TEI-9647 and TEI-9648 on $1\alpha,25$-$(OH)2D3$/VDRnuc-VDRE mediated expression of the human 25-OH-D3-24-hydroxylase gene after plasmid transfection in Saos-2 cells as evaluated by a luciferase reporter assay [13,16]. In this system, 10^{-8} M $1\alpha,25$-$(OH)2D3$ effected, after 48 hrs, a 9-fold increase in the 25-OH-D3-24-hydroxylase gene expression. 10^{-7} M TEI-9647 or TEI-9648 acting alone had no discernible effect on the 25-OH-D3-24-hydroxylase gene expression. Surprisingly, 10^{-7} M TEI-9647 and TEI-9648 respectively inhibited by 66.8% and by 33.5% the 25-OH-D3-24-hydroxylase activity induced by 10^{-8} M $1\alpha,25$-$(OH)2D3$. In contrast, 10^{-7} M TEI-9616 enhanced 5.1-fold in the 25-OH-D3-24-hydroxylase gene expression, and showed no inhibitory effect on it induced by 10^{-8} M $1\alpha,25$-$(OH)2D3$. Collectively these results described the first example of a stereo-specific vitamin D which functions as an antagonist of the VDRnuc for $1\alpha,25$-$(OH)2D3$.

4. Synthesis and biological characteristics of TEI-9647 analogues

Above data indicated that TEI-9647 and TEI-9648 were rare compounds to antagonize VDRnuc mediated HL-60 cell differentiation of $1\alpha,25$-$(OH)2D3$. On the other hand, the analogues of TEI-9647 and TEI-9648, TEI-9616 and (23S,25R)-$1\alpha,25$-$(OH)2D3$-26,23-lactone weakly but significantly induced HL-60 cell differentiation, and they did not show any inhibitory effects on HL-60 cell differentiation induced by $1\alpha,25$-$(OH)2D3$ even at 10^{-6} M. These results suggest that the vitamin D antagonistic activity of $1\alpha,25$-$(OH)2D3$-26,23-lactone analogues derives from definite structure specificity, lactone ring and double bond. So, we synthesized TEI-9647 and TEI-9648 analogues with them in their structure to investigate whether or not they show antagonistic actions to $1\alpha,25$-(OH)2D3 (Fig. 3). Among many TEI-9647 analogues, that with side chain elongeted (TEI-E00226), and those with γ-lactone converted into cyclopentanone (TEI-D2224 and TEI-D2226) showed antagonistic actions against $1\alpha,25$-(OH)2D3 inducing VDRnuc mediated HL-60 cell differentiation. The TEI-9647 and TEI-9648 analogues, (23S)- and (23R)-27-nor-1α-hydroxyvitamin D3-26,23-lactone (TEI-E00468 and TEI-E00469) which have no double bond in their structure showed no antagonistic actions to $1\alpha,25$-(OH)2D3, as we had expected. Their 25-dehydrated 24-dehydro diastereoisomers of $1\alpha,25$-(OH)2D3-26,23-lactone (TEI-D1807 and TEI-D1808) which are structurally akin to TEI-9647 and TEI-9648, indicated no inhibitory effects against $1\alpha,25$-(OH)2D3. This means they are weak agonists rather than antagonists. Amazingly, TEI-9647 and TEI-9648 analogues with γ-lactone replaced by lactam (TEI-D1715 and TEI-D1716) which we had expected would have antagonistic actions, proved to be no antagonists.

These results suggest that the vitamin D antagonistic activity of $1\alpha,25$-(OH)2D3-26,23-lactone analogues derives from definite structure specificity, γ-lactone with exo-methylene structure or cyclopentanone with exo-methylene structure might be essential to antagonistic action against $1\alpha,25$-(OH)2D3.

(A) Structures of Vitamin D Antagonists

| TEI-9647 | TEI-9648 | TEI-D2224 | TEI-D2226 | TEI-E00226 |
| (10.2%) | (7.2%) | (1.4%) | (3.5%) | (17.8%) |

(B) Structures of Vitamin D Agonists

| TEI-D1807 | TEI-D1808 | TEI-D1715 | TEI-D1716 | TEI-E00468 | TEI-E00469 |
| (0.9%) | (1.1%) | (1.4%) | (4.4%) | (0.6%) | (0.5%) |

*1; C23 stereoisomer (less polar), *2; C23 stereoisomer (more polar), *3 ; mixture of C23 stereoisomers
Binding affinities of TEI compounds to chick VDR were showed in parentheses compered to $1\alpha,25$-(OH)2D3.

Effects of TEI-9647 on nongenomic actions of $1\alpha,25$-(OH)2D3

We recently demonstrated that TEI-9647 and TEI-9648 might be antagonists of VDRnuc/VDRE-mediated genomic actions of $1\alpha,25$-(OH)2D3 [12-16]. It was

342

not clear whether these two analogues could also antagonize 1α,25-(OH)2D3-mediated nongenomic actions. The human acute promyelocytic leukemia NB4 cell differentiation induced by 1α,25-(OH)2D3 is considered to be a good model for 1α,25-(OH)2D3-mediated nongenomic actions [20]. In this system TEI-9647 and TEI-9648 did not show any inhibition of NB4 cell differentiation, while 1β,25-(OH)2D3, a specific antagonist of 1α,25-(OH)2D3-mediated nongenomic actions, effectively inhibited NB4 cell differentiation [21]. We recently found that 1α,25-(OH)2D3 induced 25-OH-D3-24-hydroxylase gene expression through VDRnuc /VDRE-mediated genomic actions in NB4 cells. In this system, 10^{-7} M TEI-9647 completely inhibited 25-OH-D3-24-hydroxylase gene expression induced by 10^{-8} M 1α,25-(OH)2D3 as shown in Fig.4. These results indicated that TEI-9647 and TEI-9648 might be the first antagonists for 1α,25-(OH)2D3/VDRnuc/VDRE-mediated genomic actions, but not for nongenomic actions.

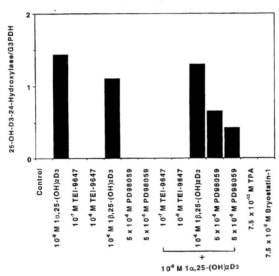

Figure 4. Effect of TEI-9647 on the 25-OH-D3-24-hydroxylase gene expression induced by 10^{-8} M 1α,25-(OH)2D3 24 hrs after the treatment in NB4 cells.

Molecular mechanism of antagonistic actions of TEI-9647

We demonstrated that TEI-9647 and TEI-9648 are antagonists of 1α,25-(OH)2D3 action, specifically VDRnuc/VDRE-mediated genomic actions. 1α,25-(OH)2D3 exerts its action via the VDRnuc through multi-step events; first it binds to the VDRnuc forming a heterodimer RXR, which is further connected to VDRE, ending in interacting with a co-activator or a co-repressor. We tried to reveal on which stage of the above process do occur the inhibitory actions of TEI-9647. To investigate the interaction between the VDRnuc and RXRα, and the VDRnuc and co-activator SRC-1, we used the modified mammalian two-hybrid system as described in Figs. 5A and 6A. 10^{-8} M 1α,25-(OH)2D3 enhanced the direct interaction between VDRnuc and RXRα 5-fold as indicated by the reporter activity (Fig. 5B). 10^{-7} M TEI-9647 remarkably inhibited the interaction between VDRnuc and RXRα induced by 1α,25-(OH)2D3 in Saos-2 cells, which is one of the key steps in expressing 1α,25-(OH)2D3 actions, indicating one mechanism of antagonistic actions of TEI-9647. Similar results were obtained in the case of the interaction between the VDRnuc and SRC-1 (Fig. 6B). In Saos-2 cells, TEI-9647 lessened the interaction between the VDRnuc and SRC-1, suggesting that the conformational change of VDRnuc elicited by the ligand differs between 1α,25-(OH)2D3 and TEI-9647 as described in recent reports [22,23].

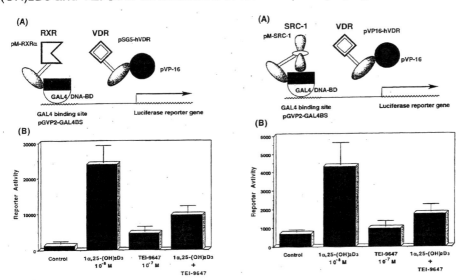

Figure 5.

Figure 5. Effect of TEI-9647 on the interaction between VDRnuc and RXR in Saos-2 cells. (A) Schematic illustration of the interaction detection method between VDRnuc and RXR. (B) The interaction between VDRnuc and RXR was examined by determining the reporter activity in Saos-2 cells transfected with pM-RXRα, pSG5-hVDRnuc and the reporter plasmin containing the GAL 4 binding site (pGVP2-GAL4BS).

Figure 6. Effect of TEI-9647 on the interaction between VDRnuc and SRC-1 in Saos-2 cells. (A) Schematic illustration of the interaction detection method between VDRnuc and SRC-1. (B) The interaction between VDRnuc and SRC-1 was examined by determining the reporter activity in Saos-2 cells transfected with pM-SRC-1, pVP16-hVDRnuc and the reporter plasmin containing the GAL 4 binding site (pGVP2-GAL4BS).

Conclusion

TEI-9647 shows inhibitory effects on the binding of 1α,25-(OH)2D3 to VDRnuc, on the heterodimer formation between VDRnuc and RXR, and on the interaction between VDRnuc and SRC-1 in Saos-2 cells. These results strongly suggest that TEI-9647 is the first antagonist of 1α,25-(OH)2D3 actions, specifically VDRnuc/VDRE-mediated genomic actions, but not nongenomic rapid actions of 1α,25-(OH)2D3.

REFERENCES

1. Haussler, M.R. (1986) Annu. Rev. Nutr. 6, 527-562
2. Bouillon, R., Okamura, W.H. and Norman, A.W. (1995) Endocr. Rev. 16, 200- 257
3. Pike, J.W. (1997) in The vitamin D receptor and its gene. Feldman, D., Glorieux, F.H. and Pike, J.W. eds. p105-125 Academic Press, San Diego
4. Haussler, M.R., Whitfield, G.K., Haussler, C.A., Hsieh, J.-H., Thompson, P.D., Selznick, S.H., Domonguez, C.E. and Juruka, P.W. (1998) J. Bone Miner. Res. 13, 325-349
5. Norman, A.W., Okamura, W.H., Hammond, M.W., Bishop, J.E., Dormanen, M.C., Bouillon, R., van Baelen, H., Ridal, A.L., Daane, E., Khoury, R. and Farach-Carson, M.C. (1997) Mol. Endocrinol. 11, 1518-1531
6. Zanello, L.P., and Norman, A.W. (1997) J. Biol. Chem. 272, 22617-22622
7. Song, X., Bishop, J.E., Okamura, W.H. and Norman, A.W. (1997) Endocrinology 139, 457-465
8. Norman, A.W., Bouillon, R., Farach-Carson, M.C., Bishop, J.E., Zhou, L.X., Nemere, I., Zhao, J., Muralidharan, K.R. and Okamura, W.H. (1993) J. Biol. Chem. 268, 20022-20030
9. Ishizuka, S., Kiyoki, M., Kurihara, N., Hakeda, Y., Ikeda, K., Kumegawa, M. and Norman, A.W. (1988) Mol. Cell. Endocrinol. 55, 77-86
10. Ishizuka, S., Kurihara, N., Hakeda, S., Maeda, N., Ikeda, K., Kumegawa, M. and Norman, A.W. (1988) Endocrinology 123, 781-786
11. Shima, M., Tanaka, H., Norman, A.W., Yamaoka, K., Yoshikawa, H., Takaoka, K., Ishizuka, S., and Seino, Y. (1990) Endocrinology 126, 832-836
12. Miura, D., Manabe, K., Ozono, K., Saito, M., Gao, Q., Norman, A.W. and Ishizuka, S. (1999) J. Biol. Chem. 274, 16392-16399
13. Ishizuka, S., Miura, D., Ozono, K., Saito, M., Eguchi, H., Chokki, M. and Norman, A.W. (2000) Steroids (in press)
14. Ishizuka, S., Miura, D., Manabe, K., Gao, Q., Sakuma, Y., Uno, H. and Ozono, K. (1997) J. Bone Miner. Res. 12 (Supplement 1) s-452 (Abstract No. s399)
15. Ozono, K., Ito, M., Miura, D., Ishizuka, S., Yanagihara, I. and Nakajima, S. (1997) J. Bone Miner. Res. 12 (Supplement 1) s-122 (Abstract No. 78)
16. Ozono, K., Saito, M., Miura, D., Michigami, T., Nakajima, S. and Ishizuka, S. (1999) J. Biol. Chem. 274, 32376-32381
17. Liu, M.,Lee, M-H., Cohen, M., Bommakanti, M., and Freedman, L.P. (1996) Genes and Dev. 10, 142-153
18. Ohyama, Y., Ozono, K., Uchida, M., Shinki, T., Kato, S., Suda, T., Yamamoto, O., Noshiro, M. and Kato, Y. (1994) J. Biol. Chem. 269, 10545-10550
19. Ishizuka, S., Miura, D., Eguchi, H., Ozono, K., Chokki, M., Kamimura, T., and Norman, A.W. (2000) Arch. Biochem. Biophys. (in press)
20. Bhatia, M., Kirkland, J.B., and Meckling-Gill, K.A. (1995) J. Biol. Chem. 270, 15962-15965
21. Miura, D., Manabe, K., Gao, Q., Norman, A.W., and Ishizuka, S. (1999) FEBS Letters 460, 297-302
22. Takeyama, K., Masuhiro, Y., Fuse, H., Endoh, H., Murayama, A., Kitanaka, S., Suzawa, M., Yanagisawa, J., and Kato, S. (1999) Mol. Cell. Biol. 19, 1049-1055
23. Peleg, S., Nguyen, C., Woodard, B.T., Lee, J-K., Posner, G.H. (1998) Mol. Endocrinol. 12, 525-535

INTESTINAL EXPRESSION DRIVEN BY THE RAT CALBINDIN-D$_{9K}$ PROMOTER IN TRANSGENIC MICE
CRUCIAL ACTIVATION BY THE HOMEOPROTEIN CDX2 AND IMPLICATION OF A NON CONVENTIONAL VITAMIN D RESPONSE UNIT

Sabine COLNOT[1,2], Béatrice ROMAGNOLO[2], Mireille LAMBERT[1], Christine OVEJERO[2], Arlette PORTEU[2], Pascal LACOURTE[1], Axel KAHN[2], Monique THOMASSET[1], Christine PERRET[2].
[1]INSERM U458 Hôpital R. Debré; [2]INSERM U129, ICGM, PARIS.

We used the Calbindin-D 9k gene as a model for intestinal transcription and tissue-specific hormonal controls. The 9kDa calcium binding protein (CaBP9k or Calbindin-D 9k), thought to be involved in intracellular calcium homeostasis, is mainly synthesized in the intestine, but also in the uterus and the lung of the rat and mouse, and in the mouse kidney. As seen in Figure 1, this synthesis is submitted to transcriptional hormonal controls, which are tissue-specific and species-specific (1-3).

	Intestine	Uterus	Lung		Kidney	
Distribution	ENTEROCYTE	MYOMETRIUM ENDOMETRIUM	ALVEOLAR TYPE II EPITHELIAL CELL		DISTAL EPITHELIAL CELL	
			Rat	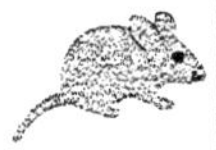 🐭	**Rat**	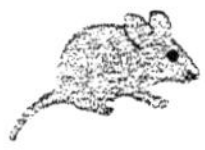 🐭
Abundance	+++++	++++	++	++	±	+++++
Hormonal control	**Vit D**	E$_2$	?	**Vit D**		**Vit D**

Figure 1 : Tissue localization and hormonal controls of rat and mouse CaBP9k

In the intestine, the highest synthesis of CaBP9k lies in the enterocytic epithelial cells, with a concentration gradient along the gastrointestinal tract (3): the CaBP9k gene is actively transcribed in the duodenum, but expression gradually decreases along the jejunum to the ileum, with no expression in the large intestine, except for the cecum. In the villus itself, the abundance of CaBP9k increases from the crypt to the upper part of the villi. In all these segments, the transcription of the gene is strongly activated by 1,25-dihydroxyvitamin D$_3$.

DNase 1 hypersensitivities have been mapped in the rat CaBP9k gene and its regulatory sequences. A cluster of five hypersensitivities (DHS) was found in the proximal promoter of the active gene (in the duodenum and the uterus), including HS4, surrounding the TATA box and major in duodenal chromatin. Another DHS called HS1 has been mapped at –3.5 kbp upstream of the start site, which is major and specific for duodenal chromatin (4).

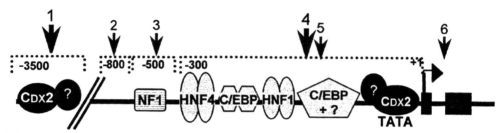

Figure 2: DNase 1 hypersensitivities and transacting factors on the rat calbindin-D 9k regulatory sequences.

We have analyzed these DHS in details and identified several transcription factors bound in the vicinity of these sites (5, 6, and Figure 2). We have found that a combination of intestine-specific (Cdx2), hepatic-enriched (HNF-1, C/EBP and HNF4), and ubiquitous (NF1) factors bind to the CabP9k regulatory sequences and may be important for the rat CaBP9k gene transcription in the intestine. As these informations brought a static view of how the CaBP9k gene is transcribed, our next goal was to use transgenic mice to define in vivo the elements responsible for the intestinal transcription and the vitamin D controlled expression of the CaBP9k gene.

Modular structure of CaBP9k gene promoter in transgenic mice (7)

We first attempted to use targeted oncogenesis to isolate molecular events implicated in the regulation of the CaBP9k gene. SV40 large T antigen was first selected as reporter gene, but some of these transgenic mice died immediately after birth. Consequently, the chloramphenicol acetyltransferase gene was used as a reporter gene. The main results of this study have shown that –117 to +365 base pairs allow a transgene expression in the uterus, that an extension of these sequences to –1011 allow to target in the kidney and the lung. But –4500 regulatory sequences were required to target a transgene expression in the intestine.

We decided to focus on the *cis*-acting elements required for the intestinal transcription of the gene, and particularly on the distal sequences in which the hypersensitive site HS1 and the Cdx2 binding site had been characterized.

The intestinal transcription of 9k transgenes in transgenic mice (5)

The active cell proliferation and turnover of the intestinal epithelium makes this tissue a good experimental model for investigating the nature of regulatory networks that control events such as cell lineage commitment and differentiation. All mature epithelial cell types found in the adult intestine are derived from a nonmigratory stem pool located at the base of the crypts of Lieberkühn. The enterocytes are the most abundant cells in the intestine, accounting for approximately 95% of the mucosal cells of the small intestine. As the enterocyte precursors migrate from the crypts, they stop proliferating and acquire differentiated functions, governed by specific patterns of gene expression, that depend on the cell lineage, state of proliferation of differentiation, and spatial location along the crypt-villus and cephalocaudal (duodenum-colon) axes.

The constructs that we micro-injected are mentioned in Figure 3. With the 9k/-4580 sequences required to target a transgene expression to the intestine, we showed by immunocytochemistry studies that the CAT protein was mainly present in the intestinal villi rather than in the crypts, as is the endogenous CaBP9k protein. The cephalocaudal gradient expression of the transgene was also similar to that of endogenous CaBP9k in the small intestine, with a peak in the duodenum, and reversed in the large intestine, with a peak in the distal colon, while the endogenous CaBP9k is synthesized in the cecum.

The 9k/-117-CAT construct did not target any detectable CAT expression in any part of the intestine. By contrast, juxtaposition of HS1 box and the minimal promoter restored CAT activity in the duodenum. In these 9k/HS1-117-CAT mice, the transgene expression was maximal in the duodenum and the cecum, which correlated more closely with the expression of the endogenous CaBP9k gene. Then, we wondered whether this HS1 region was alone responsible for the intestinal expression of the transgene, by placing this region in front of the ubiquitous promoter of Thymidine Kinase. It was not the case as no CAT activity could be observed in the four mouse lines harbouring this transgene. Thus, the distal activator HS1 acts only on its own promoter: this suggests that there must be a cooperation between the distal HS1 box and the minimal promoter to activate the CaBP9k promoter *in vivo* in the intestine.

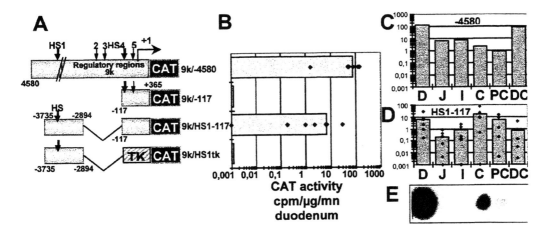

Figure 3: CAT activities of CaBP9k promoter in the intestine of transgenic mice. (A) Diagram showing the transgenes used. (B) CAT transgene expression in the duodena of transgenic mice. Bars represent the mean activities of each line, and each black diamond indicates the value of a single expressing mouse line. (C and D) CAT expression pattern along the length of the intestine D duodenum, I ileum, C cecum, PC proximal colon, DC distal colon. (E) Northern blot analysis of CaBP9k mRNA along the intestine.

A crucial implication for Cdx2 in the intestinal transcription of CaBP9k (5)

Cdx2 is one of the very few transcription factors that is active only in the adult intestinal epithelium, and it appears to be a key element controlling the differentiation of the intestinal epithelium. The functional role of Cdx2 motif *in vivo* was tested by introducing the mutated Cdx2 motif into the 9k/-4580-CAT construct (Figure 4). Six mouse lines carrying the 9k/-4580-Cdxmut-CAT fragment were obtained. Mutation of the distal Cdx2-binding site resulted in a dramatic drop of CAT activity in the duodenum to become over 100-fold decrease than in 9k/-4580-CAT mice. Thus, mutation of the distal Cdx2-binding site leads to a strong reduction of transgene expression in the duodenum. Moreover, this effect is specific for the intestine, as the expression of the transgene in the kidney is not affected by this mutation. Thus, Cdx2 plays a crucial role in the transcription of CaBP9k gene in the intestine.

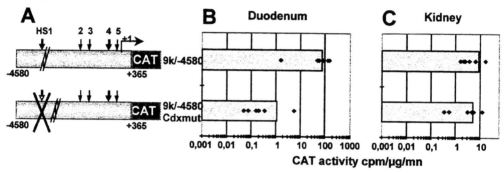

Figure 4 : CAT activity in the intestine of transgenes containing a distal mutated Cdx2 site. (A) Diagram of the transgenes used. The mutation in the Cdx2 site is shown by a black X on this site. (B and C) CAT activity of the transgenes in the duodenum (B) and in the kidney (C).

A hypothesis of transcription of CaBP9k gene in the intestine

We have now developed a working hypothesis for the intestinal transcription of the rat CaBP9k gene (figure 5), based on the two-step model for the chicken beta-globin gene (8).

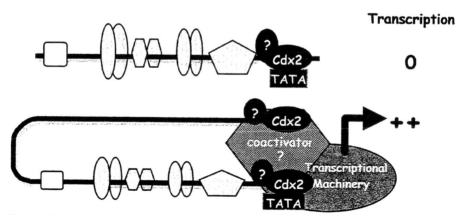

Figure 5 : A two-step hypothesis for the intestinal transcription of the CaBP9k gene.

In step 1, Cdx2 on the proximal promoter is bound to a specialized TATA-box and this impairs binding of the TATA-box Binding Protein (TBP), and blocks gene transcription. In step 2, Cdx2 on the distal promoter lifts this blockade, in cooperation with potential coactivators, and leads to transcription.

Vitamin D induction studies in transgenic mice (9)

The Vitamin D control of CaBP9k gene expression has been shown to be transcriptional (10), and requires the VDR, as shown by the drop of expression of CaBP9k in VDR-null mice (2, 11). However, no consensual VDRE has been identified by computer sequence analysis, and transient transfection assays did not allow us and others to identify a VDRE-like acitvity in CaBP9k gene regulatory sequences (12, 13).

A VDRE has been proposed for the rat CaBP9k gene (from –489 to –445) (14). It confers ony a poor responsiveness to 1,25-dihydroxyvitamin D_3 in transfection studies. Carlberg's group has proposed that the strength of the response might be greatly enhanced by adding thyroid hormone ; they suggest that heterodimerization of VDR and TR is implicated in the hormonal response (15). These data have been recently contradicted by Raval-Pandya *et al.*, who used a double hybrid approach to demonstrate that no direct interaction is possible between VDR and TR, and by Thompson *et al.*, using gel-shift and transfection studies (13, 16). However, all of these studies have been performed *in vitro* and *ex vivo*, and *ex vivo* studies are hampered by the fact that no established intestinal cell line expressing the *CaBP9k* gene is available.

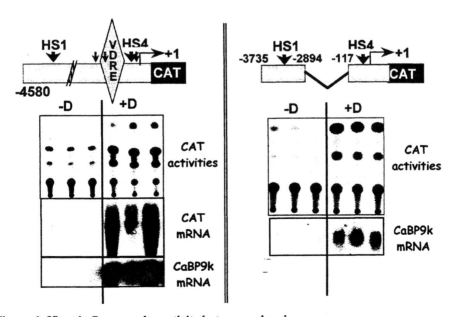

Figure 6: Vitamin D responsive activity in transgenic mice

We therefore decided to study this complex hormonal regulation using a transgenic approach. We looked for potential vitamin D responsive activity in the transgenes from mice harbouring two distinct constructs. As shown in figure 6, with the first full length construct 9k/-4580-CAT, a single injection of 1,25-dihydroxyvitamin D_3 in vitamin D deficient transgenic mice induced CAT transgene activities and mRNA expression similar to the endogenous gene. Thus, the 9k/-4580 sequences contain the elements that allow vitamin D to control CAT expression in the duodenum. The persistence of a strong vitamin D responsiveness of the transgene in the mice harbouring this second construct where an internal deletion has been performed, led us to conclude that this vitamin D responsiveness is located in a two-module region, including HS1 and HS4. This construct does not contain the putative VDRE previously described.

Thus, this hormonal control does not require the element described by Darwish & DeLuca, and is carried by a non conventional vitamin D responsive unit constituted of a two-module region.

Integration site dependence of the responses to vitamin D (9)

We next found that the responsiveness to vitamin D depended on the integration site. For the full-length construct, we assessed the same analysis on two distinct lines (Figure 7).

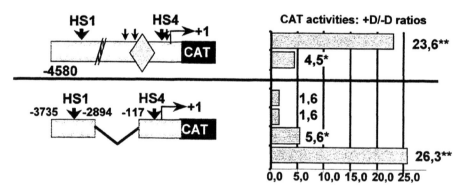

Figure 7 : Integration site dependence of the vitamin D responsiveness. Each bar represents the induction ratio for a mouse line, *p<0,05, **p<0,005

Surprisingly, the responsiveness to 1,25-dihydroxyvitamin D_3 varied greatly, depending on the line tested. Transgene activity in the 9k/-4580 construct can be induced 4-fold to 24-fold by a single injection of 1,25-dihydroxyvitamin D_3. Four distinct transgenic lines have been tested for the two-module region construct. The vitamin D response varied similarly in two lines and no significant ratio could be observed in two other lines.

In summary, the vitamin D responsiveness of CaBP9k transgenes depends greatly on the site of integration of the transgene in the host nucleus. Thus, the activity of this non conventional Vitamin D Response Unit requires interactions with other cis-acting elements, or with a permissive chromatin structure.

Analysis of a mutated putative VDRE (9)

We also tested the real implication of the putative VDRE by mutating it within the whole promoter (Figure 8). We first demonstrated that this mutation did not affect transgene activity in the duodenum or the tissue pattern of expression of the transgene along the cephalocaudal axis of the intestine, and in the kidney and the lung.

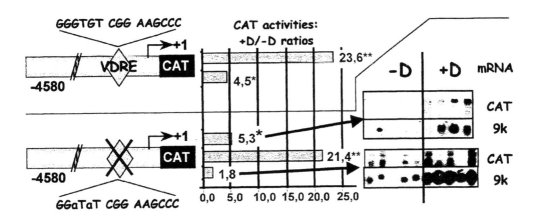

Figure 8 : Vitamin D responsive activity of a putative VDRE

A single injection of 1,25-dihydroxyvitamin D₃ to vitamin D deficient mice harbouring the putative VDRE mutated also produced the same induction of CAT activity as the wild-type construct in two mouse lines. This induction could be seen in CAT activity, as well as in the amount of CAT mRNA. However, as seen before, one mouse line harbouring the mutated VDRE, did not respond to vitamin D, either in CAT activity or in CAT mRNA, although the endogenous gene was correctly induced.

Thus, the putative VDRE in the CaBP9k promoter is not necessary for the *in vivo* response of the rat CaBP9k gene to vitamin D.

Summary

The tissue-restricted expression of CaBP9k gene is programmed by the modular structure of its promoter. We have characterized some cis-acting and trans-acting factors that are important for CaBP9k gene transcription in the intestine. Among these, Cdx2 plays a major role, acting *via* a cooperation of a distal and a proximal binding site, allowing us to define a minimal intestinal promoter.

The sequences responsible for correct crypt-villus and cephalocaudal gradients of intestinal expression have been determined. We have also shown that a two-module region acts as a vitamin D Responsive Unit, which remains to be characterized.

352

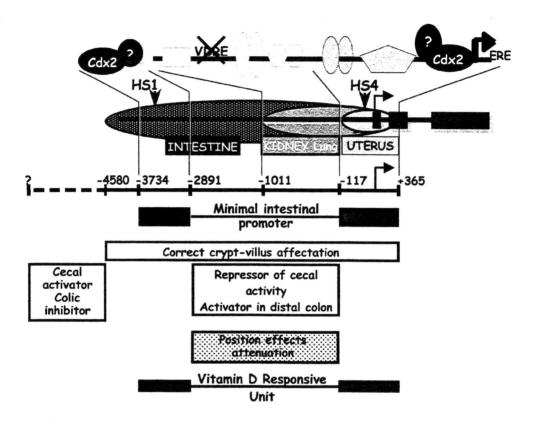

References

1. J. M. Dupret, F. L'Horset, C. Perret, J.-F. Bernaudin, M. Thomasset, *Endocrinology* **131**, 2643-8 (1992).
2. Y. C. Li *et al.*, *Proc Natl Acad Sci U S A* **94**, 9831-5 (1997); Y. C. Li, A. E. Pirro, M. B. Demay, *Endocrinology* **139**, 847-51 (1998).
3. C. Perret, C. Desplan, M. Thomasset, *Eur J Biochem* **150**, 211-7 (1985).
4. C. Perret, F. L'Horset, M. Thomasset, *Gene* **108**, 227-35 (1991).
5. S. Colnot *et al.*, *J Biol Chem* **273**, 31939-46 (1998).
6. M. Lambert *et al.*, *Eur J Biochem* **236**, 778-88 (1996).
7. B. Romagnolo *et al.*, *J Biol Chem* **271**, 16820-6 (1996).
8. M. C. Barton, N. Madani, B. M. Emerson, *Proc Natl Acad Sci U S A* **94**, 7257-62 (1997).
9. S. Colnot *et al.*, *Endocrinology* **In Press** (2000).
10. J. M. Dupret *et al.*, *J Biol Chem* **262**, 16553-7 (1987).
11. T. Yoshizawa *et al.*, *Nat Genet* **16**, 391-6 (1997).
12. C. Perret *et al.*, in *Vitamin D. A pluripotent steroid hormone: Structural studies, molecular endocrinology and clinical applications* A. Norman, R. Bouillon, M. Thomasset, Eds. (de Gruyter, Berlin, 1994) pp. 385-393.
13. P. D. Thompson *et al.*, *J Cell Biochem* **75**, 462-480 (1999).
14. H. M. Darwish, H. F. DeLuca, *Proc Natl Acad Sci USA* **89**, 603-7 (1992).
15. M. Schräder, K. M. Muller, S. Nayeri, J. P. Kahlen, C. Carlberg, *Nature* **370**, 382-6 (1994).
16. M. Raval-Pandya, L. P. Freedman, H. Li, S. Christakos, *Mol Endocrinol* **12**, 1367-79 (1998).

INTRANUCLEAR TRAFFICKING OF TRANSCRIPTION FACTORS: REQUIREMENTS FOR VITAMIN D-MEDIATED BIOLOGICAL CONTROL

Gary S. Stein*, Jane B. Lian*, André J. van Wijnen*, Janet L. Stein*, Martin Montecino[1], Je Choi[2], Jitesh Pratap*, Amjad Javed*, Kaleem Zaidi*
*Department of Cell Biology, University of Massachusetts Medical School, Worcester, Massachusetts
[1] Department of Molecular Biology, University of Concepcion, Concepcion, Chile
[2] Medical Research Institute, Kyungpook National University Hospital, Taegu, Korea

Introduction While the mechanisms that govern gene expression remain to be formally defined, there is growing awareness that fidelity of gene regulation necessitates coordination of the spatial organization of genes and regulatory proteins within the three-dimensional context of nuclear architecture. Mechanisms include transcription factor synthesis, nuclear import and retention, post-translational modifications of factors, and directing factors to subnuclear sites that support gene expression. Remodeling of chromatin and nucleosome organization to accommodate requirements for protein-DNA and protein-protein interactions at promoter elements are key to physiological control of transcription. The reconfiguration of gene promoters and assembly of specialized subnuclear domains reflect the orchestration of both regulated and regulatory mechanisms. From a biological perspective, each component of nuclear organization is linked to structure-function interrelationships that mediate transcription and processing of gene transcripts. The complexities of nuclear biochemistry and morphology provide the required specificity for physiological responsiveness to a broad spectrum of signaling pathways to modulate transcription under diverse circumstances. Equally important, evidence is accruing that modifications in nuclear architecture and nuclear structure-function interrelationships accompany and appear to be causally related to compromised gene expression under pathological conditions.

We will present an overview of the conceptual and experimental basis for involvement of multiple parameters of nuclear architecture in vitamin D-mediated transcriptional control. Pathways involved with the recruitment of factors to subnuclear sites where transcription occurs will be addressed within the context of assembly and activation of regulatory factor complexes that are required to initiate, sustain and suppress transcription of genes controlled by vitamin D. Consequences of abrogated nuclear architecture for aberrant transcription will be explored.

Multiple Levels of Nuclear Organization Support Fidelity of Gene Expression
Sequence Organization: Appreciation is occurring for the high density of information in both regulatory and mRNA coding sequences of cell growth and phenotypic genes. The osteocalcin gene promoter provides a paradigm for developmental and steroid hormone (vitamin D) responsive transcriptional control. The osteocalcin gene encodes a 10 kBa bone-specific protein that is induced in late stage osteoblasts at the onset of extracellular matrix mineralization (1,2). Transcription of the osteocalcin gene is controlled by a modularly organized promoter with proximal basal regulatory sequences

and distal hormone-responsive enhancer elements (3-12). Overlapping recognition elements expand the options for responsiveness to signaling cascades that mediate mutually exclusive protein/DNA and protein/protein interactions. Developmental and vitamin D-associated activity have been shown to involve mutual exclusive occupancy of the VDRE by the vitamin D receptor/RXR heterodimer or YY1 as well as mutual exclusive protein-protein interactions of TF2B with the vitamin D receptor or YY1 (12,13). Splice variants for gene transcripts further enhance the specificity of gene expression. However, the linear order of genes and flanking regulatory elements is necessary but insufficient to support gene expression under in vivo biological conditions. There is a requirement to integrate the regulatory information at independent promoter elements and selectively utilize subsets of promoter regulatory information to control the extent to which genes are activated and/or suppressed.

Chromatin Organization: Chromatin structure and nucleosome organization provide architectural linkages between gene organization and components of transcriptional control. Nucleosomal organization reduces distances between promoter elements that support synergism and responsiveness to multiple signaling pathways. Equally important, it has been well established that the presence of nucleosomes generally blocks the accessibility of transcription factors to their cognate binding sequences (14).

Alterations in the chromatin organization of the osteocalcin gene are functionally linked to vitamin D-dependent and phenotype-specific gene expression (15,16). Figure 1 schematically depicts modifications in chromatin structure and nucleosome organization that parallel competency for transcription and the extent to which the osteocalcin gene is transcribed. Changes are observed in response to physiological mediators of basal expression and steroid hormone responsiveness. This remodeling of chromatin provides a basis for the involvement of nuclear architecture in growth factor and steroid hormone-responsive control of osteocalcin gene expression during osteoblast phenotype development and in differentiated bone cells. Basal expression and enhancement of osteocalcin gene transcription are accompanied by two changes in the structural properties of chromatin. DNase I hypersensitivity of sequences flanking the basal, tissue-specific element and the vitamin D enhancer element are observed (15-17). Together with changes in nucleosome placement (16), accessibility of transactivation factors to basal and steroid hormone-dependent regulatory sequences can be explained. In early stage proliferating normal diploid osteoblasts, when the osteocalcin gene is repressed, nucleosomes are placed in the proximal basal domain and in the vitamin D responsive enhancer promoter sequences. Nuclease hypersensitive sites are not present in the vicinity of these regulatory elements. In contrast, when osteocalcin gene expression is transcriptionally upregulated postproliferatively and vitamin D-mediated enhancement of transcription occurs, the proximal basal and upstream steroid hormone responsive enhancer sequences

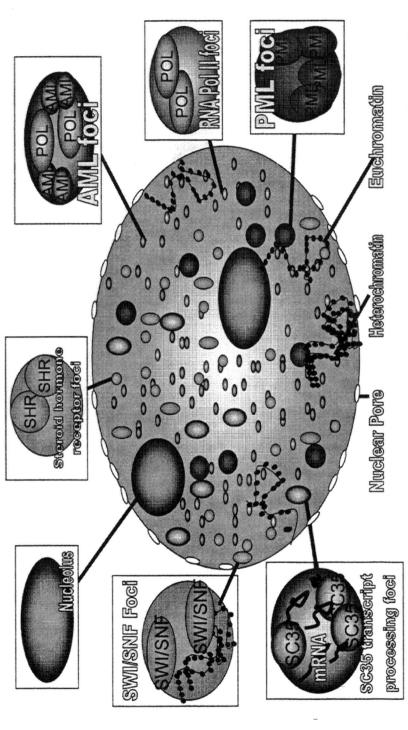

Figure 1: Multiple functionally and spatially distinct intranuclear domains support gene expression within the context of nuclear architecture. Transcription of protein-encoding genes by RNA polymerase II occurs at a large number of foci, and rRNA transcription by RNA polymerase I is restricted to one or more nucleoli. Both types of transcriptional foci are distinct from sites involved in DNA replication. Gene regulatory factors (e.g. AML, hormone receptors), chromatin-remodeling proteins (e.g. SWI/SNF), and processing factors (e.g. SC35) are organized into discrete subnuclear foci, a subset of which is associated with RNA polymerase II, depending on biological conditions. Chromatin-remodeling proteins mediate the transition between transcriptionally inactive 'closed' chromatin (heterochromatin) and active 'open' chromatin (euchromatin) through a series of enzyme-mediated regulatory steps. The nuclear pores function in the nuclear import of regulatory proteins containing nuclear localization signals (NLSs). Intranuclear trafficking of proteins through subnuclear foci associated with the nuclear matrix involves specific nuclear-matrix-targeting signals (NMTSs). PML domains are specialized subnuclear domains that are rearranged in promyelocytic leukemias. SC35 domains contain RNA-splicing factors that generate mature mRNA transcripts.

become nucleosome free and these regulatory domains are flanked by Dnase I hypersensitive sites.

We are gaining insight into mechanisms mediating chromatin remodeling of the osteocalcin gene promoter that determine competency for vitamin D-dependent transcriptional enhancement. RUNX/AML/CBFA sites that flank the VDRE have been shown by mutational analysis to be required for both steroid hormone dependent chromatin remodeling and upregulation of transcription (18). Association of RUNX/AML/CBFA with histone acetyltransferases is consistent with recruitment of factors that modify nucleosomal organization. There is growing awareness of modifications in chromatin organization that render gene regulatory sequences selectively accessible to factors that activate suppression in a physiologically responsive manner.

Intranuclear Trafficking: An understanding of interrelationships between nuclear structure and gene expression necessitates knowledge of the composition, organization and regulation of sites within the nucleus that are dedicated to replication, transcription and processing of gene transcripts. The subnuclear distribution of transcription factors appears to be important for fidelity of transcriptional control (Figure 2).

The RUNX/AML/CBFA transcription factors that support hematopoietic and bone tissue-specific gene expression have provided a paradigm for directly examining mechanisms that target regulatory factors to subnuclear sites that support transcription. We have addressed how the RUNX/AML/CBFA transcription factors are directed to nuclear matrix-associated intranuclear domains by functional biochemical and in situ immunofluorescence analysis of RUNX/AML/CBFA deletion and point mutations. Our results indicate that 1) sequences required for targeting the RUNX/AML/CBFA factors to nuclear matrix-associated sites reside in a 31 amino acid segment within the C-terminus that is physically distinct from the nuclear localization signal; 2) nuclear matrix-association of RUNX/AML/CBFA factors is independent of DNA binding activities; 3) the principal active and inactive splice variants of the RUNX/AML/CBFA transcription factors are differentially localized within the nucleus; and 4) the nuclear matrix targeting signal of RUNX/AML/CBFA factors function autonomously. A unique sequence structure based on X-ray crystallography (19,20) for the RUNX/AML/CBFA intranuclear targeting sequence is consistent with specificity for recognition of subnuclear regulatory complexes. Our findings demonstrate that at least two trafficking signals are required for subnuclear targeting of the RUNX/AML/CBFA transcription factors; the first supports nuclear import and the second mediates association with the nuclear matrix. Recent results provide insights into the functional consequences of directing transcription factors to the nuclear matrix. It has been shown that the 31 amino acid nuclear matrix targeting signal of the RUNX/AML/CBFA transcription factor targets the regulatory protein to a subnuclear domain that supports transcription. Colocalization of RUNX/AML/CBFA with transcriptionally active RNA polymerase II has been demonstrated as well as the requirements for a functional DNA binding domain

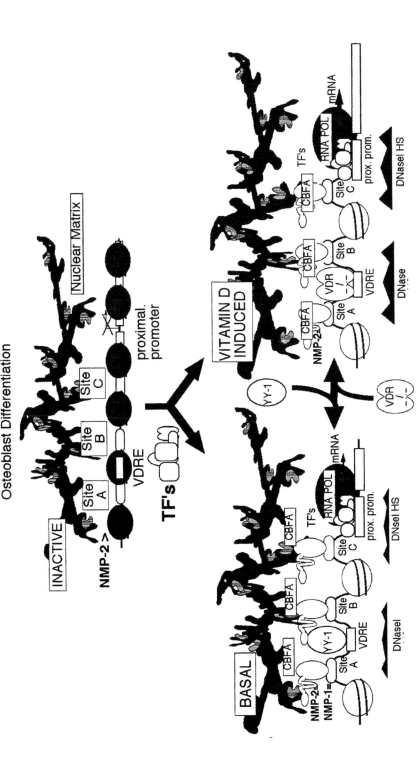

Figure 2: Schematic representation of the osteocalcin gene promoter organization and occupancy of regulatory elements by cognate transcription factors that support suppression of transcription in proliferating osteoblasts; activation of expression in differentiated cells (upper panel), or enhancement of transcription by vitamin D (lower panels). Remodeling of chromatin structure and nucleosome organization to support suppression, basal and vitamin D induced transcription of the osteocalcin gene is indicated. The location and magnitude of DNase I hypersensitive sites are designated by solid triangles. The lower panels illustrate the positioning of nucleosomes at sites within the osteocalcin gene promoter and gene-nuclear matrix interactions. The lower right panels show the three dimensional organization of the osteocalcin gene promoter under basal and steroid hormone-enhanced transcriptional control.

and ongoing transcription (21). Functional implications for nuclear matrix association of RUNX/AML/CBFA transcription factors is more directly provided by establishing that targeting to the nuclear matrix is obligatory for maximal transactivation activity (22).

Linkages of Nuclear Architecture to Pathological Control of Gene Expression

Targeting of gene regulatory factors to specific intranuclear sites may be critical for accurate control of gene expression. The acute myelogenous leukemia 8;21 (RUNX1/CBFA2/AML1/ETO) fusion protein is encoded by a rearranged gene created by the ETO chromosomal translocation. This protein lacks the nuclear matrix-targeting signal that directs the RUNX1/CBFA2/AML1 protein to appropriate gene regulatory sites within the nucleus. We observe that substitution of the chromosome 8-derived ETO protein for the multifunctional C-terminus of RUNX1/CBFA2/AML1 precludes targeting of the factor to RUNX1/CBFA2/AML1 subnuclear domains. Instead, the RUNX1/CBFA2/AML1/ETO fusion protein is redirected by the ETO component to alternate nuclear matrix-associated foci. Our results link the ETO chromosomal translocation in RUNX1/CBFA2/AML1 with modifications in the intranuclear trafficking of a key hematopoietic regulatory factor. These results indicate that misrouting of gene regulatory factors as a consequence of chromosomal translocations is an important characteristic of acute leukemias (23).

We carried out in vivo genetic mutation of the RUNX2/AML3/CBFA1 osteogenic transcription factor by introducing a stop codon into exon 7 at amino acid 376 to prevent translation of the C-terminal domain containing the intranuclear targeting signal. The mutant protein is expressed and exhibits DNA binding activity but is compromised in transactivation and subnuclear targeting. Homozygous mutant mice have skeletal abnormalities similar to those observed when the gene is completely ablated. The mutation causes prenatal lethality and complete absence of intramembranous bone as well as minimal mineralization of the ribs and limbs. Heterozygotes show complete absence of clavicles but normal development of limb and craniofacial bones. Thus, the C-terminus of RUNX2/AML3/CBFA1 is critical for in vivo bone formation. The transcriptional regulatory activity and subnuclear targeting signal within the C-terminus, apart from DNA binding, are essential for the biological function of RUNX2/AML3/CBFA1 in skeletal development.

Conclusions An inclusive model for all steps in the targeting of proteins to subnuclear sites cannot yet be proposed. However, this model must account for the apparent diversity of intranuclear targeting signals. It is also important to assess the extent to which regulatory discrimination is mediated by subnuclear domain-specific trafficking signals. Furthermore, the checkpoints that monitor subnuclear distribution of regulatory factors and the sorting steps that ensure both structural and functional fidelity of nuclear domains in which replication and expression of genes occur must be biochemically and mechanistically defined.

There is emerging recognition that placement of regulatory components of gene expression must be temporally and spatially coordinated to facilitate biological control.

The consequences of breaches in nuclear structure-function relationships are observed in an expanding series of diseases that include cancer (21,23-28) and neurological disorders (29). As the repertoire of architecture-associated regulatory factors and cofactors expands, there is increasing confidence that nuclear organization contributes significantly to control of transcription. To gain increased appreciation for the complexities of subnuclear organization and gene regulation, we must continue to characterize mechanisms that direct regulatory proteins to specific transcription sites within the nucleus so that these proteins are in the right place at the right time.

Acknowledgments The authors thank Elizabeth Bronstein for editorial assistance with the preparation of the manuscript. Studies reported were supported by grants from the National Institutes of Health (AR39588, AR45688, AR45689, DE12528, TW00990). The contents are solely the responsibility of the authors and do not necessarily represent the official views of the National Institutes of Health.

References

1. Aronow, M. A., Gerstenfeld, L. C., Owen, T. A., Tassinari, M. S., Stein, G. S., and Lian, J. B. (1990) *J.Cell.Physiol.* **143,** 213-221
2. Owen, T. A., Aronow, M., Shalhoub, V., Barone, L. M., Wilming, L., Tassinari, M. S., Kennedy, M. B., Pockwinse, S., Lian, J. B., and Stein, G. S. (1990) *J.Cell.Physiol.* **143,** 420-430
3. Hoffmann, H. M., Catron, K. M., van Wijnen, A. J., McCabe, L. R., Lian, J. B., Stein, G. S., and Stein, J. L. (1994) *Proc.Natl.Acad.Sci.USA* **91,** 12887-12891
4. Towler, D. A., Bennett, C. D., and Rodan, G. A. (1994) *Mol.Endocrinol.* **8,** 614-624
5. Tamura, M. and Noda, M. (1994) *J Cell Biol.* **126,** 773-782
6. Merriman, H. L., van Wijnen, A. J., Hiebert, S., Bidwell, J. P., Fey, E., Lian, J., Stein, J., and Stein, G. S. (1995) *Biochemistry* **34,** 13125-13132
7. Ducy, P. and Karsenty, G. (1995) *Mol.Cell.Biol.* **15,** 1858-1869
8. Banerjee, C., Hiebert, S. W., Stein, J. L., Lian, J. B., and Stein, G. S. (1996) *Proc.Natl.Acad.Sci.USA* **93,** 4968-4973
9. Bortell, R., Owen, T. A., Bidwell, J. P., Gavazzo, P., Breen, E., van Wijnen, A. J., DeLuca, H. F., Stein, J. L., Lian, J. B., and Stein, G. S. (1992) *Proc.Natl.Acad.Sci.USA* **89,** 6119-6123
10. Demay, M. B., Gerardi, J. M., DeLuca, H. F., and Kronenberg, H. M. (1990) *Proc.Natl.Acad.Sci.USA* **87,** 369-373
11. Markose, E. R., Stein, J. L., Stein, G. S., and Lian, J. B. (1990) *Proc.Natl.Acad.Sci.USA* **87,** 1701-1705
12. Guo, B., Odgren, P. R., van Wijnen, A. J., Last, T. J., Nickerson, J., Penman, S., Lian, J. B., Stein, J. L., and Stein, G. S. (1995) *Proc.Natl.Acad.Sci.USA* **92,** 10526-10530
13. Guo, B., Aslam, F., van Wijnen, A. J., Roberts, S. G. E., Frenkel, B., Green, M., DeLuca, H., Lian, J. B., Stein, G. S., and Stein, J. L. (1997) *Proc.Natl.Acad.Sci.USA* **94,** 121-126

14. Workman, J. L. and Kingston, R. E. (1998) *Annu.Rev Biochem* **67:545-79,** 545-579

15. Montecino, M., Pockwinse, S., Lian, J., Stein, G., and Stein, J. (1994) *Biochemistry* **33,** 348-353

16. Montecino, M., Lian, J., Stein, G., and Stein, J. (1996) *Biochemistry* **35,** 5093-5102

17. Breen, E. C., van Wijnen, A. J., Lian, J. B., Stein, G. S., and Stein, J. L. (1994) *Proc.Natl.Acad.Sci.USA* **91,** 12902-12906

18. Javed, A., Gutierrez, S., Montecino, M., van Wijnen, A. J., Stein, J. L., Stein, G. S., and Lian, J. B. (1999) *Mol.Cell.Biol.* **19,** 7491-7500

19. Tang, L., Guo, B., Javed, A., Choi, J.-Y., Hiebert, S., Lian, J. B., van Wijnen, A. J., Stein, J. L., Stein, G. S., and Zhou, G. W. (1999) *J.Biol.Chem.* **274,** 33580-33586

20. Tang, L., Guo, B., van Wijnen, A. J., Lian, J. B., Stein, J. L., Stein, G. S., and Zhou, G. W. (1998) *J.Struct.Biol.* **123,** 83-85

21. Zeng, C., McNeil, S., Pockwinse, S., Nickerson, J. A., Shopland, L., Lawrence, J. B., Penman, S., Hiebert, S. W., Lian, J. B., van Wijnen, A. J., Stein, J. L., and Stein, G. S. (1998) *Proc.Natl.Acad.Sci.USA* **95,** 1585-1589

22. Zeng, C., van Wijnen, A. J., Stein, J. L., Meyers, S., Sun, W., Shopland, L., Lawrence, J. B., Penman, S., Lian, J. B., Stein, G. S., and Hiebert, S. W. (1997) *Proc.Natl.Acad.Sci.USA* **94,** 6746-6751

23. McNeil, S., Zeng, C., Harrington, K. S., Hiebert, S., Lian, J. B., Stein, J. L., van Wijnen, A. J., and Stein, G. S. (1999) *Proc.Natl.Acad.Sci.U.S.A.* **96,** 14882-14887

24. Rowley, J. D. (1998) *Annu.Rev Genet.* **32:495-519,** 495-519

25. Rogaia, D., Grignani, F., Carbone, R., Riganelli, D., LoCoco, F., Nakamura, T., Croce, C. M., Di Fiore, P. P., and Pelicci, P. G. (1997) *Cancer Res.* **57,** 799-802

26. Tao, W. and Levine, A. J. (1999) *Proc.Natl.Acad.Sci.U.S.A* **96,** 3077-3080

27. Weis, K., Rambaud, S., Lavau, C., Jansen, J., Carvalho, T., Carmo-Fonseca, M., Lamond, A., and Dejean, A. (1994) *Cell* **76,** 345-356

28. Yano, T., Nakamura, T., Blechman, J., Sorio, C., Dang, C. V., Geiger, B., and Canaani, E. (1997) *Proc.Natl.Acad.Sci.U.S.A.* **94,** 7286-7291

29. Skinner, P. J., Koshy, B. T., Cummings, C. J., Klement, I. A., Helin, K., Servadio, A., Zoghbi, H. Y., and Orr, H. T. (1997) *Nature* **389,** 971-974

NUCLEAR INTERACTIONS BETWEEN STAT1α AND THE VITAMIN D RECEPTOR MEDIATE THE INHIBITORY EFFECTS Of γ-INTERFERON ON 1α,25-DIHYDROXIVITAMIN D ACTION

Marcos Vidal and Adriana S. Dusso. Renal Division, Washington University School of Medicine, St. Louis. MO. USA 63110.

Introduction The hypercalcemia of sarcoidosis, tuberculosis, and several granulomatoses is caused by high serum 1α,25-dihydroxyvitaminD (1,25D) levels, which result from an enhanced production of 1,25D by the disease-activated macrophage, and a loss of the capacity of 1,25D to suppress its own synthesis (1α–hydroxylase) and to induce its degradation (24-hydroxylase). This phenomenon can be reproduced in vitro by incubation of macrophages, monocytes or the human monocytic cell line THP-1 with the cytokine gamma interferon (γ–IFN). γ–IFN inhibits 1,25D induction of 24-hydroxylase mRNA without affecting 1,25D binding to the VDR or the stability of the 24-hydroxylase mRNA, suggesting an inhibitory effect of the cytokine on 1,25D induction of 24-hydroxylase gene transcription (1). Most transcriptional responses to γ–IFN involve activation of Stat1. Previous studies in our laboratory suggested that γ–IFN-activated Stat1-homodimer interact directly or indirectly (via CBP/p300) with the vitamin D receptor (VDR), reducing the binding of endogenous nuclear VDR/RXR heterodimer to vitamin D responsive elements (VDRE) in the 24-hydroxylase-promoter (2). In the present studies, we demonstrate a role for Stat1 in γ–IFN inhibition of VDR/RXR binding to a VDRE and show that VDR-Stat1 interactions affect Stat1-homodimer binding to γ–IFN-activation sequence (GAS).

Results & Discussion To test whether Stat1 was necessary for γ–IFN to reduce VDR/RXR binding to the VDRE, we utilized the human fribrosarcoma cell line U3A. U3A cells lack Stat1 mRNA and protein (3). Western blot analysis

362

demonstrated that U3A cells express the VDR and respond to 1,25D by increasing nuclear VDR content. Figure 1 shows the results of Electrophoretic Mobility Shift Assays (EMSA) utilizing nuclear extracts (NE) from U3A cells and the proximal 24-hydroxylase VDRE (4) as a probe. In the absence of Stat1, γ–IFN (100 IU/ml) had no effect on endogenous VDR/RXR binding to VDRE (U3A cells, compare lanes 2 and 4). Moreover, the reduction in binding of VDR/RXR to the VDRE in response to γ–IFN was restored in NE from U3A cells stably transfected with a Stat1 expression vector (compare lanes 6 and 8). Clearly, γ–IFN inhibition of VDR/RXR binding to the VDRE requires Stat1.

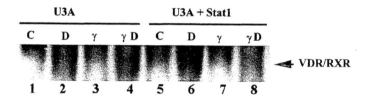

Figure 1. Stat1 mediates γ–IFN reduction of VDR/RXR binding to VDRE.

The demonstration that Stat1 mediates the reduction in VDR/RXR binding to VDRE led us to investigate whether 1,25D treatment affected the binding of Stat1 -homodimer to GAS. EMSA studies using NE from THP-1 cells and a consensus GAS sequence as a probe show (Figure 2a) that simultaneous treatment with γ–IFN (100 IU/ml) and 1,25D (50 nM) (γD) reduced the binding of Stat1-homodimer to GAS compared to that of cells treated with γ–IFN alone (γ). A higher molecular weight GAS binding complex, identified as B1, increased when cells were treated with γ–IFN and 1,25 D compared to cells treated with γ–IFN alone. Stat1-homodimer and B1 specifically bind GAS, as demonstrated by no co-migrating bands (far right lane) when utilizing a mutant GAS sequence as a probe. The binding to GAS of the B1 complex is specifically competed if

NE from γD treated cells are incubated with an excess of radioinert VDRE before GAS probe addition, which suggests that the VDR is present in B1 (Compare lanes γD and γD +VDRE in <u>Figure 1B</u>).

The B1 complex was also formed by a mixture of NE from cells treated with 1,25D only or γ–IFN only (γ+D). This suggests that independent activation of nuclear Stat1 and VDR was sufficient for B1-GAS interacting complex formation.

We utilized the EMSA coupled with immunoblot technique (5) to analyze the protein components of B1 complex. <u>Figure 1C</u> shows that both Stat1 and the VDR are part of B1 GAS-binding complex. The negative controls are pieces cut from the EMSA gel that contained no bands. The positive control is a NE from γD treated THP-1 cells.

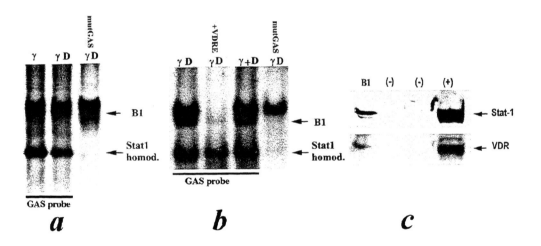

Figure 2. Effects of 1,25D treatment on the binding of Stat1 -homodimer binding to GAS.

In summary, these results suggest that nuclear interactions between ligand activated VDR and γ–IFN activated Stat1 prevent the binding of VDR/RXR heterodimers to the proximal VDRE of the human 24-hydroxylase promoter. This reduction in binding could explain the inability of 1,25D to induce its own degradation in disease-activated macrophages. On the other hand, the ability of the VDR-Stat1-containing complex to bind GAS suggests a potential for ligand activated VDR to modulate γ–IFN-regulated genes and a biological role for the increased 1,25 D production by activated macrophages in inflammatory processes.

References

1. Dusso, A.S., Kamimura, S., Gallieni, M., Zhong, M., Negrea, L., Shapiro, S. and Slatopolsky E. (1997). *J Clin Endocrinol Metab* **82**, 2222-2232.

2. Dusso, A.S.(1999). *J Bone Min Res* **14**: S168.

3. McKendy, R., John, J. Flavell, D., Muller, M., Kerr, I.M. and Stark, G.R. (1991). *Proc Natl Acad Sci USA* **24**:11455-9.

4. Chen, K.S. and DeLuca H.F. (1995) *Biochimica et Biophysica Acta* 1263:1-9.

5. Osborn, M.T., Herrin, K., Buzen, F.G., Hurlburt, B.K. and Chambers, T.C. (1999). *Biotechniques* **27**:887-892.

SELECTIVE UP- AND DOWN-REGULATION OF ENAMEL MATRIX PROTEINS BY 1α,25(OH)₂ VITAMIN D₃ IN RAT INCISOR ENAMEL

Petros Papagerakis,[*][§] Isabelle Bailleul-Forestier,[*] Martine Oboeuf,[*] Nicole Mauro,[*] Mary MacDougal,[§] and Ariane Berdal[*][‡] [*] : Laboratoire Biologie-Odontologie, Faculté de Chirurgie Dentaire, Université Paris VII, Paris, 75006, France; [§] : UTHSCSA, Pediatric Dentistry Dpt, San Antonio, Texas, USA; [‡] : Faculté de Chirurgie Dentaire, Université Paris V, Montrouge, 92120, France.

Introduction Tooth development is dependent on coordinated expression of many genes, some of which are unique to the developing tooth (1). Amelogenins and ameloblastin are both mainly expressed in the enamel-producing ameloblasts and in the developing enamel matrix (2). Immunohistochemistry of the developing enamel matrix from rat shows a specific localization of amelogenin proteins in the rod and interrod enamel and a relative absence in the sheath area which partially surrounds each enamel rod (3). In contrast, ameloblastin protein is observed specifically in the interprismatique enamel (3). Enamel dysplasia is a phenotypic trait commonly found in vitamin D-deficient and hereditary rickets (4). The present study aims to explore the potential control by 1α,25(OH)₂ vitamin D₃ (1,25(OH)₂D₃) of the major enamel proteins, i.e. amelogenins and ameloblastin, in an experimental vitamin D-deficient (-D) rat model. Our present hypothesis was that rachitic dental dysplasia is related to disturbances in the amelogenin and/or ameloblastin pathways during enamel formation.

Materials and methods Incisors and molars of vitamin D-deficient and control Spragey-Dawley rats were investigated by northern-blotting and transmission electron microscopy, as previously described (5, 6, 7). For molecular studies 3 week-old male rats (n=60) were kept for five weeks under UV light-free conditions and were given a vitamin D-deficient diet (-D rats). For ultrastructural studies vitamin D-deficient rats (n=140) were raised from vitamin D-deficient mothers, housed in a dark room and fed ad libitum with a vitamin D-deficient diet. In addition, animals (n=40), fed with a standard diet, were used as controls (+D).

Results Striking differences were observed between control (+D) and vitamin D-deficient rat (-D) enamel organs. The steady state mRNA levels were different between –D et +D animals (Fig. 1). More precisely, amelogenins mRNA expression appeared to be dramatically reduced in -D rats when compared to +D rats (Fig. 1). In contrast, ameloblastin mRNA steady state level was increased in –D animals (Fig. 1). In addition, vitamin D-deficient animals were given one intraperitoneally injection of 1,25(OH)₂D₃, and sacrificed 8 or 24 h after administration and compared to vehicle-injected animals. Quantitative analysis of 4 separate sets of pooled enamel organs showed repeated differences between different groups. More precisely, 8 and 24 hours after a single injection of 1,25(OH)$_2$D$_3$ in -D rats, an up-regulation of amelogenin mRNA levels and a down-regulation of ameloblastin mRNAs levels were observed (not shown).

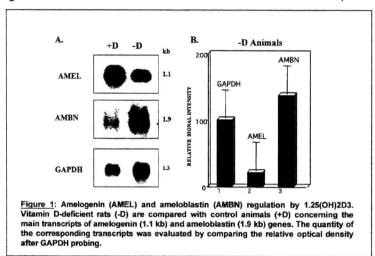

Figure 1: Amelogenin (AMEL) and ameloblastin (AMBN) regulation by 1.25(OH)2D3. Vitamin D-deficient rats (-D) are compared with control animals (+D) concerning the main transcripts of amelogenin (1.1 kb) and ameloblastin (1.9 kb) genes. The quantity of the corresponding transcripts was evaluated by comparing the relative optical density after GAPDH probing.

Furthermore, +D and -D rat enamel exhibited morphogenetic differences in the organisation of enamel prisms and distal secretory processes of ameloblasts (Fig. 2). More specifically, the intraprismatic regions of the enamel prisms were almost absent in enamel from -D rats.

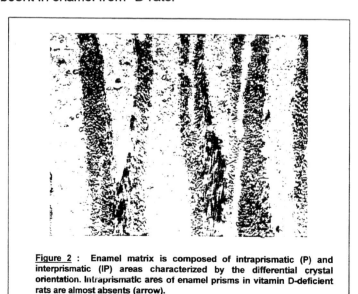

Figure 2 : Enamel matrix is composed of intraprismatic (P) and interprismatic (IP) areas characterized by the differential crystal orientation. Intraprismatic ares of enamel prisms in vitamin D-deficient rats are almost absents (arrow).

Discussion The properties of enamel are acquired through a summation of regulated expression of structural genes required for enamel formation. Thus, identifying the molecular events controlling gene expression of enamel matrix proteins is an important issue to elucidate the composition of these proteins in the enamel extracellular matrix and their potential functions.

Enamel dysplasia is commonly found in genetic diseases and also as a clinical data of many systemic disturbances, such as vitamin D rickets (4). Amelogenesis imperfecta (AI), is a clinically and genetically heterogeneous pathology showing several different types of enamel dysplasia. Alterations in the human amelogenin gene are related to several reported X-linked forms of AI (8). In addition, one autosomal-dominant form of AI was linked to a 4-megabase region on chromosome 4q21 (9), containing the ameloblastin gene (10). The enamel phenotype of these subjects shows enhanced similarities with rachitic enamel observed in rickets (4, 7). Therefore, our hypothesis was that amelogenins and ameloblastin play a key-role in the control of enamel formation by vitamin D.

Enamel is formed by the elaboration of tissue-specific extracellular matrix proteins that direct the deposition of the hydroxyapatite crystallites (3). It is critical, therefore, to investigate when and where enamel-specific proteins are expressed and secreted into the matrix and where they regulate interactions during the process of enamel biomineralization (11). Previous studies provide evidence that amelogenins are present especially in intraprismatic areas of enamel (3). On the other hand, ameloblastin seem to be accumulated in the interprismatique areas, nearby the crystal growth sites of the developing enamel (3). The function of enamel proteins during amelogenesis has been investigated in vitro and in vivo. Laboratory experiments blocking or disturbing amelogenin expression result in distinctive enamel disruptions (12, 13). All these data support the notion that amelogenins contribute to enamel prism morphogenesis and mineralization. In contrast, the nascent ameloblastin protein is hypothesized to play a role in enamel crystal formation (11). In this study, electron microscope investigation, in the vitamin D-deficient animals, identified ultrastructural enamel dysplasia involving a selective decrease in intraprismatic enamel. This finding suggest that specific dysplasia of rachitic enamel (decrease of intraprismatic enamel) is secondary to vitamin D dysregulation of amelogenins and/or ameloblastin expression at a transcriptional and/or a post-transcriptional level.

Cells devoted to enamel formation have been shown to express VDR and thus to be potentially under the control of the main metabolite, $1,25(OH)_2D_3$ (4). Matrix proteins of mineralized tissues studied so far have been shown to be sensitive to vitamin D action, for instance osteocalcin (14). Therefore, the main enamel matrix proteins have also been shown to be under the influence of vitamin D action (7, this study). Our data suggest that amelogenin and ameloblastin genes are sensitive to the hormonal control of $1,25(OH)_2D_3$, presumably via a VDR genomic pathway as shown previously for calbindin-D_{28k} in tooth (6) and in other systems (15). Other consensus sequences for the binding of transcription regulatory factors have been identified in murine (16), and bovine (17), amelogenin, suggesting that other factors regulate amelogenin expression. In addition, murine ameloblastin promoter region has been sequenced recently and evidences for regulatory regions have been shown (11).

Taken together, this data suggest that vitamin D selectively controls the expression of amelogenins and ameloblastin rat genes. In addition, functional correlations were shown between this selective up- (amelogenins) and down-(ameloblastin) regulation and the observed structure of enamel. In conclusion, this study constitutes a first analysis of tooth-specific genes regulation which extends the vitamin D targets to non-collagenous enamel proteins.

References 1. Thesleff, I., and Sharpe, P. (1997) Mech. Dev. 67, 111-123.

2. Zeichner-David, M., Vo, H., Tan, H., Diekwisch, T., Berman, B., Thiemann, F., Alcocer, M.D., Hsu, P., Wang, T., Eyna, J., Caton, J., Slavkin, H.C., and M. MacDougall. (1997) Int. J. Dev. Biol. 41, 27-38.

3. Nanci, A., Zalzal, S., Lavoie, P., Kunikata, M., Chen, W., Kresbach, P.H. Yamada, Y., Hammarstrom, L., Simmer, J.P., Fincham, A.G., Snead M.L., and Smith, C.E. (1998) J. Histochem. Cytochem. 46, 911-934.

4. Berdal, A. (1997) In Vitamin D. Feldman, D., Glorieux, F.H., and Pike, J.W., editors. Academic Press, New York. 423-435.

5. Berdal, A., Balmain, N., Cuisinier-Gleizes, P., and Mathieu, H. (1987) Arch. Oral Biol. 32, 493-498.

6. Berdal, A., Hotton, D., Pike, J.W., Mathieu, H., and Dupret, J.M. (1993) Dev. Biol. 155, 172-179.

7. Papagerakis, P., Hotton, D., Lezot, F., Brookes S., Bonass, W., Robinson, C., Forest, N., and Berdal, A. (1999) J. Cell. Biochem. 76, 194-205.

8.Hart, S., Hart, T., Gibson, C., and Wright, J.T. (2000) Arch. Oral Biol. 45, 79-86.

9. Karrman, C., Backman, B., Holmgren, G., and Forsman, K. (1996) Arch. Oral Biol. 41, 893-900.

10. MacDougall, M., DuPont, B.R., Simmons, D., Reus, B., Krebsbach, P., Karrman, C., Holmgren, G., Leach, R.J., and Forsman, K. (1997) Genomics. 41, 115-118.

11. Dhamija, S., Liu, Y., Yamada, Y., Snead, M.L., and Krebsbach, P.H. (1999) J. Biol. Chem. 274, 20738-20743.

12. Diekwisch, T., David, S., Bringas, P., Santos, V., and Slavkin, H.C. (1993) Development. 117, 471-482.

13. Lyngstadaas, S.P., Risnes, S., Sproat, B.S., Thrane, P.S., and Prydz, H.P. (1995) EMBO J. 14, 5224-5229.

14. Breen, E.C., van Wijen, A.J., Lian, J.B., Stein, G.S., and Stein, J.L. (1994) Proc. Natl. Acad. Sci. USA. 91, 2902-12906.

15. Gill, R.K., and Christakos, S. (1993) Proc. Natl. Acad. Sci. 90, 2984-2988.

16. Zhou, Y.L., and Snead, M.L. (2000) J. Biol. Chem. 275, 12273-12280.

17. Gibson, C.W., Collier, P.M., Yuan, Z-A., and Chen, E. (1998) Eur. J. Oral Sci. 106 (suppl 1), 292-298.

Analysis of the Mechanism of 1α,25(OH)$_2$D$_3$–Mediated Transcriptional Repression of the Gene for cAMP-Dependent Protein Kinase Inhibitor

B. Holmquist and H.L. Henry. Department of Biochemistry, University of California, Riverside, CA USA 92521.

Introduction

The primary mechanism by which 1α,25(OH)$_2$D$_3$ generates biological responses is alteration of the expression of target genes through binding of the ligand-activated vitamin D receptor (VDR). These changes can be regulated both tissue-specifically and developmentally.

Numerous genes have been shown to be regulated by 1α,25(OH)$_2$D$_3$, and the majority of these 1α,25(OH)$_2$D$_3$-regulated genes identified are *up*-regulated in response to ligand. However, some genes are *down*-regulated in response to 1α,25(OH)$_2$D$_3$, including the parathyroid hormone, 25-OH-1α-hydroxylase and cAMP-dependent protein kinase inhibitor (PKI). PKI is an endogenous, heat and acid stable competitive inhibitor of cAMP-dependent protein kinase (PKA).

1α,25(OH)$_2$D$_3$ decreases PKI activity in primary cultures of chick kidney cells and also decreases steady state levels of chick kidney PKI mRNA both *in vivo* and in cell culture. To further study the molecular mechanism of transcriptional repression of the PKI gene, the genomic clone of this gene was previously obtained through library screening with the PKI cDNA. A putative negative VDRE (nVDRE) was found in the PKI promoter sequence within 50 bp of the TATA box.

It is not yet clear what molecular signals (*cis*-acting elements and *trans*-acting factors) are involved in the processes by which genes are *down*-regulated by 1α,25(OH)$_2$D$_3$. It has been shown that single nucleotide mutations in the parathyroid hormone nVDRE can reverse the direction of 1α,25(OH)$_2$D$_3$ regulation from negative to positive for that gene[2]. It is very likely that variations in the nucleotide sequence of the PKI nVDRE will produce similar results.

In order to investigate the role of the PKI nVDRE sequence in negative regulation by 1α,25(OH)$_2$D$_3$, a functional assay for analyzing mutant PKI nVDRE sequences on a promoter-reporter construct was developed. In addition, differences in protein binding to the nVDRE sequence have been analyzed by electrophoretic mobility shift assays (EMSA) and by DNA-Affinity Capture (DAC).

Information gained from studying the mechanism of down-regulation of chick PKI at the transcriptional level promises to have direct relevance to other genes down-regulated by 1α,25(OH)$_2$D$_3$.

Results:

EMSA Analysis of Chick Nuclear Extract Protein Binding to the nVDRE:

Chick kidney nuclear extract (ckNE), (8 ug) was incubated for 30 minutes at room temperature with 100 fmol of the double stranded nVDRE probe (same sequence as for the DAC method), 1X EMSA binding buffer (20mM Tris pH 7.9, 1 mM EDTA, 1mM DTT, 10% glycerol, 150mM KCl, 5 ug poly [dl-dC]), and where indicated, 100-fold excess cold nVDRE sequence. Samples were electrophoresed on pre-run 4% polyacrylamide gels (1X TBE), and the gels were dried and exposed to X-ray film.

	1	2	3	4	5	6	7	8
ckNE vitamin D status:	−	−	+	+	−	−	+	+
Cold nVDRE (100X):	−	+	−	+	−	+	−	+

Lanes 1-4 demonstrate an EMSA experiment comparing the protein binding pattern for ckNE from vitamin D deficient (-D) and vitamin D replete (+D) animals. This autoradiograph shows a high degree of similarity between the -D and +D samples. Upon close examination of the data, faint bands were seen which required higher resolution in that region.

Lanes 5-8 are from a repeat experiment, with the exception that this gel was run longer to provide higher resolution of the region of interest. As can be seen from this autoradiograph, there are indeed differences between the –D (lane 5) and +D (lane 7) in the indicated region.

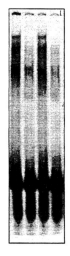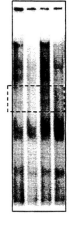

The zoomed in view of the boxed region shows two of the bands which are present in the +D (lane 7) but not the –D (lane 5) ckNE samples.

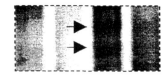

DAC Analysis of Chick Nuclear Extract Protein Binding to the nVDRE:
Biotinylated oligonucleotide were annealed and incubated in a 2:1 molar ratio with streptavidin Magnesphere particles, after which the particles were washed with binding buffer (0.1X SSC). Chick kidney nuclear extract (ckNE), 400ug was incubated with the doubled stranded DNA capture sequence:

5′-TATAAAGAAATT<u>ATGTT</u>GCTG<u>AGGTCA</u>TTGCTTTTATAAA-3′

bound to the solid support. Two reaction tubes were used in these experiments, the only difference being that one tube contained nuclear extract from vitamin D replete chick tissues (+D), and the other contained nuclear extract from vitamin D deplete chick tissues (-D). As a control for non-specific DNA binding proteins, a parallel set of binding reactions were performed using a mutated VDRE sequence instead of the wild-type VDRE sequence:

5′-TATAAAGAAATT<u>CCCTT</u>GCTG<u>AGGTCA</u>TTGCTTTTATAAA-3′.

After the binding reaction (one hour), the matrices were washed three times with 60mM KCl. The proteins were first eluted with 200mM KCl, then with 400mM KCl, and finally with 500mM KCl as a final step. All eluates (two for each reaction vessel) were analyzed via 10% polyacrylamide SDS-PAGE (Laemmeli), and silver stained. Differences in protein patterns were identified by visual examination.

As can be seen by the gel section on the left, hundreds of proteins bound to the PKI nVDRE in a $1\alpha,25(OH)_2D_3$-dependent fashion. However, most of these proteins were also present when the mutated VDRE sequence was used (rightmost section). Of the proteins which could be visualized as regulated by $1\alpha,25(OH)_2D_3$ when bound to the nVDRE sequence but not the mutated VDRE sequence, two proteins were found to be substantially regulated. The 65kD protein is present in the ciNE (chick intestinal nuclear extract), (center section) but is not regulated, whereas the 33kD protein was not present in the ciNE binding reaction.

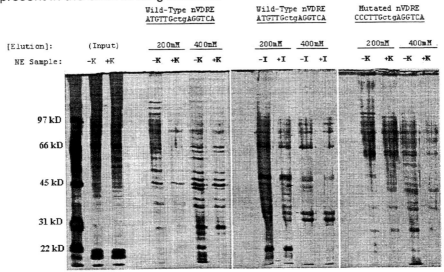

Conclusions:

- Using EMSA and DNA Affinity Capture analysis, the ckPKI nVDRE region appears to selectively bind proteins dependent on vitamin D status.
- The regulation of the protein kinase inhibitor gene provides a unique system for studying tissue-specific, $1\alpha,25(OH)_2D_3$-dependent negative gene regulation.

References:

1. Rowland-Goldsmith, M. A., B. Holmquist, and H.L. Henry. Genomic cloning, structure, and regulatory elements of the $1\alpha,25(OH)_2D_3$ down-regulated gene for cAMP-dependent protein kinase inhibitor. *Biochimica Biophysica Acta.* 1446: 414-418, 1999.
2. Koszewski, N.J., S. Ashok, and J. Russell. Turning a negative into a positive: vitamin D receptor interactions with the avian parathyroid hormone response element. *Molecular Endocrinol*ogy. 13: 455-456, 1999.
3. Rachez, C., Z. Suldan, J. Ward, C.P. Chang, D. Burakov, H. Erdjument-Bromage, P. Tempst, and L.P. Freedman. A novel protein complex that interacts with the vitamin D_3 receptor in a ligand-dependent manner and enhances VDR transactivation in a cell-free system. *Genes and Development.* 12:1787-1800, 1998.
4. Gangolli, E.A., M. Belyamani, S. Muchinsky, A. Narula, K.A. Burton, G.S. McKnight, M.D. Uhler, and R.L. Idzerda. Deficient gene expression in protein kinase inhibitor α null mice. *Molecular and Cellular Biology.* 20:3442-3448, 2000.
5. M.A. Rowland-Goldsmith and H.L. Henry. Structure and regulatory elements of the vitamin D down-regulated gene for cAMP dependent protein kinase inhibitor (PKI). In *Vitamin D: Chemistry, Biology and Clinical Applications of the Steroid Hormone.* pp. 300-301, 1997.

REGULATION OF VITAMIN D RECEPTOR BY ESTROGEN AND ANTI-ESTROGENS IN OSTEOBLASTS

Jennifer Wietzke and JoEllen Welsh, Dept. of Biological Sciences, University of Notre Dame, Notre Dame, IN 46556

Introduction

$1,25D_3$ acts through the VDR to transcriptionally regulate genes involved in calcium homeostasis, immune responses, and bone remodeling. Cellular sensitivity to $1,25(OH)_2D_3$ ($1,25D_3$) is determined, in part, by the level of functional vitamin D_3 receptor (VDR), which is in turn regulated by various agents, including $1,25D_3$ itself. Other factors such as E_2 and anti-estrogens can also regulate the VDR but this regulation may be tissue specific. Cell specific regulation of the VDR is especially important when considering SERMs and vitamin D analogs potentially being used for the prevention or treatment of diseases such as osteoporosis and breast cancer. It will be important in the drug development process to determine if SERMs act as agonists or antagonists in regulating VDR expression in breast cancer and bone cells and if so, whether the regulation is through transcriptional control of the VDR promoter. To begin analysis of control of VDR expression by E_2 in bone cells, we examined several osteoblast model systems for E_2 sensitivity. Although osteoblasts express functional ER *in vivo*, osteoblast model cell lines like MG-63 express extremely low levels of ER. The hFOB/ER4 cell line is an immortalized, normal human osteoblast cell line that stably expresses $ER\alpha$ at approximately physiological levels. Transient transfections of hFOB/ER4 cells with an ERE-luciferase construct indicate that treatments with E_2 and anti-estrogens regulate the transcriptional activity of a traditional ERE. In these studies we have used this estrogen responsive osteoblast system to examine VDR regulation by E_2 and the anti-estrogen TAM in comparison to MCF-7, a well-characterized estrogen responsive breast cancer cell line.

Materials and Methods

Cell culture: hFOB/ER4 cells were obtained from T. Spelsberg (Mayo Clinic, MN) and were grown in phenol red-free DME/F-12 1:1 mixture media, 10% charcoal stripped serum (CSS), and penicillin/ streptomycin (pen/strep). Cells were cultured at 34° C and media was changed every 2 days to alternate selection antibiotics, 100µg/ml hygromycin B and 300 µg/ml Geneticin.

MG-63 cell lines were obtained from ATCC and passaged in F-12 media and 5% fetal bovine serum (FBS). For all experiments, cells were switched to media containing 10% CSS and pen/strep.

MCF-7 cells were obtained from ATCC and passaged in αMEM media with 5% FBS. For all experiments, cells were switched to media containing 10% CSS and pen/strep.

Western Blot Analysis: Cells were plated at 1×10^6 cells in 150mm dishes and grown to 70% confluence. In various experiments, cells were treated with

374

1,25D$_3$, E$_2$, TAM, 5% FBS, or co-treated with E$_2$ and TAM, or 1,25D$_3$ and E$_2$. After 48 hours, cells were harvested, proteins were precipitated from high salt nuclear extracts, separated on SDS-PAGE gel, and transferred to nitrocellulose. The membranes were blotted with monoclonal anti-VDR (9A7) followed by horseradish peroxidase conjugated anti-rat IgG.

Transient Transfections: Control luciferase vectors were obtained from Promega and the 5' flanking region of exon 1c of hVDR (PRL-800) was constructed in our lab (Byrne, et al., Endocrinology, in press). Transfection conditions were optimized for each cell line and performed in triplicate. For transfections, all cell lines were plated at 2 x 10^5 cells per well in 6-well dishes and incubated overnight. FuGENE 6 transfection reagent was used following manufacturer's instructions to transfect either PRL-null or PRL-800 luciferase constructs along with PGL3-control vector to normalize for transfection rate. Cells were incubated overnight in media containing transfection mix, harvested, and assayed with the Dual Luciferase kit (Promega).

Results

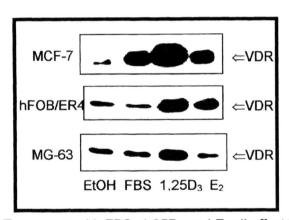

Figure 1. Treatments with FBS, 1,25D$_3$ and E$_2$ all affect VDR protein expression in three human cell lines. All three cell lines showed increased VDR when treated with 1,25D$_3$ but FBS and E$_2$ had cell specific effects. In both osteoblast cell lines, MG-63 and hFOB/ER4, there were no changes in VDR expression after treatment with FBS, compared to significant VDR up-regulation by FBS in MCF-7 cells. VDR levels increased in both MCF-7 and hFOB/ER4 cells after treatment with E$_2$, but MG-63 cells showed no increase with E$_2$ treatment.

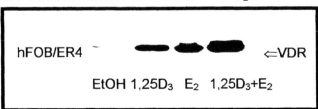

Figure 2. In hFOB/ER4 cells, treatment with either 1,25D$_3$ or E$_2$ up-regulates VDR, and simultaneous treatment with 1,25D$_3$ and E$_2$ increases the level of VDR

protein expressed above either single treatment alone. These changes in VDR expression in hFOB/ER4 cells were independent of changes in cell growth (data not shown).

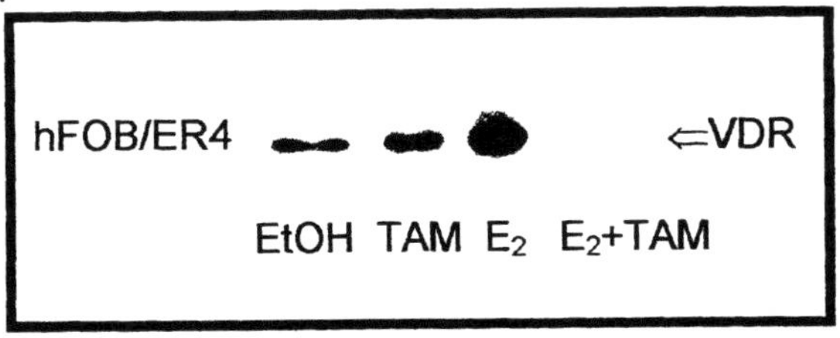

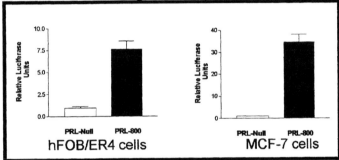

Figure 3. Treatment with E_2 increased the level of VDR in hFOB/ER4 cells, whereas treatment with the anti-estrogen TAM had no effect on VDR expression. Co-treatment with TAM and E_2 lowered VDR levels to below control, indicating that TAM was able to inhibit the E_2 stimulatory effect on VDR levels.

Figure 4. In estrogen responsive MCF-7 cells, the PRL-800 vector containing the 5' flanking region immediately upstream of exon 1c of the VDR exhibited a 30-fold increase in luciferase activity above the null vector. Activity of the PRL-800 vector in hFOB/ER4 cells is 7-fold higher than the null vector that does not contain the 5' flanking region immediately upstream of exon 1c of the VDR.

Discussion

These studies have addressed comparative aspects of hVDR expression in cell lines derived from osteoblasts or breast cancer. Our goal is to determine whether steroid hormones and growth factors differentially modulate VDR expression in a cell specific manner. We used the estrogen responsive MCF- 7 human breast cancer cell line to compare to MG-63, an osteosarcoma cell line and hFOB/ER4, a normal, human osteoblast cell line stably transfected with a vector expressing the human ERα gene.

Initial experiments (Figure 1) show that all cell lines examined, MCF-7, hFOB/ER4, and MG-63 up-regulate VDR expression after treatment with 1,25D_3, suggesting this is a general phenomen for all cells expressing VDR. This suggestion is consistent with a post-translational mechanism model such as ligand induced stabilization of VDR.

In contrast to 1,25D_3 mediated up-regulation of VDR in all cell lines, FBS stimulation only up-regulates VDR in the breast cancer cell line, MCF-7. Neither osteoblast derived cell line respond to FBS with up-regulation of VDR. While the specific components of FBS responsible for up-regulation of VDR in MCF-7 cells are not known, it appears that these factors are not linked to regulation of VDR in osteoblast cells.

Up-regulation of VDR by E_2 is observed in MCF-7 and hFOB/ER4 cell lines but not in MG-63 cells. Western blot analysis indicated that both MCF-7 and hFOB/ER4 cells express high levels of ERα, but that both ERα and ERβ are undetectable in MG-63 cells (data not shown). These data suggest that up-regulation of VDR by E_2 in bone cells is mediated by the ER. To confirm this suggestion, we examined whether the ER antagonist TAM altered basal VDR expression or modulated the up-regulation of VDR by E_2 in hFOB/ER4 cells. As demonstrated in Figure 3, TAM completely blocks the effect of E_2 on VDR expression while having no effect on basal VDR levels. These data suggest that TAM acts solely as an ER antagonist in regulation of VDR and does not mimic the effect of E_2. This is in contrast to data suggesting differential effects of TAM on cells derived from bone vs. breast.

Data from Figure 2 confirms that E_2 and 1,25D_3 up-regulate VDR in hFOB/ER4 cells. However, simultaneous treatment with both E_2 and 1,25D_3 further up-regulates the VDR above the level found with either single treatment. This suggests that E_2 and 1,25D_3 mediate VDR up-regulation through two different mechanisms. Since 1,25D_3 might be acting via a post-translational mechanism such as ligand induced stabilization of VDR, an alternative mechanism for E_2 induction of VDR might be to increase transcription through the promoter of the VDR.

Initial studies on the control of promoter activity of the VDR have focused on using a luciferase construct designed and tested in our lab. Inserted into a PRL-null vector is the 5' flanking region upstream of exon 1c of hVDR. Figure 4 compares the activity of this PRL-800 vector in MCF-7 breast cancer cells vs. hFOB/ER4 cells. Both cell lines exhibit considerable increases in activity of the PRL-800 vector compared to the activity of the PRL-null vector. It appears that activity is higher in MCF-7 breast cancer cells than in hFOB/ER4 bone cells. However, transfection rate is higher in MCF-7 cells and though normalizing with the PGL3-control vector was done, the apparent considerable difference may still be due in part to differences in transfection in the two cell lines. The question of tissue specific differences in VDR promoter activity is currently being studied through the use of other ER responsive breast cancer cell lines such as T47D. Additionally, future studies of the hormone-induced regulation of this promoter region will determine if the up-regulation of VDR protein by E_2 we observed is due to an up-regulation in exon 1c promoter activity of the VDR. These studies will also address whether E_2 and TAM have differential effects on this VDR promoter in MCF-7 breast cancer cells vs. hFOB/ER4 bone derived cells, which may identify tissue specific effects of E_2 and TAM that are not apparent by western blot analysis.

CELL DIFFERENTIATION

CELL CYCLE DEPENDENCE OF VITAMIN D RECEPTOR EXPRESSION

Kirsten Prüfer, Claudia Schröder, Attila Racz, Julia Barsony, Laboratory of Cell Biochemistry and Biology, NIDDK, National Institutes of Health, Bethesda, MD 20892 USA.

Introduction

Calcitriol regulates proliferation and differentiation in a multitude of cell types including keratinocytes (1) and several cancer cells (2,3). The antiproliferative effect of calcitriol has been correlated to the expression of its nuclear receptor, the vitamin D receptor (VDR) (4). Regulation of vitamin D receptor (VDR) expression has been studied by Northern blot analysis and either immunofluorescence or flow cytometry assays in HL60 (5) and in HC-11 mammary epithelial cells (6). Growth inhibition correlated with a decrease in VDR mRNA in HC-11 mammary cells and with a reduction of VDR protein expression in HL-60 cells. Regulation of VDR expression exists on both the pretranslational and posttranslational level. Posttranslational regulation by the proteasome has been shown for both VDR (7,8) and retinoid X receptor (RXR) expression (9). Similar to other members of the nuclear receptor family, VDR requires heterodimerization with the RXR for high affinity binding to DNA.

To study expression and trafficking of RXR and VDR we generated chimeras of yellow fluorescent protein (YFP) with RXR (YFP-RXR) and green fluorescent protein (GFP) with VDR (GFP-VDR) (10). We stably expressed YFP-RXR in CV-1 (CYR) and GFP-VDR in 293 cells (GL48). Expression of these proteins is driven by the CMV promoter and thus transcriptional regulation would not affect protein expression. This allowed us to study posttranslational regulation of VDR and RXR expression and its dependence on the cell cycle.

Methods

Plasmids

GFP-VDR was generated by cloning the human VDR cDNA (gift from Dr. J.W. Pike) C-terminal to the EGFP plasmid (Clontech). YFP-RXR was generated by cloning the human RXRα/pSVL plasmid (RXR) (gift from Dr. P. Chambon) C-terminal of the EYFP plasmid (Clontech).

Stable cell lines

293 cells were transfected with the GFP-VDR expression plasmid using Lipofectamine Plus reagents (Life Technologies) according to manufacturer's instructions. Then, G418-resistant cell clones were selected for 3-5 weeks by culturing cells in media with 1mM G418 (Life Technologies). One of the high-expressing clones (GL48) was characterized. YFP-RXR was stably expressed in CV-1 cells, and a high-expressing clone (CYR) was selected by culturing with G418.

Cell synchronization

GL48 and CYR cells were subcultured into glass coverslip chambers and the cell cycle was synchronized by serum starvation for 72h and subsequent stimulation with 10% serum. Either this method or treatment of cells with 10mM thymidine for 16h and subsequent removal of thymidine for 5h leads to accumulation of cells in S phase. In another experiment CYR cells were cell cycle arrested in G1/S transition by treatment with 10µg/ml aphidicolin for 16h.

Microscopy

Images were collected with a Zeiss Axiovert 100 fluorescent microscope equipped with an LSM 410 laser-scanning unit. The 488nm line of a krypton-argon laser was used for excitation with a long-pass 515nm emission filter.

Transactivation Assays

CV-1 cells were subcultured into 12 well plates (Costar) and transfected with both GFP-VDR (0.3µg/well) and the luciferase reporter plasmid p24OH/Luc-23 (0.07µg/well; gift, from Dr. H. F. DeLuca) using Lipofectamine Plus reagents. Transfected cells were incubated with either 10nM calcitriol or vehicle in MEM containing insulin, transferrin, selenium additive (ITS), and L-glutamin for 24h. Transcriptional activity of YFP-RXR was tested by a luciferase reporter assay. YFP-RXR or RXR (0.3µg/well) were transfected into CV-1 cells together with RXRE-Luc (0.07µg/well; gift from Dr. Karathanasis). To correct for transfection efficiency, β-galactosidase standardization plasmid pGL3 (0.7µg/well; Promega) was also cotransfected. Transfected cells were treated with either 100nM 9-cis retinoic acid or vehicle in MEM containing ITS, and L-glutamin for 24h. Then cells were lysed on the plates and both luciferase and β-galactosidase activities were determined. Luciferase activity was measured with a luminometer. β-Galactosidase activity was measured by spectrophotometry. Luminescence data were normalized with β-galactosidase values and expressed as fold induction by hormone relative to vehicle treated controls.

Cell Extracts and Immunoblotting

GL48 cells and 293 cells were grown in 162cm^2 flasks and 293 cells were transfected at 50% confluence with 5µg of plasmid DNA expressing YFP-RXR and YFP using Lipofectamine Plus. After 24h, high salt extracts were prepared from cells as described earlier (11). Samples containing either 15µg of protein (YFP-RXR and YFP extract) or 5µg protein (GL48 extract) were separated on 12% Tris-Glycine polyacrylamide gels (Novex) and electrotransfered to ECL-Hybond nitrocellulose membranes (Amersham Pharmacia Biotech). Membranes were blocked for 1h with 5% milk in PBS containing 0.1% Tween-20 (PBS-T). After incubation overnight at 4ºC with a polyclonal anti-GFP antibody (1:1000, Clontech), membranes were incubated for 1h at room temperature with the Cruz Marker compatible horseradish peroxidase-labeled anti-rabbit secondary antibody (Santa Cruz Biotechnology) (1: 2000). The Cruz Marker molecular weight standards were used. Antibodies were diluted in PBS-T with 5% milk, and washings were done with PBS-T. Blots were developed with enhanced chemiluminescence kit reagents according to the manufacturer's protocol (Amersham Pharmacia Biotech).

Results
Figure1:

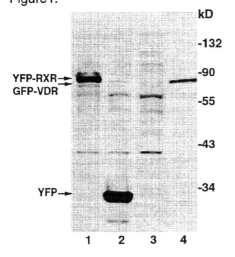

Figure 1 shows that the anti-GFP antibody detected two intact chimeric proteins, an 80kD band for the YFP-RXR (lane 1) and a 77kD band for the GFP-VDR (lane 4). As a control, we transfected cells with YFP and detected a 30kD band (lane 2). To determine whether the additional bands signify other GFP containing degradation products or represent nonspecific binding, extract from nontransfected 293 cell was also subjected to Western blot analysis (lane 3). Since all other bands showing immunoreactivity in lanes 1 and 2, are also detectable in the nontransfected cell extract, it is unlikely that they represent GFP containing proteins.

Figure 2:

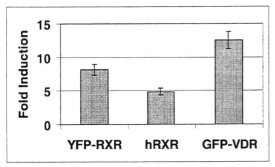

We evaluated the functionality of YFP-RXR and GFP-VDR by transactivation assays (fig. 2). The ligand 9-cis retinoic acid (100nM) caused an 8-fold induction of the RXRE-luciferase reporter activity by YFP-RXR, compared to a 5-fold induction by the untagged RXR. Calcitriol (10nM) induced 12-fold induction of a VDRE-luciferase reporter in GL48 cells by GFP-VDR.

Figure 3:

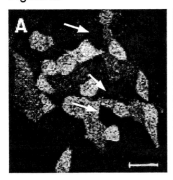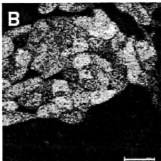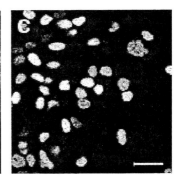

GFP-VDR partitions between the nucleus and the cytoplasm without calcitriol. The expression level varies from cell to cell in GL48 cells. In fact, in some cells GFP-VDR fluorescence is nearly undetectable (fig. 3A, arrows). Cell cycle synchronization in the S phase decreases variability of GFP-VDR expression, allowing GFP-VDR fluorescence to be visible in most GL48 cells (fig. 3B). On the other hand, YFP-RXR is predominantly nuclear, and expression variability was unaffected when cells were synchronized in S (fig. 3C) or G1 phase of the cell cycle (not shown). Bar, 25 μm

Discussion

We generated and characterized functional YFP-RXR and GFP-VDR chimeras to study the regulation of receptor expression and distribution. We demonstrated here the expression of intact tagged proteins from cell extracts and the transcriptional activities of the tagged receptors. The establishment of stable cell lines that express these chimeras provided us with a reproducible and convenient model. Fluorescence microscopy of GL48 cells showed that GFP-VDR partitions between cytoplasm and nucleus. This finding is consistent with our previous findings on transiently expressed VDR-GFP (12). YFP-RXR was predominantly nuclear in CYR cells. The uses of these stable cell lines provide many more opportunities to study receptor distribution and trafficking.

Cell to cell differences in GFP-VDR and YFP-RXR fluorescence raised the possibility that receptor expression is regulated by the cell cycle. Our studies with synchronized cells supported this hypothesis for the GFP-VDR only. These results represent regulation of GFP-VDR expression at the posttranslational level and provide a mechanism for differential regulation of VDR and RXR amounts within the cells. The results of our study are consistent with the model that posttranslational regulation of protein expression is an important way to regulate function. Several recent studies demonstrated that proteasomal degradation of signal proteins play important roles in cell differentiation and proliferation, suggesting that regulation of VDR expression could have physiological impact.

References
1. Bikle, D. D., Gee, E., and Pillai, S. (1993) *J.Invest Dermatol.* **101,** 713-718
2. Chouvet, C., Vicard, E., Devonec, M., and Saez, S. (1986) *J.Steroid Biochem.* **24,** 373-376
3. Zhuang, S. H. and Burnstein, K. L. (1998) *Endocrinology* **139,** 1197-1207
4. Hedlund, T. E., Moffatt, K. A., and Miller, G. J. (1996) *Endocrinology* **137,** 1554-1561
5. Folgueira, M. A., Federico, M. H., Katayama, M. L., Silva, M. R., and Brentani, M. M. (1998) *J Steroid Biochem.Mol.Biol.* **66,** 193-201
6. Escaleira, M. T. and Brentani, M. M. (1999) *Breast Cancer Res.Treat.* **54,** 123-133
7. vom, B. E., Zechel, C., Heery, D., Heine, M. J., Garnier, J. M., Vivat, V., Le Douarin, B., Gronemeyer, H., Chambon, P., and Losson, R. (1996) *EMBO J* **15,** 110-124
8. Masuyama, H. and MacDonald, P. N. (1998) *J Cell Biochem.* **71,** 429-440
9. Boudjelal, M., Wang, Z., Voorhees, J. J., and Fisher, G. J. (2000) *Cancer Res.* **60,** 2247-2252
10. Prufer, K., Racz, A., Lin, G. C., and Barsony, J. (2000) *J.Biol.Chem.*
11. Smith, C. L., Hager, G. L., Pike, J. W., and Marx, S. J. (1991) *Mol.Endocrinol.* **5,** 867-878
12. Racz, A. and Barsony, J. (1999) *J.Biol.Chem.* **274,** 19352-19360

ROLE OF MITOCHONDRIA AND CASPASES IN VITAMIN D MEDIATED APOPTOSIS IN MCF-7 BREAST CANCER CELLS

Carmen J. Narvaez,[1] Thomas Waterfall,[2] and JoEllen Welsh,[1] [1]Department of Biological Sciences, University of Notre Dame, Notre Dame, IN   46556; [2]Department of Biochemistry, Queens University, Kingston, Ontario   K7L3X6, Canada

Introduction   1,25-Dihydroxyvitamin D_3 (1,25-$(OH)_2D_3$), the active form of vitamin D_3, acts through the nuclear vitamin D receptor (VDR) and is a potent negative growth regulator of breast cancer cells both *in vitro* and *in vivo*. Our lab has shown that 1,25-$(OH)_2D_3$ induces morphological and biochemical markers of apoptosis (chromatin and nuclear matrix condensation, and DNA fragmentation) in MCF-7 breast cancer cells (1). The precise mechanism of how 1,25-$(OH)_2D_3$ and its nuclear receptor, the VDR, mediate apoptosis is poorly understood.

We examined the 1,25-$(OH)_2D_3$ signaling pathway downstream of the VDR in order to identify specific intracellular events involved in 1,25-$(OH)_2D_3$ mediated apoptosis and to characterize events which are blocked in MCF-7^{D3Res} cells (a vitamin D_3-resistant variant)(2).   In particular, the effects of 1,25-$(OH)_2D_3$ mediated apoptosis on mitochondrial function and caspase activity were studied and compared to the effects of TNFα. TNFα was chosen as a positive control since this cytokine induces apoptosis in MCF-7 cells by means of a well-defined pathway triggered by TNFR1, a cell surface death receptor whose signaling results in caspase activation and disruption of mitochondrial function (3). Caspases are a family of evolutionarily conserved cysteine proteases that become activated upon proteolytic cleavage, and are responsible for cell disassembly.   Mitochondria play a central role in controlling cell death. Translocation of Bax from cytosol to mitochondria, release of cytochrome *c*, and activation of caspases may initiate disruption of mitochondrial function (4,5). It may be during this mitochondrial phase that the cell makes a commitment to die. Events downstream of mitochondrial disruption are characterized by the action of caspases and nuclease activators released from mitochondria leading to the ultimate destruction of the cell.

While the role of caspases in apoptosis triggered by cell surface death receptors such as TNFR1 has been well established, it is not clear if apoptosis triggered by nuclear receptors such as the VDR is mediated via similar caspase dependent pathways.   In order to probe the mechanisms whereby vitamin D signaling modulates apoptosis in MCF-7 cells; we used a cell permeable inhibitor of caspase-related proteases (zVAD.fmk) to determine the involvement of caspase-dependent proteolysis in 1,25-$(OH)_2D_3$ mediated apoptosis.

Results and Discussion   Disruption of mitochondrial function is one of the primary events that occur during apoptosis.   Translocation of Bax to the mitochondrial outer membrane has been implicated in induction of apoptosis. Bax redistribution to mitochondria occurs in the presence of both 1,25-(OH)$_2$D$_3$ and TNFα in MCF-7 cells (Figure 1). Not only was Bax translocated to mitochondria, but it was also cleaved from 21 kDa to 18 kDa. This observation is consistent with other reports of Bax cleavage during drug-induced apoptosis (6). Bax translocation to mitochondria and apoptosis in response to TNFα can be triggered in MCF-7[D3Res] cells indicating that Bax functions appropriately during apoptosis induced by agents other than 1,25-(OH)$_2$D$_3$ (Figure 1).

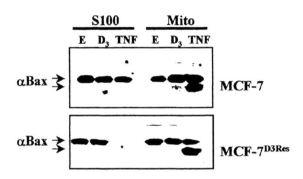

Figure 1   Subcellular distribution of Bax in MCF-7 and MCF-7[D3Res] cells after treatment with 1,25-D$_3$ or TNFα.

Translocation of Bax to mitochondria is associated with subsequent release of cytochrome c, events that are considered to be commitment points for activating apoptosis. Cytochrome c normally resides within the intermembrane space of live cells. Cytochrome c is not detected in the cytosolic fraction of vehicle treated control cells. However, 1,25-(OH)$_2$D$_3$ induces redistribution of cytochrome c from mitochondria to cytosol as early as 48 hrs in MCF-7 cells, before any morphological apoptotic events are detected. By contrast, TNFα, but not 1,25-(OH)$_2$D$_3$, induces release of cytochrome c in MCF-7[D3Res] cells.

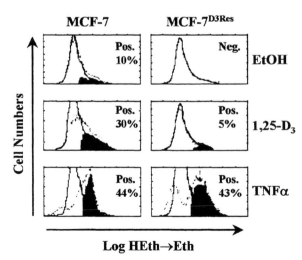

Figure 2   ROS production in MCF-7 or MCF-7[D3Res] cells after treatment with 1,25-D$_3$or TNFα.

Long term exclusion of cytochrome c from the electron transport chain can lead to impairment of proton flow, and generation of reactive oxygen species (ROS) due to incomplete reduction of molecular oxygen (7). Hence, mitochondrial generation of ROS in response to apoptotic stimuli was examined. By using flow cytometric techniques, production of superoxide anion was assessed by the degree of oxidation of hydroethidine to ethidium, a DNA stain that fluoresces red upon DNA intercalation.

MCF-7 cells, but not MCF-7^{D3Res}, produced ROS in the presence of 1,25-(OH)$_2$D$_3$, whereas TNFα induced ROS production in both cell lines (Figure 2).

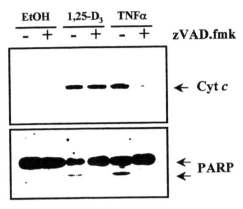

EtOH 1,25-D$_3$ TNFα
- + - + - + zVAD.fmk

← Cyt c

← PARP

Figure 3 Expression of cytochrome c and PARP in MCF-7 cells (in the presence or absence of zVAD.fmk).

Cytochrome c release into the cytosol triggers caspase activity downstream of mitochondria. In order to determine the involvement of caspase-dependent proteolysis in 1,25-(OH)$_2$D$_3$ mediated apoptosis, we used a broad-spectrum cell permeable inhibitor (zVAD.fmk) in MCF-7 cells. Proteolytic activity associated with caspases was analyzed by three different methods. First, caspase activity was detected by immunoblot analysis of the cleavage of an endogenous caspase substrate, poly (ADP-ribose) polymerase (PARP). PARP was cleaved in the presence of both 1,25-(OH)$_2$D$_3$ and TNFα. The cleavage was blocked by zVAD.fmk (Figure 3). The second and third methods utilized flow cytometry to analyze phosphatidylserine (PS) exposure and DNA fragmentation, respectively, which others have shown can be provoked by caspases (8). Annexin V-FITC is a convenient probe for monitoring changes in the distribution of PS in the plasma membrane during apoptosis. Both 1,25-(OH)$_2$D$_3$ and TNFα induced PS exposure in MCF-7 cells, which was blocked by zVAD.fmk treatment. DNA fragmentation was assessed by incorporation of bromodeoxyuridine by terminal transferase and detection by anti-bromodeoxyuridine antibody conjugated to FITC. Both 1,25-(OH)$_2$D$_3$ and TNFα induced DNA fragmentation, which was completely blocked by zVAD.fmk. However, TNFα, but not 1,25-(OH)$_2$D$_3$, induced DEVDase (caspase-3/7) cleavage activity in MCF-7 cells. This observation indicates that other, or as yet unidentified, effector caspases may be responsible for 1,25-(OH)$_2$D$_3$ mediated PARP cleavage, PS exposure, or DNA fragmentation.

Since zVAD.fmk blocked caspase activity downstream of mitochondria, we examined the effects of the caspase inhibitor on cytochrome c release and mitochondrial activity. The caspase inhibitor had no effect on 1,25-(OH)$_2$D$_3$ induced cytochrome c release (Figure 3), decrease in mitochondrial membrane potential, or ROS production. However, caspase inhibitor was able to block all mitochondrial events in response to TNFα. This demonstrates that TNFα induced cell death occurs by a caspase-dependent mechanism consistent with a role for caspase-8 in triggering cytochrome c release.

Since zVAD.fmk was unable to block cytochrome c release and mitochondrial dysfunction in response to 1,25-(OH)$_2$D$_3$, we determined the effect of caspase inhibitor on cell death and clonogenic potential. Both zVAD.fmk and zDEVD.fmk caspase inhibitors protected MCF-7 from TNFα cell death with zVAD.fmk exhibiting the greatest response. However, neither caspase inhibitor could protect MCF-7 cells from 1,25-(OH)$_2$D$_3$ mediated apoptosis since the reduction in cell number was not blocked by these inhibitors. In addition, MCF-7 cells treated with 1,25-(OH)$_2$D$_3$ lost their clonogenic potential even when they were treated in the presence of zVAD.fmk. This suggests that the activation of caspases by 1,25-(OH)$_2$D$_3$ occurs subsequent to the events that commits the cells to die.

Conclusion   This study demonstrates for the first time that 1,25-(OH)$_2$D$_3$ induces apoptosis in MCF-7 cells by disrupting mitochondrial function, which is accomplished by translocation of Bax to mitochondria, release of cytochrome *c*, production of ROS, and decrease in mitochondrial membrane potential. This is the first data that demonstrates that 1,25-(OH)$_2$D$_3$ signaling on mitochondria does not require caspase activation, since broad-spectrum caspase inhibitor zVAD.fmk was unable to block these mitochondrial events. The failure of 1,25-(OH)$_2$D$_3$ to disrupt mitochondrial function in MCF-7[D3Res] cells suggests that 1,25-(OH)$_2$D$_3$ signaling on mitochondria is a complex event requiring more than a functional VDR. Events upstream of Bax translocation to mitochondria in response to 1,25-(OH)$_2$D$_3$ are abrogated in the vitamin D3-resistant cells, and contributed to resistance to 1,25-(OH)$_2$D$_3$ mediated apoptosis. Caspases act solely as executioners by facilitating 1,25-(OH)$_2$D$_3$ mediated apoptosis, but caspase activation is not required for induction of cell death by 1,25-(OH)$_2$D$_3$ in MCF-7 cells. Although caspase inhibitor blocked all the biochemical changes associated with caspase activation occurring following perturbation of mitochondria and loss of cytochrome *c*, the commitment of MCF-7 cells to 1,25-(OH)$_2$D$_3$ mediated apoptosis is caspase independent.

References
1.   Simboli-Campbell, M., Narvaez, C. J., Tenniswood, M., and Welsh, J. (1996) *J Steroid Biochem Mol Biol* **58**, 367-76
2.   Narvaez, C. J., Vanweelden, K., Byrne, I., and Welsh, J. (1996) *Endocrinology* **137**, 400-9
3.   Budihardjo, I., Oliver, H., Lutter, M., Luo, X., and Wang, X. (1999) *Annu Rev Cell Dev Biol* **15**, 269-90
4.   Tsujimoto, Y., and Shimizu, S. (2000) *FEBS Lett* **466**, 6-10
5.   Susin, S. A., Zamzami, N., and Kroemer, G. (1998) *Biochim Biophys Acta* **1366**, 151-65
6.   Wood, D. E., and Newcomb, E. W. (2000) *Exp Cell Res* **256**, 375-382
7.   Cai, J., and Jones, D. P. (1998) *J Biol Chem* **273**, 11401-11404
8.   Thornberry, N. A., and Lazebnik, Y. (1998) *Science* **281**, 1312-6

Supported by NIH (#CA69700) & DAMD (#17-97-1-7183)

STRUCTURE-SPECIFIC CONTROL OF CELL DIFFERENTIATION AND APOPTOSIS BY 19-NOR-1α,25-DIHYDROXYVITAMIN D₃ ANALOGS IN HL-60 CELLS

Toshio Okano,[1] Kimie Nakagawa,[1] Keiichi Ozono[2] Noboru Kubodera,[3] Ayako Osawa,[4] Masahiro Terada,[4] and Koichi Mikami[4], [1]Department of Hygienic Sciences, Kobe Pharmaceutical University, Kobe 658-8558, Japan, [2]Department of Chemical Technology, Tokyo Institute of Technology, Tokyo 152-8552, Japan, [3]Chugai Pharmaceutical Co. Ltd., Tokyo 104-8301, Japan, [4]Department of Environmental Medicine, Research Institute, Osaka Medical Center for Maternal and Child Health, Osaka 594-1101, Japan

Introduction 1 α,25-dihydroxyvitamin D₃ [1α,25(OH)₂D₃] has been shown to modulate not only proliferation and differentiation but also apoptosis of malignant cells, indicating that it would be useful for the treatment of hyperproliferative diseases such as cancer and psoriasis. [1-4] Little information is available concerning structural motifs of the 1α,25(OH)₂D₃ molecule responsible for modulation of cell differentiation and apoptosis. The elucidation of the possible roles of the 1α-hydroxy group, 3β-hydroxy group, and an exocyclic methylene group at C-10 on the A-ring of 1 α,25(OH)₂D₃ might lead to the development of new drugs which are useful for the treatment of cancers and immune diseases. We evaluated the biological activities of both singly dehydroxylated A-ring analogs of 19-nor-1α,25(OH)₂D₃ and series of 19-nor-22-oxa-1α,25(OH)₂D₃ (Figure 1) [5,6] with respect to binding affinities for VDR and DBP and transactivation on target genes in transfected MG-63 cells. Surprisingly, several 19-nor analogs were found to be transcriptionally slightly less active than 1α,25(OH)₂D₃ or almost comparable to 1α,25(OH)₂D₃ despite extremely low binding affinities for VDR. To examine

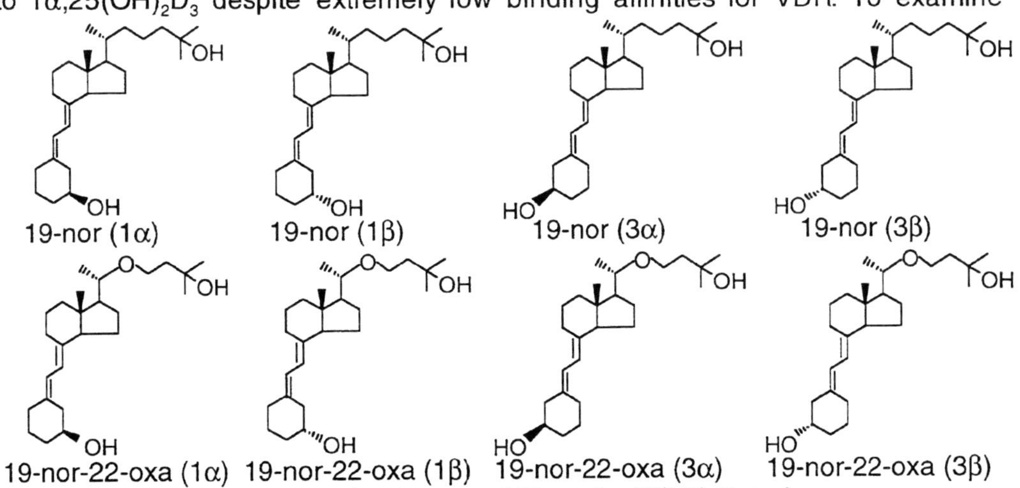

19-nor (1α)   19-nor (1β)   19-nor (3α)   19-nor (3β)

19-nor-22-oxa (1α) 19-nor-22-oxa (1β) 19-nor-22-oxa (3α) 19-nor-22-oxa (3β)

Figure 1   Chemical structure and code name of 19-nor-1 α,25(OH)2D3 and 19-nor-22oxa-1 α,25(OH)2D3 analogs.

further biological activity of the 19-nor analogs, we investigated cell cycle, differentiation and apoptosis in human promyelocytic leukemic HL-60 cells. The results revealed an inverse relationship between differentiation-inducing activity and apoptosis-stimulating activity of the 19-nor analogs. We have clearly identified the structural motifs on the basis of the stereochemistry of both hydroxyl groups at positions 1 and 3 of the A-ring of the $1\alpha,25(OH)_2D_3$ molecule responsible for the induction of differentiation and apoptosis of HL-60 cells. [7]

Results Transcriptional potencies of $1\alpha,25(OH)_2D_3$ and 19-nor analogs at 10^{-8} M on a rat $25(OH)D_3$-24-hydroxylase or human osteocalcin gene promoter in the transfected MG-63 cells are shown in Table 1. All results are expressed as percentage activity at 10^{-8}M in comparison with $1\alpha,25(OH)_2D_3$ (=100%). Of the 19-nor analogs, 19-nor(3β) and 19-nor-22-oxa(1α) exhibited approximately 50-90% potency to $1\alpha,25(OH)_2D_3$ while the other 19-nor analogs had virtually no potency. These transcriptional potencies were dependent on VDR binding and VDR/RXR heterodimerization.

Table. 1 **Relative binding affinity for DBP and VDR and transcriptional activity of 19-nor-$1\alpha,25(OH)_2D_3$ and 19-nor-22-oxa-$1\alpha,25(OH)_2D_3$ analogs .**

| Compounds | Relative binding affinity (ED50) | | Transcriptional Activity | | | |
	DBP	VDR	Rat 24-OH	Human Osteocalcin	VDR-GAL4	VDR/RXRα-GAL4
$1\alpha,25$-D_3	1.63×10^{-6}M	1.20×10^{-9}M	100	100	100	100
19-nor-Type						
19-nor (1α)	5.40×10^{-7}M	1.88×10^{-6}M	5	3	3	12
19-nor (1β)	7.46×10^{-8}M	N.R.	4	3	2	7
19-nor (3α)	3.09×10^{-7}M	2.06×10^{-6}M	6	4	4	12
19-nor (3β)	1.39×10^{-5}M	4.76×10^{-7}M	78	54	90	106
19-nor-22-oxa-Type						
19-nor-22-oxa (1α)	N.R.	3.21×10^{-7}M	86	95	113	100
19-nor-22-oxa (1β)	3.85×10^{-6}M	N.R.	4	3	1	5
19-nor-22-oxa (3α)	N.R.	1.35×10^{-6}M	3	3	1	5
19-nor-22-oxa (3β)	N.R.	N.R.	5	3	2	8

All results of transcriptional activity are expressed as percentage activity at 10^{-8}M in comparison with $1\alpha,25(OH)_2D_3$. N.R. : not reached to 50% displacement of $[^3H]$-$25(OH)D_3$ or $[^3H]$-$1\alpha,25(OH)_2D_3$.

To compare the antiproliferative effects of the analogs on HL-60 cell growth, we assayed cell cycle phase distribution of HL-60 cells treated with $1\alpha,25(OH)_2D_3$ or the 19-nor analogs. We found that like $1\alpha,25(OH)_2D_3$, 19-nor(3β) and 19-nor-22-oxa(1α) caused HL-60 cells to accumulate in the G0/G1 phase of the cell cycle. There were no significant differences in cell cycle distributions of the HL-60 cells treated with the other 19-nor analogs relative to vehicle-treated cells.

Expression of cell surface CD11b antigen is one of the major differentiation markers of HL-60 cells to monocytes/macrophages. As depicted in Figure 2-A, $1\alpha,25(OH)_2D_3$, 19-nor(3β) and 19-nor-22-oxa(1α) at 10^{-7} M, increased significantly the number of CD11b antigen-expressing cells. Other 19-nor analogs did not cause HL-60 cells to express CD11b antigen over vehicle-treated cells at any time or dose.

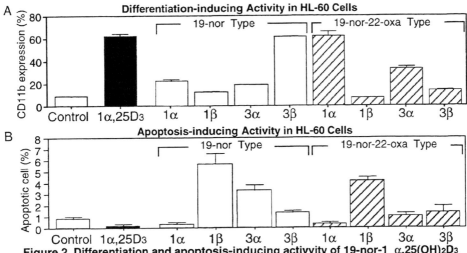

Figure 2 Differentiation and apoptosis-inducing activvity of 19-nor-1 α,25(OH)2D3 and 19-nor-22-oxa-1 α,25(OH)2D3 analogs .

To clarify whether the inhibitory effects of 1α,25(OH)$_2$D$_3$ and 19-nor analogs on HL-60 cell growth are correlated with their effects on apoptosis, the number of apoptotic HL-60 cells treated with 1α,25(OH)$_2$D$_3$ or 19-nor analogs was counted and calculated as a parcentage of 200 cells scored in each random fluoromicroscopic field of view. Figure 2-B shows that 19-nor(1β), 19-nor(3α) and 19-nor-22-oxa(1β), but not 1α,25(OH)$_2$D$_3$ or other 19-nor analogs, induced apoptosis in HL-60 cells. It has been reported that 1α,25(OH)$_2$D$_3$ itself has no apoptosis-stimulating effect on HL-60 cells, although it has an inhibitory effect on drug-induced apoptosis in HL-60 cells [8]. Our findings are consistent with these reports. Surprisingly, 19-nor(1β), 19-nor(3α), and 19-nor-22-oxa(1β) which have unnatural orientations (1 and 3 epimerization, respectively) of the hydroxyl groups at C-1 and C-3 in the A-ring, significantly increased the number of apoptotic HL-60 cells. Moreover, the apoptosis-stimulating potency of 19-nor(1β) and 19-nor(3α) bearing natural side-chains appears to be greater than those of the 19-nor(1β) and 19-nor(3α) bearing 22-oxa-type side-chains. It is possible that the orientation of the hydroxyl groups at C-1 and C-3 in the A-ring of 1α,25(OH)$_2$D$_3$ may be structural motifs responsible for controlling two signalling pathways, namely a VDR-dependent mechanism, such as cell differentiation and transactivation of target genes, and a VDR-non-dependent mechanism, such as apoptosis. Further, we studied fluoromicroscopic observation of HL-60 cells treated with 1α,25(OH)$_2$D$_3$ or 19-nor analogs using a Tdt-mediated dUTP nick end-labeling (TUNEL) method. No apoptotic cells were observed in the vehicle- or 1α,25(OH)$_2$D$_3$-treated HL-60 cells. Moreover, no apoptotic cells were observed in the 19-nor analogs bearing 1α- or 3β-hydroxyl groups in the A-ring. On the other hand, the 19-nor analogs bearing 1α- or 3β-hydroxyl groups in the A-ring exerted weak, but significant, apoptosis induction.

Discussion We previously reported that two novel 19-nor-1α,25(OH)$_2$D$_3$ analogs, 19-nor(3β) and 19-nor-22-oxa(1α) have slightly weaker or comparable abilities than 1α,25(OH)$_2$D$_3$ in stimulating rat 25-hydroxyvitamin D$_3$-24-hydroxylase gene and human osteocalcin gene promoter activity in transfected MG-63 cells, regardless of extremely low binding affinities for VDR (0.3 % and 0.1 % compared with that of 1α,25(OH)$_2$D$_3$, respectively). To clarify other possible roles of the hydroxyl groups, we further investigated the biological activities in HL-60 cells with regard to differentiation and cell cycle phase distribution and induction of apoptosis. It has been reported that 1α,25(OH)$_2$D$_3$ inhibits proliferation of HL-60 cells and promotes differentiation of HL-60 cells to macrophages without inducing apoptosis. Like 1α,25(OH)$_2$D$_3$, 19-nor(3β) and 19-nor-22-oxa(1α) also induced cell growth arrest and differentiation without inducing apoptosis, although they were much less potent. On the other hand, 19-nor(1β), 19-nor(3α) and 19-nor-22-oxa(1β), which lack VDR binding potency completely and possess an epimerized hydroxyl group at C-1 or C-3 in the A-ring, all induced apoptosis without inducing cell growth arrest and differentiation. These findings suggest that in 19-nor-1α,25(OH)$_2$D$_3$ analogs, both the 1α-hydroxyl and 3β-hydroxyl groups in the A-ring are structural motifs for the induction of monocytic differentiation in HL-60 cells, but not apoptosis, and conversely, both the 1β-hydroxyl and 3α-hydroxyl groups in the A-ring are structural motifs for the induction of apoptosis, but not monocytic differentiation. Additionally, it is interesting to note that the combination of 22-oxa side chain and 3α-hydroxyl group appears to have extremely weak VDR binding affinity and induce monocytic differentiation in HL-60 cells, but not apoptosis. These findings provide useful information not only for structure-function studies of 1α,25(OH)$_2$D$_3$ analogs but also for the development of therapeutic agents for the treatment of leukemia and other cancers.

References

1. Abe, E., Miyaura, C., Sakagami, H., Takeda, M., Konno, K., Yamazaki, T., Yoshiki, S. and Suda, T. (1981) Proc. Natl. Acad. Sci. USA 78, 4990-4994.
2. Bikle, D.D. and Pillai, S. (1993) Endocr. Rev. 14, 3-19.
3. Lemire, J.M. (1992) J. Cell. Biochem. 49, 26-31.
4. Bouillon, R., Garmyn, M., Verstuyf, A., Segaert, S., Casteels, K. and Mathieu, C. (1995) Eur. J. Endocrinol. 133, 7-16
5. Mikami, K., Osawa, A., Isaka, A., Sawa, E., Shimizu, M., Terada, M., Kubodera, N., Nakagawa, K., Tsugawa, N. and Okano, T. (1998) Tetrahedron Lett. 39, 3359-3362.
6. Okano, T., Nakagawa, K., Tsugawa, N., Ozono, K., Kubodera, N., Osawa, A., Terada, M. and Mikami, K. (1998) Biol. Pharm. Bull. 21, 1300-1305.
7. Okano, T., Nakagawa, K., Kubodera, N., Ozono, K., Isaka, A., Osawa, A., Terada, M. and Mikami, K. (2000) Chemistry & Biology 7, 173-184.
8. Wang, X. and Studzinski, G.P. (1997) Exp. Cell. Res. 235, 210-217.

CALBINDIN-D$_{28K}$ SUPPRESSES APOPTOTIC CELL DEATH BY INHIBITION OF CASPASE 3

Michael Huening*, Tamanna Patel*, Teresita Bellido[+], Stavros Manolagas[+] and Sylvia Christakos*, *Dept. of Biochemistry and Molecular Biology, UMDNJ-New Jersey Medical School and GSBS, Newark, NJ and [+]Division of Endocrinology and Metabolism, University of Arkansas for Medical Sciences, Little Rock, AR

Introduction: The calcium binding protein calbindin-D$_{28K}$ is present in mammalian kidney, brain, pancreas and osteoblasts. In kidney calbindin-D$_{28K}$ has been demonstrated to be vitamin D dependent and is thought to play a role in transcellular calcium transport (1). While calbindin in neuronal cells has not been shown to be vitamin D dependent (1), it has been reported to increase cell survival in neurons, glial cells and lymphocytes in response to a variety of insults involving calcium-dependent events. Such events include exposure to calcium ionophore (2), cAMP (2), glucocorticoid (2), IgG from amyotrophic lateral sclerosis patients (3), amyloid β peptide (4), mutant presenilin (4) and hypoglycemia (5). Studies in PC12 cells (4), glial cells (6), lymphocytes (2) and motor neuron hybrid cells (3) indicate that the type of cell death protected by calbindin is apoptotic. Recent work from our laboratory using βTC pancreatic β cells transfected with calbindin demonstrate that cytokine-mediated destruction of β cells, a cause of insulin-dependent diabetes, can also be inhibited by calbindin. Additionally, we have recently observed that stable transfection of calbindin can block apoptosis induced by tumor necrosis factor α (1nM, 24h) in osteoblastic MC3T3-E1 cells (7).

Results: In order to address the mechanism of this protective effect, we have examined the effect of calbindin on the activity of caspase 3, a common downstream effector of multiple apoptotic signaling pathways. Caspase 3 activity was assessed by measurement of the degradation of the colorimetric peptide DEVD-paranitroanilide (DEVD-pNA). The activity of caspase 3 was completely inhibited by the specific caspase 3 inhibitor peptide DEVD-CHO (DEVD) as expected. Caspase 3 activity was also markedly inhibited by 0.5 and 1.0 ug purified calbindin-D$_{28K}$ as shown in Figure 1. Lysates from calbindin-overexpressing MC3T3-E1 cells are also capable of significantly inhibiting caspase 3 activity (not shown). Other calcium binding proteins (calmodulin, S100, calbindin-D$_{9K}$ and osteocalcin) or the calcium chelator EGTA did not inhibit caspase 3 activity. Since other inhibitors of caspase 3 are cleaved by caspase 3 (8,9), we asked whether calbindin acts similarly. Calbindin did not undergo any significant cleavage in the presence of caspase 3 (Figure 2), consistent with the absence of caspase 3 consensus cleavage sites in the amino acid sequence of calbindin (10,11). These results suggest that calbindin-D$_{28K}$ does not require peptide bond hydrolysis as part of the mechanism of caspase 3 inhibition. The cytoskeletal protein gelsolin has recently been reported to be a specific substrate for caspase 3 (8). We found that in the presence of calbindin (3-5 ug) cleavage of gelsolin (3-5 ug) by caspase 3 (50 ng, 37°C for 10 min) from an apparent size of 65 kD to lower molecular weight cleavage products is blocked (Figure 2).

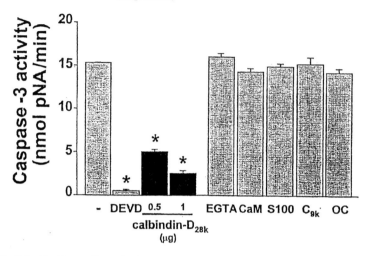

Figure 1: *Calbindin-D28K directly inhibits caspase 3 activity in a cell free system.* Thirty units of human recombinant caspase 3 were combined with 200 uM EVD-pNA in the absence or presence of 0.1uM DEVD-CHO inhibitor, or 0.5 or 1.0 ug purified calbindin-D28K, or 1 ug of the calcium binding proteins calmodulin, S100, calbindin-D9K or osteocalcin, or 1mM EGTA. Caspase 3 activity was calculated based on absorption values at 405 nm.

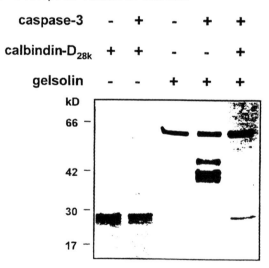

Figure 2: *Calbindin-D28K is not cleaved by caspase 3 and inhibits caspase 3 cleavage of gelsolin.* Purified calbindin-D28K and gelsolin were incubated in the absence or presence of caspase 3 (50 ng) for 10 min at 37°C. Samples were analyzed by SDS-PAGE followed by staining with Coomasie blue. Results shown are representative of four separate experiments.

Other calcium binding proteins including calretinin, parvalbumin, calmodulin and calbindin-D_{9K}, at equivalent or greater concentrations, were unable to inhibit gelsolin cleavage. Heat inactivated calbindin (boiling for 10 min) also is unable to inhibit caspase 3 activity. However, chelation of calcium by EGTA did not affect the ability of calbindin to suppress gelsolin cleavage, suggesting that the inhibitory effect of calbindin on caspase 3 activity is not due to the ability of calbindin to bind calcium. Thus, calbindin-D_{28K} blocks the degradation of both synthetic and natural substrates of caspase 3.

Discussion: While earlier work in the field has demonstrated a large body of correlative evidence associating calbindin-D_{28K} with protection from cell death and degeneration, more recent studies support the direct involvement of calbindin in protecting against cell death. Our results suggest for the first time a mechanism whereby calbindin-D_{28K}, by inhibiting caspase 3, can inhibit morphologic change during apoptosis. A further understanding of the mechanisms by which calbindin-D_{28K} protects against apoptotic cell death will have important therapeutic implications for the prevention of cellular degeneration.

References:

1. Christakos, S., Gabrielides, C., and Rhoten, W. B. (1989) *Endocr. Rev.* **10**(1), 3-26
2. Dowd, D. R., MacDonald, P. N., Komm, B. S., Haussler, M. R., and Miesfeld, R. L. (1992) *Mol. Endocrinol.* **6**(11), 1843-8
3. Ho, B. K., Alexianu, M. E., Colom, L. V., Mohamed, A. H., Serrano, F., and Appel, S. H. (1996) *Proc. Natl. Acad. Sci. U S A* **93**(13), 6796-801
4. Guo, Q., Christakos, S., Robinson, N., and Mattson, M. P. (1998) *Proc. Natl. Acad. Sci. U S A* **95**(6), 3227-32
5. Meier, T. J., Ho, D. Y., and Sapolsky, R. M. (1997) *J. Neurochem.* **69**(3), 1039-47
6. Wernyj, R. P., Mattson, M. P., and Christakos, S. (1999) *Brain Res. Mol. Brain Res.* **64**(1), 69-79
7. Bellido T, H. L., Huening M, Barger SW, Manolagas SC, Christakos S. (1998) *J. Bone Min. Res.* **23** (Supplement 1), S177
8. Kothakota, S., Azuma, T., Reinhard, C., Klippel, A., Tang, J., Chu, K., McGarry, T. J., Kirschner, M. W., Koths, K., Kwiatkowski, D. J., and Williams, L. T. (1997) *Science* **278**(5336), 294-8
9. Zhou, Q., Snipas, S., Orth, K., Muzio, M., Dixit, V. M., and Salvesen, G. S. (1997) *J Biol. Chem.* **272**(12), 7797-800
10. Hunziker, W., and Schrickel, S. (1988) *Mol. Endocrinol.* **2**(5), 465-73
11. Roy, N., Deveraux, Q. L., Takahashi, R., Salvesen, G. S., and Reed, J. C. (1997) *Embo. J.* **16**(23), 6914-25

394

$1\alpha,25(OH)_2D_3$ AND EB 1089 ARE EARLY TRIGGERS OF APOPTOTIC FEATURES IN HUMAN MCF-7 BREAST CANCER CELLS.

Christina Mørk Hansen, Dann Hansen and Lise Binderup. Dept. of Biochemistry, Leo Pharmaceutical Products, DK-2750 Ballerup, Denmark.

Introduction Substantial evidence has now emerged demonstrating that vitamin D compounds are capable of triggering apoptosis in a number of different cell types *in vitro* as well as in mammary tumours *in vivo*. In contrast to other well-known apoptosis inducers, such as TNFα, a relatively long treatment period with the vitamin D compounds seems to be required for most markers of apoptosis to be detectable. However, recent results showing that short-time pre-treatment with vitamin D analogues can potentiate the effect of TNFα- and ceramide-induced apoptosis in MCF-7 cells (1) indicate that the effect of vitamin D may be initiated within a relatively short time. In the present investigation, a series of time-course studies were performed in order to clarify whether a brief incubation with $1\alpha,25(OH)_2D_3$ or one of its analogues, EB 1089, would be sufficient to trigger the appearance of apoptotic features in human MCF-7 breast cancer cells. Apoptotic cells are characterised by a number of characteristics, including degradation of the genomic DNA. Therefore, in the present study, the level of DNA fragmentation was used as a marker of cells showing apoptotic features.

Materials The vitamin D compounds were synthesised at Leo Pharmaceutical Products, Denmark. Tumour Necrosis Factor-α (TNFα) was purchased from R&D Systems Europe Ldt. (Abington, U.K.).

The human MCF-7 breast cancer cell line was purchased from Tumorbank DKFZ (Heidelberg, Germany).

The level of DNA fragmentation was determined using the Cell Death Detection ELISA™ kit (Boehringer Mannheim GmbH, Germany). In order to correct for the growth reducing effect of the compounds, the level of DNA fragments obtained in the Cell Death Detection ELISA were normalised by directly counting cells that had been grown and treated in parallel using a Coulter Counter. The final results were calculated in relation to control cells and expressed as fold induction (OD/1000 cells).

Microscopic evaluation of apoptosis included incubation of the cells with annexin V-FITC (Pharmingen, USA), propidium iodide solution (Pharmingen, USA) and Hoechst 33342 (Molecular Probes, USA).

Results

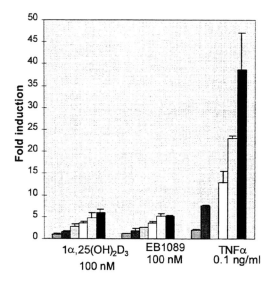

Figure 1: Time-course study showing the induction of DNA fragmentation after 1 (▨), 2(■), 3(▨), 4(□), 5( ) and 7(■) days continuous treatment of the cells with the test compounds.

As seen in **Figure 1**, a continuous treatment of MCF-7 cells with $1\alpha,25(OH)_2D_3$ or EB 1089 for up to 7 days was found to result in a time-dependent induction of DNA fragmentation, starting at day 3. In contrast, the reference compound TNFα appeared to induce a marked increase of DNA fragmentation already at day 2. Also, the level of DNA fragmentation in response to treatment of the cells with TNFα was found to be by far higher than that observed after treatment of the cells with either of the two vitamin D compounds. Interestingly, TNFα and the vitamin D compounds appeared to exert similar effects on the total number of cells, showing that other mechanisms than apoptosis are also involved in the growth inhibiting effect of the vitamin D compounds (**Table 1**).

Table 1

Effects of the test compounds on the number of cells						
Compound:	Days:					
	1	2	3	4	5	7
$1\alpha,25(OH)_2D_3$ 100nM	95±12	88±13	53±2	36±2	37±4	21±2
EB1089 100nM	102±8	92±16	54±8	31±4	33±4	18±1
TNFα 0.1ng/ml	99±5	68±5	60±7	39±8	32±7	22±1

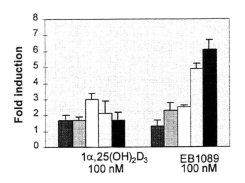

Figure 2: Time-course study showing the induction of DNA fragmentation after a 24 hours' pre-treatment of the cells with the test compounds, followed incubation in fresh medium without the test compounds for a total of 2(■), 3(▨), 4(□), 5( ) and 7(■) days.

As seen in **Figure 2**, a time-dependent induction of DNA fragmentation was seen with both compounds. The effect of EB 1089 was found to be similar to that obtained after a continuous treatment of the cells with EB 1089, while the effect of 1α,25(OH)$_2$D$_3$ showed to be slightly lower than the effect obtained after a continuous treatment with 1α,25(OH)$_2$D$_3$. This observation correlated well with the cell count data (**Table 2**).

Table 2

Effects of the test compounds on the number of cells					
Compound:	**Days:**				
	2	3	4	5	7
1α,25(OH)$_2$D$_3$ 100nM	81±7	68±4	56±5	47±4	70±7
EB1089 100nM	84±3	55±4	38±2	29±2	18±3

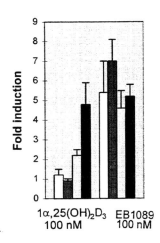

Figure 3: Induction of DNA fragmentation after 2 (□), 6 (■) or 24 ( ) hours' pre-treatment of the cells with the test compounds, followed by a total incubation time of 5 days. (■) 5 days continuous treatment.

Figure 3 shows that with EB 1089 a pre-treatment period of only 2 hours was sufficient to result in an induction of DNA fragmentation at day 5 similar to that observed after a 5 days continuous treatment with EB 1089. In contrast, pre-treatment of the cells with 1α,25(OH)$_2$D$_3$ for less than 24 hours was ineffective with respect to induction of DNA fragmentation. The total number of cells was shown to correlate with these results (**Table 3**).

Table 3.

Effects of the test compounds on the number of cells			
Compound:	2 hrs.	6 hrs.	24 hrs
1α,25(OH)$_2$D$_3$ 100nM	74±5	75±4	49±5
EB1089 100nM	31±5	26±2	29±2

Morphological evaluation of the cells, which have been treated with EB 1089 (100nM) or TNFα (0.1ng/ml) for 4 days, demonstrated that vitamin D and TNFα affect the apoptotic process in MCF-7 differently. In the EB 1089 treated cultures, cells displaying classical apoptotic features such as nuclear fragmentation, were observed. A few annexin-V positive cells (early apoptotic marker) were identified and all the cells appeared to have intact plasma membranes. In contrast, in the TNFα treated cultures, no signs of nuclear fragmentation was observed, but most cells stained strongly with annexin-V. Several cell have taken up red propidium iodide, demonstrating that the plasma membrane in these cells has become leaky (data not shown).

Conclusion

The present investigation demonstrates that a relatively brief exposure to vitamin D is sufficient to trigger DNA fragmentation in MCF-7 cells. Despite the lack of detectable DNA degradation during the first 2 days, only a short pre-treatment period appeared to be required for a significant induction of DNA fragmentation to occur at later time points. EB 1089 was found to be more efficient than 1α,25(OH)$_2$D$_3$ and also, the effect of EB 1089 appeared to be initiated earlier than that of 1α,25(OH)$_2$D$_3$. Thus, the fact that vitamin D compounds are early triggers of apoptotic features in MCF-7 cells suggests that induction of apoptosis in response to vitamin D may be a primary effect.

References

(1) Pirianov, G. Danielsson, C., Carlberg, C., James, S.Y. and Colston, K.W. (1999) Cell Death and Differentiation 6, 890-901.

1,25-DIHYDROXYVITAMIN D₃ TRIGGERS CALCIUM-MEDIATED APOPTOSIS

Igor N. Sergeev, Julie Colby and Anthony W. Norman*

*Department of Chemistry and Biochemistry, South Dakota State University, Brookings, SD 57007 and *Department of Biochemistry, University of California, Riverside, CA 92521*

Intracellular Ca^{2+} appears to be a crucial regulator of programmed cell death (apoptosis). We (1) and others (2) have shown that early and late changes in concentration of intracelluar Ca^{2+} ($[Ca^{2+}]_i$) occur in apoptosis. Mechanisms of action of intracellular Ca^{2+} in apoptotic pathways are not known and apoptosis related Ca^{2+} targets have not been identified. Our hypothesis is that a sustained increase in $[Ca^{2+}]_i$, not reaching cytotoxic levels (above 1 µM), signals the cell to enter an apoptotic pathway. This cartoon illustrates, in simplified form, how changes in $[Ca^{2+}]_i$ relate to cell fate.

Changes in $[Ca^{2+}]_i$ relate to cell fate

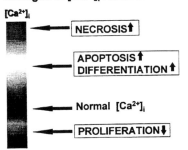

$[Ca^{2+}]_i$

NECROSIS↑

APOPTOSIS↑
DIFFERENTIATION↑

Normal $[Ca^{2+}]_i$

PROLIFERATION↓

Changes in concentration of intracellular free Ca^{2+}, $[Ca^{2+}]_i$, are regulated via Ca^{2+} channels located in cellular membranes and through intracellular Ca^{2+} buffers. 1,25-Dihydroxyvitamin D₃ [1,25(OH)₂D₃] induces a rapid increase in $[Ca^{2+}]_i$ in many cell types, as well as regulates expression of intracellular Ca^{2+} buffers (for a review see ref. 1).

Earlier we have characterized in detail regulation of intracellular Ca^{2+} in human breast cells (3, 4). Our findings show that breast cancer cells express highly permeable voltage-insensitive Ca^{2+} channels (VICC), but there was no evidence for voltage-dependent Ca^{2+} channels (VDCC) (Fig. 1 shows our new data for MCF-7 cell line). Endoplasmic reticulum is a major Ca^{2+} storage compartment, and mobilization of Ca^{2+} from the endoplasmic reticulum stores occurs through inositol 1,4,5-trisphosphate receptor, while ryanodine receptor is not expressed. We also found that 1,25(OH)₂D₃ rapidly increases Ca^{2+} influx through VICC and after a chronic treatment, depletes endoplasmic reticulum Ca^{2+} stores and significantly increases basal $[Ca^{2+}]_i$.

Early and late changes in $[Ca^{2+}]_i$ in response to 1,25(OH)₂D₃

1,25-D
mVDR

VICC

Ca^{2+}

1,25-D
mVDR

IP₃ Ca

IP₃R

ER

Ca-ATPase

This cartoon illustrates mechanisms of early and late changes in intracellular Ca^{2+} in response to 1,25(OH)₂D₃. Early changes are due to Ca^{2+} influx, and late changes result from mobilization of endoplasmic reticulum Ca^{2+} stores.

Abbreviations: VICC, voltage-insensitive Ca^{2+} channels (VICC); mVDR, membrane VDR; IP₃R, inositol trisphosphate receptor; ER, endoplasmic reticulum.

400

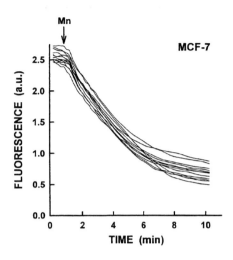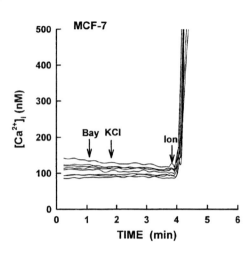

FIG. 1. Ca²⁺ entry through VICC and absence of VDCC. MCF-7 cells exhibited a pathway for Ca²⁺ influx that is permeant to Mn²⁺ ions, which quench fluorescence of the Ca²⁺ probe fura-2 (5) *(left panel)*. Depolarization with K⁺ and the agonist of VDCC Bay K8644 did not increase [Ca²⁺]ᵢ *(right panel)*.

$1,25(OH)_2D_3$ expresses significant anticancer activity, including breast cancer (6, 7). Induction of apoptosis is a particularly important event for eliminating nascent tumor cells and suppressing tumor promotion and progression. We present here results of our study indicating that $1,25(OH)_2D_3$-evoked increase in intracellular Ca^{2+} relates to induction of apoptosis in breast cancer cells.

As a model of breast cancer, we use an estrogen-receptor positive human breast cancer cell line MCF-7. This cell line also expresses VDRs (4) and vitamin D-dependent calbindin-D_{28K} (Sergeev, unpublished observations). We detected apoptosis in individual cells by fluorescent labeling of internucleosomal DNA fragments generated by an apoptotic endonuclease (TUNEL method). Additionally, we used standard morphological criteria of apoptosis: nuclear and chromatin condensation, and formation of apoptotic bodies.

Increase in intracellular Ca^{2+} with $1,25(OH)_2D_3$ did trigger apoptosis in MCF-7 cells. Fig.2 (upper panel) shows confocal images of the single nucleus of the cell labeled for fragmented DNA at the early stage of apoptosis. Middle panels of this figure show the nucleus double-labeled for total and fragmented DNA at the later stage of apoptosis, so that overlay of green and red colors indicates localization of fragmented DNA within the nucleus (on the original image; on this black and white image, those areas are seen as more transparent). Lower left panel shows compact DNA-containing apoptotic bodies at the final stage of cell death.

Importantly, significant increase in [Ca²⁺]ᵢ (measured at 4 hrs) preceded an onset of the early stage apoptosis. Moreover, breast cancer cells loaded with the cytosolic Ca²⁺ buffer BAPTA did not undergo apoptosis in response to $1,25(OH)_2D_3$. On the other hand, treatment of the cells with a Ca^{2+} ionophore similarly induced apoptosis (Fig. 2, lower right panel).

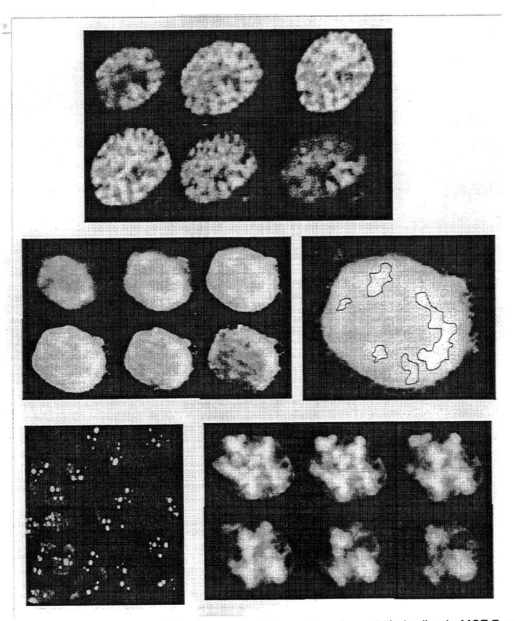

FIG 2. Confocal images of the single apoptotic nuclei and apoptotic bodies in MCF-7 cells. Apoptosis was induced by 1,25(OH)$_2$D$_3$ *(upper, middle and lower left panels)* or ionomycin *(lower right panel)*. DNA strand breaks were labeling using TUNEL method. On the middle and lower panels, the nuclei were counterstained with propidium iodide. FITC (green) and propidium iodide (red) images from optical sections 0.5 µm thick were obtained by laser scanning confocal microscopy (BioRad 1024). The overlay of green and red colors (more transparent areas on these black and white images) indicates areas of fragmented DNA within the nucleus. Similar patterns and degree of DNA fragmentation and condensation were observed in cells treated with either 1,25(OH)$_2$D$_3$ or ionomycin. Note bleb of the nuclear envelope (middle panels).

Taken together, these results show that $1,25(OH)_2D_3$ triggers apoptosis in breast cancer cells by causing an increase in Ca^{2+} entry through VICC and depletion of endoplasmic reticulum Ca^{2+} stores. The resulting elevated $[Ca^{2+}]_i$ appears to be sufficient to elicit apoptosis.

Currently, we initiated a study to investigate whether regulation of intracellular Ca^{2+} in human breast cancer cells differs from normal mammary cells with respect to regulation of intracellular Ca^{2+} (Ca^{2+} entry and Ca^{2+} mobilization pathways). Agents (e.g., certain vitamin D analogs), which stimulate highly permeable VICC characteristic for breast cancer cells, may induce a large increase in $[Ca^{2+}]_i$ and, thus, trigger apoptosis specifically in these cells. Decreasing of cytosolic Ca^{2+} buffering capacity may also increase sensitivity of breast cancer cells to apoptosis inducing signals. Understanding the Ca^{2+}- and vitamin D-mediated mechanisms of apoptotic cell death in breast cancer will help to develop more effective and selective cellular and molecular approaches, based on control of intracellular Ca^{2+}, for treatment of this disease.

Acknowledgments
Supported by NIH/NCI CA-67317 (INS).

References
1. Sergeev, I.N., Rhoten, W.B. and Spirichev, V.B. (1998). In:*Subcellular Biochemistry: Fat-Soluble Vitamins*. vol. 30, (Quinn, P and Kagan, V., eds.), Plenum Press: N.Y., p.271-297.
2. McConkey, D.J. and Orrenius, S. (1997). Biochem. Biophys. Res. Commun. 239: 357-366.
3. Sergeev, I.N. and Rhoten, W.B. (1998). *Endocrine* 9: 321-327.
4. Sergeev, I.N., Rhoten, W.B. and Norman, A.W. (1997). In:*Vitamin D: Chemistry, Biology and Clinical Applications of the Steroid Hormone* (Norman, A.W., Bouillon, R., and Thomasset, M., eds.), Univ. California Printing: Riverside, p. 473-474.
5. Sergeev, I.N. and Rhoten, W.B. (1995). *Endocrinology* 136: 2852-2861.
6. Colston, K. (1997). In: *Vitamin D* (Feldman, D., Glorieux, F.H., and Pike, J.W., eds), pp. 1107-1123, Academic Press, San Diego, CA.
7. Welsh, J., VanWeelden, K., Flanagan, L., Byrne, I., Nolan, E, and Narvaez, C.J.I (1988). In: *Subcellular Biochemistry: Fat-Soluble Vitamins*. vol. 30, (Quinn, P and Kagan, V., eds.), Plenum Press: N.Y., p.245-270.

LIGANDS FOR PPARγ AND RAR/RXR INDUCE APOPTOSIS IN BCL-2 POSITIVE HUMAN BREAST CANCER CELLS.

E. Elstner*, E.A. Williamson**, K. Possinger*, D. Heber**, and H.P. Koeffler**.
*Charité, Department of Medicine, Humboldt University, 10117-Berlin, Germany; **CSMC, Department of Medicine, UCLA, School of Medicine, Los Angeles, CA 90024, USA.

Introduction Cancers are associated with dysregulation of the balance between proliferation and apoptosis. To inhibit proliferation and/or induce apoptosis through ligands of nuclear hormone receptors (NHRs) is a recent approach to cancer therapy. The retinoic acid receptor (RAR), retinoid X receptor (RXR), and peroxisome proliferator receptor γ (PPARγ) belong to the NHR superfamily of ligand-inducible transcriptional factors that regulate gene networks involved in controlling growth, cellular differentiation, and homeostasis. Breast cancer cells express RARs and RXRs. The PPAR-γ has an important role in the differentiation of adipocytes and in fat metabolism. PPARγ ligands promote differentiation of adipocytes are including several prostanoids [15-deoxy-delta(12,14)-prostaglandin J(2) (15D-PGJ$_2$) is the most potent], members of a new class of oral antidiabetic agents, the thiazolidinediones, and a variety of non-steroidal anti-inflammatory drugs. Our recent data showed that PPARγ was expressed in breast cancer but was poorly expressed in normal breast epithelial cells suggesting these cancer cells may be a target for differentiation-based therapy with PPARγ specific ligands (1). Furthermore, ligands for PPARγ inhibited both rat mammary carcinogenesis (2) and proliferation of prostate cancer cells, renal cell carcinoma, non-small cell lung cancer, colorectal cancer and glioblastoma (3-7). Acquired alteration in the pathways required for apoptotic cell death may contribute to the failure of breast cancer to respond to therapy. Our recent data showed that the combination of troglitazone (TGZ), a member of the thiazolidinediones and ATRA synergistically and irreversibly inhibited the growth and induced apoptosis of MCF7 breast cancer cells, associated with a dramatic decrease of levels of bcl-2 protein (1). However, MCF7 is a well-differentiated cell line with low tumorigenicity having expression of wild-type p53, ERα and bcl-2. In this investigation, we have studied the effect of TGZ and retinoids on additional seven breast cancer cell lines (MDA-MB-231, BT474, MDA-MB-436, SKBR3, T47D, BT20, ZR-75-1) which have a variety of genetic defects (**Table 1**).

Results Our data showed that all breast cancer cell lines expressed PPARγ as measured by Western blot (**Table 1**). The ZR-75-1,MCF7, and MDA-MB-231 cells expressed bcl-2 protein and the BT474, MDA-MB-436 and SKBR3 cells expressed a very low level of bcl-2 protein, as measured by Western blot and immuno-histochemistry (**Table 1**). The BT20 and T47D cells were negative for bcl-2. Sensitivity of cancer cell lines to inhibition of clonal growth by NHR-ligands was measured by an effective dose (ED_{50}/ED_{90}) resulting in the inhibition of either 50% or 90% clonal growth, respectively. Each ligand (10^{-11}-10^{-5} M) or combination of TGZ (10^{-11}-10^{-5} M) with each retinoid (10^{-7} M) was studied, the results were plotted and the ED50s and ED90s were calculated. The TGZ was not a strong inhibitor of clonal proliferation of the breast cancer cell lines (ED_{50}: ranged 10^{-7} M - 10^{-5} M) and the rank order of sensitivity to inhibition of clonal growth of the breast cancer cell lines mediated by TGZ was: MCF7>MDA-MB-231>BT474>T47D=ZR-75-1>MDA-MB-436=SKBR3.   BT20 cells did not form colonies in agar. Dose-response studies with RAR-specific ligand, ATRA showed ED_{50} that ranged from 10^{-9} M to 10^{-6} M. The rank order of sensitivity to inhibition of clonal growth of the breast cancer cell lines caused by ATRA   was: MDA-MB-231>MCF7>T47D>ZR-75-1>BT474=MDA-MB-436>SKBR3. The RXR-specific ligand, LG100069 was not as potent inhibitor of clonogenic proliferation as ATRA. The RAR/RXR and RXR/RXR specific ligand, 9-cis-RA had about the same inhibitory activity as ATRA. The combination of various concentrations of TGZ together with 10^{-7} M of either ATRA or 9-cis-RA potently inhibited the clonal growth of MCF7, ZR-75-1 and T47D cells (ED_{90} for TGZ of $1-5\times10^{-11}$ M). The combination of various concentrations of TGZ with 10^{-7} M 9-cis-RA was the most potent combination with prominent inhibition of clonogenic growth of five of the cell lines. The rank order of inhibition was MCF7>ZR-75-1>T47D>MDA-MB-231>>>BT474>MDA-MB436.   Each   ligand alone did not induce apoptosis in breast cancer cells. However, the TGZ (10^{-5} M) combined with either ATRA or 9-cis-RA (10^{-7} M) for 4 days induced significant level of apoptosis ($p<0.05$) in only bcl-2 positive cell lines, MCF7, ZR-75-1 and MDA-MB-231, associated with a concomitant decreased levels of bcl-2 protein levels but expression of bax protein did not change (data not shown). Additionally, no dramatic change in the levels of wild type p53 protein was observed in MCF7 cells after their treatment with either NHR ligand or their combination (data not shown).

<u>Discussion</u>   Effective treatment of tumors is often associated with growth inhibition and/or activation of the endogenous apoptosis pathways. Our previously data showed that the combination of ligands for PPARγ- and RAR produced decreased clonal proliferation and increased apoptosis associated with a dramatic decrease of bcl-2 protein levels in ERα-positive MCF7 cells (1). Now our data showed that the combination of a PPARγ-specific ligand, TGZ with either a RAR-, RXR-, or RAR/RXR-specific ligand induced the inhibition of clonal proliferation of breast cancer cell lines, independent of their bcl-2, p53, and ERα status.

The most powerful combination was TGZ and 9-cis-RA (RAR/RXR- and RXR/RXR specific ligand). The PPARγ heterodimerizes with RXR, and each receptor can bind to its respective ligands. Previous studies have shown that the simultaneous binding of both receptors with its ligand enhances the activity of the heterodimer (9). We also found that the addition of the PPARγ ligand (TGZ) and RXR ligand (LG10069) enhanced the inhibition of clonal growth as compared to either alone. Nevertheless, we found that a RAR specific ligand (ATRA) had prominent activity suggesting that the antiproliferative effects could be mediated along several pathways. Furthermore, we made an interesting observation. Mutant occurs frequently in human breast cancers (10, 11). We showed that the breast cancer cell line, MDA-MB-231 which has a mutant p53, expressed bcl-2 protein and underwent apoptosis after treatment with TGZ and either a RAR- or RAR/RXR-specific retinoids.

Table 1. Biological profile of breast cancer cell lines.

Cell lines	ERα	ERβ[*]	p53	bcl-2[+,**]	PPARγ[+,**]
MCF7	+++	+	wt	++	+
MDA-MB-231	-	+	mut	+	+
ZR-75-1	++	-	wt	++	+
T47D	+	±	mut	-	+
BT-474	±	+	mut	±	+
MDA-MB-436	-	ND	mut	±	+
SKBR3	-	-	mut	±	+
BT-20	-	ND	mut	-	++

ND, not determined; ER, estrogen receptor; wt, wild type; mut, mutation.
*, (8); **, as measured by immunohistochemistry;
+, as measured by Western blot.

Taken together, our data showed that the combination of ligands for PPARγ and RAR/RXR induce inhibition of proliferation of breast cancer cell lines independent of their level of expression of ER, p53, and bcl-2 proteins. However, apoptosis occurred only in bcl2-positive human breast cancer cells. Therefore, the combination of these ligands may have therapeutic activity in breast cancer.

References

1. Elstner, E., Müller, C., Koshizuka, K., Williamson, E.A., Park, D., Asou, H., Shintaku, P., Said, J.W., Heber, D., Koeffler, H.P. (1998) Proc. Natl. Acad. Sci. USA 95, 8806-8811.
2. Suh, N., Wang, Y., Williams, C. R., Risingsong, R., Gilmer, R., Timothy, M., Willson, M., Sporn, M.B. (1999) Cancer Res. 59, 5671-5673.
3. Kubota, T., Koshizuka, K., Williamson, E.A., Asou, H., Said, J.W., Holden, S., Miyoshi, I., Koeffler, H.P. (1998) Cancer Res. 58, 3344-3352.
4. Copland, J.A., Sintuu, C., Wood, C.G. (2000) Proceeding AACR 41, 10 (abstr. 64).
5. Chang, T.-H., Szabo, E. (2000) Cancer Res. 60, 1129-1138.
6. Brockman, J.A., Gupta, R.A., Dubois, R.N. (1998) Gastroentology 115, 1049-1055.
7. Elstner, E., Williamson, E.A., Becker, M., Von Deimling, A., Possinger, K., Koeffler, H.P. (2000) Proceeding AACR 41, 739 (abstr. 4697).
8. Vladusis, E.A., Hornby, A.E., Guerra-Vladusic, F.K., Lakins, J., Lupu, R. (2000) Oncol. Rep. 7,157- 67.
9. Heyman, R.A., Mangelsdorf, D.J., Dyck, J.A., Stein, R.B., Eichele, G., Evans, R.M., Thaller, C. (1992) Cell 68,397-406.
10. Crawford, L.V., Pim, D.C., Lamb,P. (1984) Mol. Biol. Med. 2, 261-272.
11. Cattoretti, G., Rilke, F., Andreola, S., Dámato, L., Domenico, D. (1988) Int. J. Cancer 41, 178- 83.

HC11 MOUSE MAMMARY CELLS ARE GROWTH INHIBITED BY EB1089 AND KH1060 WITH A LATE INDUCTION OF TGF-β EXPRESSION WHEREAS HC11 HA-RAS TRANSFORMED CELLS ARE NOT AFFECTED BY THESE COMPOUNDS.

M.L.H. Katayama, M.A.A.K. Folgueira, I.M.L. Snitcovsky, E.F. Garcia, D. Apolinário, P. Bortman, R.A. Roela, M.Mitzi Brentani.
Disciplina de Oncologia, Departamento de Radiologia, Faculdade de Medicina da Universidade de São Paulo, 01246-903, São Paulo, Brazil.

Introduction Breast cancer is a public health problem throughout the world, with an estimate of 1 million new cases in 2000. In spite of recent progress in early diagnosis and drug treatment, most patients with advanced disease still die of it. Novel preventive and therapeutic approaches are urgently needed. It has long been known that breast cancer is responsive to hormonal manipulation. One such hormone which is potentially active against breast cancer is 1,25-dihydroxyvitamin D_3 [1,25(OH)$_2$D$_3$]. Although 1,25(OH)$_2$D$_3$ actions are basically modulated by nuclear vitamin D receptors (VDR), extragenomic mechanisms also exist. A major setback that limits the clinical use of 1,25(OH)$_2$D$_3$ is the induction of hypercalcemia. To circumvent this problem, 1,25(OH)$_2$D$_3$ analogs were developed and some of them, like EB1089 and KH1060, have potent anti-proliferative action and induce much less hypercalcemia (1). The molecular targets which mediate the anti-proliferative action of 1,25(OH)$_2$D$_3$ are not well defined, but a possible candidate is transforming growth factor β (TGF-β) (2). This molecule is a polypeptide produced by numerous cells that has pleiotropic effects, including growth inhibition or stimulation, cell adhesion and differentiation, depending on the context. TGF-β binds to membrane receptors (Tβ-RII), which trigger signals that end in the nucleus, modulating gene transcription. Previous work from our group has shown that 1,25(OH)$_2$D$_3$ is capable of inhibiting the growth of HC11 mouse mammary cells but not of Ha-ras transformed cells (3). These cells are an useful *in vitro* model of breast carcinogenesis. HC11 cells are derived from the breast of mid pregnant mice and retain normal features, like growth inhibition by density saturation and the potential to differentiate upon exposure to lactogenic hormones. Ha-ras transformed HC11 cells, in contrast, are not growth inhibited upon density saturation, do not differentiate and are tumorigenic when injected in nude mice (4). The objective of the present study is to test whether two 1,25(OH)$_2$D$_3$ analogs (EB1089 and KH1060) have anti-proliferative action in HC11 and HC11ras cells and to correlate this effect with variations in TGF-β1 mRNA expression.

Material and Methods
Cell culture HC11 and HC11ras cells (a kind gift from Dr. Nancy Hynes, Friedrich Miescher Inst., Basel, Switzerland) were grown in RPMI medium. Cells were induced with EB1089 10^{-9} to 10^{-7} M or KH1060 10^{-11} to 10^{-9} M (gently donated by Dr. Lise Binderup, Leo Pharmaceutical Products, Denmark) in the presence of 10% charcoal treated bovine calf serum.

<u>Growth curves</u> Disposable 8,8 cm^2 plates were seeded at an initial density of 2x10^4 cells per plate. Cells were harvested at 24-hour intervals in triplicates and counted in a Neubauer chamber. The mean cell number was plotted in monolog graph paper and cell doubling times (DT) calculated.

<u>Flowcytometric DNA content determination</u> Cells were evaluated for DNA content using the DNA intercalating agent propidium iodide. Analysis was performed in a FACSCalibur flowcytometer and percentage of cells in G0/G1, S and G2/M phases determined by the ModFit software, Becton Dickinson, USA.

<u>Northern Analysis</u> Total RNA was isolated by the guanidinium isothiocyanate/ cesium chloride method. RNA (20 μg) was separated electrophoretically and transferred to nylon membranes. Hybridization was performed with ^{32}P labeled specific probes to TGF-β1 (1.0 Kb EcoRI fragment) (5) (provided by Dr. K.H. Heldin, Uppsala, Sweden) or GAPDH (6). The resulting bands were quantified by densitometry and values expressed as the TGF-β1/GAPDH signal ratio.

<u>Indirect Immunofluorescence</u> 5x10^5 cells were incubated with anti TGFβ RII rabbit polyclonal antibody (Santa Cruz Biotechnology, USA) and then incubated with a FITC conjugated anti-rabbit IgG monoclonal antibody (Sigma, USA). Cells were analyzed in a FACSCalibur flowcytometer.

<u>Results</u> HC11control cells presented a doubling time (DT) of 30h. When these cells were exposed to EB1089 (10^{-9}, 10^{-8}, 10^{-7} M), growth inhibition was evident after a 96h treatment with 10^{-8} M, which was the minimal effective concentration. The highest EB1089 concentration (10^{-7} M) caused an early HC11 cell growth arrest. The other compound, KH 1089 (10^{-11}, 10^{-10}, 10^{-9}M), had a potent anti-proliferative action in HC11 cells, as compared to EB1089, since the minimal effective concentration was lower (10^{-9} M). HC11 cell DT more than doubled (from 30 to 66h) after exposure to KH1089 10^{-9} M. HC11ras cells, in contrast, had a shorter DT (12h) and were resistant to the anti-proliferative effect of EB1089 as well as to KH1089 (<u>Figure 1</u>).

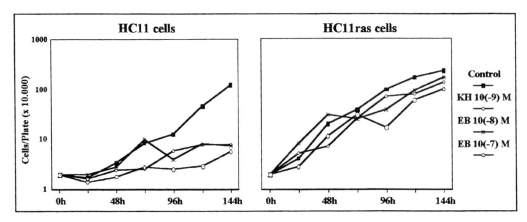

Figure 1: Growth curves of HC11 and HC11ras cells exposed or not (control) to EB1089 (EB) 10^{-8} M, EB1089 10^{-7} M or KH1060 (KH) 10^{-9} M, as described in material and methods. Two independent assays were performed in triplicate and mean values are represented.

Cell cycle distribution was then determined in HC11 cells exposed or not to EB1089 10^{-7} M or KH1060 10^{-9} M. Both inducers caused, after a 96h exposure, a shift to G0/G1 (from 60 to 81%), with a corresponding fall in the S phase fraction. On the other hand, HC11ras cells were not growth inhibited upon these treatments and the S phase fraction remained high. To verify whether growth inhibition could be mediated by TGF-β induction, HC11 and HC11ras cells were exposed to EB1089 10^{-7} M or KH1060 10^{-9} M and TGF-β1 mRNA expression examined. TGF-β1 mRNA was not expressed by HC11 cells grown for 24, 72 or 120hs. Exposure to EB1089 10^{-7} M or KH1060 10^{-9} for the same periods led to a late (120h) induction of TGF-β1 mRNA (shown only 120h). In HC11ras cells, TGF-β1 mRNA expression was constitutive at 24, 72, 96 or 120h and exposure to EB1089 10^{-7} M or KH1060 10^{-9} M for the same periods did not change it (shown only 24 and 72h) (Figure 2).

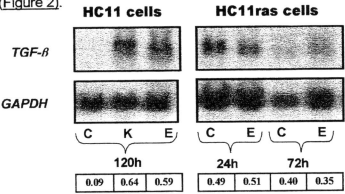

Figure 2: Expression of TGF-β1 mRNA (2.5 Kb) in HC11 (left) and HC11ras cells (right), grown without (C, control) or in the presence of EB1089 10^{-7} M (E) or KH1060 10^{-9} M (K) for different time periods. GAPDH mRNA (1.2 Kb) expression is also shown. The ratio of TGF-β1 transcripts standardized to GAPDH, as determined by densitometric readings, appears on the table below.

In addition, we have also determined Tβ-RII expression in HC11 parental and Ha-ras transformed cells and verified that only a low fraction of both cells (10%) present this molecule (Figure 3).

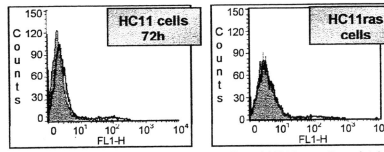

Figure 3: Histograms of Tβ-RII expression in HC11 (left) and HC11ras cells maintained in culture medium for 72 hours. Cell number appears on the y-axis and fluorescence channel on x-axis, the filled area represents the unspecific staining and the open area represents cells specifically labeled with anti Tβ-RII antibody.

Discussion HC11 cells were growth inhibited by the 1,25(OH)$_2$D$_3$ analogs, EB1089 and KH1060, in contrast with HC11ras cells. These results are in accordance to those obtained with the parent compound, 1,25(OH)$_2$D$_3$. HC11ras cells resistance could in part be explained by the lower VDR content found in these cells (3). We also observed that HC11ras cells constitutively expressed 25(OH)D$_3$–24 hydroxilase, a 1,25(OH)$_2$D$_3$ metabolizing enzyme, which could lead to a lower intracellular concentration of the inducers (data not shown). Another possibility is that Ha-ras expression could preclude VDR/RXR heterodimerization by phosphorylating RXRα, impairing the transactivating capacity of this complex (7). In HC11 cells exposed to the inducers, there was a late (120h) induction of TGF-β1 expression, that took place after cells were growth arrested and hence, did not seem related to their anti-proliferative effects. Furthermore, TGF-β receptors, critical elements in this pathway, were detected in only 10% of HC11 cells and our preliminary data in 1,25(OH)$_2$D$_3$ treated cells, revealed no variations on the expression of these receptors. In addition, in HC11ras cells TGF-β1 expression was constitutive, unrelated to growth inhibition. Previous studies have shown that in keratinocytes harboring a mutated Ha-ras, TGF-β synthesis was higher than that observed in normal cells (8). Furthermore, mammary cells showing mutated ras lose the anti-proliferative response to TGF-β (9). We hypothesize an anomalous role for the TGF-β pathway in HC11ras cells, as proliferation persisted unchecked, and only 10% of these cells expressed TGF-β receptors. In summary, EB1089 and KH1060 inhibit the growth of HC11 cells independent of TGF-β1 expression.

References
1.Carlberg, C., Mathiasen, I.S., Saurat, J-H. and Binderup, L. (1994) J. Steroid Biochem. Molec. Biol. 51, 137-142.
2.Mercier, T., Chaumontet, C., Gaillard-Sanchez, I., Martel, P. and Heberden, C. (1996) Biochemical Pharmacology 52: 505-510, 1996.
3.Escaleira, M.T.F. and Brentani. M.M. (1999) Breast Cancer Res. Treatment, 54, 123-134.
4.Happ, B., Hynes, N.E. and Groner, B. (1993) Cell Growth & Differentiation 4, 9-15.
5.Derynck, R., Jarret, J.A., Chen, E.Y., Eaton, D.H., Bell, J.R., Assoian, R.K., Roberts, A.B., Sporn, M.B. and Goeddel, C.V. (1985) Nature 316, 701-705.
6.Fort, P., Piechaczyk, M., Sabrouty, S.E., et al. (1985) Nucl. Acid Res. 13, 1431-1442.
7.Solomon, C., White, J.H. and Kremer, R. (1999) J. Clin. Invest. 103: 1729-1735.
8.Fahey, M.S., Paterson, I.C., Stone, A., Collier, A.J., Heung, Y.L., Davies, M., Patel, V., Parkinson, E.K. and Prime, S.S. (1006) Br. J. Cancer 74, 1074-1080.
9.Kretzschmar, M., Doody, J., Timokhina, I. and Massague J. (1999) Genes Dev. 13, 804-816.

This work was supported by FAPESP grant n°98/16066-9

MCF-7 CLONAL HETEROGENEITY IS RESPONSIBLE FOR A DIFFERENTIAL SENSITIVITY TO THE ANTIPROLIFERATIVE EFFECTS OF 1a,25-DIHYDROXYVITAMIN D3.

Simon Skjøde Jensen[*#], Mogens W. Madsen[*], Jiri Bartek[#], Lise Binderup[*].
[*] LEO Pharmaceutical Products, DK-2750 Ballerup, and [#] Dept. of Cell Cycle and Cancer, The Danish Cancer Society, DK-2100 Copenhagen Ø.
Correspondance:Simon.Jensen@LEO-pharma.com

Introduction: 1α,25-dihydroxyvitamin D3 (VD$_3$) exhibits antiproliferative effects in most mammalian cells in vitro as well as in vivo. The molecular mechanisms responsible for these effects have been described in a variety of model systems including cancer cell lines and non transformed cells like keratinocytes. It is our observation that heterogeneity of the human breast cancer cell line MCF-7 is responsible for a biphasic antiproliferative response to VD$_3$. We have isolated four MCF-7 clones which are either hypersensitive or nearly resistant to VD$_3$ treatment.

Results and discussion:
Our MCF-7 cell line responds to VD$_3$ by decreased S phase entry (measured by Brd U incorporation) up to 8 days of VD$_3$ treatment (Fig 1). From day 8 to day 14, Brd U incorporation increased slightly again. This phenomenon could be the result of a selection and/or acquisition of resistant cells in the total cell pool. In order to develop a model system, in which the antiproliferative response to VD$_3$ was stronger and more homogeneous, we isolated 40 clones from the parental MCF-7 cell line, and analyzed the relative response of each clone to VD$_3$ treatment (Fig. 2). The ratio between control and VD$_3$ treated cells were scored, with parental cells showing a proliferative indeks (P.I.) of 5 (control cells are five times more numerous relative to VD$_3$ treated cells). The P.I. of selected clones are shown in Fig. 2, with two VD$_3$ hypersensitive (clones 22 and 44) and two nearly resistant clones (clones 3 and 4). Taken together, Fig. 2 indeed shows that the parental MCF-7 cells consists of a very heterogeneous pool of cells.
Clones 3, 4, 22 and 44 were selected for further characterization. In a proliferation assay over 6 days, clone 22 indeed showed a strong response to VD$_3$ compared to clone 3 which was only weakly affected by VD$_3$ (Fig. 3). Clone 22 decreased significantly in cell number from 4 to 6 days of VD$_3$ treatment, strongly indicating that clone 22 respond to VD$_3$ by increased apoptosis.
Dose-response experiments performed by thymidine incorporation assays after 3 days of VD$_3$ treatment of the selected clones, showed a strong response in clones 22 and 44, whereas clones 3 and 4 responded rather weakly (Fig. 4). The IC$_{50}$ values were 10 times lower for clones 22 ($1,4\times10^{-8}$ M) and 44 ($2,1\times10^{-8}$ M), relative to parental cells ($1,9\times10^{-7}$ M).
The phosphorylation status of the retinoblastoma tumor suppressor protein

412

(pRb) is an indicator of cell cycle state, with the hypophosphorylated and faster migrating species of pRb indicative for cells arrested in G_1 phase. Biochemical

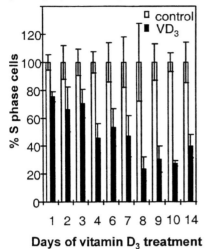

Figure 1. Brd U incorporation in parental MCF-7 cells, showing decreased S phase entry up to 8 days of treatment, and weak increase from day 8 to 14.

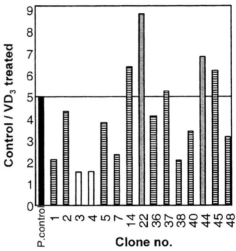

Figure 2. The response of selected clones to VD_3. After 5 days of treatment parental cells had a P.I. of 5 (Black bar), whereas clones 3 and 4 were nearly resistant (white bars), and clones 22 and 44 were hypersensitive (gray bars).

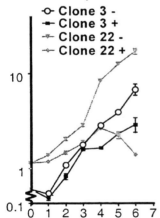

Figure 3. Representative proliferation assay over 6 days comparing clone 22 (hypersensitive), and clone 3 (resistant). Clones 44 and 4 responded like clone 22 and 3 respectively.

analysis of the phosphorylation status of pRb in clone 22 showed accumulation of the hypophosphorylated pRb upon VD_3 treatment (Fig. 5), whereas clone 3 after 96 h of exposure to VD_3 still contained large amounts of hyperphosphorylated pRb (denoted pRb^{pp}).Phosphorylation of pRb is mediated by a group of cyclin dependent kinases (cdk). Cdk2 is important for the cell cycle progression of G_1 and S phase, and is a key target for cell cycle inhibition induced by VD_3. The differential phosphorylation status of pRb in clone 3 and 22 (Fig. 5), indicates that cdk2 is regulated in different manner in sensitive versus resistant

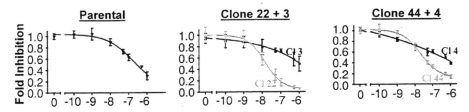

Figure 4. Proliferation assay measured by thymidine incorporation after 3 days of VD$_3$ treatment.

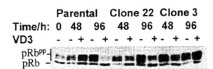

Figure 5. Western blot of pRb in clones treated as indicated, showed accumulation of hypophosphorylated pRb in clone 22, whereas clone 3 was not affected similarly.

clones. Cdk2 *in vitro* kinase assays using a recombinant GST-pRb protein as substrate showed fast and effective inhibition of cdk2 in clones 22 and 44, whereas cdk2 from clone 3 treated for 96 h did not show any significant inhibition even after 96 h treatment (data not shown). Collectively, biochemical analysis of key cell cycle regulators in the clones correlate with the differential response to VD$_3$ identified by proliferation assays. Our data indicate that the four clones are deregulated in pathways upstream of pRb phosphorylation and cdk2 inhibition. Candidate mechanisms for a differential response to VD$_3$ could be either loss or inactivation of the VD$_3$ receptor (VDR). We investigated the mRNA for VDR in each clone by RT- PCR (Fig. 6). Clone 22 showed slightly elevated levels of the VDR mRNA, whereas the other clones contained similar levels of the VDR mRNA. We analyzed if VDR was activated to the same extent after 24 h VD$_3$ treatment in each clone. VDR activation correlates with strong induction of the 24-hydroxylase gene, and indicates if VDR activation and cofactor requirements are deregulated in the respective clones. The 24-hydroxylase was strongly induced in all clones, similar to parental cells, again with slightly higher levels in clone 22 (Fig. 7). The antiproliferative effects mediated by VD$_3$ and retinoic acid affects similar cell cycle components like cdk2, p21$^{CIP1/WAF1}$ and pRb phosphorylation. Since retinoic acid also activate nuclear receptors similar to VDR, we speculated if the clones would respond to all-trans-retinoic acid (R.A.) in the characteristic hypersensitive and resistant manner as shown above for VD$_3$. Dose-response experiments with R.A. showed that clone 3 was resistant also to R.A. (data not shown), suggesting that clone 3 could be aberrant in components shared by both VD$_3$ and R.A. signaling pathways, e.g. cofactors required for transcriptional regulation or in the pathway(s) leading to cell cycle arrest.

414

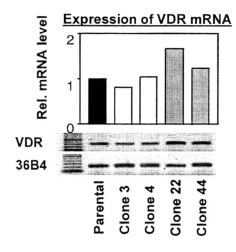

Expression of VDR mRNA　　　**Induction of 24-hydroxylase**

Figure 6. Expression of VDR mRNA detected by RT-PCR in exponentially growing cells.

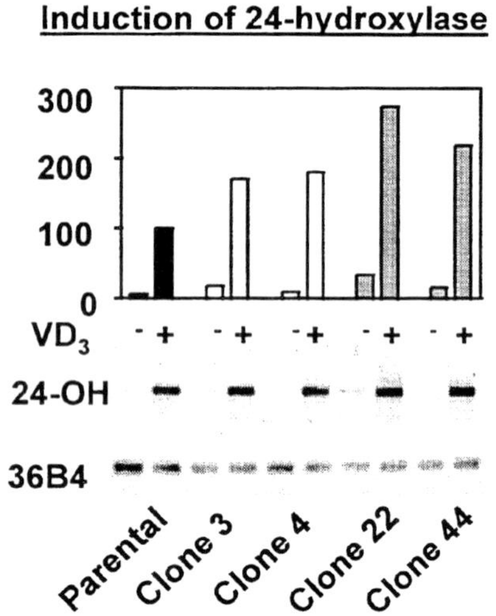

Figure 7. Induction of 24-hydroxylase mRNA after 24 h VD₃ treatment, detected by RT-PCR.

Clones 4, 22 and 44 responded to R.A. like parental cells, suggesting that the different response to VD_3 in these clones is due to aberrations in pathways independently of R.A. signaling.

Conclusion:

Our data show that the parental MCF-7 cell line is very heterogeneous in the antiproliferative response to VD_3. We have selected four MCF-7 clones which respond to VD_3 in either hypersensitive of almost resistant manners.

Biochemical characterization correlates with the proliferation assays, showing strong inhibition of cdk2 kinase activity and lack of pRb phosphorylation in hypersensitive clones, whereas resistant clones are nearly unaffected at the level of cell cycle regulation.

We have investigated why these clones behave differently to VD_3, and where in the VD_3 signaling pathway(s) leading to cell cycle arrest the clones are deregulated. Our studies indicate that resistance is not due to loss of VDR or its ability to regulate transcription.

Increased sensitivity to VD_3 could occur by increased VDR levels and activation, as identified in clone 22, but if and how this is linked to increased cell cycle arrest remains elusive.

We are currently investigating if the differential sensitivity to VD_3 could be a consequence of aberration in the non-genomic signaling pathway(s) recently identified for VD_3. Alternatively, the clones could be deregulated in pathways leading to either apoptosis or differentiation.

VITAMIN D AND HOMEOGENE CROSS-TALKS IN DENTAL CELLS IN VIVO AND IN VITRO.

A. Berdal[1], F. Lézot[1], C. Blin[1], P. Papagerakis[1], M. MacDougall[2] and Y. Kato[3].
[1]University Paris 7, EA 2380, Cordeliers Institute, Paris, France ; [2]UTHSC, Dpt Ped. Dentistry, San-Antonio, TX, USA and [3]Genetic Unit, Tokyo, Japan.

Introduction   Previous investigations on nutritional rickets have shown that vitamin D may control tooth morphogenesis, differentiation and biomineralization (1). More specifically, the epithelial-mesenchymal interactions leading tooth development were proposed to be affected, based on the site-specific defects of cell differentiation. These interactions involve up- and down-regulation of the expression of several transcription factors by diffusible growth and differentiation factors (2). The paradigm for these cell-cell interactions is the signalling cascade of the bone morphogenetic proteins BMP2-BMP4 and homeoproteins encoded by divergent homeogene Msx (Muscle Segment Homeobox gene) and Dlx (Distaless Segment Homeobox gene). Furthermore, Msx and Dlx homeoproteins have been shown to control the expression of bone matrix proteins such as osteocalcin, an established vitamin D-target (3). Preliminary studies suggest that these homeogenes may also contribute to the control of dental formation and biomineralization (4, 5). Our general hypothesis is that vitamin D acts on dental cells by controlling this epigenetic cascade which would regulate early development and biomineralization. These homeogenes were investigated in null mutants for the nuclear vitamin D receptor (6) as an experimental model system for the vitamin D-resistant rickets.

The developmental expression pattern of the nuclear vitamin D receptor is characterized by successive up- and down-regulation in the epithelial and mesenchymal dental cells, which follows the developmental stages of the Msx/Dlx epigenetic cascade. Therefore, our second hypothesis was that the transcription factors Msx and Dlx may reversely control the developmental expression pattern of the nuclear vitamin D receptor.

Results

Vitamin D action on homeogenes in vivo. Msx1, Msx2, Dlx2 and Dlx5 transcripts were screened in microdissected teeth by RT-PCR (3 to 56 day-old wild-type mice). The involvement of each homeogene varied according to the tissue-type (epithelial and mesenchymal) and anatomical site (incisors versus molars).

The developmental pattern of Dlx2 expression was investigated in a transgenic mice bearing a construct including the 3.7 kb Dlx2 promoter and a reporter gene lacZ (4, 5). This homeogene was expressed during late biomineralization, i.e. in the epithelial cels during the diffrent stages of amelogenesis (Figure 1) and cementogenesis (Figure 2).

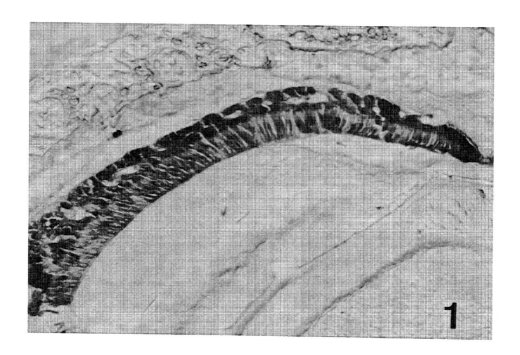

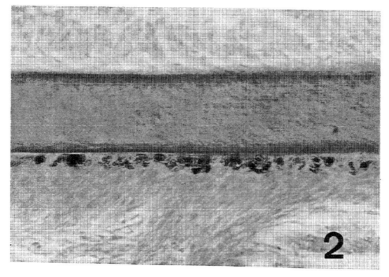

The effects of the nuclear vitamin D receptor annulation (VDR -/-) were analyzed at 56 days. Msx/Dlx expression was affected in VDR -/- teeth. There, morphogenetic disruptions were also identified by histological analysis, at the same age and earlier before weaning. These defects varied depending on the tissue-type and anatomical site, accordingly to the Msx/Dlx expression patterns and as previously reported in nutritional rickets.

Homeogene actions on VDR and vitamin D-dependent osteocalcin in vitro. Msx1, Msx2, and Dlx5 (expression vectors from S. Harris and C Abate-Shen) were transiently overexpressed in immortalized MO6-G3 dental cells. The steady-state levels of an established target of vitamin D, osteocalcin, and the vitamin D receptor were analyzed after single or co-transfections and $1\alpha,25(OH)_2$ vitamin D_3 addition. The data show that each transfected homeogene and $1\alpha,25(OH)_2$ vitamin D_3 jointly inhibited osteocalcin expression. Msx/Dlx co-transfection annuled their effects, supporting that they antagonise through Msx/Dlx heterodimer formation. Msx/Dlx homeogenes appeared to also modulate VDR, in conjunction with $1\alpha,25(OH)_2$ vitamin D_3.

Discussion Thus, cross-talks of Msx, Dlx homeogenes and VDR were identified in dental cells. These same homeogenes control site-specific growth in cranio-facial bone (for instance Msx-1 and the basal outgrowth of the mandible ; Orestes-Cardoso et al., submitted). All these data highlight the morphogenetic role of vitamin D in teeth and cranio-facial skeleton, as they jointly derive from Msx/Dlx-dependent neural crests in contrast to the mesodermal skeleton which patterning is governed by the archetypal Hox homeogenes.

References

1. Berdal, A., Balmain, N., Cuisinier-Gleizes, P. and Mathieu, H. (1987) Arch. Oral. Biol. 32, 493-498.
2. Thesleff, I. and Sharpe, P. (1997) Mech. Dev. 67, 111-123.
3. Bidder, M., Latifi, T. and Towler , D.A. (1998) J. Bone Miner. Res. 13, 609-619.
4. Lézot, F., Thomas, B., Hotton, D., Forest, N., Orestes-Cardoso, S., Robert, B., Sharpe, P. and Berdal, A. (2000a) J. Bone Min. Res. 15, 430-441.
5. Lézot, F., Davideau, J.L., Thomas, B., Sharpe, P., Forest, N. and Berdal, A. (2000b) J. Histochem. Cytochem. 48(2), 2777-283.
6. Yoshigawa, T., Handa, Y., Uematsu, Y., Takeda, S., Sekine, K., Yoshihara, Y., Kawakami, T., Arioka, K., Sato, H., Uchiyama, Y., Masushige, S., Fukamizu, A., Matsumoto, T. and Kato, S. (1997) Nature Genet. 16, 391-396.

IMMUNOCYTOCHEMICAL, ELECTRON-MICROSCOPE AND BIOCHEMICAL INVESTIGATIONS OF MO6-G3 ODONTOBLASTS IN VITRO.

C. Mesgouez[1], N. Forest[1], M. MacDougall[2], M. Oboeuf[1], S. Monteiro[1], H. Mansour[1], S. Christakos[2], and A. Berdal[1], [1]University Paris 7, EA-2380, Cordeliers Institute, IFR-058, Paris, France ; [2]UTHSC, Department of Pediatric Dentistry, San Antonio, Texas, USA.

Introduction Odontoblasts are characterized by their morphodifferentiation into polarized secretory cells and the acquisition of their biochemical phenotype (1). They produce a set of matrix proteins. Some of them are common to bone and dentin, for instance collagen type I and osteocalcin. Two matrix proteins have been described to be dentin-specific : the dentin phosphoprotein or phosphophoryn and dentin sialoprotein. These two proteins are encoded by a single gene, DSPP (2). Odontoblasts also express several proteins involved in calcium and phosphate handling : calbindins (3) and alkaline phosphatase (4).

Dentinogenesis may be controlled by several environmental variables such as vitamin D (5) and fluoride supplementation (6). Experimental approaches *in vivo* and in organotypic cultures *in vitro* are difficult to interpret regarding the direct effects of these agents on odontoblasts because of 1°) the known epithelial-mesenchymal interactions leading odontoblast activity and 2°) cell heterogeneity within the dental mesenchyme.

The establishment of cell lines which reproduces *in vitro* the functions of odontoblasts, may therefore be used to more specifically study the effects of intrinsic and extrinsic factors on the physiology of these cells. The aim of the present study is to analyze an odontoblast cell line after immortalization with a viral transformation by SV 40 (7). Cells were studied by immunolocalization of type I collagen, histoenzymatic staining and biochemical investigation of alkaline phosphatase (AP) and by transmission electron microscopy. Furthermore, the action of fluoride was tested in these culture systems.

Materials and Methods The cells were cultured as previously described (7) for up to 42 days. Sodium Fluoride was added extemporary by dilution with culture medium to obtain the following concentrations : 50 µM and 1 mM. Fluoride was added at day 11 and investigations realized 48 hours later.

Polyclonal rabbit antibodies directed against type I collagen (Institut Pasteur, Lyon, France) were used at dilutions of 1/50. Monoclonal murine primary antibodies specific for rat TNAP (M. Vogel, G. Rodan, Merck Research Laboratories, West Point, PA) was used at dilution of 1/50. Cells were examined under a Leitz-Orthoplan fluorescence microscope.

At day 11 Alkaline phosphatase activity was determined with 15 mM paranitrophenyl-phosphate as substrate and compared with a p-nitrophenol standard solution (Sigma). Protein concentrations were measured by the BCA protein assay reagent (Pierce, Rockford, II, USA). The enzymatic activity was expressed as nmol released p-nitrophenol (PNP) per minute per milligram of protein at 37°C.

Alkaline phosphatase histoenzymatic localization was determined as outlined by Osbody and Caplan (1981) and the samples were studied microscopically.

At day 3, cells were fixed, scraped off and post-fixed and dehydrated in a graded series of ethanol. Then, the cells were embedded in Epon-Araldite. Semi-thin sections were cut with a diamond knife, mounted on glass slides and stained with methylene blue-Azur II. Ultra-thin sections were collected on copper grids and stained with 2.5% uranyl acetate in absolute ethanol and lead citrate. All sections were examined using a Philips CM-12 transmission electron microscope.

Results

Survey of cellular kinetics Phase contrast microscopy allowed to identifiy the behaviour of MO6-G3 cell lines. After 11 days, they formed multiple layers (Figure 1).

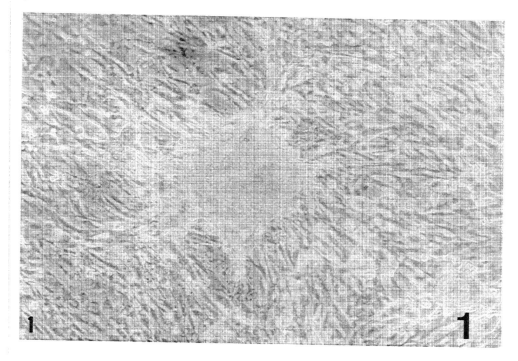

Analysis of odontoblast phenotype Immunolocalization for AP and type I collagen were performed at 3, 7 and 11 days of culture. Immunolocalization with collagen type I antibodies (Figure 2) showed cytoplasmic staining for the two types of cell lines throughout the culture, as well as in the extracellular network appearing at 7 days.

Alkaline phosphatase was analyzed through three different methods : immunolabeling, histoenzymology and analysis of enzymatic activity

The AP immunolocalization was positive on the two lines. AP activity appeared significant at 11 days by histoenzymology. Aggregates of AP-active cells and isolated AP-positive cells were randomly distributed in the cell layer. Furthermore, the effects of fluoride were also identified. The effects of 50 μM and 1 mM fluoride were significant at 11 days.

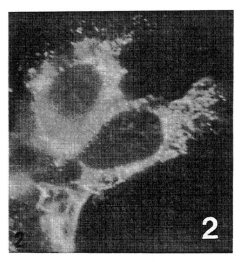

Electron microscope observations The rough endoplasmic reticulum and Golgi apparatus appeared well developped, confirming the secretory character of these cells.

Discussion The dynamic evolution of the specific markers of differentiation has been defined in MO6-G3 cell lines (This study, 7). Major protein of the extracellular matrix expressed by odontoblasts is type I collagen. However, this phenotypic marker is not very characteristic, since this protein is also found in the fibroblasts, osteoblasts and also cementoblasts. Dentin contains two tissue-specific proteins : dentin phosphoprotein (DPP) and dentin sialoprotein (DSP). They are encoded by from the same gene (2). Immunolocalization of the DPP in MO6-G3 (7) allows to affirm that these cells are, indeed, odontoblastic-type cells. It as been suggested that ALP is implicated in mineralization process of bone and dental tissues (8). It is, therefore, an important phenotype marker of the formative cells of hard tissues. This enzyme has been widely used as a marker for odontoblastic type cells (9, 10), and also of bone cells (11) in vitro. It seemed particularly interesting that, at a time when fluoride is so extensively used in preventive and conservative dentistry, we could be also able to study its role in certain metabolic odontoblastic activities.

In conclusion, immortalized odontoblasts may be useful experimental system to investigate the effects of fluoride and vitamin D on odontoblast activity.

References

1. Ruch, J.V. (1998) Biochem. Cell. Biol. 76, 923-38.
2. MacDougall, M., Simmons, D., Xianghon, G.L., Nydegger, J., Feng, J. and Gu, T.T. (1997) J. Biol. Chem. 272(2), 835-842.
3. Berdal, A., Hotton, D., Saffar, J.L., Thomasset, M. and Nanci, A. (1996) J. Bone Miner. Res. 11, 768-779.
4. Hotton, D., Mauro, N., Lézot, F., Forest, N. and Berdal A. (1999) J. Histochem. Cytochem. 47, 1541-1552.
5. Berdal A. (1997) In : vitamin D. Feldman D., Glorieux F.H., Pike J.W.(Eds). New York, Academic Press, pp. 423-435.
6. Bronckers, A.L.J.J., Jansen, L.L. and Wöltgens, J.H.M. (1984) Archs. Oral Biol. 29, 803-810.
7. MacDougall, M., Thiemann, F., Ta, H., Hsu, P., Chen, L.S. and Snead, M.L. (1995) Connec. Tissue Res. 33, 97-103.
8. Beertsen, W., Van Den Bos, T. and Everts, V. (1999) J. Dent. Res. 78, 1221-1229.
9. Kasugai, S., Adachi, M. and Ogura, H. (1988) Archs. oral Biol. 33(12), 887-891.
10. Nakashima, M. (1991) Archs. oral Biol. 36(9), 655-663.
11. Wlodarski, K.H. and Reddi, A.H. (1986) Calcif. Tissue Int. 39, 382-385.

VITAMIN D ANALOGS MODULATE DIFFERENTIATION OF CULTURED RAT BONE MARROW TO OSTEOBLASTS AND THEIR RESPONSE TO GONADAL STEROIDS.

Somjen D.[1], Offer M.[2], Kaye A.M.[3] and Bleiberg I.[2].
[1]Inst. of Endocrinology, Tel-Aviv Sourasky Med. Ctr., [2]Dept. of Histology and Cell Biology the Sackler faculty of Medicine, Tel-Aviv Univ., Tel-Aviv and [3]Dept. Of Molecular Genetics, The Weizmann Inst. of Science, Rehovot, Israel.

Introduction: We have demonstrated previously that skeletal tissues and cells from different sources show sex-specific response to gonadal steroids and selective estrogen receptor modulators (SERMS) in the stimulation of the specific activity of the BB isozyme of creatine kinase (CK) (1-3). This response can be modulated by manipulation of the endocrine environment during early postnatal development (4-6). Moreover pretreatment with vitamin D analogs upregulated the responsiveness and sensitivity to gonadal steroids and SERMS with no effect on the sex-specificity (7-10). We also found that $1,25(OH)_2D_3$ (1,25D) can modulate the differentiation of bone marrow from mice in culture to osteoblast-like cells, resulting in increased alkaline phosphatase activity and acquisition of sex-specific responsiveness to gonadal steroids when CK is assayed (11). Mice femoral bone marrow, when cultured in the presence of Dexamethasone (Dex), 1,25D or both, show CK responsiveness to gonadal steroids with augmented responsiveness and sensitivity in the presence of both (12). In the present study we used bone marrow from the rat and we used the nonhypercalcemic side chain modified analogs of vitamin D CB 1093 (CB), EB 1089 (EB) and MC 1288 (MC) (7,9). We analyzed both the sex-specificity and the age dependence of the differentiation process.

Materials and Methods:
Cell culture: Wistar derived rats at the age of 2 months (young) or > 6 month (old) were sacrificed and femoral bone marrow was collected and cultured as described for the mice (11,12). For differentiation into osteoblast-like cells, Dex (10nM) or 1,25D (4nM) or CB (1nM) or the combinations of Dex with the analogs were added for the whole culturing period.
Hormonal treatment: Subconfluent cell cultures were treated with either estradiol-17β (E_2, 30nM) or raloxifene (Ral 3000nM) for 24 hours.
CK extraction and assay: After hormonal treatment, cells were collected, homogenized and CK extract was obtained and assayed as described previously (1,11).

Results:
1.Sex and age dependency: When bone marrow from male or female rats was cultured in the presence of Dex, the differentiated cells respond sex-specifically to E_2 and to DHT. Male derived cells responded to DHT only and female derived cells to E_2 only. When bone marrow from young or old females was cultured with Dex, the sex-specific response of the cells from young animals was significantly higher than that of the cells derived from older animals (60 and 39%, respectively). 1,25D replacing Dex had the same effect (50 and 35%, respectively). When both were

applied the response was very much augmented in both age groups (130 and 71%, respectively) (fig. 1.).

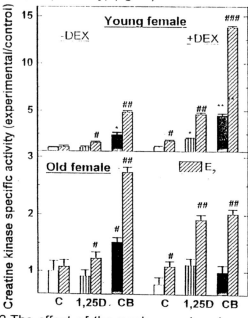

Fig: 1. The effect of Dex., 1,25D or CB at 1nM, or their combinations on basal CK activity and on its response to E_2 in bone marrow cultures derived from either young or old rats female. # t-test of E_2 treatment vs. its C and * t-test of the vitamin D treatment vs. C. Details are given in Materials and Methods.

2. The effect of the nonhypercalcemic analogs of vitamin D: When CB was used instead of 1,25D at 1nM, it was much more effective in both old and young derived bone marrow. CB caused an increase in CK activity of 130% in young and 50% in old bone marrow, EB and MC had similar effects compared to 1,25D 4% and -10% respectively. (fig.1.). They also caused responsiveness to E_2; in young after CB by 103% and in old bone marrow by 80%. CB also augmented in the presence of Dex the response to E_2 by 207% in young and by 104% in old bone marrow. EB and MC had also similar effects compared to 1,25D which by itself increased CK by 101% and augmented E_2 response by 130% in the young and 12% and 71% in the old bone marrow (fig. 1.). Moreover, the nonhypercalcemic analogs were also effective in augmenting E_2 effect at 1pM; CB by 40 and 103%, EB by 1.5 fold in both and MC by 1.65 fold in both compared to 1,25D by 1.06 fold in both young and old bone marrow.

3. The effect of the 1,25 $(OH)_2D_3$ on the response to Ral: When 1,25D was used in young or old female derived bone marrow, the differentiated cells responded to E_2 (by 66% and 55%, respectively) and to Ral (both by 50 and 32%) and this response was also augmented when they were used together with Dex. (to E_2 by 130 and 85% and to Ral by 96 and 87%, respectively) compared to Dex alone (E_2 by 72 and 56% and to Ral by 60% in both age groups, fig. 2.).

Discussion: Culturing rat bone marrow in the presence of Dex, resulted in osteoblast-like cells which acquire sex-specific responsiveness to gonadal steroids and to SERMS when CK activity was assayed (12, fig. 1 and 2.). The results indicated that 1,25D can replace Dex and moreover when applied together with

Dex, augmented the sex-specific response to the hormones. The new side chain modified nonhypercalcemic analogs of vitamin D can be used instead of 1,25D more efficient at 1nM and effective even at 1000 fold lower concentrations (fig. 1.). The vitamin D analogs were effective in upregulating the response of bone marrow from both age groups although their basal activity and the basal response in the young was significantly higher (fig. 1. and 2.). The 1,25D also upregulated the response to Ral (fig. 2.). The analogs were not equally potent but the order of activity was CB> MC> EB> 1,25D. The age difference in the response to either gonadal steroids or to Ral might be due to changes in the level of estrogen receptors (ER) and/or differences in the coactivators or corepressors in the cells (2,14,15). This is similar to other systems (2,16) a possibility, which is under investigation. We can therefore suggest that the vitamin D analogs can either control the differentiation or promote selective proliferation of osteoprogenitor cells, which preferentially respond to gonadal steroids and/or regulate the genes involved in the synthesis of the relevant receptors for gonadal steroids.

In summary this culture system for differentiation of bone marrow into osteoblast-like cells, is a relevant model to investigate the differentiation process, the role of vitamin D in the process and the mechanism of the role of vitamin D in the induction of cellular receptors for gonadal steroids. This system may also be applied to human bone marrow and might be of use in studying the induction of osteoblasts formation from bone marrow for helping in metabolic bone diseases.

Acknowledgment: We would like to thank Dr. L. Binderup from the Leo Company for providing the nonhypercalcemic analogs of vitamin D.

References:
1.Somjen D, Weisman Y, Harell A, Berger E and Kaye A M (1989) Proc. Natl. Acad. Sci. 86; 3361-3365.
2.Fournier B, Haring S, Kaye AM and Somjen D (1996) J. Endocrinol, 150; 275-285.
3.Katzburg S, Ornoy A, Hendel D, Lieberherr M, Klein B, Kaye AM and Somjen D (1997) Abst. Annual Meeting of The Israel Calcified Tissues Res. Soc., Jerusalem, December 1997.
4.Weisman Y, Cassorla F, Molozowski S, Kreig Jr RJ, Goldray D, Kaye AM and Somjen D (1993) Steroids 8; 379-388.
5.Somjen D, Kaye AM, Harell A and Weisman Y (1989) Endocrinology 125; 1870-1876.
6.Somjen D, Harell A, Weisman Y and Somjen D (1990) J. Steroid Mol. Biol. 37; 491-499.
7.Somjen D, Waisman A, Weisman Y and Kaye AM (2000) J. Steroid Mol. Biol 72; 79-88.
8.Berger E, Frisch B, Lifschitz-Mercer B, Weisman Y and Somjen D (1999) Abst. 11th Inter. Workshop on Calcif. Tiss. Res., Eilat, Israel, February 7-11,1999,p. 106.
9.Somjen D, Waisman A, Weisman Y and Kaye AM (1998) Steroids 63; 340-343.
10. Somjen D, Katzburg S, Knoll E, Waisman A, Kaye AM, Weisman Y and Stern N (1999) Abst. 1st Intl. Conf. On Chemistry and Biology of vitamin D

426

analogs, Providence, RI. USA, September 26-28, 1999.

11. Berger E, Bleiberg I, Weisman Y, Lifschitz-Mercer B, Leider-Trecho L, Harell A, Kaye AM and Somjen D (2000) Bone and Miner. Res. (submitted for publication).

12.Berger E, Bleiberg I, Weisman Y, Harell A, Kaye AM and Somjen D (2000) J. Steroid Mol. Biol. (submitted for publication).

13.Bradford MM (1976) Analyt. Biochem. 72; 248-254.

14.Glass C K, Rose MG and Rosenfeld MG (1997) Curr. Opin. Cell Biol. 9; 222-232.

15. Horwitz KB, Jackson TA, Bain DL, Richer JK, Takimoto GS and Tung L (1996) Mol. Endocrinol. 1167-1177.

16. Somjen D, Kohen F, Amir-Zaltsman Y, Knoll E and Stern N (1999) Amer. J. Hypertension (in press).

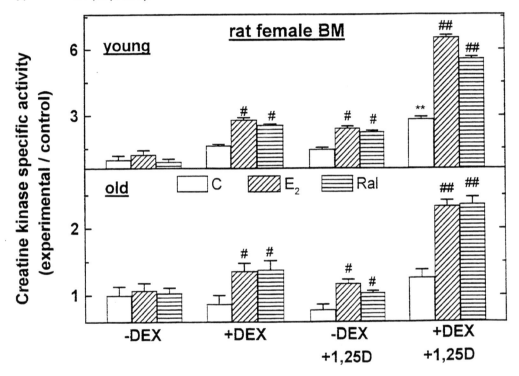

Fig. 2. The effect of Dex., 1,25D, or their combination on basal CK activity and on its response to E_2 and to Ral in bone marrow cultures from young or old rats. # t-test of E_2 treatment vs. its C and * t-test of the vitamin D treatment vs. C. Details are given in Materials and Methods.

1,25-DIHYDROXYVITAMIN D₃ AND RANKL POTENTLY STIMULATE OSTEO-CLAST FORMATION *IN VITRO* THROUGH DIRECT ACTIONS ON OSTEOCLAST PRECURSORS.

N. K. Shevde, K. M. Dienger, A. C. Bendixen and J. W. Pike, Department of Molecular and Cellular Physiology, University of Cincinnati, Cincinnati, Ohio, USA 45267

Introduction The bone resorbing osteoclast is derived from myelomonocytic precursor cells through the actions of a variety of soluble and stromal cell membrane-linked cytokines and growth factors (1). While a number of bone marrow derived factors play important roles in osteoclast precursor development and/or maturation, recent studies have defined a key factor that is essential for osteoclast differentiation, fusion, and activation. This factor, termed receptor activator of NFκB ligand (RANKL)/TRANCE/OPGL, belongs to the TNF family of regulatory molecules (2-4). It induces signals through receptor activator of NFκB (RANK), a membrane receptor that is related to the TNF receptor family and which is expressed by stroma as well as cells of the immune system (3). RANKL, together with M-CSF are essential to the formation of osteoclasts from its proximal precursors.

$1,25(OH)_2D_3$ plays an important role in bone, both as an inducer of calcium and phosphorus absorption via the intestine and as a remodeler in bone (5). The latter action implies both anabolic and catabolic functions. The apparent absence of significant bone defects in the vitamin D receptor (VDR) null mouse (VDR $^{-/-}$) following administration of a high calcium and phosphorus diet (6), as observed earlier in patients with hereditary $1,25(OH)_2D_3$ resistant rickets (7), suggests that $1,25(OH)_2D_3$ plays an essential role in the intestine but a redundant role in bone. $1,25(OH)_2D_3$ regulates the growth and activity of the osteoblast. $1,25(OH)_2D_3$ also regulates the expression of RANKL from stromal cells and osteoblasts (8), providing an explanation for the requirement for $1,25(OH)_2D_3$ in osteoclast differentiation assays that are carried out in the presence of stromal cells or osteoblasts. These and other studies do not, however, exclude the possibility that the vitamin D hormone can act on osteoclast precursors and facilitate osteoclast differentiation through direct actions. Indeed, receptors for $1,25(OH)_2D_3$ have been demonstrated in osteoclast precursors as well as in mature osteoclasts themselves (9). That $1,25(OH)_2D_3$ can act directly on hematopopietic cells is supported by the activity of $1,25(OH)_2D_3$ in macrophage differentiation (10), by the responsiveness of isolated monocytes to $1,25(OH)_2D_3$ and through the observation that osteoclast precursors derived from patients with Paget's Disease exhibit an enhanced sensitivity to $1,25(OH)_2D_3$ (11). These and other studies suggest the possibility of a direct role for $1,25(OH)_2D_3$ in osteoclast differentiation.

Soluble recombinant versions of the extracellular domain of RANKL can induce the formation of osteoclasts from precursors independent of supportive cells such as stroma, monocytes and other immunoregulatory cell types (2-4). This technical advance has enabled a variety of studies aimed at assessing the role of steroid hormones and other regulatory molecules in osteoclast formation, activity and survival that is independent of supportive cells. In addition, while isolated bone marrow mononuclear cells have provided excellent models for studying osteoclast differentiation, myelomonocyte-derived cell lines such as murine RAW264.7 have recently been discovered that permit not only direct studies of cytokine, growth factor, and lipophilic hormone action, but also permit molecular dissection of the mechanisms involved (4,12). We show here using RAW264.7 cells as a model that RANKL and M-CSF can induce the formation of functional osteoclasts. In addition, we show that in the presence of RANKL, $1,25(OH)_2D_3$ can substitute for M-CSF, and directly induce osteoclast formation. The "M-CSF-like" role of $1,25(OH)_2D_3$ does not appear to involve stimulation of M-CSF expression in RAW264.7 cells. It suggests that M-CSF and $1,25(OH)_2D_3$ may induce a common subset of genes essential to osteoclast precursor cell maturation through signaling mechanisms that appear at present to be unrelated.

Methods Osteoclast Differentiation. The murine monocytic cell line RAW264.7 was plated in 48 well dishes at a density of 2×10^3 cells/well and cultured in phenol red-free α-MEM supplemented with 10% charcoal-stripped FBS. Factors were introduced at the beginning of culture and during a medium change on day 3. Osteoclast formation was assessed by counting the total number of multinucleated (>3 nuclei), tartrate-resistant acid phosphatase (TRAP)-positive cells present per well on day 5. Osteoclast-like cells generated from RAW264.7 cells were also characterized for vitronectin receptor expression using antibodies to the αV integrin. Finally, the ability of RAW264.7 cell-derived osteoclasts to resorb bone was assessed by stimulating osteoclast formation on synthetic bone discs (Millenium Biologix Inc., Canada) for 6 days with M-CSF and RANKL, and then removing the adherent cells and examining the discs for the presence of resorption lacunae using dark field microscopy.

Results The murine cell line RAW264.7 was used as a model to evaluate whether $1,25(OH)_2D_3$ could act directly to modulate osteoclast formation. RAW264.7 cells express RANK and are known to differentiate into osteoclasts in the present of RANKL and M-CSF. Indeed, treatment with murine M-CSF (mM-CSF, 10 ng/ml) and soluble human RANKL (shRANKL, 30 ng/ml) for 5 days led to a profound differentiation of this monocyte-macrophagic cell line into multi-nucleated (>3 nuclei), tartrate-resistant acid phosphatase (TRAP)-positive osteoclast-like cells. As observed in Fig. 1, over 700 osteoclast-like cells were routinely formed in response to RANKL and M-CSF from an initial concentration of 2×10^3 RAW264.7 cells/well; only a few osteoclasts were formed with either factor alone. These cells also expressed the $\alpha V \beta 3$ integrin ((4,12) and data not shown). Most importantly, RANKL-induced differentiation of these cells on artificial bone slices resulted in the formation of numerous resorption lacunae not present in cultures stimulated with M-CSF alone ((4,12) and data not shown). The results indicate that the multinucleated cells produced from RAW264.7 cells exhibit not only relevant morphological, biochemical and enzymatic characteristics of osteoclast-like cells but crucial functional properties as well.

We treated RAW264.7 cells with RANKL and M-CSF together with either dexamethasone or $1,25(OH)_2D_3$. As seen in Figure 1, although neither steroid was effective in stimulating osteoclast formation individually above that induced by RANKL and M-CSF, $1,25(OH)_2D_3$ was able to completely replace M-CSF as a co-inducer of osteoclast formation when RANKL was present. This effect of $1,25(OH)_2D_3$ was concentration-dependent, ranging from 1 pM to 10 nM (data not shown). This finding suggests that $1,25(OH)_2D_3$ is capable of a direct action on osteoclast precursors to promote differentiation and fusion into mature osteoclasts and appears to be capable of substituting for the essential growth factor M-CSF.

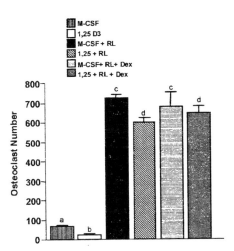

Figure 1: Effects of $1,25(OH)_2D_3$ on osteoclast formation. 2×10^3 RAW264.7 cells/well were plated and treated with M-CSF (10 ng/ml), RANKL (50 ng/ml), $1,25(OH)_2D_3$ (10 nM), dexamethasone (10 nM) or combinations thereof for 5 days. Multinucleated (>3 nuclei), TRAP-positive osteoclasts were then quantitated using a numbered grid. Mean ± SE, n = 3. (c & d are significant vs a & b at p< 0.05)

Although monocytes do not normally produce M-CSF, the RAW264.7 cell line is transformed and therefore potentially able to express this hematopoietic growth factor in response to $1,25(OH)_2D_3$. We tested this possibility by treating cells with RANKL and $1,25(OH)_2D_3$ in the presence of neutralizing antibody to M-CSF. While this antibody blocked the formation of osteoclasts from RAW264.7 cells when exogenous RANKL and M-CSF was added, it was only weakly able to block osteoclast formation in the presence of RANKL and $1,25(OH)_2D_3$ (data not shown). This experiment suggests that the actions of $1,25(OH)_2D_3$ are independent of M-CSF activity.

Discussion Soluble RANKL and M-CSF induce the formation of osteoclasts from myelomonocytic precursors as well as from murine RAW264.7 cells in the absence of stroma. Osteoclasts derived from these cells are multinucleated, TRAP- and $\alpha V\beta 3$-positive, and are capable of forming resorption lacunae when cultured on synthetic bone discs. Treatment of RAW264.7 cells with RANKL and $1,25(OH)_2D_3$ also induces the formation of multinucleated, TRAP-positive osteoclasts. While it is possible that $1,25(OH)_2D_3$ simply induced the expression of M-

CSF, neutralizing antibodies to murine M-CSF failed to block the stimulatory effect of $1,25(OH)_2D_3$ (in combination with RANKL) on osteoclast formation, suggesting that this mechanism of action is unlikely. We conclude that $1,25(OH)_2D_3$ exerts a direct action on osteoclast precursors independent of its ability to stimulate the expression of RANKL from stromal or osteoblastic cells. Thus, $1,25(OH)_2D_3$ acts at the dual level of both the osteoblast and the osteoclast to regulate bone remodeling. We speculate, as observed in the model in Fig. 2, that M-CSF and $1,25(OH)_2D_3$ regulate a similar subset of genes that participate in the progression and maturation of the monocyte that is required for RANKL-induced differentiation of precursors into fully functional osteoclasts.

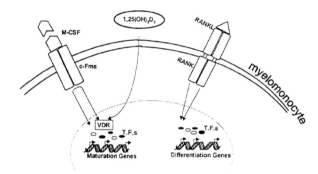

Figure 2: Model for $1,25(OH)_2D_3$-induced osteoclast formation. M-CSF and $1,25(OH)_2D_3$ induce a common or equivalent set of genes within osteoclast precursors (maturation genes) that are essential for RANKL activation of osteoclast differentiation.

References

1. Suda, T., et al. Endocr. Rev. 20, 345-357 (1999)
2. Lacey, D., et al. Cell 93, 165-176 (1998)
3. Yasuda, H., et al. Proc. Natl. Acad. Sci. USA 9a5, 3597-3602 (1998)
4. Hsu, H., et al. Proc. Natl. Acad. Sci. USA 96, 3540-3545 (1999)
5. Feldman, D., Glorieux, F., and Pike, J.W. (1997) Vitamin D. Academic Press. San Diego, CA
6. Amling, M., et al. Endocrinology. 140, 4982-4987 (1999)
7. Mallow, P.J., Pike, J.W., and Feldman, D. Endor. Rev. 20, 156-188 (1998)
8. Ytsukii, K., et al. Biochem. Biophys. Res. Commun. 246, 337-341 (1998)
9. Mee, A.P., et al. Bone 18, 295-299 (1996)
10. Mangelsdorf, D.J., et al. J. Cell Biol. 98, 391-398 (1984)
11. Menaa, C., et al. J Bone Min. Res. 15, 228-236 (2000)
12. Shevde, N.K., et al. Proc. Natl. Acad. Sci. USA, in press

EFFECTS 0F 1,25-DIHYDROXYCHOLECALCIFEROL ON CYTOSKELETON ORGANIZATION OF AORTAL SMOOTH MUSCLE CELLS IN PRIMARY CULTURE

Cecylia Tukaj[#], Jerzy Bohdanowicz* Jolanta Kubasik-Juraniec[#], [#]Laboratory of Electron Microscopy, Medical University of Gdańsk,
*Dept. of Genetics and Cytology University of Gdańsk, Poland

Introduction The phenotypic transition of smooth muscle cells (SMCs) from the differentiated „contractile" to the immature „synthetic" state appears to be an early critical event in the pathogenesis of atherosclerosis (1). This process includes a prominent structural reorganization with partial loss of myofilaments and formation of a large endoplasmic reticulum and Golgi complex. During the development of atherosclerosis SMCs become able to divide and to secrete extracellular matrix components. A numerous observations suggest that an active metabolite of vitamin D_3 [1,25(OH)$_2$cholecalciferol= calcitriol] is a growth regulatory factor, which plays an important role in maintaining normal cardiovascular function through its receptors in cardiac muscle or in arterial SMCs (2). Calcitriol induces development of experimental atherosclerosis in rats causing changes restricted to the tunica media.

Materials and Methods SMCs were obtained from aortas of newborn Wistar rats after digestion of collagenase 1A (Sigma). The cells were seeded on cover-slips in Petri dishes at a density of 2×10^5 cells/dish and cultured at 37^0C in a humidified, 5% CO_2 and 95% air atmosphere. The culture medium was changed every second day, and each time 1.2 μM of 1,25(OH)$_2$D$_3$ in 95% ethanol was added to the medium.
The cultures of SMCs were fixed and prepared for transmission electron microscopy (TEM), scanning electron microscopy (SEM) and for freeze–etching. Specimens were examined with the JEM1200EX II electron microscope and PHILIPS XL 30 scanning microscope. Direct immunofluorescence was performed on cell cultures that were washed with PBS, fixed by immersion in absolute methanol for 5 minutes at -20^0C and air dried. The culture was rehydrated in PBS and incubated for 30 minutes with the monoclonal antibody anti-α-smooth muscle actin and anti-tubulin FITC (Sigma). The cells were examined using a Nicon Eclipse 800 Optiphot microscope.

Results and Discussion The cells attached to the Petri dishes were spread out after 1-2 days in culture and began to proliferate after the third day. Thereafter they grew logarithmically up to the ninth day of the culture. Non-treated SMCs grew in a focally multilayered fashion – thickening appeared as mounds surrounded by monolayers. Cells in thickened regions were rather small, elongated, spindle shaped, and not well spread out; whereas cells from monolayers were larger, polygonal, and well spread out. SMCs treated by calcitriol formed a more abundant multilayer with flattened configuration.

432

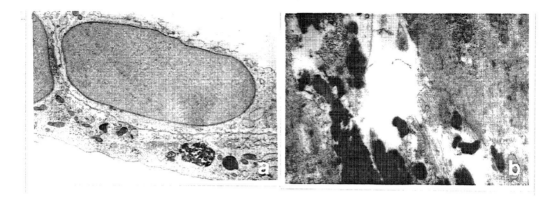

Fig.1. SMCs in primary culture stained with lead citrate and uranyl acetate:
a) cell in control culture exhibiting the "synthetic" phenotype,
b) cell in calcitriol–treated culture exhibiting "contractile" phenotype. The large part of cytoplasm densely filled with thin myofilaments forming dense areas at some sites. Large amount of amorphous elastin visible in extracellular space.

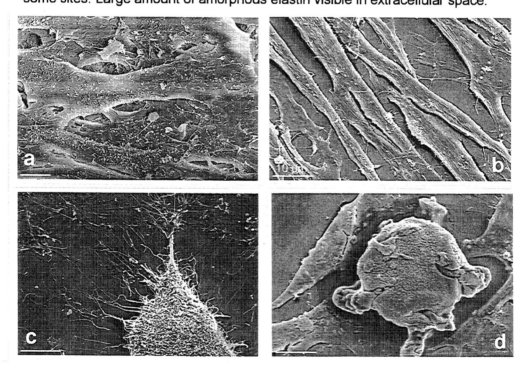

Fig.2. SMCs attached to the cover-slip: a) control culture, b) calcitriol-treated culture, c) SMC during mitosis, d) apoptosis in SMC indicated by the cell shrinkage, loss of pericellular adhesion, and outpouching of membrane segments.

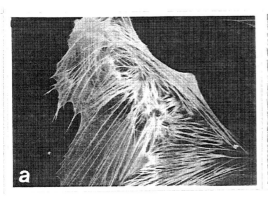
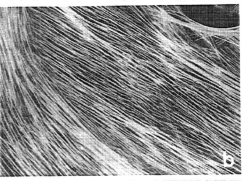

Fig.3. Immunostaining with antibodies against smooth muscle α-actin in SMCs.:
a) three-dimensional network of filaments and positive staining in ruffling zones
b) actin filaments running parallel to the major axis of cell

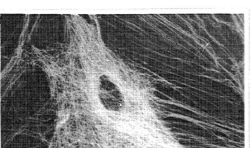
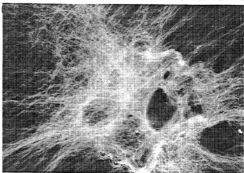

Fig.4. Immunostaining with antibodies against tubulin in SMCs.

The results show that calcitriol promoted the initial rate of phenotypic transition from contractile to synthetic state, resulting in increased cell proliferation in log–phase. TEM analysis revealed smooth muscle „synthetic" phenotype determined by: increase in membranous organelles such as prominent Golgi apparatus, abundant rough endoplasmic reticulum, mitochondria, free rybosomes; and decrease in intracytoplasmic myofilaments (3). After a high mitotic activity calcitriol-treated SMCs clearly differentiated, loosing their features of synthetic activities (4).
SEM electron microscopic observations confirmed our light microscopic findings about heterogeneity of SMCs in culture. Apoptotic cells were characterized by loss of pericellular adhesion, shrinkage and outpouching of membrane segments. Compared to control cells, calcitriol-treated SMCs showed resistance to apoptosis (5).

To investigate changes in three-dimensional microfilament architecture of SMCs during phenotypic modulation we examined immunofluorescence using antiserum specific for the differentiation marker α-actin. SMCs expressed the different organization of various components of the contractile apparatus. In the cells which modulate toward the "synthetic" phenotype, poor staining for smooth muscle α-actin was noted. Densely growing cells after calcitriol treatment displayed prominent linear myofilament bundles throughout the cytoplasm. The freeze–etching technique demonstrated cytoplasmic matrix with several organelle profiles and areas of plasma membrane faces with numerous globular particles.

References
1. Ross R. (1993) Nature 362, 801-809
2. Haussler M.R., Jurutka P.W., Hsieh J.C.,et al. (1995) Bone 17, 33S-38S
3. Tukaj C., Wrzolkowa T., (1996) Toxicol in vitro 10, 701-717
4. Mitsuhashi R., Curtis M.R., Ives H.E. (1991) J. Clin. Inv. 87, 1989-1895
5. Bennet M.R. (1999) Cardiovascular Res. 41, 361-368

CELL DIFFERENTIATION AND BONE PROTEIN SYNTHESIS IN THE AORTA AND LUNG CAUSED BY PLANTS INDUCED HYPERVITAMINOSIS D.

M.S. Gomar, E.L. Portiansky, M.E. Dallorso*, S.S Barros** and E.J. Gimeno Department of Pathology, School of Veterinary Sciences, La Plata, Argentina; *Zootecnic Pathology and Hygiene, School of Agricultural Sciences, National University of Lomas de Zamora, Buenos Aires, Argentina; **Department of Pathology, Veterinary Faculty, Federal University of Pelotas, Pelotas, Brazil

Introduction. Enzootic calcinosis (EC) are chronic plant poisonings of grazing livestock characterized by calcification of soft tissues and loss of body condition. Different calcinogenic plants have been identified worldwide (1). *Solanum glaucophyllum* (*Sg*) (synonym: *S. malacoxylon*) causes EC in cattle and sheep in Argentina, Brazil, Paraguay and Uruguay (2). *Nierembergia veitchii* (*Nv*) causes EC to sheep in Southern Brazil (3). These plants contain high levels of 1,25-dihydroxyvitamin D_3 as glycoside derivative (4). The effects of vitamin D are not only important in calcium homeostasis but also in immune regulation, cell growth and differentiation (5). Sheep aortas and lungs of spontaneous *Nv* induced EC and the same organs of *Sg* experimentally poisoned rabbits were studied with electron microscopy, immunohistochemistry and image analysis in order to determine the patterns of cell differentiation and bone protein synthesis.

Materials and methods. Experimental design: Three Corriedale sheep were bleeding to white under deep anesthesia at the beginning of the EC clinical signs. The animals were grazing on a pasture with abundant quantities of *Nv*. Six white New Zealand rabbits received 300 mg of powered *Sg* per via oral daily, during 9 days. Two other rabbits were used as control. They were sacrificed at 9 days after intoxication. All the animals were carefully necropsied. Tissues were fixed in 10% neutral formaldehyde.

Inmunohistochemistry: Tissue samples were embedded in paraffin, sectioned at 5 μm, and stained with hematoxylin-eosin and von Kossa stain. All the sections were mounted on slides coated with 3-aminopropyltriethoxy-silane (Sigma Diagnostics, St. Louis, MO, USA), deparaffinized with xylene, passed through graded alcohol, and rinsed three folds in deionized water and phosphate buffered saline (PBS). Osteocalcin (1:400) (clone OC1, Biodesign International, Kennebunk, ME, USA), osteonectin (1:800) (clone N50, Biodesign International, Kennebunk, ME, USA) and osteopontin (1:500) (clone MPIIIB10, Developmental Studies Hybridoma Bank, Iowa, USA) were used as primary monoclonal antibodies. The catalized signal amplification (CSA) system (Dako® CSA, HRP) was used as the immunohistochemical (IHC) detection system.

Image processing and analsysis: The histological images were evaluated using this technique. Briefly, the histological images were captured from the microscope (Olympus BX50 system microscope, Tokyo, Japan) with an objective magnification of 40x, through an attached video camera (Sony DXC-151A CCD color video camera, Tokyo, Japan) and digitized with a 24 bits true color TIFF format through a frame grabber (Flashpoint 128, Integral Technologies Inc, Indianapolis, IN, USA) attached to an high performance personal computer using the Image-Pro Plus for Windows v4.1 (Media Cybernetics, Silver Spring, MA, USA) software. The grid matrix was set to 500 x 300 pixel as to give a yield of 0.32 μm/pixel. Immunohistochemically stained slides were used to separate the immunostain (brown stain) from the hematoxylin stain (blue stain). The brownish stain was selected with a sensitivity of 4 (maximum 5). A mask was then applied in order to make a permanent separation of colors. The images were then transformed into a 8 bit gray scale TIFF format. After spatial and intensity of light calibration of the images the immunohistochemically stained area (IHCSA) and the optical density (OD) of the labeled reaction, defined by the antigen-antibody complex (6), was obtained. Histomorphometric measurements were carried out in different sections. No less than 10 images were obtained for each determination from every microscopic slide. Values obtained from the histograms were exported to a spreadsheet in order to perform the statistical analysis.

Statistical analysis: The analysis of variance was used to evaluate differences between experimental groups. The Tuckey's method was used as a post hoc test. Significant differences between the selected retrieval methods were defined as those with an error probability < 0.05. Highly significant differences were defined as those with a P value < 0.01. To determine the significance of the OD data the student t test of the differences between paired groups was applied.

Results. Clinical signs: All the intoxicated animals showed anorexia as early as 24 hours after the administration of the first dose. Decrease in body weight was, in consequence, observed. Some of them presented diarrhea and rhinitis.

Post mortem findings: At necropsy soft tissue mineralization was evident in the heart, aorta and lungs but also in other organs like arteries, kidneys and ligaments. The bones were extremely hard. Lungs were mildly emphysematous and small areas of calcification were detected by palpation in the diafragmatic lobes.

Histological findings: Microscopically, there were areas with distended alveoli which walls were thickened by loose connective tissue and large areas of mixoid appearance with spindle shaped, branched or stelated cells within an eosinophylic extracellular matrix with collagen fibers and deposition of von Kossa positive material. The bronchial cartilage was strongly calcified and lymphocytes, macrophages and multinucleated giant cells infiltrated the peribronchial tissue. Macrophages and multinucleated giant cells were also seen in the interstitium. The bone proteins osteocalcin, osteopontin, and osteonectin, were detected in the cytoplasm of activated fibroblast, in modified smooth muscle cells and in the extracellular matrix.

Ultrastructure: in the interstitium and in the mixoid areas, irregular shaped well delimited formations were early detected, in which calcium precipitation were found as amorphous or acicular crystals arranged in concentric bands of electron lucent and electron dense material (Fig. 1). Activated fibroblasts and modified smooth muscle cells were associated to these mineralized areas and in some places to abundant collagen fibers. Macrophages and multinucleated giant cells, some of them with calcium crystals free in their cytoplasm, were observed in areas of mineralization.

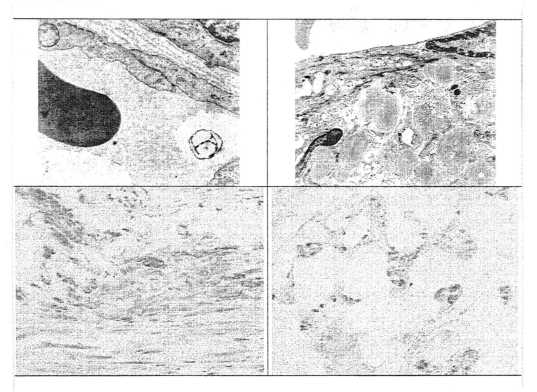

Upper left. Lung capilar. Modified smooth muscle cell and replication of basal lamina. 24.000 X.

Upper right. Interalveolar space with proliferation of collagen fibers and areas of mineralization. Cytoplasm of modified smooth muscle cell, with numerous synthetic organoids and decrease of myofibers. 12.000 X.

Lower left. Aorta. Osteopontin detected by inmunohistochemistry in the cytoplasm of activated mesenchymal cells, multinucleated cells and in the extracellular matrix. 200 X.

Lower right. Osteocalcin detected by immunohistochemistry in lung. 200 X.

Discussion. Calcification and bone metaplasia of soft tissues is a hallmark feature of EC. Morphological, morphometrical and histochemical analysis have demonstrated alterations of the elastic fibers, accumulation of proteoglycans and deposits of calcium salts. Additionally, the development of cartilage and bone tissue have been repeatedly reported (1,2,7). These metaplastic changes are preceded by proliferation of mesenchymal cells (8). Macrophages and multinucleated giant cells were seen in the interstitium and peribronchial tissue of the lungs of sheep with EC. The presence of a great number of cells of the mononuclear phagocytic system in the lungs of sheep with EC could result from the

438

action of 1,25(OH)$_2$D$_3$ as was proposed by Vasconcelos *et al.,* 1998 in the arteries of sheep with EC (9). The giant cells could be the response to mineralized tissue, but the presence of some cells in areas without calcium precipitation reinforced the hypothesis of a participation of 1,25(OH)$_2$D$_3$. Fibroblasts and smooth muscle cells change to secretory cells, a modification that has also been observed in the arteries of animals with experimental (8) and spontaneous EC (10). It is known that noncollagenous bone matrix proteins, osteocalcin, osteonectin and osteopontin play a pivotal role in the processes of cell differentiation, cell activation and normal tissue mineralization (10). Our results could indicate a specific differentiation effect of the 1,25(OH)$_2$D$_3$ on mesenchymal cells. The expression of noncollagenous matrix proteins by activated fibroblasts or smooth muscle cells is partially coincident with membranous ossification.

In conclusion, the mineralization of soft tissues in EC is complex process. The morphological and biochemical modifications could be attributed to specific genomic effects of 1,25(OH)$_2$D$_3$. It is suggested that 1,25 dihydroxyvitamin D$_3$ in *Sg* induce the cellular differentiation and the synthesis of a calcificable matrix. Differentiation related changes should, therefore, be included in the pathology and pathogenesis of the enzootic calcinosis.

References

1. Morris, K.L.M. (1982). Vet. and Human Toxicol.: 24: 34-48.
2. Worker, N.A. and Carrillo, B.J. (1967). Nature, 215: 72-74.
3. Riet-Correa, F., Schild, A.L., Mendez, M.C., Wasserman, R. and Krook, L. (1987). Pesq. Vet. Brasil. 7: 85-95
4. Wasserman, R.H., Henion, J.D., Haussler, M.R. and Mc Cain, T.A. (1976). Science 194: 853-855.
5. Walters, M.R. (1992). End. Rev. 13: 719-764.
6. Wells WA, Rainer RO, Memoli VA (1993). Am. J. Clin. Pathol. 99: 48-56.
7. Puche, R.C., Faienza, H.Q., Valenti, J.L., Juster, G., Osmetti, G., Hayase, J. and Dristas, J.A. (1980). Calcif. Tiss. Res. 40: 378-381.
8. Barros, S.S., Tabone, E., Dos Santos, M., Andujar, M. and Grimaud, J.A. (1981). Virchow Archives (Cell Pathology) 35: 167-175.
9. Sommer, B., Bickel, M., Hofstetter, W. and Wetterwald, A. (1996). Bone 4: 371-380.
10. Vasconcelos, R.O., Barros, S.S, Russowski, D., Grando, S.M. and Irigoyen, L.F. (1998). Pesq. Vet. Brasil. 18: 9-15.

Acknowledgements

ELP and EJG are Research Career Members of CONICET (National Scientific Council)

INHIBITORY RESPONSE TO 1α,25-DIHYDROXYVITAMIN D3 IS RESTORED IN HC11-RAS CLONE TRANSFECTED WITH VDR-POP13 EXPRESSION VECTOR

Simone Maistro, Ana L. B. Cabral[#], Vilma R. Martins[#], M. Mitzi Brentani, Miriam H. H. Federico, Departamento de Radiologia, Faculdade de Medicina de São Paulo, 0126-903, São Paulo, Brazil;
[#] Centro de Pesquisa e Tratamento do Hospital do Câncer, São Paulo, Brazil.

Introduction 1α,25-dihydroxyvitamin D_3 (1,25D_3), the active form of vitamin D_3, plays an important role in the proliferation as well as in the differentiation process of several normal and malignant cells (1). Its action is thought to be mediated primarily through binding to the vitamin D receptor (VDR), a member of the superfamily of nuclear transcription factors, which includes the steroid, retinoid, and thyroid hormone receptors (2). VDR appears to be essential for hormonal action in several cancer cells including colon, ovarian and breast cancer cells. Response to 1,25D_3 correlates with receptor number in breast cancer cell lines (3). HC11 cells, a mammary epithelial lineage established from a midpregnant BALB/c mice, differentiate in culture producing the milk protein β-casein when pre-treated with epidermal or basic fibroblast growth factors followed by the lactogenic hormones dexametasone, insulin and prolactin. The expression of β-casein is abolished in HC11ras, the Ha-ras transfected form of HC11, along with the acquisition of tumorigenic properties (4). Escaleira & Brentani (5) have previously demonstrated higher VDR mRNA expression together with higher VDR protein content in HC11 cells as compared to HC11ras, determined by Northern analysis and immunofluorescence assays respectively. In contrast to HC11ras, HC11 parental lineage was strongly growth inhibited, presenting with high percentage of cells arrested in G0/G1 phase of cell cycle when exposed to 1,25D_3. In this work we asked whether or not the lack of response of the HC11ras cells to 1,25D_3 should be ascribed to the low VDR content in those cells. In order to clarify the role played by VDR in HC11ras growth kinetcs, we tested the effect of 1,25D_3 treatment upon HC11ras clones generated by using HC11 VDR cDNA pOP13 as an expression vetor.

Material and Methods.
Cell culture HC11 and HC11ras (donated by Dr. Nancy Hynes from Friedrich Miescher Inst., Basel, Switzerland), maintained in RPMI medium, were exposed to 1,25D_3 10 nM in the presence of 10% of heat-inactevated fetal bovine serum. Growth curves 2×10^4 cells per plate were seeded in 8,8 cm^2 plates and experiments done in triplicates. Cells harvested at 24 hour intervals were counted by using a Neubauer chamber. The mean cell number was plotted in monolog paper and the doubling times (DT) were calculated.

<u>VDR expression vector</u> Mouse VDR DNA fragment was amplified by PCR using HC11 cDNA as template. Total RNA from HC11 cell line was reverse transcribed using the Super Script II. The oligonucleotides, linked with Not I site were: antisense downstream sequence 5'-GAGGCGGCCGCAAGAGCACCCT TGGGC TCTAC-3' and the sense upstream sequence 5'-AGAGCGGCCG CACAGGCAC CACTGTGGGCCACC-3'. PCR produts (1354 pb fragments) were introduced into the multiple cloning site of the pUC18 plasmid. Ampicillin-resistant clones were screened for the presence of VDR cDNA using PCR and automatic sequencing. VDR cDNA then rescued by restriction with Not I and ligated to operator vector, pOP13CAT (Lac Switch System, Stratagene) cleaved with Not I. The plasmid was tested for the diretion of VDR insertion by HindIII and AvaI. A large scale plasmid preparation of a clone containing the insert in the sense orientation was done.

<u>Generation of VDR expressing clones transfection</u> HC11ras cells were cultured in DMEM medium supplemented with 10% heat-inactivated FBS. Transfection of the subconfluent monolayers with the VDR cDNA expression vector (VDRpOP13) and p3'SS vector was carried out with the calcium phosphate method. Cells were selected in medium containing geneticin at 200 µg/ml and hygromicin B at 250 µg/ml for two weeks.

<u>Indirect immunfluorescence</u> 5×10^5 cells were incubated with the biotinilated anti-VDR monoclonal antibody (VD2F12) (6). Cells were then incubated with 2,5 µg/ml fluoresceinated avidin. The cells were analysed in FACScalibur flow cytometer (Becton Dickinson, USA). Results were presented as the percentage of cells reacting with the monoclonal antibody, and positive cells were defined as cells showing greater expression of the antigen than that measured on 99% of cells labeled only with the second antibody.

<u>Flowcytometric DNA content determination</u> Cells were evaluated for DNA content using the DNA intercalating agent propidium iodide (PI) as described elsewhere (7). The cells were analysed in FACScalibur flow cytometer and percentage of cells in G0/G1, S and G2/M phases was evaluated using the ModiFitLT software (Becton Dickinson, USA).

<u>RNA isolation and Northern analysis</u> Total RNA was isolated by guanidinium isothiocyanate/cesium chloride method. RNA (20 µg) was electrophoresed on 1% agarose-formaldehyde gels, transferred to Hybond membranes. Hybridization was done with ^{32}P labeled probes recognizing mouse VDR: 1.3 kb Not I fragment isolated from plasmid pOP13VDR and rRNA 18S. Bands were quantified by densitometry and the values expressed as the VDR/18S signal ratio.

<u>Results</u> We first reverse transcribed total RNA obtained from HC11 parental lineage. VDR cDNA was then amplified and cloned into the Not-1 site of the pOP13 expression vector. Using hygromycin B and geneticin, we selected 16 VDR-transfected HC11ras clones expressing variable amount of VDR. Clone 1 expressed higher percentage of VDR positive cells as measured by using anti-VDR MoAb and

flow cytometry (64% ± 8.2% VDR positive cells) as compared to HC11ras (35.93% ± 15.10% VDR+) and similar to parental HC11 lineage (85.5% ± 14.0% VDR+). VDR expression in clones 7 and 13 were similar to that presented by HC11ras (clone 7: 29.28% ± 10.62%; clone 13: 31.11% ± 27.2%). When exposed to 10nM 1,25D$_3$ during 72 hours, clone 1 presented an upward trending in doubling time which increased from 17.28h ± 1.98h to 28.48h ± 7.02h (p=0.056), whereas HC11ras doubling time did not change after the same treatment (control: 18.24h vs treated: 19.92h), as shown in Table 1. The G0/G1 phase fraction, as determined by flow cytometry, increased in clone 1 after exposure to 1,25D$_3$, from 79.54% ± 1.3 to 91.01% ± 2.66, p < 0,005, as shown in Figure 1. In keeping with these data, clones 7 and 13 presenting with low VDR content, were not growth inhibited.

	Control Cells	1,25D$_3$ Treated Cells	n	P
Clone 1	17.28 ± 1.98	28.48 ± 7.02	3	0.056
Clone 7	17.52 ± 3.91	21.52 ± 4.93	3	0.3
Clone 13	26.76	31.56	2	
HC11	18.64 ± 0.79	33.12 ± 4.31	3	0.002
HC11 ras	18.24	19.92	1	

Table 1: The effect of 1,25D$_3$ exposure on the growth kinetics of HC11 cells. Doubling time in each cell was determined as described in material and methods. The mean cell number was plotted in monolog paper and doubling times (DT) calculated. Statistical significance was evaluated by ANOVA test as compared to corresponding untreated cells. Results were considered as the mean ± SD of triplicates in each experiment.

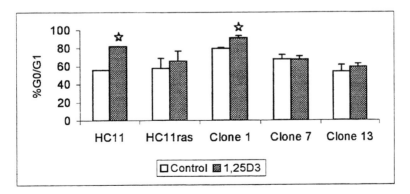

Figure 1 . The effect of 1,25D$_3$ exposure on the G0/G1 cell fraction in HC11, HC11ras cells, clones 1, 7 and 13. Cells were stained with propidium iodide and analysed by flow cytometry as described in material and methods. ☆ denotes significant difference as compared to corresponding untreated control (p< 0.005, ANOVA test).

<u>Discussion</u> In accordance with previous reports showing that $1,25D_3$ affects the proliferation rate of HC11 mammary cell line but not of HC11ras by increasing the percentage of cells arrested in G0/G1 (5), we describe here that Clone 1, expressing high VDR content was growth inhibited when treated with $1,25D_3$ in contrast to Clone 7 and 13, expressing low VDR content, which were not growth inhibited. Our results are in agreement with previous data showing that ras transformed keratinocytes are resistant not only to the growth inhibitory effects of $1,25D_3$, but also to its transcriptional influences (8). Taking into consideration the effect of VDR replacement in clone 1, restoring HC11 susceptibility to $1,25D_3$ treatment, we suggest that, in HC11ras, the $1,25D_3$ resistant phenotype might be attributed to the lower VDR content in those cells. Furthermore, our results suggest the assessment of VDR in primary breast cancer may be used to select patients responsive to $1,25D_3$ treatment.

Supported by FAPESP 96/6253-0, FAPESP 93/4373-0

References
1- Bouillon, R., Okamura, W.H. and Norman A.W. (1995) Endocrine Rev. 16, 200-256.
2- MacDonald, P.N., Dowd, D.R., and Haussler, M.R. (1994) Sem. Nephrol 14, 101-118.
3- Buras, R.R., Schumaker, L. M, Dovoodi, F., Brenner, R.V., Shabahand, M., Nauta, R.J. and Evans, S.R.T. (1994) Breast Cancer Res. Treat. 31, 191-202.
4- Happ, B., Hynes, N.E. and Groner, B. (1993). Cell growth Differ. 4, 9-15.
5- Escaleira, M.T.F. and Brentani, M.M. (1999) Breast Cancer Res. Treat. 54, 123-134.
6- Dame, M.C., Pierce, E.A., Prahl, J.M., Hayes, C.E., DeLuca, H.F. (1986) Biochemistry 25, 4523-4534.
7- Vindelov, L.L. and Christensen. I.J. (1990) Cytometry 11, 753-770.
8- Solomon, C., Sebag, M., White, J. H., Rhim, J., Kremer, R. (1998) J. Biol. Chem. 273, 17573-17578.

CANCER

PROSTATE CANCER AND VITAMIN D: FROM CONCEPT TO CLINIC. A TEN-YEAR UPDATE.

Gary G. Schwartz, Departments of Cancer Biology and Public Health Sciences, Wake Forest University School of Medicine, Winston-Salem, NC 27157, USA.

Introduction Prostate cancer is the most commonly diagnosed (non-skin) cancer among American men and the second most fatal, accounting for approximately 32,000 deaths per year. Mortality rates for prostate cancer vary over 20-fold worldwide and are highest in American blacks and in northern Europe, and lowest in Asia. Despite the high costs of prostate cancer in terms of morbidity and mortality, its etiology remains obscure.

A unique feature of prostate cancer is the high prevalence of "incidental" (also known as "subclinical" or "autopsy") cancer. Autopsy data indicate that approximately 30% of men over the age of 50 have histological prostate cancer. The prevalence of these incidental cancers reaches 60% in men over the age of 80 and continues to increase with age (1). Histologically, these incidental cancers are indistinguishable from prostate cancers that are potentially life-threatening and are considered to be at an earlier stage in their natural history. Unlike prostate cancer mortality rates, incidental prostate cancer is ubiquitous among elderly men regardless of race or geography. The discrepancy between the occurrence of clinical and incidental prostate cancer suggests that clinical prostate cancers result from the effects of some factor(s) that governs the growth of the subclinical cancers. What might these factors be?

In 1990, we noted that the major descriptive features of the epidemiology of clinical prostate cancer (increasing incidence with age, black race, and residence at northern latitudes), all are associated with low levels of vitamin D. We argued that these features could be understood if vitamin D restrained the progression of subclinical cancers to clinical cancer. This idea has become known as "the vitamin D hypothesis" for prostate cancer and, in the course of a decade, has progressed from the proverbial "dark horse" to a leading candidate in the race to understand the etiology of prostate cancer (2). Here we review some key developments in the vitamin D hypothesis and their implications for prostate cancer therapy.

Risk Factor	Explanation by D-deficiency hypothesis
Age	The elderly receive little exposure to ultraviolet light and consequently are vitamin D-deficient.
Race	
Blacks	Melanin inhibits the synthesis of Vitamin D.
Asians	Traditional diet high in fish protects against clinical cancer. Protection wanes as migrants adopt a more Western diet.
Geography	U.S. mortality rates show a strong negative association with ultraviolet radiation.

Table 1. Risk factors for prostate cancer and their interpretation (from Ref. 2).

446

Because the major source of vitamin D is casual exposure to ultraviolet radiation, in 1992 we studied the geographic distributions of ultraviolet radiation and of age-adjusted prostate cancer mortality rates among Whites in all 3,073 counties of the contiguous U.S. We demonstrated that ultraviolet radiation and prostate cancer mortality are inversely correlated (P<0.0001), and exhibit opposite geographic trends (Figures 1 and 2). Exposure to ultraviolet radiation is a well known determinant of vitamin D status in normal populations. Thus, these data suggest that vitamin D may protect against clinical prostate cancer at the population level (3) .

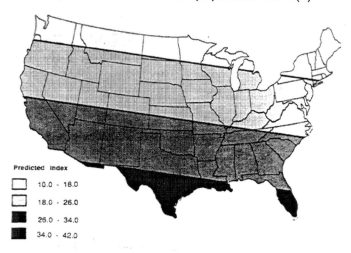

Figure 1. Linear trend surface map of ultraviolet radiation.

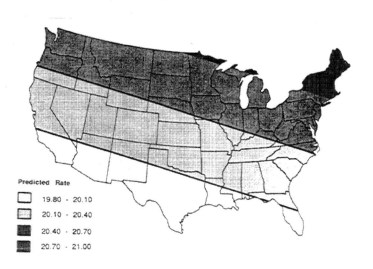

Figure 2. Linear trend surface map of prostate cancer mortality (age-adjusted) among White men, 1970-1979. Figures 1 and 2 are reproduced with permission from Cancer, 1992, 70:2861-2869.

Although these results are consistent with the vitamin D hypothesis, the mechanism of the protective effect of ultraviolet radiation on prostate cancer mortality was unclear. That is, although systemic levels of 25-Hydroxyvitamin D (25-OHD), the major circulating vitamin D metabolite, are known to be dependent on exposure to ultraviolet radiation, 25-OHD has little biologic activity. Conversely, in normal individuals, systemic levels of the hormonally active metabolite, 1,25(OH)$_2$D, are very tightly regulated and generally are not correlated with systemic levels of 25-OHD (4) (5). Thus, how could increased levels of ultraviolet radiation result in decreased risk of prostate cancer? This puzzle was not resolved until 1998, when we demonstrated that prostatic cells can synthesize 1,25(OH)$_2$D from 25-OHD.

1,25(OH)$_2$D Has Antiproliferative and Anti-metastatic Effects in Prostate Cancer

The vitamin D hypothesis has stimulated many laboratory investigations. The first laboratory study on the role of 1,25(OH)$_2$D in prostate cancer was published in 1992 by Miller and colleagues and utilized the LNCaP human prostate cancer cell line. Miller et al. demonstrated high-affinity binding sites for 1,25(OH)$_2$D (vitamin D receptors, or VDR) in LNCaP cells and showed that exposure of these cells to 1,25(OH)$_2$D inhibited their proliferation and increased the secretion of Prostate Specific Antigen (PSA), a differentiation marker. This finding, they concluded, "is consistent with the hypothesis of Schwartz and Hulka in that physiological concentrations of vitamin D$_3$ promote the differentiation of prostatic carcinoma cells" (p. 519) (6). Subsequently receptors for 1,25(OH)$_2$D were demonstrated in seven well-characterized human prostate cancer cell lines and 1,25(OH)$_2$D was shown to inhibit their proliferation (7) (8) (9) (10).

Because with advancing age, virtually all men have foci of subclinical carcinoma within their prostate glands, but relatively few men have invasive, clinical prostate cancer, the vitamin D hypothesis predicts that 1,25(OH)$_2$D should inhibit prostate cancer invasiveness. This is a critical issue, both theoretically and clinically, because prostate cancer that is invasive, i.e., that has penetrated the prostate capsule, is rarely curable. We investigated the effects of 1,25(OH)$_2$D on the invasive behavior of DU 145 human prostate cancer cells, an androgen-insensitive cell line. DU 145 cells were plated on Amgel, an artificial basement membrane composed of human amnions, and were treated with increasing doses of 1,25(OH)$_2$D. 1,25(OH)$_2$D inhibited the ability of prostate cancer cells to invade through the basement membrane in a time-and dose-dependent manner. This anti-invasion effect was apparent at physiological concentrations of 1,25(OH)$_2$D and was accompanied by a decrease in the expression of the collagenases MMP-2 and MMP-9, enzymes critical to the metastatic cascade (11).

We extended these in vitro findings to study the inhibition of metastasis in vivo, using a rodent prostate cancer model (MATLylu cells). Like DU 145 cells, MATLylu cells are androgen-insensitive, and thus are a model of the type of cancer that ultimately proves fatal in men. We showed that 1,25(OH)$_2$D and the 1,25(OH)$_2$D-analogue EB 1089 profoundly inhibited the occurrence of lung metastases from MATLylu cells (12). Thus, in addition to its antiproliferative and differentiating effects on prostate cells, 1,25(OH)$_2$D is anti-invasive and anti-metastatic. However, before 1,25(OH)$_2$D or 1,25(OH)$_2$D-analogues can be useful clinically, the effects of these drugs on elevating serum calcium levels must be minimized. In the present study, EB 1089 was as effective as $1,25(OH)_2D$ in inhibiting metastases but was significantly less calcemic (see Figure 3). Drugs which retain (or improve upon) the anticancer effects of $1,25(OH)_2D$ but with even less calcemic effects may herald the next era of anticancer drugs in prostate cancer.

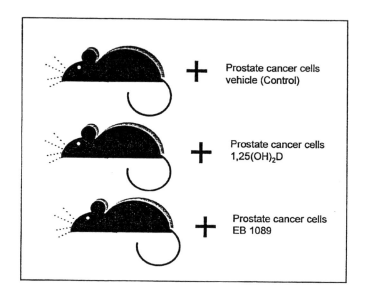

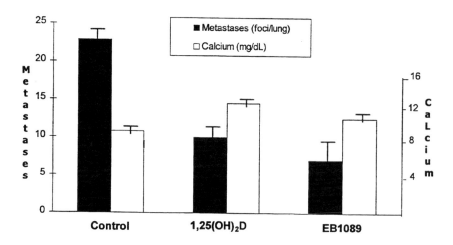

Figure 3. Effects of $1,25(OH)_2D$ and EB 1089 on lung metastases and serum calcium levels in Copenhagen rats inoculated with MATLylu prostate cancer cells.

Clinical Trials of 1,25(OH)₂D in Prostate Cancer The dramatic effects of $1,25(OH)_2D$ and $1,25(OH)_2D$ analogues in inhibiting prostate cancer proliferation and metastasis have led several groups to investigate the role of $1,25(OH)_2D$ in men with prostate cancer. The first of these trials treated men with advanced, androgen-independent prostate cancer with oral $1,25(OH)_2D_3$ at a dose that escalated to 1.5µg/day (13). These men had high PSAs, reflective of their metastatic disease (average PSA 220, range, 20--980). Two of the 13 men experienced sustained decreases in PSA corresponding to 25 and 45% of their initial values–e.g., a drop in PSA from 800 to 500. These effects are unlikely to be chance or placebo effects because the PSA values increased when the drug was withdrawn (due to hypercalcemia), and decreased when $1,25(OH)_2D_3$ was reintroduced (once serum calcium levels had normalized). Similarly, Gross et al. treated men with early recurrent prostate cancer (men with very low levels of PSA following definitive treatment) with oral $1,25(OH)_2D_3$. Treatment of these men caused a drop in the rate of rise of PSA in 6 of 7 men (14). However, as in our trial, dose-escalation was limited by the drug's calcemic effects.

New Developments in the Search for Non-Calcemic forms of 1,25(OH)₂D for Prostate Cancer How, then, can we preserve the antitumor and differentiating effects of $1,25(OH)_2D$ while limiting its calcemic ones? There are at least two potential solutions to this problem. The first of these is the use of non- or less-calcemic analogues of $1,25(OH)_2D$. For example, 19-nor-$1,25(OH)_2D_2$ (Zemplar) is a $1,25(OH)_2D_3$ analogue that has recently been approved for human use (for the treatment of secondary hyperparathyroidism). Recent clinical trials have demonstrated that Zemplar is essentially non-calcemic (i.e., its calcemic effects were identical to those of a placebo) (15). The structural similarity between 19-nor-$1,25(OH)_2D_2$ and $1,25(OH)_2D_3$ led us to hypothesize that prostatic cells would also respond to19-nor-$1,25(OH)_2D_2$. We have recently shown that Zemplar is as potent as $1,25(OH)_2D$ in transactivating the VDR in prostate cancer cells and inhibiting cell proliferation in primary cultures of human prostate cancer cells (16). However, because Zemplar is far less calcemic than $1,25(OH)_2D$, Zemplar can be given at higher doses, potentially making Zemplar safer and more effective than $1,25(OH)_2D$ in treating prostate cancer.

The second potential solution exploits our discovery of the autocrine synthesis of $1,25(OH)_2D$ by prostatic cells. Although the kidney is the major source of $1,25(OH)_2D$, the enzyme that converts 25-OH-D to $1,25(OH)_2D$, 1-α-hydroxylase, is also present in a number of non-renal cells, e.g., activated macrophages and keratinocytes (17) (18). We have recently demonstrated that human prostate cancer cell lines in culture and cells derived from normal prostates and prostates with benign prostatic hypertrophy possess 1-α-hydroxylase activity and synthesize $1,25(OH)_2D$ from 25-OHD. Thus, the prostate is an extrarenal source of $1,25(OH)_2D$ (Figure 4). The levels of $1,25(OH)_2D$ produced by prostatic cells in culture are likely to be physiologically significant for the prostate gland because they are comparable to the levels of $1,25(OH)_2D$ produced by renal tubular cells, the "classic" source of $1,25(OH)_2D$. Furthermore, because the $1,25(OH)_2D$ that is produced by prostatic cells is localized within the cell, the $1,25(OH)_2D$ that is produced locally will not contribute to systemic $1,25(OH)_2D$ levels and thus should not cause hypercalcemia (19).

450

We tested the antiproliferative effects of 25-OHD on prostate cancer cell lines and on primary cultures of human prostate epithelial cells (20). 25-OHD inhibited growth in a time- and dose-dependent manner that was not significantly different from the effects of 1,25(OH)$_2$D. These data have important implications for prostate cancer therapy and chemoprevention. For example, they suggest that prostatic tumors that express 1-α-hydroxylase could be treated with 25-OHD, which is far less calcemic than 1,25(OH)$_2$D. Conversely, tumors that do not express 1-α-hydroxylase could be treated with drugs like Zemplar. Both 25-OHD and Zemplar will soon be in clinical trials for prostate cancer. Finally, because 25-OHD is produced endogenously from exposure to vitamin D, our findings raise the exciting possibility that vitamin D itself (i.e., cholecalciferol and/or ergocalciferol), which is very inexpensive and relatively nontoxic, may be useful in the chemoprevention of clinical prostate cancer.

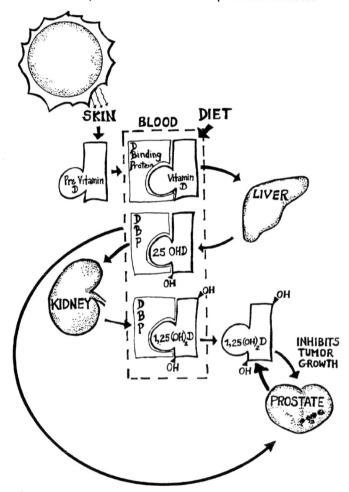

Figure 4. Current understanding of the prostate-vitamin D endocrine system. Vitamin D undergoes sequential hydroxylations in the liver and kidney to form 1,25(OH)$_2$D. The prostate also synthesizes 1,25(OH)$_2$D from 25-OHD. Because the prostate both synthesizes and responds to 1,25(OH)$_2$D, 1,25(OH)$_2$D is an autocrine hormone in the prostate. (Figure modified from (21)).

Acknowledgements

This work was supported by R01 CA68565 from the National Cancer Institute.

1. Breslow N, Chan CW, Dhom G, et al. (1998) Int. J. Cancer. 20, 680-8.

2. Schwartz GG, Hulka BS. (1990) Anticancer Res. 10. 1307-1311.

3. Hanchette CI, Schwartz GG. (1992) Cancer 70, 2861-2869.

4. Chesney, RW, Rosen, JF, Hanstra, AJ, Smith, C, Mahaffey, K., DeLuca, H.F. (1981) J. Clin. Endocrin. Metab. 53, 139-143.

5. Dusso, A, Finch, J, Delmez, J, Rapp, H, Lopez-Hilker, S, Brown, A, Slatopolsky, E. (1990). Kidney Internat. 38(Suppl. 29): S36-S40.

6. Miller GJ, Stapleton GE, Ferrara JA, Lucia MS, Pfister S, Hedlund, TE, Upadhya P. (1992) Cancer Res. 52, 515-520.

7. Skowronski RJ, Peehl DM, Feldman D. (1993) Endocrinology. 32, 1952-60.

8. Miller GJ, Stapleton GE, Hedlund TE, Mofatt KA. (1995) Clin. Cancer Res.1, 997-1003.

9. Hsieh, T, Ng, C, Mallouh C, Tazaki H, Wu, JM. (1996) Biochem. Biophys. Res. Comm.223,141-146.

10. Schwartz GG, Oeler TA, Uskokovic MR, Bahnson RR. (1994) Anticancer Res. 14,1077-81.

11. Schwartz GG, Wang, M-H, Zhang, RK, Siegal, GP. (1997) Cancer Epidemiol. Biomark. Prev. 6, 727-732.

12. Lokeshwar, BL., Schwartz GG, Selzer, M, Burnstein K, Zhuang S-H, Block N, Binderup, L. (1999). Cancer Epidemiol. Biomark. Prev. 8, 241-248.

13. Osborn JL, Schwartz GG, Smith DC, Bahnson RR, Day R, Trump DL. (1995) Urologic Oncology. 1,195-198.

14. Gross C, Stamey T, Hancock S, Feldman D. (1998) J. Urol., 1998;159, 2035-2040.

15. Llach F, Keshav G, Goldblat MV, Lindberg JS, Sadler R, Delmez J, Arruda J, Lau A, Slatopolsky E. (1998) Am. J. Kidney Dis. 32, Suppl 2, S48-S54.

16. Chen TC, Schwartz GG, Burnstein KL, Lokeshwar BL, Holick, MF. (2000) Clin. Cancer Res. 6, 901-908.

17. Barbour GL, Coburn JW, Slatopolsky E, Norman AW, Horst RL. (1989) N. Eng. J. Med. 305, 440-443.

18. Bikle DD, Nemanic MF, Gee E, Elias P. (1986) J. Clin. Invest. 78, 557-566.

19. Schwartz GG, Whitlatch LW, Chen TC, Lokeshwar BL, Holick MF. (1998) Cancer Epidemiol. Biomark. Prev. 7, 391-395.

20. Barreto AM, Schwartz GG, Woodruff R, Cramer SD. (2000) Cancer Epidemiol. Biomark. Prev.9, 265-270.

21. Schwartz GG. Prostate cancer and the Vitamin D Hypothesis.(1996) In M. Holick & E. Jung (Eds.,) Biologic Effects of Light 1995. Walter de Gruyter, pp. 309-316.

VITAMIN D₃ AND ITS RECEPTOR IN MAMMARY GLAND: FROM NORMAL DEVELOPMENT TO BREAST CANCER.

JoEllen Welsh, Department of Biological Sciences, University of Notre Dame, Notre Dame, IN 46556

Introduction

The VDR is a nuclear receptor which modulates gene expression when complexed with its ligand, 1,25 dihydroxyvitamin D_3 (1,25D), derived from vitamin D_3. We propose that VDR induces genes which suppress proliferation and maintain or induce differentiation in normal mammary gland and in breast cancer cells. Mechanistic studies indicate that 1,25D inhibits estrogen and growth factor (EGF, IGF-1) driven proliferation of human breast cancer cells via induction of growth arrest and apoptosis. One of the major goals of our lab has been to identify the mechanism by which 1,25D signals the apoptotic process in breast cancer cells. This work has been facilitated by the development of several subclones of MCF-7 cells which are resistant to the growth inhibitory effects of 1,25D and its analogs. One of these resistant cell lines, MCF-7[DRes] cells, has been characterized with respect to function of the VDR and sensitivity to 1,25D and its analogs both *in vitro* and *in vivo* (1-4).

Effect of vitamin D₃ compounds on MCF-7 breast cancer cells and tumors

In estrogen receptor (ER) positive MCF-7 cells, treatment with 1,25D or bioactive analogs such as EB1089 dose dependently induces growth arrest and apoptosis over a fairly prolonged time course (2-4 days). Growth arrest is associated with up-regulation of p21, which has been identified as a direct transcriptional target of 1,25D, dephosphorylation of the retinoblastoma (Rb) protein and cell cycle arrest in G_0/G_1. Similar effects of 1,25D and EB1089 have been observed in ER negative cell lines, such as SUM159PT (5). Induction of apoptosis by 1,25D is characterized by cell shrinkage and condensation, translocation of bax to mitochondria, redistribution of cytochrome c, generation of reactive oxygen species and DNA fragmentation (6,7). In MCF-7[DRes] cells, neither growth arrest or apoptosis is induced by 1,25D or its analogs (1,2). However, MCF-7[DRes] cells undergo growth arrest *in vitro* in response to other agents, including anti-estrogens, phorbol esters, TNFα, ceramide, retinoids and calcium ionophores. These findings indicate that the MCF-7[DRes] cells display a selective resistance to 1,25D and structural analogs.

To examine whether vitamin D mediated growth arrest and apoptosis of human breast cancer cells could be demonstrated *in vivo*, we have employed the nude mice xenograft system with the MCF-7 and MCF-7[DRes] cell lines (4). Treatment of mice bearing established (>200mm³) MCF-7 tumors with 45pmole EB1089 injected ip three times per week effectively reduces tumor volume within four weeks (8). Daily injections of 60pmole EB1089 are more effective, with reductions in tumor volume noted within 2 weeks (4), however at this dose,

454

EB1089 induces calcemia and weight loss. EB1089 adminstered at 25 pmole EB1089 three times per week also inhibits tumor growth but with less efficacy. This series of *in vivo* studies indicates that the effect of EB1089 on inhibition of human breast tumors is dose dependent. For routine studies, we use 45pmole EB1089 administered ip three times per week, which reproducibly induces >60% reduction in tumor volume compared to vehicle treated control mice after five weeks of treatment.

Histological analysis of tumors after five weeks indicated that EB1089 treatment decreases the epithelial to stromal ratio due to epithelial cell death by apoptosis. Quantitation of mitotic and apoptotic indices on tumor sections indicated that EB1089 decreases epithelial cell proliferation by 2-3 fold, and increases apoptosis by 6-10 fold. Thus, both *in vitro* and *in vivo* studies consistently demonstrate that vitamin D_3 compounds coordinately regulate both proliferation and apoptosis of human breast cancer epithelial cells.

MCF-7^{DRes} cells are capable of forming estrogen dependent tumors in nude mice, but the growth rate is slower than that of parental MCF-7 tumors. Treatment of tumor bearing mice with EB1089 (45pmole three times per week) does not modulate growth of tumors derived from MCF-7^{DRes} cells (4). Tumors derived from MCF-7^{DRes} cells display a distinct morphology from tumors derived from MCF-7 cells. MCF-7^{DRes} tumors are extremely well differentiated and the epithelial cells form circular ductal-like structures which are surrounded by stroma. Parental MCF-7 tumors are composed of pleomorphic, undifferentiated epithelial cells with very little organization and diffuse stroma. Futher studies are necessary to determine the basis of this phenotypic difference between tumors derived from MCF-7 and MCF-7^{DRes} cells, and its significance.

To determine whether the growth inhibitory effects of EB1089 on human breast tumors *in vivo* were comparable to that of an established breast cancer treatment, we compared the efficacy of EB1089 with that of the anti-estrogen tamoxifen. Tamoxifen is the most commonly prescribed drug for human breast cancer and has shown efficacy in breast cancer prevention trials. The data (8) indicate that EB1089 is as effective as tamoxifen in inhibiting growth of MCF-7 tumors. To determine if additive or synergistic effects of EB1089 and tamoxifen could be demonstrated, the effects of combination therapy in the MCF-7 tumor model was employed. Even at sub-maximal doses of EB1089

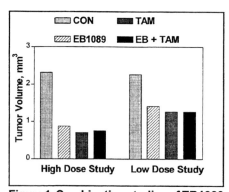

Figure 1. Combination studies of EB1089 and Tamoxifen in MCF-7 xenografts. Mice bearing established MCF-7 tumors were treated with placebo, EB1089, Tamoxifen (TAM) or both for 5 weeks. EB1089 was given at either 45 (high dose study) or 25 (low dose study) pmole 3x/wk. Tam was given as implanted pellets designed to deliver either 15mg (high dose) or 7.5mg (low dose) over 42 days. *See text for details.*

(25pmole/day three times per week) and tamoxifen (7.5mg continuous release pellet), combination therapy did not enhance the effectiveness of either drug alone (Figure 1). Similar results were observed when the pure anti-estrogen ICI182,780 instead of tamoxifen was used in combination with EB1089. These results were un-expected since additive effects of EB1089 with both anti-estrogens can be demonstrated *in vitro* (3,9). These data suggest that anti-estrogens and vitamin D$_3$ analogs might antagonize each others actions *in vivo*.

Interactions between ER and VDR signaling

One potential mechanism for antagonism between anti-estrogens and vitamin D$_3$ analogs in tumor growth regulation is at the level of their cognate receptors, the ER and the VDR. Numerous studies have shown that 1,25D decreases expression of ER, and a functional vitamin D response element has recently been characterized in the ER promoter (10). If EB1089 down-regulates ER in MCF-7 tumors *in vivo*, this would de-sensitize cells to anti-estrogen therapy. Conversely, we have found that anti-estrogens down regulate, and estrogens up-regulate, the VDR in MCF-7 cells (Figure 2). Thus, anti-estrogen therapy would be predicted to de-sensitize tumor cells to the actions of EB1089. Further studies to characterize the interactions between ER and VDR signaling pathways in relation to control of breast cancer cell growth will be necessary

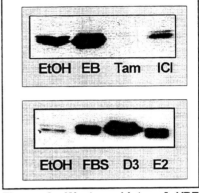

Figure 2. Western blots of VDR expression in MCF-7 cells. *Top,* cells growing in media containing FBS were treated with ethanol vehicle (EtOH), 100nM EB 1089 (EB), tamoxifen (TAM) or ICI 182,780 (ICI) for 72 hrs. *Bottom,* cells growing in charcoal stripped serum were treated with ethanol (EtOH), 5% FBS, 100nM 1,25D (D3) or 10nM estradiol (E2) for 48 hrs.

to determine if such interactions underlie the failure of combination therapy to exert additive effects *in vivo*.

Studies to address the mechanism by which estrogen modulates VDR expression have examined transcriptional regulation of a novel promoter we have characterized in the 5' flanking region of exon 1c in the VDR (11). This putative hVDR promoter exerts significant basal activity in MCF-7 and other breast cancer cell lines in transient transfections of luciferase reporter gene assays. Reporter gene activity is up-regulated in a dose dependent manner by estradiol treatment (0.1-100nM estradiol) in estrogen responsive breast cancer cells such as MCF-7. The induction of the hVDR promoter is not observed in ER negative breast cancer cells such as SUM159PT. In MCF-7 cells, tamoxifen is able to completely block the estradiol mediated increase in hVDR promoter activity. These data suggest the possibility that the effects of estrogen on up-regulation of the VDR in MCF-7 cells may, at least partially, be at the transcriptional level. These are the first studies to demonstrate hormonal responsiveness of a VDR promoter region and provide the basis for studies to examine the mechanism and significance of estradiol regulation of the VDR in different cell types.

To determine whether estrogen up-regulation of the VDR enhances the actions of 1,25D in MCF-7 cells, we examined 1,25D mediated transcriptional activation of a 24-hydroxylase luciferase promoter construct in MCF-7 cells which had been pre-treated with estrogen (24h, 10nM) or ethanol (vehicle control). These data indicate that estrogen pre-treatment markedly enhances 1,25D mediated reporter gene activity in MCF-7 cells (Figure 3). Further studies are necessary to determine whether this enhanced sensitivity to 1,25D correlates with changes in VDR expression, and whether anti-estrogens block the ability of estradiol to up-regulate 1,25D mediated transcription. In addition, it will be of interest to assess whether estradiol enhances 1,25D mediated transcription in other estrogen responses tissues such as bone.

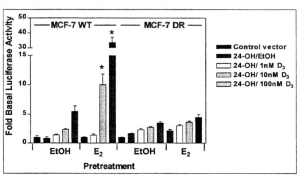

Figure 3. Activity of 24-hydroxylase promoter in parental and vitamin D resistant MCF-7 cells. MCF-7^{WT} and MCF-7^{DRes} cells growing in charcoal stripped serum were pre-treated for 24h with 10nM estradiol (E2) or ethanol vehicle (EtOH) and transiently transfected with the native 24-hydroxylase luciferase reporter plasmid. Reporter gene assays were conducted after 24hrs treatment with increasing doses of 1,25D. *Significantly different, E2 vs. EtOH pretreatment values.

The activity of the 24-hydroxylase promoter in MCF-7^{DRes} cells in the absence and presence of estradiol pre-treatment is also shown in Figure 3. In the absence of estradiol pre-treatment, the induction of the 24-hydroxylase promoter is reduced in MCF-7^{DRes} cells compared to MCF-7 cells. This is particularly obvious with the highest dose of 1,25D. Relative to ethanol treated cells, 100nM 1,25D induced reporter gene activity more than five fold by 1,25D in parental MCF-7 cells, in contrast to less than three fold induction in the MCF-7^{DRes} cells. Furthermore, estrogen pre-treatment did not enhance the sensitivity of MCF-7^{DRes} cells to 1,25D. These data clearly implicate a defect in VDR transcriptional activation in MCF-7^{DRes} cells which may underlie their resistance to the growth inhibitory effects of 1,25D. The VDR is present in MCF-7^{DRes} cells, and can bind 1,25D and synthetic VDREs *in vitro* comparably to the VDR from the parental MCF-7 cells (1). In addition, we have found no differences in the VDR sequence between MCF-7 and MCF-7^{DRes} cells. Further studies are underway to determine the underlying basis for the impaired 1,25D mediated transcriptional regulation in MCF-7^{DRes} cells.

Summary

The studies reviewed here demonstrate that vitamin D_3 analogs are effective in modulating growth of human breast cancer cells both *in vitro* and *in vivo*. In MCF-7 tumors *in vivo*, the analog EB1089 is as effective in growth inhibition as the anti-estrogen tamoxifen, the standard therapy for hormone responsive breast cancer in human patients. Although combination therapy of EB1089 with chemotherapeutic drugs has been reported, no additive effects are observed in MCF-7 tumors treated simultaneously with anti-estrogens and vitamin D_3 analogs. We speculate that the failure of combination therapy to exert additive effects *in vivo* is due to antagonism between ER and VDR signaling. We show that estradiol markedly enhances the sensitivity of MCF-7 cells to 1,25D mediated transcriptional activation, suggesting that anti-estrogens might interfere with the actions of 1,25D and its analogs. The sensitivity to 1,25D is not enhanced by estradiol in MCF-7[DRes] cells which have been selected for resistance to the growth inhibitory effects of 1,25D. Although we have demonstrated that resistance to vitamin D_3 analogs occurs, tumors derived from MCF-7[DRes] cells were not more aggressive than tumors derived from parental MCF-7 cells, as MCF-7[DRes] tumors grow slower and exhibit a distinct, differentiated morphology compared to MCF-7 tumors.

Model

Based on the studies discussed above, we propose a simplified model for the interactions of vitamin D_3 and estrogen signaling pathways in the regulation of breast cancer cell growth (Figure 4). Estrogen and other growth factors (such as EGF and IGF-1) induce proliferation and promote survival of mammary epithelial cells. Estrogens (and possibly other growth factors) up-regulate the VDR co-incident with enhancing proliferation, thus enhancing cellular sensitivity to circulating 1,25D. The 1,25D-VDR complex then acts to induce genes, such as p21, which effectively limit cell proliferation in response to estrogens and growth factors. 1,25D also transcriptionally down-regulates ER, further de-sensitizing cells to estrogen driven proliferation. The end result is cell cycle arrest in G_0/G_1 and a reduction of cells in S phase. As noted on the left side of the model, dysregulation of vitamin D_3 signaling (due to lack of 1,25D, mutations in the VDR or disruption of VDR target genes)

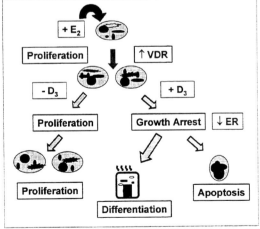

Figure 4. Model for interactions between estradiol (E_2) and 1,25Dihydroxyvitamin D_3 (D_3) in regulation of mammary epithelial cell proliferation, differentiation and apoptosis. *ER*, estrogen receptor, *VDR*, vitamin D receptor. *See text for details.*

would lead to un-opposed proliferation of undifferentiated cells (hyperplasia), which may pre-dispose to transformation.

As depicted on the right side of the figure, we propose that continued exposure to 1,25D will either induce terminal differentiation (in cells which are inherently capable of differentiation), or induce apoptosis (in cells that are not). It is well known that MCF-7 cells are heterogeneous, and we have observed considerable heterogeneity in cellular sensitivity to 1,25D in different MCF-7 clones. Thus, a certain percentage of cells will undergo apoptosis after cell cycle arrest, and a certain percentage will undergo differentiation. Continuous exposure to 1,25D eliminates (via apoptosis) cells unable to undergo differentiation, resulting in a more differentiated cell population (typified by the MCF-7^{DRes} cells). This model proposes that the end result (and the major function) of 1,25D is to oppose estrogen (and growth factor) driven proliferation and to induce/maintain mammary epithelial cell differentiation. Although not shown in this model, effects of estradiol and 1,25D on mammary stromal cells are likely to impact on mammary epithelial cell biology via cell-cell interactions and/or secretion of soluble growth factors and cytokines. This simplified model also does not emphasize that mammary cell differentiation involves coordination of a complex network of signals, and vitamin D_3 signaling is only one player. A challenge for the future will be to clarify how 1,25D and the VDR interact with other known players in this network.

Relevance to normal mammary gland function

Although most of our work to date has been in breast cancer cells, we propose that the model presented in Figure 4 is equally applicable to the functions of 1,25D and the VDR in normal mammary gland. We propose that in normal mammary gland, the VDR also induces genes which suppress proliferation and maintain differentiation, and consequently, that dysregulation of VDR target genes will predispose mammary epithelial cells to transformation. Extensive preclinical and clinical data indirectly support this concept. In animal models, vitamin D_3 negates the effects of dietary fat and chemical carcinogens on mammary tumorigenesis. In clinical studies, low serum levels of 1,25D correlate with increased breast cancer risk, disease progression and metastasis. Data from the NHANES I epidemiological study suggest that optimal vitamin D_3 nutrition affords protection against breast cancer. Genetic studies have identified specific alleles of the VDR which correlate with an increased risk for sporadic breast cancer and with more aggressive metastatic disease.

Despite these consistent data supporting an important protective role for vitamin D_3 and its receptor in breast cancer, it has been difficult to demonstrate that lack of vitamin D_3 directly affects the mammary gland *in vivo*. Dietary vitamin D_3 deficiency has profound effects on calcium and bone homeostasis, confounding interpretation of the role of the VDR in mammary gland differentation. In recent studies, we examined the role of the VDR in mammary gland development and function using the VDR knockout mouse developed by Marie Demay (12). In the VDR knockout mouse model, complications such as hypocalcemia can be prevented by provision of a high calcium/high phosphate/high lactose diet. VDR null mice are fertile and can lactate, indicating that mammary gland function is not grossly abnormal in the absence of the vitamin D_3 endocrine system. However, recent data indicate that VDR knockout mice exhibit subtle defects in mammary gland differentiation during the early pubertal period (13). Compared to VDR wild type (+/+) mice, mammary glands from VDR knockout (-/-) mice have increased numbers of undifferentiated terminal end bud structures at the critical pubertal period of development. It is at this time that the mammary gland is most susceptible to tumorigenesis because the terminal end bud, with its high rate of proliferation, is the target for chemical carcinogens such as DMBA. Thus, the persistance of terminal end buds at this stage of development in the VDR knockout mouse may have functional significance in relation to transformation potential. This notion is supported by studies by Mehta et al (14) who reported that 1,25D inhibits the development of pre-neoplastic lesions in explants of mammary gland derived from pubertal mice. Studies are currently underway to determine whether lack of the VDR in mammary gland enhances sensitivity to chemically induced carcinogenesis, and if so, whether mammary tumors which lack VDR exhibit more aggressive behavior than tumors expressing VDR.

Acknowledgements

The work described in this paper reflects a team effort of current and former members of the Welsh lab: Ian Byrne, Manjula Donepudi, Louise Flanagan, Judy Narvaez, Elizabeth Nolan, Kathryn Packman, Saraa Romu, Maura Simboli-Campbell, Sarah Smyczek, Jennifer Wietzke and Glendon Zinser. Special thanks to Dr. Marie Demay for supplying the VDR knockout mice breeding pairs and to Dr. John Omdahl for the 24-hydroxylase promoter luciferase construct. Funding for our work has been received from the National Cancer Institute, the American Institute for Cancer Research, the USDA CREES program and the Department of Defense Breast Cancer Research Program.

References

1. Narvaez CJ, VanWeelden K, Byrne I and Welsh JE (1996) *Endocrinology* 137, 400-409

2. Narvaez CJ, and Welsh JE (1997) *Endocrinology* 138, 4690-4698

3. Nolan E, Donepudi M, VanWeelden K, Flanagan L, and Welsh JE (1998) *Molecular and Cellular Biochemistry* 188, 13-20

4. VanWeelden K, Flanagan L, Binderup L, Tenniswood M, and Welsh JE (1998) *Endocrinology* 139, 2102-2110

5. Flanagan L, VanWeelden K, Ammerman C, Ethier S, and Welsh JE (1999) *Breast Cancer Research and Treatment* 58, 193-204

6. Simboli-Campbell M, Narvaez CJ, Tenniswood M and Welsh JE (1996) *Journal of Steroid Biochemistry and Molecular Biology* 58, 367-376

7. Narvaez CJ and Welsh JE (2000) *Proceedings of the Eleventh Workshop on Vitamin D* (this volume)

8. Packman K, Flanagan L, Zinser G, Mitsch R, Tenniswood M and Welsh JE (2000) *Proceedings of the Eleventh Workshop on Vitamin D* (this volume)

9. Welsh J, VanWeelden K, Flanagan L, Byrne I, Nolan E, and Narvaez CJ *(1998) Subcellular Biochemistry* 30, 245-270

10. Stoica, A, Saceda M, Fakhro A, Solomon H, Fenster B and Martin MB (1999) *Journal of Cell Biochemistry* 75, 640-651

11. Byrne I, Flanagan L, Tenniswood M and Welsh JE (2000) *Endocrinology*, in press (see also Byrne et al, this volume)

12. Li Y, Pirro A, Amling M, Delling G, Baron R, Bronson R, and Demay M (1997) *Proceedings of the National Academy of Science USA* 94, 9831-9835

13. Zinser G, Packman K and Welsh J (2000) *Proceedings of the Eleventh Workshop on Vitamin D* (this volume)

14. Mehta R, Moriarty R, Mehta R, Penmasta R, Lazzaro G, Constantinou A, and Guo L (1997) *J. National Cancer Institute* 89, 212-218

1,25 DIHYDROXYCHOLECALCIFEROL (CALCITRIOL) AS AN ANTICANCER AGENT: PRECLINICAL STUDIES.

Candace S. Johnson, Pamela A. Hershberger, Ruth A. Modzlewski, Ronald J. Bernardi, Terence F. McGuire, Robert M. Rueger, Wei-Dong Yu, Kent E. Blum and Donald L. Trump.

Departments of Pharmacology, Medicine and Urology, University of Pittsburgh Cancer Institute, Pittsburgh, PA, USA, 15213.

Vitamin D is a steroid hormone, which modulates calcium homeostasis through actions on kidney, bone and the intestinal tract (1). In addition to classical effects on bone and mineral metabolism, calcitriol is also involved in the proliferation and differentiation of a variety of different cell types and tissues (1-18). The VDR is found, not only in classical target organs (intestinal tract, kidney, and bone), but also in many other epithelial and mesenchymal cells as well as leukemic cells, osteosarcoma, breast and colon carcinoma, melanoma, glioma, lung and prostate carcinoma, and other malignant cell types (1, 2). Initial *in vivo* studies focused on the use of calcitriol in murine leukemia models where calcitriol has anti-proliferative and differentiating effects (5, 10). Calcitriol inhibits growth *in vitro* and *in vivo* in murine and human breast and colon cancer models (6, 9, 19, 20). Calcitriol has also been investigated in prostate cancer where anti-proliferative activity has been observed with established human prostate cell lines (8, 21-23). PSA secretion and androgen receptor (AR) expression are enhanced in LNCaP cells in response to calcitriol, which also inhibits LNCaP proliferation, in a dose-dependent manner (44, 45).

Anti-tumor effects *in vitro/in vivo*. In a variety of model systems (murine syngeneic SCC VII/SF, metastatic Dunning rat prostate adenocarcinoma and the human xenograft PC-3 prostate), We have demonstrated that calcitriol has significant anti-proliferative effects both *in vitro* and *in vivo* (3, 4, 11). In the metastatic rat Mat-LyLu (MLL) model, calcitriol resulted not only in an inhibition of tumor volume, but also a significant reduction in the number and size of lung metastases (4). Calcitriol also significantly arrests tumor cells in G_0/G_1 and is associated with altered expression of cell cycle regulatory proteins (4, 12). In SCC *in vitro* calcitriol treatment results in decreased expression of $p21^{Waf1/Cip1}$ (p21) mRNA and protein, and increased expression of $p27^{Kip1}$ (p27) mRNA and protein and Rb dephosphorylation (13). *In vivo*, a decrease in SCC tumor volume induced by calcitriol correlates with a significant decrease in the intratumoral p21 expression.

Apoptotic cell death occurs through the activation of caspases, which result in specific cleavage of key cellular proteins including poly(ADP-ribose) polymerase or PARP (24, 25). The bcl-2 protein, which is over-expressed in many tumors, suppresses apoptosis; whereas the bax protein promotes apoptotic cell death (55-57). Calcitriol induces apoptosis in MCF-7 breast and HL-60 leukemic cell lines (58-60). We demonstrated by Western blot that calcitriol induced 90-100% PARP cleavage in MLL cells treated with 10 µM of calcitriol (half the IC50) (11). Induction of apoptosis was confirmed using annexin binding as a measure of phosphatidylserine exposure. The caspase inhibitors, ZVAD-fmk and DEVD-fmk had no effect alone but were capable of significantly inhibiting a calcitriol-mediated increase in annexin binding. In addition, when bax and bcl-2 protein expression was examined, bax was unchanged and bcl-2 was decreased with a significant at 24 hr in MLL treated with calcitriol resulting in an increased bax/bcl-2 ratio, which favors death. Calcitriol did not alter Fas or Fas ligand.

Calcitriol enhancement of chemotherapeutic efficacy. Using *in vitro* clonogenic assays, pretreatment with calcitriol or the calcitriol analogue R023-7553 significantly enhances cisplatin, carboplatin, paclitaxel, and docetaxel mediated cytotoxicity compared to cytotoxic agents alone (12). In the *in vivo* excision clonogenic assay where tumors are removed 24 hr after cytotoxic drug treatment and plated in a 7 day clonogenic assay, pretreatment with calcitriol markedly enhances platinum and taxane-mediated clonogenic tumor cell kill, even at low doses of cytotoxic drug. Similarly, a significant decrease in fractional tumor volume and an increase in regrowth delay are observed with calcitriol in combination with these drugs as compared to any agent alone. Schedule and timing of calcitriol administration are critical to optimal anti-tumor efficacy. The optimal effects are seen when tumor-bearing animals are treated with calcitriol daily for 3 days and the cytotoxic agent administered with calcitriol on day 3. In addition, to our surprise, this sequence of administration of calcitriol and a taxane reduces hyper-calcemia. Figure 1 illustrates the effects of calcitriol, dexamethasone (dex) and docetaxel therapy in nude mice bearing human prostate cancer (PC-3) xenografts. We have shown previously that dex alone has little effect on tumor cell growth. Similar results were obtained with paclitaxel.

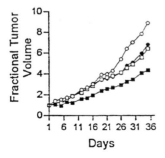

Figure 1. Fractional tumor volume (mean ± SD) of PC-3 tumor bearing mice (8-10 per group) either untreated (o), treated with a single dose of docetaxel (1 mg/kg) with dex (9 µg/mouse, daily x 4; -1, 1, 2, 3) (•), or pre-treated with calcitriol (0.5 µg/day x 3 days)/dex (same as above) (□) and in combination (■)

As noted above we also observed that tumor-bearing animals treated with the combination of calcitriol and paclitaxel were not as hypercalcemic as animals treated with calcitriol alone (26). Peak serum calcium and duration of hypercalcemia (calcium >12mg/dL) were significantly reduced in calcitriol/paclitaxel treated animals as compared to calcitriol alone (Table 1).

Table 1: Effect of Paclitaxel and Zoledronic Acid on Calcitriol-Induced Hypercalcemia and Hypercalciuria in C3H/HeJ Mice following Calcitriol Treatment

	Serum Calcium[E] (mg/dL)	24 hr Urinary Calcium[F] (mg/dL)
Control	9.5 ±0.2	7.5 ± 0.1
DDD[A]	16.9 ± 0.7	40.2 ± 0.8
DDD[B] T	13.4 ± 1.0	6.4 ± 0.3
DDD[C] T	9.9 ± 1.5	—
T[D]	9.6± 0.2	—
Zoledronic acid+ DDD[G]	12.8 ± 0.3	—
Zoledronic acid	9.5 ± 0.5	—

A=calcitriol 0.75µg/kg/d, Day 1,2,3; B=calcitriol 0.75µg/kg/d, Day 1,2,3 + paclitaxel (20mg/kg) Day1;
C = calcitriol 0.75µg/kg/d, Day 1,2,3 1,2,3+paclitaxel (20mg/kg) day3; D= paclitaxel (20mg/kg), E = calcium measured on day 3 immediately after calcitriol is administered; F= 24 hour urine calcium measured over the first 24 hours of therapy; G=zoledronic acid 10µg/kg on day -1, calcitriol 1,2,3.

Serum creatinine and blood urea nitrogen (BUN), a reflection of dehydration or the nephrotoxic effects of hypercalcemia, were elevated in animals treated with calcitriol alone but not in animals treated with calcitriol/paclitaxel. These data indicate that paclitaxel blocks the only known toxicity of calcitriol and that taxane antitumor effects are substantially augmented by calcitriol. Other agents which disrupt microtubule function, such as colchicine have been shown to modify cellular transport of calcium. Studies are underway to determine the mechanisms by which taxanes modify calcitriol-induced hypercalcemia. Bisphosphonates have been reported to modify calcitriol-associated hypercalcemia. We have demonstrated that the potent, third generation bisphosphonate zoledronic acid (Zometa®, Aventis) [Table 1] substantially reduces calcitriol-associated hypercalcemia in normal and tumor-bearing mice. Studies exploring the mechanisms and clinical application of these interactions are underway.

464

The mechanism(s) of calcitriol-mediated enhancement of chemotherapeutic efficacy are yet to be determined. As shown in Fig. 2, we have demonstrated that the combination of calcitriol and paclitaxel results in 100% PARP cleavage at 12 hr. as compared to 24 hr. for calcitriol alone (11). We also have evidence that down modulation of p21 with calcitriol may sensitize tumor cells cytotoxic drug-mediated cytotoxicity (15.) Clinical trials have been initiated based on these pre-clinical data to examine the combinations of calcitriol and bisphosphonates and taxanes and carboplatin.

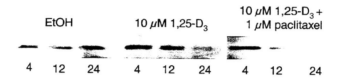

Figure 2. Paclitaxel (100μM) ± calcitriol (5μM) treatment of MLL prostatic adenocarcinoma cells and time to induction of PARP cleavage.

The antiproliferative activity of calcitriol in squamous cell carcinoma is associated with decreased $p21^{Waf1/Cip1}$ (p21) expression in vitro and in vivo (13). Recent studies indicate p21 suppression increases sensitivity to paclitaxel (27, 28). We have examined the molecular accompaniments of paclitaxel cytotoxicity with and without calcitriol in the human prostatic adenocarcinoma, PC-3 (63, see attached). The *in vitro* effects of calcitriol and paclitaxel on p21, Bcl-2, caspase-3, and PARP in PC-3 were evaluated by Western blot. Treatment *in vitro* with calcitriol resulted in a decrease in p21 expression in PC-3. Paclitaxel induced apoptosis in PC-3 as evidenced by the time-dependent loss of procaspase-3 and full-length PARP. Paclitaxel caused increase of p21 and loss of Bcl-2. None of the molecular alterations induced by paclitaxel were further modulated by calcitriol. Thus, calcitriol and paclitaxel each have antitumor effects in PC-3; antiproliferative effects are greatly increased by combining these agents. Optimal activity is observed when cells are pre-treated with calcitriol followed by paclitaxel. In PC-3, calcitriol does not modulate the apoptosis-inducing ability of paclitaxel suggesting that calcitriol and paclitaxel function through separate pathways to inhibit tumor growth.

Effect of calcitriol and dex on anti-tumor activity and VDR ligand binding.
We demonstrated that dex significantly enhanced calcitriol anti-tumor efficacy both *in vitro* and *in vivo* (18). In PC-3, dex was able to significantly enhance *in vitro* and *in vivo* clonogenic cell kill as compared to either agent alone. This combination was also effective at inducing significant tumor regression in this model system. We demonstrated that dex significantly increased VDR receptor content (number) without changing the affinity (Kd) (18). To further examine the effects of steroids on calcitriol-mediated anti-tumor effects, treated cells

were examined for changes in VDR protein by Western blot analysis. The combination of calcitriol and dex resulted in a significant increase in VDR protein as compared to calcitriol alone, which itself increases the VDR, or dex alone. This increase was maximal at 48 hours and correlates with an increase in VDR ligand binding. As previously described, dex alone did not result in significant induction of VDR protein (18). To determine whether dex mediates its effects through an increase in mRNA levels for the VDR, we isolated RNA from tumor cells treated *in vitro* with calcitriol with and without dex. By Northern blot analysis, no significant increase in mRNA levels was observed in any of the treatment groups (date not shown). Treatment with calcitriol alone or other agents that enhance VDR protein do not significantly increase VDR mRNA expression in a number of cell types (29).

We also examined whether changes could be observed *in vivo* in animals treated with calcitriol. Tumor-bearing mice were treated for 3 days with calcitriol and tumors harvested 4 hrs. later (Figure 3). Tumors were homogenized and while cell extracts were analyzed by Western blot. At 4 hours after the last injection of calcitriol, VDR protein, especially the upper band of the doublet, was induced in the animals treated with calcitriol. Modulation of VDR demonstrated the presence of calcitriol in the tumor and we demonstrated that enhanced VDR in the tumor correlated with an increase in antitumor efficacy.

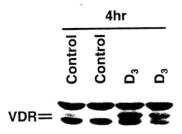

Fig. 3. Western blot analysis of VDR in whole cell extracts from SCC tumor-bearing animals treated with calcitriol (1μg) daily x3 and harvested 4 hrs. after the last injection.

Effects of calcitriol and dex on activated MAPK. The anti-tumor effects of calcitriol were significantly enhanced by treatment with dex. *In vitro*, exponentially growing tumor cells express significant levels of phosphorylated/ activated mitogen-activated protein kinases (MAPKs; i.e. Erk1 and Erk2) which are known to transduce mitogenic and survival signals to the nucleus in response to a number of extra cellular stimuli (30, 31). We have examined the effects of calcitriol alone and in combination with dex on MAPK activity in tumor cells. Treatment with calcitriol alone at 10 nM demonstrated no inhibition of MAPK activity after 4 hrs, modest inhibition after 24hrs, and strong inhibition after 48

466

hrs. An increase in vitamin D receptor (VDR) expression accompanied the loss of MAPK activity in calcitriol-treated cells. At both 24 and 48 hrs, treatment of cells with calcitriol and dex (0.5 μM) demonstrated a further increase in VDR expression and an inhibition of activated MAPK as compared to treatment with calcitriol or dex alone. Similar effects were observed even at lower dose of calcitriol (1 nM) and dex (0.01 – 0.02 μM). Importantly, Erk-1 and Erk-2 protein levels were unchanged in any of the treatment groups. These results suggest that calcitriol exert its growth inhibitory effects on tumor cells by inhibiting the mitogenic signaling pathway at a point upstream of MAPK.

Summary. We have demonstrated that calcitriol and its analogues have significant anti-proliferative activity, arrest cells in G_0/G_1, modulate expression of the cell cycle related proteins p27 and p21, induce PARP cleavage and pre-treatment with calcitriol enhances the anti-tumor activity of cisplatin, carboplatin, paclitaxel and docetaxel. Dex enhances calcitriol-mediated anti-proliferative effects and decreases $1,25D_3$ induced hypercalcemia. These activities are mediated through effects on the VDR. In a phase II trial in hormone-refractory prostate cancer using high dose (12μg/day QDx3, weekly) oral calcitriol and dex (4 mg QDx4, weekly), we observed a partial response (PR) as defined as greater than a 50% reduction in prostate specific antigen (PSA) in 28% of the patients and no hypercalcemia. We are also conducting two phase I trials of calcitriol + cytotoxics: carboplatin (AUC=5) Q28 days + escalating doses of calcitriol QD x 3 Q28 days and paclitaxel (80 *mg/m2* weekly x 6) + escalating doses of calcitrive, QDx3 weekly x 6. These trials continue to enroll patients with no observable toxicity. These studies form the basis to examine the mechanisms of $1,25D_3$-mediated anti-proliferative and cell-cycle effects both pre-clinically in vitro and in vivo animal tumor models and clinically.

References

1. Bikle DD, Pillai S. Vitamin D, calcium, and epidermal differentiation. Endocrine Rev (1993) 14 3-19.
2. Reichel H, Koeffler HP, Norman AW. The role of the vitamin D endocrine system in health and disease. New Engl J Med (1989). 320, 980-981
3. McElwain MC, Dettelbach MA, Modzelewski RA, Russell DK, Uskokovic MR, Smith DC, Trump DL, Johnson, CS. Antiproliferative effects in vitro and in vivo of 1,25-dihydroxyvitamin D3 and a vitamin D3 analog in a squamous cell carcinoma model system. Mol Cell Diff (1995) 3(1), 31-49.
4. Getzenberg RH, Light BW, Lapco PE, Konety BR, Nangia AK, Acierno JS, Dhir R, Shurin Z, Day RS, Trump DL, Johnson CS. Vitamin D inhibition of prostate adenocarcinoma growth and metastasis in the Dunning rat prostate model system. Urology (1997) 50, 999-1006.

5. Mangelsdorf DJ, Koeffler HP, Donaldson CA, Pike JW, Hanssler MR. 1,25-Dihydroxyvitamin D3 induced differentiation in a human promyelocytic leukemia cell line HL-60: receptor mediated maturation to macrophage-like cells. J Cell Biol (1984) 98, 391-398.

6. Colston KW, Chander SK, Mackay AG, Coombes RC. Effects of synthetic vitamin D analogues on breast cancer cell proliferation in vivo and in vitro. Biochem Pharmacol (1993) 44, 693-702.

7. Shabahang M, Buras RR, Davoodi F, Schumaker LM, Nauta RJ, Uskokovic MR, Brenner RV, Evans SRT. Growth inhibition of HT-29 human colon cancer cells by analogues of 1,25-dihydroxyvitamin D3. Cancer Res (1994) 54, 4057-4064.

8. Peehl DM, Skowronski RJ, Leung GK, Wong ST, Stamey TA, Feldman D. Antiproliferative effects of 1,25-dihydroxyvitamin D_3 on primary cultures of human prostatic cells. Cancer Res (1994) 54, 805-810.

9. Eisman JA, Barkla DH, Tutton PJM. Suppression of in vivo growth of human cancer solid tumor xenografts by 1,25-dihydroxyvitamin D3. Cancer Res (1987) 47, 21-25.

10. Zhou JY, Norman AW, Chen DL. 1,25-dihydroxy-16-ene-23-yne-vitamin D3 prolongs survival time of leukemic mice. Proc Natl Acad Sci USA (1990) 87, 3929-3932.

11. Modzelewski RA. Apoptotic effects of paclitaxel and calcitriol in rat dunning MLL and human PC-3 prostate tumor cells *in vitro*. Proc Amer Assoc Cancer Res (1999) 40, 580.

12. Light BW, Yu W-D, McElwain MC, Russell DM, Trump DL, Johnson CS. Potentiation of cisplatin anti-tumor activity using a vitamin D analogue in a murine squamous cell carcinoma model system. Cancer Res (1997) 57, 3759-3764.

13. Hershberger PA, Modzelewski RA, Shurin ZR, Rueger RM, Trump DL, Johnson CS. *In vitro* and *in vivo* modulation of p21[Wafl/Cip1] and p27[Kip1] in squamous cell carcinoma in response to 1,25-dihydroxycholecalciferol (1,25-D3). Cancer Res (1999) 59, 2644-2649.

14. Light BW, Potentiation of paclitaxel-mediated anti-tumor activity with 1,25-dihydroxycholecalciferol (1,25-D₃). Proc amer Assoc Cancer Res (1998) 39, 308.

15. Hershberger PA Yu WD, Modzelewski RA, Rueger RM, Shurin ZR, Johnson CS, Trump DL. Enhancement of paclitaxel antitumor activity in squamous cell carcinoma and prostatic adenocarcinoma by 1,25-dihydroxycholecaciferol (1,25-D₃) Cancer Res (submitted).

16. Smith DC, Johnson CS, Freeman CC, Muindi J, Wilson JW, Trump DL. A phase I trial of subcutaneous calcitriol (1,25- dihydroxycholecalciferol) in patients with advanced malignancy. Clin Cancer Res (1999) 5, 1339-1345.

468

17. Johnson CS Effects of high dose calcitriol (1,25-dihydroxyvitamid D_3) on the pharmacokinetics of paclitaxel of carboplatin: results of two phase I studies. Amer Soc Oncol (2000) 19, 210.

18. Yu W-D, McElwain MC, Modzelewski RA, Russell DM, Trump DL, Johnson CS. Potentiation of 1,25-dihydroxyvitamin D3-mediated anti-tumor activity with dexamethasone. J Natl. Cancer Inst (1998) 90 134-141.

19. Frappart L, Falette N, Lefebvre MF, Bremond A, Vauzelle JL, Saez S. In vitro study of effects of 1,25-dihydroxyvitamin D3 on the morphology of human breast cancer cell line BT.20. Differentiation (1989) 40 63-69.

20. Shabahang M, Buras RR, Davoodi F, Schumaker LM, Nauta RJ, Uskokovic MR, Brenner RV, Evans SRT. 1,25-dihydroxyvitamin D3 receptors as a marker of human colon carcinoma cell line differentiation and growth inhibition. Cancer Res (1993) 54: 4057-4064.

21. Miller GJ, Stapleton GE, Ferrara JA, Lucia MS, Pfister S, Hedlund TE, Upadya P. The human prostatic carcinoma cell line LNCaP expresses biologically active, specific receptors for 1,25-dihydroxyvitamin D3. Cancer Res (1992) 52, 515-520.

22. Skowronski RJ, Peehl DM, Feldman D. Vitamin D and prostate cancer: 1,25-dihydroxyvitamin D3 receptors and actions in human prostate cancer cell lines. Endocr (1993) 132, 1952-1959.

23. de Vos S, Holden S, Heber D. Effects of potent vitamin D3 analogs on clonal proliferation of human prostate cancer cell lines. Prostate (1997) 31, 77-83.

24. Biggs JR, Kraft AS. Inhibitors of cyclin-dependent kinase and cancer. J Mol Med (1995) 73, 509.

25. Henkart PA. ICE family proteases: mediators of all apoptotic cell death? Immunity (1996) 4, 195.

26. Rueger RM. The ability of paclitaxel to significantly decrease vitamin D mediated hypercalcemia. Proc Amer Assoc Cancer Res (1999) 40, 162.

27. Barboule N, Chadebach P., Baldin V, Vidal S, Valette A. Involvement of p21 in mitotic exi after paclitaxel treatment in MCF-7 breast adenocarcinoma cell line. Oncogene (1997) 15 ,2867-2967.

28. Stewart ZA, Mays D., Pietenpol JA. Defective G.-S cell cycle control checkpoint function sensitizes cells to microtubule inhibitor-induced apoptosis. Cancer Res (1999) 59, 3831-3837.

29. Hisham Darwish, Hector F. Deluca. Vitamin D-regulated Gene Expression. Critical Reviews in Eukaryotic Gene Expression, (1993) 3(2),: 89-116.

30. Paul A, Wilson S, Belham CM, et al. Stress-activated protein kinases: activation, regulation and function. Cell Signal (1997) 96, 403.

31. Lewis TS, Shaprio PS, Ahn NG. Signal transduction through MAP kinase cascades. Advances in Cancer Res (1998) 49.

Clinical Development of Calcitriol and Calcitriol Analogues as Anticancer Agents

Donald L. Trump, M.D., Pamela A. Hershberger, Ph.D., Ruth A. Modzelewski, Ph.D., Ronald J. Bernardi, Josephia Muindi, M.D., Ph.D, Robert M. Rueger, Wei-Dong Yu, Merrill J. Egorin, M.D., Kent E. Blum and Candace S. Johnson,Ph.D.

Departments of Medicine, Pharmacology and Urology, The University of Pittsburgh Cancer Institute Pittsburgh, PA 15213, USA

Vitamin D or 1,25 dihydroxycholecalciferol (calcitriol), a central factor in bone and mineral metabolism, is also a potent anti-proliferative agent in a wide variety of malignant cell types (1-4). Many investigators have demonstrated that calcitriol has significant anti-tumor activity *in vitro* and *in vivo* in murine, rat and human xenograph systems. (1-5). Initial *in vivo* studies focused on the use of calcitriol in murine leukemia models where calcitriol has anti-proliferative and differentiating effects. Calcitriol inhibits growth *in vitro* and *in vivo* in murine and human breast and colon cancer models. Calcitriol has also been investigated in prostate cancer where anti-proliferative activity has been observed with established human prostate cell lines (5,6). PSA secretion and androgen receptor (AR) expression are enhanced in LNCaP cells in response to calcitriol, which also inhibits LNCaP proliferation, in a dose-dependent manner. In many of these systems, calcitriol has been shown to induce G_0/G_1 arrest with a decrease of cells in S phase, modulate p27[Wafi/Cip1], the cyclin dependent kinase (cdk) inhibitor implicated in G_1 arrest. Calcitriol induces PARP cleavage, phosphatidlyserine exposure and increases bax/bcl-2 ratio, all early markers of apoptosis. Several investigators have shown that calcitriol significantly enhances the anti-tumor efficacy of cisplatin, carboplatin and paclitaxel (6-9). Our group has shown that dexamethasone potentiates the anti-tumor effect of calcitriol and decreases calcitriol-induced hypercalcemia (8). Both *in vitro* and *in vivo*, dexamethasone significantly increases vitamin D receptor (VDR) ligand binding in the tumor and decreases binding in the intestinal mucosa. While the mechanisms underlying these effects are incompletely delineated, many investigators have explored approaches for the development of calcitriol and calcitriol analogues as anticancer agents. The following reviews the work of many investigations in this field focusing particularly on work with calcitriol since development of analogues for anticancer indications is just beginning.

Calcitriol has been utilized in a number of clinical trials. The majority of these were in leukemia and myelodysplasia. Although some evidence of response was seen, the results were largely disappointing (14). Most investigators have argued that the propensity of calcitriol to cause hypercalcemia is a major limitation in the application of calcitriol as an anticancer drug. This has led to considerable efforts to develop calcitriol analogues which retain the anticancer activities of the parent compound but are less potent in inducing hypercalcemia. There are three vitamin D analogues currently being developed in the clinic as anticancer agents:

1. ILX23-7553

This agent (1,25-dihydroxy-16-ene-23-yne vitamin D_3) was originally developed by Hoffman LaRoche as Ro23-7553. It has been extensively tested in preclinical models and reported to be 30-50 fold less potent than calcitriol in mediating gastrointestinal absorption of calcium and mobilizing bone calcium stores and 4-12 fold more potent than calcitriol in inhibiting cell growth and inducing differentiation in leukemia models. ILEX Oncology has recently initiated clinical trials with ILX23-7553. Phase one trials in patients with advanced cancer have just begun. The agent will be studied following oral administration on a QD X5, every other week schedule and on a QD X3, weekly with and without dexamethasone by investigators at Robert Wood Johnson School of Medicine/Memorial Sloan-Kettering Cancer Center and the University of Pittsburgh, respectively. As these studies have just begun, there are no data regarding toxicity, maximum tolerated dose, biologic effects or antitumor responses.

2. EB 1089

This analogue (1(S), 3(R)-dihydroxy-20(R)-(5'-ethyl-5'-hydroxy-hepta-1'(E),3'(E)-dien-1'-yl)-9,10-secopregna-(Z),7(E),10(19)-triene)) is also active in preclinical systems at doses which do not appear to induce hypercalcemia. Phase 1 trials of this agent have been completed in Europe. The dose limiting toxicity of EB1089 is hypercalcemia which was seen in all patients receiving 15-25μg/sqm/d. The dose "estimated to be tolerable" for most patients was 15-25μg/sqm/d. Phase II and III trials are underway in Europe. No published data are available regarding antitumor efficacy of EB1089.

3. 1 alpha D_2

This analogue is also reported to retain antitumor activity at doses which do not induce hypercalcemia in experimental animals. The drug is being developed by Bone Care International and phase I and II studies are being conducted by Dr.George Wilding at the University of Wisconsin. The maximum tolerated dose of 1 alpha D_2 is 15μg/sqm QD. Dr. Wilding and colleagues have described antitumor activity in a small number of patients with prostate cancer. Development of this drug through phase II and III trials is being dexpored in prostate cancer. Data currently available indicate that this agent is less active in inducing hypercalcemia and preliminary data suggest that antitumor activity is present in a minority of patients with prostate cancer.

4. Calcitriol (1,25 dihydroxycholecalciferol)

Gross et al have reported potential beneficial effects of calcitriol administered as a single agent to men with prostate cancer in whom the prostate specific antigen (PSA) is rising following local therapy (prostatectomy or irradiation. In men with rising PSA the rate of rise was diminished with a dose of 1.5-2.0µg calcitriol per day. This study was halted due to the development of hypercalciuria in most men treated but indicates that calcitriol itself may have antitumor activity in individuals with cancer.

Our group has been interested in evaluating new schedules of calcitriol administration, hypothesizing that schedule modification and the use of "adjunctive" medications may permit administration of considerable doses of this agent without limiting toxicity. Our extensive data indicate that this hypothesis is correct.

We have completed a study to evaluate the pharmacokinetics and MTD of calcitriol following subcutaneous (sc) QOD administration (15). Thirty-six patients were entered at doses ranging from 2 µg to 10 µg QOD; dose limiting toxicity (hypercalcemia) occurred in 3 of 3 patients entered at the 10 µg QOD dose. Hypercalciuria occurred at all dose levels examined. No other toxicity was seen. Assessment of serum calcitriol concentrations by a radioimmunoassay revealed a decrease in concentration-time curves on the seventh day compared to the first day of therapy. A dose dependent increase in peak serum level and estimated area under the curve (AUC) were seen; the maximum serum levels occurred at the 10 µg QOD dose: 288 ± 74 pg/mL and 321 ± 36 pg/mL days 1 and 7 respectively. The normal range of calcitriol serum concentrations using this assay is 16-56 pg/mL. Serum calcitriol levels were maintained at near peak concentrations for at least 8 hours following sc. injection. This study indicates that substantial doses of calcitriol can be administered via this route with tolerable toxicity. After completion of this phase I trial of calcitriol alone we explored the effect of glucocorticoids on the MTD of calcitriol using the every other day schedule. Patients were treated concurrently with either sc calcitriol and dexamethasone or calcitriol and prednisone. Neither dexamethasone at 4 mg QOD nor prednisone at 40 mg QOD with calcitriol allowed further dose escalation. The tolerable dose was 8 µg QOD sc whether calcitriol was given alone or with glucocorticoids. It should be emphasized that our pre-clinical studies in which we demonstrated that dexamethasone potentiates calcitriol anti-tumor activity and reduces hypercalcemia have administered dexamethasone before and during calcitriol administration Schedule and timing of administration of dexamethasone and calcitriol appear critical to optimal effects Calcitriol + Glucocorticoids: Prostate Cancer.

Our first study of calcitriol in androgen independent prostate cancer (AIPC) was a straight forward phase II study of "replacement doses" of calcitriol [0.5µg QD, po x 7d, 1.0 µg QD x 7d and 1.5 µg po QD continuously thereafter]. No therapeutic affects were seen and 3 of 13 (23%) had hypercalcemia. As our preclinical data indicated that dose escalation of calcitriol was important and that dexamethasone potentiates calcitriol antitumor effects and blocks hypercalcemia, we initiated a phase II study of calcitriol and dexamethasone in AIPC. Calcitriol and dexamethasone are administered according to the following schedule: calcitriol 8µg Monday, Tuesday and Wednesday (MTW) weekly X4, then if no toxicity was seen the dose was escalated to 10µg MTW for one month. If no toxicity occurred the dose of calcitriol was increased to 12µg MTW weekly for the duration of the study. Dexamethasone is administered orally 4mg Sunday MTW each week. We sought to administer the highest dose of calcitriol possible in this study, but were concerned that this novel and intensive dosing schedule of calcitriol may be poorly tolerated. Thirty-two patients have or are currently receiving 12 µg MTW and no patient has required dose reduction because of hypercalcemia. The only calcitriol related toxicity in this trial has been the development in 2 patients of urinary tract stones; in one man this was an asymptomatic renal stone, detected by ultrasound and in the second it was a symptomatic bladder stone. All patients undergo pretreatment and every three month renal ultrasound to monitor for nephrolithiasis. Twenty-nine patients are evaluable at this time; 8 experienced a 50% reduction in PSA (28%) and patients with bone pain at study entry have experienced pain relief. Eighty percent of patients have experienced a slowing in the rate of PSA rise and 34% have had stable disease or decrease in PSA (>50% reduction). While the role of calcitriol in the antitumor effects seen in this trial is difficult to assign, independent of dexamethasone, this trial does very clearly indicate that substantial does of calcitriol can be administered on a QD X3, weekly schedule with dexamethasone without substantial toxicity.

We are conducting two phase I trials of calcitriol + cytotoxics:

1. carboplatin (AUC=5) Q28 days + escalating doses of calcitriol QDx3 Q28 days. Calcitriol starting dose was 4µg QDx3. Studies are designed such that in each patient, carboplatin is given on day 1 before calcitriol in one of the first two cycles of treatment and on day 3 after two days

of high dose calcitriol on the other. This permits comparison of AUC of carboplatin in the same patient before and after pretreatment with calcitriol. Dose-limiting toxicity has not been encountered in this trial; current doses of calcitriol are 13µg po QDX3, Q4 week with carboplatin. The AUC of carboplatin is higher in patients treated with calcitriol before carboplatin (mean AUC = 7.8 µg/ml.hr ± 1.3, carboplatin Day 3 versus AUC = 6.7µg/ml.hr ± 1.5, carboplatin Day 1). While no dose limiting toxicity has been seen, myelosuppression (%change in platelet count) following the sequence carboplatin→calcitriol was consistently less than that following calcitriol →carboplatin, consistent with the change in AUC. No clinically detectable renal impairment has been seen with either sequence. These data indicate that potentiation of carboplatin by calcitriol may in part be related to reduced carboplatin clearance (16).

2. We are conducting a phase I study of paclitaxel (80mg weekly x 6, Q8 weeks) + escalating doses of calcitriol. Starting dose of calcitriol was 4µg po QDX3, weekly and we are currently entering patients at 22µg po QDX3, weekly. No limiting toxicity has been encountered. The study design calls for administration of paclitaxel on day 1 cycle 1 of therapy prior to any calcitriol therapy and on day 3 with the third dose of calcitriol week two and all subsequent weeks. This permits evaluation of the effect of calcitriol on paclitaxel pharmacokinetics – week 1 vs week 2. No changes in peak concentration, AUC or T 1/2 have been noted. PSA responses have occurred in 2 of 4 patients with AIPC entered in the study.

Our studies indicate that modification in the schedule and route of administration of calcitriol and dexamethasone and paclitaxel permit dose escalation of this agent.

Daily Dose	14 Day Dose Intensity	Limiting Hypercalcemia
10µg QOD subq	70µg/14 d	100%
1.5µg QD po	21µg/14d	30%
12µgQD x 3 po	72µg/14d	0%
22µgQD x 3 po, weekly + paclitaxel	102µg/14d	0%

474

Conclusion

Preclinical data that clearly indicate that calcitriol and analogues have antitumor effects as single agents and potentiate the effects of a number of cytotoxic agents – particularly taxanes and platinum analogues. Early clinical data clearly indicate that calcitriol and analogues (EB1089, ILX23-7553 and 1 alpha D_2) can be given safely in humans. Dose escalation of calcitriol appears to be possible by considering schedule and concomitant medication approaches. Substantial doses of calcitriol can be given safely and indications of antitumor activity in prostate cancer have been demonstrated. These preliminary data strongly support the further development of vitamin D analogues as antitumor agents.

References

1. McElwain MC, Dettelbach MA, Modzelewski RA, et al. Antiproliferative effects *in vitro* and *in vivo* ov 1,25-dihydroxyvitamin D3 and a vitamin D3 analog in a squamous cell carcinoma model system. Mol Cell Diff <u>3</u> (1) 31 (1995).
2. Getzenberg RH, Light BW, Lapco PE, et al. Vitamin D inhibition of prostate adenocarcinoma growth and metastasis in the Dunning rat prostate model system. Urology 50 999 (1997).
3. Mangelsdorf DJ, Koeffler HP, Donaldson CA, et al. 1,25-Dihydroxyvitamin D3 induced differentiation in a human promyelocytic leukemia cell line HL-60: receptor mediated maturation to macrophage-like cells. J Cell Biol <u>98</u> 391 (1984).
4. Colston KW, Chander SK, Mackay AG, et al. Effects of synthetic vitamin D analogues on breast cancer cell proliferation *in vivo* and *in vitro*. Biochem Pharmacol <u>44</u> 693 (1993).
5. Modzelewski RA. Apoptotic effects of paclitaxel and calcitriol in rat dunning MLL and human PC-3 prostate tumor cells *in vitro*. Proc Amer Assoc Cancer Res <u>40</u> 580 (1999).
6. Peehl DM, Skowronski RJ, Leung GK, et al. Antiproliferative effects of 1,25-dihydroxyvitamin D_3 on primary cultures of human prostatic cells. Cancer Res <u>54</u> 805 (1994).
7. Shabahang M, Buras RR, Davoodi F, et al. 1,25-dihydroxyvitamin D3 receptors as a marker of human colon carcinoma cell line differentiation and growth inhibition. Cancer Res <u>53</u> 3712 (1993).
8. Yu W-D, McElwain MC, Modzelewski RA, et al. Potentiation of 1,25-dihydroxyvitamin D3-mediated anti-tumor activity with dexamethasone. J Natl Cancer Inst <u>90</u> 134 (1998).
9. Hershberger PA Yu WD, Modzelewski RA, et al. Enhancement of paclitaxel antitumor activity in squamous cell carcinoma and prostatic adenocarcinoma by 1,25-dihydroxycholecaciferol (1,25-D_3) Cancer Res (submitted).
10. Smith DC, Johnson CS, freeman CC, et al. A phase I trial of subcutaneous calcitriol (1,25-dihydroxycholecalciferol) in patients

with advanced malignancy. Clinical Cancer Research 5 1339 (1999).

11. Light BW, Yu W-D McElwain MC, et al. Potentiation of cisplatin anti-tumor activity using a vitamin D analogue in a murine squamous cell carcinoma model system. Cancer Res 57 3759 (1997).

12. Light BW, YuBW, Shurin ZR et al. Potentiation of paclitaxel-mediated anti-tumor activity with 1,25-dihydroxycholecalciferol (calcitriol). Proc Amer Cancer Res 39 308 (1998).

13. Yu W-D, McElwain MC, Modzelewski RA, et al. Potentiation of 1,25-dihydroxyvitamin D3-mediated anti-tumor activity with dexamethasone. J Natl Cancer Inst 90 134 (1998).

14. Koeffler HP, Hirji K, Iltri L, et al. 1,25-Dihydroxyvitamin D3: in vivo and in vitro effects on human preleukemic and leukemic cells. Cancer Treat Rep 69 1399 (1985).

15. Smith DC, Johnson CS, freeman CC, et al. A phase I trial of subcutaneous calcitriol (1,25-dihydroxycholecalciferol) in patients with advanced malignancy. Clinical Cancer Research 5 1339 (1999).

16. Johnson CS, Egorin MJ, Zuhowski R, et al. Effects of high dose calcitriol (1,25 dihydroxyvitamin D3) on the pharmacokinetics of paclitaxel of carboplatin: results of two phase I studies. Amer Soc Oncol 19 210a (2000).

NON-CLASSICAL ACTIONS OF VITAMIN D: MECHANISMS AND CLINICAL ASPECTS

Kay Colston, Grisha Pirianov, Janine Mansi, Department of Oncology/GEM, St George's Hospital Medical School, London, UK

Introduction Vitamin D is essential for the maintenance of a healthy sketeton. Without vitamin D, children develop rickets and adults develop osteomalacia. Casual exposure to sunlight is the major source of vitamin D for most individuals: vitamin D_3 is formed in the skin by the action of ultraviolet light on a precursor molecule, 7-dehydrocholesteronl. Once vitamin D_3 is formed in the skin or ingested in the diet, it must be hydroxylated in the liver and kidney to form 1,25-dihydroxyvitamin D_3 [1,25 $(OH)_2D_3$].The active metabolite. It has been recognised for nearly two decades that a wide variety of tissues and cells, both those involved in calcium transport and others apparently unrelated to calcium metabolism, are targets for 1,25 $(OH)_2D_3$. 'Noncalcemic' tissues that possess receptors for 1,25 $(OH)_2D_3$ respond to the hormone in a variety of ways ("non-classical" actions). In this regard, 1,25 $(OH)_2D_3$ has been shown to possess both immunomodulatory actions and effects on cell proliferation and differentiation. Thus it has been suggested that 1,25 $(OH)_2D_3$ and it analogs could have wide clinical application in such diverse disorders as psoriasis, immune disease and certain malignancies. The extent to which this latter therapeutic potential can be realized will depend in part on the successful dissociation between calcaemic and antiproliferative effects in the development of new synthetic analogs. While 'vitamin D' formulations, both topical and systemic, have already proved useful as a new approach to treatment of psoriasis, trials of vitamin D analogs given systemically are now underway in patients with malignant disease.

The first observation relating vitamin D to cancer was the demonstration that cultured human breast cancer cells contain the receptor for vitamin D (1). Subsequently, the first demonstration that 1,25 $(OH)_2D_3$ is capable of inhibiting the growth of human cancer cells was made with malignant melanoma cells (2), and later in murine leukaemia cells, in which induction of differentiation was also reported (3). Such observations led to suggestions that conventional vitamin D metabolites could have therapeutic potential in certain haematological malignancies. Initial clinical trials suggested that oral administration of 1,25 $(OH)_2D_3$ or alfacalcidol may be of benefit in myelofibrosis, myelodysplastic syndromes and non-Hodgkin's lymphoma(4). However, clinical use of these compounds is limited by calcaemic side effects. The development of synthetic vitamin D analogs with potent effects on cell growth and decreased calcaemic activity have presented the opportunity to further evaluate the therapeutic potential of vitamin D compounds in hyperproliferative disorders.

The analog MC903 (calcipotriol) has been evaluated in patients with locally advanced or metastatic breast cancer. In this trial, 19 patient with evaluable cutaneous lesions were treated topically with calcipotriol ointment. All were normocalcaemic at entry and 14 completed 6 weeks of treatment. Of these 3 showed a partial and 1 a minimal response (5).

Given systemically, MC903 is rapidly inactivated with a serum half-life of only a few minutes. However, other analogs have been developed which display increased antiproliferative effects relative to calcaemic activity and are less rapidly metabolized. Such compounds have been shown to have potent effects on inhibition of cancer cell growth and a number have been reported to promote differentiation of myeloid leukemia cells (6). An example is the analog EB 1089 (Leo Pharmaceuticals). This compound has been demonstrated to inhibit the growth of a number established human cancer cell lines *in vitro*. In addition, studies with animal models of breast cancer have shown that treatment with this analog leads to tumor regression. Thus substantial regression of both carcinogen-induced rat mammary tumors and MCF-7 xenografts have been demonstrated (7). Laboratory studies have demonstrated that, in some cancer cell types, vitamin D analogs can both inhibit cell growth and promote apoptosis (programmed cell death). A number of laboratories have demonstrated induction of DNA fragmentation (a key feature of apoptosis) in breast cancer cells treated with vitamin D analogs. Evidence of induction of apoptosis *in vivo* as indicated by the TUNEL staining method have also been described in experimental mammary tumours following treatment with these compounds (8).

The mechanisms by which vitamin D analogs promote active cell death are not clear but could involve suppression of cell survival signals and/or induction of pathways that stimulate apoptosis. The susceptibility of a cell to undergo apoptosis depends in part on the relative expression of a family of proteins which display anti-apoptotic activty (eg bcl-2) and those family members having apoptotic activity (eg bax). Cleavage and activation of the cell death proteases (caspases) is considered essential to the execution stage of the apoptotic process, leading to cleavage of death substrates, fragmentation of chromosomal DNA and formation of apoptotic bodies. The disregulation of normal programmed cell death mechanisms play an important role in the pathogenesis and progression of breast cancer as well as the response of tumors to therapeutic intervention. Overexpression of antiapoptotic members of the bcl-2 family such as bcl-2 or bclx$_L$ has been implicated in cancer chemoresistance whereas high levels of proapoptotic proteins, such a bax promote apoptosis and sensitize tumor cells to various anticancer therapies.

Although the mechanisms by which bcl-2 family proteins regulate apoptosis are diverse, ultimately they govern decision steps that determine whether certain caspases remain quiescent or become active. Recently, it has became clear that alterations leading to disfunction of mitochondria are decisive events in the apoptotic process. Opening of the mitochndrial pore, which is regulated by the bcl-2 family and other factors, can lead to loss of membrane potential and liberation of intermembrane proteins, such as cytochrome c and Apaf-1, resulting in activation of caspases. Bcl-2 can block caspase activation by preventing the release of cytochrome c (Fig 1). Although apoptosis can be induced by engagement of cell death receptors, a deficiency of essential survival factors also has become well recognised as an important trigger for apoptosis. In breast cancer cells, the most important serum growth factor appears to be the insulin-like growth factor-I. IGF-I receptors are overexpressed in many breast cancer cells and there is evidence for a relationship between circulating IGF-I levels and risk of breast cancer (9). There is substantial evidence that IGF-I is not only a potent mitogen in breast cancer cells but also promotes cells survival by prevention or delay of apoptosis induced by a variety of stimuli.

Stimulation of IGF-IR by its agonists leads to activation of the ras/raf/MAPK protein cascade and the PI3K signalling pathway which appears to be an essential step in the survival effect. Inhibitors of PI3K prevent IGF-I mediated cell survival. The downstream target of PI3K is Akt/PKB which phosphorylates BAD, a proapoptotic protein. Phosphorylation prevents BAD translocation to the nucleus where it would neutralize effects of bcl-2 in its ability to prevent cytochrome c release (10).

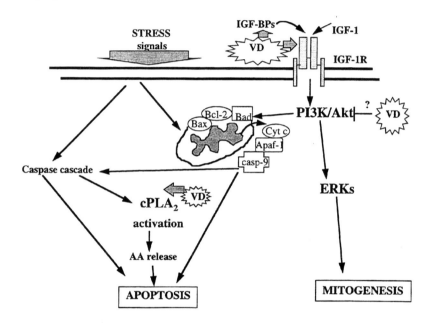

Figure 1: Potential interactions of IGF-I and vitamin D signalling pathaways.

Results and Discussion Established human breast cancer cell lines are a good model to evaluate the antiapoptotic effects of IGF-I and potential interactions with vitamin D analogs. Serum deprivation induces apoptosis in MCF-7 cells as assessed by loss of cell viability and induction of DNA fragmentation. IGF-I alone (4 nM) for 4 days can completely prevent the induction of apoptosis due to serum factor deprivation. Thus these cells are dependent upon IGF-I only for their survival. However, treatment with the vitamin D analogs CB1093 and EB1089 can prevent cell survial in response to IGF-I. Therefore the vitamin D analogs abrogate anti-apoptotic effects of IGF-I in these cells (11).

To address to role of caspases in the ability of vitamin D analogs to abrogate IGF-I effects we have utilised the broad spectrum caspase inhibitor z-VAD-fmk. Over the 4 day incubation period, 50 µM z-VAD-fmk reduced induction of DNA fragmentation in response to serum deprivation to an extent similar to that seen with IGF-I resupplementation. Co-treatment with CB1093 in serum-free conditions reversed this effects of IGF-I. However, the ability of CB1093 to abrogate IGF-I-induced cell survival was not prevented by z-VAD-fmk suggesting that caspase activation is not required for the vitamin D analog CB1093 to mediate anti-IGF-I effects (Fig 2a). Furthermore, co-incubation with the caspase inhibitor did not prevent loss of cell viability in response to CB1093 in MCF-7 cells incubated in 1% serum-containing medium. These results suggest that induction of apoptosis by vitamin D analogs in MCF-7 cells is not dependent on activation of a known caspases (Fig 2b).

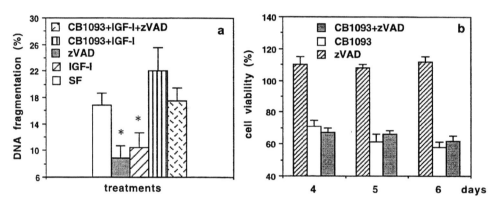

Figure 2: Vitamin D analogue CB1093 inhibits IGF-I survival signals and induces cell death in a caspase-independent manner in MCF-7 cells. a) Cells were pretreated with z-VAD-fmk (50 µM) for 3 h and finally co-treated with CB1093 (100 nM) and IGF-I (4 nM) in serum-free medium (SF) for 4 days. DNA fragmentation was assessed as previously described (12). (*p<0.005). b) MCF-7 cells were pre-incubated with or without z-VAD-fmk (50 µM for 3 h) and co-treated with CB1093 (100 nM for 6 days). Cell viability was assessed by MTS assay as previously described (13).

Activation of cytosolic phospholipase A_2 (cPLA2) and release of arachidonic acid (AA) in TNFα-induced apoptosis can be attenuated by inhibitors of cPLA2.in breast cancer cells (14). The role of AA release in cell death is not clear but may be associated with generation of reactive oxygen species or may target down stream effectors involved in the execution stage of apoptosis. We have identified cPLA2 activation as a mechanism by which vitamin D analogs potentiate TNFα-mediated apoptosis in breast cancer cells (15). In order to assess the role of cPLA2 activation in the induction of cell death by vitamin D analogs, cells were incubated with CB1093 in the presence or absence of the cPLA2 inhibitor MAFP. The inhibitor prevented cPLA2 activation and partially protected against loss of cell viability (Fig 3a,b) in contrast to the caspase inhibitor z-VAD-fmk where no protection was evident (Fig 2b).

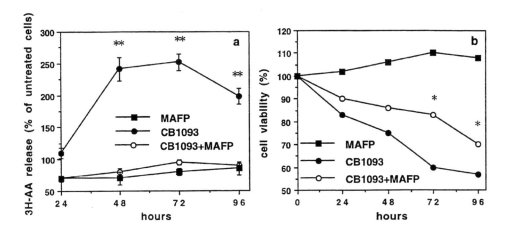

Figure 3: CB1093 promotes release of AA and MAFP partially prevents CB1093-induced loss of MCF-7 cell viability. a) Cells were pre-treated with 5 µM MAFP for 3 h and finally treated with CB1093 (100 nM for 96 h). Release of [3H]-AA was assessed as previously described (16). b) Replicate cultures were assessed for cell viability determined by MTS assay (13). ($p^*<0.005$ and $p^{**}<0.001$).

cPLA2 activation is also apparent in MCF-7 cells induced to undergo apoptosis due to serum starvation or IGF-I deprivation. Figure 4 contrasts the time course of cPLA2 activation in serum-deprived cells and cells treated with CB1093 in serum-containing medium. cPLA2 activation in response to serum starvation is inhibited by z-VAD-fmk, the cPLA2 inhibitor MAFP and IGF-I. Addition of CB1093 prevented IGF-I inhibition of cPLA2 activation (Fig 4).

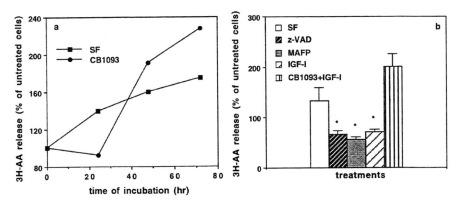

Figure 4: Effects of CB1093 and IGF-I on cPLA2 activation in MCF-7 cells: role of inhibitors. Cells were pre-treated with or without 5 µM MAFP or 50 µM z-VAD-fmk for 3 h and finally exposed to IGF-I (4 nM) alone or co-treated with CB1093 (100 nM) in serum-free medium (SF). cPLA2 activation was assessed by [3H]-AA release (16). ($p^*<0.005$).

These studies indicate that cPLA$_2$ activation is a feature of apoptosis induced by vitamin D analogs and serum deprivation. Failure of IGF-I to prevent cPLA$_2$ activation in the presence of CB1093 indicates that release of AA may play a role in the interactions of vitamin D and IGF-I signalling. Furthermore vitamin D analogs may be useful agents to identify the nature of caspase-independent pathways leading to abrogation of IGF-I survival signals. Since it has been suggested that inhibition of IGF-I action could be a useful adjunct to cytotoxic chemotherapy, these agents may have a role in combination with antiestrogens or taxanes in the treatment of patients with breast cancer.

The analog EB1089 (Seocalcitol) has been evaluated in a phase I trial in patients with advanced breast and colorectal carcinoma. 36 patients received EB1089 in doses between 0.15 and 17mg/m^2 daily for 5 days. 21 patients received compassionate treatment for between 10 and 234 days. 10 patients developed hypercalcaemia which was reversed by discontinuing or reducing therapy. No complete or partial responses were seen. Six patients showed stabilization of disease in excess of 3 months (17).

Pancreatic carcinoma is an increasingly common malignancy five year survival is less than 5%. Surgery is the only curative treatment and chemotherapy is of limited value. 5-fluorouracil is the standard cytotoxic drug but response rates are reported to be less than 20%. Gemcitobine treatment is associated with improved 1 year survival and preclinical trials have indicated synergistic effects between this drug and cisplatin. Immunocytochemical studies have suggested that tumors of the exocrine pancreas may be VDR positive and established pancreatic carcinoma cells show growth inhibition when exposed to active vitamin D analogs both *in vitro* and when grown as tumor xenografts in immunodeficient mice (18). Thus analogs of vitamin D could be considered as a potential new therapeutic approach in pancreatic carcinoma. *In vitro* studies with a number of established pancreatic carcinoma cell lines suggest that pretreatment of cells with vitamin D analogs potentiates effectiveness of chemotherapeutic agents (Fig 5).

A phase I/II trial of seocalcitol in patients with inoperable pancreatic carcinoma has been utertaken in which 42 patients were enrolled. Dose of the vitamon D analog was individually escalated until hypercalcaemia developed. Survival ranged from 13-887 days (median 107). Hypercalcaemia was reversed by discontinuing or reducing therapy. No responses were seen with regard to tumour measurement. In patients survived more than 2 years and from 2 more than 6 months. The potential benefit of combination therapy with cytotoxics or other agents in this malignancy is worthy of consideration.

Studies have revealed an important role for the IGF-I pathway in growth and survival of breast cancer cells and this may have relevance to other cell types. Synthetic analogs of vitamin D have been found irreversibly to prevent ant-apoptotic effect of IGF-I. It is therefore important to gain a clear inderstanding of the mechanisms by which vitamin D analogs abrogate IGF-I-mediated survival. An improved understanding of these interactions could ultimately lead to indentification of new preventative or therapeutic targets.

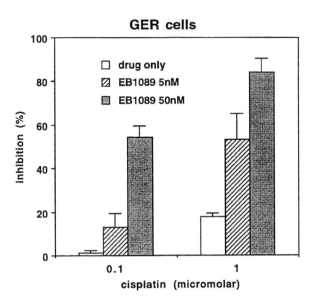

GER cells

Figure 5 Effects of EB1089 and cisplatin in GER pancreatic carcinoma cells. Cells were pre-treated for 2 days with EB1089 and pos-treated with cisplatin for 3 days. Results are expressed as % inhibition of cell growth relative to control cultures.

References
1. Elsman, J.A., MacIntyre, I., Martin, T,J., Moseley, J.M. (1979) Lancet 2, 1335-1336.
2. Colston, K.W., Colston, M.J. and Feldman, D. (1981) Endocrinology 108, 1083-1086.
3. Abe, E., Miyaura, C., Sakagami, H., Takeda, M., Konno, K., Yamazaki, T., Yoshiki, S. and Suda T. (1981) Proc Natl Acad Sci USA 78, 4990-4995.
4. Cunningham D, Gilchrist NL, Cowan RA. and Soukup K. (1985) Brit Med J 291, 1153-1155.
5. Bower, M., Colston, K.W., Stein, R.C., Hedley, A., Gazet, J.C., Ford, H,T and Coombes, R.C. (1991) Lancet 337, 701-702.
6. Binderup L. (1992) Biochem Pharmacol 43, 1885-1892.
7. Danielsson C., Mathiasen, I.S., James, S., Nayeri, S., Bretting, C., Mork Hansen, C., Colston, K.W. and Carlberg, C. (1997) Cell Biochem 66, 552-565.
8. James, S.Y., .Mercer, E., Brady, M., Binderup, L. and Colston KW. (1998) Brit J Pharmacol 125, 953-962.
9. Hankinson, S.E., Wilett, W.C., Colditz, G.A., Hunter, D.J., Michaud, D.S., Deroo, B,, Rosner, B. and Pollak M. (1998) Lancet 351, 1393-1396.
10. Datta, S.R., Dudek, H., Tao, X., Master, S., Fu, H., Gotoh, Y. and Greenberg, M.E. (1997) Cell 91, 231-241.
11. Xie, S.P., Pirianov, G. and Colston, K.W. (1999) Eur J Cancer 35, 1717-1723.

12. Duke, R.C. and Cohen, J.J. (1992) in Current protocols in immunology (Coligan, J.E. ed) Green/Wiley, New York, pp3.17.1-3.17.6.
13. Cory, A.H., Owen, T.C., Barltrop, J.A. and Cory, J.G. (1991) Cancer Comm 3, 207-212.
14. Wissing, D., Mousitzen, H., Egeblad, M., Poirer, G. and Jaattela, M. (1997) Proc Natl Acad Sci USA 94, 5073-5077.
15. Pirianov, G., Danielsson, C., Carlberg, C., James, S.. and Colston, K.W. (1999) Cell Death Diff 6, 890-901.
16. Wu, Y., Jiang, X., Lillinngton, D., Allen, P., Newland, A. and Kelsley, S. (1998) Cancer Res 58, 633-640.
17. Gulliford, T., English, J., Colston, K.W., Menday, P., Moller, S. and Coombes, R.C. (1998) Brit J Cancer 78, 6-13.
18. Colston, K.W., James, S.Y., Ofori-Kuragu., Binderup, L. and Grant, A.G. (1997) Brit J Cancer 76, 1017-1020.

SEOCALCITOL (EB1089) - CLINICAL EXPERIENCE TO DATE

T R J Evans[1], K J Hamberg[2], T Skov[2], H L O Haahr[2], P Menday[3], C Bay[2], L Binderup[2].
[1.] Beatson Oncology Centre, University of Glasgow, Glasgow, UK.
[2.] Leo Pharmaceutical Products, Copenhagen, Denmark.
[3.] Leo Laboratories Ltd, Princes Risborough, UK.

It is well established that the metabolically active form of vitamin D, 1 α, 25-dihydroxyvitamin D_3, plays a key role in regulating calcium metabolism in the body. In addition vitamin D_3 can exert potent cell regulatory effects in many cell types not directly involved in calcium homeostasis, including cancer cells. Most of these effects are mediated through the binding of vitamin D_3 to a specific, high affinity receptor, the vitamin D receptor (VDR). However, a number of investigations have indicated the presence of another, non-genomic pathway through which various biological responses can be initiated.

Vitamin D receptors are expressed in numerous types of cancer cell, including cells derived from cancers of the breast, prostate, pancreas, colon, bladder, cervix, thyroid, pituitary, skin, as well as melanoma, glioma, neuroblastoma, leukaemia and lymphoma cells, and hepatocellular carcinoma cells. Vitamin D_3 is able to inhibit growth and stimulate differentiation of tumour cells in vitro, although it's use in vivo is limited by its tendency to cause hypercalcaemia.

EB1089 (seocalcitol) is a synthetic analogue of vitamin D which is 50 - 200 times more potent than vitamin D_3 in the regulation of cell growth and differentiation but with a calcaemic effect in vivo in rats which is approximately 50% weaker than that of vitamin D_3 (1,2). Furthermore, EB1089 induces apoptosis, reduces invasiveness and inhibits angiogenesis in a range of cancer cells in vitro, and many of the genetic events associated with these cellular responses have been described. Based on these encouraging in vitro data, numerous in vivo experiments have been carried out which have demonstrated that EB1089 can cause regression of established tumours, prevent the development of metastases, and prolong survival time in tumour-bearing animals (3-7). Moreover, significant inhibition of tumour progression can be achieved at doses that do not cause significant hypercalcaemia (4), and can also induce apoptosis in both breast and prostatic tumours in vivo (3,5). Consequently, this agent has now been evaluated in early clinical trials.

Initially, EB1089 was evaluated in 13 healthy volunteers, with one subject receiving treatment over 4 consecutive days at one of 7 dose levels ranging from 7 - 40 μg per day. Subsequently 3 subjects were treated at each of 2 higher dose levels (60μg and 80μg per day). All subjects had a constant dietary calcium intake, and daily measurements of serum calcium, urinary calcium excretion and serum, creatinine, phosphate and PTH were performed.

Treatment was continued until hypercalcaemia, defined as albumin-corrected serum calcium of >2.80 mmol/l occurred. Two patients developed hypercalcaemia: one at 60μg/day on day 4, and one on day 3 at 80μg/day. Other drug-related toxicities were mild and infrequent, and included headache and nausea at the higher dose levels. All events, including the hypercalcaemia resolved within 10 days of stopping the medication.

Subsequently EB1089 was evaluated in 36 patients with advanced cancer, either breast (n=25), or colorectal (n=11) cancer (8). Patients (28 female, 8 male) of age 31 - 80 years with adequate renal, hepatic and haematological function, and with albumin-corrected serum calcium <2.65 mmol/l, were included. Eleven patients received a single dose followed by the 5-day repeated dosing period at dose level of 0.15 - 0.6μg/m^2/day. Twenty-five patients received only the 5-day repeated dosing at dose levels of 0.9 - 17μg/m^2/day. Hypercalcaemia was defined as a corrected serum calcium >2.65 mmol/l, severe hypercalcaemia as a corrected serum calcium >2.80 mmol/l (or 2 consecutive values of >2.75 mmol/l) and hypercalcuria as a 24 hour urine calcium excretion >7.5 mmol/l. Neither hypercalcaemia or hypercalcuria occurred during the single day dosing. Eleven patients developed hypercalcaemia during the 5-day repeated dosing, of whom 4 had severe hypercalcaemia at doses of 0.45, 12.5, and 17 (2 patients) μg/m^2/day. Twenty one patients received compassionate treatment for between 10 and 234 days (mean 90 ± 62 days). Ten patients developed hypercalcaemia (severe in 6) and this usually resolved within 7 days of stopping treatment. On the basis of this study, the estimated MTD was 7μg/m^2/day for prolonged use. Other side-effects were mild and infrequent and included nausea, vomiting and dizziness. Eighteen patients received compassionate treatment for at least 30 days. Although no objective responses were seen, 6 patients had disease stabilisation for ≥ 3 months (4 breast, 2 colorectal cancer). Subsequently several phase II studies have been completed or are in progress, and have been reported in abstract form.

Preliminary data from these phase II studies have been reported in abstract form and include studies in Myelodysplasia (MDS) (9), colorectal, pancreatic (10) and hepatocellular cancer (11). Again, these studies have indicated that EB1089 is well tolerated with dose limiting hypercalcaemia the only consistently reported adverse event, usually mild and resolving within 1 week of stopping the drug.

Ten patients with myelodysplastic syndromes were treated with EB1089 at a starting dose of 10μg/day and the dose escalated weekly based on the serum calcium levels. Two patients were withdrawn within 21 days and the remaining 8 patients completed the planned 3 months of therapy at doses of 20 μg/day (1 patient), 10μg/day (6) and 7μg/day (1 patient). Three patients went on to receive compassionate EB1089 (range 5 months to >3 years). No response were seen in terms of transfusion dependency or the neutrophil count. Two patients had a rise in platelet counts from 20 to 48 and from 87 to 115 & $10^9/l$. There were no changes in bone marrow blast counts apart from one patient who relapsed.

Twenty seven patients with inoperable colorectal cancer (24 metastatic, 3 locally advanced) were treated with EB1089, starting at 10μg/day and escalating 2-weekly. Tolerated doses ranged from 5-35μg/day. Although no complete or partial responses were observed, a large liver metastasis decreased by 30% and then subsequently progressed after 12 months of treatment, and a similar decrease in local disease was observed in another patient which was sustained for 8 months. The median progression-free survival was 83 days. Forty-two patients with non-resectable adeno-carcinoma of the exocrine pancreas (25 metastatic, 17 locally advanced) were treated at a starting dose of 15μg/day and which was escalated 2-weekly. The mean dose was 15μg/day (range 5 - 30 μg/day). Thirteen patients had received previous palliative chemotherapy and 7 patients were withdrawn prior to starting therapy, mainly due to rapid disease progression highlighting the poor prognosis of this tumour. Although no objective responses were observed, two patients survived for >6 months, and a further 2 patients survived over 2 years for a median survival of 107 days (range 13 - 887).

Preliminary results are also available from a study evaluating the safety and efficacy of EB1089 in 22 patients with inoperable hepatocellular carcinoma (HCC). The median tolerated dose was 15μg/day (range 10 - 40 μg/day) and there have been 2 objective responses observed. One patient had a complete response (CR) after 6 months then developed a new lesion after 10 months, probably due to non-compliance. The patient remained in the study and a new CR was noted 5 months later, and this patient remains disease free at 78 weeks. The other patient achieved a PR after 6 months treatment, and is now a CR after 30 months treatment. EB1089 is currently being evaluated in phase III clinical trials in HCC.

In conclusion, EB1089 is well tolerated with the main toxicity being reversible hypercalcaemia and has evidence of activity in HCC. Furthermore, EB1089 is a cytostatic and as such the conventional end-point of objective tumour response may not be applicable in phase II clinical trials of this agent, and may underestimate its anti-tumour activity. Future phase II studies should incorporate a surrogate marker of anti-tumour activity such as imaging for metabolic changes within the tumour during treatment, for example by using PET scanning technology.

488

References

1. Kissmeyer, A.M., Binderup, E., Binderup, L., Hansen, M.C., Andersen, N.R., Makin, H.L., Schroeder, N.J., Shankar, V.N. and Jones, G. (1997) Biochem. Pharmacol. 53, 1087-1097.

2. Hansen, C.M. and Maenpaa, P.H. (1997) Biochem. Pharmacol. 54, 1173-1179.

3. James, S.Y., Mercer, E., Brady, M., Binderup, L. and Colston, K.W. (1998) Br. J. Pharmacol. 125, 953-962.

4. Colston, K.W., Mackay, A.G., James, S.Y., Binderup, L., Chander, S., Coombes, R.C., (1992) Biochem. Pharmacol. 44, 2273-2280.

5. Nickerson, T. and Huynh, H. (1999) J. Endocrinol. 160, 223-229.

6. Lokeshevar, B.L., Schwartz, G.G., Selzer, M.G., Burnstein, K.L., Zhuang, S.H., Block, N.L. and Binderup, L. (1999) Cancer Epidemiol. Biomark. Prev. 8, 241-248.

7. Colston, K.W., James, S.Y., Ofori-Kuragu, E.A., Binderup, L. and Grant, A.G. (1997) Br. J. Cancer 76, 1017-1020.

8. Gulliford, T., English, J., Colston, K.W., Menday, P., Moller, S. and Coombes, R.C. (1998) Br. J. Cancer 78, 6-13.

9. Pakkala, S., Sprogel, P., Remes, K., Nousiainen, T., Koivunen, E., Pelliniemi, T-T., Ruutu, T. and Elanen, E. Blood (1997), 90 (suppl 1) 508A (abstract).

10. Evans, T.R.J., Mansi, J.L., Lofts, F.J., Gogas, H., Anthoney, D.A., de Bono, J.S., Colston, K.W., Menday, P., Moller, S. and Hamberg, K.J., Proc. Am. Soc. Clin. Oncol. (1999) 18, 1085 (abstract).

11. Dalhoff, K., Astrup, L., Bach-Hansen, J., Burcharth, F., Haahr, H.L.O., Hamberg, K.J., Evans, T.R.J., Lofts, F., Moller, S., Ranek, L., Skovsgaard, T. and Steward, W. Hepatology (1998), 28 (4) 227-A (abstract).

ANTI-PROLIFERATIVE MECHANISMS OF $1\alpha,25(OH)_2D_3$ IN HUMAN PROSTATE CANCER CELLS

Xiao-Yan Zhao and David Feldman, Division of Endocrinology, Stanford University School of Medicine, Stanford, CA 94305

Introduction

$1\alpha,25$-Dihydroxyvitamin D_3 [$1,25$-$(OH)_2D_3$] exerts antiproliferative effects on many cancer cells including prostate cancer. The induction of cell cycle arrest and programmed cell death (apoptosis) are among the events triggered by $1,25$-$(OH)_2D_3$ (1-5). However, the complete mechanism by which $1,25$-$(OH)_2D_3$ inhibits prostate cancer cell growth has not yet been defined. Here we describe three additional pathways or mechanisms by which $1,25$-$(OH)_2D_3$ may inhibit prostate cancer cell growth.

Results and Discussion

A. Vitamin D Metabolism.

$1,25$-$(OH)_2D_3$ inhibits the proliferation of many prostate cancer cells in culture but not the aggressive human prostate cancer cell line DU 145 (6-7). We postulated that the $1,25$-$(OH)_2D_3$-resistant phenotype in DU 145 cells might result from the high levels of expression of 25-hydroxyvitamin D-24-hydroxylase (24-hydroxylase) induced by treatment with $1,25$-$(OH)_2D_3$ (6-7). Since this P450 enzyme initiates $1,25$-$(OH)_2D_3$ inactivation, we presumed that a high level of enzyme induction would limit the effectiveness of the antiproliferative action of $1,25$-$(OH)_2D_3$. To examine this hypothesis we explored combination therapy with liarozole fumarate (R85,246), an imidazole derivative that had been tested in trials for efficacy in treating prostate cancer. Since imidazole derivatives are known to inhibit P450 enzymes (8), we postulated that this drug would inhibit 24-hydroxylase activity, increasing $1,25$-$(OH)_2D_3$ half-life, thereby enhancing $1,25$-$(OH)_2D_3$ antiproliferative effects on DU 145 cells.

Cell growth was assessed by measurement of viable cells using the MTS assay. When used alone, neither $1,25$-$(OH)_2D_3$ (10 nM) nor liarozole (1 μM) inhibited DU 145 cell growth. However, when added together, $1,25$-$(OH)_2D_3$ (10 nM) plus liarozole (1 μM) inhibited growth 65% at 4 days of culture (Figure 1). We used a thin layer chromatography method to assess 24-hydroxylase activity and demonstrated that liarozole (1-100 μM) inhibited this P450 enzyme in a dose-dependent manner. Moreover, liarozole treatment caused a significant increase in $1,25$-$(OH)_2D_3$ half-life from 11 to 31 h. In addition, it is

490

known that 1,25-(OH)2D3 can cause homologous up-regulation of the VDR (9). In the presence of liarozole, this effect was amplified thus enhancing 1,25-(OH)2D3 activity (10). Western blot analyses demonstrated that DU 145 cells treated with 1,25-(OH)2D3 plus liarozole showed greater VDR up-regulation than with either drug alone (10). In summary, our data demonstrate that liarozole augments the ability of 1,25-(OH)2D3 to inhibit DU 145 cell growth. The mechanism appears to be due to inhibition of 24-hydroxylase activity leading to increased 1,25-(OH)2D3 half-life and augmentation of homologous up-regulation of VDR. We raise the possibility that combination therapy using 1,25-(OH)2D3 and liarozole or other inhibitors of 24-hydroxylase, both in non-toxic doses, might serve as an effective treatment for prostate cancer.

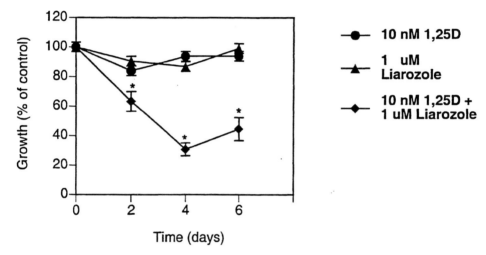

Figure 1. Effect of 1,25-(OH)2D3, liarozole and the combination on DU 145 cell growth over a time course of 6 days. Cells were plated at approximately 2000 cells/well in 96-well tissue culture plates in 200 ul medium with the indicated concentrations of hormone. Media were changed every 2 days. Cell proliferation was estimated using an MTS assay. Data are expressed as the mean ± SD (n=3).

B. Regulation of Androgen Receptor.

We have shown recently that 1,25-(OH)2D3 significantly inhibits the proliferation and increases the secretion of prostate specific antigen (PSA) in LNCaP cells, an androgen-responsive human prostate cancer cell line (11-16). The present study was designed to investigate whether the actions of 1,25-(OH)2D3 and androgens on LNCaP cells are interdependent. LNCaP cell growth was inhibited by 1,25-(OH)2D3 (60% inhibition at 10 nM) when cells were cultured in medium supplemented with 5% fetal bovine serum (FBS medium). 1,25-(OH)2D3-treated cells showed a 5-fold increase in PSA secretion, similar to the increase seen in dihydrotestosterone (DHT)-treated cells. In combination, 1,25-(OH)2D3 and DHT synergistically enhanced PSA secretion 22-fold. This synergistic effect was even greater when cells were cultured in medium supplemented with charcoal-stripped serum (CSS medium), where endogenous steroids are substantially depleted (Figure 2). Western blot analyses showed that the androgen receptor (AR) content was increased significantly by 1,25-(OH)2D3 at 48 h. When cells were grown in CSS medium (devoid of endogenous hormones), 1,25-(OH)2D3 alone no longer inhibited cell growth or induced PSA secretion. Titration experiments revealed that the addition of DHT at 1 nM to the medium restored the antiproliferative activity of 1,25-(OH)2D3. Conversely, an anti-androgen, bicalutamide (Casodex), completely blocked 1,25-(OH)2D3 actions in FBS medium (11). To test if the regulatory effect of 1,25-(OH)2D3 on the AR gene expression is specific to the prostate, we also extended these studies to breast cancer cells. No change in AR gene expression was detected with 1,25-(OH)2D3 treatment in the human breast cancer cell lines MCF-7 and T47D. In summary, these results demonstrate that the ability of 1,25-(OH)2D3 to inhibit LNCaP cell growth and stimulate PSA is dependent upon androgen action. 1,25-(OH)2D3 increases AR gene expression in LNCaP cells, and the AR up-regulation by 1,25-(OH)2D3 likely contributes to the mechanism of the synergistic activity of 1,25-(OH)2D3 and DHT.

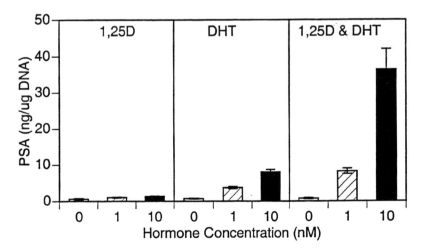

Figure 2. Synergistic interactions of 1,25-(OH)2D3 (1,25D) and DHT on PSA secretion. LNCaP cells were cultured in RPMI-1640 medium containing charcoal-stripped fetal bovine serum (CSS medium) and were treated with either 1,25-(OH)2D3 or DHT or both at concentrations of 0, 1, and 10 nM. The conditioned media were collected and the PSA levels were measured by radioimmunoassay. The data are expressed as ng of PSA per μg of DNA for each well, a mean of three samples ± *SEM*.

Subsequently, we have investigated the mechanism by which 1,25-(OH)2D3 regulates AR gene expression and the involvement of AR in the 1,25-(OH)2D3 -and 9-cis retinoic acid (RA)-mediated growth inhibition of LNCaP cells. Northern blot analyses demonstrated that the steady-state mRNA level of AR was significantly increased by 1,25-(OH)2D3 in a dose-dependent manner. Time course experiments revealed that the increase of AR mRNA by 1,25-(OH)2D3 exhibited delayed kinetics. In response to 1,25-(OH)2D3, AR mRNA levels were first detected to rise at 8 h and reached a maximal induction of 10-fold over the untreated control at 48 h; the effect was sustained at 72 h. Furthermore, the induction of AR mRNA by 1,25-(OH)2D3 was completely abolished by incubation of cells with cycloheximide, a protein synthesis inhibitor. 1,25-(OH)2D3 was unable to induce expression of an AR promoter-luciferase reporter. These findings indicate that the stimulatory effect of 1,25-(OH)2D3 on AR gene expression was indirect. Western blot analyses showed an increase of AR protein in 1,25-(OH)2D3-treated cells. This increased expression of AR was followed by an inhibition of growth in LNCaP cells by 1,25-(OH)2D3. Similar to 1,25-(OH)2D3, 9-cis RA also induced AR mRNA expression and the effect of both hormones was additive (13). Moreover, 1,25-(OH)2D3 and 9-cis RA acted synergistically to inhibit LNCaP cell growth (13). The anti-proliferative effects of 1,25-(OH)2D3 and 9-cis RA, alone or in combination were blocked by the pure AR antagonist, Casodex. In conclusion, our results demonstrate that growth inhibition of LNCaP by 1,25-(OH)2D3 and 9-cis RA is mediated by an AR-dependent mechanism and preceded by the induction of AR gene expression. This finding that differentiating agents such as vitamin D and vitamin A derivatives are potent inducers of AR may have clinical implications for the treatment of prostate cancer.

C. IGFBP-3.

One way in which 1,25-(OH)2D3 may bring about an antiproliferative effect is through regulation of insulin-like growth factor (IGF) binding protein-3 (IGFBP-3), which has been shown to block IGF action and inhibit prostate cancer growth. In addition to binding and sequestering the IGFs, IGFBP-3 has been shown to mediate IGF-independent actions which are antiproliferative (17). Using the LNCaP cell line, we demonstrated that 1,25-(OH)2D3 is capable of inducing both IGFBP-3 mRNA and protein (Boyle et al. unpublished data). In addition, we showed that exogenous IGFBP-3 administration results in LNCaP growth inhibition. Importantly, we used antisense oligonucleotides that block IGFBP-3 production or immunoneutralizing antibodies that block IGFBP-3 action, to show that 1,25-(OH)2D3 -mediated growth inhibition is abrogated by interfering with IGFBP-3. Our findings provide strong evidence that IGFBP-3 mediates 1,25-(OH)2D3 -induced growth inhibition in LNCaP cells. Furthermore, we demonstrated that p21/WAF-1, a protein established as one mechanism of action of 1,25-(OH)2D3 in growth inhibition (18), is induced by IGFBP-3. We also found that immunoneutralization of IGFBP-3 abolishes p21 induction by 1,25-(OH)2D3. Taken together, these data strongly suggest that 1,25-(OH)2D3-induced growth inhibition in LNCaP cells is dependent upon IGFBP-3.

In conclusion, multiple pathways are involved in the antiproliferative actions of 1,25-(OH)2D3 in prostate cancer cells. It is hoped that understanding these mechanisms will yield new therapeutic approaches to the treatment of prostate cancer.

References

1. Feldman, D., Zhao, X.Y. and Krishnan, A.V. (2000) Endocrinology 141,5-9.
2. Miller, G. (1999) Cancer Met Rev 17,353-360.
3. Blutt, S. and Weigel, N. (1999) Proc Soc Exp Biol Med 221:89-98
4. Konety, B.R., Johnson, C.S., Trump, D.L., and Getzenberg, R.H. (1999) Semi Urolog Oncol 17,77-84.
5. Ruijter, E., Van De Kaa, C., Miller, G., Ruiter, D., Debruyne, F., and Schalken, J. (1999) Endocr Rev 20,22-45.
6. Skowronski, R.J., Peehl, D.M. and Feldman, D. (1993) Endocrinology 132,1952-1960.
7. Miller, G.J., Stapelton, G.E., Hedlund, T.E., and Moffatt, K.A. (1995) Clinc Cancer Res. 1, 997-1003.
8. Feldman, D. (1986) Endo Endocr Rev 7,409-420.
9. Krishnan, A. and Feldman, D (1997) In Feldman, D., Glorieux, F.H., Pike, J.W. (eds) Vitamin D. Academic Press, San Diego, pp 179-200.
10. Ly, L.H., Zhao, X.Y., Holloway, L. and Feldman, D. (1999) Endocrinology 140,2071-2076.
11. Zhao, X.Y., Ly, L.H., Peehl, D.M. and Feldman, D. (1997) Endocrinology 138,3290-3298.
12. Zhao, X.Y., Ly, L.H., Peehl, D.M. and Feldman, D. (1999) Endocrinology 140,1205-1212.
13. Zhao, X.Y., Boyle, B., Krishnan, A.V., Navone, N.M., Peehl, D.M. and Feldman, D. (1999) J Urology 162,2192-2199.
14. Zhao, X.Y., Peehl, D.M., Navone, N.M. and Feldman, D. (2000) Endocrinology (in press).
15. Zhao, X.Y. and Feldman, D. (2000) Steroids (in press).
16. Zhao, X.Y., Eccleshall, T.R., Krishnan, A.V., Gross, C. and Feldman, D. (1997) Mol Endocrinol 11,366-378.
17. Rajah, R., Valentinis, B., and Cohen, P. (1997) J. Biol. Chem. 272, 12181.
18. Liu, M., Lee, M.H., Cohen, M., Bommakanti, M., and Freedman, L.P. (1996) Genes Dev. 10, 142-153.

VITAMIN D COMPOUNDS AND COLORECTAL CANCER: A RATIONALE FOR THEIR USE IN PREVENTION AND THERAPY

Heide S. Cross, Harald Hofer, Petra Bareis, Giovanna Bises, Gary H. Posner[*], Meinrad Peterlik, Department of Pathophysiology, University of Vienna Medical School, Austria, and [*]Department of Chemistry, Johns Hopkins University, Baltimore, MD 21218

Introduction Large bowel cancer is a major cause of morbidity and mortality in Western industrialized countries. Epidemiological and in vitro evidence suggests that vitamin D3 obtained from dietary sources and by sunlight exposure, has a protective potential against the development of colorectal cancer (1). The active metabolite of vitamin D, the secosteroid 1α,25-dihydroxyvitamin D3 (1,25-D3) is, besides maintaining calcium and phosphate homeostasis, an important regulator of growth and differentiation of a large number of cell types (2). Potent antimitogenic properties of vitamin D and of its sidechain-modified analogs have been demonstrated in normal and in tumor cells in multiple in vitro and in vivo studies. In particular, the mechanism of action of 1,25-D3 and of various vitamin D analogs on human colorectal cancer cell lines and primary cultures derived from human colorectal tissue were investigated by our laboratory (3, 4, 5, 6, 7, 8). However, therapeutic use of such compounds in adjuvant treatment of human colorectal cancer is still not possible due to the hypercalcemia ensuing from doses which have strong antimitogenic and prodifferentiating effects. For this reason, efforts have been made in the past decade to design analogs with low or no hypercalcemic, but pronounced growth inhibitory action.

However, applicability of such substances for human cancer therapy may also largely depend on the intrinsic presence of the nuclear vitamin D receptor (VDR) in tumor cells: 1,25-D3 exerts its biological effects on growth control via the nuclear VDR and, apparently, levels of VDR expression determine effectiveness of 1,25-D3 on growth control (9). This prompted us to determine initially the presence and regulation of the two components of the active vitamin D system, namely expression of 25-D3-1α-hydroxylase and of the VDR in human colorectal normal and malignant tissue.

Hulla et al. (10) presented evidence that in human colon adenocarcinoma-derived cells the antimitogenic action of 1,25-D3 occurred independently of c-myc down-regulation, which was postulated as a mechanism of action in human leukemia cells. Tong et al. (11) rather found reduced expression of cyclin D1, a key mediator of the G1 to S phase transition of the cell cycle, in colon cells under 1,25-D3 treatment. Among the three D-type cyclins, cyclin D1 is the most strongly implicated during the multistage process of colon tumorigenesis. In this respect it is interesting that Weinstein et al. (12) found reversion of the malignant phenotype in colon cancer cells after introduction of an antisense cyclin D1. We therefore also determined expression levels of this cell cycle regulator during colon tumor progression. In addition, we evaluated, parallel to the VDR, expression of cytokeratin 20, a marker for differentiated intestinal cells (13), in human neoplastic and normal colon tissue.

Methods Colorectal tissue from 60 patients was used for evaluation. For non-malignant colon we used mucosa from diverticulitis patients after stoma reoperation. Adenomas, and tumors of different stages (TNM system) were obtained. Histological grading was low, medium and high (G1-G3), with the majority of patients presenting with medium to high grading, i.e. moderate to poor differentiation and high proliferation of colon cells. Adjacent mucosa outside the tumor border from the same patients was used as internal "normal" mucosal control. For RNA preparations, snap frozen surgical specimen were minced in liquid nitrogen and subsequently homogenized. Total RNA was isolated with Trizol. The OD at 260/280 was measured to determine the concentration and purity of RNA (ratio 1.7-1.9). First strand cDNA was reverse transcribed from total RNA using the superscript^{TM} preamplification system for first strand cDNA synthesis.

For primer design, DNA sequences of the mRNA for human VDR, human cyclin D1, and human β–actin were found using National Center for Biotechnology Information *Entrez* Nucleotide Query software. Primers were designed and checked for 3'-terminal dimer formation. β-actin was used as an internal control in multiplex RT-PCR with 4 primers in one amplification assay. The β-actin primers were designed to cross a 112 bp intron which would result in a 318 bp band if there was genomic contamination of the sample. None of the samples used for PCR showed this band. To test for proper amplification gel bands, after visualization, were cut out and DNA was extracted, sequenced and matched with gene bank data.

VDR (HUMVDR, 4604 bp, accession No. J03258)
Primer sequence length: 23 base pairs
Forward primer: starts at bp 1193: 5' TCCAACACACTGCAGACGTACAT 3'
Reverse primer: starts at bp 1723: 5' ATCAGTCAGCAGCCACTTAGGCA 3'
Expected band: 530 base pairs

Cyclin D1 (HUMCYCD1;1325 bp, accession No. M64349)
Primer sequence length: 20 base pairs
Forward primer start at bp 235. Sequence 5' ATGCTGAAGGCGGAGGAGAC 3'
Reverse primer start at bp 848. Sequence 5' TGGAGAGGAAGCGTGTGAGG 3'
Expected band: 614 base pairs

Beta-actin (HSAC07,1761 bp, accession No. X00351, J00074, AM10278)
Primer length: 23 base pairs
Forward primer at bp 921. Sequence 5′TACGCCAACACAGTGCTGTCTGG 3′
Reverse primer at bp 1126. Sequence 5′TACTCCTGCTTGCTGATCCACAT 3′
Expected band: 205 base pairs

Results

VDR and cyclin D1 expression: Fig. 1 shows a histogram based on densitometric evaluation of RT-PCR for VDR (left) and cyclin D1 (right) mRNA. Data are referred to the density of the internal control β-actin band obtained during the same amplification. While in mucosa from non-cancer patients both VDR and cyclin D1 mRNA expression is rather low, both mRNA species are obviously elevated significantly in adenomas. In patients with low to medium grade (G1-G2) of tumors, i.e. well to moderately differentiated cells, high expression of VDR and cyclin D1 mRNA is observed in tumor tissue. In the tumor-adjacent normal colon mucosa from the same patients, VDR and cyclin D1 mRNA is present, but at levels similar to that in non-cancer patients. When high-grade (G3) tumors (dedifferentiated cells with high proliferative capacity) are evaluated a striking decrease of VDR mRNA expression becomes apparent, which is paralleled, to a lesser extent, by cyclin D1 mRNA expression.

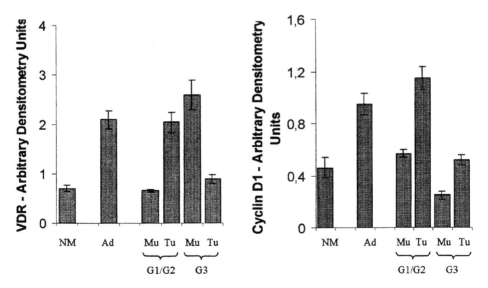

Fig 1. Evaluation of VDR and Cyclin D1 mRNA by RT-PCR and subsequent densitometry. NM, mucosa from a non-tumor patient, Ad, adenoma tissue, Mu, normal-appearing mucosa outside the tumor border, Tu, tumor tissue

We were able to verify this decrease of VDR mRNA by evaluating VDR protein expression in various human colon tumors by immunohistochemistry (not shown): actually in very malignant carcinomas of the colon, for instance signet ring carcinomas, VDR protein expression is totally eliminated. We also observed heterogeneous distribution of the nuclear VDR protein in tumor epithelial cells similar to that found by Tong et al. (7) in primary cultured colonocytes. This, and our data on cyclin D1 expression indicate, that VDR expression is associated with certain growth conditions and cell cycle distribution. In this context we would like to point out that expression of the epidermal growth factor receptor (EGFR) mRNA, when evaluated parallel to the VDR by in situ hybridization, appears to be regulated in a similar manner (Table 1): statistical evaluation of cells with positive grains shows that there is low expression of VDR and relatively low expression of EGFR mRNA in normal human colorectal tissue, whereas in low grade G1 and G2 colon carcinomas both mRNA species are increased. In G3, i.e. poorly differentiated cancers, VDR expression drops significantly, whereas abundance of EGFR mRNA is not altered.

Table 1. VDR and EGFR mRNA expression in human normal and cancerous colon tissue

Tissue	Mean in situ hybridization reactivity score	
	VDR	EGFR
Normal adjacent mucosa (n=5)	13.5	57.3
Adenocarcinoma, low grade (n=5)	129.3	123.0
Adenocarcinoma, high grade (n=3)	46.2	144.5

Data are means from n samples per group, and were calculated by multiplying the percentage of receptor-positive cells by the average signal intensity.

Our data therefore indicate, that raised VDR mRNA and protein expression (cf. 14, see also Fig. 2) appears to be a hallmark of enhanced proliferation, however only in tumors of relatively low grade, i.e. in well to moderately differentiated carcinomas. On the other hand, Shabahang et al. (15) and Hulla et al. (10) both demonstrated in a panel of colon cancer cell lines, that the higher the differentiation level, the higher VDR was expressed. In order to further test this assumption in human colonic tissue we evaluated by Western blotting VDR and cytokeratin 20 (CK20) protein distribution. CK8, 18, 19 and 20 are typical epithelial markers for simple epithelia present in the intestine. Whereas some of these cytoskeletal proteins are mainly found in fetal or proliferative colonocytes, CK20 is a marker for highly differentiated cells only at the villus respectively crypt top (16). During advancing malignancy in the colon a decrease of its expression occurs (13). In parallel, markers for highly proliferative cells (such as PCNA) are increasingly expressed (manuscript in preparation). Figure 2 demonstrates immunoblots for evaluation of VDR and CK20 expression in mucosa derived from non-cancerous and cancerous human colon. While there is little VDR found in normal colonocytes, and increased expression during early malignancy, the steroid hormone receptor is reduced strongly during high grade cancer similar to the observed mRNA regulation. CK20 however is highly expressed in normal tissue, whereas there is already a decrease in G1 and G2 (well to moderately differentiated) tumor cells, with total disappearance in G3 tumors.

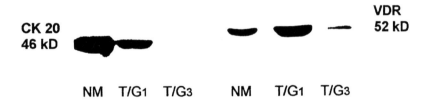

Fig. 2 Immunoblot of CK20 (left) and VDR protein. NM, mucosa from a non-cancer patient, T, Tumor (G1 and G3).

Discussion and Therapeutic Aspects Colon cancer cells may apparently respond to stimulation of tumor cell proliferation by increased expression of the vitamin D receptor which is known to mediate the antimitotic and prodifferentiating effects of the steroid hormone. This however is only valid for carcinomas which are at least moderately differentiated. This is very suggestive of a physiological defense mechanism against further proliferation and progression, if endogenous 1,25-D3 is present in sufficient amounts. During progression into high grade malignancy apparently this defense mechanism becomes downregulated as evidenced by reduced amounts of VDR mRNA and protein.

Activation of VDR expression may be a valid therapeutic approach against tumor progression. Analogs of 1,25-D3 with high antimitotic, but low hypercalcemic activity could be employed to up-regulate expression of the VDR.

For therapy of low to medium grade cancers, when presence of the VDR is actually increased over that of normal cells, substances could be used which, by virtue of their 1-α-hydroxylation, bind strongly to the VDR, but due to sidechain modification gain particularly strong antimitotic and prodifferentiating potential (up to a 100fold higher than 1,25-D3). As a result of this, lower concentrations could be used in vivo, with less hazard of hypercalcemia (see e.g. 6).

On the other hand, new analogs could be used, which contain an A ring modification: apparently substitution of the 1α-hydroxy by a 1β-hydroxymethyl group yields hybrid analogs that combine weak calcemic activity with a still high growth regulatory potential, although (or because) they do not bind well to the nuclear VDR (17). These analogs could conceivably be used in patients with high grade colorectal tumors, with low expression of the VDR.

To test this hypothesis in vitro, we employed the spontaneously differentiating human colon adenocarcinoma-derived cell line Caco-2. Table 2 demonstrates data obtained with 1,25-D3 and the sidechain modified analog 1α,25-$(OH)_2$-16-ene,23-yne-D_3 (Ro 23-7553) (courtesy Dr. Milan R. Uskokovic), and two 1β-hydroxymethyl analogs, 1ß-(hydroxymethyl)-3α,25-dihydroxy-22,24-diene-26,27-dihomo vitamin D_3 (MCW-EE) and 1ß-(hydroxymethyl)-3α,25-dihydroxy-16-ene,24-oxovitamin D_3 (JK-1624-2) (courtesy Dr. Gary H. Posner).

Table 2. Effect of Vitamin D Compounds on Proliferation, Differentiation, VDR and Cyclin D1 Protein Expression

	Proliferation	Differentiation	VDR	Cyclin D1	
		(Percent of Vehicle Control)			
				24 h	96 h
1,25-D3	73	162	150	100	60
Ro23-7553	75	142	130	80	75
MCW-EE	80	110	75	42	70
JK-1624-2	75	126	80	40	75

Data were obtained from evaluation of [^{3}H]thymidine incorporation, alkaline phosphatase activity, and immunoblotting for VDR and cyclin D1 ($n \leq 12$).

Data collated in Table 1 demonstrate a similar antiproliferative effect on human colon adenocarcinoma-derived Caco-2 cells regardless whether 10 nM 1α–hydroxy substances or 1β-hydroxymethyl compounds were used. Interestingly, the degree of differentiating activity is lower in the latter. Since also osteoclast differentiating activity of 1β-hydroxymethyl compounds is much reduced (8) this could underlie their low hypercalcemic activity observed in vivo. It is striking that VDR expression is distinctly increased after 48 h exposure to 1α-hydroxy compounds, whereas VDR expression is actually decreased after exposure to 1β–hydroxymethyl compounds. When cyclin D1 expression was evaluated at two time points we found that the cell cycle regulatory protein was not affected after 24 h exposure to 1,25-D3 and the side chain modified compound, whereas there was a fast and very strong reduction in expression of cyclin D1 by the 1β-hydroxymethyl compounds. Only after 96 h exposure the 1α compounds reached their highest effectiveness in downregulation of cyclin D1, whereas the effectiveness of 1β-hydroxymethyl compounds was already attenuated, but still strong. This comparison suggests to us that the 1β-hydroxymethyl compounds may be faster acting and could actually also be active for a more extended time span than the 1α substances. In addition they are less hypercalcemic, and, importantly at late stages and high grade of colorectal tumors, are less dependent on VDR expression. We therefore suggest that 1β-hydroxymethyl vitamin D analogs could have therapeutic relevance for treatment of patients with high grade colorectal tumors with low VDR expression.

Acknowledgement We thank the Austrian National Bank for financial support (projects no. 6152 and 7111) and the University of Vienna Medical School for a grant from the Maria Buss/Josefine Hirtl bequest. G. H. Posner acknowledges support from the NIH (CA 44530). We also thank Ms. Theresa Manhardt and Erika Bajna for excellent technical support.

References
1. Garland, C.F. and Garland, F.C. (1989) Int. J. Epidemiol. 9, 227-231.
2. Studzinski, G.P., McLane, J.A. and Uskokovic, M.R. (1993) Crit. Rev. Eukar. Gene Expr. 3, 279-312.
3. Cross, H.S., Pavelka, M., Slavik, J. and Peterlik, M. (1992) J. Natl. Cancer Inst. 84, 1355-1357.
4. Cross, H.S., Farsoudi, K.H. and Peterlik, M. (1993) Naunyn-Schmiedeberg's Arch. Pharmacol. 347, 105-110.

5. Cross, H.S., Hulla, W., Tong, W.-M. and Peterlik, M. (1995) J. Nutr. 125, 2004-2008.
6. Bischof, M.G., Redlich, K., Schiller, C., Chirayath, M.V., Uskokovic, M., Peterlik, M. and Cross, H.S. (1995) J. Pharmacol. Exp. Therap. 275, 1254-1260.
7. Tong, W.-M., Bises, G., Sheinin, Y., Ellinger, A., Genser, D., Pötzi, R., Wrba, F., Wenzl, E., Roka, R., Neuhold, N., Peterlik, M. and Cross, H.S. (1998) Int. J. Cancer 75, 467-472.
8. Hofer, H., Ho, G.M., Peterlik, M., Uskokovic, M.R. Lee, J.K., White, M.C., Posner, G.H. and Cross, H.S. (1999) J. Pharm. Exp. Ther. 291, 450-455.
9. Miller, G.J., Stapleton, G.E., Hedlund, T.E. and Moffatt, K.A. (1995) Clin. Cancer Res. 1, 997-1003.
10. Hulla, W., Kallay, E., Krugluger, W., Peterlik, M. and Cross, H.S. (1995) Int. J. Cancer 62, 711-716.
11. Tong, W.-M., Hofer, H., Peterlik, M. and Cross, H.S. (1999) Oncology Res. 11, 77-84.
12. Weinstein, I.B., Begeman, M., Zhou, P., Han, E.K., Sgambato, A., Doki, Y., Arber, N., Ciaparrone, M. and Yamamoto, H. (1997) Clin. Cancer Res. 3, 2696-2702.
13. Cross, H.S. Bajna, E., Bises, G., Genser, D., Kallay, E., Pötzi, R., Wenzl, E., Wrba, F., Roka, R. and Peterlik M. (1996) Anticancer Res. 16, 2333-2338.
14. Sheinin, Y., Kaserer, K., Wrba, R., Wenzl, E., Kriwanek, S., Peterlik, M. and Cross, H.S. (2000) Virchows Archive, in press.
15. Shabahang, M., Buras, R.R., Davoodi, F., Schumaker, L.M., Nauta, R.J. and Evans, S.R. (1993) Cancer Res. 53, 3712-3718.
16. Quaroni, A., Calnek, D., Quaroni, E. and Chandler, J.S. (1991) J. Biol. Chem. 266, 11923-11931.
17. Peleg, S., Nguyen, C., Woodard, B.T., Lee, J.-K. and Posner, G.H. (1998) Mol. Endocrinol. 12: 525-535.

VITAMIN D RECEPTOR (VDR) EXPRESSION IS NOT A PROGNOSTIC FACTOR IN BREAST CANCER

Leyla Rafi[1], Jörg Reichrath[2], Roland Meyberg[1], Wolfgang Tilgen[2], Werner Schmidt[1], Michael Friedrich[1]. Departments of [1]Gynecology and [2]Dermatology, University Hospital of Saarland, D-66421 Homburg/Saar, Germany.

Introduction: Epidemiologic studies have shown a negative correlation between sunlight exposure and breast cancer death rates, indicating that vitamin D might have a protective role against breast cancer (1). The expression of the vitamin D receptor (VDR) in breast cancer was first demonstrated in the human breast cancer cell line MCF-7 (2). Further studies have shown VDR in normal breast and breast tumor tissue (3). It was shown that VDR is expressed in about 80% of human breast tumor specimens. Two studies reported that the VDR status in breast carcinomas correlated positively with disease-free interval (4,5). Additionally, a relationship between VDR level and growth inhibition has been suggested for breast cancer cells (6). The aim of this study was to analyze, whether VDR status in breast cancer correlates with prognostic factors (staging, grading, histological type of breast cancer, lymphangiosis, hemangiosis, metastases, expression of ER, PR).

Material and Methods: *Breast specimens:* Biopsies from normal breast tissue (n=62) were obtained from patients that underwent surgery for macromasty (hyperplasia) of the breast. Histological examination by a certified pathologist confirmed normality. Biopsies from breast carcinomas (n=228) were obtained from patients that underwent surgery for breast tumors. Usually, a breast preserving surgery was performed. Biopsies were taken from macroscopically visible tumor areas. Histological examination by a certified pathologist confirmed diagnosis. All breast specimens were immediately embedded in OCT-Tissue-Tek II (Miles Laboratories, Naperville, Illinois, U.S.A.), snap frozen in melting isopentane, precooled in liquid nitrogen and stored at -80°C.
Primary antibodies: VDR was detected by mAb 9A7γ (Dianova, Hamburg, Germany) whose preparation and specificity was described previously. To assess the expression of estrogen and progesterone receptors in breast tissue, we used rat mAbs directed against estrogen- and progesterone receptors (ER-ICA- and PR-ICA-Kits, Abbott Laboratories, Chicago, USA). P53-protein was detected by mouse *m*Ab directed against p53 protein (clone D0-7, Dakopatts, Copenhagen, Denmark). Proliferation was investigated applying mouse mAb Ki-67 directed against the Ki-67 antigen (clone Ki-67, Dakopatts, Copenhagen, Denmark).
Preparation of sections and fixation: Serial sections (5 μm) were cut on a cryostat (Reichert-Jung, Heidelberg, Germany), mounted on glass slides and fixed in 3,7% paraformaldehyde (Merck 4005, Darmstadt, Germany) in phosphate buffered

saline (PBS, 10 min, room temperature [RT]), incubated in methanol (Merck 6009, 3 min, -20°C), acetone (Merck 22, -20°C, 1 min), and transferred into PBS.

In situ detection of primary antibodies: The incubation steps were performed in a moist chamber at RT, covering the sections with 100 µl of the respective reagents. To reduce nonspecific staining, the slides were incubated with heat-inactivated normal rabbit serum (20 min, RT). The slides were then incubated (19 h, 4°C) with the different primary antibodies (anti-VDR 1 : 1000; anti-p53 1 : 100; Ki-67 1 : 100) or as control with polyclonal mouse IgG1 (Dakopatts) at similar concentrations. After intermediate washing steps (TBS, 2 x 5 min), the sections were incubated with biotin-labeled rabbit anti-mouse IgG (Dakopatts, 1 : 400, 30 min, RT) and incubated with streptavidin-peroxidase complexes (Dakopatts, 1 : 400, 30 min, RT). After washing in PBS, the sections were incubated for 6 min with 3-amino-9-ethylcarbazole (AEC, Sigma A 5754, München, Germany) to visualize the peroxidase reaction.

Semi-quantitative analysis of immunoreactivity: Microscopic analysis was performed by two independent observers (J. R. and M. F.). VDR-, p53-, ER- and PR-staining intensity (VDR-SI, p53-SI, ER-SI, PR-SI), percentage of VDR-, p53-, ER- and PR-positive tumour cells (VDR-PP, p53-PP, ER-PP, PR-PP) and an immunreactive VDR-, p53-, ER- and PR-score (IRS; negative: 0-1; weak immunoreactivity: 2-3; moderate immunoreactivity: 4-6; strong immunoreactivity: 8-12) were assessed as described previously for estrogen and progesterone receptors (15). Sections stained for Ki-67 were assessed by counting the number of Ki-67 positive and negative cells in the strongest stained tumour area (magnification x 400, at least 200 tumour cells were counted).

Flow-Cytometry: For all flow-cytometry examinations (FACScan, Becton & Dickinson), frozen sections were used. Serial section (45µm) were cut on a cryostat. The determination of the S-phase fraction was performed with the standard software "Cellfit" (Becton & Dickinson).

Statistical Analysis: Statistical analysis was performed by using Mann-Whitney U-Wilcoxon Rank Sum W-test, Kruskal-Wallis-H-test and Chi-Square-test. Statistical significance was defined as $p < 0.05$.

Results: *Increased Expression of VDR in Breast Cancer:* The expression of VDR was statistically significantly increased in breast cancer compared to normal breast tissue (table I). We did not find a correlation comparing VDR expression with the proliferation marker Ki-67 or with prognostic factors in breast cancer (staging, grading, histological type of breast cancer, lymphangiosis, hemangiosis, metastases, expression of ER, PR and p53) (tables II-IV).

Table I: Increased expression of VDR in breast cancer compared to normal breast tissue.

	VDR-SI	VDR-PP	VDR-IRS
Benign breast Tissue (n=62)	1,0+/-1,0	35,6%+/-34,1	3,0+/-3,0
Breast cancer (n=228)	2,1+/-0,7	83,8%+/-9,4	7,9+/-3,0
	p<0,001*	p<0,0001*	p<0,0001*

*Mann-Whitney-U-Test

No correlation between the Expression of VDR and Staging and Grading: No statistically significant correlation between VDR expression and parameters for staging and grading in breast cancer was found (table II).

Table II: No correlation between VDR-expression and staging and grading in breast cancer.

p-values	pT	pN	G	M	Hem.	Lym.	Hist. type
VDR-SI	0,71**	0,51**	0,99**	0,91**	-	-	0,93**
VDR-PP	0,19*	0,61*	0,84*	0,50***	-	-	0,06*
VDR-IRS	0,15*	0,95*	0,95*	0,75***	0,27**	0,15***	0,98*

*Kruskal-Wallis-H-test, **Chi-Square-test, *** Mann-Whitney-U-test

No correlation between the Expression of VDR and the Tumorsuppressor p53: No statistically significant correlation between the expression of VDR and the tumor suppressorgen p53 was detected in breast cancer (VDR-IRS: r=0.08, p=0.26; VDR-SI: r=0.09, p=0.23; VDR-PP: r=0.06, p=0.39; Spearman-correlation).

Table III: VDR- and p53-expression in breast cancer

	p53-SI	p53-PP	p53-IRS
VDR-SI	0.61*	-	-
VDR-PP	-	0.63**	-
VDR-IRS	-	-	0.55**

*Chi-Square-test; **Kruskal-Wallis-H-test

No correlation between the Expression of VDR and Parameters of Proliferation: No statistically significant correlation was found comparing VDR expression and the Ki-67-index (VDR-SI: r=0.04; p=0.56; VDR-PP: r=-0.02; p=0.82; VDR-IRS: r=-0.01; p=0.93   Spearman-correlation). Furthermore, no statistically significant correlation was seen comparing expression of VDR and Ki-67-positivity (VDR-SI: p=0.35   Chi-Quadrat-Test; VDR-PP: p=0.28   Mann-Whitney-U-Test; VDR-IRS: p=0.47   Mann-Whitney-U-Test). 67.4% of the tumors showed aneuploidy. There was no significant correlation between ploidy and VDR-expression (VDR-SI: p=0,30; Chi-Quadrat-test VDR-PP: aneuploidy: mean VDR-PP: 85,4%+/-6,9; diploidy: mean VDR-PP: 86,3%+/-3,2; p=0,06; Mann-Whitney-U-test; VDR-IRS: aneuploidy: mean VDR-IRS: 7,8+/-2,9; diploidy: mean VDR-IRS: 8,2+/-3,2;

p=0,50; Mann-Whitney-U-test). The S-phase fracture was not significantly correlated to the expression of VDR (VDR-SI: p=0.45 Chi-Square-test; VDR-PP: p=0.45 Kruskal-Wallis-H-Test; VDR-IRS: p=0.59 Kruskal-Wallis-H-Test).

No correlation between Expression of VDR, Estrogen and Progesterone Receptors: There was no statistically significant correlation between the expression of VDR and ER or PR (table IV).

Table IV: Expression of VDR and ER/PR in breast cancer.

	ER-SI/PR-SI*	ER-PP/PR-PP**	ER-IRS/PR-IRS**
VDR-SI	0.64/0.82	-	-
VDR-PP	-	0.63/0.72	-
VDR-IRS	-	-	0.69/0.96

* Chi-Square-test; ** Kruskal-Wallis-H-test

Discussion: We show that vitamin D receptor protein-level is increased in breast carcinomas compared to benign breast tissue. The strong expression of VDR in breast cancer identifies breast carcinomas as potential targets for adjuvant or palliative treatment with vitamin D analogues. We did not find a correlation comparing VDR expression with the proliferation marker Ki-67, indicating that upregulation of VDR in breast cancer is not exclusively regulated by the altered proliferative activity of these tumor cells but by different, unknown mechanisms. Additionally, we could not detect a correlation comparing VDR protein expression with prognostic factors in breast cancer (staging, grading, histological type of breast cancer, lymphangiosis, hemangiosis, metastases, expression of ER, PR and p53), indicating that VDR status is not a prognostic factor in breast cancer.

References:
1   Gorham, E.D., Garland, F.C., and Garland, C.F. (1990) Int. J. Epidemiol. 19: 820-824.
2   Eisman, J.A., Martin, T.J., MacIntyre, I., and Moseley J.M. (1979) Lancet 2: 1335-1336.
3   Eisman, J.A. 1,25-Dihydroxyvitamin D_3 receptor and role of 1,25-$(OH)_2D_3$ in human cancer cells. In: Vitamin D Metabolism: Basic and Clinical Aspects. Kumar R, ed. The Hague: Martinus Nijhoff, 1984; 365-382.
4   Berger, U., McClelland, R.A., Wilson, P., Greene, G.L., Haussler, M.R., Pike, J.W., Colston, K., Easton, D., and Coombes R.C. (1991) Cancer Res. 51:239-244.
5   Colston, K.W., Berger, U., and Coombes, R.C. (1989) Lancet 1: 188-191.
6   Buras, R.R., Schumaker, L.M., Davoodi, F., Brenner,R.V., Shabahang, M., Nauta, R.J., and Evans, S.R.T. (1994) Breast Cancer Res. Treatment 31: 191-202.

TWO NOVEL 14-EPI-ANALOGS OF 1,25-DIHYDROXYVITAMIN D$_3$ INHIBIT THE *IN VITRO* GROWTH OF HUMAN BREAST CANCER CELLS.

L. Verlinden[1], A. Verstuyf[1], K. Sabbe[2], X. Zhao[2], P. De Clercq[2], M. Vandewalle[2], C. Mathieu[1], R. Bouillon[1]. [1]
Lab. Exp. Med. and Endocrinology (LEGENDO), KU Leuven, 3000 Leuven, Belgium.
[2]Department of Organic Chemistry, Ghent University, 9000 Ghent, Belgium.

Introduction Intensive research has led to the development of analogs of 1α,25(OH)$_2$D$_3$ characterized by a clear dissociation of the antiproliferative and prodifferentiating capacity from the calcemic effects (1). Due this dissociation these analogues can be used not only for the treatment of bone disorders but also for non-classical applications such as treatment of psoriasis, cancer and autoimmune disorders (2). The knowledge of the precise molecular mechanism underlying the growth inhibitory effect of 1,25(OH)$_2$D$_3$ and its analogs remains fragmentary. In the present study we have examined the antiproliferative effect of two novel 14-epi-1α,25(OH)$_2$D$_3$ analogs (TX 522, TX 527) on breast cancer cells and the cell cycle regulatory genes involved.

Methods Studies on cell proliferation were performed on human breast cancer cells (MCF-7, SK-BR-3, T47D). Proliferation was assessed after 72 h of culture in the presence of 1,25(OH)$_2$D$_3$, analogs or vehicle by measurement of [^{3}H]thymidine incorporation. Cell cycle analysis was performed with a FACSort flow cytometer (Becton Dickinson, Lincoln Park, NJ) using the CellFit program after incubating the cells with propidium iodide/RNase A. Regulation of the expression of apoptosis regulator genes, bcl-2, bcl-xl and bax by 1,25(OH)$_2$D$_3$ or its analogs was measured using real time quantitative reverse transcriptase PCR. The activity of caspase 3 was assayed fluorometrically by the CaspACE^{TM} Assay System (Promega, Madison, Mi). The proportion of Annexin V positive cells was measured using flow cytometry, utilizing a commercially available apoptosis detection kit from Clontech (ApoAlert^{TM} Annexin V Apoptosis kit, Palo Alto, CA). Induction of DNA strand breaks was investigated using the in situ cell death detection kit from Roche (Palo Alto, CA) and analyzed by flow cytometry. Morphological features of programmed cell death have been studied on cytospins stained with hemaluin-eosine. Western blotting was performed to investigate cyclin D, cyclin C, p15, p19, p21, p27.

Results and Conclusions Proliferation of MCF-7 cells was dose-dependently inhibited by 1,25(OH)$_2$D$_3$ and was characterized by an EC$_{50}$ value of approximately 5×10^{-8} M (Fig.2A). The EC$_{50}$ value of both 14-epi analogs was however 10 times lower than that of the parent molecule. Cell cycle analysis revealed that a 72-h treatment with 10^{-8} M 1,25(OH)$_2$D$_3$ caused a significant increase in the percentage of cells in the G1 phase (64% vs. 55% in control cultures, p<0,01) while the proportion of S phase cells decreased (14% vs. 24% in control cultures, p<0,01) (Fig. 2B). This shift in cell cycle distribution was more pronounced when MCF-7 cells were treated with 10^{-8} M TX 522 or TX 527; 75% of cells were found in the G1 phase of the cell cycle (p<0,01) and the percentage of actively proliferating cells was decreased to 6% of the total population (p<0,01) (Fig. 2B).

508

Figure 1: Chemical structure of 14-epi-1α,25(OH)₂D₃ analogs

TX 522   TX 527

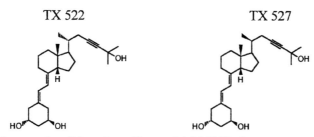

Figure 2: In vitro antiproliferative effects of 1,25(OH)₂D₃ and 14-epi analogs on MCF-7 cells

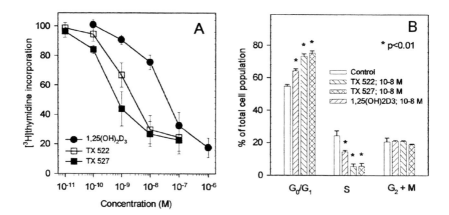

(A) ^{3}[H]thymidine incorporation of MCF-7 cells incubated for 72 h with 1,25(OH)₂D₃ (●), TX 522 (□) or TX 527 (■). (B) Cell cycle distribution of MCF-7 cells incubated for 72 h in presence of 10^{-8} M 1,25(OH)₂D₃; TX 522; TX 527.

A 70% decrease in cyclin D1 protein levels was observed in MCF-7 cells that were incubated during 120 h in presence of 10^{-7} M 1,25(OH)₂D₃ (Fig. 3A). A similar downregulation was found when cells were incubated in presence of the 14-epi-analogs. Furthermore, protein levels of the G1/S specific cyclin C were hardly affected by 1,25(OH)₂D₃ but were clearly decreased (50%, $p<0.01$) after treatment with 10^{-7} M TX 522 or TX 527 (Fig. 3A). No induction of the cdk-inhibitors p15 and p19 proteins could be observed after a 72-h incubation with 10^{-7} M 1,25(OH)₂D₃, TX 522 or TX 527. A significant 4-fold and 6-fold increase in p21 protein production (Fig. 3B) was observed when MCF-7 cells were treated with 1,25(OH)₂D₃ and TX 522, respectively ($p<0.01$).

Figure 3: Effect of 1,25(OH)₂D₃ (10⁻⁷ M) and 14-epi analogs (10⁻⁷ M) on the regulation of cell cycle genes in MCF-7 cells.

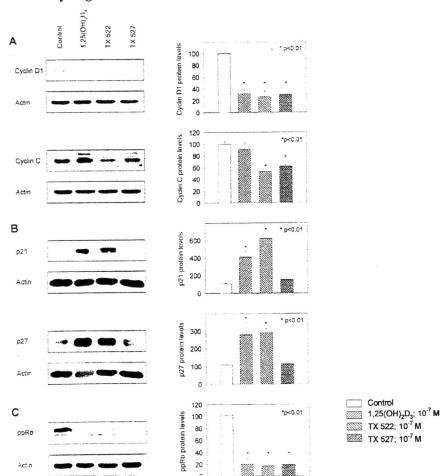

A) Protein levels of cyclin D1 and cyclin C measured after a 120- and 72-h incubation period, respectively. (B) Protein levels of p21 and p27 measured after a 72-h incubation period. (C) The amount of highly phosphorylated Rb after a 72-h incubation period

Surprisingly, p21 protein levels, measured at regular time points during a 120 h incubation with the analog TX 527 were significantly different from that of control cultures. This inability to upregulate p21 seemed to be cell-type specific because TX 527 was as potent as 1,25(OH)₂D₃ and TX 522 in inducing p21 protein levels in normal keratinocytes (3-fold) and in SK-BR-3 breast cancer cells (4-fold) (data not shown). Protein levels of p27 were also significantly enhanced by a 72 h incubation period with 10⁻⁷ M 1,25(OH)₂D₃ or TX 522 (Fig. 3B). However the degree of induction was lower than that of p21 (p<0.01). Again, the analog TX 527 was not able to induce an enhanced production of p27. However, no induction of p27 by 1,25(OH)₂D₃ or any other analogs was found neither in the

SK-BR-3 nor in the T47D cell line (data not shown). Treatment with either 10^{-7} M 1,25(OH)$_2$D$_3$, TX 522 or TX 527 led to a similar reduction (5-fold) in the amount of highly phosphorylated Rb (p<0.01). Different protocols were used to analyze the possible induction of programmed cell death. In a first approach no significant alterations in the expression of bcl-2- and bax- related genes were found in MCF-7 cells that were incubated with 1,25(OH)$_2$D$_3$ or analogs (10^{-7} M) at any time point investigated (24, 48, 72 and 120 h) (data not shown). Secondly, no induction of the effector caspase 3 could be detected in lysates of MCF-7 cells that were treated with vehicle, 1,25(OH)$_2$D$_3$ or its analogs during different time periods (24, 48, 72 and 120 h) (Fig.4A). Thirdly, the proportion of annexin V-positive cells was slightly increased in MCF-7 cells after a 72-h incubation period with either 10^{-7} M 1,25(OH)$_2$D$_3$ or analogs (Fig. 4B). This increase did not reach significance for treatment with 10^{-7} M 1,25(OH)$_2$D$_3$ whereas it did for treatment with 10^{-7} M TX 522 and TX 527 (from 3% in control cultures to 7% in cultures treated with TX 522 or TX 527). The same tendency was observed after a 120-h incubation period. Fourthly, neither 1,25(OH)$_2$D$_3$ nor these 14-epi-analogs were able to induce DNA strand breaks (data not shown). Finally, no significant differences could be found in the number of cells displaying morphological characteristics of programmed cell death.

Figure 4: Effect of 1,25(OH)$_2$D$_3$ and 14-epi-analogs on apoptotic features.

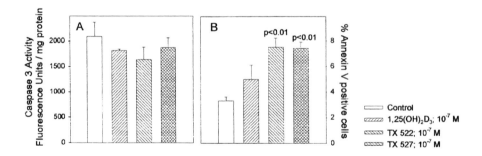

MCF-7 cells were incubated for 72 h in presence of 10^{-7} M 1,25(OH)$_2$D$_3$, TX 522 or TX 527. Caspase 3 activity (A) and the proportion of annexin V positive cells (B) were measured by flow cytometry.

In conclusion, these new structural analogs of vitamin D appear to possess enhanced antiproliferative activity compared to 1,25(OH)$_2$D$_3$ and seem to be of particular interest as potential anticancer drugs.

References

1. Bouillon, R., Okamura, W.H. and Norman, A.W. (1995) Endocr. Rev. 16, 200-257.
2. Verstuyf, A., Segaert, S., Verlinden, L., Bouillon, R. and Mathieu, C. (2000) Exp.Opin. Invest. Drugs 9, 443-455.

COMBINATION TREATMENT OF MCF-7 XENOGRAFTS WITH THE VITAMIN D₃ ANALOG EB1089 AND ANTIESTROGENS.

K. Packman, L. Flanagan, G. Zinser, R. Mitsch, M. Tenniswood, and J. Welsh
Department of Biological Sciences, University of Notre Dame, Notre Dame, IN

Introduction Our lab has shown antiestrogens have an additive effect on EB1089 induced apoptosis in MCF-7 cells *in vitro*. In the present studies, the ability of combined therapy with antiestrogens to potentiate the anti-tumor effects of EB1089 *in vivo* was investigated. A breast cancer model was utilized with established, rapidly growing tumors in the continuous presence estradiol throughout treatment. Combined treatment of MCF-7 xenografts with EB1089 and either the partial ER agonist tamoxifen or the pure ER antagonist ICl182,780 was compared. Previous studies with xenografts derived from MCF-7^{D3Res} cells demonstrated the tumors were resistant to the growth inhibitory properties of EB1089. Studies of MCF-7^{D3Res} cells *in vitro* demonstrated that although MCF-7^{D3Res} cells were resistant to EB1089, they were sensitive to antiestrogens, and antiestrogen induced apoptosis was potentiated by co-incubation of cells with EB1089. The current studies examined whether tumors derived MCF-7^{D3Res} cells exhibited comparable sensitivity to antiestrogen induced apoptosis *in vivo,* and whether combined treatment of MCF-7^{D3Res} xenografts with EB1089 and tamoxifen or ICI 182,780 would produce additional anti-tumor effects.

Materials and Methods In all studies, ovariectomized NCr nu/nu mice were implanted sc with 1.7 mg 17ß-estradiol sustained release pellets (Innovative Research). Mice were inoculated sc in the flank region with approximately 5×10^6 MCF-7 or MCF-7^{D3Res} cells suspended in 0.3 ml Matrigel/ αMEM.   After three weeks, mice bearing tumors with volumes averaging approximately 200 mm³ were randomized for treatment. Treatments and duration for each experiment are located in the corresponding figures or figure legends.

After treatment was completed, tumors were removed from mice, formalin-fixed, paraffin embedded, and sectioned at 5 μM. Mitotic index and apoptotic index were assessed by quantitative morphometric analysis of proliferating cell nuclear antigen (PCNA) expression and in situ terminal transferase mediated fluorescein dUTP nick end labeling (TUNEL), established markers of proliferation and apoptosis. PCNA expression and TUNEL were quantitated by viewing and photographing four random fields of each tissue section with a brightfield microscope and 40x objective. Photographs were taken with a digital camera, and were analyzed with the Zeiss KS 300 Imaging Analysis software. To detect vitamin D receptor (VDR) expression tissue sections were incubated with an anti-VDR (clone 9A7) monoclonal antibody. To detect estrogen receptor (ER) or progesterone receptor (PR) expression, sections were incubated with an anti-ER (clone 6F11) or anti-PR (clone 1A6) monoclonal antibody. The ABC technique was used to develop VDR, ER, or PR staining followed by the substrate DAB. ER, PR, and VDR expression were evaluated by utilizing a qualitative scale with sections receiving a score from (++++) for highest staining, to (-) for no staining.

512

Tumor growth data are expressed as the mean ± SE. Differences between means were considered significant when p<0.05. Statistical comparisons were performed using the Kruskal-Wallis ANOVA. Post-test comparisons between groups were made using the Dunn test.

Results

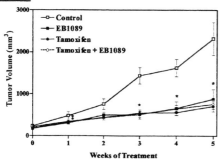

Figure 1. Effect of EB1089, tamoxifen, or combination treatment, on MCF-7 tumor volume. Tumor volume of MCF-7 xenografts treated with either vehicle + placebo (control) (n=8) 45 pmol EB1089 3x/ week (n=10), 15 mg/ 35 days tamoxifen (n=7), or both EB1089 and tamoxifen (n=10), *p<0.05 for EB1089, tamoxifen, and EB1089 + tamoxifen, compared to control.

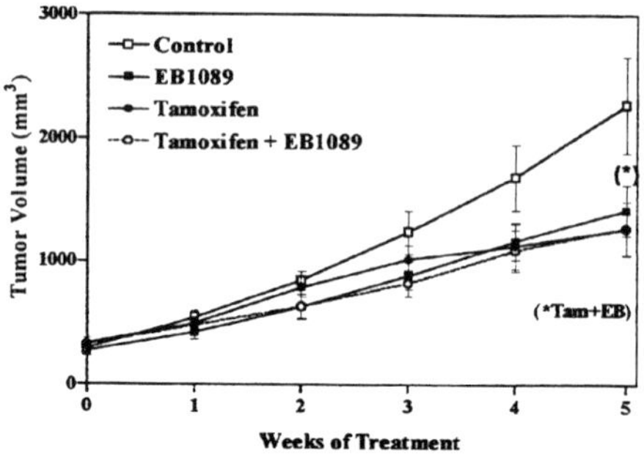

Figure 2. Effect of EB1089, tamoxifen, or combination treatment, on MCF-7 tumor volume. Tumor volume of MCF-7 xenografts treated with either vehicle + placebo (control) (n=9) 25 pmol EB1089 3x/ week (n=11), 7.5 mg/ 42 days tamoxifen (n=10), or both EB1089 and tamoxifen (n=12), *p<0.05 for EB1089 + tamoxifen, compared to control.

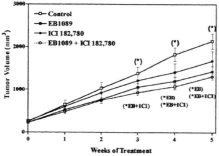

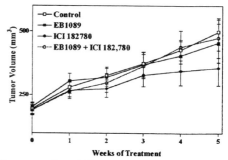

Figure 3. Effect of EB1089, ICI 182,780, or combination treatment, on MCF-7 tumor volume. Tumor volume of MCF-7 xenografts treated with either vehicle + placebo (control) (n=11) 25 pmol EB1089 3x/ week (n=11), 10 mg/ 35 days ICI 182,780 (n=8), or EB1089+ ICI 182,780 (n=14), *p<0.05 for EB1089, and EB1089 + ICI 182,780, compared to control.

Figure 4. Effect of EB1089, ICI 182,780, or combination treatment, on MCF-7^{D3Res} tumor volume. Tumor volume of MCF-7^{D3Res} xenografts treated with either vehicle + placebo (control) (n=13) 25 pmol EB1089 3x/ week (n=13), 10 mg/ 35 days ICI 182,780 (n=13), or both EB1089 and ICI 182,780 (n=12).

% Cells	Control	EB1089	Tamoxifen	EB + Tam
A. PCNA	66.11 ± 3.26 n=6	62.97 ± 1.26 n=8	61.54 ± 2.71 n=9	45.08 ± 4.38* n=10
TUNEL	2.35 ± .40 n=9	29.74 ± 4.9* n=10	15.89 ± 3.12* n=9	23.70 ± 4.13* n=10
% Cells	Control	EB1089	ICI 182,780	EB + ICI
B. PCNA	67.15 ± 2.91 n=10	55.65 ± 3.06 n=10	54.63 ± 3.22 n=10	35.97 ± 2.35*[a] n=10
TUNEL	3.31 ± 1.09 n=10	21.37 ± 6.33* n=10	25.48 ± 4.09* n=10	15.16 ± 4.08* n=10

Table 1. *Quantitation of PCNA expression and DNA fragmentation in MCF-7 tumors.* Data are expressed as percentage of cells positive for PCNA or DNA fragmentation. *A.* Tumor sections from mice treated with vehicle, 25 pmol EB1089 3x/wk, 7.5 mg/ 42 days tamoxifen, or EB1089 + tamoxifen for 6 weeks. *B.* Tumor sections from mice treated with vehicle, 25 pmol EB1089 3x/wk, 10 mg/ 35 days ICI 182,780, or EB1089 + ICI 182,780 for 5 weeks. *p<0.05 compared to control. [a]p<0.05 compared to EB1089 and ICI 182,780.

VDR	++++	+++	++	VDR	++++	+++	++
A. Control	22%	67%	11%	B. Control	31%	54%	15%
EB1089	55%	36%	9%	EB1089	45%	36%	18%
Tamoxifen	50%	40%	10%	ICI182,780	30%	50%	20%
EB1089 + Tamoxifen	27%	64%	9%	EB1089 + ICI182,780	29%	36%	36%

Table 2. *Effect of EB1089, antiestrogen, or combination treatment, on relative VDR expression in MCF-7 xenografts.* Data are expressed as percentage of tumors with relative VDR expression. *A.* MCF-7 xenografts were treated for 6 weeks with either vehicle (n=9), 25 pmol EB1089 3x/ week (n=11), 7.5 mg/ 42 days tamoxifen (n=10), or both EB1089 and tamoxifen (11). *B.* MCF-7 xenografts were treated for 5 weeks with either vehicle (n=13), 25 pmol EB1089 3x/ week (n=11), 10 mg/ 35 days ICI 182,780 (n=10), or both EB1089 and ICI 182,780 (n=14).

ER	+++	++	+	PR	+++	++	+	+/-	-
A. Control	56%	22%	22%	A. Control	56%	22%	22%	0%	0%
EB1089	36%	45%	18%	EB1089	36%	18%	9%	9%	27%
Tamoxifen	50%	40%	10%	Tamoxifen	30%	40%	10%	10%	10%
EB1089 + Tamoxifen	50%	42%	8%	EB1089 + Tamoxifen	42%	33%	8%	0	17%
B. Control	64%	21%	14%	B. Control	43%	21%	14%	14%	7%
EB1089	42%	42%	17%	EB1089	33%	25%	8%	17%	17%
ICI182,780	46%	39%	15%	ICI182,780	31%	31%	8%	8%	23%
EB1089 + ICI182,780	36%	43%	21%	EB1089 + ICI182,780	21%	21%	21%	0%	36%

Table 3. *Effect of EB1089, antiestrogen, or combination treatment, on relative ER and PR expression in MCF-7 xenografts.* Data are expressed as percentage of tumors with relative ER or PR expression. *A.* MCF-7 xenografts were treated for 6

weeks with either vehicle (n=9), 25 pmol EB1089 3x/ week (n=11), 7.5 mg/ 42 days tamoxifen (n=10), or both EB1089 and tamoxifen (n=12). *B.* MCF-7 xenografts were treated for 5 weeks with either vehicle (n=14), 25 pmol EB1089 3x/ week (n=12), 10 mg/ 35 days ICI 182,780 (n=13), or both EB1089 and ICI 182,780 (n=14).

Discussion   Our previous studies have shown that both the partial agonist tamoxifen and the pure antagonist ICI 182,780 can potentiate EB1089 induced apoptosis in MCF-7 and MCF-7[D3Res] cells *in vitro.* We have also demonstrated that EB1089 exerts anti-tumor effects in MCF-7 tumors by inducing apoptosis. In the current studies, we demonstrated that EB1089 is as effective as antiestrogens, the endocrine therapy of choice, in MCF-7 tumor growth inhibition. In contrast to *in vitro* studies however, results of combination studies *in vivo* indicated that additive effects on MCF-7 and MCF-7[D3Res] tumors could not be observed with EB1089 in combination with either tamoxifen or ICI 182,780. Mitotic index demonstrated some enhancement of anti-tumor effect with EB1089 + antiestrogens over single treatments alone in MCF-7 tumors however, the relevance of these small differences is questionable, since overall changes in tumor volume and weight were minimal.   Regardless of how these small differences are interpreted, a much larger effect on anti-tumor activity was anticipated with combination treatment based on *in vitro* studies.

Studies of ER and PR expression in MCF-7 xenografts after treatment with EB1089 and antiestrogens implicated down-regulation of the ER growth regulatory pathway as a mechanism of action for EB1089. Comparison of ER and VDR regulation with combination treatment *in vitro* and *in vivo* indicates that ER down-regulation is maintained *in vivo*, whereas VDR up-regulation is absent *in vivo.* Thus, upregulation of VDR with combination treatment may be necessary for additive anti-tumor effects. *Supported by AICR 98A100 and DAMD17-97-1-726.*

Selected References
1. VanWeelden, K., Flanagan, L., Tenniswood, M., Binderup, L., and Welsh, J. (1998) Apoptotic regression of MCF-7 xenografts in nude mice treated with the vitamin D_3 analog EB1089. *Endocrinology* 139, 2102-2110
2. Narvaez, C.J., VanWeelden, K., Byrne, I., and Welsh, J. (1996) Characterization of a Vitamin D_3 Resistant MCF-7 cell line. *Endocrinology* 137, 400-409
3. Welsh, J., VanWeelden, K., Flanagan, L., Byrne, I., Nolan, E. and Narvaez, C.J. (1997) The role of vitamin D_3 and antiestrogens in modulating apoptosis of breast cancer cells and tumors. *In: Subcellular Biochemistry, Vol. 30, Fat Soluble Vitamins.* (Quinn PJ and Kagan VE, eds.) Plenum Press, pp. 245-270.
4. Nolan, E., Donepudi, M., VanWeelden, K., Flanagan, L., and Welsh, J. (1998) Dissociation of vitamin D_3 and antiestrogen mediated growth regulation in MCF-7 breast cancer cells. *Molecular and Cellular Biochemistry* 188, 13-20

VITAMIN D AND METASTATIC BREAST CANCER

Louise Flanagan [1,2], Brian Juba [2] and JoEllen Welsh [2], University College Dublin, Belfield, Ireland [1]; University of Notre Dame, IN 46556 USA [2].

Breast cancer is one of the leading causes of death among women in North America and Western Europe despite intense efforts to develop more effective chemo- and hormonal therapies. Although five-year survival rates for localized and regionally spread breast cancer have improved, the survival rate for women with distant metastases is only 20%. The development of a metastatic, hormone independent, and drug resistant phenotype is largely responsible for the high percentage of treatment failures among breast cancer patients. Although understanding the molecular mechanisms of cancer is crucial for the design of effective, novel therapeutic strategies, progress has been limited by the lack of appropriate experimental models for the study of metastatic breast cancer. In these studies, we describe and characterize, *in vitro* and *in vivo*, the growth of a novel estrogen independent human breast cancer cell line, SUM-159PT and examine the effects of vitamin D_3 compounds on its growth and invasion.

Our studies have shown that ER protein was not detected in SUM-159PT cells or tumors, correlating with lack of estradiol binding. Furthermore SUM-159PT cells were tumorigenic in ovariectomized nude mice in the absence of estradiol supplementation, consistent with estrogen independence. Our work has shown that the SUM-159PT cell line is epithelial in origin, as determined by expression of cytokeratin 18 by western blot. However, the levels of cytokeratin 18 expression were considerably lower (10-fold) than those observed in the estrogen-dependent MCF-7 cells. We demonstrated that approximately 45% of SUM-159PT cells are capable of invading through an 8µM Matrigel invasion chamber whilst exhibiting a stellate morphology in the Matrigel outgrowth assay. In contrast, the non-invasive MCF-7 cells formed smooth spherical colonies in Matrigel and were minimally invasive *in vitro*. These results correlate well with previous data indicating that poorly differentiated cell lines express cytokeratins at low levels, and are highly invasive in *in vitro* chemoinvasion assays.

To investigate metastatic markers in SUM-159PT cells, we examined the expression of vimentin and E-cadherin, proteins that have been strongly implicated in the transition of carcinoma cells to a metastatic phenotype. SUM-159PT cells and xenografts were found to express vimentin, which has been associated with poor prognosis, low differentiation, lack of ER, high invasive capacity and shorter disease–free interval. In contrast, the well-differentiated MCF-7 cells did not express vimentin. In breast cancer, loss of E-cadherin expression has been observed in high-grade tumors and correlates with increased invasiveness and significantly shorter disease-free interval. E-cadherin was expressed in the MCF-7 cells, but no expression was observed in the invasive, vimentin-positive SUM-159PT cells. We also report an inverse relationship between the levels of the putative anti-metastatic protein nm23 and tumor aggressiveness. Little or no nm23 expression was observed in the invasive SUM-159PT xenografts, in contrast to high expression detected in well-differentiated MCF-7 tumors.

Thus SUM-159PT cells can be categorized with other poorly-differentiated fibroblastic-like breast cancer cell lines (1). Use of SUM-159PT cells as an *in vitro* model of estrogen-independent human breast cancer will be useful for molecular studies on the mechanisms of invasion and for testing the effectiveness of potential therapeutics in advanced breast cancer cells.

Our lab and others have shown that the vitamin D metabolite $1,25(OH)_2D_3$ induces growth arrest and apoptosis in MCF-7 cells *in vitro* (2). In ER-positive breast cancer cells, the effects of $1,25(OH)_2D_3$ are similar to those induced by anti-estrogens in that $1,25(OH)_2D_3$ mediated cell death in MCF-7 cells is preceded by down regulation of the ER. These finding have led to the hypothesis that, at least in MCF-7 cells, the effects of $1,25(OH)_2D_3$ may in part be related to disruption of estrogen related survival signals. If so, then sensitivity to $1,25(OH)_2D_3$ mediated growth arrest and apoptosis could be reduced in estrogen independent breast cancer cells. Our studies have demonstrated that both $1,25(OH)_2D_3$ and its analog EB1089 caused a significant 60-70% reduction in SUM-159PT cell number after a six day time course relative to that of EtOH control. We have shown that SUM-159PT cells express the VDR which is capable of binding $1,25(OH)_2D_3$ and VDREs and its protein expression is upregulated or stabilized upon treatment with $1,25(OH)_2D_3$ or EB1089. Because previous work has demonstrated that MCF-7 cells treated with $1,25(OH)_2D_3$ or EB1089 arrest in G_0/G_1, we examined the effects of these agents on cell cycle regulatory proteins (p21 and p27) and the M phase cdc2p34 protein kinase in the estrogen independent SUM-159PT cell line. SUM-159PT cells treated with $1,25(OH)_2D_3$ or EB1089 exhibited an early increase (48 h) in both p27 and p21 expression compared to EtOH controls. It has been previously shown that a block in the M-phase is imposed by inhibiting the cdc2p34 protein kinase. In SUM-159PT cells treated with $1,25(OH)_2D_3$ little or no downregulation of cdc2p34 was observed. In contrast, a significant downregulation of cdc2p34 was observed when SUM-159PT cells were treated with EB1089 for 72 h. We also examined expression of the lysosomal protein, cathepsin B thought to be involved in the apoptotic pathway, and found an increase in the processed, mature form of cathepsin B in SUM-159PT cells treated with $1,25(OH)_2D_3$ or EB1089. Furthermore, using the TUNEL method, positive nuclear staining indicative of DNA fragmentation was detected in SUM-159PT cells treated with $1,25(OH)_2D_3$ or EB1089 for four days, similar to that observed in MCF-7 cells.

To further elucidate the apoptotic pathway in the SUM-159PT cells we analyzed the expression and subcellular distribution of several proteins that have recently been implicated in apoptotic signaling (3). In SUM-159PT cells, the proapoptotic protein bax was translocated to the mitochondrial fraction upon treatment with $1,25(OH)_2D_3$ or etoposide. This translocation of bax to the mitochondria was concominant with the release of cytochrome c from the mitochondria into the cytosol after 96 h treatment with $1,25(OH)_2D_3$ or 48 h with etoposide. To exclude mitochondrial contamination in the cytosol fractions, cytochrome oxidase expression was assessed and found to be present only in the mitochondrial fractions. To determine whether caspase activation was involved in apoptosis of SUM-159PT cells, we assessed the cleavage of PARP, a substrate of caspase 3 and 7. SUM-159PT cells treated with $1,25(OH)_2D_3$ for 96 h or etoposide for 48h were analyzed with an antibody that recognizes both intact PARP (116 kDa) and the apoptotic cleavage product (85 kDa). SUM-159PT cells treated with $1,25(OH)_2D_3$ or etoposide exhibited cleavage of PARP to generate the 85kDa fragment, whereas no PARP cleavage was detected in EtOH treated cells.

Thus, while the downregulation of the ER observed in MCF-7 cells may be a contributing factor to the apoptotic and growth inhibitory effects of $1,25(OH)_2D_3$, the effects of $1,25(OH)_2D_3$ are not dependent upon estradiol signaling, as both the growth inhibitory and apoptotic effects of $1,25(OH)_2D_3$ and EB1089 were observed in the ER-negative SUM-159PT cells.

To determine whether the vitamin D analog EB1089 could modulate growth and/or apoptosis of estrogen independent breast tumors, ovariectomized nude mice bearing either subcutaneous or orthotopic tumors were implanted with pellets designed to release 120 pmoles EB1089 per day. A similar reduction in tumor volume was observed upon treatment with EB1089 in either subcutaneous or orthotopic tumors. In mice implanted with EB1089 pellets, tumor volumes decreased gradually over the four weeks of treatment. Tumor volumes after four weeks was significantly ($P<0.001$) lower in the EB1089 treated groups (99.7 ± 61.3 mm^3) than in the control placebo group (656.5 ± 321.05 mm^3). In addition, several tumors completely regressed in response to EB1089 treatment. Morphological analysis of SUM-159PT tumors from mice treated with 120 pmole EB1089 or placebo was accomplished after staining with hematoxylin and eosin. Tumors from placebo treated mice were primarily composed of dense tumor epithelial cells, with small amounts of mouse-derived stroma, frequent blood cells and numerous mitotic figures. In contrast, tumors from mice treated with 120pmoles EB1089/day displayed an increased percentage of stroma, loss of epithelial cells, few mitotic figures and in many areas, epithelial cells with classic apoptotic morphology were observed. To determine whether the changes in SUM-159PT tumor morphology induced by EB1089 were associated with alterations in mitotic or apoptotic index, we examined expression of PCNA as a marker of proliferation and DNA fragmentation (assessed as TUNEL-positive cells) as a marker of apoptosis. Analyses of DNA fragmentation indicated that tumors from EB1089 treated mice exhibited apoptotic morphology and an increased number of TUNEL-positive cells compared with tumors from control mice. In addition to induction of apoptosis, EB1089-treated tumors exhibited a decrease in proliferation, as measured by PCNA. Our data demonstrating induction of apoptosis and decrease in proliferation in EB1089 treated SUM-159PT tumors correlates with our *in vitro* data that $1,25(OH)_2D_3$ and EB1089 induce apoptosis and cell cycle arrest in SUM-159PT cells.

Our data are the first to show apoptotic tumor regression of ER-independent breast tumors by the vitamin D analog EB1089, and are consistent with previous reports of tumor regression and apoptosis in the ER-dependent MCF-7 tumors (4). Our work also shows that sensitivity of breast tumors to the vitamin D analog EB1089 *in vivo* is not diminished during progression to estrogen independence.

Our *in vivo* studies further demonstrated that SUM-159PT cells were metastatic after inoculation into the mammary fat pad of ovariectomized nude mice, consistent with the expression of metastatic markers and *in vitro* invasiveness. Micro-metastases were observed in the lymph nodes, muscle area surrounding the mammary fat pad, lungs and liver, Metastatic spread was not observed when SUM-159PT cells were inoculated subcutaneously. Therefore, implantation of tumor cells into anatomically appropriate (orthotopic) sites, rather than subcutaneously, allowed for the metastatic potential of SUM-159PT cells.

Very few studies have addressed the potential effects of vitamin D compounds on invasion and metastases in any cancer type but in the few studies that have been carried out, vitamin D compounds have been implicated in the regulation of angiogenesis, invasion and metastasis (5). In SUM-159PT cells $1,25(OH)_2D_3$ and EB1089 induced 65% and 80% reductions respectively in invasive potential compared to EtOH treated cells. These effects were independent of the anti-proliferative effects of the compounds. Our results have further demonstrated a reduction in the numbers of mice exhibiting secondary tumors after treatment with EB1089, indicating a direct effect of EB1089 on metastases. Further investigation on the effects of EB1089 in preventing SUM-159PT metastases *in vivo* would clearly be of interest.

These data demonstrate that vitamin D compounds may inhibit both growth of primary tumors and metastasis of breast cancer cells, and may in the future prove to be highly useful in the clinical setting, alone or in conjunction with other agents, in the treatment of metastatic breast cancer.

References
1. Sommers, C. L., Byers, S. W., Thompson, E. W., Torri, J. A., and Gelmann, E. P. (1994) Breast Cancer Res Treat 31(2-3), 325-335
2. Simboli-Campbell, M., Narvaez, C. J., Van Weelden, K., Tenniswood, M., and Welsh, J. (1997) Breast Cancer Res Treat 42(1), 31-41
3. Budihardjo, I., Oliver, H., Lutter, M., Luo, X., and Wand, X. (1999) Annu. Rev. Cell Dev. Biol. 15, 269-90
4. Van Weelden, K., Flanagan, L., Binderup, L., Tenniswood, M., and Welsh, J. (1998) Endocrinology 139, 2102-2110
5. Schwarz, G., Lokeschwar, B. L., Selzer, M. G., Block, N. L., and Binderup, L. (1997) Vitamin D: Chemistry, Biology and Clinical Applications of the Steroid Hormone (489-490)

1,25-DIHYDROXYVITAMIN D_3 ENHANCES CELL DEATH AND CELLULAR SIGNALING INDUCED BY REACTIVE OXYGEN SPECIES IN HUMAN BREAST CANCER CELLS

Amiram Ravid, Efrat Zuck, Carmela Rotem, Dafna Rocker, Uri A. Liberman and Ruth Koren. The Felsenstein Medical Research Center, Tel Aviv University, Beilinson Campus, Petah Tikva, Israel, 49100.

Introduction: In addition to its direct effects on cell proliferation and viability, $1,25(OH)_2D_3$ increased the susceptibility of cancer cells to the cytotoxic action of TNF, doxorubicin and menadione (1,2). A common mechanistic feature in the anti cancer action of these agents is the excessive intracellular formation of superoxides. These reactive molecules are further converted by the action of superoxide dismutases to H_2O_2 and via the Fenton reaction to the toxic OH radical. The potentiating effect of $1,25(OH)_2D_3$ on the cytotoxic action of these anti cancer agents was markedly inhibited by the addition of antioxidants (2,3), and the combined action of $1,25(OH)_2D_3$ and TNF resulted in increased oxidative stress manifested by a decrease if reduced glutathione levels (3). Taken together, these findings support the notion that the interaction between the hormone and the cytotoxic agents is mediated by reactive oxygen species (ROS). The effect of $1,25(OH)_2D_3$ could be due to increase in intracellular ROS formation or/and increase in the cytotoxic potential of pre-formed ROS. This study aimed to directly examine the second alternative by assessing the effect of $1,25(OH)_2D_3$ on the cytotoxicity of exogenous H_2O_2.

Results: We found that pretreatment of MCF-7 breast cancer cells with $1,25(OH)_2D_3$ increased their susceptibility to the cytotoxic action of H_2O_2 (assessed by neutral red uptake) time and dose dependently (apparent after 48 hours and at 10 nM). By following the degradation of H_2O_2 in the culture medium of MCF-7 cells and by employing specific inhibitors, we established that this process is fully accounted for by the combined action of the enzymes catalase and glutathione peroxidase. Using this experimental system that $1,25(OH)_2D_3$ did not affect the action of either enzyme. This finding rules out the possibility that the potentiation of H_2O_2 cytotoxic activity stems from increased intracellular ROS levels due to inhibition of H_2O_2 degradation. In addition to their direct oxidative damage to key cellular macromolecules, ROS can induce and modulate signal transduction pathways leading to programmed cell death. For instance, ROS can oxidize an essential cysteine residue in the active site of tyrosine phosphatases, inhibit their activity and consequently bring about an increase in protein tyrosine phosphorylation. The association between reduced tyrosine phosphatase activity and cell death is inferred from previous findings that the known tyrosine phosphatase inhibitor, vanadate, enhances ROS-induced cell death. Overall tyrosine phosphorylation of proteins from whole cells extracts of MCF-7 cells was unaffected by treatment with $1,25(OH)_2D_3$ alone or by exposure of the cells to 0.2 mM H_2O_2 for 10-20 minutes. However, tyrosine phosphorylation was markedly enhanced in cells pretreated with $1,25(OH)_2D_3$ and than exposed to H_2O_2. Activation of the stress-activated protein kinases, in particular c-Jun N-terminal kinase (JNK), is thought to play an important role in the signaling that links exogenous stimuli, including exposure to ROS, with programmed cell death. The level of the dually phosphorylated active JNK was not altered by a 48 h hour treatment with $1,25(OH)_2D_3$ alone or by a 10-45 minute exposure to H_2O_2 (0.2 mM). However, a marked increase in JNK activation occurred in $1,25(OH)_2D_3$-treated cultures exposed to H_2O_2.

Conclusions and discussion: These results demonstrate that the increased susceptibility of $1,25(OH)_2D_3$-treated cells to the cytotoxic action of H_2O_2 is manifested at the earliest stages of ROS signaling and thus is probably not due to modulation of the cell execution machinery or to impairment of repair mechanisms. Traditionally ROS were thought of as harmful molecules, the unwanted and toxic by-products of living in an aerobic environment. However, sufficient evidence has accumulated to suggest that, under normal conditions, molecules such as H_2O_2 can and do function in signal transduction in mammalian cells. Stimulation of a wide variety of cell types with growth factors, hormones and cytokines results in an increase of intracellular ROS. It remains to be shown whether $1,25(OH)_2D_3$ increases also the effectiveness of ROS action as modulators of different signaling pathways mediated by tyrosine phosphorylation. If this is proven, such insight could suggest that the diverse and sometimes opposite effects of $1,25(OH)_2D_3$ in various biological systems originate from this common mechanism.

Bibliography
1. Rocker, D., Ravid, A., Liberman, U.A., Garach-Yehoshua, O. and Koren, R. (1994) *Mol. Cell. Endocrinol.* 106, 157-162.
2. Ravid, A., Rocker, D., Machlenkin, A., Rotem, C., Hochman, A., Kessler-Icekson, G., Liberman, U.A. and Koren, R. (1999) *Cancer Res.* 59, 862-867.
3. Koren, R., Rocker, D., Kotestiano, O., Liberman, U.A., Ravid, A. (2000) *J. Steroid Biochem. Molec. Biol.* (in press).

VITAMIN D RECEPTOR EXPRESSION IS NOT A PROGNOSTIC FACTOR IN CERVICAL CANCER

Roland Meyberg[1], Michael Friedrich[1], Leyla Rafi[1], Wolfgang Tilgen[2], Werner Schmidt[1], and Jörg Reichrath[2]. Departments of [1]Gynecology and [2]Dermatology, University Hospital of Saarland, D-66421 Homburg/Saar, Germany.

Introduction: Carcinomas of the uterine cervix represent approximately 4.5% of all malignancies of the female genital tract (1). Therapeutical procedures include surgery, such as radical hysterectomy, and radiotherapy. Survival time of responders to palliative chemotherapy is approximately 4-6 months (1). New therapies for the treatment of patients with tumour progression or metastasizing disease are desirable. Succesfull endocrine therapy regimens are not known so far. Epidemiological studies have suggested the association of 1,25-dihydroxyvitamin D_3 ($1,25(OH)_2D_3$) deficiency with an increased risk of various malignancies including colon and breast cancer (2,3). The molecular mechanisms involved in this phenomenon are still unknown. It has been shown that nuclear receptors for $1,25(OH)_2D_3$ (VDR) are almost ubiquitiously expressed in human tissues (4,5,6). We have recently demonstrated expression of VDR in cervical carcinomas and in normal cervical tissue (7). *In vitro* studies have demonstrated that $1,25(OH)_2D_3$ suppresses proliferation and induces differentiation in various cell types, including epithelial cells (8,9). Such studies prompted the suggestion of the use of calcitriol analogues in the treatment of certain malignancies. However, the biological function of VDR in normal cervical tissue and in cervical carcinomas is not completely understood. The aim of this immunohistochemical study was to analyze semi-quantitatively expression of VDR in normal cervical tissue and in cervical carcinomas and to compare VDR expression with the staining pattern of the proliferation marker Ki-67 and with parameters of staging and grading to analyze whether VDR expression may be a prognostic factor in cervical carcinomas.

Materials and Methods: *Cervical specimens:* Biopsies from normal Cervical tissue (n=15) were obtained from patients that underwent surgery for uterine leiomyomas. Histological examination by a certified pathologist confirmed normality. Biopsies from Cervical carcinomas (n=50) were obtained from patients that underwent surgery after the tumour was diagnosed histologically. Usually, a radical hysterectomy was performed. Biopsies were taken from macroscopically visible tumor areas. Histological examination by a certified pathologist confirmed diagnosis. All Cervix specimens were immediately embedded in OCT-Tissue-Tek II (Miles Laboratories, Naperville, Illinois, U.S.A.), snap frozen in melting isopentane, precooled in liquid nitrogen and stored at -80 C.
Primary antibodies: VDR was detected by mAb 9A7γ (Dianova, Hamburg, Germany) whose preparation and specificity was described previously (9,10). This antibody (IgG2b) was raised against chicken intestinal VDR and cross-reacts with human, mouse, and rat VDRs, but does not bind to glucocorticoid, progesterone, or estrogen receptors. The epitope has been determined to reside between residues 90 and 104 of the human VDR, a location which is just C-terminal to the DNA-binding fingers. 9A7γ perturbs, but does not inhibit, the receptor-DNA interaction. P53-protein was detected by mouse *m*Ab directed

against p53 protein (clone D0-7, Dakopatts, Copenhagen, Denmark). Proliferation was investigated applying mouse mAb Ki-67 directed against the Ki-67 antigen (clone Ki-67, Dakopatts, Copenhagen, Denmark).

Preparation of sections and fixation: Serial sections (5 μm) were cut on a cryostat (Reichert-Jung, Heidelberg, Germany), mounted on glass slides and fixed in 3,7% paraformaldehyde (Merck 4005, Darmstadt, Germany) in phosphate buffered saline (PBS, 10 min, room temperature [RT]), incubated in methanol (Merck 6009, 3 min, -20°C), acetone (Merck 22, -20°C, 1 min), and transferred into PBS.

In situ detection of primary antibodies: The incubation steps were performed in a moist chamber at RT, covering the sections with 100 μl of the respective reagents. To reduce nonspecific staining, the slides were incubated with heat-inactivated normal rabbit serum (20 min, RT). The slides were then incubated (19 h, 4°C) with the different primary antibodies (anti-VDR 1 : 1000; anti-p53 1 : 100; anti-Ki-67 1 : 100) or as control with polyclonal mouse IgG1 (Dakopatts) at similar concentrations. After intermediate washing steps (TBS, 2 x 5 min) the sections were incubated with biotin-labeled rabbit anti-mouse IgG (Dakopatts, 1 : 400, 30 min, RT) and incubated with streptavidin-peroxidase complexes (Dakopatts, 1 : 400, 30 min, RT). After washing in PBS, the sections were incubated for 6 min with 3-amino-9-ethylcarbazole (AEC, Sigma A 5754, München, Germany) to visualize the peroxidase reaction.

Semi-quantitative analysis of immunoreactivity: Microscopic analysis was performed by two independent observers (J. R. and M. F.). VDR-, p53 -staining intensity (VDR-SI, p53-SI), percentage of VDR-, p53 -positive tumour cells (VDR-PP, p53-PP) and an immunreactive VDR-, p53-score (VDR-IRS: VDR negative: 0-1; weak VDR-immunoreactivity: 2-3; moderate VDR-immunoreactivity: 4-6; strong VDR-immunoreactivity: 8-12; p53-IRS) were assessed as described previously for estrogen and progesterone receptors. Sections stained for Ki-67 were assessed by counting the number of Ki-67 positive and negative cells in the strongest stained tumour area (magnification x 400, at least 200 tumour cells were counted).

Statistical Analysis: Statistical analysis was performed by using Mann-Whitney U-Wilcoxon Rank Sum W-test, Kruskal-Wallis-H-test and Chi-Square-test after Pearson. Statistical significance was defined as $p < 0.05$.

Results: *Increased Expression of VDR in Cervical Cancer compared to Normal Cervical Tissue:* The expression of VDR was statistically significantly increased in cervical cancer compared to normal cervical tissue (table I). There was no statistically significant correlation between VDR expression in cervical cancer and parameters for staging and grading in cervical cancer (table II). Additionally, no statistically significant correlation between the expression of VDR and the expression of the tumor suppressor p53 (table III) or the proliferation marker Ki-67 were detected in cervical cancer.

Table I: Increased expression of VDR in cervical cancer compared to normal cervical tissue.

	VDR-SI	VDR-PP	VDR-IRS
Benign Cervical Tissue (n=62)	1.0+/-0.9	9.0%+/-13.5	1.2+/-1.0
Cervical cancer (n=228)	2.2+/-0.8	76.5%+/-18.5	8.2+/-3.7
	p<0,001*	p<0,0001*	p<0,0001*

*Mann-Whitney-U-Test

No Correlation between Expression of VDR and Staging or Grading in Cervical Cancer: There was no statistically significant correlation between VDR expression in cervical cancer and parameters for staging and grading in cervical cancer (table II).

Table II: No correlation between VDR-expression and staging and grading in cervical cancer.

p-values	pT	pN	G	Hist. type
VDR-SI	0.24**	0.99**	0.69**	0.91**
VDR-PP	0.62*	0.74*	0.59*	0.78*
VDR-IRS	0.21*	0.96*	0.47*	0.98*

*Kruskal-Wallis-H-test, **Chi-Square-test, *** Mann-Whitney-U-test

No Correlation between Expression of VDR and Expression of the Tumorsuppressor p53 in Cervical Cancer: No statistically significant correlation between the expression of VDR and the expression of the tumor suppressor p53 were detected in cervical cancer (VDR-IRS: r=-0.12, p=0.40; VDR-SI: r=-0.13, p=0.35; VDR-PP: r=-0.13, p=0.39; Spearman-correlation).

Table III: No correlation between VDR- and p53-expression in cervical cancer

	p53-SI	p53-PP	p53-IRS
VDR-SI	0.15*	-	-
VDR-PP	-	0.56**	-
VDR-IRS	-	-	0.22**

*Chi-Square-test; **Kruskal-Wallis-H-test

No Correlation between the Expression of VDR and Parameters of Cell Proliferation in Cervical Cancer: There were no statistically significant correlations comparing VDR expression and Ki-67-index (VDR-SI: r=0.14; p=0.32; VDR-PP: r=-0.002; p=0.99; VDR-IRS: r=0.11; p=0.45 Spearman-correlation). Furthermore, no statistically significant correlation was seen comparing the expression of VDR and Ki-67 (VDR-SI: p=0.43 Chi-Quadrat-Test; VDR-PP: p=0.54 Mann-Whitney-U-Test; VDR-IRS: p=0.45 Mann-Whitney-U-Test).

Discussion: We show that the vitamin D receptor is expressed in cervical cancer and that VDR protein-levels are increased in cervical carcinomas compared to benign cervical tissue. We found no correlation of VDR immunoreactivity with staining pattern of the proliferation marker Ki-67, indicating that VDR upregulation in cervical cancer is not exclusively regulated by the increased proliferative activity in these tumor cells. Additionally, we demonstrate that VDR protein level is not a prognostic factor in cervical cancer. VDR status in cervical carcinomas analyzed was independent from staging, grading, histological type of cervical cancer, or p53 status. The strong expression of VDR in cervical cancer and in benign cervical tissue identifies these tissues as potential targets for preventive, adjuvant or palliative treatment with vitamin D analogues.

References:
1   Gorham, E.D., Garland, F.C., and Garland, C.F. (1990) Int. J. Epidemiol. 19:820-824.
2   Eisman, J.A., Martin, T.J., MacIntyre, I., and Moseley J.M. (1979) Lancet 2: 1335-1336.
3   Eisman, J.A. 1,25-Dihydroxyvitamin D_3 receptor and role of 1,25-$(OH)_2D_3$ in human cancer cells. In: Vitamin D Metabolism: Basic and Clinical Aspects. Kumar R, ed. The Hague: Martinus Nijhoff, 1984; 365-382.
4   Berger, U., McClelland, R.A., Wilson, P., Greene, G.L., Haussler, M.R., Pike, J.W., Colston, K., Easton, D., and Coombes R.C. (1991) Cancer Res. 51:239-244.
5   Colston, K.W., Berger, U., and Coombes, R.C. (1989) Lancet 1: 188-191.
6   Friedrich, M., Rafi, L., Tilgen, W., Schmidt, W., Reichrath, J. (1998) J Histochem Cytochem
7   Reichrath, J., Rafi, L., Tilgen, W., Schmidt, W., Friedrich, M. (1998) Histochem J
8   Krishnan, A.V., and Feldman, D. (1991) J. Bone Miner. Res. 6: 1099-1107.
9   Buras, R.R., Schumaker, L.M., Davoodi, F., Brenner,R.V., Shabahang, M., Nauta, R.J., and Evans, S.R.T. (1994) Breast Cancer Res. Treatment 31: 191-202.

ENHANCEMENT OF 25-HYDROXYVITAMIN D-1α-HYDROXYLASE ACTIVITY IN PROSTATE CELLS BY GENE TRANSFECTION: A NOVEL APPROACH FOR THE TREATMENT OF PROSTATE CANCER.

TC Chen, L Whitlatch, M Young, J Flanagan, GG Schwartz, BL Lokeshwar, X Kong, X Zhu and MF Holick. Boston Univ. School of Medicine, Boston, MA, 02118, Cancer Ctr of Wake Forest Univ., Winston-Salem, NC, 27157, Univ. of Miami School of Medicine, Miami, FL, 33101.

Introduction: There is considerable experimental data supporting a role for $1\alpha,25$-dihydroxyvitamin D_3 [$1\alpha,25(OH)_2D_3$] in the growth regulation of prostate cells (1). Vitamin D receptor [VDR] is present in several cell lines derived from prostate carcinoma as well as in non-transformed primary cultures of prostatic cells, and $1\alpha,25(OH)_2D_3$ and its analogues exert antiproliferative and differentiating effects on these cells both *in vitro* and *in vivo*. These results clearly indicate a potential role for $1\alpha,25(OH)_2D_3$ and its analogues in prostate cancer prevention and therapy.

In 1992, Schwartz and colleagues demonstrated that mortality rates from prostate cancer were correlated ($p<0.0001$) inversely with the availability of ultraviolet radiation (2). The north-south gradient in prostate cancer mortality, and the high incidence in Blacks, is reminiscent of the vitamin D deficiency disease, rickets, suggesting that one cause of prostate cancer may be vitamin D insufficiency (2).

The serum levels of $1\alpha,25(OH)_2D$ are mainly derived from the action of renal 1α-OHase, which is tightly regulated by calcium, phosphorus and parathyroid hormone [PTH] and do not fluctuate significantly with changing levels of serum 25-hydroxyvitamin D [25(OH)D] under normal physiological conditions (3). Therefore, it was difficult to associate vitamin D deficiency with low circulating levels of 25(OH)D with prostate cancer mortality rates (2). One explanation for this dilemma is that prostatic cells have their own 25(OH)D-1α-hydroxylase [1α-OHase] that can convert $25(OH)D_3$ to $1\alpha,25(OH)_2D_3$. To test this hypothesis, we investigated three human prostate cancer cell lines (LNCaP, DU145 and PC-3) and primary cultures of cells derived from normal, and benign prostatic hyperplasia [BPH] for their ability to synthesize $1\alpha,25(OH)_2D_3$. We found that all those cells studied except LNCaP had 1α-OHase activity (4). In this report, we investigated (i) whether there was difference in enzyme activity among cultures obtained from normal, BPH, and cancerous prostatic cells, and (ii) whether an increase in enzyme activity by transfecting LNCaP cells with 1α-OHase cDNA plasmid would retard the cancer cell growth in the presence of $25(OH)D_3$.

Methods:

Cell cultures: Primary cultures of human prostatic epithelial cells were grown in a serum-free-defined medium PrEGM BulletKit [Clonetics, San Diego, CA] (4). The exact identity of whether the prostate sample obtained represents either, normal, BPH or cancerous tissue was determined by the final pathologic sectioning of a biopsy taken from the same region of the prostate. Prostatic cancer line LNCaP cells were cultured in DMEM medium supplemented with 5% FBS.

<u>1α-OHase activity determination</u>: 1α-OHase enzyme activity was determined on monolayer cultures in the presence of 50nM of ^{3}H-25(OH)D$_3$ containing 0.1 μCi radioactivity and 10 μM 1,2-dianilinoethane (DPPD), an anti-oxidant which prevents the free radical, non-enzymatic auto-oxidation of 25(OH)D to 1α,25(OH)$_2$D. ^{3}H-1α,25(OH)$_2$D$_3$ was separated from ^{3}H-25(OH)D$_3$ by HPLC using methylene chloride/isopropanol (19:1) solvent system and an Econosphere silica column (5μ particle size, 250 x 4.6 mm) with a flow rate of 0.5 ml/min as described previously (4).

<u>Cell proliferation assay</u>: ^{3}H-Thymidine incorporation and counting cell number were performed in the presence of 1α,25(OH)$_2$D$_3$ or 25(OH)D$_3$ as described (5).

<u>1α-OHase-cDNA plasmid construction and LNCaP cell transfection</u>: PCR mutagenesis was used to generate the 1α-OHase-GFP fusion construct from 1α-OHase cDNA as described (6). First, 1α-OHase(-stop) fragment was generated, and ligated into pCR3.1 T/A cloning vector, followed by ligating 1α-OHase(-stop).pCR3.1 to pEGFP vector (Invitrogen, San Diego, CA, USA). Transfection of 1α-OHase cDNA to cells was performed using liposome-mediated transfection kit (Lipofect AMINE PLUS, Cat. No. 10964-013, Life Technologies, Gaithersburg, MD). Twenty-four hrs after transfection, cells were dosed with 25(OH)D$_3$ and the biological effect of 25(OH)D$_3$ was studied by ^{3}H-thymidine proliferation assay. Controls without cDNA (mock-transfection), or vector (lipid control), or liposome were also performed.

Results and Discussion: A comparison of different primary cultures obtained from prostate cancer cells [CaP], BPH and three prostate cancer cell lines [LNCaP, DU145 and PC-3] with primary cultures from normal prostate cells illustrated that the normal prostates had higher 1α-OHase activity than cells from BPH, which in turn had higher 1α-OHase activity than prostate cancer cells (Figure 1). No activity could be detected in LNCaP cells.

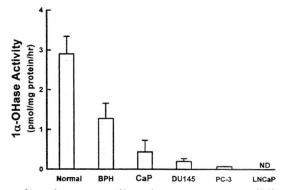

Figure 1. Synthesis of 1α,25(OH)$_2$D$_3$ by the primary cultures of normal, BPH, and prostate cancer cells (CaP), and by human prostate cancer cell lines, DU145, PC-3 and LNCaP cells. Bars shown are standard errors of 2-4 primary cultures from different donors.

Previously, we showed that 1α,25(OH)$_2$D$_3$ caused a dose-dependent inhibition in primary cultured prostate cells and prostate cancer cell line, LNCaP (5). We also showed that when primary cultures of prostate cancer cells were treated with 25(OH)D$_3$ or 1α,25(OH)$_2$D$_3$, the two compounds were equipotent in inhibiting the proliferation of prostate cancer cells at 10^{-7} M. If prostate cells had 1α-OHase activity, 25(OH)D$_3$ should be converted to 1α,25(OH)$_2$D$_3$ and cause an inhibition in prostate cell proliferation. Because 25(OH)D$_3$

has only 1/500 to 1/1000 of binding affinity for VDR as compared to $1\alpha,25(OH)_2D_3$, the most likely explanation of the results is that $25(OH)D_3$ was converted to $1\alpha,25(OH)_2D_3$ by 1α-OHase present in prostate cancer cells during the incubation.

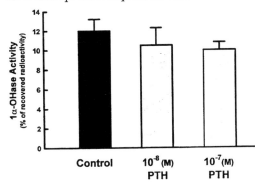

Figure 2. Regulation of 1α-OHase activity in the primary cultures of normal human prostate epithelial cells by PTH.

When primary cultured prostate cells were treated with PTH at 10^{-8} and 10^{-7} M for 24 hours, no significant effect on the 1α-OHase activity was observed (Figure 2), suggesting that the prostate 1α-OHase enzyme activity was not regulated by PTH.

In order to visualize and estimate the transfection efficiency, a human 1α-OHase-green fluorescence protein (GFP) fusion construct was transfected into LNCaP cells to examine the expression and the appearance of cellular distribution of the 1α-OHase-GFP fusion protein using scanning laser confocal microscopy. The fluorescence of the 1α-OHase-GFP protein in live transfected LNCaP cells showed a mitochondrial distribution, consistent with the location of the cytochrome P_{450}-1α-OHase (Data not shown).

Table 1. Effect of transfection of 1α-OHase cDNA into LNCaP cells on the conversion of ^{3}H-25(OH)D$_3$ to ^{3}H-$1\alpha,25(OH)_2D_3$ and ^{3}H-thymidine incorporation into DNA in the presence of 25(OH)D$_3$. *Means±SE of 3 determinations, ** Means±SE of 8 determinations.

Treatment	% Conversion ^{3}H-25(OH)D$_3$ to ^{3}H-$1\alpha,25(OH)_2D_3$*	^{3}H-Thymidine Incorporation** (% of control in the absence 10^{-8} M of 25(OH)D$_3$)
pCR 3.1 Vector or Antisense 1α-OHase cDNA	<1 %	100 ± 3 %
Sense 1α-OHase	36 ± 5 %	65 ± 6 %

To determine whether the expressed 1α-OHase-GFP was functional, we examined the efficiency in the conversion of ^{3}H-25(OH)D$_3$ to ^{3}H-$1\alpha,25(OH)_2D_3$ in LNCaP cells transfected with 1α-OHase cDNA plasmid and ^{3}H-thymidine incorporation into DNA in the presence of 25(OH)D$_3$. Table 1 demonstrates that LNCaP had little or no 1α-OHase activity and 25(OH)D$_3$ had no antiproliferative activity in LNCaP cells. However, there was more than 35-fold increase in the conversion of ^{3}H-25(OH)D$_3$ to ^{3}H-$1\alpha,25(OH)_2D_3$ in LNCaP cells transfected with 1α-OHase-cDNA plasmid compared to less than 1% conversion by LNCaP cells mock-transfected with pCR 3.1 vector alone. The LNCaP cells transfected with 1α-OHase-GFP showed similar conversion of ^{3}H-25(OH)D$_3$ to ^{3}H-$1\alpha,25(OH)_2D_3$ as the cells transfected with 1α-OHase-cDNA gene alone without the GFP tag (Data not shown). After we established that LNCaP cells transfected with 1α-OHase or 1α-OHase-GFP had enhanced the 1α-OHase activity, we evaluated whether the increased conversion of 25(OH)D$_3$ to 1α,25(OH)$_2$D$_3$ would result in an increased sensitivity to the antiproliferative effects of 10^{-8} M 25(OH)D$_3$. In Table 1, transfection with sense 1α-OHase cDNA plasmid into LNCaP cells caused a significant decrease in ^{3}H-thymidine incorporation (35±6% inhibition), compared to no inhibition in LNCaP cells transfected with antisense 1α-OHase cDNA (control).

In summary, the 1α-OHase activity in the prostate primary cultures showed a marked decrease from normal prostate to BPH to cancerous prostate cells. Unlike renal 1α-OHase, the 1α-OHase activity in prostate cells was not regulated by PTH. Confocal microscopy of live LNCaP cells transfected with 1α-OHase-GFP plasmid illustrated granualar appearance, consistent with the mitochondrial localization of the cytochrome P-450-1α-OHase. Furthermore, transfection of 1α-OHase cDNA into LNCaP cells enhanced the conversion of 25(OH)D$_3$ to 1α,25(OH)$_2$D$_3$, and therefore increased the antiproliferative activity of 25(OH)D$_3$. Thus, the results suggest that a defect in 1α-OHase activity and/or expression might be involved in the progression and metastatic potential of human prostate cancer. Increases in systemic levels of 25(OH)D could result in increased local production of 1α,25(OH)$_2$D in prostate, without producing hypercalcemia. The introduction of 1α-OHase gene to prostate cancer cells could offer a novel and less toxic approach for treating prostate cancer with vitamin D and 25(OH)D.

References:

1. Feldman D, Zhao XY, Krishnan AV. Vitamin D and prostate cancer. Endocrinology 141: 5-9, 2000.
2. Hanchett CL and Schwartz GG. Geographic patterns of prostate cancer mortality: Evidence for a protective effect of ultraviolet radiation. Cancer 70, 2861-2869, 1992.
3. Holick MF Vitamin D: photobiology, metabolism, and clinical applications. In:DeGroot L, Besser H, Burger HG, et al (eds) Endocrinology, 3rd Ed. W.B. Saundrs, Philadelphia, PA, U.S.A. pp.990-1013, 1995.
4. Schwartz GG, Whitlatch LW, Chen TC, Lokeshwar BL, Holick MF. Human prostate cells synthesize 1,25-dihydroxyvitamin D$_3$ from 25-hydroxyvitamin D$_3$. Cancer Epidemiol, Biomark & Prev. 7:391-395, 1998.
5. Chen TC, Schwartz GG, Burnstein KL, Lokeshwar BL, Holick MF. The in vitro evaluation of 25- hydroxyvitamin D$_3$ and 19-nor-1α,25-dihydroxyvitamin D$_3$ as therapeutic agents for prostate cancer. Clin Cancer Res 6:901-908, 2000.
6. Kong XF, Zhu XH, Pei YL, Jackson DM, Holick MF. Molecular cloning, characterization, and promoter analysis of the human 25-hydroxhvitamin D$_3$-1α-hydroxylase gene. Proc Natl Acad Sci 96:6988-6993, 1999.

Acknowledgements
This work was supported in part by grants 4118PP1017 and 41210067006 from The Commonwealth of Massachusetts, MO1RR00533, RO1CA68565, R01CA63108 from NIH and DAMD 17/98/8526 from US Army.

ANALYSIS OF 1,25-DIHYDROXYVITAMIN D3 RECEPTORS (VDR) IN SQUAMOUS CELL CARCINOMAS OF HUMAN SKIN

Arnold Wagner[1], Jörg Reichrath[1], Jörn Kamradt[1], Michael Friedrich[2], Wolfgang Tilgen[1], Michael F. Holick[3]. Departments of Dermatology and [2]Gynecology, University of Saarland, Homburg/Saar, Germany and [3]Vitamin D, Skin and Bone Research Laboratory, Boston University Medical Center, Boston, MA, U.S.A.

Introduction: Vitamin D3 is photochemically synthesized in the skin, that itself is a target for the active vitamin D metabolite 1,25-dihydroxyvitamin D3 (1). In vitro, $1,25(OH)_2D_3$ reduces the proliferation and regulates the terminal differentiation of cultured human keratinocytes (2). Additionally, this potent hormone acts on the immune system and has been shown to be effective in the treatment of hyperproliferative skin diseases such as psoriasis (3). Genomic actions of $1,25(OH)_2D_3$ are mediated through a nuclear vitamin D receptor (VDR) (4). The VDR belongs to the retinoid/thyroid/vitamin D subfamily of the steroid receptor superfamily of trans-acting transcriptional regulatory factors. Expression of VDR in significant amounts has been shown in many cell types present in human skin, including keratinocytes, Langerhans cells, monocytes/macrophages and activated T and B lymphocytes (5). The rat monoclonal antibody 9A7γ has been successfully applied for the immunohistochemical detection of VDR in frozen sections of many tissues including human skin (5). The aim of the present study was to analyze immunohistochemically expression of VDR in squamous cell carcinomas of human skin. For VDR is a major regulator of keratinocyte growth, it may be of importance for tumorigenesis and growth characteristics of squamous cell carcinomas (SCC). Additionally, combination of 1,25-dihydroxyvitamin D3 and isotretinoin was reported to be highly effective in the chemotherapy of precancerous and cancerous skin lesions (6).

Materials and Methods: *Skin specimens:* Normal human skin was obtained from the arms of eight patients (no history of skin disease), squamous cell carcinomas were obtained from 24 patients with informed consent. Histologic diagnosis was confirmed by a certified pathologist. All freshly excised specimens were embedded in OCT-Tissue Tek II (Miles Laboratories, Naperville, Illinois, U.S.A.), snap frozen in melting isopentane precooled in liquid nitrogen and stored at -80° C. *Immunohistochemical staining procedure:* VDR were visualized immunohistochemically using mAb 9A7γ. Additionally primary antibodies directed against Ki-67 protein and cytokeratin 10 were used. *Preparation of sections and fixation:* Serial sections (7 μm) were cut on a cryostat and mounted on glass slides that were derivatized by incubation with triethoxysilylpropylamin in dimethyl-sulfoxid and activated by 2% (v/v) glutardialdehyde. All frozen sections were fixed in 4% paraformaldehyde in PBS (10 min, room temperature [RT], rinsed in PBS (1 x 5 min), incubated in methanol (3 min, -20°C) and in acetone (1 min, -20°C), and transfered into PBS. *Immunohistochemical staining:* VDR were detected using a highly specific streptavidine peroxidase technique as described previously (7) or using Cy3[TM]-conjugated secondary antibodies for confocal laser scanning microscopy (Zeiss, Oberkochen, Germany, equipped with a helium-neon-laser [543 nm]).

530

Results: *Epidermis:* Epidermal VDR immunoreactivity was found in normal human skin that was absent when polyclonal rat IgG at the same concentration was used as a control. Immunoreactivity was found in nuclei of all cell layers of the viable epidermis. VDR-labelling was pronounced in lower epidermal cell layers, where almost every nucleus was VDR-positive. In upper epidermal cell layers (upper stratum spinosum, stratum granulosum) density of VDR-labelled cells appeared to be reduced. Isolated non specific staining in stratum corneum was noticed. *Epidermal appendages:* Strong VDR immunoreactivity was detected in the nuclei of cells of the pilosebaceous apparatus. VDR immunoreactivity was pronounced in the nuclei of the outer root sheath keratinocytes and heterogeneous in the keratinocytes of the inner root sheath. A majority of the eccrine sweat gland cells and sebaceous gland cells were VDR positive. *Dermis:* Skin immune cells, fibroblasts and cells of the cutaneous microvasculature were particularly VDR immunoreactive. *Squamous cell carcinomas:* VDR immunoreactivity was observed in all SCCs analyzed. Almost all tumor cells revealed consistently strong nuclear labeling for VDR. There was no visual difference comparing staining pattern for VDR in the different types of SCCs analyzed. In general, VDR expression was less pronounced in central tumor areas that revealed strong cytokeratin 10 immunoreactivity. VDR staining intensity was markedly pronounced in SCCs as compared to adjacent unaffected epidermis of the same section or as compared to normal human skin. Double staining experiments using VDR and Ki-67 antibodies revealed no comparable staining patterns.

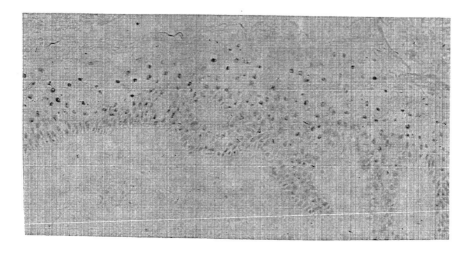

Figure 1:

Immunohistochemical demonstration of VDR (mAb 9A7γ) in normal human skin using streptavidin-peroxidase technique. Notice strong VDR-immunoreactivity in nuclei of all cell layers of the viable epidermis.

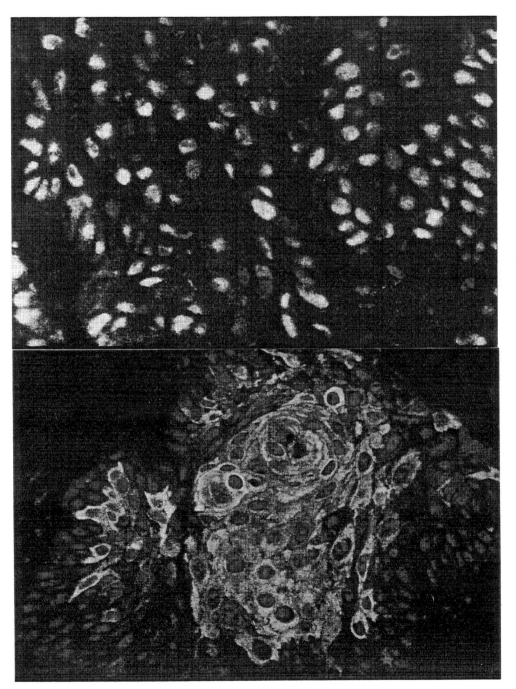

Figure 2:
Immunohistochemical demonstration of VDR (mAb 9A7γ, red label) and Ki-67 protein (up, green label) or cytokeratin 10 (down, green label) in SCCs using confocal laser scanning microscopy.

Discussion: To our knowledge, this is the first report analyzing immunohistochemically VDR expression in SCC of human skin. Interestingly, VDR staining intensity was much stronger in SCC as compared to unaffected epidermis of the same section or normal human skin, indicating upregulation of VDR expression in these tumor cells. Expression of VDR may be related to the growth of SCCs. Regulation of differentiation and proliferation by 1,25-dihydroxyvitamin D_3 and its corresponding receptor has been demonstrated in various cell types, including keratinocytes. Combination of 1,25-dihydroxyvitamin D_3 and isotretinoin was reported to be highly effective in the chemotherapy of precancerous and cancerous skin lesions, including actinic keratoses, cutaneous T-cell lymphomas, basal cell carcinomas and SCCs (6). The steroid hormone responsiveness is directly proportional to the number of corresponding receptors. Because VDR mediates the biological effects of 1,25-dihydroxyvitamin D_3 on cell proliferation and differentiation in target cells, VDR upregulation in SCCs indicates that new vitamin D analogues that exert less calcemic side effects may be effective in the treatment of these tumors

References:

1. HOLICK. M.F., SMITH, E., PINCUS S. (1987) *Arch. Dermatol.* **123,** 1677-1683

2. SMITH, E.L., WALWORTH, N.C., HOLICK, M.F. (1986) *J. Invest. Dermatol.* **86**, 709-14

3. HOLICK, M. F., (1987) *Arch. Dermatol.* **125,** 1692-1697

4. DARWISH, H., DeLuca, H.F.(1993) *Crit. Rev. Eukaryot Gene Expr.*3, 89-116

5. MILDE, P., HAUSER, U., SIMON, T., MALL, G., ERNST, V., HAUSSLER, M. R., FROSCH, P., RAUTERBERG, E. W. (1991) *J. Invest. Dermatol.* **97**, 230-39

6. MAJEWSKI, S., SKOPINSKA, M., BOLLAG, W., JABLONSKA, S. (1994) *Lancet* **344**, 1510-1511.

7. KAMRADT, J., REICHRATH, J. (1996) J Histochem Cytochem **44**, 1415-1420.

INTERACTION OF VITAMIN D ANALOG CB 1093 WITH BISPHOSPHONATES AND DEXAMETHASONE ON HUMAN MULTIPLE MYELOMA CELLS

SG Senaratne and KW Colston. Dept. Oncology, Gastroenterology, Endocrinology and Metabolism, St George's Hospital Medical School, London, UK

INTRODUCTION

Multiple myeloma is a form of human cancer caused by an accumulation of neoplastic plasma cells and is frequently associated with bone disease involving osteolytic lesions, osteoporosis, pathological fractures and hypercalcaemia. The treatment of multiple myeloma has not progressed significantly over recent years. In addition to the use of cytotoxic chemotherapy, treatment options include glucocorticoids and bisphosphonates. Novel analogs of vitamin D inhibit growth and promote apoptosis in number of cancer cell types. Little is known about effects of vitamin D as a therapeutic agent for multiple myeloma. Since malignant plasma cells express the vitamin D receptor (1). we investigated whether the novel vitamin D analog CB 1093 could directly reduce viability of myeloma cells. Treatment with bisphosphonates has been reported to provide significant protection against skeletal complications and improve quality of life in patients with advanced multiple myeloma (2). Both pamidronate and the novel bisphosphonate YM175 have been shown to cause cell cycle arrest and apoptosis in human myeloma cells in vitro (3). Therefore we investigated whether CB 1093 could enhance apoptosis in combination with bisphosphonates (pamidronate and zoledronate) in multiple myeloma cells. Glucocorticoids (dexamethasone) are among the most effective agents in treating myeloma (4). Although dexamethasone has a clear anti-tumoral effects on multiple myeloma, some patients do not responds to this treatment. It has been suggested that Interleukin-6 (IL-6) may counteract the anti-proliferative effects of dexamethasone (5). Therefore we determined whether CB 1093 could potentiate the cytotoxic effects of dexamethasone alone and in the presence of IL-6.

MATERIALS AND METHODS

Compounds: Pamidronate (APD) and zoledronate were obtained from Novartis Pharmaceuticals Limited. CB 1093 was a gift from Leo Pharmaceutical Products. Dexamethasone and Interleukin-6 were obtained from Sigma Chemical Co. Bisphosphonates were dissolved in PBS. CB 1093 and dexamethasone were dissolved in absolute ethanol and IL-6 was dissolved in PBS containing 0.1% BSA. The human myeloma cell line RPMI 8226 was obtained from the ECACC. _Cell cultures:_ The myeloma cell line was maintained in RPMI 1640 supplemented with 100 U/ml penicillin, 100mg/ml streptomycin and 10% FCS. _MTS assay:_ Cell viability was determined by MTS dye-reduction assay measuring mitochondrial respiratory function (6). Myeloma cells (1×10^3/ well) were plated in 96 well plates and treated with or without the reagents. Cells were incubated with MTS dye for 2h. _Western blotting for bcl-2 and PARP:_ Myeloma cell cultures treated with APD (50µM), CB 1093 (25nM) alone or in combination were harvested and lysed in lysis buffer.

534

Equivalent protein extracts (15 µg) from each sample were electrophoresed on 10% SDS-PAGE mini gels. Total protein was quantitated by the method of Bradford (7). Mouse monoclonal antibodies against bcl-2 giving a protein band at 28kD (Santa Cruz) and a rabbit polyclonal antibody to PARP (Boehringer Mannheim) was used. Bcl-2 was detected by horseradish peroxidase-conjugated secondary antibodies to anti-mouse immunoglobulins and for PARP cleavage secondary antibodies to anti-rabbit immunoglobulins. *DNA fragmentation assay:*

Myeloma cells were incubated with [^{3}H-*methyl*]-thymidine (0.1mCi/ml) for 9 to 16 h to label DNA and then washed before exposure to the indicated treatment. Cells were lysed with lysis buffer (10mM Tris (pH 7.4), 10mM EDTA and 0.2% Triton-x100) and, fragmented double stranded DNA was separated from chromosome-length unfragmented DNA by centrifugation followed by TCA precipitation (8). Incorporated radiolabel was determined by liquid scintillation counting using the formula:% fragmented DNA=100 x (fragmented/fragmented + intact chromatin) (8).

RESULTS

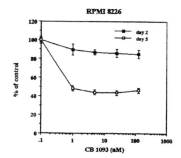

Figure 1. Effects of CB 1093 on cell viability of RPMI 8226 cells.

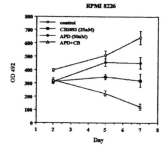

Figure 2. Combined effect of APD And CB 1093 on cell viability.

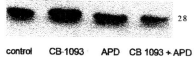

control   CB-1093   APD   CB 1093 + APD

Figure 3. Combined effect of APD and CB1093 on expression of bcl-2 protein

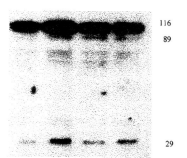

cont   CB1093 APD   CB 1093+APD

Figure 4. Identification of the proteolytic cleavage of PARP.

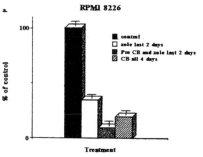

Figure 5a. Effects of pretreatment with CB 1093 reduction of cell viability.

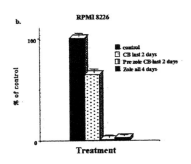

Figure 5b. Effects of pretreatment with zoledronate on reduction of cell viability

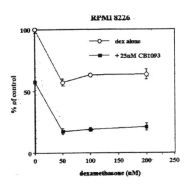

Figure 6. Effects CB1093 and dexamethasone on cell viability.

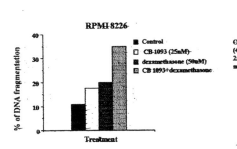

Figure 7. Combined effect of CB 1093 and dexamethasone on induction of DNA fragmentation.

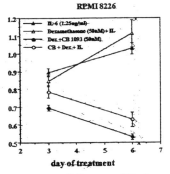

Figure 8. Effects of IL-6 on cell viability of RPMI 8226 cells treated with 50nM dexamethasone and 25nM CB 1093.

RPMI 8226 cells were treated with 1, 5, 25 and 125nM of CB 1093 for up to 5 days. A significant dose dependent reduction in cell viability was seen at day 5 (Figure 1). RPMI 8226 cells were treated with or without 50µM APD, 25nM CB 1093 and both treatments together for up to 7 days respectively. CB 1093 and APD reduced cell viability and an enhanced effect was observed with combined treatment (Figure 2). To assess the effects of combined bisphosphonate and vitamin D analog treatment on expression of the oncoprotein bcl-2 in myeloma cells, RPMI 8226 cells were treated for up to 3 days with 50µM APD, 25nM CB 1093 alone and in combination. Level of expression of bcl-2 protein was determined by Western analysis. APD treatment led to a decrease in bcl-2 expression which was enhanced by co-treatment with CB 1093 (Figure 3). Proteolytic cleavage of PARP as a consequence of activation of caspases is a key feature of apoptosis (9). PARP cleavage consistent with caspase activation was observed in extracts of RPMI 8226 cells incubated with 50µM APD, 25nM CB 1093 and also with combined treatment. Cells were incubated with the agents for 3 days and cleavage of the 116kD molecule was determined by Western analysis. We demonstrate a decrease in the 116kD intact PARP and an appearance of a 29kD fragment in all three treatments *(Figure 4)*. Two groups of RPMI 8226 cells were a) pre-treated with or without 25nM CB 1093 for the first 2 days and the last 2 days one group was in addition treated with 50µM zoledronate. b) pre-treated with or without 50µM zoledronate for the first 2 days and the last 2 days one group was in addition treated with 25nM CB 1093. The most effective treatment regimen was pre-treatment with zoledronate followed by the combined treatment for the last two days *(Figure 5b)*. RPMI 8226 cells were treated with increasing concentrations of dexamethasone with or without 25nM CB 1093 for 3 days. CB 1093 significantly enhanced the inhibition effect of dexamethasone on viability of myeloma cells *(Figure 6)*. To assess the effects of combined vitamin D analog and dexamethasone treatment on induction of DNA fragmentation in myeloma cells, RPMI 8226 cells were treated for 4 days with 25nM CB 1093, 50nM dexamethasone alone and in combination. In RPMI 8226 cells, CB 1093 and dexamethasone induced DNA fragmentation and an enhanced effect was observed with combined treatment *(Figure 7)*. RPMI 8226 cells were treated with 1.25ng/ml IL-6, with 50nM dexamethasone, 50nM CB 1093 with 50nM dexamethasone and IL-6 with both CB 1093 and dexamethasone for up to 6 days. IL-6 completely prevented the inhibitory effects of dexamethsone on myeloma cell viability. However the resistance to dexamethasone induced apoptosis in the presence of IL-6 was prevented by co-treatment with CB 1093 *(Figure 8)*.

CONCLUSIONS
The vitamin D analog CB 1093 has direct inhibitory effects on RPMI 8226 myeloma cells by significantly reducing the cell viability. CB 1093 induces apoptosis in RPMI 8226 myeloma cells and potentiates effects of APD. Apoptosis is associated with the down regulation of bcl-2 protein and cleavage of PARP, suggesting involvement of caspases. Pre-treatment with either CB 1093 or zoledronate potentiated combined effects of these agents. Pre-treatment with zoledronate for 2 days followed by zoledronate/CB 1093 treatment for further 2 days is the most effective treatment regimen. CB 1093 potentiates the cytotoxic effects of dexamethasone and attenuated the inhibitory effects of IL-6 on dexamethasone induced apoptosis. This study suggests that the vitamin D analogs could have therapeutic potential in multiple myeloma, particularly if combined with glucocorticoids or bisphosphonates.

REFERENCES
1. Rossi JF, Durie BG, Duperray C, et al (1988). Cancer Res. 48 (5):1213-6.
2 Berenson JR, Lichtenstein A, Poter L, et al (1996) N Engl J Med 334 (8):488-93.
3. Shipman CM, Rogers MJ, Apperley JF, et al (1997) Br J Haematol. 98: 665-672
4. Salmon SE, Shadduck RK, Schilling A. (1967). Cancer Chemother Rep. 51:179.
5. Puthier D, Bataille R, Barille S et al. (1996) Blood 88(12): 4659-66.
6. Cory AH, Owen TC, Barltrop JA, Cory JG. (1991).Cancer Commun 3(7):207-12.
7. Bradford M, (1976) Analyt Biochem. 72:248-54.
8. Duke RC, et al (eds). (1992) Current protocols in Immunology (suppl.3) 3.17. 1-3.17.16. New York: Green/Wiley.

EFFECTS OF 1,25-DIHYDROXYVITAMIN D$_3$ [1,25(OH)$_2$D$_3$] AND ITS ANALOGUES (EB1089 AND ANALOG V) ON CANINE ADENOCARCINOMA (CAC-8) IN NUDE MICE.

S. Kunakornsawat[1], T.J. Rosol[1], C.C. Capen[1], G.S. Reddy[2], L. Binderup[3], and N. Inpanbutr[1]. [1]Dept. of Veterinary Biosciences, OH. [2]School of Medicine, Brown University, RI. [3]Leo Pharmaceutical Products, Ballerup, Denmark.

Introduction Recently the active form of vitamin D, 1,25(OH)$_2$D$_3$, and its synthetic analogues have been shown to exert anti-tumor effects both *in vitro* and *in vivo* (1-2). However, most studies have been done in human tumors. There is little information on the effects of 1,25(OH)$_2$D$_3$ on tumors in other species. This study examined the effects of 1,25(OH)$_2$D$_3$ and its analogues [22,24-diene-24a,26a,27a-trihomo-1α,25-dihydroxyvitamin D$_3$ (EB1089) and 1,25-dihydroxy-16ene-23-yne-vitamin D$_3$ (analog V)] on canine adenocarcinoma (CAC-8) in nude mice. It is well documented that parathyroid hormone-related protein (PTHrP) causes hypercalcemia in dogs with this carcinoma (3). The inhibitory effect of 1,25(OH)$_2$D$_3$ and its analogues on PTHrP production thus for have reported on both normal human cells (4) and human tumor cells (5). In order to achieve the inhibitory effect of 1,25(OH)$_2$D$_3$ on PTHrP production, high doses and/or prolonged treatment with this potent active vitamin D metabolite most likely will be needed, which has the potential to enhance the hypercalcemia. In order to minimize this potential toxic effect vitamin D analogues have been synthesized with noncalcemic effect. Among these noncalcemic analogues, EB1089 and analog V, have been extensively studies on tumor growth (1-2,6). The objectives of this study were to (a) investigate the distribution of the 1,25(OH)$_2$D$_3$ receptor (VDR) in the CAC-8 carcinoma; (b) evaluate effects of 1,25(OH)$_2$D$_3$ and its analogues on tumor growth and body weight; (c) determine plasma ionized calcium; and (d) examine bone resorption and number of osteoclasts/mm of endosteal surface in lumbar vertebrae of nude mice-bearing the CAC-8 adenocarcinoma.

Methods Thirty-seven male nude mice were injected subcutaneously between the scapulae with CAC-8 tumor tissues. Two weeks after injections, mice were divided into 5 groups (Grps) and injected intraperitoneally 3 times per week with 5 different substances. Grp I was nontumor-bearing mice injected with vehicle (0.1 ml/mouse). Grps II to V were all tumor-bearing mice injected with these following substances; II — vehicle (0.1 ml/mouse), III — analog V (1.5 µg/mouse), IV — 1,25(OH)$_2$D$_3$ (0.05 µg/mouse), and V — EB1089 (0.01 µg/mouse) for up to 4 weeks. Tumor size and body weight were determined 3 times per week. After euthanasia tissues were analyzed for 1,25(OH)$_2$D$_3$ receptor (VDR), bone resorption and number of osteclasts. Blood plasma was analyzed for ionized calcium.

Results **Histopathology.** Histologic evaluation of CAC-8 revealed a bimorphic pattern in the adenocarcinoma with the formation of glandular acini containing eosinophilic secretory material interspersed with solid area of neoplastic cells. There were no histopathologic differences in CAC-8 between groups of animals. Mineralization at the corticomedullary region of the kidney was present in some mice, but was not limited to any particular group. Microscopic lesions or tumor metastases were not found in the liver and lung, or elsewhere.

VDR distribution in the CAC-8 adenocarcinoma: Immunohistochemical staining of CAC-8 with VDR-antibody demonstrated positive peroxidase reaction in nuclei of carcinoma cells (Figures 1A, 1B).

Tumor volume. Tumor volumes of CAC-8-bearing mice treated with $1,25(OH)_2D_3$ and its analogues were numerically smaller than vehicle-treated CAC-8-bearing mice; however, the differences in tumor volume (%change) were not statistically significant ($P<0.05$) (Figure 2).

Body weight The body weights (% change) of CAC-8-bearing mice were significantly lower than those of nontumor-bearing mice ($P<0.05$) (Figure 3). There was a significant difference in body weight gain between control CAC-8-bearing mice treated with vehicle and CAC-8-bearing mice treated with EB1089 at Day 14 (Figure 3). CAC-8-bearing mice treated with analog V maintained their body weight better than CAC-8-bearing mice treated with either vehicle, $1,25(OH)_2D_3$, or EB1089 (Figure 3).

Hypercalcemia: The plasma level of ionized calcium [$Ca^{++}(mg/dl)$] was greater in all tumor-bearing mice (Grp II = 8.9±0.87, Grp III = 9.02±1.38, Grp IV = 9.34±1.64, Grp V = 9.0±1.41) compared to nontumor-bearing mice (Grp I = 4.89±0.14) (Table 1).

Bone resorption: Histomorphometric evaluation of lumbar vertebrae stained for tartrate-resistant acid phosphatase showed a significant increase in bone resorption and number of osteoclasts/mm of endosteal surface in CAC-8-bearing mice as compared to nontumor-bearing mice ($P<0.001$) (Table 2, Figures 4A, 4B). There were no significant differences in bone resorption and number of osteoclasts/mm of endosteal surface in all CAC-8-bearing mice treated with vehicle, analog V, $1,25(OH)_2D_3$ and EB1089 ($p<0.05$) (Table 2).

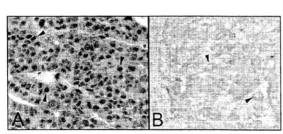

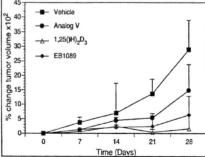

Figure1 (A) Immunoperoxidase labeling of $1,25(OH)_2D_3$ receptor (VDR) from CAC-8 adenocarcinoma transplanted mouse treated with vehicle. The tumor section was stained with monoclonal anti-VDR demonstrated a positive labeling in all nuclei of tumor cells (arrowheads), (B) Control section was reacted with non-specific antiserum in place of a specific primary antibody. The absence of reaction product in the nuclei of tumor cells (arrowheads) indicates the reaction observed with anti-VDR is due to the presence of authentic VDR. Original magnification x 300

Figure 2 Percent change in tumor volume of CAC-8-bearing mice administered intraperitoneally (per mouse) 3 times per week (4 treatments) vehicle at 0.1ml, analog V at 1.5 µg, $1,25(OH)_2D_3$ at 0.05 µg, or EB1089 at 0.01 µg. Each point represents the mean ± standard error of the mean (SEM).

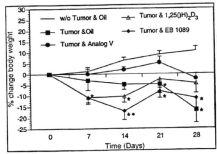

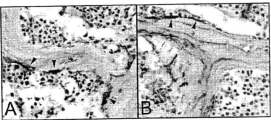

Figure 3 Percent change in body weight gain in mice administered 1,25(OH)₂D₃ and its analogues (EB1089 and analog V). Normal nontumor-bearing mice were injected with vehicle alone. Results are expressed as percent change from Day 0. Each time point represents the mean ± standard error of the mean (SEM). Significant differences in mice body weight from control nontumor-bearing mice at each time point are represented by asterisks (* p< 0.05). A significant difference in mice body weight from control CAC-8-bearing mice treated with vehicle is represented by period (• p< 0.05).

Figure 4 Lumbar vertebrae from nude mice stained for tartrate-resistant acid phosphatase-positive osteoclasts (TRAP). (A) CAC-8-bearing nude mouse administered EB1089 for 4 weeks. Note the numerous osteoclasts on the endosteal surface (arrowheads), (B) Nontumor-bearing control nude mouse. There are few osteoclasts on the endosteal surfaces (arrowheads).

TREATMENT	Plasma Ionized Calcium (mg/dl) (Mean ± SD)
Nontumor-bearing mice + Vehicle	4.89 ± 0.14
CAC-8-bearing mice + Vehicle	8.99 ± 0.87
CAC-8-bearing mice + Analog V	9.02 ± 1.38
CAC-8-bearing mice + 1,25(OH)₂D₃	9.34 ± 1.64
CAC-8-bearing mice + EB1089	9.00 ± 1.41

Table 1 Plasma levels of ionized calcium levels in CAC-8-bearing and nontumor-bearing mice either administered Vitamin D analogues or vehicle.

Group	Endosteal perimeter (mm)	Osteoclast perimeter (mm)	% Resorptive perimeter (%)	Osteoclasts /mm
Nontumor-bearing mice controls (n=5)	7.82±1.9	0.34±0.07	4.68±0.8	1.63±0.3
CAC-8-bearing mice + Vehicle (n=6)	5.7±0.9	1.05±0.2	18.44±1.5	5.1±0.5
CAC-8-bearing mice + Analog V (n=6)	7.01±1.0	1.14±0.2	16.68±2.7	3.85±0.6
CAC-8-bearing mice+1,25(OH)₂D₃ (n=4)	6.97±1.8	1.49±0.4	21.72±1.6	5.35±0.5
CAC-8-bearing mice + EB1089 (n=8)	7.58±0.8	1.67±0.2	21.53±1.4	5.46±0.4

Table 2 Histomorphometric evaluation of lumbar vertebrae from CAC-8-bearing mice, and nontumor-bearing mice either administered Vitamin D analogues or vehicle (mean ± SEM).

<u>Discussion</u> The results of the current study demonstrated a numerical reduction of tumor volume in CAC-8-bearing mice treated with 1,25(OH)₂D₃ and its analogues (EB1089 and analog V). CAC-8-bearing mice treated with analog V maintained body weight gain better than other CAC-8-bearing groups with hypercalcemia. These mice also were more active than other CAC-8-bearing groups and did not have the toxic side effects of hypercalcemia despite an increase in plasma ionized calcium comparable to nontumor-bearing mice (Table 1). In addition, only a single mouse from the analog V-treatment group (Grp III) became clinically ill and had to be sacrificed because of weight loss, anorexia, depression, and dehydration. In contrast, mice from other CAC-8-bearing groups had to be sacrificed at days 11 (from Grps II and V) and at days 14 and 18 (from Grps IV and V). A previous study reported that analog V (1.6μg/mouse)-treated mice with myeloid leukemia had a significantly longer survival time than those

treated with $1,25(OH)_2D_3$ (0.1µg/mouse) with a diminished hypercalcemic effect (1). The same study reported that $1,25(OH)_2D_3$ and its analogues also inhibited leukemia cell growth and differentiation *in vitro* (1). Analog V may need to be administered at a higher dose for a longer interval in order to achieve a significant reduction in tumor volume. In the present study, EB1089 and analog V failed to lower plasma ionized calcium concentration. In contrast, a previous study reported that treatment with EB1089 (0.05 µg/kg/day) in rats with nitrosomethylurea-induced tumors significantly inhibited tumor growth without changing serum calcium levels. It appears that effective treatment of neoplasms with noncalcemic vitamin D analogues relys on many factors, including the type of tumor, dosage of analogue, route of administration, and duration of treatment. The specific mechanism by which $1,25(OH)_2D_3$ and its analogues inhibit tumor growth at present is unclear. Therefore, it is possible that feeding a low calcium diet during the experimental period in future studies will permit the use of a higher dose of vitamin D analogues for longer intervals and obtain a greater inhibitory effect on tumor growth.

Humoral hypercalcemia of malignancy has been reported to be associated with increased osteoclastic bone resorption and hypercalcemia (2,7). In our study we also found a significant increase in percent resorption perimeter and number of osteoclasts/mm of endosteal surface in lumbar vertebral of tumor-bearing mice with hypercalcemia as compared to nontumor-bearing controls (P<0.001). The results of our study revealed that $1,25(OH)_2D_3$ and its noncalcemic analogues did not decrease osteoclastic bone resorption on CAC-8-tumor-bearing mice.

In conclusion, this study demonstrated that CAC-8-bearing mice treated with analog V had a greater effect in maintaining body weight and were more active than other CAC-8-bearing groups. Analog V-treated mice also showed no toxic side effects of hypercalcemia despite an increase in plasma ionized calcium comparable to nontumor-bearing mice. Tumor volumes of CAC-8-bearing mice treated with $1,25(OH)_2D_3$ and its analogues were smaller than vehicle-treated CAC-8-bearing mice, suggesting an inhibitory effect on tumor cell growth.

References
1. Zhou, J.Y., Norman, A.W., Dan-Lin, C., Guo-wen, S., Uskokovic, M. and Koeffler, H.P. (1990) Proc. Natl. Acad. Sci. USA 87, 3929-3932.
2. Haq, M., Kremer, R., Goltzman, D. and Rabbani, S.A. (1993) J. Clin. Invest. 91, 2416-2422.
3. Rosol, T.J., Nagode, L.A., Couto, C.G., Hammer, A.S., Chew, D.J., Peterson, J.L., Ayl, R.D., Steinmeyer, C.L. and Capen, C.C. (1992) Endocrinology 131, 1157-1164.
4. Sebag, M., Henderson, J., Goltzman, D. and Kremer, R. (1994) Am. J. Physiol. 267, C723-C730.
5. Falzon, M. and Zong, J. (1998) Endocrinology 139, 1046-1053.
6. Colston, K.W., Mackay, A.G., James, S.Y., Binderup, I. Chander, S. and Coombes, R.C. (1992) Biochem. Pharmacol. 44, 2273-2280.
7. Rosol, T.J., Capen, C.C., Weisbrode, S.E. and Horst, R.L. (1986) Lab. Invest. 54, 679-688.

VITAMIN D₃ AND ANALOGUES INHIBIT THE DIFFERENTIATION OF HUMAN MONOCYTE-DERIVED DENDRITIC CELLS

Kejian Zhu#, Ulrich Zügel*, and Ulrich Mrowietz#, #Department of Dermatology, University of Kiel and *Department of Experimental Dermatology, Schering AG, Berlin, Germany

Introduction Dendritic cells (DC) represent a population of cells crucial for presentation of antigen and for initiation and stimulation of an antigen-specific immune response. These cells develop from CD34-positive myeloid progenitor cells or from peripheral blood monocytes after treatment with granulocyte macrophage-colony stimulating factor (GM-CSF) and interleukin 4 (IL-4) (1). Monocyte-derived dendritic cells (MoDC) are also termed immature or inflammatory-type DC. They can be further differentiated into mature DC by stimuli such as tumor-necrosis-factor alpha, or lipopolysaccharide (LPS). Antigen-specific immune responses against foreign or auto-antigens are the basis for a number of human disorders such as diabetes, rheumatoid arthritis or multiple sclerosis (2). In transplant patients the rejection of allografts depend mostly on the activity of antigen-presenting cells (APC) and subsequent immune responses leading to graft rejection. In psoriasis, a common inflammatory and hyperproliferative cutaneous disorder, the T-cell dominated immune response is thought to be mediated by antigen-presenting DC (3). Since these cells do not proliferate in situ, the influx of monocytes with subsequent differentiation into MoDC may be responsible for initiation and maintenance of the immune response. Vitamin D₃ is a secosteroid hormone and its active metabolite, calcitriol, is crucial for the regulation of calcium and phosphate homeostasis. It has been shown, that calcitriol is able to induce differentiation and to inhibit proliferation in various cell types such as leukemia cells, keratinocytes and lymphocytes (4,5). In peripheral blood mononuclear cells (PBMC) calcitriol was shown to potently inhibit mitogen-stimulated lymphocyte proliferation (6). Recently, calcitriol was found to be therapeutically effective in animal models for multiple sclerosis and heart transplant rejection (7;8). Furthermore, vitamin D₃ analogues are widely used for topical treatment of psoriasis (9). We have addressed the question whether calcitriol may interfere with the differentiation of monocytes into DC.

Material and Methods

Generation of DC MoDC were generated by incubation of highly purified human monocytes obtained by counterflow centrifugation elutriation in medium RPMI 1640 with 10% FCS, GM-CSF (100 U/ml) and IL-4 (10 ng/ml) for 5 days.

Vitamin D₃ and analogues Calcitriol $(1,25(OH)_2D_3)$, its analogues calcipotriol and tacalcitol, as well as the low-affinity vitamin D-receptor agonist $24,25\ (OH)_2D_3$ were dissolved in ethanol and added to the monocyte cultures from the beginning. Calcitriol was used in concentrations from 10^{-8} to 10^{-13} mol/l, the other compounds were used at 10^{-8} mol/l. An ethanol solvent control (0.1%, v/v) was always included.

Flow cytometry analysis The expression of surface molecules on MoDC was taken as a phenotypic marker for DC differentiation. Antibodies against the following epitopes were used: CD1a, CD14, CD86, HLA-DR. The expression of these markers was measured by single fluorescence staining using a Coulter Epics XL flow cytometer.

Mixed lymphocyte reaction To determine the antigen-presenting capacity of MoDC as a functional activity of DC development the mixed lymphocyte reaction (MLR) was used with allogeneic as well as autologous responder cells. MoDC after 5 days of culture were mixed with allogeneic PBMC obtained after Ficoll-Paque centrifugation of human venous blood using a MoDC:PBMC ratio of 1:2. After four days of co-culture cells were pulsed with [^{3}H]thymidin and lymphocyte proliferation measured after 24hours in a scintillation counter as incorporation of radioactive thymidin.

Results

Effect of vitamin D_3 and analogues on the phenotype of MoDC The expression of the surface markers CD1a and CD14 was used as a read-out for DC differentiation. GM-CSF/IL-4 treatment of monocytes for 5 days up-regulated CD1a- and down-regulated CD14-expression as shown in fig. 1. Addition of calcitriol during the time of culture completely inhibited this effect (fig. 1). The solvent ethanol and 24,25(OH)$_2$D$_3$ were without effect. Furthermore, expression of CD86 and HLA-DR was also decreased after calcitriol treatment (fig. 1). In fig. 2 the dose-dependent effect of calcitriol, its analogues calcipotriol and tacalcitol are shown. All three compounds inhibited CD1a- and up-regulated CD14-expression with an IC$_{50}$ of 10^{-10} mol/l. The solvent ethanol was without effect.

Effect of calcitriol on the MLR To assess the antigen-stimulating capacity of MoDC an allogeneic MLR was performed. After 5 days of culture with GM-CSF/IL-4 MoDC were able to induce lymphocyte proliferation as measured by [^{3}H]thymidin-incorporation (fig. 3). After treatment with calcitriol a dose-dependent decrease in lymphocyte proliferation was noted indicating a reduced antigen-presenting capacity. Calcitriol and tacalcitol equally inhibited MLR as compared to calcitriol.

Discussion Beside its function as regulatory hormone for calcium and phosphate homeostasis, calcitriol was shown to have a number of activities on immunological processes. Our results demonstrate, that calcitriol as well as its analogues calcipotriol and tacalcitol completely inhibit the GM-CSF/IL-4-induced differentiation of human monocytes into DC. This was indicated by the inhibition of CD1a-expression, a marker for DC development, and for the up-regulation of the monocyte/ macrophage marker CD14, the ligand for the complex of LPS and LPS-binding protein. The effect of calcitriol was dose-dependent with an IC$_{50}$ as low as 10^{-10} mol/l. Calcipotriol and tacalcitol, vitamin D_3 analogues used effectively in the topical treatment of psoriasis, showed the same effect. The expression of CD86 (B7-2) and HLA-DR were also found to be decreased by calcitriol. However, the low-affinity VDR-agonist 24,25(OH)$_2$D$_3$ as well as the solvent ethanol did not inhibit MoDC-differentiation.

The effect of vitamin D_3 and analogues on the phenotype of MoDC was paralleled by functional changes as measured by the ability of MoDC to stimulate lymphocyte proliferation in the MLR. Calcitriol dose-dependently inhibited the antigen-stimulating capacity of MoDC resulting in a decreased lymphocyte proliferation as compared to the medium and ethanol control. APC are crucial for initiation and regulation of specific immune responses. In disease states foreign or auto-antigens are often responsible for tissue or organ damage. DC are the most potent antigen-presenting cells. In vitro they can be differentiated from peripheral blood monocytes after stimulation with GM-CSF and IL-4 (10). Inhibition of DC development is an effective measure to decrease T-cell dominated immune responses. Since calcitriol was shown to be effective in animal models of autoimmune encephalitis, inflammatory joint disease as well as in transplant models our data seem to indicate that the effect of this compound is due to the inhibition of DC differentiation and subsequent inhibition of T-cell mediated immune responses.

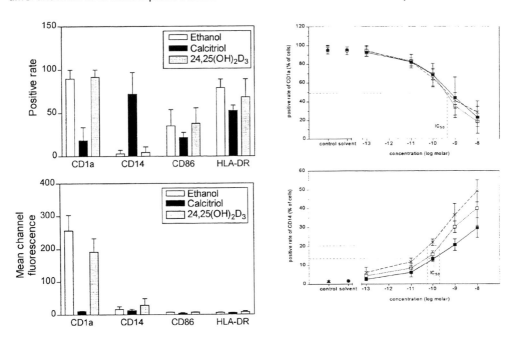

Figure 1: Expression of surface molecules CD1a, CD14, CD86 and HLA-DR in human MoDC treated with calcitriol 10^{-8} mol/l, $24,25(OH)_2D_3$ 10^{-8} mol/l and ethanol (0.1%, v/v) after 5 days of culture as determined by single fluorescence flow cytometry. Mean and SD, n=5.

Figure 2: Concentration-dependent down-regulation of CD1a- and up-regulation of CD14- expression in MoDC by calcitriol, calcipotriol and tacalcitol. Monocytes were cultured for 5 days in the prescence of a solvent (ethanol) control or various concentrations of calcitriol and its analogues. The IC_{50} of calcitriol, calcipotriol and tacalcitol is about $5x$ 0^{-10} mol/l for CD1a and about 10^{-10} mol/l for CD14. Mean and SD, n=5. - ■ - Calcitrol, - □ - Calcipotriol, - X - Tacalcitol.

544

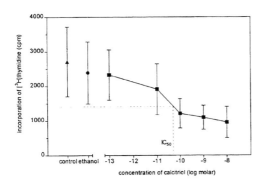

Figure 3: Proliferation of allogeneic lymphocytes after three days of co-culture with MoDC treated with calcitriol (10^{-8} to 10^{-13} mol/l), ethanol (0.1%, v/v) or medium alone for 5 days prior to the addition of PBMC. results are expressed as counts per minute (cpm). Mean and SD, n=3.

Literature

1. Steinman, R.M. (1991). Annu Rev Immunol. 9:271-296.
2. Drakesmith, H., Chain, B. and Beverley, P. 2000. Immunol Today. 21:214-217.
3. Nestle, F.O, Turka, L.A. and Nickoloff, B.J. 1994. J. Clin. Invest. 94:202-209.
4. Munker, R., Kobayashi, T., Elstner, E., Norman, A.W., Uskokovic, M., Zhang, W., Andreeff, M. and Koeffler, H.P. 1996. Blood. 88:2201-2209.
5. Bikle, D.D. 1996. J. Invest. Dermatol. Symp. Proc. 1:22-27.
6. Rigby, W.F., Stacy, T. and Fanger, M.W. 1984. J. Clin. Invest. 74:1451-1455.
7. Cantorna, M.T., Woodward, W.D., Hayes, C.E. and DeLuca, H.F. 1998. J. Immunol. 160:5314-5319.
8. Hullett, D.A., Cantorna, M.T., Redaelli, C., Humpal-Winter, J., Hayes, C.E., Sollinger, H.W. and DeLuca, H.F. 1998. Transplantation. 66:824-828.
9. Van de Kerkhof, P.C. 1998. Skin Pharmacol. Appl. Skin Physiol.11:2-10.
10. Peters, J.H., Gieseler, R., Thiele, B., Steinbach, F. 1996. Immunol. Today 17:273-278.
11. Penna, G. and Adorini, L. 2000. J. Immunol. 164:2405-2411.
12. Griffin, M.D., Lutz, W.H., Phan, V.A., Bachman, L.A., McKean, D.J. and Kumar, R. 2000. Biochem. Biophys. Res. Commun. 270:701-708.

Note After the abstract for this poster was submitted Penna and Adorini (11) as well as Griffin et.al. (12) fully confirmed our data using human monocytes and murine macrophages, respectively.

IMMUNOLOGY

INHIBITION OF ALLO AND XENOGRAFT REJECTION BY 1,25-DIHYDROXYVITAMIN D₃ AND THE ANALOGUE Ro 26-2198

Silvia Gregori[1], Mara Casorati[2], Giuseppe Penna[1], Susana Amuchastegui[1], Simona Smiroldo[1], Federico Bertuzzi[2], Milan Uskokovic[3], Alberto M. Davalli[2] and Luciano Adorini[1]

[1]Roche Milano Ricerche; [2]Department of Internal Medicine, Vita-Salute University School of Medicine, H San Raffaele, I-20132 Milan, Italy; [3]Hoffmann-La Roche, Nutley, NJ 07110, USA

Introduction 1,25-dihydroxyvitamin D_3 [1,25(OH)$_2$D$_3$], the activated form of vitamin D_3, not only has a central role in bone and calcium metabolism, but also modulates the immune response via specific receptors expressed in antigen-presenting cells (APCs) and activated T cells (1). 1,25(OH)$_2$D$_3$ inhibits antigen-induced T cell proliferation (2) and cytokine production (3), preventing Th1 cell development (4). APCs and in particular dendritic cells (DCs), are primary targets for the immunosuppressive activity of 1,25(OH)$_2$D$_3$. 1,25(OH)$_2$D$_3$ inhibits the differentiation and maturation of human DCs in vitro, leading to down-regulated expression of costimulatory molecules and to the inhibition of alloreactive T cell activation (5,6). Based on these results, we have analyzed the ability of 1,25(OH)$_2$D$_3$ and the analog 1,25-dihydroxy-16,23Z-diene-26,27-hexafluoro-19-nor vitamin D_3 (Ro 26-2198), administered alone or in combination with mycophenolate mofetil (MMF), an inhibitor of both T and B cell proliferation to mitogenic and allogenic stimulation (7), to inhibit the rejection of allogenic and xenogenic grafts.

1,25(OH)$_2$ D$_3$ Ro 26-2198

Inhibition of costimulatory pathways for T cell activation by 1,25(OH)$_2$D$_3$ and Ro 26-2198 Optimal activation of naïve T cells requires engagement of the TCR complex by peptide-MHC ligands and a second signal provided by costimulatory molecules expressed on activated APCs (8). Failure to deliver a costimulatory signal during antigen presentation induces a state of T cell anergy. The two major costimulatory pathways for T cell activation depend on the engagement of CD28 and CD154 on T cells by CD80/CD86 and CD40, respectively, expressed on activated APCs (8,9). Blockade of the CD80/CD86-CD28 costimulatory pathway with the fusion protein CD152-Ig induces long-term allograft survival in rodents (10), although it is less effective in prolonging islet allograft survival in non-human primates (11). Blocking the CD40/CD154 pathway with anti-CD154 mAb has been demonstrated to prevent rejection of heart, skin (12) and islet (13) allografts in rodents. Moreover, administration of anti-CD154 prevents acute renal allograft rejection (14) and induces long-term survival of islet allografts (15,16) in non-human primates. Simultaneous blockade of the CD28 and CD40 pathways most effectively promotes long-term graft survival and inhibits the development of chronic rejection (12). These findings, and the complications associated with anti-CD154 treatment in clinical trials (17), have stimulated the search for low molecular weight compounds able to disrupt costimulatory pathways.

$1,25(OH)_2D_3$ is an immunomodulator inhibiting not only autoimmune diseases but also allograft rejection in different models (18). We have recently shown that $1,25(OH)_2D_3$ inhibits alloreactive T cell activation by targeting APCs (5). Compared to other immunosuppressive agents targeting T cells, like mycophenolate mofetil (MMF), $1,25(OH)_2D_3$ was more potent in the inhibition of IFN-γ production (Fig. 1). The inhibitory effect on T cell responses appeared to be indirect because T cell activation by plate-bound anti-CD3, with or without costimulation by anti-CD28, was scarcely affected by $1,25(OH)_2D_3$. This indicates that $1,25(OH)_2D_3$ inhibits the ability of APCs to induce alloreactive T-cell activation, rather than directly inhibiting T cells. Ro 26-2198 was 6-8 fold more potent than $1,25(OH)_2D_3$ in the inhibition of IFN-γ production (Fig. 1).

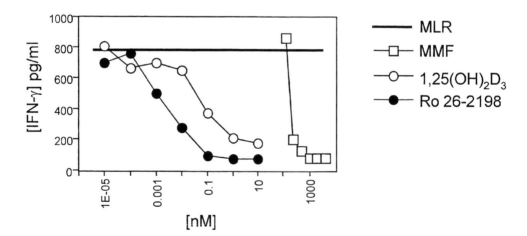

Figure 1. Inhibition of antigen presenting cell function by $1,25(OH)_2D_3$ and Ro 26-2198. Allogeneic PBMCs from 2 different donors ($3x10^5$ cells/well each) were co-cultured in 96-well flat-bottom plates in the presence of the indicated concentrations of MMF, CsA or $1,25(OH)_2D_3$. After 5 days, IFN-γ secretion was

measured. The solid line indicates the control response obtained in the absence of immunosuppressive drugs.

1,25(OH)$_2$D$_3$ inhibits the differentiation, maturation and activation of DCs in vitro while promoting their apoptosis (5). DCs matured in the presence of 1,25(OH)$_2$D$_3$ display reduced levels of MHC class II and CD40, CD80 and CD86 costimulatory molecules, and induce hyporesponsiveness in alloreactive T cells (5). Ro 26-2198 is over 5 times more potent than 1,25(OH)$_2$D$_3$, as judged by the reduction in mean fluorescence intensity, in inhibiting the expression of CD40, a key costimulatory molecule, during DC maturation (Fig. 2).

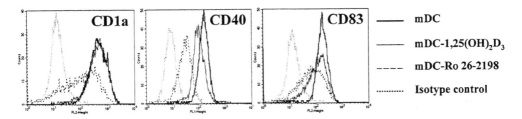

Figure 2. Inhibition of DC maturation and CD40 expression by 1,25(OH)$_2$D$_3$ and Ro 26-2198. Maturation was induced by incubation of immature DCs with LPS (200 ng/ml) for 48h. The staining profile of matured DCs (mDC) for the indicated surface molecules is shown. Stippled lines refer to isotype controls.

Transplantation tolerance induced by combined treatment with MMF and 1,25(OH)$_2$D$_3$ We first analyzed the ability of 1,25(OH)$_2$D$_3$ and MMF, administered alone or in combination, to inhibit islet allograft rejection. Pancreatic islets isolated from C57BL/6 (B6) mice were transplanted under the kidney capsule of BALB/c mice rendered diabetic by a single injection of streptozotocin. Recipient mice were treated from day −1 to 30 with MMF (100 mg/Kg p.o. daily) and/or 1,25(OH)$_2$D$_3$ (5 μg/Kg p.o. 3x/week). The mean rejection time in vehicle-treated recipients was 23±3 days. MMF and 1,25(OH)$_2$D$_3$ administered alone prolonged islet graft survival, but only in about 50% of the recipients. Conversely, over 80% of the mice treated with both drugs showed long-term (>70 days) islet graft acceptance (Fig. 3a). Analysis of CD45[+] cells, isolated from islet grafts 15 days after transplantation, revealed that mice treated with MMF and 1,25(OH)$_2$D$_3$ had a significant reduction of CD4[+] T cells, macrophages and DCs compared to vehicle-treated mice (data not shown). Conversely, the percentage of CD8[+] and B cells was similar in both groups. These results were confirmed by immunohistology (data not shown).

Next, we challenged BALB/c recipients showing long-term (>70 days) allograft acceptance with i.p. injection of 10[6] donor-type B6 spleen cells. Recipient mice treated with peri-transplant administration of anti-CD4 mAb accommodated the islet graft but were not tolerant, because all mice rejected the graft after challenge with a mean survival time of 14±2.4 days (Fig. 3b). Indeed, induction of transplantation tolerance in fully-mismatched combinations by anti-CD4 mAb has been found to require additional treatments, such as CD152-Ig (19) or donor-specific transfusion (20). Forty percent of allografts accepted under the cover of MMF alone were resistant to rejection upon challenge, confirming the tolerogenic properties of MMF in this model (21), and 1,25(OH)$_2$D$_3$ even had superior activity. Combined treatment with MMF and 1,25(OH)$_2$D$_3$ resulted in resistance to rejection upon challenge in 73% of allografts (Fig. 3b). Mice that continued to show islet graft function for 4 weeks after the challenge were transplanted, 100 days after the initial islet graft, with a vascularized heart from B6 (donor-type) or C$_3$H (third-party) mice. Naive BALB/c mice rejected B6 heart grafts in 10 days, whereas only one tolerant mouse out of five rejected the heart graft 25 days after transplant. In contrast, tolerant BALB/c mice rejected a third-party heart in 10-12 days. Thus, a short-term treatment of recipient mice with MMF and 1,25(OH)$_2$D$_3$ leads to long-term islet allograft acceptance and donor-specific tolerance induction.

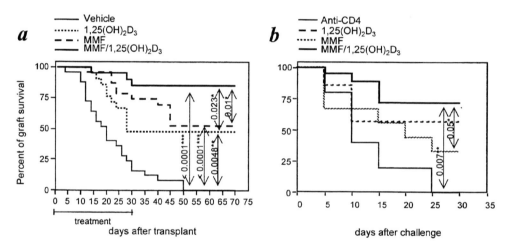

Figure 3. Tolerance induction by combined MMF and 1,25(OH)$_2$D$_3$ treatment. *a.* Long-term islet allograft survival induced by MMF and 1,25(OH)$_2$D$_3$ treatment. BALB/c mice rendered diabetic by a single injection of streptozotocin (250 mg/Kg i.v.) were transplanted with 350 C57BL/6 islets. Recipient mice were treated with MMF (100 mg/Kg p.o. daily) and/or (1,25(OH)$_2$D$_3$ 5 µg/Kg p.o. 3x/week) from day -1 to day 30. *b.* Percent islet graft survival after B6 spleen cell challenge. Recipient mice were treated with MMF (100 mg/Kg p.o. daily) and/or 1,25(OH)$_2$D$_3$ (5 µg/Kg p.o. 3x/week) from day -1 to day 30. Alternatively, recipient mice were treated at day -1, 0, 1 and 2 with anti-CD4 mAb i.p. (10 mg/Kg/d). Mice with functioning islet grafts 70 days after transplantation were injected i.p. with 10^6 B6 spleen cells. The function of islet allografts was monitored 2x/week by blood glucose measurement. P values were determined by Fisher's exact test.

Inhibition of discordant xenograft rejection by treatment with MMF and 1,25(OH)$_2$D$_3$ or Ro 26-2198 As shown above, the combination of MMF and 1,25(OH$_2$)D$_3$ is able to disrupt APC-T cell costimulatory pathways and induce transplantation tolerance to islet allografts. We have also analyzed the capacity of MMF and 1,25(OH)$_2$D$_3$ or Ro 26-2198 to prevent human to mouse islet xenograft rejection. Recipient mice rendered diabetic by streptozotocin administration were transplanted with 2000 human islets under the kidney capsule and treated with MMF and 1,25(OH$_2$)D$_3$ or Ro 26-2198. This treatment prolonged the survival of islet xenografts, as indicated by the increased frequency of normoglycemic mice assessed either randomly or after fasting (Fig. 4). Ro 26-2198-treated mice showed a response to intravenous glucose challenge comparable to that of normal mice, indicating a preserved β-cell mass. Cytofluorimetric analysis of leukocytes recruited in the islet xenograft area 15 days after transplantation revealed a marked reduction in CD4, CD8 and B cells in treated mice compared to controls, probably mostly due to the inhibitory activity of MMF on lymphocyte proliferation. Conversely, the reduced numbers of macrophages and dendritic cells associated with the xenografts could be ascribed to the immunomodulatory capacity of vitamin D$_3$ analogues, with a more pronounced effect of Ro 26-2198 compared to 1,25(OH$_2$)D$_3$ (Fig. 5). In terms of CD45$^+$ cell percentage, Ro 26-2198 was also more effective than 1,25(OH$_2$)D$_3$ in reducing the levels of xenograft-associated macrophages and dendritic cells (Fig. 5).

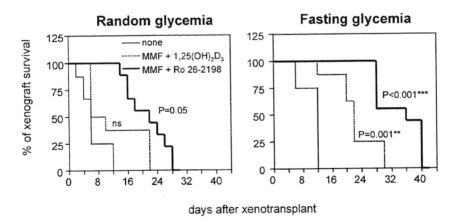

Figure 4. Prolongation of xenograft survival by treatment with MMF and 1,25(OH)$_2$D$_3$ or Ro 26-2198. BALB/c mice were rendered diabetic by a single injection of streptozotocin (200 mg/Kg i.v.) were transplanted with 2000 human islet cultured for 7 days at 25°C. Recipient mice were treated with MMF (100 mg/Kg p.o. daily) and non-hypercalcemic doses of 1,25(OH)$_2$D$_3$ (5 μg/Kg p.o. 3x/week) or Ro 26-2198 (0.03 μg/Kg p.o. 5x/week) from day -1 to day 30. The function of islet xenografts was monitored 2x/week by random and fasting (6 h after food withdrawal) blood glucose measurements. P values were determined by Fisher's exact test.

552

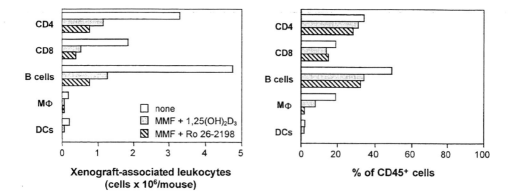

Figure 5. Cytometric analysis of xenograft-associated leukocytes. Graft-associated cells isolated from recipient mice treated with MMF (100 mg/Kg p.o. daily) and $1,25(OH)_2D_3$ (5 µg/Kg p.o. 3x/week) or Ro 26-2198 (0.03 µg/Kg p.o. 5x/week) from day -1 to day 30, were stained with mAbs specific for the indicated surface molecules and analyzed by flow cytometry. Acquisition was performed on CD45[+] cells. Analysis was performed 15 days after xenotransplantation.

Thus, inhibition of APC recruitment in the site of transplantation by $1,25(OH_2)D_3$ and its analogs can be detected not only in allografts, but also in discordant xenografts, and is associated with extended graft survival. We are currently trying to further delay islet xenograft rejection by adding to the protocol a peri-transplant treatment with anti-IL-2 receptor mAb.

Summary Costimulation blockade by biological agents such as CD152-Ig and anti-CD154 antibodies can induce transplantation tolerance. We now report that co-administration of mycophenolate mofetil and 1,25-dihydroxyvitamin D₃, an immunomodulator that can down-regulate costimulatory molecules on dendritic cells and macrophages, induces tolerance to fully-mismatched islet allografts and prolongs the survival of discordant islet xenografts. Tolerance to islet allografts is associated with massive peri-transplant lymphomononuclear cell infiltration, characterized by CD4[+] cells with a memory resting phenotype and a reduced proportion of antigen-presenting cells, expressing down-regulated costimulatory molecules. Alloreactive T cells from tolerant mice, rather than being deleted, mount a higher response to donor-type antigen-presenting cells compared to acutely rejecting mice. Interestingly, spleen cells from tolerant mice transfer tolerance to islet grafts with an alloantigen-specific active tolerogenic mechanism, leading to impaired development of IFN-γ-producing type 1 CD4[+] and CD8[+] cells in the recipient. Understanding the mechanisms leading to long-lasting costimulation blockade and to transferable transplantation tolerance by MMF and $1,25(OH)_2D_3$ treatment will help in implementing appropriate clinical protocols for the prevention of graft rejection, potentially able to induce tolerance allografts. This, coupled with the identification of a $1,25(OH)_2D_3$ analogue with enhanced immunosuppressive activity and reduced effects on the calcium/phosphate metabolism may lead to an effective prevention of human allograft rejection.

References

1. Bouillon, R., Garmyn, M., Verstuyf, A., Segaert, S., Casteels, K., and Mathieu, C. (1995) *Eur J Endocrinol* **133,** 7-16
2. Bhalla, A. K., Amento, E. P., Serog, B., and Glimcher, L. H. (1984) *J Immunol* **133,** 1748-54
3. Rigby, W. F., Denome, S., and Fanger, M. W. (1987) *J Clin Invest* **79,** 1659-64
4. Mattner, F., Smiroldo, S., Galbiati, F., Muller, M., Di Lucia, P., Poliani, P. L., Martino, G., Panina-Bordignon, P., and Adorini, L. (2000) *Eur J Immunol* **30,** 498-508
5. Penna, G., and Adorini, L. (2000) *J. Immunol* **164,** 2405-2411
6. Piemonti, L., Monti, P., Sironi, M., Fraticelli, P., Leone, B. E., Dal Cin, E., Allavena, P., and Di Carlo, V. (2000) *J Immunol* **164,** 4443-51
7. Allison, A. C., and Eugui, E. M. (1996) *Clin Transplant* **10,** 77-84
8. Lenschow, D. (1996) *Annu Rev Immunol* **14,** 233-258
9. Grewal, I. S., and Flavell, R. A. (1998) *Annu Rev Immunol* **16,** 111-35
10. Lenschow, D., Zeng, Y., Thistlethwaite, J., Montag, A., Brady, W., Gibson, M., Linsley, P., and Bluestone, J. (1992) *Science* **257,** 789-792
11. Levisetti, M. G., Padrid, P. A., Szot, G. L., Mittal, N., Meehan, S. M., Wardrip, C. L., Gray, G. S., Bruce, D. S., Thistlethwaite, J. R., Jr., and Bluestone, J. A. (1997) *J Immunol* **159,** 5187-91
12. Larsen, C. P., Elwood, E. T., Alexander, D. Z., Ritchie, S. C., Hendrix, R., Tucker-Burden, C., Cho, H. R., Aruffo, A., Hollenbaugh, D., Linsley, P. S., Winn, K. J., and Pearson, T. C. (1996) *Nature* **381,** 434-8
13. Rossini, A. A., Parker, D. C., Phillips, N. E., Durie, F. H., Noelle, R. J., Mordes, J. P., and Greiner, D. L. (1996) *Cell Transplant* **5,** 49-52
14. Kirk, A. D., Burkly, L. C., Batty, D. S., Baumgartner, R. E., Berning, J. D., Buchanan, K., Fechner, J. H., Jr., Germond, R. L., Kampen, R. L., Patterson, N. B., Swanson, S. J., Tadaki, D. K., TenHoor, C. N., White, L., Knechtle, S. J., and Harlan, D. M. (1999) *Nat Med* **5,** 686-93
15. Kenyon, N. S., Fernandez, L. A., Lehmann, R., Masetti, M., Ranuncoli, A., Chatzipetrou, M., Iaria, G., Han, D., Wagner, J. L., Ruiz, P., Berho, M., Inverardi, L., Alejandro, R., Mintz, D. H., Kirk, A. D., Harlan, D. M., Burkly, L. C., and Ricordi, C. (1999) *Diabetes* **48,** 1473-81
16. Kenyon, N. S., Chatzipetrou, M., Masetti, M., Ranuncoli, A., Oliveira, M., Wagner, J. L., Kirk, A. D., Harlan, D. M., Burkly, L. C., and Ricordi, C. (1999) *Proc Natl Acad Sci U S A* **96,** 8132-7
17. Kawai, T., Andrews, D., Colvin, R. B., Sachs, D. H., and Cosimi, A. B. (2000) *Nat Med* **6,** 114
18. Casteels, K., Bouillon, R., Waer, M., and Mathieu, C. (1995) *Curr Opin Nephrol Hypertens* **4,** 313-8

19. Yin, D., and Fathman, C. G. (1995) *J Immunol* **155,** 1655-9
20. Bushell, A., Niimi, M., Morris, P. J., and Wood, K. J. (1999) *J Immunol* **162,** 1359-66
21. Hao, L., Calcinaro, F., Gill, R. G., Eugui, E. M., Allison, A. C., and Lafferty, K. J. (1992) *Transplantation* **53,** 590-5

IN VITRO AND IN VIVO ANALYSIS OF THE IMMUNE SYSTEM OF VDR-KO MICE.

Chantal Mathieu [1], Evelyne van Etten [1], Shigeaki Kato [2], Annemieke Verstuyf [1], Jos Laureys [1], Jos Depovere [1], Dirk Valckx [1], Roger Bouillon [1].

[1] Laboratory of Experimental Medicine and Endocrinology (LEGENDO), Catholic University of Leuven, Belgium.
[2] Institute of Molecular and Cellular Biosciences, University of Tokyo, Japan.

Introduction.

Important immunomodulatory effects have been described in vitro and in vivo for the active form of vitamin D, $1,25(OH)_2D_3$ (1). These immunomodulatory actions are however only observed upon exposure to supraphysiological levels of the molecule, necessitating the use of less calcemic analogs of $1,25(OH)_2D_3$ or combinations with other immunomodulators at subtherapeutical levels in order to avoid side effects on calcium and bone metabolism (2,3).

Several data also point towards $1,25(OH)_2D_3$ as a physiological local immunomodulator in the natural immune system. Many authors have demonstrated that important immune defects exist in situations of vitamin D deficiency, in humans as well as in experimental animals (4, 5). In these conditions mainly defects in macrophage and neutrophil function (especially chemotactic capacity) and decreased cellular immunity have been described. Also the fact that receptors for vitamin D (VDR) and the machinery for final activation of the molecule (the enzyme 1-α-hydroxylase) are present in immune cells, points towards a physiological role for vitamin D or at least its active form, $1,25(OH)_2D_3$, in the immune system. Our group has recently demonstrated at the molecular level that the 1-α–hydroxylase present in macrophages corresponds to the enzyme present in kidney cells, but is regulated in a different manner: especially immune stimuli such as interferon-γ stimulate the enzyme while no down-regulation by $1,25(OH)_2D_3$ can be observed in macrophages (6). Interestingly, in macrophages of autoimmune diabetic NOD mice, a defect in up-regulation of 1-α-hydroxylase upon stimulation with different immune stimuli was observed, suggesting a possible role of this defect in the pathogenesis of autoimmunity.

An important question remains whether the vitamin D system is vital for the immune system. The aim of the present study was to investigate the in vitro and in vivo effects of disruption of the VDR in the immune system by studying VDR-knock out (VDR-KO) mice.

556

Materials and methods.

VDR-KO mice.

Mice were a kind gift of S. Kato (University of Tokyo, Japan) (7). They were bred under conventional conditions using heterozygous (+/-) mice as breeders. The phenotype was determined at 2 weeks of age when mice were identified using ear clips. For this purpose, a piece of tail was lysed overnight at 57°C using proteinase K. Afterwards, the enzyme was inactivated by incubating the lysate at 98°C for 10 minutes. DNA analysis for VDR (forward primer: aaagaactgccacccactctcc; reverse primer: ctgccattgcctccatcc; Probe: ctatgctgaaggtgccagctccttttg) and Neo (forward primer: gtgctcgacgttgtcactgaa; reverse primer: caaggtgagatgacaggagatcc; Probe: cgggaagggactggctgctattgg) was performed using real time PCR (ABI-prism 7700 sequence detector, PE Biosystems, Foster city, CA). Phenotypes of mice corresponded to the ones described previously. Mice were fed a standard mouse chow diet (Muracon G, Carfil-Huybrechts, Oud Turnhout, Belgium).

In vitro immune testing was performed at 90 days of age, in vivo testing was performed at 120 days of age. Calcium levels in these animals were 9.4 ± 1.2 mg/dl in wild type mice compared to 6.7 ± 1.1 mg/dl in VDR-KO mice (p<0.001). Levels of $1,25(OH)_2D_3$ were 60.0 ± 11.9 pg/ml in wild types versus 4001 ± 1539 pg/ml in VDR-KO mice (p<0.001).

In vitro macrophage function analysis.

Macrophages were isolated from the mouse peritoneum as described previously (6). Briefly, mice were injected intraperitoneally with 5 ml sterile medium (RPMI supplemented with Glutamax-I and 25 mM HEPES). After withdrawal of the needle, mice were rested for 1 minute. Then cells were harvested by puncturing the peritoneum using an 18G needle. Medium containing macrophages was collected and kept immediately on ice. By using this procedure, a macrophage purity of >90% was reached, as assessed by FACS analysis (FACSsort, Becton Dickinson, Erembodegem, Belgium). Per mouse, a mean of 2×10^6 macrophages was harvested. Cells were resuspended in a final volume of 10 ml ice cold PBS (pooled per 2 mice) and counted. Living cells were identified by Trypan blue exclusion. Cells were then centrifuged during 5 minutes at 930 g (4°C) and resuspended in medium (RPMI supplemented with Glutamax-I, 25 mM HEPES, 20% AB serum, 100 U/ml penicillin and 100 µg/ml streptomycin) at a final concentration of 10^6 cells/ml.

For phagocytosis evaluation, fluorescein-labeled Zymosan particles (Saccharomyces cerevisiae, Molecular Probes Europe, Leiden, The Netherlands) were used (8). Briefly, the fluoresceinated particles were added to 1 ml of the cell suspension (1-100 particles zymosan/cell). After a 2 h incubation at 37°C, cells were washed and dissolved in 100 µl Trypan blue. After exactly 1 minute, 1 ml PBS was added. Cells were then washed 3 times, centrifuged during 5 minutes at 930 g (4°C) and resuspended in 0.5 ml paraformaldehyde 2%. Fluorescein staining was analyzed using a FACSsort. Phagocytosis was expressed as percent fluorescein positive cells.

For evaluation of oxidative burst capacity, the burst-test kit of Orpegen Pharma (Heidelberg, Germany) was used. Briefly, to activate the macrophages, 20 µl unlabeled opsonized bacteria (E. coli) was added to 100 µl cell-suspension containing 10^6 cells. After 10 minutes incubation at 37°C, 20 µl fluorogenic substrate was added. After another 10 minutes incubation at 37°C, 2 ml lysing solution was added to stop the reaction and fixate the cells. Tubes were kept at room temperature for 20 minutes and then washed. At least 200 µl DNA staining solution was added to exclude aggregation artifacts of bacteria or cells. The percentage of cells having produced reactive oxygen radicals was then analysed using the FACSsort. Oxidative burst capacity was expressed as percent fluorescein positive cells.

Chemotaxis capacity of macrophages was evaluated by measuring the ability to bind casein and fnlpntl as described previously (9). Briefly, 50 µl of a standardized solution of fluorescein-labeled casein or fnlpntl (formyl-Nle-Leu-Phe-Nle-Tyr-Lys fluorescein derivative) (Molecular probes Europe, Leiden, The Netherlands) was added to 100 µl of the cell-suspension. After incubation for 1 h at 4°C, cells were washed with PBS and dissolved in 0.5 ml paraformaldehyde 2%. Fluorescein staining was analyzed using a FACSsort. Chemotactic capacity was expressed as percent fluorescein positive cells.

In vivo low dose streptozotocin diabetes model.

Diabetes was induced in mice (wild type and VDR-KO) by intraperitoneal injection of streptozotocin (50 mg/kg, Sigma, St. Louis, MO) maximum 15 minutes after it is dissolved in citrate buffer (25 mM, pH 4.5) on 5 consecutive days. Mice were monitored for diabetes incidence by daily glucosuria measurement starting 3 days after the last streptozotocin injection and ending 40 days later. Diabetes was defined as positive glucosuria (Clinistix, Bayer Diagnostics, Tarrytown, NY) on two consecutive days an a consequently determined glycemia of >200 mg/dl (Glucocard, Menarini, Firenze, Italy).

Statistics.

Statistical analysis of the in vitro macrophage results was performed using unpaired Student's *t*-test. Results were expressed as mean ± standard deviation. For comparing the in vivo diabetes incidence, the *chi-square* test was used.

Results and discussion.

Macrophage function is illustrated in table 2. No differences in fagocytosis and burst forming capacity of macrophages were observed between wild types and VDR-KO mice. However, a clear defect in chemotactic capacity of VDR-KO macrophages was observed, irrespective of the used stimulus (casein or fnlpntl). These data are in complete concordance with the observations in vitamin D deficient animals.

Table 2: In vitro macrophage function of VDR-KO compared tot their wild types expressed as mean ± SD.

	Wild Types	VDR-KO	
Fagocytosis (%)	76 ± 11	79 ± 13	NS
Respiratory burst (%)	86 ± 15	89 ± 19	NS
Casein chemotaxis (%)	33 ± 19	21 ± 11	P<0.05
Fnlpntl chemotaxis (%)	34 ± 16	21 ± 13	P<0.05

In contrast to data in vitamin D deficient animals, however, we have up to now not been able to identify defects in cellular immunity. We have analyzed T cell subsets in thymus and peripheral lymphoid organs, such as spleen, and found no differences. Also the proliferative capacity of T lymphocytes upon stimulation with lectins (PHA or Con A) or antigen (MLR) was normal. No defects in natural killer cell function could be observed.

In vivo, a clear difference in sensitivity to diabetes induced by low doses of streptozotocin, a model of experimental autoimmune diabetes, was observed between wild type and VDR-KO mice (figure 1). Whereas an expected diabetes incidence was observed in wild type mice (65%), VDR-KO mice were nearly completely protected against the disease (5%, p<0.001), indicating defects in cellular immunity in vivo.

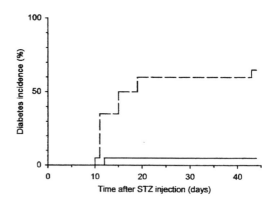

Figure 1: Streptozotocin (STZ) induced diabetes incidence of VDR-KO mice (———) compared to their wild types (- - - -).

We conclude that VDR-KO mice, fed a normal chow diet, display severe hypocalcemia and high levels of $1,25(OH)_2D_3$, as described previously. In these circumstances they display important defects in macrophage function in vitro and in cellular immunity in vivo.

At present it is, however, not fully clear whether these defects are a direct consequence of the VDR disruption or can be attributed to the severe metabolic dysregulation, especially hypocalcemia.

References.

1. Casteels K, Bouillon R, Waer M, Mathieu C (1995). Curr. Opin. Nephrol. Hypertens. 4, 313-318.
2. Bouillon R, Okamura WH, Norman AW (1995). Endocr. Rev. 16, 200-256.
3. van Etten E, Branisteanu DD, Verstuyf A, Wear M, Bouillon R, Mathieu C (2000). Transplantation 69, 1932-1942.
4. Lorente F, Fontan G, Jara P, Casas C, Garcia-Rodriguez MC, Ojeda JA (1976). Acta Paediatr. Scand. 65, 695-699.
5. Yang S, Smith C, Prahl JM, Luo X, DeLuca HF (1993). Arch. Biochem. Biophys. 303, 98-106.
6. Overbergh L, Decallonne B, Valckx D, Verstyuf A, Depovere J, Laureys J, Rutgeerts O, Saint-Arnaud R, Bouillon R, Mathieu C (2000). Clin. Exp. Immunol. 120, 139-146.
7. Yoshizawa T, Handa Y, Uematsu Y, Masushige S, Fukamizu A, Mastumoto T, Kato S (1997). Nature genetics 16, 391-396.
8. Galis ZS, Sukhova GK, Libby P (1995). FASEB J. 9, 974-980.
9. Lewis SL, Van Epps DE (1983). Inflammation 7, 363-375.

IMMUNOMODULATORY EFFECTS OF A 14-EPI-1α,25(OH)$_2$D$_3$ ANALOG IN COMBINATION WITH IFNβ AND CYCLOSPORIN A IN AN ANIMAL MODEL OF SYNGENEIC ISLET TRANSPLANTATION.

Evelyne van Etten, Conny Gysemans, Jos Laureys, Annemieke Verstuyf, Roger Bouillon, Chantal Mathieu.

Laboratory of Experimental Medicine and Endocrinology (LEGENDO), K.U.Leuven, Belgium.

Introduction.

Type I diabetes results from a specific autoimmune destruction of the pancreatic islet β-cells. Although the precise etiology of type I diabetes remains unclear, it has been demonstrated that an imbalance in the immune system contribute to the pathogenesis of this disease. 1,25(OH)$_2$D$_3$ and its analogs are immunomodulators restoring this immune imbalance by down-regulation T-helper1 mediated immune responses and by decreasing antigen presentation . We have demonstrated that 1,25(OH)$_2$D$_3$ and its analogs can prevent diabetes as well as the recurrence of diabetes after syngeneic islet transplantation in the nonobese diabetic (NOD) mouse . Synergistic immunomodulatory effects with other immunomodulators, such as cyclosporin A (CsA), are also demonstrated for 1,25(OH)$_2$D$_3$ and its analogs in animal models for this and other autoimmune diseases (1). Interferon(IFN)β is currently the most used immunomodulatory treatment in multiple sclerosis, an organ-specific autoimmune disease of the central nervous system. After treatment with IFNβ, a shift towards T-helper2 mediated immune responses is induced (2), restoring the immune imbalance seen in organ-specific autoimmune diseases.

In the present study we investigated if combinations of the 19-nor-14,20-bisepi-23-yne-1,25α(OH)$_2$D$_3$ analog of 1,25(OH)$_2$D$_3$ (TX527) with IFNβ or CsA resulted in cooperative immunomodulatory effects after syngeneic islet transplantation in spontaneously diabetic NOD mice.

Materials and methods.

Syngeneic transplantations of 500 NOD islets were performed under the left kidney capsule of male and female spontaneously diabetic NOD mice. Treatment was initiated the day before transplantation and was continued until 20 days (CsA and IFNβ) or 30 days (TX527) after transplantation or until recurrence. All drugs were administered intraperitoneally. Control mice were treated with vehicle only. Single-drug treatments were: 5 µg/kg/d TX527, 1 x 10^5 IU/d IFNβ and 7.5 mg/kg/d CsA. Combination treatments were: 5 µg/kg/d TX527 + 1 x 10^5 IU/d IFNβ, 5 µg/kg/d TX527 + 7.5 mg/kg/d CsA and 1 x 10^5 IU/d IFNβ + 7.5 mg/kg/d CsA. Three times weekly, mice were tested for recurrence of diabetes through detection of random non-fasting blood glucose levels by tail vein puncture. Mice were considered diabetic upon experiencing hyperglycemia

(<200 mg/dl) on two consecutive days. Upon disease recurrence blood was collected by heart puncture under ether anesthesia. Serum calcium was determined as a parameter of calcium metabolism.

Results and discussion.

All control mice showed disease recurrence within 2 weeks after transplantation with a mean graft survival time (MST) of 11 days (Table 1). Treatment with TX527, IFNβ or CsA alone only resulted in a minor prolongation of the MST. When combinations of TX527 and CsA were used, MST could be significantly prolonged to 31 days, approximately the time that CsA treatment was arrested. Mice treated with TX527 and IFNβ showed a significantly delayed MST to 62 days, long after IFNβ treatment was ended. However, combination of IFNβ with CsA did not prolong graft survival.

No severe calcemic side effects could be observed with the TX527, IFNβ or CsA treatments (Table 1).

Table 1: Effects of TX527, IFNβ and CsA on mean graft survival time (MST) and on calcium metabolism.

Groups (n)	MST ± SD (days)	serum calcium (mg/dl)
Control (n=6)	11 ± 3	9.4 ± 1.0
TX527 (n=4; 5 µg/kg/d)	15 ± 3	10.1 ± 0.9
IFNβ (n=4; 1 x 10^5 IU/d)	21 ± 14	9.5 ± 1.2
CsA (n=5; 7.5 mg/kg/d)	20 ± 8 ($p<0.03$)	10.6 ± 1.1
IFNβ+CsA (n=4; 1 x 10^5 IU/d + 7.5 mg/kg/d)	13 ± 4	8.2 ± 1.1
TX527+IFNβ (n=5; 5 µg/kg/d + 1 x 10^5 IU/d)	62 ± 20 ($p<0.0001$)	8.9 ± 1.2
TX527+CsA (n=6; 5 µg/kg/d + 7.5 mg/kg/d)	31 ± 12 ($p<0.009$)	8.4 ± 1.1

In conclusion, we demonstrate that combinations of non-toxic doses of the $1,25(OH)_2D_3$ analog TX527 with CsA and especially with IFNβ result in specific cooperative immunomodulatory effects responsible for a significant delay of the autoimmune diabetes recurrence. We therefore propose that clinical trials using analogs of $1,25(OH)_2D_3$ in combination with IFNβ in type I diabetes can be taken under serious consideration.

References.

1. van Etten E, Branisteanu DD, Verstuyf A, Waer M, Bouillon R, Mathieu C. (2000) Transplantation 69, 1932-1942.
2. Yong VW, Chabot S, Stuve O, Williams G. (1998) Neurology 51, 682-689.

VDR-KO MICE HAVE NORMAL INSULIN SECRETION IN VITRO AND NORMAL GLUCOSE TOLERANCE IN VIVO.

Evelyne van Etten[1], Shigeaki Kato[2], Annemieke Verstuyf[1], Jos Laureys[1], Roger Bouillon[1], Chantal Mathieu[1].

[1] Laboratory of Experimental Medicine and Endocrinology (LEGENDO), Catholic University of Leuven, Belgium.
[2] Institute of Molecular and Cellular Biosciences, University of Tokyo, Japan.

Introduction. The vitamin D receptor (VDR) is not only present in tissues responsible for calcium homeostasis and bone remodeling (bone, intestine, kidney and parathyroid glands) but also in many other tissues and cell types not primarily connected with mineral metabolism such as pancreatic β cells. Vitamin D deficient rats have an impaired glucose-mediated insulin response that can be reversed by $1,25(OH)_2D_3$ repletion (1). It has been postulated that $1,25(OH)_2D_3$, through a VDR-mediated modulation of one or more signal transduction pathways, controls calcium handling in the β cells, which in turn affects insulin release. We hypothesized that mice lacking the VDR might have, beside impaired bone formation, uterine hypoplasia and growth retardation (2), an impaired insulin response to glucose stimulation. Therefore, we investigated in this study in vitro insulin synthesis and secretion of β cells and in vivo glucose metabolism in VDR-/- mice.

Materials and methods. For the in vitro insulin synthesis and secretion of β cells, islets isolated from VDR -/-, VDR +/+ and VDR +/- mice were incubated for 2 hours with different concentrations of D-(+)-glucose (0-30 mM; 5 islets/300μl Hanks' balanced salt solution). Insulin levels in both supernatant (insulin secretion) and islet homogenate (insulin synthesis) were measured using a radioimmunoassay for rat insulin. Initial insulin contents, reflecting in vivo produced reserves, were also measured. In vivo, glucose tolerance tests were performed by injecting D-(+)-glucose (3g/kg body weight) intraperitoneally in VDR -/-, VDR +/+ and VDR +/- mice. Glycemia was measured in tail vein blood of fasting mice at different time points until 2 hours after glucose challenge.

Results and discussion.

Table 1: Insulin content of islets from VDR -/-, VDR +/- and VDR +/+ mice after in vitro incubation with different concentrations of D-(+)-glucose.

glucose conc.	VDR-/-	VDR+/-	VDR+/+
0 mM	12.5 ± 0.1 pmol/islet	10.3 ± 0.1 pmol/islet	10.0 ± 2.3 pmol/islet
1.5 mM	11.3 ± 0.1	12.6 ± 2.3	8.7 ± 3.5
5 mM	12.9 ± 3.7	14.2 ± 7.0	8.4 ± 3.3
10 mM	14.1 ± 6.8	14.0 ± 6.7	10.1 ± 2.2
20 mM	11.0 ± 3.5	13.1 ± 4.2	10.2 ± 3.6
30 mM	11.0 ± 0.1	11.4 ± 0.6	9.3 ± 1.6

In vitro, initial insulin contents were comparable between all groups (NS). After stimulation with various concentrations of glucose, no significant difference in insulin synthesis or secretion between VDR -/-, VDR +/- and VDR +/+ mice could be observed (table 1 and 2). In vivo, again no significant difference in glycemia could be observed between knock-out and wild type mice after glucose challenge (table 3).

Table 2: Insulin secretion by islets of VDR -/-, VDR +/- and VDR +/+ mice after in vitro incubation with different concentrations of D-(+)-glucose.

glucose conc.	VDR-/-	VDR+/-	VDR+/+
0 mM	0.37 ± 0.31 pmol/300µl	0.47 ± 0.16 pmol/300µl	0.37 ± 0.01 pmol/300µl
1.5 mM	0.22 ± 0.10	0.33 ± 0.06	0.18 ± 0.04
5 mM	0.39 ± 0.10	0.31 ± 0.08	0.34 ± 0.02
10 mM	1.40 ± 1.00	0.94 ± 0.38	0.89 ± 0.08
20 mM	6.72 ± 1.36	6.61 ± 0.86	5.06 ± 1.70
30 mM	7.33 ± 1.24	8.10 ± 0.85	6.43 ± 0.55

Table 3: Glycemia in VDR -/-, VDR +/- and VDR +/+ mice at different time points after D-(+)-glucose monohydrate challenge.

time after glucose	VDR-/-	VDR+/-	VDR+/+
0 min	150 ± 13 pmol/islet	141 ± 20 pmol/islet	142 ± 20 pmol/islet
15 min	301 ± 52	283 ± 47	267 ± 64
30 min	223 ± 36	201 ± 43	200 ± 31
60 min	187 ± 20	177 ± 25	187 ± 30
90 min	201 ± 33	174 ± 27	182 ± 28
120 min	165 ± 32	160 ± 26	172 ± 35

In summary, these results show that no abnormalities in glucose metabolism could be detected in VDR -/- mice compared to wild types. This may be explained by a redundancy of the vitamin D_3 and calcium system in the glucose metabolism of this VDR-/- mouse model since these knock out mice did have severe hypocalcemia at the time of experiments (6.7 ± 1.1 vs. 9.4 ± 1.2 in +/+ animals, $p<0.001$). The discrepancy with the previously described abnormalities in rachitic mice may be attributed to other deficiencies in the rachitic diet.

References.
1. Bourlon PM, Billaudel B, Faure-Dusset A (1999). J. Endocrinol. 160,87-95.
2. Yoshizawa T, Handa Y, Uematsu Y, Takeda S, Sekine K, Yoshihara Y, Kawakami T, Arioka K, Sato H, Uchiyama Y, Masushige S, Fukamizu A, Matsumoto T, Kato S (1997). Nature genetics 16, 391-396.

NFAT-MEDIATED TRANSACTIVATION IN ACTIVATED T CELLS OF VITAMIN D RECEPTOR NULL MUTANT MICE: LACK OF REGULATION BY 1α, 25-DIHYDROXYVITAMIN D₃

Atsuko Takeuchi[1], Surendra Sharma[2], Mariko Yoshikawa[1], Tatsuya Yoshizawa[3], Shigeaki Kato[3] and Toshio Okano[1]
[1]Department of Hygienic Sciences, Kobe Pharmaceutical University, Kobe, Japan 658-8558, [2]Department of Pediatrics, Women and Infants' Hospital, Brown University, Providence, RI, USA 02905, [3]Institute of Molecular and Cellular Bioscience, The University of Tokyo, Japan 113-8657.

Introduction

Activated lymphocytes express the vitamin D_3 receptor (VDR) (1) and $1\alpha,25(OH)_2D_3$ treatment of activated T cells results in partial growth inhibition as well as in transcriptional repression of cytokine genes (2,3). $1\alpha,25(OH)_2D_3$ interacts with VDR, which acts as a transcription factor and binds to its specific response element (VDRE). The binding of VDR to VDRE is usually regulated by its heterodimerization with the retinoid X receptor (RXR). Recently, $1\alpha,25(OH)_2D_3$ has been shown to control expression of several cytokine genes which do not contain classical VDREs in their regulatory regions (4-7). Nuclear factor of activated T cells (NFAT) is a member of growing family of transcription factors which cooperatively bind with Fos and Jun family members. Cyclosporin A (CsA) and FK506 target NFAT activity by inhibiting calcineurin, a Ca^{2+}-activated serine /threonine phosphatase necessary for nuclear translocation of cytoplasmic NFAT proteins. The protein plays a key role in the inducible expression of cytokine genes, such as IL-2, IL-4, TNF-α, GM-CSF and IFN-γ, in T cells. We have previously reported that $1\alpha,25(OH)_2D_3$-mediated suppressive effects on the inducible expression of cytokine genes in human T cells may, in part, be due to diminished activity of the transcription factor NFAT (7). The vitamin D_3 receptor (VDR) and its heterodimeric partner retinoid X receptor α (RXRα) specifically bound to the distal NFAT site in the human IL-2 promoter, and this binding was abolished by mutating unique regions in the NFAT oligonucleotide. *In vitro* inhibition of NFAT complex formation was noted when VDR-RXRα heterodimers were added to DNA binding reactions containing nuclear extracts from activated B or T cells, whereas *in vitro* NFκB complex formation was not significantly influenced. Furthermore, $1\alpha,25(OH)_2D_3$ treatment of activated T cells resulted in decreased formation of NFAT complexes detected upon incubation of nuclear extracts from these cells with ^{32}P-labeled probe. Transient expression of both VDR and RXRα but not of a single component was capable of inhibiting expression of a NFAT-driven reporter gene in stimulated Jurkat cells in a ligand dependent manner. These results suggest that NFAT plays a crucial role in

566

1α,25(OH)$_2$D$_3$-mediated immunosuppressive activity. Herein, we attempted to examine the properties of NFAT-responsive immune system and immunomodulatory effects by 1α,25(OH)$_2$D$_3$ in VDR null mutant (VDR-KO) mice (8).

Results and discussion

I. Comparison of NFAT-responsive immune system between wild type and VDR-KO mice

We first examined the population of CD4 and CD8 positive cells in thymus and spleen of wild type and VDR-KO mice using the flow cytometry technique. As shown in Fig. 1, there were no significant differences in CD4 and CD8 cell compartments from both thymus and spleen of wild type and VDR-KO mice.

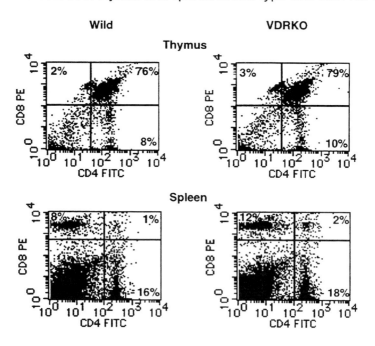

Fig.1 Comparison of the population of CD4 and CD8 positive cells in thymus and spleen cells between wild type and VDRKO mice

Dephosphorylation of a cytoplasmic component of NFAT complex by calcineurin results in its cytoplasmic-to-nuclear translocation. Nuclear translocated NFAT molecules form functional NFAT complex with Fos and Jun proteins. Using the same cell system, we next examined the levels of NFAT protein and dephosphorylation of NFAT protein in stimulated T cells by Western blot analysis. The amounts of NFATp protein observed in thymus and spleen of VDR-KO mice were similar to those of wild type mice, respectively (Fig.2). Moreover, to test the

NFATp phosphorylation-dephosphorylation status, thymus and spleen cells from wild type and VDR-KO mice were activated with ionomycin and cell extracts were analyzed by Western blotting. Treatment with ionomycin for 10 min resulted in similar but significant dephosphorylation as determined by faster migrating NFAT band (data not shown). These results suggest

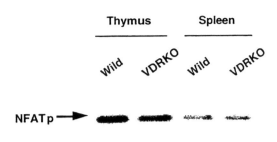

Fig.2 Comparison of NFATp protein in thymus and spleen cells between wild type and VDRKO mice

that there are no differences in the levels of NFATp protein and dephophorylation of NFATp protein in cells derived from wild type and VDR-KO mice. We also examined subcellular localization of NFATp in cells from freshly isolated thymus and spleen using immunocytochemical fluorometric method. NFATp mainly localized in the cytoplasm in unstimulated cells. Stimulation with ionomycin resulted in the translocation of NFATp into the cell nucleus. These results suggest that cytoplasmic-to-nuclear translocation of NFAT protein is not defective in VDR-KO mice. From these results, it is suggested that intrinsic immunomodulatory and biochemical properties of NFAT were independent of $1\alpha,25(OH)_2D_3$.

II. Comparison of $1\alpha,25(OH)_2D_3$–mediated immunosuppressive effects between wild type and VDR-KO mice

We have previously shown that $1\alpha,25(OH)_2D_3$ treatment of activated T cells does not influence nuclear translocation of NFATp, however, VDR/RXR heterodimer directly binds to the IL-2 distal NFAT site (7). This is accompanied by inhibition of NFAT complex formation, attenuation of NFAT-mediated transactivation and partial inhibition of T cell growth.

As rapid and efficient means of evaluating $1\alpha,25(OH)_2D_3$-mediated effects on NFAT, we performed electrophoretic mobility shift assays (EMSA) using a synthetic oligonucleotide corresponding to the distal NFAT binding site in the IL-2 promoter. Although nuclear extracts from activated T cells from wild type and VDR-KO mice readily formed a DNA-protein complex with ^{32}P-labeled NFAT probe, the complex formation was significantly inhibited only in $1\alpha,25(OH)_2D_3$-treated cells of wild type mice (Fig.3).

Next, we examined the effect of $1\alpha,25(OH)_2D_3$ on NFAT-driven transcription in transient transfection assays. Treatment of cells with ionomycin and PMA significantly induced luciferase expression by endogenous NFAT activity in both types. As expected, $1\alpha,25(OH)_2D_3$ treatment inhibited the transcriptional activity in wild type mice (~70%), whereas failed to inhibit NFAT functions in VDR-KO mice.

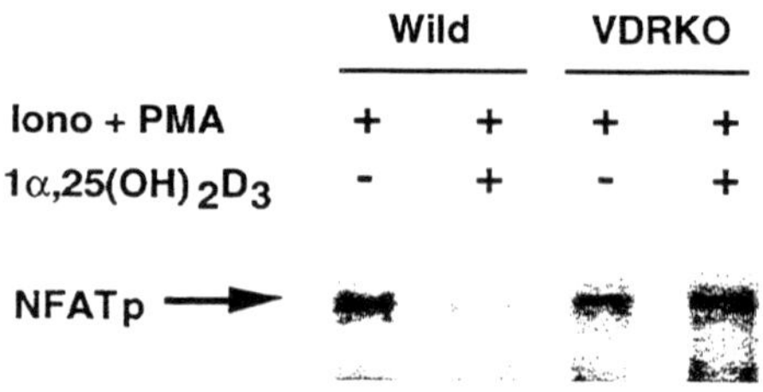

We also examined the effect of $1\alpha,25(OH)_2D_3$ on growth of activated T cells. DNA synthesis was monitored by ^{3}H-thymidine incorporation. As shown in Fig.4, $1\alpha,25(OH)_2D_3$ inhibited growth of T cells from wild type mice in a dose-dependent manner, but not from VDR-KO mice. However, inhibition of activated T cell proliferation by CsA was dose-dependent in both types (data not shown) (9).

	Wild		VDRKO	
Iono + PMA	+	+	+	+
$1\alpha,25(OH)_2D_3$	-	+	-	+

Fig.3 Comparison of $1\alpha,25(OH)_2D_3$-mediated effect on DNA-NFATp protein complex formation in thymus cells between wild type and VDRKO mice

Conclusion

These results suggest that the expression of T cell growth factors, such as IL-2 and other cytokines, is suppressed by CsA, but not by $1\alpha,25(OH)_2D_3$ in VDR-KO mice. Taken together, these results demonstrate that, in VDR-KO mice, NFAT-responsive immune system is normal, while $1\alpha,25(OH)_2D_3$-mediated immune system is impaired.

References

(1) Provvedini, D.M., Tsoukas, C.D., Deftos, L. and Manolagas, S. (1983) Science **221**, 1181-1183.
(2) Bhalla, A.K., Amento, E.P., Serog, B. and Glimcher, L.H. (1984) J. Immunol. **133**, 1748-1754.
(3) Rigby, W.F.C., Denome, S. and. Fanger, M.W. (1987) J. Clin. Invest. **79**, 1659-1664.
(4) Alroy, I., Towers, T.L. and Freedman, L.P. (1995) Mol. Cell. Biol. **15**, 5789-5799.
(5) Towers, T.L. and Freedman, L.P. (1998) J. Biol. Chem. **273**, 10338-10348.
(6) Cippitelli, M. and Santoni, A. (1998) Eur. J. Immunol. **28**, 3017-3030.
(7) Takeuchi, A., Reddy, G.S., Kobayashi, T., Okano, T., Park, J. and Sharma, S. (1998) J. Immunol. **160**, 209-218.
(8) Yoshizawa, T., Handa, Y. Kato, S. (1997) Nat. Genet. **16**, 391-396.
(9) Mathiu, C., Wear, M., Laureys, J., Rutgeerts, O. and Bouillon, R. (1994) Transplantation Proceedings **26**, 3048-3049.

DOWN-REGULATION OF TNFα EXPRESSION BY 1 ,25-DIHYDROXYVITAMIN D$_3$ AND 1,24(S)-DIHYDROXYVITAMIN D$_2$ IN HUMAN MACROPHAGES FROM CAPD PATIENTS

Shraga Shany, Merav Cohen-Lahav, Cidio Chaimovitz[1] and Amos Douvdevani.
Departments of Clinical Biochemistry and Nephrology,[1] Soroka University Medical Center and Ben-Gurion University of the Negev, Beer Sheva 84101, Israel.

Introduction: Convincing evidence has been gathered indicating that 1α,25-dihydroxyvitamin D$_3$ (1α,25(OH)$_2$D$_3$) is an important immune response regulator at inflammatory sites [1,2]. Such a property of 1α,25(OH)$_2$D$_3$ may find expression in the special microenvironment of the peritoneal cavity characteristic of the continuos ambulatory peritoneal dialysis (CAPD) technique used in the treatment of end stage uremic patients. We have previously demonstrated that peritoneal macrophages of CAPD patients are capable of converting 25-hydroxyvitamin D$_3$ (25-OH-D$_3$) into 1α,25(OH)$_2$D$_3$ and that 1α,25(OH)$_2$D$_3$ accumulates in the dialysis fluid of these patients [3-5]. We have demonstrated earlier that 1α,25(OH)$_2$D$_3$ significantly increases superoxide generation and bactericidal activity of peritoneal macrophages [5]. It is noteworthy, however, that in CAPD treated patients, the capacity of macrophages to phagocyte microorganisms is limited due to the diluting effect of the infused dialysis solution on the peritoneal macrophage population. Consequently, the contribution of the peritoneal macrophages in combating bacterial invasion relies mainly on their ability to secrete inflammatory cytokine effectors, such as IL-1 and TNFα. The present study was designed to investigate the regulatory effect of 1α,25(OH)$_2$D$_3$ and of some vitamin D$_2$ analogs on the generation of TNFα by peritoneal macrophages of CAPD treated patients. We believe such an investigation could be of particular clinical value since in the peritoneal environment there is a simultaneous up-regulation of TNFα production and 1α,25(OH)$_2$D$_3$ synthesis in response to bacterial invasion.

Materials and Methods:

Materials: 1α,25(OH)$_2$D$_3$ and 25-OH-D$_3$ were kindly provided by Hoffman La-Roche, Basel. 1α,24(S)-dihydroxyvitamin D$_2$ (1α,24(S)(OH)$_2$D$_2$) and 1α-dihydroxyvitamin D$_2$ (1α-OH-D$_2$) were kindly provided by Bone Care International Co. Madison WI. Each compound was dissolved in ethanol and stored in a concentrated solution at -20°C, protected from light. Vitamin D compounds were freshly diluted in the appropriate culture medium before each experiment. The final ethanol concentration did not exceed 0.1%.

Cell preparation: Human peritoneal macrophages (HPM) were obtained from effluent dialysates of patients in end-stage renal disease undergoing CAPD treatment. Isolation of macrophages from the dialysate fluides was performed as described elsewhere [3,6]. Briefly, complete dialysate effluent was centrifuged at 2000 rpm × 15 minutes (Hettich, Rotanta/RP). Cells were washed with Hanks' solution and re-centrifuged. Then the cells were washed twice in RPMI-1640 medium and re-suspended in same medium, which contained 10% fetal calf serum

(FCS), 2mM L-glutamin, 100 U/ml penicillin, 10 □g/ml streptomycin and 12.5 U/ml nistatine. Cells were plated into a plastic flask and incubated for 90 minutes at 37°C in humidified atmosphere of 5% CO_2 and 95% air. Non-adherent cells were removed by discarding the medium and replacing it with fresh medium. The adherent cells were released, cells were counted by a hemocytometer and adjusted to 1×10^6 cells/ml. Viability of more than 99% was determined in the isolated HPM Preparations, by trypan blue exclusion.

Incubation of HPM: One ml portions of HPM primary cultures (1×10^6 cells/tube) were seeded in plastic tissue culture tubes (12.4×75 mm) and incubated as monolayers overnight. Treatments were performed in triplicate that were incubated in RPMI-1640 medium containing 2% FCS with various concentrations of $1\alpha,25(OH)_2D_3$ (10^{-10} to 10^{-7} M), or vitamin D_2 analogs, for 16 h. The cells were then exposed to 1 μg/ml of lipopolysaccharide (LPS), for 6 h for protein expression or for 2.5 h for mRNA expression. Following the incubation period, tubes were placed on ice and supernatants were collected and stored at -20°C for TNFα protein determination. Cells were subjected to mRNA extraction procedure.

TNFα mRNA analysis: At the end of each incubation, the isolated cells were lysed with 0.75 ml Tri Reagent. TNFα mRNA determination was performed according to the methods of Bouaboula et al [7], using a quantitative RT-PCR procedure. This method uses internal standard RNA obtained from synthetic DNA construct containing TNFα primer sites identical to the primer sites of native TNFα mRNA. A synthetic RNA mixture (0.0325 ng) and a RT reaction mixture including 1 μl dNTP (2.5 nmol/μl of each nucleotide) were added to each RNA sample for cDNA production. Co-amplification of the synthetic TNFα cDNA (370 bp) together with native TNFα cDNA (427 bp) and of β-actin (263 bp) was carried out by PCR using specific primers. PCR was performed at 30 cycles for TNFα and at 25 cycles for β–actin. Eight μl of each sample containing amplified cDNA of the two kinds of TNFα, together with 8 μl of the corresponding sample containing amplified cDNA of β–actin, were loaded on an agarose gel (2%) containing ethidium bromide (0.5 μg/ml). PCR products were quantified by a video densitometry with the UV GDS 5000 system. The TNFα results were calculated for each treatment by the ratios of native TNFα / synthetic TNFα to compensate differences in RT and PCR efficiency. these results were normalized according to β-actin levels to compensate differences in mRNA between the various samples. Results were compared to those of LPS stimulated HPM.

TNFα protein determination: TNFα protein levels were measured in the supernatants of HPM cultures in triplicate by an ELISA for human TNFα using a commercially available paired antibodies assay (R&D Systems, Minneapolis, MN, USA), as per the protocol of the manufacturer.

Statistical analysis: Results are presented as mean ± standard error of the mean (S.E.). Student's t-test was used to compare TNFα levels between treatments. P values below 0.05 were considered significant.

Results:

The effect of 1α,25(OH)₂D₃ on TNFα mRNA levels: RT-PCR of total RNA from HPM yielded a band of mRNA for TNFα at the expected size of 427 bp (**Fig 1**). The RT-PCR products of the synthetic RNA of TNFα yielded cDNA at the expected size of 370 bp. The synthetic RNA of TNFα accompanied each treatment in order to normalize the differences in loading amounts. As shown in **Fig 1** TNFα mRNA was detected in untreated primary HPM cultures only at minimal levels (first lane). However, TNFα expression was found to be significantly inducible by LPS (second lane). On the other hand, pre-incubation with increased concentrations of 1α,25(OH)₂D₃ (10^{-10}- 10^{-7} M) before the addition of LPS, induced a significant dose-dependent decrement in TNFα mRNA expression.

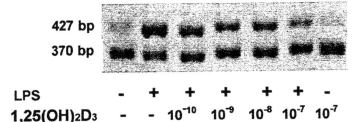

427 bp						
370 bp						
LPS	-	+	+	+	+	+	-
1,25(OH)₂D₃	-	-	10^{-10}	10^{-9}	10^{-8}	10^{-7}	10^{-7}

Fig 1: Dose response of increased concentrations of 1α,25(OH)₂D₃ (10^{-10}- 10^{-7} M) on TNFα mRNA production by LPS stimulated HPM.

The effect of 1α,25(OH)₂D₃ and vitamin D₂ analogs on TNFα Protein levels: TNFα protein expression was examined in HPM media using a specific ELISA. Pre-incubation of HPM for 16 hours with increasing concentrations of 1α,25(OH)₂D₃, or of the vitamin D₂ analogs (1α,24S(OH)₂D₂ and 1α-OH-D₂), followed by activation with LPS for additional 6 hours, induced a dose-related decrement in TNFα protein concentrations (**Fig 2**). TNFα production was down regulated significantly (P< 0.01) even in the presence of physiological concentrations of 1α,25(OH)₂D₃ (10^{-10}M) and reached a maximal effect at 10^{-8}M (**Fig 2a**). The results in **Fig 2b** summarize the effect of the synthetic vitamin D₂ analog, 1α,24(S)(OH)₂D₂ on TNFα production. This effect was found to be dose dependent similarly to that of 1α,25(OH)₂D₃. A similar trend was observed also by incubating HPM with 1α-OH-D₂ (data not shown).

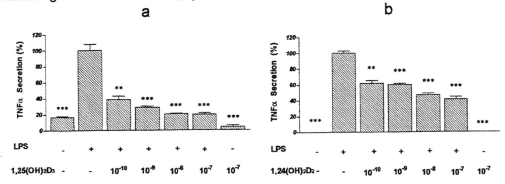

Fig 2: Dose response of increased concentrations of 1α,25(OH)₂D₃ and 1α,24(S)(OH)₂D₂ (10^{-10}- 10^{-7} M) on TNFα protein secretion from LPS stimulated HPM.

Discussion: In recent years, there has been increasing evidence showing that beyond its role in divalent ion homeostasis, $1\alpha,25(OH)_2D_3$ may also affect immune cells and thus function as an important regulatory agent at sites of inflammation [6]. The present data showing a regulatory role of $1\alpha,25(OH)_2D_3$ on TNFα production by HPM further emphasize this contention. We found that $1\alpha,25(OH)_2D_3$ induced a marked suppression of TNFα production by LPS-stimulated peritoneal macrophages. Incubation of HPM with $1\alpha,25(OH)_2D_3$ prior to exposure to LPS caused a significant inhibition of TNFα expression by these cells. This inhibition of TNFα expression by $1\alpha,25(OH)_2D_3$ was observed on both mRNA and protein levels and was found to be dose dependent. During peritonitis in CAPD treated patients, peritoneal macrophages secrete TNFα which has a pro-inflammatory effect in the peritoneal cavity. However, we have shown earlier that under these conditions, peritoneal macrophages will up-regulate $1\alpha25(OH)_2D_3$ synthesis. Due to the present results, we can hypothesize that $1\alpha25(OH)_2D_3$ have an important role in moderating the magnitude and the extent of the inflammatory response of the peritoneum to invading microorganisms. In many cases, the inflammation is suppressed by dexamethasone treatment, often at the price of side effects. Although the present results may suggest the therapeutic advantage of $1\alpha,25(OH)_2D_3$ as an anti-inflammatory agent, practically its use is restricted due to its hypercalcemic activity. However, it was found in the present study that incubation of HPM with vitamin D_2 analogs such as $1\alpha,24(S)(OH)_2D_2$ and 1α-OH-D_2, revealed a significant down-regulation of TNFα expression. Since $1\alpha,24(S)-(OH)_2D_2$ is less calcemic than $1\alpha,25(OH)_2D_3$ [8], its potential pharmaceutical application as an anti-inflammatory agent seems to be safer *in vivo* and appears to be superior to that of $1\alpha,25(OH)_2D_3$.

References:

1. Shany S, Levy R, Chaimovitz C. (1995) *Nephron* 69:367-370

2. Rigby WF. (1988) The immunobiology of vitamin D. *Immunol Today* 9:54-58.

3. Shany S, Rapoport J, Zuili I, Gavriel A, Lavi N, Chaimovitz C. (1991) *Kidney Int* 39:1005-1011.

4. Aloni Y, Shany S, Chaimovitz C. (1983) *Miner Electrolyte Metab* 9:82-86.

5. Deutsch A, Chaimovitz C, Nagauker-Shriker O, Zlotnik M, Shany S, Levy R. . (1995) *J Am Soc Nephrol* 6:102-109.

6. Levy R, Klein J, Rubinek T, Alkan M, Shany S, Chaimovitz C. (1990) *Kidney Int* 37:1310-1315.

7. Bouaboula M, Legoux P, Pessegue B, Delpech B, Dumont X, Piechaczyk M, Casellas P, Shire D. (1992) *J Biol Chem* 267:21830-21838.

8. Knutson JC, LeVan LW, Valliere CR, Bishop CW. (1997) *Biochem Pharmacol* 53:829-837,

IMMUNOMODULATORY EFFECTS OF VITAMIN D_2 AND D_3 ON ADENOSINE METABOLISING ENZYMES OF PERITONEAL MACROPHAGES.

Tatjana Jevtovic-Stoimenov[1], Predrag Vlahovic[2], Gordana Kocic[1], Vidosava B.Djordjevic[1], Dusica Pavlovic[1], Vojin Savic[2], 1 Institute of Biochemistry, 2 Institute of Nephrology and Hemodialisys, Faculty of Medicine, University of Nis, Serbia, Yugoslavia

Introduction   Vitamins D_2 (ergocalciferol) and D_3 (holecalciferol) are biologically inactive prohormons. Following hydroxylation, first in liver and than in kidney, they become activated ($1,25(OH)_2 D_3$) in order to exert their function via specific vitamin D receptors (VDR) at target tissues. In past two decades it has been shown that macrophages (Mϕ) are very important extrarenal sources of calcitriol ($1,25(OH)_2 D_3$)(1). Since Mϕ shows 1-α-hydroxylase activity as well as constitutively express VDR, calcitriol was promoted as an autocrine and paracrine cytokine and immunomodulator (2).

The importance of purine metabolism is based on purine nucleotide function in cells and tissues. The association of deficiency of purine metabolic enzymes with immunodeficiency diseases has stimulated the research in purine metabolism of lymphoid cells, especially Mϕ. The investigation of purine metabolism in intact and activated Mϕ showed that metabolism of adenosine was predominant purine metabolic pathway (3). High catabolic activity of purines seems to be in correlation with the biological function of Mϕ. On the other hand, the salvage pathway plays an important role in delivery of the purine nucleotides in Mϕ, being considered as the only source of nucleotides in these cells. 5'-nucleotidase (5'-NT) as adenosine producing enzyme and adenosine deaminase (ADA) adenosine degrading enzyme, are not important only for adenosine metabolism but they are also considered as biochemical parameters of Mϕ function and activity (4,5). Since Mϕ are one of the target immune cells during adjuvant calcitriol immune therapy, it is of great clinic interest to investigate the activity of 5'-nucleotidase and ADA during Mϕ immunosuppression and stimulation.

The aim of this study was to investigate the effects of vitamin D_2 and D_3 on 5'-NT and ADA activity in the culture of peritoneal macrophages. The obtained results show significant elevation of 5'-NT activity together with the significant decrease of ADA activity during treatment with vitamins D_2 and D_3. Since 5'-NT is the enzyme necessary for adenosine production, it might be proposed that the accumulation of adenosine in macrophages could be one of immunomodulating mechanisms of vitamin D action.

Materials and methods

In vitro experimental study The culture of peritoneal macrophages was prepared by the method of Mosier (6). Macrophages were isolated from peritoneal cavity of 5 male Wistar rats weighing 200-250g, 4 days after intraperitoneal injection of 5ml Brewer's thyoglycollate medium. The cells were collected after injection of 20ml of

Hanks' balanced salt solution (HBSS) containing 50IU sodium heparin, 50IU/ml penicillin and 50µg/ml streptomycin. The collected fluids were then centrifuged at 1800 rpm for 10min at 4°C and the cell pellet was washed twice with tissue-culture medium, counted and resuspended. The cells were plated in 35mm dishes at a density of 1.5-2.5 x 10^6 per dish containing 2ml of medium. The isolated peritoneal macrophages were divided into 9 groups: Group 1, 2, 3, and 4 for dose dependent effects of vitamin D_2 (10^{-5}, 10^{-7}, 10^{-9}, and 10^{-11}M/ml of reaction mixture); groups 5, 6, 7, and 8 for dose-dependent effects of vitamin D_3 (10^{-5}, 10^{-7}, 10^{-9}, 10^{-11}, M/ml of reaction mixture): and group 9 was control one. Each of the investigated groups had 4 samples and peritoneal macrophage samples were incubated in PC incubator for 48 h.

Biochemical methods The activity of 5'-nucleotidase was measured according to the method of Wood and Williams (7) and the activity of ADA was measured according to the method of Pederson and Barry (8). Cell protein content was determined by the method of Lowry (9), using bovine serum albumin as standard. The enzyme activity was expressed as U/g proteins and as a percent of control value.

Results: When the culture of thyoglicolate-elicited M φ was treated with increased doses of vitamin D_2 and D_3 (10^{-11}, 10^{-9}, 10^{-7}, 10^{-5} M/ml of reaction mixture for 48 h), the activity of 5'-NT was significantly elevated (Fig 1).

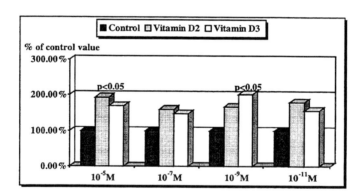

Figure 1. The activity of 5'-NT of Mφ treated with vitamins D_2 and D_3

Maximum activity was found during treatment with D_3 in a dose of 10^{-9}M (202.8% of control value) and with D_2 in a dose of 10^{-5}M (198.3% of control value). Contrary to 5'-NT, the activity of ADA was significantly decreased during in vitro incubation of elicited peritoneal Mφ with different doses of D_2 and D_3 (Fig 2). Maximum reduction was seen in cell culture treated with D_3 in a dose of 10^{-5}M (51.4% of control value) and with D_2 in a dose of 10^{-9}M/ml of reaction mixture (46.88% of control value).

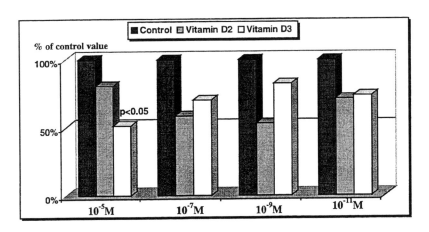

Figure 2. The activity of ADA Mφ treated with vitamins D_2 and D_3

Discussion Evidence obtained during the last fifteen years has revealed that vitamin D, in addition to playing a major role in mineral and skeletal homeostasis, is involved in the regulation of immune phenomena. It is well established that calcitriol promotes the differentiation of leukemic, normal myeloid stem cells and peripheral blood monocytes toward the Mφ phenotype, enhances the cytotoxic function of Mo/Mφ and exhibits enhanced phagocytosis and killing mycobacteria (10).

5'-nucleotidase (EC 3.1.3.5.) (5'-NT) is an extracellular enzyme anchored to the cell membrane through a glycosyl phosphatidylinositol linkage. The enzyme catalyses the reaction of hydrolytic dephosphorilation of purine and pyrimidine monophosphate nucleotides to the corresponding nucleosides. The most important product of 5'-nucleotidase activity is adenosine. Although this enzyme is present in all mammalian tissues it appears to play a major role in the development and function of lymphoid tissue especially in Mφ. The activity of 5'-NT and ADA in peritoneal Mφ should be discussed from different aspects. 5'-NT is established as a marker of immune cells maturity and differentiation (11) and the increase that was observed after calcitriol treatment could be explained in terms of its effects on differentiation.

There is considerable evidence demonstrating the ability of calcitriol to suppress immune cells proliferation (12). The importance of this effect is reflected in its possible application in the treatment of high proliferative malignancies (13). Decreased activity of ADA, known as a parameter of proliferative activity in cells(14), could be explained by antiproliferative properties of vitamin D.

It has been apparent that adenosine plays an important role in the regulation of the immune system. Mostly, the reports have pointed the general immunosuppressive and anti-inflammatory properties of adenosine. For example, in macrophages adenosine inhibited process of normal hemotaxis and phagocytosis (15,16). In LPS activated Mφ adenosine stimulated production of IL-

10 and IL-6 and suppressed production of TNF-α and NO (17). Accumulated adenosine in PMA activated peritoneal Mϕ decreased the generation of toxic oxygen metabolites thereby preventing further injury (18). These findings point out an overall suppressive effects of adenosine that may be relevant to both cell-mediated and inflammatory immune responses.

Given the strong immunosuppressive activity of adenosine it seems likely that the variability in 5'-NT expression among lymphoid cell population (19) has functional significance.

CONCLUSION: The elevated activity of 5'-NT and reduced activity of ADA in peritoneal Mϕ lead to the extracellular and intracellular accumulation of adenosine. Since adenosine is well known immunosuppressive local metabolite the immunomodulatory effects of vitamin D could be mediated by adenosine immunosuppressive action.

Literature

1. Adams, J.S. and Gacad, M.A. (1985) J. Exp. Med. 161,755-765.
2. Adams, J.S. and Ren, S.Y. (1996) Endocrinology 137, 4514-4517.
3. Barankiewicz, J. and Cohen, A.(1984) Adv. Exp. Med. Biol. 165, 227-232.
4. Edelson, P.J, and Cohn, Z.A.(1976) J. Exp. Med. 144, 1581-1595.
5. Fischer, D., Van der Weyden, M.B., Snyderman, R. and Kelley, W.N. (1976) J. Clin. Invest. 58, 399-407.
6. Mosier, D.E. (1984) Methods in enzymology 108, 294-297.
7. Wood, R.J., and Williams, D.G. (1981) Clin. Chem. 27, 464-465.
8. Pederson, R.C. and Berry, AJ.(1977) Clin. Chem. 23, 1726-1733.
9. Lowry, O.H., Rosebrough, N.J., Farr, A.L. and Randall, R.J.(1951) J. Biol. Chem. 193, 265-275.
10. Manolagas, S.C., Hustmayer, F.G., Yu Xiao-Peng. (1989) Proc. Soc. Exp. Biol. Med. 191, 238-243.
11. Resta, R., Yamashita, Y. and Thompson, L.H. (1989) Immunol. Rew. 161, 95-109.
12. Suda, T.(1989) Proc. Soc. Exp. Biol. Med. 191, 214-220.
13. Nagakura, K., Abe, E., Suda, T., Nayakawa, M., Nakamura, H. and Tazaki, H. (1986) Kidney. Int. 29, 834-840.
14. Gan,T.E., Dadonna, P.E. and Mitchell, B.S.(1987) Blood 69,1376-80.
15. Feng, Y.X., Liu, F., Bian, D., Hu, J.(1994) Chung. Kuo. Yao. Hsueh. Pao. 15, 473-6.
16. Zalavary, S. and Bengtsson, T.(1998) Eur. J. Cell. Biol. 75, 128-39.
17. Hasko, G., Szabo, C., Nemeth, Z.H., Kvetan, V., Pastores, S.M.and Vizi, E.S.(1996) J. Immunol. 157, 4634-40.
18. Shen, H., Wiederhold, M.D., Ou, D.W.(1995) Immunopharmacol. Immunotoxicol.17, 301-9.
19. Thompson, L.F., Resta, R.(1994) Med. Immunol. 27, 247-258.

ABNORMAL VITAMIN D METABOLISM IN HYP MICE WAS RESCUED BY SYNGENEIC BONE MARROW TRANSPLANTATION.

Hiroyuki Tanaka, Takako Miyamura, Mayu Shinohara, Yoshiki Seino, Department of Pediatrics, Okayama University Medical School, Okayama, Japan

Introduction   X-linked hypophosphatemic vitamin D resistant rickets (XLH) is an inherited disorder of phosphate homeostasis characterized by severe renal phosphate wasting. In 1995, the gene responsible for XLH was identified as *PHEX* (Phosphate regulating gene with homology to Endopeptidase on the X-chromosome)(1), and the responsible gene for hypophosphatemic mouse (Hyp) was also identified as the murine homolog of *PHEX*. It has been reported that the *PHEX/Phex* mRNA is detected in osteoblasts but not in kidney(2). This expression pattern led us the idea that introduction of normal gene into XLH/Hyp osteoblast may correct their abnormal phenotypes including rickets, hypophosphatemia and abnormal vitamin D metabolism. Bone marrow cells contain not only hematopoietic stem cells but also progenitors of several cell types including osteoblast(3). Therefore, we performed syngeneic bone marrow transplantation to introduce normal gene into Hyp osteoblast.

Materials and Methods   We established and have maintained a homozygous Hyp strain. Tibiae and femora were dissected from donor mice, and bone marrow was flushed out with phosphate buffered saline and was resuspended at $2 \times 10^6/0.1$ ml. Syngeneic bone marrow transplantation was performed by peritoneal injection to each recipient within 24 hours after birth. Recipients were newborn female Hyp mice (C57BL/6J *Hyp/Hyp*). Donrs were 8 to 10 weeks old male wild type mice (WH group; experiment group) and male Hyp mice (HH group; control group). All recipient mice were killed at 8 weeks after injection and their phenotypes were evaluated.

Results   Chimerism, which was evaluated by detection of male specific gene *Sry* in female organs, was detected in bone marrow, spleen, thymus and isolated osteoblasts. Chimeric efficiency, which was evaluated as the ratio of the relative *Sry* gene dosage corrected by the dose of GAPDH, was 4.80 ± 1.01 %. The serum inorganic phosphorus levels were significantly increased in the WH group compared with the HH group (7.10 ± 0.21 mg/dl vs 4.32 ± 0.10 mg/d, $p<0.001$). Moreover, the serum inorganic phosphorus levels showed a linear correlationship to the chimeric efficiencies. In WH group, renal expression of murine *Npt-2* mRNA was 1.84 times higher than that in HH group (fig.1). Along with these improvements of the phosphate metabolism, the serum ALP levels were significantly decreased after bone marrow transplantation (14.0 ± 1.71 pmol/min in WH group vs 33.8 ± 2.14 pmol/min in HH group) and bone mineral contents were also significantly increased in WH group.

Fig.1 Effects of Bone Marrow Transplantation

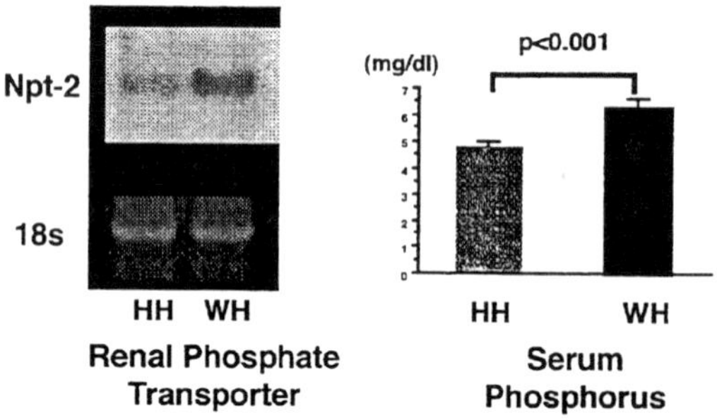

Renal Phosphate Transporter

Serum Phosphorus

Fig.2

24 OHase

18S

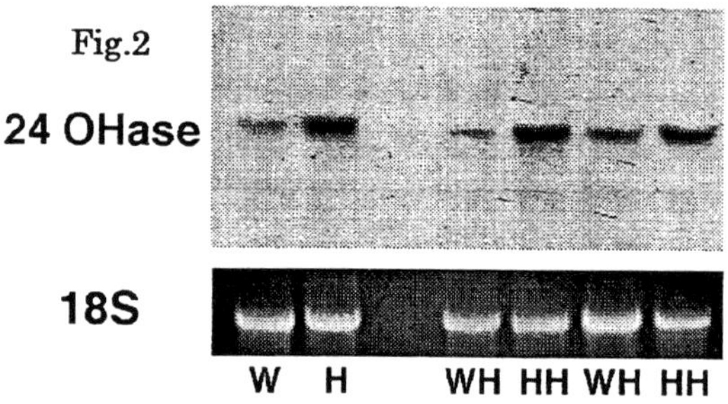

Fig.3 The Expression of 1 α hydroxylase in Kidneys

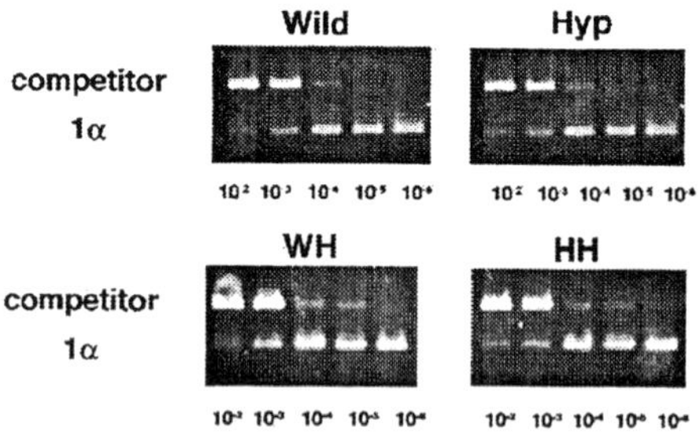

It has been reported that Hyp mice exhibit increased vitamin D 24-hyroxylase gene expression(4). The expression of the untreated Hyp mice was increased by an average 3.8 times compared with that of wild type mice (fig.2). Bone marrow transplantation from wild type mice suppressed it almost half level. On the other hand, renal 1α-hydroxylase gene expression, which was evaluated by competitive PCR, did not show any differences among untreated Hyp, wild type, HH group and WH group mice (fig 3).

Discussion The introduction of the normal bone marrow cells to Hyp mice corrected all phenotypes in a dose dependent manner. This result strongly supports the circulating phosphaturic factor theory in the pathogenesis of XLH/Hyp. Moreover, the results suggest that abnormal vitamin D metabolism in XLH/Hyp may not be secondary to the abnormal phosphate metabolism but due to the loss of function in PHEX. Because bone marrow transplantation could not induce any change in the expression of the renal 1α-hydroxylase gene, which may modulated by serum phosphorus levels.

Our data also suggest the usefulness of the bone marrow transplantation in the gene delivery system to the bone.

Conclusion   The abnormal vitamin D metabolism in XLH/Hyp may not be secondary to the abnormal phosphate metabolism but due to the loss of function of the *PHEX* gene product.

References
(1) The HYP consortium (1995) Nature Genetics. 11, 130-136
(2) Ruchon, F.R., Marcinkiewicsz, M., Siegfried, G., Tenenhouse, H.S., DesGroseillers, L., Crine, P., Boileau, G. (1998) J. Histochem. Cytochem. 99, 1200-1209
(3) Pereira R.F., Halford, K.W., O'Hara, M.D., Leeper, D.B., Sokolov, B.P., Pollard, M.D., Bagasra, O., Prockop, D.J. (1995) Proc. Natl. Acad. Sci. USA. 92, 4857-4861
(4) Tenenhouse, H.S., Yip, A., Jones, G. (1988) J. Clin. Invest. 81, 461-465

DERMATOLOGY

EPIDERMAL KERATINOCYTES AS SOURCE AND TARGET CELLS FOR VITAMIN D

Siegfried Segaert[1,2] and Roger Bouillon[1], [1]Laboratory for Experimental Medicine and Endocrinology and [2]Department of Dermatology, University of Leuven, Belgium.

The epidermis as a source of vitamin D and active vitamin D metabolites

The cutaneous photosynthesis of vitamin D_3 represents the main source of vitamin D in humans. It is formed from 7-dehydrocholesterol (7DHC or provitamin D_3), which is present in large amounts in cell membranes of keratinocytes of the basal and spinous epidermal layers (1). By the action of ultraviolet B light (UVB light with a wavelength of 290-315 nm) the B ring of 7DHC can be broken to form previtamin D_3. Previtamin D_3 has very low or no affinity for vitamin D binding protein, precluding its entrance into the circulation. In the lipid bilayer of membranes, the unstable previtamin D_3 is further isomerized to vitamin D_3 by thermal energy (1). The conformational change due to this isomerization can project vitamin D_3 into the circulation, where it is caught by vitamin D binding protein and transported to the liver and kidney for further metabolization to $1\alpha,25$-dihydroxyvitamin D_3 [$1,25(OH)_2D_3$] (1).

The production of previtamin D_3 is a non-enzymatic photochemical reaction which is not subject to regulation other than substrate (7DHC) availability or intensity of UVB irradiation. 7DHC is the last precursor in the de novo biosynthesis of cholesterol. The enzyme 7DHC Δ^7-reductase (or sterol Δ^7-reductase) catalyzes the production of cholesterol from 7DHC. Inactivating mutations of the recently cloned 7DHC Δ^7-reductase gene (2) are the hallmark of the autosomal recessive Smith-Lemli-Opitz syndrome, characterized by high tissue and serum 7DHC levels and multiple anomalies including craniofacial dysmorphism and mental retardation, due to the lack of cholesterol synthesis (3). These patients exhibit increased vitamin D_3 and 25-hydroxyvitamin D_3 ($25OHD_3$) serum concentrations (4). Likewise, animals which are pre-treated with a specific sterol Δ^7-reductase inhibitor, also exhibit an augmented vitamin D_3 synthesis following UVB irradiation (5). In a similar fashion, the high incidence of Smith-Lemli-Opitz syndrome may be explained by the heterozygote advantage, provided by increased production of vitamin D_3 in carriers of a dysfunctional 7DHC Δ^7-reductase gene (2). To keep its provitamin D_3 levels elevated, skin in vivo exhibits low sterol Δ^7-reductase activity, probably by the presence of an endogenous inhibitor of the enzyme (6). With increasing age however, the cutaneous stores of provitamin D_3 decrease together with photoproduction of vitamin D_3 (1). In some animals like cats, the high cutaneous sterol Δ^7-reductase activity hampers photoproduction of vitamin D, making it a true vitamin in these animals (7). Taken together, the activity of 7DHC Δ^7-reductase is highly correlated with dependence on nutritional sources of vitamin D. Therefore the regulation of its activity may represent a future pharmacological target for influencing the magnitude of the cutaneous 7DHC stores and vitamin D_3 production in response to sunlight.

Apart from substrate (7DHC) availability, the photochemical synthesis of vitamin D_3 in the skin largely depends on the amount of UVB photons that strike the basal epidermal layers. Glass, sunscreens, clothes and skin pigment absorb UVB and blunt vitamin D_3 synthesis (1). Latitude, time of day and season are factors that influence the intensity of solar radiation and the cutaneous production of vitamin D_3. Therefore there is a risk for shortage of vitamin D supplies during and after winter (1).

Nature has built in a few feedback mechanisms to minimize the risk that prolonged sun exposure would cause vitamin D intoxication. Cutaneous previtamin D_3 and vitamin D_3 are photosensitive and will be photodegraded to inactive sterols, when they are not translocated to the circulation (1). This makes that only a maximum of 10 to 15% of the provitamin D_3 will be converted to vitamin D_3. Sunlight induced melanin synthesis, acting as a natural sunscreen, provides an additional negative feedback (1). In addition, $1,25(OH)_2D_3$ downregulates its own biosynthesis and induces its own catabolism by regulating 1α- and 24-hydroxylase activity (8). Finally, UVB suppresses the expression of the vitamin D receptor (VDR) in a dose-dependent fashion (9), maybe further adding to this feedback.

Epidermal keratinocytes not only produce vitamin D_3, they also possess vitamin D receptors, rendering them responsive to $1,25(OH)_2D_3$ treatment (8). Furthermore they express $CYP1\alpha$ very abundantly, enabling them to convert $25OHD_3$ to $1,25(OH)_2D_3$ (10). Cutaneous 1α-hydroxylase activity is under tight feedback control by $1,25(OH)_2D_3$ (8). The mitogenic growth factors EGF and $TGF\alpha$ stimulate production of $1,25(OH)_2D_3$ (11) whereas the triggering of keratinocyte differentiation by density arrest or calcium exerts the opposite effect (8). The generation of calcitriol thus appears to be restricted to actively cycling cells, suggesting its involvement in epidermal growth and differentiation. The regulation of keratinocyte 1α-hydroxylase by the cytokines $TNF\alpha$ and $IFN\gamma$ (8), which may be released by infiltrating inflammatory cells, maybe refers to a function for vitamin D in local immunomodulation in the skin.

In addition to 1α-hydroxylase, recent evidence indicates the cutaneous presence of CYP27 (12,13) as well as 25-hydroxylase activity in epidermal cells (14,15). The combined presence of vitamin D production, 25-hydroxylase, 1α-hydroxylase and VDR in the epidermis suggests the existence of a unique vitamin D intracrine system in which keratinocytes may supply their own needs for $1,25(OH)_2D_3$ (Figure). In support of this hypothesis, Lehmann (unpublished) demonstrated production of calcitriol following UVB irradiation of 7DHC supplemented keratinocytes. In addition, our unpublished data indicate that UVB-irradiated keratinocytes, when pretreated with a 7DHC Δ^7-reductase inhibitor, secrete $1,25(OH)_2D_3$ and exhibit a marked upregulation of the expression of 24-hydroxylase (the most sensitive vitamin D-responsive gene).

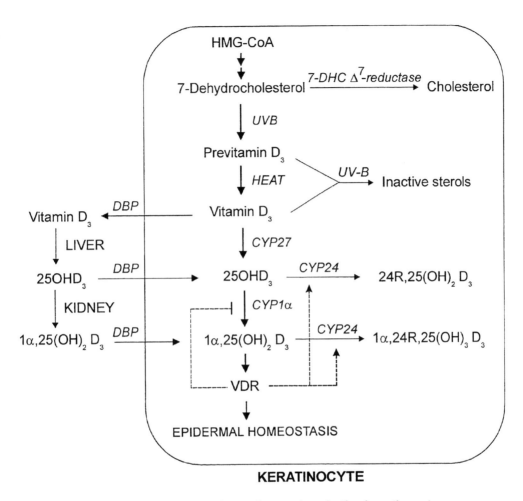

Figure: Putative vitamin D intracrine system in the keratinocyte

The epidermal keratinocyte as a target cell for 1,25(OH)$_2$D$_3$

Since the discovery of vitamin D receptors in the skin, numerous research groups have focused on investigating 1,25(OH)$_2$D$_3$ effects on keratinocyte function. Calcitriol at pharmacological concentrations is a potent inducer of keratinocyte growth arrest and differentiation (8). These properties were the basis for the application of vitamin D analogues in the treatment of psoriasis (16). Although various vitamin D regulated genes have been identified in keratinocytes (Table), the primary mechanism of action for vitamin D induced cell cycle arrest remains elusive. Calcitriol treated keratinocytes fail to progress from the G$_1$ to the S phase of the cell cycle, leaving retinoblastoma protein in its dephosphorylated growth suppressive state (17). Keratinocyte transformation by the adenovirus E1A gene product confers resistance to the growth inhibitory effects of 1,25(OH)$_2$D$_3$, further suggesting that E1A binding proteins such as retinoblastoma family members (and/or the transcriptional co-integrator p300/CBP) are required for the vitamin D action (18). The suppression of phosphorylation of the retinoblastoma protein by vitamin D is preceded by induction of the cyclin-dependent kinase inhibitors p21^{WAF1} and p27^{KIP1} (17), which prevent the activity of G$_1$ cyclin-dependent kinases on retinoblastoma. p21^{WAF1} is a transcriptional target for 1,25(OH)$_2$D$_3$ (19) but it is presently unknown to which extent this direct vitamin D effect contributes to the growth suppression. Indeed, the effects of calcitriol on p21^{WAF1} accumulation and on cell cycle kinetics take 24h to several days (17) and are preceded by changed expression of immediate early genes such as c-myc and c-fos (20,21) and by upregulation of phospholipase C with increased phosphoinositide turnover (22). Indirect effects through autocrine or paracrine growth factors such as TGF β1 and β2 (17,23), TNFα (24) and PTHrP (25) are also likely to contribute to the antimitotic vitamin D effect together with induction of 17β-hydroxysteroid dehydrogenase causing changes in local oestrogen metabolism (26). Increased differentiation is illustrated by induction of type I transglutaminase and cornified envelope precursors such as involucrin (8). A stimulatory effect on stratification by translocation of E-cadherin to assembling adherens junctions (27) will enhance the prodifferentiative actions of calcitriol, which further require a functional protein kinase C (27,28). The increased secretion of extracellular matrix molecules such as fibronectin and osteopontin in vitamin D treated keratinocytes (23,29) may prove beneficial for wound healing but also enhances anchorage-independent growth and possibly invasiveness of transformed keratinocytes (29).

Most of the studies concerning growth and differentiation were carried out with rather high pharmacological concentrations of 1,25(OH)$_2$D$_3$ and may not add to knowledge about the physiological role of vitamin D in the epidermis. Indeed, some reports indicated that (low concentrations) of calcitriol might exert mitogenic activity rather than a growth inhibiting effect on keratinocytes (30,31). These proproliferative effects were most obvious in cells that were committed to differentiate (30) and correlate with activation of the mitogen activated protein kinase pathway (32). Increased proliferation was also observed following application of vitamin D compounds to normal mouse skin (33). In contrast, hyperproliferative epidermis (in psoriasis or induced by application of hyperplasiogens) responds to vitamin D derivatives with growth arrest (16,34). With respect to the prodifferentiating actions of vitamin D, paradoxical negative effects have also been reported (35). These observations indicate that the activation state of the keratinocyte (non cycling versus actively cycling) appears to determine the vitamin D effects with respect to proliferation and differentiation. This may be explained by the regulation of VDR expression by environmental factors that determine the proliferation and differentiation state of the cells such as interaction with the extracellular matrix (36), cell density, extracellular calcium concentration, growth factors (37), and ultraviolet B irradiation (9).

Target gene	mRNA	Protein/Activity	VDRE	Reference
Proliferation associated genes				
c-fos	↗		+	(21,51)
c-myc	↘			(17,20)
Cyclin D1	↘			(Unpublished)
p21^{WAF1}	↗	↗	+	(17)
p27^{KIP1}		↗		(17)
TGF β1 and 2	↗	↗	+(β2)	(17,23)
PTHrP	↘	↘	+	(25)
IGF binding protein 3		↗		(52)
PDGF-AB		↗		(53)
ErbB1 (EGFR), ErbB 2 and 3		↗		(31)
Phospholipase C β, γ and δ	↗	↗	+ (γ1)	(22)
Phospholipase D-1	↗	↗		(54)
Differentiation related genes				
Involucrin	↗	↗		(8)
Transglutaminase I	↗	↗		(8)
Vitamin D / calcium metabolism related genes				
Vitamin D receptor	↗↘	↗		(17,55)
24-hydroxylase	↗	↗	++	(8,36,37)
1α-hydroxylase	=	↘		(8,unpublished)
Calcium receptor	↗			(56)
Inflammation related genes				
TNFα	↗	↗	+	(24,51)
IL-1α		↘		(57)
IL-6	↘	↘		(Unpublished)
IL-8		↘		(38,57)
RANTES		↘		(38)
IL-10 receptor	↗			(39)
Miscellaneous				
Osteopontin	↗		+	(29)
Fibronectin	↗		+	(23,51)
Metallothionein	↗	↗		(49,50)
17β-OH-steroiddehydrogenase	↗	↗		(26)
Urokinase	↘	↘		(58)
Tissue plasminogen activator		↘	+	(58)

Table: vitamin D regulated genes in keratinocytes.

Keratinocytes that are activated by pro-inflammatory cytokines such as IL-1, TNFα and IFNγ are known to participate in the cutaneous inflammation process by the production of cytokines, chemokines and cell adhesion molecules that allow communication with infiltrating immune cells. Many of these functions are also targeted by vitamin D: the release of the chemokines RANTES and IL-8 is inhibited by tacalcitol (38) and the pro-inflammatory cytokine IL-6 is also negatively regulated by active vitamin D (own unpublished data). The receptor for the immunosuppressive cytokine IL-10 is upregulated (39) and IL-10 release was also stimulated in calcipotriol treated psoriatic skin (40), although its cellular source was not investigated.

Like in other target tissues, autoregulation of the vitamin D system also takes place in epidermal keratinocytes. 1,25(OH)$_2$D$_3$ exerts a strong negative feedback on its own production (8), in spite of the maintenance of CYP1α mRNA levels (Bikle, unpublished; Segaert, unpublished): (post-)translational regulation or targeting of cytochrome p450 cofactors (ferridoxin or ferridoxinreductase) conceivably might explain this discrepancy. In contrast, 24-hydroxylase activity is strongly induced by 1,25(OH)$_2$D$_3$ (8) via a very potent upregulation of CYP24 mRNA levels (36,37). Finally, keratinocyte VDR protein is stabilized by its ligand in the absence of overt regulation of its mRNA (17).

Physiological function of the epidermal vitamin D system

Despite the numerous studies that describe the effects of vitamin D derivatives on cultured skin cells or on normal or diseased skin, the exact physiological function of 1,25(OH)$_2$D$_3$ and VDR in the epidermis remains elusive. The alopecia in VDR deficient mice or patients (41,42,43), which cannot be cured by normalization of mineral ion homeostasis (44), firmly indicates a direct role for VDR in hair follicle function. However, the underlying mechanisms as well as the vitamin D target cells or target genes in the hair follicle apparatus remain to be identified. The early appearance of cutaneous VDR in the phylogenetic tree (with high levels observed in frog skin) may refer to an initial role for VDR in cutaneous calcium absorption in aquatic animals (45). Although the developmental role of VDR (if any) remains to be delineated (as demonstrated by normal development in VDR knockout mice), VDR is also expressed early during ontogeny, with the skin as one of the first organs for VDR to appear (46). Moreover, during the neonatal period, when high proliferative activity in epidermis and hair follicles is manifest, there is a sharp increase in cutaneous VDR levels, before a similar rise is seen in the gut (47). An association between VDR expression and proliferation was also noticed in cultured keratinocytes (36,37). Together with the mitogenic effects of 1,25(OH)$_2$D$_3$ on normal skin (33) these data raise the hypothesis that 1,25(OH)$_2$D$_3$ and VDR may participate in the maintenance of keratinocyte proliferation in the epidermis. A preliminary study demonstrating higher p21^{WAF1} in VDR -/- murine keratinocytes is in support of this view (48). The paradoxical antiproliferative and pro-differentiative pharmacological effects of vitamin D analogues in hyperproliferative conditions such as psoriasis or cultured keratinocytes (8,16) may be explained by increased VDR expression under these circumstances (36,37). Finally, in view of the close interplay between UVB and the generation of vitamin D (and calcitriol), active vitamin D compounds may serve as an endogenous defense mechanism against harmful events caused by UVB. Indeed, we (unpublished) and others recently identified a strong photoprotective effect of calcitriol against UVB mediated events in cultured keratinocytes, that may be related to its capability to induce metallothionein, a protein with antioxidant properties (49,50).

References

1. Holick, M.F. (1994) in Modern nutrition in health and disease, eds. Shils, M.E., Olson, J.A., and Shike M. (Lea & Febiger, USA) pp. 308-325.
2. Kelley, R.I. (1998) Am. J. Hum. Genet. 63, 322-326.
3. Cunniff, C., Kratz, L.E., Moser, A., Natowicz, M.R. and Kelley, R.I. (1997) Am. J. Med. Genet. 68, 263-269.
4. Chen, T.C., Lu, Z., Shao, Q., Tint, G.S., Matsuoka, L., Wortsman, J. and Holick, M.F. (1995) Photodermatol. Photoimmunol. Photomed. 11, 63.
5. Bonjour, J.-P., Trechsel, U., Granzer, E., Klöpffer, G., Müller, K. and Scholler, D. (1987) Pflügers Arch. 410, 165-168.
6. Pillai, S., Bikle, D.D. and Elias, P.M. (1988) Skin Pharmacol. 1, 149-160.
7. Morris, J.G. (1999) J. Nutr.129, 903-908.
8. Bikle, D.D. and Pillai, S. (1993) Endocr. Rev. 14, 3-19.
9. Courtois, S.J., Segaert, S., Degreef, H., Bouillon, R. and Garmyn, M. (1998) Biochem. Biophys. Res. Commun. 246, 64-69.
10. Fu, G.K., Lin, D., Zhang, M.Y.H., Bikle, D.D., Shackleton, C.H.L., Miller, W.L. and Portale, A.A. (1997) Mol. Endocrinol. 11, 1961-1970.
11. Lehmann, B. (1997) J. Invest. Dermatol. 108, 78-82.
12. Ichikawa, F., Sato, K., Nanjo, M., Nishii, Y., Shinki, T., Takahashi, N. and Suda, T. (1995) Bone 16, 129-135.
13. Lehmann, B., Tiebel, O. and Meurer, M. (1999) Arch. Dermatol. Res. 291, 507-510.
14. Lehmann, B., Pietzsch, J., Kampf, A. and Meurer, M. (1998) J. Dermatol. Sci. 18, 118-27.
15. Lehmann, B., Rudolph, T., Pietzsch, J. and Meurer, M. (2000) Exp. Dermatol. 9, 97-103.
16. Fogh, K. and Kragballe, K. (1997) Clin. Dermatol. 15, 705-713.
17. Segaert, S., Garmyn, M., Degreef, H., and Bouillon, R. (1997) J. Invest. Dermatol. 109, 46-54.
18. Park, K., Bae, H., Heydemann, A., Roberts, A.B., Dotto, P., Sporn, M.B. and Kim, S.-J. (1994) Cancer Res. 54, 6087-6089.
19. Liu, M., Lee, M.-H., Cohen, M., Bommakanti, M. and Freedman, L.P. (1996) Genes Dev. 10, 142-153.
20. Matsumoto, K., Hashimoto, K., Nishida, Y., Hashiro, M. and Yoshikawa, K. (1990) Biochem. Biophys. Res. Commun. 166, 916-923.
21. Sebag, M., Gulliver, W. and Kremer, W. (1994) J. Invest. Dermatol. 103, 323-329.
22. Xie, Z. and Bikle, D.D. (1997) J. Biol. Chem. 272, 6573-6577.
23. Kim, H.-J., Abdelkader, N., Katz, M. and Mc Lane, J.A. (1992) J. Cell. Physiol. 151, 579-587.
24. Geilen, C.C., Bektas, M., Wieder, T., Kodelja, V., Goerdt, S. and Orfanos, C.E. (1997) J. Biol. Chem. 272, 8997-9001.
25. Kremer, R., Karaplis, A.C., Henderson, J., Gulliver, W., Banville, D., Hendy, G.N. and Goltzman, D. (1991) J. Clin. Invest. 87, 884-893.
26. Hughes, S.V., Robinson, E., Bland, R., Lewis, H.M., Stewart, P.M. and Hewison, M. (1997) Endocrinology 138, 3711-3718.
27. Gniadecki, R., Gajkawska, B. and Hansen, M. (1997) Endocrinology 138, 2241-2248.

28. Ohba, M., Ishino, K., Kashiwagi, M., Kawabe, S., Chida, K., Huh, N.-H. and Kuroki, T. (1998) Mol. Cell. Biol. 18, 5199-5207.
29. Chang, P.-L. and Prince, C.W. (1993) Cancer Res. 53, 2217-2220.
30. Gniadecki, R. (1996) J. Invest. Dermatol. 106, 510-516.
31. Garach-Jehoshua, O., Ravid, A., Liberman, U.A. and Koren, R. (1999) Endocrinology 140, 713-721.
32. Gniadecki, R. (1996) J. Invest. Dermatol. 106, 1212-1217.
33. Gniadecki, R. and Serup, J. (1995) Biochem. Pharmacol. 49, 621-624.
34. Sato, H., Sugimoto, I., Matsunaga, T., Tsuchimoto, M., Ohta, T., Uno, H. and Kiyoki, M. (1996) Arch. Dermatol. Res. 288, 656-663.
35. Lu, B., Rothnagel, J.A., Longley, M.A., Tsai, S.Y. and Roop, D.R. (1994) J. Biol. Chem. 269, 7443-7449.
36. Segaert, S., Garmyn, M., Degreef, H. and Bouillon, R. (1998) J. Invest. Dermatol. 111, 551-558.
37. Segaert, S., Garmyn, M., Degreef, H. and Bouillon, R. (2000) J. Invest. Dermatol. 114, 494-501.
38. Fukuoka, M., Ogino, Y., Sato, H., Ohta, T., Komoriya, K., Nishioka, K. and Katayama, I. (1998) Br. J. Dermatol. 138, 63-70.
39. Michel, G., Gaillis, A., Jarzebska-Deussen, B., Müschen, A., Mirmohammadsadegh, A. and Ruzicka, T. (1997) Inflamm. Res. 46, 32-34.
40. Kang, S., Yi, S., Griffiths, C.E.M., Fancher, L., Hamilton, T.A. and Choi, J.H. (1998) Br. J. Dermatol. 138, 77-83.
41. Yoshizawa, T, Handa, Y., Uematsu, Y., Takeda, S., Sekine, K., Yoshihara, Y., Kawakami, T., Arioka, K., Sato, H., Uchiyama, Y., Masushige, S., Fukamizu, A., Matsumoto, T. and Kato, S. (1997) Nat. Genet. 16, 391-396.
42. Li, Y.C., Pirro, A.E., Amling, M., Delling, G., Baron. R., Bronson, R. and Demay, M.B. (1997) Proc. Natl. Acad. Sci. U.S.A. 94, 9831-9835.
43. Malloy, P.J., Pike; J.W. and Feldman, D. (1999) Endocr. Rev. 20, 156-188.
44. Li, Y.C., Amling, M., Pirro, A.E., Priemel, M., Meuse, M., Baron, R., Delling, G. and Demay, M.B. (1998) Endocrinology 139, 4391-4396.
45. Li, Y.C., Bergwitz, C., Jüppner, H. and Demay, M.B. (1997) Endocrinology 138, 2347-2353.
46. Johnson, J.A., Grande, J.P., Roche, P.C. and Kumar, R. (1996) J. Bone Miner. Res. 11, 56-61.
47. Horiuchi, N., Clemens, T.L., Schiller, A.L. and Holick, M.F. (1985) J. Invest. Dermatol. 84, 461-464.
48. Sakai, Y and Demay, M.B. (1999) J. Bone Miner. Res. 14, S302.
49. Hanada, K., Sawamura, D., Nakano, H. and Hashimoto, I. (1995) J. Dermatol. Sci. 9, 203-208.
50. Lee, J.-H. and Youn, J.I. (1998) J. Dermatol. Sci. 18, 11-18.
51. Carlberg, C. and Polly, P. (1998) Crit. Rev. Eukar. Gene Expr. 8, 19-42.
52. Chen, T.C., Rosen, C.J. and Holick, M.F. (1997) In Vitamin D, chemistry, biology and clinical applications of the steroid hormone, eds. Norman, A.W., Bouillon, R., Thomasset, M. (University of California, Riverside) pp. 569-570.
53. Zhang, J.-Z., Maruyama, K., Ono, I. and Kaneko, F. (1995) J. Dermatol. 22, 305-309.
54. Griner, R.D., Qin, F., Jung, E., Sue-Ling, C.L., Crawford, K.B., Mann-Blakeney, R., Bollag, R.J. and Bollag, W.B. (1999) J. Biol. Chem. 274, 4663-4670.
55. Sølvsten, H., Svendsen, M.L., Fogh, K. and Kragballe, K. (1997) Arch. Dermatol. Res. 289, 367-372.
56. Ratnam, A.V., Bikle, D.D. and Cho, J.K. (1999) J. Cell. Physiol. 178, 188-196.
57. Zhang, J.-Z., Maruyama, K., Ono, I., Iwatsuki, K. and Kaneko, F. (1994 J. Dermatol. Sci. 7, 24-31.
58. Koli, K. and Keski-Oja, J. (1993) J. Invest. Dermatol. 101, 706-712.

ALOPECIA IN VITAMIN D RECEPTOR NULL MICE.

Marie B. Demay and Yoshiyuki Sakai. Endocrine Unit, Massachusetts General Hospital and Harvard Medical School, Boston MA 02114, USA.

The biological effects of 1,25-dihydroxyvitamin D3 are mediated by a nuclear receptor, the vitamin D receptor (VDR) which is a member of the nuclear receptor superfamily(1). Targeted ablation of the VDR in mice results in hypocalcemia, hypophosphatemia, hyperparathyroidism, rickets, osteomalacia and alopecia(2,3). Normalization of mineral ion homeostasis by a diet high in calcium (2.0%), phosphorus (1.25%) and lactose (20%) prevents these abnormalities with the exception of the alopecia(4). Alopecia has been observed, as a variable manifestation, in humans with mutations of the VDR(5). Alopecia is not a feature of profound vitamin D deficiency in humans or animals, nor is it seen in kindreds with mutations of the 25-hydroxyvitamin D 1-α hydroxylase.

Hair follicle development occurs during embryogenesis(6,7). Signals from the dermal mesenchyme induce epidermal placode formation by the epithelium. In response to a signal from the epidermal cells, mesenchymal condensation occurs and signals are sent back to the epithelial compartment to initiate hair growth. Mice are born with immature hair follicles that begin to produce hair within the first six days of life.

Postnatally, the hair follicle undergoes cycles of growth (anagen), regression (catagen) and rest (telogen) (8,9). Factors thought to originate from the dermal papilla act on cells of the follicular epidermis which respond by growing deep into the dermis to form the full length anagen follicle. These cells then begin to differentiate and form the hair shaft. A signal, whose cell of origin is presently unclear, initiates catagen, characterized by apoptosis of the lower part of the hair follicle. The hair cycle then enters the telogen or resting phase, until anagen is re-initiated.

Whether the same signals responsible for folliculogenesis *in utero* are responsible for normal hair cycling postnatally is not known. It is known, however, that continued reciprocal interactions between the dermal papilla and the epithelium of the follicle are critical for both development of hair follicles and maintenance of a normal hair cycle.

Several investigators have demonstrated that 1,25-dihydroxyvitamin D plays a role in keratinocyte proliferation and differentiation(10-15). VDR expression has also been shown to vary with the hair cycle. Mouse anagen follicles and dermal papilla cells have been shown to have strong nuclear VDR immunoreactivity (16). This immunoreactivity decreases during catagen and is present at very low levels during telogen. Because the VDR has been shown to have important effects on keratinocyte proliferation and differentiation, and because it is expressed in a hair cycle-dependent fashion, we undertook studies in primary keratinocytes isolated from neonatal VDR null mice to determine if a keratinocyte abnormality could explain the alopecia observed.

Primary keratinocytes were isolated from 2 to 3 day old VDR null mice and control littermates. Cells were cultured in 8% CO_2 at 34^0C(17). After achieving 80% confluence, the cells were plated in low calcium medium before addition of 10^{-8} M 1,25-dihydroxyvitamin D_3 and / or inducing differentiation with high calcium medium(18).

Tritiated thymidine incorporation was used to assess the basal proliferation rate of the keratinocytes(19). Interestingly, 10^{-8} M 1,25-dihydroxyvitamin D_3 decreased the proliferation of the wild-type keratinocytes cultured in low calcium medium by approximately 30% but had no effect on the proliferation of wild-type keratinocytes induced to differentiate by the addition of high calcium media. The proliferation rate of the VDR null keratinocytes was identical to that of keratinocytes isolated from wildtype littermates under both proliferating and differentiating culture conditions. Addition of 10^{-8} M 1,25-dihydroxyvitamin D_3 did not affect the proliferation of the VDR null keratinocytes under either of these culture conditions. Proliferating cell nuclear antigen immunoreactivity of keratinocytes in skin sections obtained at 4 days of age, confirmed that VDR ablation did not have a significant effect on proliferation *in vivo*.

The expression of mRNAs encoding selected keratinocyte differentiation markers was assessed in both keratinocyte cultures as well as in neonatal mouse skin(20). Results of these *in vivo* and *in vitro* analyses demonstrated that expression of Keratin 1, involucrin and loricrin was not altered in the VDR null mice.

These data suggest that keratinocytes isolated from VDR null mice have the same proliferative and differentiation potential as those isolated from wild-type littermates.

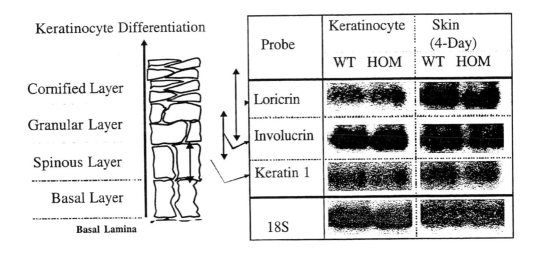

Expression of Markers of Keratinocyte Differentiation.
      Keratinocytes were grown to 80 % confluence in 0.05 mM calcium, then induced to differentiate in 2.0 mM calcium. Cells were harvested after 40 hours. Total RNA was also isolated from the skin of 4 days old mice. Three µg of total RNA were used for northern analysis of keratinocyte mRNA and 15 ug of skin RNA was used. Membranes were sequentially hybridized with mouse keratin 1, involucrin and loricrin cDNA probes. 18S ribosomal RNA signals were used to normalize for RNA loading. Data is representative of at least four independent experiments performed with keratinocytes or skin isolated independently from at least four mice of each genotype. WT, Wild type; HOM, homozygous.

PTHrP is expressed in a wide variety of tissues, including epidermal keratinocytes. This hormone has been implicated in keratinocyte differentiation(21) and forced overexpression of PTHrP in keratinocytes interfered with normal hair follicle development(22). In addition, an antagonist of the PTH/PTHrP receptor has been shown to increase hair growth in mice(23). Because the expression of PTHrP is suppressed by vitamin D(24), and because of its purported negative effects on hair growth, we postulated that overexpression of PTHrP in the absence of a functional VDR could play a role in the pathogenesis of the alopecia in the VDR null mice. However, levels of PTHrP mRNA in the keratinocytes of the VDR null mice did not differ from those of wild-type control keratinocytes.

Because these studies failed to reveal an intrinsic keratinocyte defect in the VDR null mice, we performed studies to determine if an abnormality in mesenchymal – epithelial communication could explain the alopecia observed. Since the factors involved in development of the initial hair coat are largely thought to be distinct from those that contribute to the normal cycling of hair, *in vivo* studies were performed to assess whether the alopecia in the VDR null mice could be secondary to impaired anagen initiation. In the C57BL-6 background, following anagen initiation, progressive skin pigmentation and thickening is seen within 6 days, correlating with marked proliferation of the cells of the anagen follicle. Mature follicles, with hair shafts are present by 10 days post anagen induction.

BrdU incorporation was marked in the follicle keratinocytes of the wild-type mice after anagen initiation and hair growth was clearly evident within 10 days. The VDR null mice failed to initiate anagen. Abnormalities in the knockout mice included absence of anagen follicle formation, lack of skin pigmentation and lack of skin thickening(25).

These data suggest that the alopecia in the VDR null mice is not a consequence of an intrinsic keratinocyte defect, but rather is secondary to an abnormality in the mesodermal - epithelial interactions that are required for the maintenance of a normal hair cycle.

(These studies were supported by RO1-DK46974 to MBD)

References.

1.	Haussler MR, W. G., Haussler CA, Hsieh JC, Thompson PD, Selznick SH, Dominguez CE, Jurutka PW. (1998) *J Bone Min Res* **13**(3), 325-49

2.	Li, Y. C., Pirro, A. E., Amling, M., Delling, G., Baron, R., Bronson, R., and Demay, M. B. (1997) *Proc Natl Acad Sci U S A* **94**(18), 9831-5

3.	Yoshizawa, T., Handa, Y., Uematsu, Y., Takeda, S., Sekine, K., Yoshihara, Y., Kawakami, T., Alioka, K., Sato, H., Uchiyama, Y., Masushige, S., Fukamizu, A., Matsumoto, T., and Kato, S. (1997) *Nat Genetics* **16,** 391-396

4.	Li, Y. C., Amling, M., Pirro, A. E., Priemel, M., Meuse, J., Baron, R., Delling, G., and Demay, M. B. (1998) *Endocrinology* **139**(10), 4391-6

5.	Malloy, P. J., Pike, J. W., and Feldman, D. (1999) *Endocr Rev* **20**(2), 156-88

6.	Paus, R., and Cotsarelis, G. (1999) *N Engl J Med* **341**(7), 491-7

7.	Hardy, M. H. (1992) *Trends Genet* **8**(2), 55-61

8.	Stenn KS, C. N., Eilersten KJ, Gordon JS, Pardinas JR, Parimoo S, Prouty SM. (1996) *Derm Clinics* **14**(4), 543-558

9.	Messenger, A. G. (1993) *J Invest Dermatol* , 4S-9S

10.	Arase, S., Sadamoto, Y., Kuwana, R., Nakanishi, H., Fujie, K., Takeda, K., and Takeda, E. (1991) *J Dermatol Sci* **2**(5), 353-60

11.	Bikle, D. D., and Pillai, S. (1993) *Endocr Rev* **14**(1), 3-19

12.	Bollag, W. B., Ducote, J., and Harmon, C. S. (1995) *J Cell Physiol* **163**(2), 248-56

13.	Sebag, M., Gulliver, W., and Kremer, R. (1994) *J Invest Dermatol* **103**(3), 323-9

14.	Sorensen, S., Solvsten, H., Politi, Y., and Kragballe, K. (1997) *Skin Pharmacol* **10**(3), 144-52

15.	Su, M. J., Bikle, D. D., Mancianti, M. L., and Pillai, S. (1994) *J Biol Chem* **269**(20), 14723-9

16.	Reichrath, J., Schilli, M., Kerber, A., Bahmer, F. A., Czarnetzki, B. M., and Paus, R. (1994) *Br J Dermatol* **131**(4), 477-82

17.	Hennings, H., Michael, D., Cheng, C., Steinert, P., Holbrook, K., and Yuspa, S. H. (1980) *Cell* **19**(1), 245-54

18.	Hennings, H., and Holbrook, K. A. (1983) *Exp Cell Res* **143**(1), 127-42

596

19.   Puzas JE, B. J. (1986) *Calcif Tissue Int* **39,** 104-108

20.   Dlugosz, A. A., and Yuspa, S. H. (1993) *J Cell Biol* **120**(1), 217-25

21.   Foley, J., Longely, B. J., Wysolmerski, J. J., Dreyer, B. E., Broadus, A. E., and Philbrick, W. M. (1998) *J Invest Dermatol* **111**(6), 1122-8

22.   Wysolmerski, J. J., Broadus, A. E., Zhou, J., Fuchs, E., Milstone, L. M., and Philbrick, W. M. (1994) *Proc Natl Acad Sci U S A* **91**(3), 1133-7

23.   Holick, M. F., Ray, S., Chen, T. C., Tian, X., and Persons, K. S. (1994) *Proc Natl Acad Sci U S A* **91**(17), 8014-6

24.   Kremer, R., Karaplis, A. C., Henderson, J., Gulliver, W., Banville, D., Hendy, G. N., and Goltzman, D. (1991) *J Clin Invest* **87**(3), 884-93

25.   Sakai, Y., and Demay, M.B. (2000) *Endocrinology***141**(6),2043-2053

THE ROLE OF PHOSPHOLIPASE C-γ1 IN 1α,25-DIHYDROXYVITAMIN D REGULATED KERATINOCYTE DIFFERENTIATION

Zhongjian Xie and Daniel Bikle. Department of Medicine, Veterans Affairs Medical Center and University of California, San Francisco, CA, USA

Background.   Phospholipase C (PLC) enzymes play critical roles in intracellular signal transduction pathways (1). These enzymes hydrolyze phosphatidylinositol bisphosphate (PIP2), generating two second messengers, inositol trisphosphate (IP3) and diacylglycerol (DAG). Diacylglycerol is a physiologic activator of protein kinase C, and IP3 induces the release of calcium from internal stores. Calcium mobilization and protein kinase C activation are essential for many cellular functions including cell proliferation and differentiation. A number of distinct PLC isoenzymes have been cloned from a variety of mammalian tissues. Comparison of the deduced amino acid sequences has indicated that PLCs are divided into three types (PLC-β, PLC-γ, and PLC-δ), and each type contains several subtypes (1,2). The various PLC isoenzymes appear to be activated by distinct mechanisms that initiate the cascade of molecular events leading to various cellular responses. Among the isoenzymes, PLC-γ1 has attracted attention because PLC-γ1 is activated by growth factors such as platelet-derived growth factor (3), epidermal growth factor (3,4), fibroblast growth factor (5), and nerve growth factor (6). These growth factors increase the activity of PLC-γ1 in several types of cultured cells. PLC-γ1 is overexpressed in human breast cancer carcinoma (7), human colorectal cancer (8), familial adenomatous polyposis (9), human epidermis in hyperproliferative conditions (10), and squamous carcinoma cell lines (11). Microinjection of PLC-γ1 into NIH3T3 cells causes a dose-dependent transformation, whereas injection of PLC-γ1 antibody blocks serum- or ras-induced transformation (12,13). PLC-γ1 may also play a role in the regulation of cell differentiation in that PLC-γ1 and δ1 protein expression increase in calcium induced differentiation of murine keratinocytes (14). Our studies have focused on the role of PLC-γ1 in mediating 1,25(OH)$_2$D and calcium regulated keratinocyte differentiation.

Induction of PLC by 1,25-dihydroxyvitamin D.   An acute increase in IP$_3$, DAG and intracellular calcium after 1,25-dihydroxyvitamin D [1,25(OH)$_2$D] administration has been reported by some but not all investigators (15-21). We (22) observed that treatment of keratinocytes with 1,25(OH)$_2$D results in potentiation of the intracellular calcium response of these cells to ATP. This potentiation required at least 4h, was maximal by 24h, was inhibitable with cycloheximide, was unaccompanied by a change in total intracellular calcium pools, and was associated with an increase in basal IP$_3$ levels and ATP-stimulated IP$_3$ production (22). These results suggested an effect of 1,25(OH)$_2$D on PLC activity; we (22) subsequently determined that 1,25(OH)$_2$D could increase the protein and mRNA levels of phospholipase C isoenzymes (Figure 1).

598

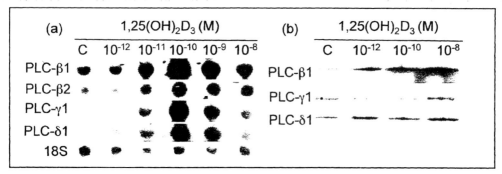

Figure 1: Induction of PLC-β1, -β2 -γ1 and -δ1 mRNA (a) and protein (b) expression by 1,25(OH)$_2$D in human keratinocytes. Cells were treated for 24 hr with 0 (C) or 10^{-12} to 10^{-8} M 1,25(OH)$_2$D in the presence of 0.07 mM calcium for 24 hr. mRNA levels were determined by northern analysis using 18S ribosomal RNA as control; protein levels were determined by western analysis with the appropriate antibodies.

VDRE in PLC-γ1 is a DR6. We then investigated the mechanism by which 1,25(OH)$_2$D induced the PLC family, focusing on PLC-γ1 because it is the most abundant PLC in keratinocytes and potentially the most important with respect to mediating the effects of 1,25(OH)$_2$D and calcium on proliferation and differentiation. The 5'-flanking region of the human PLC-γ1 gene was isolated from a human P1 genomic library. S1 nuclease mapping and primer extension analysis revealed that there is a single transcriptional start site located 135 bases upstream from the translation start site (23). The DNA sequence around the transcriptional start site is very GC rich and contains no TATA box (23). We then subcloned a fragment from -135 to -877 bp into the pGL3 luciferase reporter vector and demonstrated its responsiveness to 1,25(OH)$_2$D. Deletion and mutation studies of this fragment demonstrated a vitamin D-responsive element (VDRE) that contains a motif arranged as two direct repeats separated by 6 bases (DR6) (5'-**AGGTCA**gaccac**TGGACA**-3') between −786 and −803 bases (23). Incubation of the oligonucleotide containing the DR6 with keratinocyte nuclear extracts produced a specific protein-DNA complex. This binding could be blocked with an oligonucleotide containing the native DR6 from the PLC-γ1 promoter (W) or the DR3 from the 24-hydroxylase promoter (H), but not with an oligonucleotide that contained a mutated DR6 (M) (Figure 2a) (23). The addition of an antibody to VDR shifted the complex to a higher molecular weight form indicating the presence of VDR in the complex (Figure 2a) (23). Subsequently, we determined that the DR6 in the PLC-γ1 promoter also bound the retinoic acid receptor (RAR) but not the retinoid X receptor (RXR) indicating that for this VDRE, the VDR couples to RAR (Figure 2b) (11). All trans retinoic acid (tRA) potentiated the ability of 1,25(OH)$_2$D to stimulate not only the PLC-γ1 VDRE in transfected keratinocytes but also the mRNA levels for PLC-γ1 in normal keratinocytes (Figure 3) (11). In contrast, the VDRE from the 24-hydroxylase promoter is a

DR3 (3 nucleotide spacing between the 2 half sites) and has been shown by others as well as ourselves to bind VDR and RXR but not RAR (data not shown). We (11) made constructs with the PLC-γ1 and 24-hydroxylase promoters and confirmed that although both promoters responded to 1,25(OH)₂D, only the PLC-γ1 promoter responded to all trans retinoic acid (Figure 4).

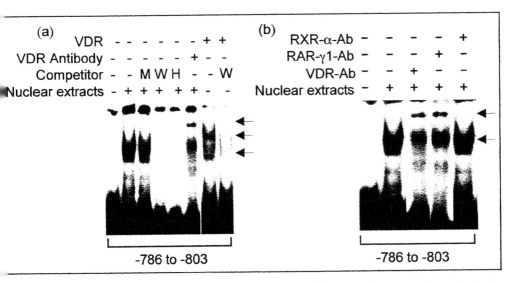

Figure 2: The binding of VDR and RAR in normal human keratinocytes with the fragment -786 to -828 containing the DR6 type VDRE in the human PLC-γ1 gene. A ³²P-labeled oligonucleotide representing the DR6 type VDRE was incubated with nuclear extracts isolated from normal human keratinocytes treated with 1,25(OH)₂D. Unlabeled competitors (M, W, H) were added at the preincubation step (a). In the super gel shift reaction (a,b), a VDR antibody (a,b), RARγ1 antibody (b), or RXRα antibody (b) was added to the DNA-protein reaction. DNA-protein complexes were resolved on a 6% polyacrylamide gel. The arrows indicate VDR-DNA or RAR-DNA and antibody-VDR or RAR-DNA complexes. H is an oligonucleotide containing the DR3 VDRE at bp-152 to -172 in the human 24-hydroxylase promoter; W is an oligonucleotide containing the native DR6 of the PLC-γ1 promoter from bp-786 to -828; M is an oligonucleotide containing a mutated form of W in which the DR6 half site sequences AGGTCA and TGGACA were replaced by TAGGTA and ATGCAT.

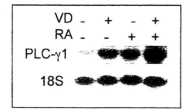

Figure 3: The effect of 1,25 (OH)₂D on PLC-γ1 mRNA in normal keratinocytes. The cells were grown to near confluence in KGM containing 0.03 mM calcium, at which point $1,25(OH)_2D_3$ (VD), all-trans RA (RA), or vehicle (ethanol) was added. The cultures were maintained for 24 hours, and the cells harvested for RNA. The RNA was isolated, electrophoresed and blotted on to a membrane. The membrane was hybridized with the probes for human PLC-γ1 and 18S RNA.

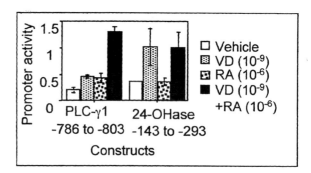

Figure 4: The effect of $1,25(OH)_2D$ and all-trans RA on the VDRE in the human PLC-γ1 promoter in normal keratinocytes. The fragment -768 to -803 in the human PLC-γ1 promoter was ligated to the SV40 promoter and luciferase gene in a pGL-3-promoter vector. The construct was transfected into keratinocytes, and luciferase activities were measured following 24 hours exposure to 10^{-9} M $1,25(OH)_2D_3$ (VD), 10^{-6} M all-trans RA (RA) or vehicle. The results are normalized to β-galactosidase activity. A construct containing the vitamin D responsive region at -143 to -293 in the human 24-hydroxylase gene (24-OHase) was used as a control.

Role of PLC-γ1 in keratinocyte differentiation. Having shown that PLC-γ1 is regulated by $1,25(OH)_2D$ and calcium, we sought to determine whether PLC-γ1 plays an essential role in the regulation of keratinocyte differentiation by $1,25(OH)_2D$ and calcium. To address this issue, we blocked expression of PLC-γ1 in human keratinocytes by transfecting cells with an antisense human PLC-γ1 cDNA construct. These cells demonstrated a specific reduction in PLC-γ1 protein levels compared to the empty vector-transfected cells and a marked reduction in the mRNA and protein levels of the differentiation markers involucrin and transglutaminase following administration of calcium (24) or $1,25(OH)_2D$ (Xie and Bikle, unpublished) (Figure 5). Similarly, cotransfection of antisense PLC-γ1 constructs with a luciferase reporter vector containing involucrin or Transglutaminase promoters led to a substantial reduction in calcium stimulated involucrin and transglutaminase promoter activities (Figure 6) (24). Similar results were seen following treatment with a specific PLC inhibitor U73122 (24). To determine whether PLC-γ1 regulated differentiation by controlling intracellular calcium (Cai), we examined the ability of antisense PLC-γ1 to block the calcium induced rise in Cai and found that it could (Figure 7) (46). These findings indicate that calcium and $1,25(OH)_2D_3$ require PLC-γ1 to induce differentiation in keratinocytes, presumably via the ability of PLC-γ1 to generate the second messengers, IP3, DAG, and Cai, required for the differentiation response.

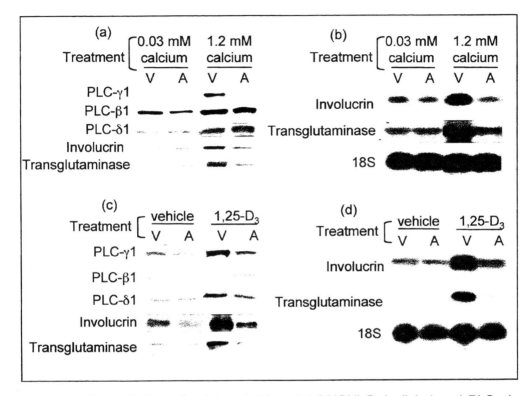

Figure 5: The inhibition of calcium (a,b) and 1,25(OH)₂D (c,d) induced PLC-γ1, involucrin, and transglutaminase protein (a,c) and mRNA (b,d) levels by antisense PLC-γ1 cDNA in normal keratinocytes. The antisense PLC-γ1 construct was made by inserting 4.2 kb human PLC-γ1 cDNA fragments containing the ATG start codon in an antisense orientation into the *Bam*HI site in a pcDNA3.1(+) (Invitrogen) vector which expresses a neomycin (G418) resistance gene. Keratinocytes isolated from neonatal human foreskin were transfected in suspension with the antisense PLC-γ1 (A) or pcDNA3.1(+) vector (V) using a polybrene/glycerol method and incubated in KGM with 0.03 calcium. The transfected cells were selected by G418 48 hours after transfection. Cells were harvested 48 hours after addition of 1.2 mM calcium (a,b) or 10^{-9} M 1,25(OH)₂D₃ (c,d). The PLC isozymes and differentiation markers were quantitated by western analysis and northern analysis.

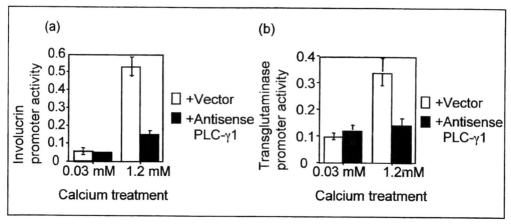

<u>Figure 6:</u> The inhibition of involucrin and transglutaminase promoter activities by antisense PLC-γ1 cDNA in calcium-induced human keratinocytes. The antisense PLC-γ1 construct or the empty vector (described in Figure 5 legend) was transfected into second passage human keratinocytes cultured in KGM medium containing 0.03 mM calcium along with the involucrin promoter-luciferase construct (a) or transglutaminase promoter-luciferase construct (b) and the β-galactosidase expression vector. Cell lysates were prepared, and the luciferase and β-galactosidase activities were measured at 48 hours after addition of 1.2 mM calcium. The data were normalized to β-galactosidase activity.

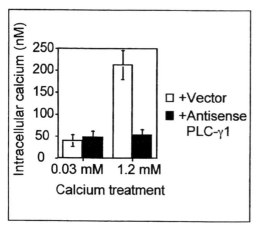

<u>Figure 7:</u> Reduction of keratinocyte intracellular Ca^{2+} by antisense PLC-γ1. NHK were transfected with the antisense PLC-γ1 or pcDNA3.1(+) vector according to the method described in the Fig 5 legend. The cells cultured on glass coverslips in KGM with 0.03 mM or 1.2 mM Ca^{2+} were loaded with Fura-2 and Pluronic and the fluorescence measured using a dual-wavelength fluorescence imaging system.

In summary, our studies have demonstrated that $1,25(OH)_2D$ induces PLC-γ1 through an unusual VDRE consisting of a DR6 to which VDR and RAR but not RXR bind. The critical role of PLC-γ1 in mediating the ability of $1,25(OH)_2D$ to induce keratinocyte differentiation is demonstrated by the inability of $1,25(OH)_2D$ or calcium to induce the differentiation process when PLC-γ1 production or activity are inhibited. Thus PLC-γ1 plays a critical role in the prodifferentiating response of normal keratinocytes to $1,25(OH)_2D$.

References

1. Rhee S.G., Suh P.G., Ryu S.H., Lee S.Y. (1989) *Science* **244**:546-550
2. Rhee, S.G. and Choi, K. D. (1992) *Adv. Second Messenger Phosphoprotein Res.* **26**: 35-61
3. Meisenhelder J., Suh P.G., Rhee S.G., Hunter T. (1989) *Cell* **57**:1109-1122
4. Margolis B., Rhee S.G., Felder S., Mervic M., Lyall R., Levitzki A., Ullrich A., Zilberstein A., Schlessinger J. (1989) *Cell.* **57**:1101-1107
5. Burgess W.H., Dionne C.A., Kaplow J., Mudd R., Friesel R., Zilberstein A., Schlessinger J., Jaye M. (1990) *Mol. Cell. Biol.* **10**: 4770-4777
6. Kim U.H., Fink D. Jr., Kim H.S., Park D.J., Contreras M.L., Guroff G., Rhee S.G. (1991) *J. Biol. Chem.* **266**:1359-1362
7. Arteaga C.L., Johnson M.D., Todderud G., Coffey R.J., Carpenter G., and Page D.L. (1991) *Proc. Natl. Acad. Sci. USA* **88**:10435-10439
8. Park J.-G., Lee Y.H., Kim S.S., Park K.J., Noh D.-Y., Ryn S.H., and Suh P.-G. (1994) *Cancer Res.* **54**:2240-2244
9. Noh D.-Y., Lee Y.H., Kim S.S., Kim Y.I., Ryu S.-H., Suh P.-G., and Park J.G. (1994) *Cancer* **73**:36-41
10. Nanney L.B., Gates R.E., Todderud G., King L.E. Jr., and Carpenter G. (1992) *Cell Growth Diff.* **3**:233-239
11. Xie Z. and Bikle D.D. (1998) *J. Invest. Dermatol.* **110**(5):730-733
12. Smith M.R., Ryu S.H., Suh P.G., Rhee S.G., Kung H.F. (1989) *Proc. Natl. Acad. Sci. USA* **86**:3659-3663
13. Smith M.R., Liu Y.L., Kim H., Rhee S.G., Kung H.F. (1990) *Science* **247**:1074-1077
14. Punnonen K., Denning M., Lee E., Li L., Rhee S.G., Yuspa S.H. (1993) *J. Invest. Dermatol.* **101**:719-726
15. McLaughlin J.A., Cantley L.C., and Holick M.F. (1990) *J. Nutr. Biochem.* **1**:81-87
16. Bittiner B., Bleehen S.S., MacNeil S. *Br.* (1991) *J. Dermatol.* **124**:230-235
17. Jaken S., and Yuspa S.H. (1988) *Carcinogenesis* **9**:1033-1038
18. Lee E., and Yuspa S.H. (1991) *J Cell Physiol.* **148**:106-115
19. Yada Y., Ozeki T., Meguro S., Mori S., Nozawa Y. (1989) *BBRC*, **163**:1517-1522

20. Tang W., Ziboh V.A., Isseroff R.R., Martinez D. (1987) *J. Cell Physiol.* **132**:131-136

21. McLaughlin J.A., Cantley L.C., Holick M.F. (1990) *J. Nutr. Biochem.* **1**:81-87

22. Pillai S., Bikle D.D., Su M.J., Ratnam A., Abe J. (1995) *J Clin. Invest.* **96**:602-609

23. Xie Z. and Bikle D.D. (1997) *J. Biol. Chem.* **272**:6573-6577

24. Xie Z. and Bikle D.D. (1999) *J. Biol. Chem.* **274**:20421-20424

1,25DIHYDROXYVITAMIN D CONTRIBUTES TO PHOTOPROTECTION IN SKIN CELLS.

Rebecca S Mason and Carolyn J Holliday. Department of Physiology and Institute for Biomedical Research, University of Sydney. NSW 2006 Australia

Introduction: Although vitamin D3, 1,25dihydroxyvitamin D3 (1,25(OH)2D3) and possibly 25hydroxyvitamin D3 are made in skin cells, their function in skin is not fully understood. 1,25(OH)2D3 probably contributes to normal differentiation of keratinocytes (1), to hair follicle development (2) and, under some circumstances, can enhance pigmentary responses (3). In cell culture studies, we had earlier shown that treatment with 1,25(OH)2D3 resulted in increased cornified envelope formation in keratinocytes (4) and, under some circumstances, increased melanogenesis in melanocytes (5). Since increased cornification of keratinocytes and increased pigment production by melanocytes are features of the normal cellular responses to UVR _in vivo_ as well as _in vitro_ (6), we were interested in the responses of skin cells to UVR in the presence of 1,25(OH)2D3.

Ultraviolet irradiation (UVR) interacts with 7-dehydrocholesterol to form pre-vitamin D3 which, at body temperature, converts to vitamin D3. UVR also results in DNA damage in skin cells through direct interaction with DNA causing, for example, pyrimidine dimer formation and through oxidative DNA damage with increase in markers such as 8-hydroxyguanosine. The DNA damage, as well as general cellular damage due to oxidative stress, in turn activate repair mechanisms and, in part through up regulation of the tumor suppressor gene p53, may also activate apoptosis. Agents such as tocopherol which are effective antioxidants have been shown to provide some protection from UVR-induced skin cell damage (7).

Methods: Keratinocytes were cultured from human skin explants in low calcium media (DMEM) with epidermal growth factor, cholera toxin and hydrocortisone as previously described (6). Melanocytes were cultured from a skin cell suspension in DMEM with phorbol ester and cholera toxin then changed to MCDB 153 media without these additives for at least 2 days before experiments (8). The UV source consisted of an FS20T12 UVB lamp and an FL20SBL UVA lamp filtered through cellulose acetate to remove wavelengths below 290nm. Irradiance was $0.08mJ/cm^2$ UVB and $0.19mJ/cm^2$ UVA. In some studies an F3S solar simulator was used (6). For experiments cells were plated in multiwell plates and allowed to attach before treatment with ethanol vehicle (0.1%) or 1,25(OH)2D3 at $10^{-8}M$ unless otherwise stated. Pre-treatment was for 24h unless otherwise indicated. Media was changed to phosphate-buffered saline before irradiation. After irradiation, cells were maintained in normal medium with vehicle or 1,25(OH)2D3 for 24h, when remaining viable cells were counted. Sham-irradiated cells were subjected to similar procedures but were covered with black cardboard during the irradiation. In some studies, skin cells were treated with doxorubicin 20μM (Adriamycin) instead of UVR. The procedure was similar, except that after the pre-treatment period cells were

606

changed to media containing doxorubicin or its vehicle, water, and maintained in that for the following 24h before counting.

Results: Both keratinocytes and melanocytes from different donors were damaged by UVR. Twenty-four hours after exposure to $62mJ/cm^2$, keratinocyte numbers were reduced by 10 to 42% compared with sham-irradiated controls (fig 1) while melanocyte numbers were reduced by 16 to 56%, depending on donor (fig 1). When either keratinocytes or melanocytes were pre-treated with $10^{-8}M$ 1,25(OH)2D3, cell losses were reduced to between 6 and 34% for keratinocytes and between 0 and 37% for melanocytes (fig 1).

Figure 1. Effect of pretreatment with 1,25(OH)2D3 on skin cell numbers after UVR

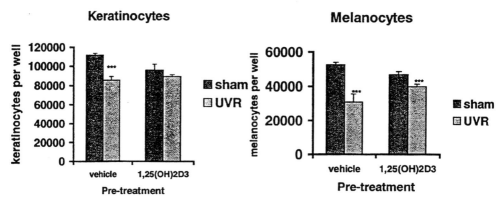

In experiments with keratinocytes from 9 different donors the average percentage cell loss after UVR with vehicle was 19.5±9.5 while it was only 11.6±8.8% after pre-treatment with $10^{-8}M$ 1,25(OH)2D3 (p<0.05). With melanocytes from 10 different donors the average UVR-induced cell loss was 35.5±13.6% with vehicle and 13.1±11.8% in the presence of 1,25(OH)2D3. In both cases the reduction in cell loss after UVR was dose-dependent (fig 2).

. Figure 2. Reduction in cell loss after UVR by 1,25(OH)2D3 – dose response

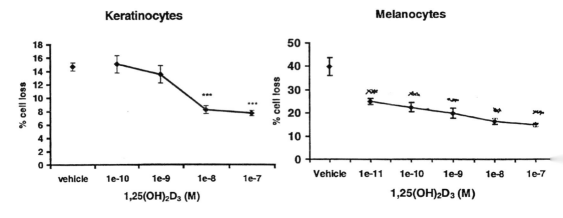

In comparison to melanocytes incubated with vehicle, where cell losses were 27±3.6%, pre-treatment with 10^{-8}M 1,25(OH)2D3 for 0.2h reduced cell loss to 12.7±1%, to 2.7±0.7% after 3h, to 1.5±0.7% after 5h and to 0.5±0.1% after 24h pre-treatment. In contrast to the cell survival promoting properties of 1,25(OH)2D3, retinoic acid at 10^{-6}M reduced keratinocyte losses significantly in only 1 of 4 experiments and reduced melanocyte losses in only 1 of 5 separate experiments.

Since much of the cell damage produced by UVR has been ascribed to oxidative damage, we tested whether 1,25(OH)2D3 would protect cells from the damage induced by the agent doxorubicin which is anti-neoplastic based on its inhibition of topoisomerase II, but which causes cardiotoxicity due to oxidative stress. Pre-treatment with 1,25(OH)2D3 reduced both keratinocyte and melanocyte losses after treatment with doxorubicin. In one experiment, keratinocyte numbers were decreased 14.3±2.3% by doxorubicin 20µM in the presence of vehicle and by 7.9±3% in the presence of 1,25(OH)2D3 (p<0.01). A dose response for the effect in melanocytes is shown in figure 3.

Figure 3. Effect of 1,25(OH)2D3 on melanocyte loss after doxorubicin

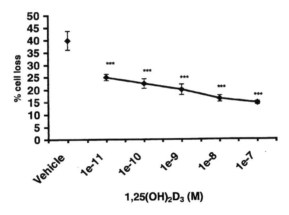

Figure 4: Comparison of protective effect of 1,25(OH)2D3 on cell loss.

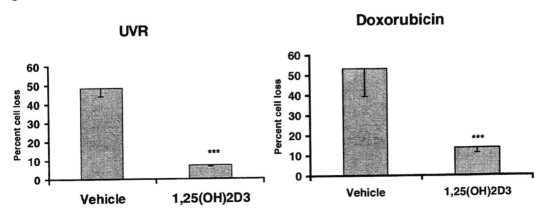

Figure 4 shows that when protection by 1,25(OH)2D3 against UVR and doxorubicin were compared in a single experiment, the reduction in cell loss after UVR was remarkably similar to the protection from doxorubicin.

Discussion: Both melanocytes and keratinocytes are prone to cell damage after UVR, resulting to some extent in apoptotic cell death. 1,25(OH)2D3 reduces cell losses after UVR and after treatment of cells with doxorubicin. The effect is dose-dependent in both keratinocytes and melanocytes and can be conferred after relatively short pre-treatment times.

The protection from doxorubicin-induced cell death shows that 1,25(OH)2D3 cannot merely be acting as a UV absorber. Both UVR and doxorubicin can cause cell death through oxidative stress (7,9). Considering that the 1,25(OH)2D3-induced protection from cell death is similar in both UVR- and doxorubicin-related damage, it may be postulated that the vitamin D compound in some way enhances cellular defences against oxidative damage. One possible candidate pathway is through an increase in metallothionein expression. Metallothionein is a transition metal-binding protein which is induced by heavy metals such as cadmium and by 1,25(OH)2D3 (10). Metallothionein induction by cadmium has been shown to protect against both UVR damage and doxorubicin-induced cardiotoxicity (9) and increased staining for metallothionein has been reported by Youn and Lee (11) in the skin of mice treated with 1,25(OH)2D3. Sunburn cell formation was also reduced in these mice (11). Other pathways such as upregulation of other cellular antioxidant defences, the IGF-1 – IGF-receptor pathway, or induction of heme-oxygenase remain possible candidates.

There is good evidence for the existence of 1α-hydroxylase in skin cells (1) and some evidence for 25-hydroxylase activity (12). In data not shown, we have demonstrated that the parent compound, vitamin D3, also protects skin cells from UVR and doxorubicin. It is possible that in addition to its other functions, the vitamin D system is part of the skin's natural defences against UVR.

References:
1. Bikle DD (2000) *In* Kragballe K ed-Vitamin D in Dermatology. Marcel Dekker p75-110
2. Reichrath J (2000) *In* Kragballe K-Vitamin D in Dermatology. Marcel Dekker p111- 123.
3. Mason RS (2000) *In* Kragballe K-Vitamin D in Dermatology. Marcel Dekker p123-132.
4. Holliday C & Mason RS (1997) *In* Norman AW, Bouillon R and Thomasset M eds - Vitamin D, Chemistry, Biology and Clinical Applications of the Steroid Hormone p95-96.
5. Ranson M, Posen S, Mason RS (1988) J Invest Dermatol 91:593-598.
6. Dissanayake N, Greenoak G, Mason RS (1993) J Cell Physiol 157:119-127.
7. Lopez-Torres M, Thiele JJ, Shindo Y, Han D et al. (1998) Brit J Dermatol 138:207-215.
8. McLeod SD, Smith C, Mason RS (1995) J Endocrinol 146:439-447.
9. Kang YJ (1999) Proc Soc Exptl Biol Med 222:263-2739
10. Karasawa M, Hosoi J, Hashiba H, Nose K et al. (1987) PNAS USA 84:8810-8813
11. Youn JH & Lee JI (1998) J Dermatol Sci 18:11-18.
12. Lehmann B, Tiebel O, Meurer M (1997) Arch Dermatol Res 291:507-510

NEW ASPECTS FOR THE VITAMIN D₃ PATHWAY IN HUMAN SKIN

Bodo Lehmann, Thurid Genehr, Thomas Rudolph, Sören Dreßler, Peter Knuschke, Oliver Tiebel*, Wolfgang Sauter[§], Jens Pietzsch* and Michael Meurer, Department of Dermatology, *Institute of Clinical Chemistry and Laboratory Medicine, [§]Department of Neurology, *Institute & Policlinic of Clinical Metabolic Research, Carl Gustav Carus Medical School, Dresden University of Technology, D-01307, Germany.

Introduction   Cutaneous vitamin D_3 (D_3) is generated by UVB-induced photolysis of 7-dehydrocholesterol (7-DHC). Once formed, D_3 is translocated into the dermal blood circulation and transported via a vitamin D-binding protein to the liver where it is metabolized to calcidiol (25-hydroxyvitamin D_3, 25OHD$_3$) which is further metabolized in the kidney to calcitriol (1α,25-dihydroxyvitamin D_3, 1α,25(OH)$_2$D$_3$) the hormonally active form of D_3. It is postulated that isomerization of previtamin D_3 (pre-D_3) to D_3 is the last step in D_3 metabolism in human skin. However, it was shown that cultured keratinocytes can convert exogeneous 25OHD$_3$ to 1α,25(OH)$_2$D$_3$ suggesting the presence of 1α-hydroxylase in keratinocytes. In addition, we were able to demonstrate that cultures of human keratinocytes can convert both the synthetic D_3 analogue 1α-hydroxyvitamin D_3 (1α-OHD$_3$) and exogeneous D_3 to 1α,25(OH)$_2$D$_3$ (1, 2). These experiments gave first evidence for the action of functionally active 1α- and 25-hydroxylases in epidermal cells. In more recent studies, we were interested to see whether the UVB-induced photolysis of 7-DHC can directly initiate the production of 1α,25(OH)$_2$D$_3$ in epidermal cells *in vitro* and possibly *in vivo*.

Results and Discussion   The rates of the enzyme-catalyzed hydroxylations of 25OHD$_3$, 1α-OHD$_3$ and D_3 to 1α,25(OH)$_2$D$_3$ in cultured keratinocytes show the following substrate range order: 25OHD$_3$ (app. $K_m = 5.4 \times 10^{-8}$ M, Bikle et al. (3)) > 1α-OHD$_3$ (app. $K_m = 6.6 \times 10^{-7}$ M, Lehmann, unpublished result) > D_3 (app. $K_m = 2.3 \times 10^{-6}$ M, Lehmann et al. (2)). Calcitriol produced co-migrated with synthetic ^{3}H-1α,25(OH)$_2$D$_3$ in NP- and RP-HPLC systems. The displacement curves obtained in a radioreceptor assay by competitive binding of ^{3}H-1α,25(OH)$_2$D$_3$ and increasing concentrations of newly formed calcitriol or of unlabeled standard 1α,25(OH)$_2$D$_3$ to the calf thymus receptor were found to be identical. Studies of the TMS derivatives of synthetic and generated calcitriol by GC-MS demonstrated identical retention times. The full-scan EI mass spectra of the TMS derivatives of standard and produced calcitriol were in essential accordance. The hydroxylation at the C-1α and C-25 position of 25OHD$_3$, 1α-OHD$_3$ and D_3 in cultured keratinocytes is inhibited by ketoconazole, indicating the participation of P450-mixed function oxidases (Figure 1). Human keratinocytes constitutively express 1α-hydroxylase activity. Using RT-PCR we detected vitamin D_3 25-hydroxylase (CYP27) mRNA in keratinocytes which supports our biochemical concept that both 1α- and 25-hydroxylase are active in keratinocytes. Notably, CYP27 mRNA is not constitutively expressed in keratinocytes but induced both by D_3 and by UVB irradiation (4).

610

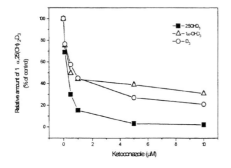

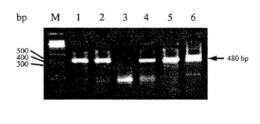

Figure 1: Inhibitory effect of ketoconazole on hydroxylation of 25OHD3, 1α-OHD3 and D3 in HaCaT keratinocytes. Culture medium supplemented with 1% BSA and 37.5 nM 25OHD3, 300 nM 1α-OHD3 or 750 nM D3 were incubated with various concentrations of ketoconazole (0.5-10 μM) or ethanol (control) and further incubated for 2 h (25OHD3) or 6 h (1α-OHD3 and D3) at 37°C. Concentrations of 1α,25(OH)2D3 are depicted as mean values of two independent experiments compared to the control.

Figure 2: RT-PCR analyses of mRNA encoding for vitamin D3 25-hydroxylase (CYP27). HepG2 cells were treated for 4 h with control vehicle (6 μl EtOH) (lane 1), vitamin D3 (780 nM) (lane 2); RT-PCR products from HSE underlying the same treatment are shown at lane 3 and 4, respectively; HSE preincubated with 7-DHC (25 μM) (lane 5) and control (lane 6) both irradiated with UVB at 300 nm (30 mJ x cm^{-2}) followed by incubation at 37° for 16 h. DNA size markers (100 bp) are shown at lane M.

In vitro experiments using the HaCaT cell line and *in vivo*-like human skin equivalents (HSE) consistently demonstrated the partial UVB-induced conversion of 7-DHC via pre-D3 and D3 to 1α,25(OH)2D3 in these cells. The rate of formation of 1α,25(OH)2D3 depends on the UVB wavelength used for irradiation and is very similar to that of D3 and showing maxima at around 302 nm. This finding points to a linkage between UVB-induced D3 synthesis and formation of 1α,25(OH)2D3. Fractions (No 1-25) obtained after NP-HPLC (eluent 2) of extracts of irradiated HSE (300 nm; dose: 30 mJ x cm^{-2}; irradiance: 0.23 mW x cm^{-2}) and of unirradiated controls were analyzed for calcitriol (Figure 3).The peak in fractions 20-22 is identical with calcitriol as shown by co-migration with synthetic ^{3}H-1α,25(OH)2D3 in NP- and RP-HPLC systems. The peak occurring after 17 min represents an unidentified D3 metabolite. No calcitriol was detectable in analogous fractions obtained after NP-HPLC of unirradiated controls. Studies of the TMS derivatives of synthetic and generated calcitriol by GC-MS demonstrated identical retention times as well as full-scan EI mass spectra. The GC-MS analysis of pooled fractions collected between 6 and 8 min provided a mass spectrum with identical mass fragments obtained from synthetic 25OHD3. This finding strongly argues for the generation of 25OHD$_3$ as an intermediary metabolite during the UVB- induced conversion of 7-DHC to 1α,25(OH)$_2$D$_3$.

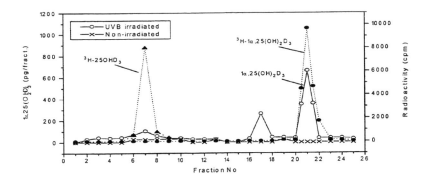

<u>Figure 3:</u> Quantification of calcitriol in extracts of irradiated and non-irradiated HSE after separation by NP-HPLC. Cultures containing 25 µM 7-DHC were irradiated at 300 nm (dose: 30 mJ x cm^{-2}) or not irradiated (control) and further incubated for 16 h. Extracts of cultures were separated by NP-HPLC (eluent 2) and fractionated (1ml/min). Fractions 1-25 were analyzed for calcitriol by a radioreceptor-assay.

Ketoconazole dose-dependently inhibited the UVB induced generation of calcitriol when the inhibitor was added to HSE immediately after irradiation (<u>Figure 4</u>). In contrast, the radical scavanger and antioxidant 1,2-dianilinoethane showed only marginal inhibitory effects on the generation of 1α,25(OH)$_2$D$_3$. This finding indicates an enzymatically catalyzed pathway of D$_3$ to 1α,25(OH)$_2$D$_3$ as previously found after exogeneous addition of D$_3$ to cultured keratinocytes. Calculations show that maximal 0.013 to 0.015% of the UVB irradiated 7-DHC (30 nmol/dish) is converted to 1α,25(OH)$_2$D$_3$ in HSE. The percentage turnover of photosynthesized D$_3$ (≈625 pmol/dish) to 1α,25(OH)$_2$D$_3$ amounts to maximal 0.78%. For comparison, the percentage turnover of exogeneously added D$_3$ (625 pmol/dish) amounts to only 0.3%. Finally, we have been able to show in preliminary experiments that the UVB-induced formation of calcitriol at 300 nm in human skin can be demonstrated using a microdialysis technique (<u>Figure 5</u>). Calcitriol concentrations in the dialysate were at a maximum 12 to 18 h after UVB irradiation and increased with rising UVB doses up to 28 mJ x cm^{-2} (equal to 1.4 MED).

<u>Conclusions</u> The metabolism of D$_3$ to 1α,25(OH)$_2$D$_3$ in keratinocytes is obviously catalyzed by P450 mixed function oxidases. Our findings indicate that keratinocytes *in vitro* convert D$_3$ to substantial amounts of 1α,25(OH)$_2$D$_3$, in particular, when D$_3$ is photochemically formed from 7-DHC added to the cell culture. Preliminary *in vivo* experiments using a microdialysis technique suggest synthesis of calcitriol in human skin irradiated with UVB light at 300 nm in

612

therapeutical doses. These findings are of potential importance for known genomic and non-genomic effects of calcitriol on keratinocytes. In particular one could speculate whether the proven therapeutical effect of UVB in hyperproliferative skin

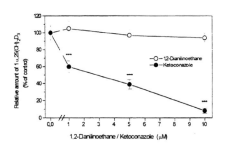

Figure 4: Inhibitory effect of ketoconazole or 1,2-dianilinoethane on hydroxylation of D_3 created after irradiation with UVB to $1\alpha,25(OH)_2D_3$ in HSE. Cultures containing 25 µM 7-DHC were irradiated at 300 nm (dose: 30 mJ x cm^{-2}). Immediately after irradiation, various concentrations of ketoconazole (1,2-dianilinoethane) (1 µM, 5 µM and 10 µM) or ethanol (control) were added to the cultures, and further incubation for 16 h at 37°C was done in the dark. Concentrations of $1\alpha,25(OH)_2D_3$ are depicted as mean ± S.D. of three independent experiments ***P < 0.001 compared to control.

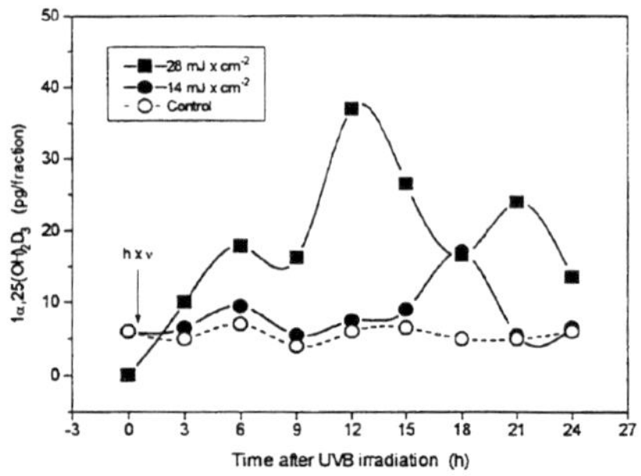

Figure 5: Microdialysis probe for cutaneous monitoring of $1\alpha,25(OH)_2D_3$ after UVB irradiation of human skin. Skin was irradiated at 300 nm at 14 mJ x cm^{-2} or 28 mJ x cm^{-2} (equal to 0.7 and 1.4 MED, respectively) and not irradiated (control). Flow rate of dialysis fluid: 0.3 µl/min, volume of fraction: 54 µl/3 h, total duration of microdialysis: 27 h. Calcitriol was determined in 50 µl dialysate. Data are depicted as mean values of two independent experiments.

diseases such as psoriasis may be directly related to the action of epidermally synthesized calcitriol.

References

(1) Lehmann, B., Pietzsch, J., Kämpf, A. and Meurer, M. (1998) J. Dermatol. Sci. 18, 118-127.
(2) Lehmann, B., Rudolph, T., Pietzsch, J. and Meurer, M. (2000) Exp. Dematol. 9, 97-103.
(3) Bikle, D.D., Nemanic, M.K., Gee, E. and Elias, P. (1986) J. Clin. Invest. 78, 557-566.
(4) Lehmann, B., Tiebel,O. and Meurer, M. (1999) Arch. Dermatol. Res. 291, 507-510.

UVB-INDUCED CONVERSION OF 7-DEHYDROCHOLESTEROL TO 1α,25-DIHYDROXYVITAMIN D₃ IN ORGANOTYPIC CULTURES OF HUMAN KERATINOCYTES

Thurid Genehr, Bodo Lehmann, Peter Knuschke, [§]Jens Pietzsch and Michael Meurer, Department of Dermatology, [§] Institute and Policlinic of Clinical Metabolic Research, Carl Gustav Carus Medical School, Dresden University of Technology, D-01307, Germany.

Introduction At present it is not clear whether the isomerization of previtamin D_3 (pre-D_3) to vitamin D_3 (D_3) is the last step in the D_3 metabolism in human skin or whether calcitriol ($1\alpha,25(OH)_2D_3$) the hormonally active form of D_3 can be generated by hydroxylation of D_3 within the epidermis. Previous findings have shown that cultured human keratinocytes can convert biologically inactive D_3 to the hormone $1\alpha,25(OH)_2D_3$ (1, 2). The aim of this study was to investigate (i) the generation of $1\alpha,25(OH)_2D_3$ in organotypic cultures of human keratinocytes (OTC) after UVB-induced transformation of provitamin D_3 (7-dehydrocholesterol, 7-DHC) via pre-D_3 into D_3; and (ii) the wavelengths of UVB involved.

Materials and Methods: OTC: Fibroblasts were embedded in rat tail collagen type 1 lattices two days before second-passage keratinocytes were inoculated onto the gel matrix (seed density: 4×10^4 / cm^2) in the culture dishes ($\varnothing$ 30 mm). Cultivation was carried out in KGM (Clonetics). After achieving preconfluence (equal to $0.45 - 0.60 \times 10^6$ cells / dish) fresh KBM (1.2 ml) supplemented with 1.0% (w/v) of BSA was added. The viability of the cells was $\geq 92\%$. Incubations: 7-DHC dissolved in 10µl ethanol, was added to the cultures. Controls were carried out using (i) solvent alone or (ii) medium containing substrate without cells. Irradiation: Monochromatic UVB light (Dermolum, Müller, Germany) at wavelengths ranging from 285 to 315 nm (bandwidth 2.5 nm) was used. The distance between the light source and culture dish without dish lid was 2 mm. After irradiation, followed by several periods of incubation the medium and detached cells were extracted with methanol:chloroform (1:1). The chloroform phase was used for the determination of pre-D_3, D_3, 7-DHC and $1\alpha,25(OH)_2D_3$. HPLC analysis: NP-HPLC: Merck/Hitachi; column: LiChroCART 250-4, Superspher Si 60, 5 µm; eluent 1 (n-hexane:2-propanol = 95:5 (v/v); flow rate: 0.5 ml/min; UV-detection at 265 nm) for the determination of pre-D_3, D_3, and 7-DHC; eluent 2 (n-hexane:2-propanol:methanol = 87:10:3 (v/v/v); flow rate: 1.0 ml/min) for fractionation of calcitriol. Calcitriol was analyzed using a radioreceptor assay (Nichols Institute). GC-MS analysis: D_3 metabolites were derivatized to TMS-derivatives. The derivatized sample (1 µl) was analyzed by a 5890/II gas chromatograph interfaced with a model 5989A MS-Engine (Hewlett-Packard, Palo Alto, CA, USA).

Results and Discussion In a preliminary study we tested the UVB-induced conversion of 7-DHC via pre-D_3 to D_3 in OTC at different incubation times (0.17 h - 16 h) after irradiation at 297 nm (dose: 30 mJ x cm^{-2}): The isomerization of pre-D_3 to D_3 was completed after 8 h in presence of cells and after 16 to 24 h in KBM without cells. There was a shift of the wavelength related to the maximum synthesis rate of D_3 from 294 nm in absence of cells to 302 nm in presence of cells. Fractions (No 1-25) obtained after HPLC (eluent 2) from extracts of irradiated OTC (300 nm; dose: 30 mJ x cm^{-2}; irradiance: 0.23 mW x cm^{-2}, 16 h incubation) and of unirradiated controls were analyzed for calcitriol (Figure. 1). The peak in fractions 20-22 is identical with calcitriol as demonstrated by NP- and RP-HPLC systems as well as by GC-MS. In pooled fractions collected between 6 and 8 min, a substance with a very similar mass spectrum to that obtained from authentic 25OHD₃ was detectable by GC-MS. Therefore, It is assumed that 25OHD$_3$ possibly acts as an intermediary metabolite on the way to calcitriol in our system. The minor peak at 17 min is unidentified yet. No calcitriol was detectable in analogous fractions obtained after NP-HPLC of unirradiated controls.

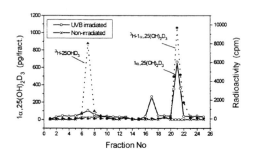

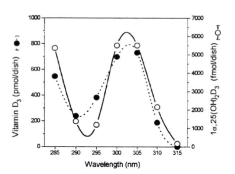

Figure 1: Determination of calcitriol in extracts of irradiated and non-irradiated OTC after separation by NP-HPLC (eluent 2) OTC in the presence of 25 µM 7-DHC were irradiated at 300 nm (30 mJ x cm^{-2}) or not irradiated (control) and further incubated for 16 h. Fractions 1 - 25 were analyzed for calcitriol by a radioreceptor-assay.

Figure 2: Relationship between wavelengths of UVB light and the generation of D$_3$ and 1α,25(OH)$_2$D$_3$ in OTC. Cultures preincubated with 25 µM 7-DHC were irradiated at several wavelengths between 285 nm and 315 nm (dose: 30 mJ x cm^{-2}) followed by 16 h-incubation. The datapoints represent means of two experiments.

OTC preincubated with several concentrations of 7-DHC (3.15 - 35 µM), irradiated at 300 nm (30 mJ x cm^{-2}) followed by a 16 h incubation period showed a clear dependence of the concentrations of D$_3$ and 1α,25(OH)$_2$D$_3$ on the dose of 7-DHC. Ketoconazole, a known P450 oxidase inhibitor, dose-dependently decreased the generation of calcitriol when the inhibitor was added to OTC immediately after irradiation. The time course indicates that the maximal synthesis rate of D$_3$ was reached after 8 h whereas that of calcitriol continously increased up to 16 h. The UVB doses showed a close correlation with D$_3$ levels and the respective amounts of calcitriol up to 30 mJ x cm^{-2} at 16 h-incubation. While the D$_3$ levels increase linear to the UVB doses the calcitriol synthesis is maximal near a dose of 30 mJ x cm^{-2} and decreases at higher UV doses. The relation between UVB wavelength and the generation of D$_3$ and calcitriol in OTC preincubated with 25 µM 7-DHC is depicted in Figure 2. There was a similar course of the synthesis rates of both D$_3$ and calcitriol in dependence on the wavelength with maxima at approximately 302 nm and minima around 292 nm. We were unable to detect D$_3$ and calcitriol at wavelengths $\geq$ 315 nm. These results show that UVB radiation efficiently induces the transformation of 7-DHC via pre-D$_3$ and D$_3$ into the hormone calcitriol in OTC. These findings are of potential iimportance for biological and therapeutical effects of 1α,25(OH)$_2$D$_3$ in the skin under the influence of UVB.

References
(1) Lehmann, B., Pietzsch, J., Kämpf, A. and Meurer, M. (1998) J. Dermatol. Sci. 18, 118-127.
(2) Lehmann, B., Rudolph, T., Pietzsch, J. and Meurer, M. (2000) Exp. Dematol. 9, 97-103.

PRECLINICAL PROFILE OF THE CYCLOHEXANEDIOL RO 65-2299, A POTENTIAL ORAL ANTIPSORIATIC

F.W. Bauer, P. Barbier, P. Mohr, T. Pfister, W. Pirson and F-P. Theil
F. Hoffmann-La Roche Ltd, Pharma Research, CH-4070 Basel, Switzerland

Introduction Psoriasis is characterised by an increased epidermal proliferation and abnormal differentiation of keratinocytes coupled with inflammation and complex immune disturbances. Calcitriol and vitamin D congeners, known to counteract these deviations, have indeed shown anti-psoriatic activities in the clinic (1,2,3). However because of the calcium liabilities of this class, up to now only topical preparations have been marketed. We have screened *in vivo* for compounds with epidermal effects after oral administration combined with a reduced calcaemic risk. From some 400 vitamin D analogs, we have selected the cyclohexanediol Ro 65-2299 for development as an oral anti-psoriatic. Ro 65-2299, a cyclohexanediol, is an atypical vitamin D analog lacking the CD ring.

Ro 65-2299   calcitriol

Methods   *Activation of vitamin D receptor:* A transcription activation assay was used with COS cells cotransfected with the human VDR (expressed in pSG5), a reporter gene containing 3 response elements (VDRE3) from rat osteocalcine gene, the thymidine kinase basal promoter, and the luciferase reporter gene. *Inhibition of keratinocyte proliferation:* The immortalized human cell line HaCaT was used. ^{3}H-thymidine incorporation was measured in exponentially growing cells with vitamin D derivatives present for 6 days of culture. *Differentiation of HL-60 cells:* The differentiated cells were determined by measuring their oxidative burst potential via the reduction of NBT (Nitro-blue-tetrazolium). *Inhibition of T-cell proliferation:* ^{3}H-thymidine incorporation was determined for the last 6 h of the culture with human T-cells on day 3 of culture in presence of vitamin D derivatives. *Inhibition of INF-γ production in T-cells:* Interferon-γ in the supernatant of cultured human T-cells was determined by ELISA on day 3 of culture in presence of vitamin D analogs.

Background for in vivo methods: *Many compounds or treatments, which inhibit epidermal proliferation in psoriatic lesions, elicit hyperproliferation of normal skin, after topical or oral administration. Orally administered vitamin D analogs can lead to epidermal hyperproliferation in mice and mini-pigs. This apparent paradox may be explained by a in vitro study with keratinocytes: calcitriol either inhibits keratinocyte proliferation if growth is already optimal (psoriasis) or activates their growth if keratinocytes are slowly growing in a depleted medium without activating growth factors (normal skin) (4).*

Mouse model: The model allows to identify analogs with an improved ratio between effects on the target tissue (epidermis) and unwanted systemic effects (hypercalcaemia). Weight loss was used as a surrogate parameter for hypercalcaemia, and the highest tolerated dose without weight loss was determined (HTD). Hairless mice were orally treated for 4 days, skin biopsies were taken at day 5. *Mini-pig model:* Mini-pigs received daily administrations for 7 days of Ro 65-2299 in arachis oil. On day 8 bromodeoxyuridine (BrdU) was injected s.c., and 2 hours later a skin biopsy was taken. BrdU labeled cells were detected immunohistochemically. The labeling index (BrdU index), a measure of epidermal proliferative activity, is the number of labeled epidermal cells/ mm length along the surface. The effective dose (ED) is defined as the dose that causes an increase of at least 50% above the labeling index of control pigs. *IL-12 dependent septic shock model:* A septic shock was induced in C57BL/6 mice by i.p. injection of LPS (Salmonella abortus-equi) (5). Ro 65-2299 or calcitriol were orally administered 72 h, 48 h, 24 h, and 1 h prior to LPS. INF-γ (ELISA) and calcium levels were determined in serum obtained 6 h after LPS application.

Results Pharmacology in vivo   Mouse model The epidermis reacts with hyperproliferation both to calcitriol and to Ro 65-2299 which is associated with weight loss, a surrogate parameter for hypercalcaemia. Calcitriol leads to epidermal thickening only at extremely toxic dosage, which the mice can survive for no more than 3 days (Fig.1c). In contrast to calcitriol, Ro 65-2299 induces epidermal proliferation at well-tolerated dosages (Fig. 1d,e).

Figure 1. Skin histology of mice after oral treatment

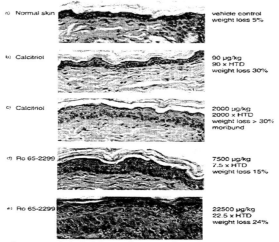

Ro 65-2299 is superior to calcitriol by a factor of 67 based on the shift in the index skin effect/calcaemic effect:

compound	skin effect ED_{50} µg/kg	non-toxic dose HTD p.o. µg/kg	index ED_{50}/HTD	shift in index compared to calcitriol
65-2299	7500	1000	7.5	67
calcitriol	500	1	500	1

Mini-pig model Ro 65-2299 was able to induce epidermal hyperproliferation (increased BrdU index) at all doses even in the normocalcaemic dose range.

Experiment 1			Experiment 2		
Dose µg/kg	BrdU Index	Ca mmol/L	Dose µg/kg	BrdU Index	Ca mmol/L
100	11.4	2.60	61.7	9.0	2.55
300	11.0	2.71	185	8.3	2.57
900	12.5	2.69	556	5.3	2.69
2700	18.4	2.78	1667	8.5	3.24
8100	9.5	3.07			

Control values: BrdU Index: 4.4 ± 0.9 (n=22)

The hypercalcaemic dose (values >3.0 mmol/L Ca) is ~1500-5000 µg/kg. Therefore, the lowest effective dose is at least 15-50 times lower than the hypercalcaemic dose. We estimated the shift versus calcitriol as very large: >100-350. Therefore, we expect the therapeutic window of 65-2299 in psoriasis to be much better than that of calcitriol:

compound	Rel. shift in mice	Effective dose µg/kg	Calcaemic dose µg/kg	TI Ratio Cal./Eff.	Rel. shift in minipig
calcitriol	1	>22.5	~3	<0.15	1
65-2299	67	<100	1500-5000	>15-50	>100-350

IL-12 dependent septic shock model IL-12 mediates Th-1 lymphocyte maturation and concomitant INF-γ production. IL-12 is increased in psoriatic plaques (6). Since psoriasis is Th-1 driven, a drug's potential to inhibit IL-12 may contribute to its antipsoriatic effect. Ro 65-2299 shows in a mouse septic shock model an inhibition of IL-12 mediated INF-γ production. This occurs, similar to calcitriol, in a normo-calcaemic dose range. These results indicate that Ro 65-2299 has a similar immunosuppressive effect as calcitriol in this in vivo model.

Results Pharmacology in vitro The in vitro data characterise Ro 65-2299 as a weak vitamin D congener. Except from being weaker, the overall in vitro profile of the compound is similar to calcitriol (EC_{50} /IC_{50} nM): VDR activation: 120 vs 2.2; HaCaT proliferation: 965 vs 43; HL-60 differentiation: 2420 vs 11; T-cell proliferation: 400 vs 1.4: T-cell INF-γ: 196 vs 0.7.

Pharmacokinetics and Metabolism   The results from mice, rats rabbits, mini-pigs and dogs indicate a moderate plasma clearance of 5-19 ml/min/kg for 4 species (mouse, rat, rabbit, dog), a moderate volume of distribution (1-3 L/kg), high bioavailability (55-100%), high protein binding (~99%). The extrapolation from animal experiments predicts a high oral bioavailability in man and a once a day treatment. The metabolic profile is very similar in mouse, rat, pig, dog, and man. The elimination occurs exclusively by metabolism via oxidative metabolism (CYP 3A4) and glucuronidation. In summary, there appears not to be any critical DMPK issue.

Toxicology   The expected class-specific calcium liability was observed with calciuria and hypercalcaemia as primary effects, body weight decrease, renal damage (tubular nephrosis), and tissue calcification as secondary effects. The no-effect-levels (NOEL) in 4 weeks treatment was 25 µg/kg for the rat and 50 µg/kg in the dog. Preliminary reprotox studies revealed no selective teratogenic potential (embryo-fetal toxicity related to maternal hypercalcaemia) in rats. Neither genotoxic/mutagenic and phototoxic potential was found nor effects on the circulatory, respiratory, renal function, and on the central nervous system.

Summary   Ro 65-2299 has *in vitro* pharmacology typical of a weak agonist of the vitamin D receptor. It has an overall *in vitro* profile similar to calcitriol with respect to a number of biological properties such as inhibition of keratinocyte proliferation, differentiation potential and immuno-modulation. *In vivo*, Ro 65-2299 exerts skin effects typical for vitamin D analogs after oral administration with a clear indication of less calcaemic liability than calcitriol. Further *in vivo* pharmacology in mice showed an inhibition of IL-12 mediated INF-γ production indicating an immunosuppressive property similar to calcitriol. Based on these data, Ro 65-2299 is expected to have a potential for the treatment of psoriasis with a large therapeutic window. Studies for DMPK did not reveal critical issues and toxicological investigations did not show any other toxicity than that associated with hypercalcaemia. Ro 65-2299 is being developed for oral treatment of psoriasis vulgaris.

References:
1. Guilhou, J.J. (1998) Exp. Opin. Invest. Drugs 7, 77-84.
2. Perez ,A., Raab, R., Chen, T.C., Turner, A., Holick, M.F. (1996) Br J Dermatol. 134, 1070-1078.
3. Morimoto, S., Yoshikawa, K., Kitano, Y., Imanaka, S., Fukuo, K., Koh, E., Kumahara, Y. (1986) Br J Dermatol. 115, 421-429.
4. Gniadecki, R. (1996) J Invest Dermatol. 3, 510-516.
5. Mattner, F., Ozmen, L., Podlaski, F.J., Wilkinson, V.L., Presky, D.H., Gately, M.K., Alber, G. (1997) Infect. Immun. 65, 4734-4737.
6. Yawalkar, N., Karlen, S., Hunger, R., Brand, C.U., Braathen, L.R. (1998) J Invest Dermatol. 111, 1053-1057.

1,25-DIHYDROXYVITAMIN D$_3$ ENHANCES PROLIFERATION AND MITOGENIC SIGNALING MEDIATED BY FIBROBLAST GROWTH FACTORS IN HUMAN KERATINOCYTES

Anat Gamady, Amiram Ravid, Dina Ron, Uri A. Liberman and Ruth Koren. The Felsenstein Medical Research Center, Tel Aviv University, Beilinson Campus, Petah Tikva, Israel, 49100.

Introduction: Keratinocyte proliferation and re-epithelialization during wound healing depend on a network of autocrine and paracrine growth factors. While a number of EGF receptor ligands are predominant among the autocrine growth factors, members of the FGF growth factor family play a major role in the paracrine network. Basic and acidic FGF (bFGF, aFGF) and keratinocyte growth factor (KGF) are produced by inflammatory cells and fibroblasts during wound healing. They interact with four types of tyrosine kinase receptors that display overlapping affinities for the various FGFs. Unique among them is the KGF receptor that binds KGF, aFGF and bFGF, but is the only receptor for KGF.

This study aimed to investigate the effect of 1,25(OH)$_2$D$_3$ on mitogenic signaling of FGFs in keratinocytes. To this end we established an experimental system in which signaling by FGFs could be studied with no interference from signaling mediated by other growth factor receptors. We used the immortalized human keratinocytes, HaCaT cells, that in contrast to primary keratinocyte cultures that require a complex growth medium can proliferate in culture in the absence of exogenous growth factors. We have previously shown that this autonomous proliferation is mediated by autocrine proteoglycan dependent EGF receptor ligands and that it can be abolished by the addition of the specific EGF receptor tyrosine kinase inhibitor AG 1478 (1). Under these conditions HaCaT cell cultures are completely dependent for both survival and proliferation on the presence of exogenous growth factors.

Results: HaCaT keratinocytes growth arrested by inhibition of the EGFR tyrosine kinase could be stimulated to proliferate by the addition of either bFGF, aFGF or KGF. This experimental system was employed to study the modulation of FGF mitogenic signaling by 1,25(OH)$_2$D$_3$. The relative mitogenic efficacy of the FGFs was: KGF=aFGF>bFGF, in correlation with their known affinities for the KGF receptor. The expression of this receptor in HaCaT cells was verified by RT-PCR.

48 hour co-treatment with 1,25(OH)$_2$D$_3$ enhanced bFGF, aFGF and KGF-driven cell proliferation. This effect was dose dependent and apparent at 1 nM. The synthetic, non calcemic, vitamin D analogs, EB1089, CB1093 and MC1288 were even more potent than the parent hormone in this system.

Activation of MAP kinase cascade plays a major role in the determination of cell fate. Activation of ERK 1/2 is usually associated with increased mitogenesis whereas activation of stress activated kinases, such as c-Jun N-terminal kinase (JNK) is asociated with cell cycle arrest and cell death. The extent of enzyme activation was assessed by semi-quantitative determination of the dually phosphorylated enzymes by Western blot analysis. Both MAP kinases, ERK1/2 and JNK, were activated in the presence of AG 1478 and FGFs. Under these conditions treatment of HaCaT kerainocytes with 1,25(OH)$_2$D$_3$ increased the activation of ERKs and concomitantly decreased that of JNK, thus shifting the balance between the two signaling cascades and increasing the net mitogenic effect. Treatment of KGF dependent cultures with 1,25(OH)$_2$D$_3$ resulted in increased levels of KGF receptor (assessed by immunoblotting). This effect was observed in cultures treated with FGFs but not in autonomously proliferating cultures. These findings are consistent with the assumption that the increase in KGF receptor levels is due to inhibition of growth factor-induced receptor down regulation.

Conclusions: 1,25(OH)$_2$D$_3$ enhances FGFs driven proliferation in keratinocytes. This effect is associated with a shift in the balance between different MAP kinase pathways (increased activation of ERK ½ and decreased activation of c-Jun N-terminal kinase) and increased cellular levels of the KGF receptor. Keratinocyte proliferation in vivo is regulated by various autocrine and paracrine growth factors, FGFs play a significant role during tissue repair following damage to the integrity of the epidermis. These findings may therefore be relevant under conditions of wound healing and epidermal atrophy.

Bibliography
1. Garach-Jehoshua, O., Ravid, A., Liberman, U.A. and Koren, R. (1999) *Endocrinology* 140, 713-721.

1,25-DIHYDROXYVITAMIN D$_3$ INHIBITS THE ACTIVATION OF C-JUN N-TERMINAL KINASE BY PHYSIOLOGICAL AND ENVIRONMENTAL STRESSES IN KERATINOCYTES

Ruth Koren, Efrat Rubinstein, Anat Gamady, Uri A. Liberman and Amiram Ravid. The Felsenstein Medical Research Center, Tel Aviv University, Beilinson Campus, Petah Tikva, Israel, 49100.

Introduction: Being the barrier between the individual and the environment, the skin prevents entry of microorganisms, blocks radiation and prevents water loss. Epidermal cells may thus be exposed to environmental stressors that affect the cellular redox state and osmotic balance. Cells within the skin are also exposed to physiological stressors such as immune cells that produce various active mediators including inflammatory cytokines. The activation of the stress-activated protein kinases, notably the c-Jun N-terminal kinase (JNK) and p38, is an early cellular response to stress signals and a major determinant of cell fate. Activation of these enzymes is closely associated with induction of apoptosis in various experimental systems. This work was undertaken to assess whether 1,25(OH)$_2$D$_3$ affects keratinocyte response to stress as reflected by reduction of cell number and by activation of the SAPK cascades. To this end we used as an experimental model the HaCaT cell line of spontaneously immortalized human keratinocytes. In contrast to keratinocyte primary cultures that require a complex growth medium with various active mediators known to activate MAP kinases, HaCaT cells can proliferate in culture in the absence of exogenous growth factors. We have previously shown that this autonomous proliferation is mediated by autocrine EGF receptor ligands and is enhanced by 1,25(OH)$_2$D$_3$ (1).

Results: Treatment of HaCaT human keratinocytes with agents that perturb the cellular redox state, both oxidants and antioxidants, reduced cell number as judged by crystal violet staining and culture DNA content. Treatment with 1,25(OH)$_2$D$_3$ protected HaCaT cells from the damaging effect of the thiol antioxidant N-acetylcysteine (NAC) or the OH radical quenchers, dimethylsulfoxide (DMSO) and dimethylthiourea. $1,25(OH)_2D_3$ also protected HaCaT cells from the damage induced by hydrogen peroxide. Treatment of HaCaT cells with various stressors induced a marked activation of JNK isoenzymes and p38 as assessed by immunoblotting of the dually phosphorylated, activated enzymes. The stressors employed were: (1), perturbation of the redox state by exposure to the antioxidants NAC and DMSO, and the oxidant H_2O_2; (2), tumor necrosis factor; (3), hyperosmotic shock caused by exposure to sorbitol (200 mM). 48 hour pretreatment with $1,25(OH)_2D_3$ caused a marked inhibition of JNK activation in response to all these stressors. In parallel experiments the activation of the other stress activated protein kinase, p38, by the same stressors was only marginally affected by $1,25(OH)_2D_3$. HaCaT cells, in the absence of exogenous growth factors, were also exposed to the specific EGF receptor tyrosine kinase inhibitor, AG 1478. Treatment with this agent results in inhibition of mitogenic signaling via the EGF receptor leading to blockage of the autonomous proliferation mediated by autocrine ligands. The consequent activation of both JNK and p38 was markedly inhibited by $1,25(OH)_2D_3$. This finding also implies that inhibition of stressor-induced signaling by $1,25(OH)_2D_3$ is not mediated by the EGF receptor.

Conclusions: $1,25(OH)_2D_3$ invariably inhibits signaling induced by various environmental and physiological stresses that lead to activation of stress activated protein kinases. This action of the hormone may confer protection against cell death resulting from these stresses. This novel activity of $1,25(OH)_2D_3$ may be related to previous reports of a protective effect of vitamin D receptor agonists on skin damage following exposure to UV irradiation and may suggest novel applications of active vitamin D metabolites and analogs as protective agents under various conditions leading to skin atrophy.

Bibliography

1. Garach-Jehoshua, O., Ravid, A., Liberman, U.A. and Koren R. (1999) *Endocrinology* 140, 713-721.

REQUIREMENT OF VITAMIN D RECEPTOR IN EPIDERMAL DIFFERENTIATION AND HAIR FOLLICLE RECYCLING

Z. Xie*, L. Komuves*, D. C. Ng*, C. Leary*, T. Yoshizawa*, S. Kato* and D. D. Bikle*, *Endocrine Unit, Veterans Affairs Medical Center, University of California, San Francisco, CA, USA; *Institute of Molecular and Cellular Biosciences, The University of Tokyo, Bunkyo-Ku, Tokyo, Japan

Introduction The active form of vitamin D, $1\alpha,25$-dihydroxyvitmin D ($1\alpha,25(OH)_2D$), mediates its action by binding with high affinity to specific vitamin D receptors (VDR) located in the nucleus of target cells (1-3). VDR is a member of the nuclear hormone receptor super family and acts as a ligand-inducible transcription factor, which activates vitamin D-responsive genes (4). While classic vitamin D target tissues include intestine, kidney and bone, where it acts to maintain serum calcium levels and to build and preserve bone (1), compelling evidence has emerged in recent years that vitamin D is also critical for the differentiation and proliferation of a large number of normal and malignant cells including epidermal cells (5). Keratinocytes, the most abudant cells of the epidermis, are the source of 7-dehydrocholesterol, necessary for the photochemical production of the parent vitamin D. They possess both the 24- and 1α-hydroxylase enzymes, and thus can produce endogenous $1\alpha,25(OH)_2D$ (6, 7). Keratinocytes contain VDR (8-9) and so can respond to the $1\alpha,25(OH)_2D$ produced (6, 7, 10). Most likely the $1\alpha,25(OH)_2D$ produced by keratinocytes serves an autocrine or paracrine function to regulate the proliferation and differentiation of the keratinocytes. The importance of this differentiation effect of $1\alpha,25(OH)_2D_3$ in vivo is difficult to assess. However, the alopecia that is variably found in the patients with hereditary VDR deficiency (vitamin D-dependent rickets type II, VDDR-II), suggests a biological role for the VDR in the epidermis. To investigate the physiologic role of $1\alpha,25(OH)_2D_3$ in mediating epidermal differentiation and hair follicle growth, we examined the tissue histology and expression of differentiation markers in the epidermis of VDR-deficient mice generated by gene targeting at different stages of postnatal development.

Results The VDR-deficient mouse was generated by gene targeting at the exon 2 encoding the first Zn finger motif in the DNA binding domain essential for the biological functions of VDR. The homozygous VDR knockout (VDRKO) mouse showed normal growth after birth until weaning (at 3 weeks). After weaning, the VDRKO mice showed modest growth retardation and developed rickets. The skin and hair looked normal after birth until about 12 weeks. After 12 weeks, the VDRKO mouse showed progressive alopecia which led to nearly total hair loss by 8 months. Hematoxylin-eosin (H & E) staining of the skin of the homozygous littermates showed normal morphology at birth until weaning. After weaning, the H & E staining revealed dilation of the hair follicles with formation of dermal cysts. These cysts increased in size and number with age. The hair sheathes of homozygous knockout mice are markedly thinner than wild type mice. The enlarged hair follicles contain no hair shafts. The proliferating cell nuclear antigen (PCNA) staining in aborted hair follicles and dermal cysts did not show a marked increase in the homozygous knockout mouse. Epidermal differentiation markers including involucrin, profilaggrin and loricrin detected by immunostaining showed decreased expression levels in the homozygous knock-out mouse by one week after birth. However, these differences in immunostaining at least for involucrin and loricrin became less apparent by 3 months between the homozygous knockout mouse and the wild type mouse.

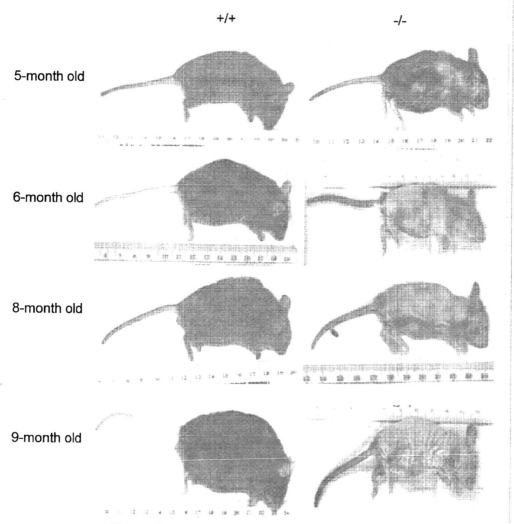

Figure 1: Appearance of VDRKO mice at age of 5, 6, 8, 9 months old. +/+, wild type mice; -/+, VDRKO homozygous mice.

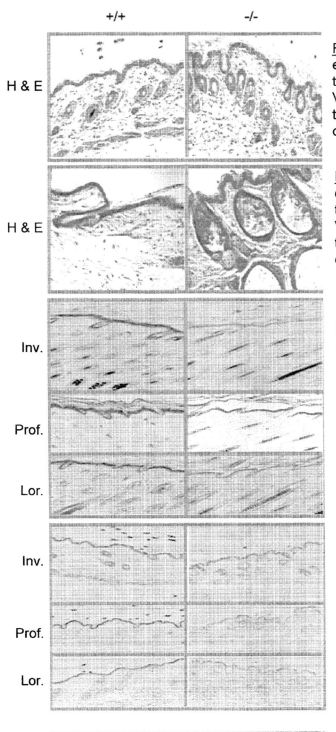

+/+   -/-

H & E

H & E

Inv.

Prof.

Lor.

Inv.

Prof.

Lor.

Figure 2: Hematoxylin-eosin (H & E) section through the skin of VDRKO (-/-) *versus* wild type (+/+) mice at the age of 3 weeks.

Figure 3: Hematoxylin-eosin (H & E) section through the skin of VDRKO (-/-) *versus* wild type (+/+) mice at the age of 3 months.

Figure 4: Involucrin (Inv), profilaggrin (Prof.) and loricrin (Lor.) expression in the epidermis of VDRKO (-/-) *versus* wild type (+/+) mice at the age of 1 week, detected by immunocytochemistry.

Figure 5: Involucrin (Inv), profilaggrin (Prof.) and loricrin (Lor.) expression in the epidermis of VDRKO (-/-) *versus* wild type (+/+) mice at the age of 3 weeks, detected by immunocytochemistry.

Discussion   These data indicate that VDR is critical for epidermal differentiation and hair recycling in vivo. The reduced expression of epidermal differentiation markers was seen by 1 week after birth, whereas changes in the hair follicles were seen by 3 weeks. The timing of these changes indicate that prenatal development of the epidermis and hair growth do not require VDR, whereas the development of the adult skin including normal hair follicle recycling does. VDR is not only expressed in epidermal keratinocytes, but also in the outer root sheath keratinocytes and dermal papilla cells of hair follicles (11, 12). This mouse model provides an excellent means by which vitamin D acting on the epidermis including the hair follicle can be studied in vivo.

References

1.   Bouillon, R., Okamura, W. H., and Norman, A. W. (1995) *Endocrine Reviews* **16**(2), 200-57
2.   Reichel, H., Koeffler, H. P., and Norman, A. W. (1989) *New England Journal of Medicine* **320**(15), 980-91
3.   Darwish, H., and DeLuca, H. F. (1993) *Critical Reviews in Eukaryotic Gene Expression* **3**(2), 89-116
4.   Mangelsdorf, D. J., and Evans, R. M. (1995) *Cell* **83**(6), 841-50
5.   Bikle, D. D., and Pillai, S. (1993) *Endocrine Reviews* **14**(1), 3-19
6.   Hosomi, J., Hosoi, J., Abe, E., Suda, T., and Kuroki, T. (1983) *Endocrinology* **113**(6), 1950-7
7.   Smith, E. L., Walworth, N. C., and Holick, M. F. (1986) *Journal of Investigative Dermatology* **86**(6), 709-14
8.   Stumpf, W. E., Sar, M., Reid, F. A., Tanaka, Y., and DeLuca, H. F. (1979) *Science* **206**(4423), 1188-90
9.   Pillai, S., Bikle, D. D., and Elias, P. M. (1988) *Journal of Biological Chemistry* **263**(11), 5390-5
10.   Pillai, S., and Bikle, D. D. (1991) *Journal of Cellular Physiology* **146**(1), 94-100
11.   Stumpf, W. E., Clark, S. A., Sar, M., and DeLuca, H. F. (1984) *Cell and Tissue Research* **238**(3), 489-96
12.   Reichrath, J., Schilli, M., Kerber, A., Bahmer, F. A., Czarnetzki, B. M., and Paus, R. (1994) *British Journal of Dermatology* **131**(4), 477-82

Autocrine role for vitamin D and PTHrP during differentiation of rat new born keratinocytes.

Amina Errazahi, Zhor Bouizar*, Brigitte Grosse, Michèle Lieberherr, Marthe Rizk-Rabin. UPR 1524, CNRS Paris France, *Unit 349, INSERM, Paris France

Introduction: A paracrine role for vitamin D during keratinocyte differentiation has been previously suggested (1). PTHrP is another factor enhancing the differentiation of the epidermal cells and its synthesis in keratinocytes is regulated by vitamin D. However the precise site of its production in the epidermis and the possibility of an autocrine role for PTHrP in this tissue remain an open question. To investigate this hypothesis, the expression of PTHrP and PTH/PTHrP receptor was analyzed in keratinocytes derived from rat new born skin. Separation and isolation of the epidermal keratinocytes in subpopulations according to their state of differentiation allowed precise investigation of the cells producing PTHrP and of those responding to the peptide. Messenger RNA and protein expression of PTHrP and PTH/PTHrP receptor were examined using RT-PCR, immunocytochemistry and western blot.

VDR expression was analyzed in parallel using similar techniques in order to determine whether vitamin D can locally control the PTHrP production via its specific receptor.

Finally, in order to evaluate the function of the PTHrP receptor in the keratinocytes, we investigated in these cells the intracellular signalling pathways in response to various exogenous PTHrP peptides: the N-terminal (1-34), Mid region (67-89) and C-terminal (107-139) fragments

Materials and Methods: Keratinocytes of new born rat skin were separated according to their size in four different subpopulations as previously described (2). Immunocytochemistry and western blotting using specific antibodies were performed to study the protein expression of VDR, PTHrP and PTHrP receptor Polymerase chain reaction was used to analyze the mRNA expression of the three corresponding genes. Specific pairs of oligonucleotides primers were used: -1) a 280 bp fragment including both the bases 41-60 as sense primer and bases 301-320 as antisense primer of the reported rat VDR cDNA sequence; -2) a fragment of 611 bp corresponding to exons 3-4 of the rat PTHrP cDNA; -3) two fragments of 643 bp and 913 bp corresponding to exons M-T and exons E-M, respectively, of the rat PTH/PTHrP receptor cDNA. Adenylate cyclase response was analyzed in primary culture of total keratinocytes. Cells were incubated with IBMX for 20 min and then for 10 min with different concentrations of PTHrP peptides; cAMP was extracted by incubation with ethanol, and measured by the protein assay of Lust . Calcium measurement : confluent keratinocytes were loaded with 1μM Fura 2/AM for 30min. The effects (1min) of the different PTHrP fragments on intracellular [Ca^{2+}] were tested at different concentrations.

Results:

Epidermal keratinocytes from new born rat were separated by unit gravity sedimentation into poorly differentiated cells (pop1), more differentiated slow cycling cells (pop2), actively proliferating cells (pop3) and terminally differentiating subpopulations (pop4).Table 1

Expression of the PTHrP protein in keratinocytes was restricted to populations 2 to 4, with a peak expression in actively proliferative cells from population 3. PTHrP mRNA expression correlated well with the immunocytochemical localization of the PTHrP protein.

VDR expression was found in all keratinocyte populations. But its nuclear expression was clearly more frequent in cells from populations 3 and 4 .

The PTH/PTHrP receptor mRNA was expressed in keratinocytes whatever their state of differentiation. This expression of PTHrP receptor was observed using RT-PCR. Both transcripts shared homologies with the Type I PTH/PTHrP receptor as they hybridized with the full length cDNA of rat PTH/PTHrP receptor, R15B.

Studies using the PTH/PTHrP receptor rat antibody revealed several protein bands by western blotting, as in renal membrane extracts. However the major band size was larger in keratinocytes, about 95 kDa, than in renal extracts, 90-85kDa. The presence of PTHrP receptor was also confirmed by immunostaining of keratinocytes. Membrane localisation of PTHrP receptor was absent in the slow cycling cells (pop1) but uniformely expressed in the other populations (pop 2,3 and 4).

Percentage of cells	population 1	population 2	population 3	population 4
in G0/G1	30	32	20	20
in S,G2/M	15	20	47	45
% stained cells				
VDR	11.05± 1.2	10.25± 1.1	25.7±2.3	26.34±1.7
PTHrP	2.5± 0.5	32 ±10.2	69±12.5	32± 7.5
PTHrP receptor	1±0.5	25± 5.6	27±4.3	35±7.5

Table 1. Results are mean ± 1 SE of 3 to 5 separate cell smears

The study of the signal transduction pathways involved in the response of keratinocytes to the different PTHrP peptides showed a clear response to PTHrP (1-34) via both the stimulation of cAMP production and a rise in intracellular calcium (Table 2). Cells only responded to the C -terminal peptide by enhancing intracellular calcium. No response was observed to the Mid region fragment.

PTHrP (100 nM)	cAMP response (percent of controls)	(Ca+)i response nM
basal	-	149.7 ±4.9
PTHrP (1-34)	180±16**	297.5±18.7**
Mid-Region(67-89)	115±4	147.1±3.9
Cterminal (107-139)	79±7	319.3±40.8**
bPTH (100 nM)		
basal	-	152.2±10.5
bPTH (1-34)	136±13**	228.8±16.4**

Table 2. Results are mean ± 1 SD of 3 to 6 different experiments in triplicate. **: $p < 0.01$ (ANOVA)

In conclusion: We have localized PTHrP production in the actively proliferative keratinocytes and shown the presence of a functional PTH/PTHrP receptor in the same cells by RT PCR, immunoblotting and biological assays. These findings demonstrate an autocrine function for PTHrP in new born rat epidermis. The observed calcium response to the C-terminal fragment of PTHrP suggests the presence of additional PTHrP receptors in keratinocytes.The colocalization of VDR and PTHrP and the different distribution of PTH/PTHrP receptor suggests complex implication of both hormones in the proliferation / differentiation equilibrium of the epidermis.

References
1.Rizk-Rabin, M., Rougui, Z., Zhor, B., Garabedian, M., Pavlovitch, JH. (1994). J of Cell Physiol. 159,131-141.
2. Pavlovitch, JH., Rizk-Rabin, M., Gervaise, M., Metezeau, P. and Grunwald, D. (1989) Am J Physiol . 256,C977-C986.

CALCIUM TRANSPORT

THE EPITHELIAL CALCIUM CHANNEL, ECAC, FUNCTIONS AS GATE-KEEPER OF ACTIVE CALCIUM (RE)ABSORPTION

Joost G.J. Hoenderop[1], Dominik Müller[1], Carel H. van Os[1], Rudi Vennekens[2], Bernd Nilius[2] and René J.M. Bindels[1].
[1]Department of Cell Physiology, University of Nijmegen, The Netherlands.
[2]Department of Physiology, University of Leuven, Belgium.

Introduction.
The maintenance of the body Ca^{2+} balance is of crucial importance for many vital physiological functions including neuronal excitability, muscle contraction and bone formation, and is tightly controlled by a concerted action of kidney, intestine and bone (1,2,9). The Ca^{2+} absorbing activity of intestine and kidney determine the net intake and excretion of Ca^{2+} for the entire body and, therefore, the Ca^{2+} balance. In normal adults, the renal excretion of Ca^{2+} is critically balanced by gastrointestinal absorption. On the other hand, the distribution of Ca^{2+} within the body is determined by exchanges of Ca^{2+} between interstitium and bone. These Ca^{2+} pathways are primarily regulated by vitamin D_3 metabolites and parathyroid hormone. Alterations in these regulatory processes are present in many (patho)physiological states including idiopathic hypercalciuric syndromes, chronic renal failure, aging-related Ca^{2+} malabsorption and vitamin D intoxication.

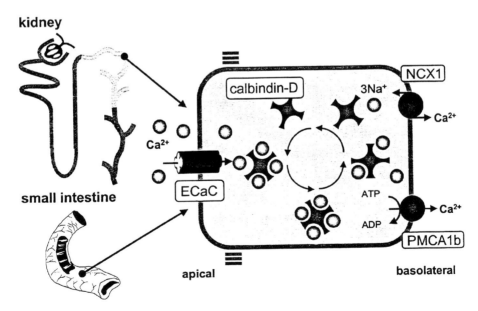

Figure 1: Process of transcellular Ca^{2+} transport in polarized epithelia present in kidney and intestine. 1. apical Ca^{2+} entry via the epithelial Ca^{2+} channel (ECaC); 2. binding of Ca^{2+} to calcium-binding proteins (calbindin-D) and subsequent diffusion to the basolateral membrane; 3. basolateral extrusion of Ca^{2+} via Ca^{2+}-ATPase (PMCA1b) and/or Na^+- Ca^{2+} exchange (NCX1).

In kidney and intestine Ca^{2+} is absorbed via a paracellular and transcellular pathway. As shown in figure 1, this transcellular transport is realized in three steps consisting of Ca^{2+} entry across the apical plasma membrane, followed by cytosolic diffusion of Ca^{2+} bound to calbindin-D (CaBP) and then extrusion across the basolateral membrane by a Na^+-Ca^{2+} exchanger (NCX) and/or a Ca^{2+}-ATPase (PMCA) (13). A major breakthrough in completing the molecular details of this pathway was the recent identification of an epithelial Ca^{2+} channel, named ECaC. Recent functional and morphological analysis indicated that this Ca^{2+} channel constitutes the rate-limiting step in transcellular Ca^{2+} transport (10,11,14,28). It is the prime target for hormonal control of active Ca^{2+} flux from the intestinal lumen or urine space to the blood compartment.

Structural identification of ECaC.
The unidentified molecular nature of the Ca^{2+} influx mechanism has seriously hampered our understanding of transcellular Ca^{2+} transport. We applied an expression cloning strategy in *Xenopus laevis* oocytes to identify this Ca^{2+} influx protein. This resulted in cloning of the epithelial Ca^{2+} channel (ECaC) which exhibits the defining characteristics of transepithelial Ca^{2+} transport. ECaC consists of six transmembrane domains including a putative pore-forming region between transmembrane segments 5 and 6 and shares its topology with the recently cloned capsaicin receptors, the growth-factor-regulated channel and the group of transient receptor potential channels (TRP's) (figure 2) (5,6,15,25,29).

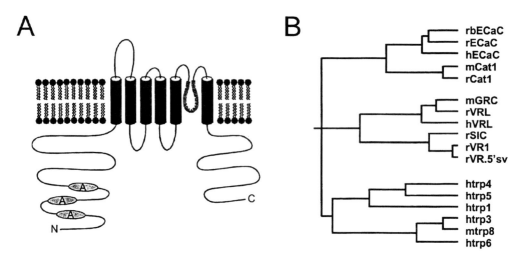

Figure 2: A) Predicted topology of ECaC. **B)** Phylogram based on full-length sequences of rabbit ECaC (AJ133128), rat ECaC (AB032019), human ECaC (AJ271207), mouse CaT1 (AB037373), rat CaT1 (AF029310), mouse GRC (AB021665), rat VRL (AF129113), humanVRL (AF103906), rat SIC (AB015231), rat VR1 (AF029310), rat VR.5'sv (AF158402), human trp4 (AF175406), human trp5 (NM012471), human trp1 (U47050), human trp3 (NM003305), mouse trp8 (NM012035) and human trp6 (AF080394).

This classical ion channel structure has been presented for other nonhomologues ion channels, like the shaker potassium channel (16), and voltage-gated Ca^{2+} channels (7). It has been demonstrated for some of these structurally-related channels that the ion channel "core" is formed by the co-assembly of four homologues subunits. For example, the shaker potassium channel family (16), and the inward rectifying K^+ channel (20) are composed of four subunits, while voltage-gated Na^+ and Ca^{2+} channels form concatomers composed of four internal repeats (4,7). The oligomeric structure of these channels implies that functional ECaC pores must also be composed of four subunits, but this remains to be shown.

The ECaC sequence has now been identified from three different species including rabbit, rat and human. The obtained sequences exhibit an overall homology of about 85%. Recently, the ECaC family has been extended. Peng *et al.* identified a Ca^{2+} transporter (CaT1) from rat small intestine (18). This new Ca^{2+} channel is a rat homologue of ECaC and should therefore be renamed ECaC2. Strikingly, some domains are completely conserved within this growing family. For instance, the putative pore-forming regions of ECaC and CaT1 are identical among different species. Furthermore, in rbECaC two combined putative phosphorylation sites for cAMP- and cGMP-dependent kinase (S669 and T709) were originally identified (10). However, these predicted phosphorylation sites are not conserved in other species and in CaT1. This is in strong contrast to the putative protein kinase C phosphorylation sites of which three are conserved within the complete ECaC family. These findings corroborate the recently postulated role of protein kinase C (PKC) in hormone-stimulated Ca^{2+} reabsorption (12). In addition, ECaC contains ankyrin repeat domains in the N-terminal region of the channel, which are also present in a diverse range of receptors and ion channels including the TRP family and the vanilloid receptor family.

Functional characteristics of ECaC.
Immunohistochemical analysis showed that in rabbit kidney ECaC positive staining was found along the apical membrane of the connecting tubules (10,14) (Figure 3A). In rabbit intestine ECaC was abundantly present in brush border membranes of duodenum (Figure 3B). Importantly, ECaC colocalized in these immunopositive cells with the other Ca^{2+} transport proteins including CaBP28, NCX and PMCA, and thus completes the family of Ca^{2+} transport proteins involved in transepithelial Ca^{2+} transport. Our studies indicate that, at least in rabbit, these Ca^{2+} transport proteins are absent from the distal convoluted tubule. The distal convoluted tubule is, therefore, functionally dissociated from the connecting tubule implying that thiazide-sensitive NaCl cotransport and $1,25(OH)_2D_3$-regulated Ca^{2+} reabsorption are localized to different cells (8,14). It is important to investigate the intrarenal distribution of ECaC in other species, including human, to examine whether this functional dissociation is a general phenomenon.

636

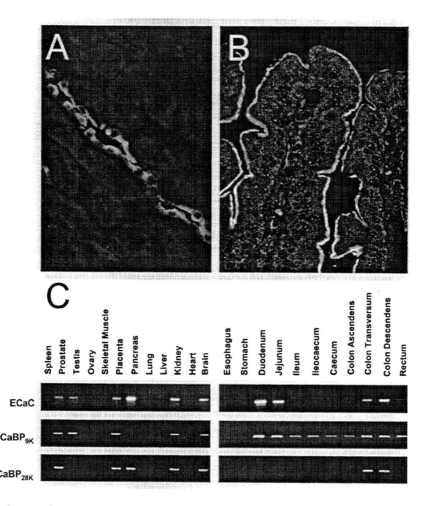

Figure 2: Immunofluorescence staining for ECaC of rabbit kidney cortex **(A)** and duodenum **(B)**. **C)** Localization of the human ECaC family using a cDNA tissue panel.

In addition to duodenum and kidney, ECaC was highly expressed in pancreas (Figure 3C). At present the function of ECaC in the latter tissue remains unknown since the localization has not yet been determined. However, the recent observation that calbindin-D_{28K} knockout mice suffer from a diminished insulin release is interesting in this respect and could indicate that ECaC participates in the process of insulin release (24). Interestingly, ECaC is not expressed in tissues lacking calbindin suggesting a functional interaction between these two Ca^{2+} transporting proteins. The distinctive properties of ECaC include a constitutively activated Ca^{2+} permeability at physiological membrane potentials, a high selectivity for Ca^{2+}, an anomalous mole-fraction behavior and hyperpolarization-stimulated and Ca^{2+}-dependent feedback regulation of channel activity.

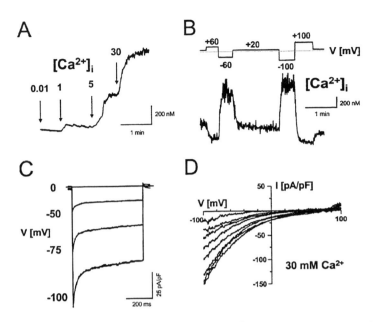

Figure 4: A) Representative traces of the changes in [Ca²⁺]ᵢ in ECaC expressing HEK 293 cells which were voltage clamped at +20 mV and exposed to different [Ca²⁺]ₑ, administered at the the times of indicated by aroows. **B)** Changes in [Ca²⁺]ᵢ in ECaC expressing HEK 293 cells clamped at various potentials at an extracellular Ca²⁺ concentration of 1.5 mM. **C)** Current at steps from +20 mV holding potential to -100, -75, and -50 mV, respetively. Extracellular Ca²⁺ concentration was 30 mM. **D)** Rundown of the current through ECaC in the presence of 30 mM Ca²⁺. Voltage ramps were applied every 5s (ramps of 400 ms, from −100 to +100 mV, holding potential +20 mV).

Evidence that ECaC forms a constitutively active Ca²⁺ entry pathway was obtained from experiments showing a close correlation between the level of intracellular Ca²⁺ ([Ca²⁺]ᵢ) and the electrochemical Ca²⁺ gradient in ECaC-expressing HEK 293 cells. The driving force for Ca²⁺ entry was modified by changing extracellular Ca²⁺ ([Ca²⁺]ₑ) from 0 to 30 mM in cells clamped at +20 mV which resulted in a markedly increase in the [Ca²⁺]ᵢ (Figure 4A). Depolarization of the membrane potential from +20 mV to +60 mV decreased [Ca²⁺]ᵢ while hyperpolarization from +20 mV to −100 mV increased [Ca²⁺]ᵢ (Figure 4B). ECaC-expressing HEK 293 cells displayed large inward currents which were strongly dependent on extracellular Ca²⁺ and reversed at high positive membrane potentials (28). The current-voltage relationship showed prominent inward rectification.

Under unstimulated physiological conditions when the membrane potential is typically around −70 mV in the distal nephron (9), ECaC constitutes a substantial Ca²⁺ conductance permitting basal Ca²⁺ influx. Stimulatory and inhibitory hormones could effectively control this apical influx and, thereby, transepithelial Ca²⁺ transport by, respectively, hyperpolarization or depolarization of the apical membrane. In addition, the presence of multiple conserved putative phosphorylation sites for PKC suggests phosphorylation-dependent regulation of ECaC activity. Obviously, further studies are required to delineate these putative regulatory mechanisms.

ECaC channel activity is regulated by intrinsic feedback control mechanisms which is illustrated by the following observations (11,28). ECaC mediated currents rapidly inactivate during hyperpolarizing voltage steps (Figure 4C). This inactivation was eliminated when Ba^{2+} or Sr^{2+} were used as charge carriers, suggesting that ECaC activity is controlled by Ca^{2+}-dependent feedback. Fast binding, high affinity Ca^{2+} buffers such as BAPTA, attenuated this feedback action of permeating Ca^{2+} ions but were unable to completely abolish it. This data suggests the involvement of a selective Ca^{2+} binding site in the channel mouth facing a microdomain of elevated Ca^{2+} levels. In addition, the current response slowly vanished during repetitive activation (Figure 4C). This rundown or desensitization was significantly diminished when Ca^{2+} was replaced by Ba^{2+} as charge carrier and abolished when extracellular Ca^{2+} was lowered to 1 nM, again indicating that a Ca^{2+}-operated process inhibits ECaC activity.

The electrophysiological experiments clearly demonstrate that ECaC exhibits the defining properties of a Ca^{2+} channel, including a positive reversal potential and anomalous mole fraction behavior (28). ECaC shares these properties with the extensively studied L-type Ca^{2+} channels. However, the above outlined auto-regulatory properties of ECaC together with the anticipated small conductance in the presence of divalent cations will make further biophysical analysis of single channel events extremely difficult. This notion could also explain the inability to register single channel events of CaT1 heterologously expressed in *Xenopus* oocytes (18). Since ECaC and CaT1 are highly homologous proteins that display remarkably similar macroscopic kinetic properties, it seems appropriate to consider both proteins as the first members of a new ECaC family. The definitive nomenclature will dependent on the future validation whether both proteins are splice variants of a single gene or duplicate genes derived from a common ancestor.

The Ca^{2+} entry mechanism that is located in the apical membrane of the distal part of the nephron has been extensively studied by several methods (3,9,12,26,27). The prevailing picture emerging from these latter studies is that the putative Ca^{2+} channels are highly sensitive to dihydropyridines. This is a notable difference with the fact that ECaC is insensitive to classical Ca^{2+} channel blockers such as felodipine and verapamil, which has also been reported for transepithelial Ca^{2+} transport in primary cultures of renal connecting tubule cells (3). The functional role of these other described Ca^{2+} channels in the distal part of the nephron has never been established, but they may be involved in store-operated Ca^{2+} entry which is an important part of Ca^{2+} signaling in nonexcitable cells.

Implications for Ca^{2+} homeostasis-related disorders
The identification of ECaC and its human homologue may shed new light on Ca^{2+} metabolism under pathophysiological circumstances. The treatment with vitamin D

which has been proven to be beneficial for various situations (e.g. the prevention of rickets during infancy) could find now its molecular target. Primary or secondary involvement of ECaC can be expected for several pathological conditions. Among those, conditions associated with hypercalciuria are certainly of interest due to the dominant localization in kidney and small intestine. Closely related to hypercalciuria is Ca^{2+}-related kidney stone disease that has, due to its high prevalence, a considerable socio-economic impact. Intensive investigations have, therefore, been performed in the past to clarify the responsible mechanisms (1,21). Recent studies imply that the pathogenesis is rather heterogeneous since different molecular pathways have been causally related to this disease (17). Interest of research has also centered around defective regulation of Ca^{2+} homeostasis and closely related vitamin D metabolism. Potential candidate genes have been screened for their involvement but several genes (e.g. 1-α-hydroxylase) have been excluded (23). Alternatively, dysregulation of the process of active transcellular Ca^{2+} transport, that occurs in kidney and intestine and that controls partly the Ca^{2+} flux into the blood compartment, could participate in the pathogenesis of Ca^{2+}-related kidney stone disease.

Conclusions

ECaC constitutes the rate-limiting step in transcellular Ca^{2+} transport and is, therefore, the prime target for hormonal control of the Ca^{2+} flux into the "milieu interior". Studying the regulation of ECaC is a novel activity and will give insight in the physiological role of these Ca^{2+} channels in Ca^{2+} homeostasis in general and in particular in vitamin D_3-regulated Ca^{2+} transport processes and Ca^{2+} homeostasis-related disorders. The future generation of ECaC knockout mice will in potency be a powerful tool to study ECaC function *in vivo*. The obtained knowledge using (tissue-specific) ECaC knockout mice will not only substantiate the role of ECaC under (patho)physiological conditions, but could ultimately also give way to the development of pharmacological strategies to treat Ca^{2+}-related disorders.

References

1   Asplin, J.R., Favus M.J. and Coe F.L. (1996) Nephrolithiasis. In: The Kidney, 5th ed., ed. Brenner BM, Philadelphia, WB Saunders, 1893-1935.
2   Bindels R.J.M. (1993) J. Exp. Biol. 184, 89-104.
3   Bindels, R.J.M., Hartog A., Abrahamse S.L. and Van Os C.H. (1994) Am. J. Physiol. 266, F620-F627.
4   Birnbaumer L., Zhu X., Jiang M., Boulay G., Peyton M., Vannier B., Brown D., Platano D., Sadeghi H., Stefani E. and Birnbaumer M. (1996) Proc. Natl. Acad. Sci. U.S.A. 93:15195-15202.
5   Caterina M.J., Schumacher M.A., Tominaga M., Rosen T.A., Levine J.D. and Julius D. (1997) Nature 389:816-824.
6   Caterina M.J., Rosen T.A., Tominaga M., Brake A.J. and Julius D. (1999) Nature 398:436-441.
7   Catterall W.A. (1998) Cell Calcium 24:307-323.
8   Bachmann S., Velázquez H., Obermüller N., Reilly R.F., Moser D. and Ellison D.H. (1995) J. Clin. Invest. 96:2510-2514.

9   Friedman P.A. and Gesek F.A. (1995) Physiol. Rev. 75:429-471.

10   Hoenderop J.G.J., van der Kemp A.W.C.M., Hartog A., van de Graaf S.F.J., Van Os C.H., Willems P.H.G.M. and Bindels R.J.M. (1999) J. Biol. Chem. 274:8375-8378.

11   Hoenderop J.G.J., van der Kemp A.W.C.M., Hartog A., Van Os C.H., Willems P.H.G.M. and Bindels R.J.M. (1999) Biochem. Biophys. Res. Commun. 261:488-492.

12   Hoenderop J.G.J., de Pont J.J.H.H.M., Bindels R.J.M. and Willems P.H.G.M. (1999) Kidney Int. 55:225-233.

13   Hoenderop J.G.J., Willlems P.H.G.M. and Bindels R.J.M. (2000) Am. J. Physiol. 278:F352-F360.

14   Hoenderop J.G.J., Hartog A., Stuiver M., Doucet A., Willems P.H.G.M. and Bindels R.J.M. (2000) J. Am. Soc. Nephrol. in press (July).

15   Kanzaki M., Zhang Y.Q., Mashima H., Li L., Shibata H. and Kojima I. (1999) Nature Cell. Biol. 1:165-170.

16   Kreusch A., Pfaffinger P.J., Stevens C.F. and Choe S. (1998). Nature 30:945-948.

17   Lloyd S.E., Pearce S.H., Fisher S.E., Steinmeyer K., Schwappach B., Scheinman S.J., Harding B., Bolino A., Devoto M., Goodyer P., Rigden S.P., Wrong O., Jentsch T.J., Craig I.W. and Thakker R.V. (1996) Nature 379:445-449.

18   Peng J.B., Chen X.Z., Berger U., Vassilev P.M., Tsukaguchi H., Brown E.M. and Hediger M. (1999) J. Biol. Chem. 274:22739-22746.

19   Poujoul P., Bidet M. and Tauc M. (1995) Kidney Int. 48:1102-1110.

20   Raab-Graham K.F. and Vandenberg C.A. (1998) J. Biol. Chem. 273:19699-19707.

21   Scheinman S.J. Nephrolithiasis. Seminars in Nephrology 19:381-388.

22   Schumacher M.A., Moff I., Sudanagunta S.P. and Levine J.D. (2000) J Biol Chem 275:2756-2762.

23   Scott P., Ouimet D., Proulx Y., Trouvé M.L., Guay G., Gagnon B., Valiquette L. and Bonnardeaux A. (1998) J. Am. Soc. Nephrol. 9:425-432.

24   Sooy K., Schemerhorn T., Noda M., Surana M., Rhoten W.B., Meyer M., Fliescher N., Sharp W.G. and Christakos S. (1999) J. Biol. Chem. 274:34343-34349.

25   Suzuki M., Sato J., Kutsuwada K., Ooki G. and Imai M. (1999) J. Biol. Chem. 274:6330-6335.

26   Tan S., Lau K. (1993) J. Clin. Invest. 1993; 92:2731-2736.

27   Taniguchi J., Takeda M., Yoshitomi K. and Imai M. (1994) J. Membr. Biol. 140:123-132.

28   Vennekens R., Hoenderop J.G.J., Prenen J., Stuiver M., Willems P.H.G.M., Droogmans G., Nilius B. and Bindels R.J.M. (2000) J. Biol. Chem. 275:3963-3969.

29   Zhu X. and Birnbaumer L. (1999) NIPS 13: 211-217.

EXPRESSION OF THE APICAL MEMBRANE CALCIUM TRANSPORTER IN HUMAN DUODENUM IS REGULATED BUT VITAMIN D INDEPENDENT: IMPLICATIONS IN THE UNEXPLAINED VARIABILITY IN FRACTIONAL CALCIUM ABSORPTION.

Natalie F Barley, Alison Howard, Stephen Legon, Julian RF Walters.
Gastroenterology Section, Imperial College School of Medicine, Hammersmith Campus, London W12 0NN, UK.

Vitamin D-independent variability of human calcium absorption

Dietary calcium is inefficiently and variably absorbed. There are considerable individual differences in intake of calcium containing foods, with different biological availabilities. Numerous nutritional studies have looked at effects on the absorption of calcium, and how these may correlate with subsequent pathological events, such as osteoporotic fractures or urinary calcinosis, and physiological measurements, including peak bone mass, bone mineral density, and urinary calcium excretion. Therapeutic studies indicate that calcium supplements have benefits in the prevention of osteopenia and osteoporotic fractures. However, all these studies are confounded by the large, inherent variability in the individual efficiency of intestinal calcium absorption.

The active hormonal form of vitamin D, 1,25-dihydroxycholecalciferol $(1,25(OH)_2D_3)$, is well established in humans and in animal models as having a significant role in the regulation of calcium absorption. Vitamin D-dependent genes have been identified and abnormal vitamin D-receptor function, in humans and in knock-out mice, leads to major impairment in calcium absorption. In many disease states, vitamin D therapy improves calcium absorption.

However, studies in normal humans have repeatedly shown there is wide variability in fractional calcium absorption, ranging from 15 to 50%, much of which is vitamin D-independent. Many studies (3,8,9) have demonstrated that $1,25(OH)_2D_3$ and absorption are significantly correlated, but as the correlation coefficients are of the order of $r = 0.5$ (or less), this association will account for only 25% of the variability. Vitamin D receptor polymorphisms and differences in expression, intestinal resistance to vitamin D, and effects of ageing or oestrogens are among the other factors studied – with no consistent finding on fractional calcium absorption. One study looking at sources of the variation in calcium absorption in normal individuals (1), found that the various known factors accounted for only about a half of the variability. In that study, the effects of $1,25(OH)_2D_3$ were insignificant. The variability in absorption is physiological, and consistent in differing experimental situations (4), suggesting that there must be other factors, currently unrecognised that influence calcium absorption.

Molecular mechanisms for calcium absorption

Absorption of calcium by the enterocyte comprise three steps: (i) ionic calcium must first enter the cell down a large gradient at the apical, brush-border membrane, (ii) cross the cytoplasm without raising the submicromolar free calcium concentration, and then (iii) be actively extruded at the basolateral membrane. We have previously characterised the cytoplasmic and basolateral calcium transport molecules in humans (6,7). Calbindin-D9k is the vitamin D-dependent calcium binding protein in the cytoplasm, and the calcium-pumping ATPase, PMCA1, is the active transport step at the basolateral membrane. We studied the expression of transcripts for these two molecules in duodenal biopsies from normal subjects. showing that $1,25(OH)_2D_3$ was weakly (r = 0.40), but significantly correlated with calbindin-D9k, whereas no significant correlation was found overall with PMCA1 (11). The mechanisms for the effects of vitamin D on transcription of the human calbindin-D9k gene are unclear in our studies (2).

The molecular basis for calcium entry at the brush-border membrane was unknown until 1999, when apical membrane calcium channels were described in the rabbit and rat (5,10). These two sequences were unlike other previously described calcium channels and were shown to have the electrophysiological properties expected for an epithelial apical calcium channel. The rabbit sequence, known as ECaC (for epithelial calcium channel) was expressed in kidney as well as in proximal intestine and placenta. The rat sequence, CaT1 (for calcium transporter) was not found in kidney.

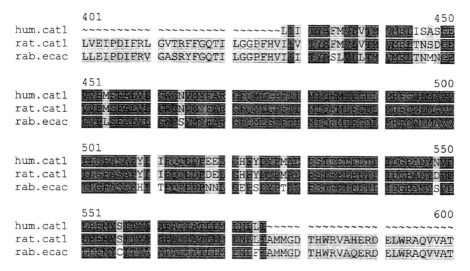

Figure 1. Comparison of amino acid sequences of the partial human apical calcium transporter (hum.cat1), the rat CaT1 (rat.cat1) and the rabbit ECaC (rab.ecac). Numbering is that of rat CaT1.

The human apical calcium transport protein
We have now identified the human homologue of rat CaT1 using a strategy of mixed primer PCR with conserved regions of the rat and rabbit sequences and human duodenal cDNA. In the 446bp of this partial cDNA sequence (AJ277909), there is greater identity with the rat sequence than with the rabbit ECaC sequence. This is particularly apparent at the amino acid level (Fig.1). The region shown comprises part of the predicted transmembrane domains (3, 4, 5 and 6) and includes the putative pore region. Based on these identities, we consider that this human sequence should be named CaT1. We have also isolated and mapped a genomic clone to chromosome 7q34-7q35.

Using this cDNA probe, we have shown that a 3kb transcript is expressed in duodenum, pancreas and placenta, but not in ileum, colon or kidney. Larger transcripts are found in pancreas, placenta and brain. Its expression in this latter tissue, which is supported by the data in the rat [Peng}, makes it inappropriate to identify it as an epithelial transporter.

We studied the expression of human CaT1 in normal duodenal biopsies from 20 subjects, part of the set we studied previously (11). Human CaT1 expression varied considerably, by a factor of 10, after correction for differences in loading and blotting. No correlation was found with $1,25(OH)_2D_3$ or with $25(OH)$ vitamin D. CaT1 was weakly associated with the vitamin D-dependent calcium-binding protein calbindin RNA ($r = 0.48$, $p < 0.05$). There was a strong, unexpected correlation with PMCA1 expression ($r = 0.83$, $p < 0.001$), suggesting there may be co-regulation of the genes for calcium entry and exit.

Implications
These findings imply that the variable expression of the human calcium apical transporter in duodenum could be a major factor in the observed differences in the efficiency of intestinal calcium absorption. The close correlation of CaT1 expression with that for the exit step, PMCA1, suggests that the wide variation in expression is physiological and not due to experimental reasons. The individual variation in calcium entry into the enterocyte would be coupled with calcium transport into the circulation at the baso-lateral membrane. The expression of the genes for calcium entry (CaT1) and exit (PMCA1) appear to show no vitamin D-dependence, in humans at least, suggesting that the transcriptional effects of $1,25(OH)_2D_3$ are principally those to increase calbindin-D9k expression.

One can postulate that those with the greatest CaT1 expression would have the greatest calcium absorption and possibly absorptive hypercalciuria. Conversely, those with lowest CaT1 expression would have the lowest fractional calcium absorption and might have the lowest bone mineral mass, being at risk for the subsequent development of osteoporosis. Experiments are now in progress to determine the relationship between CaT1 expression and fractional calcium absorption, and to indicate mechanisms that might govern CaT1 expression.

References:

1. Barger-Lux, M. J., Heaney, R. P., Lanspa, S. J., Healy, J. C., and DeLuca, H. F. (1995) *J Clin Endocrinol Metab* **80,** 406-411
2. Barley, N. F., Prathalingam, S. R., Zhi, P., Legon, S., Howard, A., and Walters, J. R. F. (1999) *Biochem J* **341,** 491-500
3. Gallagher, J. C., Riggs, B. L., Eisman, J., Hamstra, A., Arnaud, S. B., and DeLuca, H. F. (1979) *J Clin Invest* **64,** 729-736
4. Heaney, R. P., Weaver, C. M., Fitzsimmons, M. L., and Recker, R. R. (1990) *J Bone Miner Res* **5,** 1139-1142
5. Hoenderop, J. G. J., Van Der Kemp, A. W. C. M., Hartog, A., Van De Graaf, S. F. J., Van Os, C. H., Willems, P. H. G. M., and Bindels, R. J. M. (1999) *J Biol Chem* **274,** 8375-8378
6. Howard, A., Legon, S., Spurr, N. K., and Walters, J. R. F. (1992) *Biochem Biophys Res Commun* **185,** 663-669
7. Howard, A., Legon, S., and Walters, J. R. F. (1993) *Am J Physiol* **265,** G917-G925
8. Kinyamu, H. K., Gallagher, J. C., Prahl, J. M., DeLuca, H. F., Petranick, K. M., and Lanspa, S. J. (1997) *J Bone Miner Res* **12,** 922-928
9. Morris, H. A., Need, A. G., Horowitz, M., O'Loughlin, P. D., and Nordin, B. E. C. (1991) *Calcif Tissue Int* **49,** 240-243
10. Peng, J. B., Chen, X. Z., Berger, U. V., Vassilev, P. M., Tsukaguchi, H., Brown, E. M., and Hediger, M. A. (1999) *J Biol Chem* **274,** 22739-22746
11. Walters, J. R. F., Howard, A., Lowery, L. J., Mawer, E. B., and Legon, S. (1999) *Eur J Clin Invest* **29,** 214-19

RAPID RESPONSES OF CALCIUM AND PHOSPHATE ABSORPTION IN DUODENUM OF YOUNG PIGLETS AS AFFECTED BY CALCITRIOL

Bernd Schroeder, Ulrike Nurnus and Gerhard Breves, Department of Physiology, School of Veterinary Medicine, Bischofsholer Damm 15/102, D-30173 Hannover, Germany, bernd.schroeder@tiho-hannover.de

Introduction Earlier studies suggested lack of classical calcitriol dependent mechanisms for stimulation of active absorption of calcium (Ca^{2+}) and inorganic phosphate (P_i) from upper small intestines during early postnatal life of pigs, and it appears that the onset of these mechanisms including genomic pathways does not occur before weaning time (1-3). This study was performed to investigate the potential existence of non-genomic calcitriol actions (4) which could play a significant role in controlling intestinal Ca^{2+} and/or P_i absorption during early postnatal life.

Methods For the studies we used duodenal tissues from newborn and weaned piglets (<1 and >6 weeks post natum, respectively). Measurements of Ca^{2+} and Pi flux rates across intact epithelial tissues from stripped duodenum were performed using the in vitro Ussing chamber technique as described in detail previously (2). The unidirectional mucosal to serosal (J_{ms}) and serosal to mucosal (J_{sm}) flux rates of Ca^{2+} and P_i were measured simultaneously in Ussing-type chambers with an exposed serosal area of 1.13 cm^2. The tissues were incubated on both sides with 10 ml of a buffer solution (pH 7.4) containing (mmol·l^{-1}) 125.4 NaCl, 5.4 KCl, 1.2 $CaCl_2$, 21 $NaHCO_3$, 0.3 Na_2HPO_4, 1.2 NaH_2PO_4, and 0.01 indomethacin. In addition, the serosal solution contained 10 mmol·l^{-1} glucose and the mucosal solution contained 10 mmol·l^{-1} mannitol. All buffers were continuously circulated and gassed with carbogen at 39°C. About 20 min after mounting the tissues, for double isotope labelling 185 KBq $^{45}CaCl_2$ (1.14 MBq·mg^{-1}; DuPont NEN, Bad Homburg, Germany) and equal amount of [^{32}P]orthophosphate (370 MBq·ml^{-1}, Amersham Buchler, Braunschweig, Germany) were added to one of either side of the mucosa. After an initial equilibrium period of 20 min flux rates were calculated from the rate of tracer appearance on the unlabeled side. Therefore samples were taken in three 10 min intervals (basal conditions) and after serosal application of

500 pg·ml^{-1} calcitriol (mean of 3 x 10 min flux periods beginning 15 min after treatment). All measurements were performed in the absence of electrochemical gradients which allows to interpret significant net flux rates as active transport process.

Results As shown in Figure 1 in both groups mucosal-to-serosal flux rates of Ca^{2+} in duodenum exceeded respective flux rates in the opposite direction resulting in significant positive net flux rates indicating active Ca^{2+} absorption. Only in weaned piglets calcitriol rapidly stimulated net flux rates of Ca^{2+} by about 20 %: 61.6 ± 11.3 (basal) versus 74.3 ± 12.2 (calcitriol) nmol·cm^{-2}·h^{-1} ($\bar{x}$ ± SEM, n = 6). This effect could not be observed in newborn piglets (74.8 ± 9.8 versus 77.3 ± 13.4 nmol·cm^{-2}·h^{-1}; n=5).

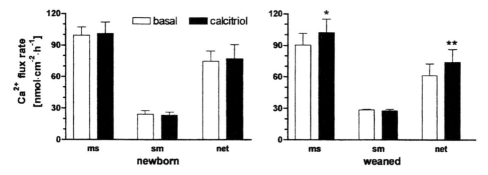

Figure 1: Rapid response of unidirectional (ms mucosal-to-serosal, sm serosal-to-mucosal) and net (net = ms-sm) flux rates of Ca^{2+} in duodenum of newborn (n=5) and weaned (n=6) piglets to calcitriol (500 pg·ml^{-1}, serosal side). ($\bar{x}$ ±SEM, * P<0.05, ** P<0.01, Student's t-test for paired observations)

Similarily, in both groups mucosal-to-serosal flux rates of P$_i$ exceeded serosal-to-mucosal flux rates (Figure 2) resulting in significant positive net flux rates of 95.9 ± 11.6 nmol·cm^{-2}·h^{-1} in newborn piglets (n = 5) and 64.6 ± 3.4 nmol·cm^{-2}·h^{-1} in weaned animals (n = 4). Serosal application of calcitriol revealed significant increases of ms and net P$_i$ flux rates in both groups. Net flux rates of P$_i$ in newborn and weaned animals reached 116.8 ± 9.0 and 77.3 ± 3.1 nmol·cm^{-2}·h^{-1}, respectively.

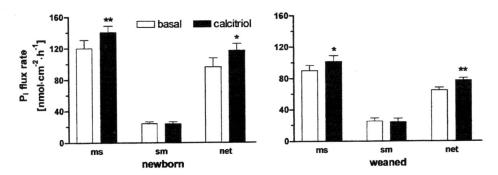

Figure 2: Rapid response of unidirectional (ms mucosal-to-serosal, sm serosal-to-mucosal) and net (net = ms-sm) flux rates of P_i in duodenum of newborn (n=5) and weaned (n=4) piglets to calcitriol (500 pg·ml^{-1}, serosal side). ($\bar{x}$ ±SEM, * P<0.05, ** P<0.01, Student's t-test for paired observations)

To examine the potential contribution of an intact cytoskeleton in transepithelial Ca^{2+} movement as it has been proposed for chick (5) we used colchicine (1 mmol·l^{-1}, mucosal side) as an antagonist of cytosolic microtubule functions (2). As shown previously (2), in contrast to weaned animals application of colchicine significantly inhibited active Ca^{2+} absorption in newborn piglets by about 25%. This effect seems to be rather specific since simultaneously recorded P_i net absorption remained unaffected. Rapid stimulation of active duodenal Ca^{2+} and P_i absorption in weaned piglets could completely be blocked in the presence of colchicine.

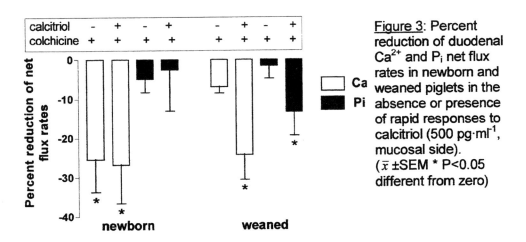

Figure 3: Percent reduction of duodenal Ca^{2+} and P_i net flux rates in newborn and weaned piglets in the absence or presence of rapid responses to calcitriol (500 pg·ml^{-1}, mucosal side). ($\bar{x}$ ±SEM * P<0.05 different from zero)

<u>Conclusions</u> In conclusion, our findings again support the assumption of calcitriol-independent mechanisms for active duodenal Ca^{2+} and P_i absorption during early postnatal life. Functioning microtubules appear to be relevant for transepithelial Ca^{2+} movement in newborn piglets. Non-genomic, rapid stimulations of both Ca^{2+} and P_i transport by calcitriol in duodenum of weaned piglets may also be mediated by microtubules. Weaned piglets may be a good model to study mechanisms and regulation of calcitriol-induced rapid responses of intestinal Ca^{2+} absorption in future studies.

References

(1) Schröder, B., Kaune, R., Schlumbohm, C., Breves, G., Harmeyer, J. (1993) Calcif. Tissue Int. 52, 305-309.

(2) Schröder, B., Dahl, M.R., Breves, G. (1998) Am. J. Physiol. 275, G305-G313.

(3) Schröder, B., Hattenhauer, O., Breves, G. (1998) Endocrinology 139, 1500-1507.

(4) Norman, A.W. (1997) In: Feldman, D., Glorieux, F.H., Pike, J.W. (eds): Vitamin D. Academic Press, New York, 233-256.

(5) Nemere, I., Norman, A.W. (1990). Miner. Electrolyte Metab. 16, 109-114.

THE INFLUENCE OF ESTROGEN ON CALCIUM METABOLISM IN THE INTACT AND OVARIECTOMIZED RAT.

M. Dijkgraaf-ten Bolscher[1], J.C. Netelenbos[1], R. Barto[2], W.J.F. van der Vijgh[2*]
[1]Dept. Endocrinology, [2]Clin. Res. Lab. Int. Med., University Hospital Vrije Universiteit, De Boelelaan 1117, 1081 HV Amsterdam, The Netherlands e-mail : wjf.vandervijgh@azvu.nl

Introduction: The mechanism of ovarian hormones to modulate bone mass is not fully understood. Menopause is often associated with intestinal malabsorption of calcium [1] and increased renal excretion of calcium [2]. Reduced intestinal calcium absorption has been attributed to reduced levels of $1,25(OH)_2$vitamin D [3] or appeared to be related to intestinal resistance to $1,25(OH)_2$vitamin D [4] or to decreased $1,25(OH)_2$vitamin D receptor expression [5]. In addition, it is quite possible that estrogen itself acts directly on intestinal cells to stimulate calcium absorption rather than through $1,25(OH)_2$vitamin D [6]. The ovariectomized (OVX) rat is considered to be the best animal model for postmenopausal osteoporosis [7]. Whether the changes in calcium metabolism after OVX in rats are similar to those observed in postmenopausal women is not evident. Questions remain about intestinal calcium absorption in OVX rats because intestinal calcium absorption has been reported to increase [8], decrease [9], or to remain unchanged [10]. The effect of OVX on urinary calcium excretion is also controversial: an increase [11], a decrease [12] and no effect [13] has been reported. It has also been described that ovariectomy causes an increase in intestinal calcium secretion leading to an impaired calcium balance [14]. Therefore, the purpose of this study was to investigate whether a) OVX has an influence on calcium metabolism, b) calcitriol stimulates intestinal calcium absorption (positive control), c) estrogen modulates calcium metabolism.

Methods: Using an OVX rat model, we examined the consequences of OVX on calcium metabolism (absorption, fecal and urinary elimination) after an oral and intravenous [45]calcium administration [15]. Subsequently, the rat model was validated by checking the positive effect of $1,25(OH)_2$vitamin D_3 (=calcitriol) on the bioavailability of calcium. After that, the effect of estrogen administration on calcium metabolism was examined. Rats were treated with estrogen by two regimes. To examine the short-term effects of estrogen, rats were treated with a pharmacological dose of estrogen during 2 days prior to the test. To mimic long-term estrogen replacement therapy, as usual in postmenopausal women, the effect of sustained release of estrogen from Alzet osmotic mini-pumps on calcium metabolism was investigated.

The experimental design of the studies is depicted in Table 1. Each study consisted of 4 tests performed with 6 OVX and 6 SHAM rats at 8 weeks after operation (day 0). Tests 3 and 4 were performed after intervention i.e. A= 12.5 ng/100 g calcitriol administered 48 and 24 hours prior to the test (*study 1*), B= 7.5 µg/100 g estradiol-benzoate administered 48 and 24 hours prior to the test (*study 2a*), C= 1 µg/100 g estradiol-benzoate per day administered by osmotic mini-pump during 28 days (*study 2b*).

Table 1: Experimental design of the study.

Day	Test	Intervention	Ca Route (µmol/100 g b.w.)
0	1	No	Oral (4.0)
14	2	No	Iv (2.25)
42	3	A, B or C	Oral (4.0)
56	4	A, B or C	Iv (2.25)

Data analysis and statistics The plasma concentration-time (C-t) curves of calcium were analyzed by non-compartmental pharmacokinetic analysis using the computer program Topfit 2.0. The following variables were calculated: area under the curve from t=0 to infinity ($AUC^{0-\infty}$, µmol.L^{-1}.h), clearance (Cl, ml/min), volume of distribution at steady state ($V_{d,ss}$, L), mean residence time (MRT, h) and the final half-life ($t_{\frac{1}{2}}$,h) from 24h to 240h after administration. The bioavailability (f) was calculated from the ratio of the $AUC_{po}^{0-\infty}$ and the $AUC_{iv}^{0-\infty}$, in which both areas were normalized for the dose:

$$f(\%) = \frac{AUC_{po}^{0-\infty}}{AUC_{iv}^{0-\infty}} \times \frac{Dose_{iv}}{Dose_{po}} \times 100$$

The bioavailability assessed in this way corresponds with the true absorption of calcium i.e. the amount absorbed from the intestine into the general circulation, because the ratio of the AUCs is supposed to be independent of distribution and excretion.

Results: OVX did not influence calcium metabolism. In the OVX and SHAM rats, $AUC_{po}^{0-\infty}$ and bioavailability nearly doubled (P<0.0001) after treatment with 1,25-dihydroxyvitamin D$_3$, indicating that the rat can be used as a model for studying modulation of calcium metabolism. Short-term estrogen treatment significantly increased $AUC_{po}^{0-\infty}$ in OVX and SHAM rats (76%, P<0.0001 and 72%, P<0.005, respectively). During long-term estrogen treatment $AUC_{po}^{0-\infty}$ only significantly increased in the OVX rats (83%, P<0.0001). However, after short- and during long-term estrogen treatment, also $AUC_{iv}^{0-\infty}$ increased in both OVX and SHAM rats (30%-65%). Therefore bioavailability did not increase significantly. Besides, long-term estrogen treatment significantly increased endogenous fecal calcium excretion in both OVX and SHAM rats (68% and 60%, respectively, both P<0.0001).

Conclusions: Our data showed that OVX had no influence on calcium metabolism. Estrogen treatment increased $AUC_{po}^{0-\infty}$, but $AUC_{iv}^{0-\infty}$ also increased and therefore bioavailability did not significantly increase. The lack of effect of OVX on intestinal calcium absorption may suggest that the present endogenous estrogen levels do not contribute to intestinal calcium absorption in the adult rat.

References:
1   Heaney, R.P., Recker, R.R. and Saville, P.D. (1978) J Lab Clin Med 92,953-963.
2   Prince, R.L. and Dick, I. (1997) Osteoporos Int 7,S150-S154.
3   Gallagher, J.C. (1990) Bone Miner 9,215-227.
4   Gennari, C., Agnusdei, D., Nardi, P. and Civitelli, R. (1990) J Clin Endocrinol Metab 71,1288-1293.
5   Liel, Y., Shany, S., Smirnoff, P. and Schwartz B (1999) Endocrinology 140,280-285.
6   Bolscher ten M., Netelenbos, J.C., Barto, R., Van Buuren, L.M. and Van der Vijgh, W.J.F. (1999) J Bone Miner Res 14,1197-1202.
7   Kalu, D.N. (1991) Bone Miner 15,175-192.
8   Hope, W.G., Buns, M.E.H. and Thomas, M.L. (1992) Proc Soc Exp Biol Med 200,528-535.
9   Kalu, D.N., Liu, C.C., Hardin, R.R. and Hollis, B.W. (1989) Endocrinology 124,7-16.
10 Miller, S.C., Bowman, B.M., Miller, M.A and Bagi, C.M. (1991) Bone 12,439-446.
11 Morris, H.A., O'Loughlin, P.D., Mason, R.A. and Schulz, S.R. (1995) Bone 17,169S-174S.
12 Colin, E.M., Van den Bemd, G.J.C.M., Van Aken, M., Christakos, S., De Jonge, H.R., DeLuca, H.F., Prahl, J.M., Birkenhager, J.C., Buurman, C.J., Pols, H.A.P. and Van Leeuwen, J.P.T.M. (1999) J Bone Miner Res 14,57-64.
13 O'Loughlin, P.D. and Morris, H.A. (1998) J Physiol 511,313-322.
14 O'Loughlin, P.D. and Morris, H.A. (1994) J Nutr 124,726-731.
15 Sips, A.J.A.M., Barto, R., Netelenbos, J.C. and Van der Vijgh WJF (1997) Am J Physiol 272, E422-E428.

EFFECTS OF DIETARY CALCIUM RESTRICTION ON RADIOCALCIUM ABSORPTION AND TRABECULAR BONE STRUCTURE IN THE RAT

AJ Moore, HA Morris, R Larik, PD O'Loughlin

Division of Clinical Biochemistry, Institute of Medical and Veterinary Science, Frome Road, Adelaide, South Australia 5000

INTRODUCTION

Dietary calcium restriction leads to bone loss in the rat (1), and also triggers an adaptive mechanism to increase the efficiency of intestinal calcium absorption. This has been shown to involve increased renal production of 1,25 dihydroxyvitamin D (2). Calcium supplements increase bone density and reduce fracture risk as well as affecting other calcium and bone related variables. For example, we have shown that serum 1,25 dihydroxyvitamin D levels are markedly reduced with increased dietary calcium in the rat. However, it is not known whether the rise in circulating 1,25 D has an effect on trabecular architecture. The present study demonstrates the effects of dietary calcium restriction on circulating levels of 1,25 dihydroxyvitamin D, intestinal radiocalcium absorption and trabecular architecture in the distal femur.

MATERIALS AND METHODS

Five groups of 6 ovary-intact rats (4.5 months) were ad-libitum fed either standard rat chow (1.0 % calcium) or one of 4 semi-synthetic diets containing between 0.05 % and 1 % calcium (syn0.05, syn0.2, syn0.4 or syn1.0) for seven weeks. Radiocalcium absorption was estimated at seven weeks from a blood sample taken 30 minutes after gavage with ^{45}Ca 18.5kBq in 1 ml H_2O and was corrected for body weight and expressed as circulating calcium relative to the administered dose (%AD). 1,25 dihydroxyvitamin D was determined by radioimmunoassay (IDS) of the 30 minute blood sample.

Fluorochrome labels (declomycin and calcein) were injected at 6 and 2 days prior to death. Rats were subsequently killed and distal femora were prepared for quantitative histomorphometry using established resin embedding techniques. Quantitative bone histomorphometry was performed on 5-micron thick sections of distal femur stained with either a modified Von Kossa (VK) or a Von Kossa and Haematoxylin and Eosin (VK/H&E) stain. Trabecular bone volume (BV/TV), Trabecular Thickness (Tb.Th) and Trabecular Number (Tb.N) were calculated in both the epiphysis and the metaphysis using a Quantimet 500 image analysis system. In addition, unstained sections were prepared for double fluorochrome labelled surface measurements. Statistical analysis was performed using analysis of variance (ANOVA) and Tukeys post hoc test at a significance level of $P < 0.05$.

RESULTS

Intestinal ^{45}Ca uptake was highest in syn0.05 (mean $\pm$ sem:12.5 $\pm$ 1.8 % AD) and lowest in syn1.0 (3.5 $\pm$ 0.66 % AD) ($P < 0.001$). The effect of dietary calcium level on circulating 1,25D showed high levels of 1,25 D in syn0.05 (189 $\pm$ 20 pmol/l) and low levels in syn1.0 (11 $\pm$ 1.0 pmol/l) ($P < 0.001$). There was a significant relationship between circulating ^{45}Ca

654

and serum 1,25D ($r^2 = 0.69$, P < 0.001) that was best described by the logarithmic function: 45Ca = 3.13 $\log_n$ (1,25D)-3.74.

Figure 1 show the effects of diet on double-labelled surface in the epiphysis. A reduction in osteoblastic activity is observed in the epiphysis in rats fed high levels of dietary calcium. A decrease in double-labelled surface is also observed in the metaphysis where mechanical loading is significantly decreased (Figure 2). Osteoclast surface was also observed to decrease as dietary calcium increased (Table 1). Changes in cell activity were also accompanied by changes in trabecular bone structure. Although no changes in BV/TV were observed in the epiphysis (Figure 3), a reduction in BV/TV in the syn0.05 group was observed in the metaphysis (Figure 4). This occurred as a result of a reduction in Tb.N (Table 1).

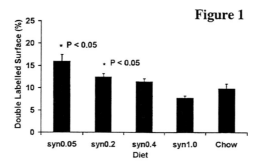

Percentage double-labelled surface in the epiphysis in ovary intact rats fed various levels of dietary calcium P < 0.05 compared with chow and syn1.0

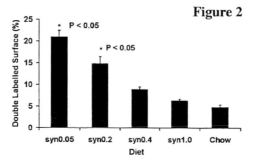

Percentage double-labelled surface in the metaphysis in ovary intact rats fed various levels of dietary calcium P < 0.05 compared with chow and syn1.0

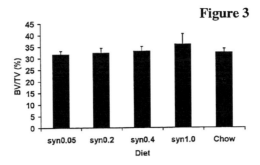

BV/TV in the epiphysis in ovary intact rats fed
various levels of dietary calcium. No significant
differences detected.

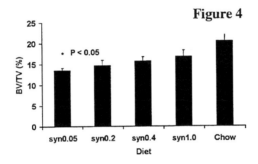

BV/TV in the metaphysis in ovary intact rats fed
various levels of dietary calcium. P < 0.05
compared with chow.

Table 1

| | Epiphysis | | | Metaphysis | |
	Tb.Th	Tb.N	Oc.Surf.	Tb.Th	Tb.N
Syn0.05	0.096 ± 0.004	3.30 ± 0.14	38.38 ± 2.45*	0.080 ± 0.003	1.82 ± 0.27*
Syn0.2	0.100 ± 0.004	3.12 + 0.12	33.29 + 1.42	0.079 ± 0.003	1.83 ± 0.13
Syn0.4	0.095 ± 0.006	3.52 + 0.19	29.09 + 1.96	0.076 ± 0.004	2.10 ± 0.18
Syn1.0	0.102 ± 0.011	3.49 ± 0.20	30.99 + 1.62	0.080 ± 0.006	2.13 ± 0.21
Chow	0.096 ± 0.002	3.35 ± 0.11	26.78 + 1.86	0.076 ± 0.004	2.68 ± 0.30

Femoral bone histomorphometric and osteoclast surface data
Data presented as mean ± SEM. Oc Surf. = Osteoclast surface *P < 0.05 compared to chow
Tb.Th = Trabecular Thickness. Tb.N = Trabecular Number *P < 0.05 compared to chow

DISCUSSION

The percentage of the administered dose of ^{45}Ca in the circulation 30 minutes after gavage is strongly determined by circulating 1,25D. Circulating 1,25D levels may also be determined by dietary calcium. Dietary calcium has been shown to significantly modulate bone remodelling activity. However, in ovary intact rats, calcium adaptation is sufficient to maintain trabecular architecture except at specific sites with the syn0.05 diet. Trabecular bone in the metaphysis experiences reduced mechanical loading compared with the epiphysis (3). It appears that this mechanical loading can protect bone against increased remodelling activity of calcium restriction.

REFERENCES

(1)   Shen, V., Birchman, R., Xu R, Lindsay, R., Dempster, D.W. (1995).
        Bone. 16 (1), 149-156.

(2)   Rader, J.I., Baylink, D.J., Hughes, M.R., Safilian, E.F., Haussler, M.R.
        (1979). Am.J.Physiol. 236, 1396-1404.

(3)   Westerlind, K.C., Wronski, T.J., Ritman, E.L., Luo, Z.P., An, K.N., Bells,
        N.H., Turner, R.T. (1997). Proc.Natl.Acad.Sci. 94, 4199-4204.

HYPOCALCEMIA LOWERS THE "CAPACITATIVE/SOTRE-OPERATED Ca^{2+} ENTRY" THRESHOLD

Marielle Gascon-Barré and Jean-Luc Petit, Centre de recherche, Hôpital Saint-Luc, Centre hospitalier de l'Université de Montréal and Department of Pharmacology, Faculty of Medicine, Université de Montréal, Montréal, Québec, Canada.

Introduction   Following agonist stimulation linked to IP$_3$ Ca^{2+} mobilisation, Ca^{2+} influx through the plasma membrane, the "capacitative calcium entry mechanism", is dependent upon the repletion state of the intracellular Ca^{2+} ([Ca^{2+}]$_c$) pools (1-6). It has already been suggested that vitamin D (D) depletion influences the handling of [Ca^{2+}]$_c$ pools (7,8) and perturbs several cellular functions most specifically those associated with compensatory liver growth following partial hepatectomy (9-14). These observations lead us to put forward the hypothesis that the sub-optimal state of the cellular Ca^{2+} pools induced by D depletion *in vivo* should be linked to an increased sensitivity in the regulatory mechanism(s) responsible for Ca^{2+} entry from the external compartment.

Aims   The aims of the present studies was to investigate, using an *in vivo* model, the influence of calcium deficiency on the mechanism responsible for calcium entry following agonist stimulation, the mechanism known as "capacitative Ca^{2+} entry/store-operated Ca^{2+} entry" (5,15,16).

Materials and Methods   Hepatocytes, a cell type well characterized for its cellular Ca^{2+} response and its ability to be maintained in primary culture at extracellular Ca^{2+} concentration ([Ca^{2+}]$_e$) similar to that prevailing *in vivo* was chosen for all studies. Hepatocytes isolated from Normal (N), or calcium-deficient hypocalcemic D depleted rats (Ca-) were maintained in primary culture at Ca^{2+} concentration similar to that prevailing *in vivo* as previously described (8). Cells were subjected to protocols aimed at studying *i*) Ca^{2+} mobiliazation from IP$_3$ sensitive stores, *ii*) the state of the IP$_3$-sensitive Ca^{2+} pools, and *iii*) Ca^{2+} entry following agonist stimulation linked to Ca^{2+} mobilization from IP$_3$-sensitive pools in order to investigate the sensitivity of the "capacitative calcium entry" process. The intracellular Ca^{2+} signal was analysed using Fura-2AM in single hepatocytes while the IP$_3$-sensitive Ca^{2+} pools were evaluated in permeabilized cells (10^7/mL) using the Fura-2 free acid as probe as previously described (8,17,18).

Results and Discussion   Figure 1 presents typical Ca^{2+} mobilization traces induced by phenylephrine, an α_1 adrenergic agonist as well as by the V$_1$ receptor agonist vasopressine. As illustrated, Ca^{2+} mobilization by both agonists was significantly decreased by calcium deficiency clearly indicating that the response to agonists linked to Ca^{2+} signaling is impaired by calcium deficiency. In order to investigate the locus responsible for the decreased cellular response to agonists linked to Ca^{2+} mobilization in hypocalcemia, the size of the IP$_3$-sensitive Ca^{2+} pools was probed in permeabilized hepatocytes (Fig. 2). As illustrated, Ca^{2+} mobilization induced by 10 μM IP$_3$ was significantly lower in cells obtained from Ca- compared to that obtained in cells isolated form N animals. Ca^{2+}

mobilization could be blocked by heparin, a blocker of the IP$_3$R. These data indicate that the size of the hormone-sensitive cellular Ca^{2+} pools is decreased by calcium deficiency. Collectively our data illustrate that calcium deficiency *in vivo* significantly influences the response to agonists linked to IP$_3$ Ca^{2+} mobilization as well as the state of the IP$_3$-sensitive cellular Ca^{2+} pools.

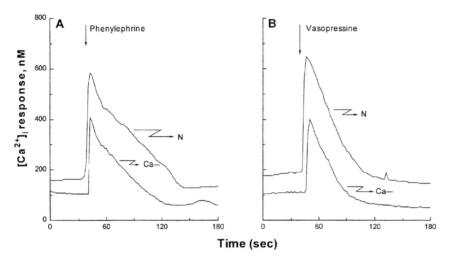

FIGURE 1. Influence of calcium deficiency *in vivo* on the [Ca^{2+}]$_c$ response to phenylephrine (A) and vasopressine (B) in single hepatocytes obtained from hypocalcemic and normal rats. The response to agonists was measured in Ca^{2+}-free medium.

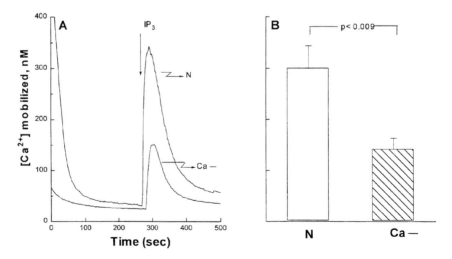

FIGURE 2. Influence of calcium deficiency *in vivo* on the IP$_3$-induced Ca^{2+} mobilization from cellular pools. IP$_3$ was used at a concentration of 10 µM in permeabilized hepatocytes.

To study whether the depletion state of the IP_3-sensitive Ca^{2+} pools led to an increased sensitivity of the mechanism(s) involved in Ca^{2+} entry form the extracellular compartment, cells were stimulated with phenylephrine and then exposed to an extracellular Ca^{2+} gradient (300 nM to 3 mM Ca^{2+}) and the intracellular Ca^{2+} ($[Ca^{2+}]_c$) response was measured (Fig. 3).

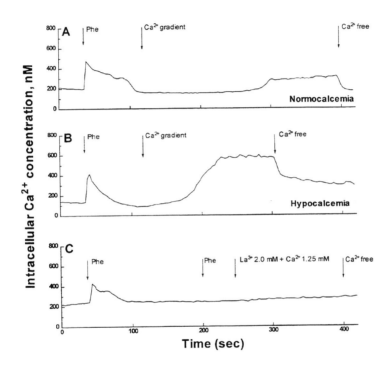

FIGURE 3. Influence of calcium deficiency *in vivo* on Ca^{2+} entry during application of an extracellular Ca^{2+} gradient following phenylephrine stimulation in Ca^{2+}-free medium in single hepatocytes obtained from normal (A) or calcium deficient (B) rats. Ca^{2+} entry could be blocked in both groups by the La^3, a blocker of "capacitative Ca^{2+} entry".

Studies on the Ca^{2+} entry reveal that calcium deficiency shifted to the left the $[Ca^{2+}]_e$ needed to elicit Ca^{2+} entry into the cell. The Ca^{2+} entry curves were also accompanied by steeper slopes and higher maximum increases in $[Ca^{2+}]_c$ as illustrated in Figure 3. Ca^{2+} entry could be blocked by La^3, a blocker of the CRAC channel (19-21). These observations indicate that the threshold for Ca^{2+} entry is significantly lowered by a state of calcium deficiency *in vivo*. These data clearly demonstrate that the sensitivity of the capacitative calcium entry mechanism is increased by a state of calcium deprivation *in vivo*. They also suggest that cellular calcium replenishment would occur with increased efficiency when extracellular Ca^{2+} is made available.

Conclusion   Our data, thus, show that calcium deficiency significantly influences the handling of cellular Ca^{2+} by decreasing the response to agonists linked to IP_3-dependent Ca^{2+} mobilization, decreasing the luminal Ca^{2+} content, and by lowering the threshold for Ca^{2+} entry following emptying of the IP_3-sensitive Ca^{2+} pools. The latter observation is the first indication that calcium deficiency *in vivo* accelerates the development of the "capacitative Ca^{2+} entry mechanism".

References

1. Douglas, J. D. (1993) *Acad. Med.* **68**, S77-S83

2. Putney, J. W.,Jr. (1977) *J. Physiol.* **268**, 139-149

3. Zweifach, A. and Lewis, R. S. (1993) *Proc. Natl. Acad. Sci. USA* **90**, 6295-6299

4. Clementi, E., Scheer, H., Zacchetti, D., Fasolato, C., Pozzan, T., and Meldolesi, J. (1992) *J. Biol. Chem.* **267**, 2164-2172

5. Montero, M., Garcia-Sancho, J., and Alvarez, J. (1994) *J. Biol. Chem.* **269**, 3963-3967

6. Hofer, A. M., Fasolato, C., and Pozzan, T. (1998) *J. Cell Biol.* **140**, 325-334

7. Gascon-Barré, M., Petit, J. L., Éthier, C., and Bilodeau, S. (1997) *Cell Calcium* **22**, 343-356

8. Mailhot, G., Petit, J. L., Demers, C., and Gascon-Barré, M. (2000) *Endocrinology* **141**, 891-900

9. Rixon, R. H., Isaacs, R. J., and Whitfield, J. F. (1989) *J. Cell. Physiol.* **139**, 354-360

10. Youdale, T., Whitfield, J. F., and Rixon, R. H. (1985) *Can. J. Biochem. Cell Biol.* **63**, 319-324

11. Youdale, T., Frappier, L., Whitfield, J. F., and Rixon, R. H. (1984) *Can. J. Biochem. Cell Biol.* **62**, 914-919

12. Sikorska, M., Whitfield, J. F., and Rixon, R. H. (1983) *J. Cell. Physiol.* **115**, 297-304

13. Éthier, C., Kestekian, R., Beaulieu, C., Dubé, C., Havrankova, J., and Gascon-Barré, M. (1990) *Endocrinology* **126**, 2947-2959

14. Goupil, D., Éthier, C., Zarnegar, R., and Gascon-Barré, M. (1997) *J. Hepatol.* **26**, 659-668

15. Putney, J. M.,Jr. (1986) *Cell Calcium* **7**, 1-12

16. Putney, J. W.,Jr (1990) *Cell Calcium* **11**, 611-624

17. Grynkiewicz, G., Poeni, M., and Tsien, R. Y. (1986) *J. Biol. Chem.* **260**, 3440-3450

18. Missiaen, L., Taylor, C. W., and Berridge, M. J. (1991) *Nature* **352**, 241-244

19. Waldron, R., Short, A. D., and Gill, D. L. (1997) *J. Biol. Chem.* **272**, 6440-6447

20. Fasolato, C., Innocenti, B., and Pozzan, T. (1994) *TiPS* **15**, 77-83

21. Preuss, K. D., Noller, J. K., Krause, E., Gobel, A., and Schulz, I. (1997) *Biochem. Biophys. Res. Commun.* **240**, 167-172

EXPRESSION OF THE EXTRACELLULAR CALCIUM-SENSING RECEPTOR IN VITAMIN D RECEPTOR KNOCK-OUT MICE

Enikö Kállay, Meinrad Peterlik, Heide S. Cross, Department of Pathophysiology, University of Vienna Medical School, A-1090 Vienna, Austria.

Introduction   Epidemiological data suggest a protective role of calcium and vitamin D against development of colorectal tumors in humans (1). In this respect, Lipkin and Newmark (2) showed that increased intake of oral calcium can prevent a lumen-ward shift of the proliferative compartment of the colonic crypt in patients already at high risk for familial colon cancer. This suggests that changes in luminal calcium concentration have profound effects on cell kinetics in colonic crypts. Extracellular calcium (Ca^{2+}_0) itself can act as if it were a calciotropic "hormone" by binding to a specific plasma membrane calcium-sensing receptor (CaR). Previous studies from our laboratory demonstrated the presence of the parathyroid-type CaR also in various types of human colon epithelial cells and thereby furnished evidence for the involvement of the CaR in regulation of colonocyte proliferation and differentiation (3, 4).

1,25-dihydroxyvitamin D_3 (1,25-D_3), the hormonally active metabolite of vitamin D, plays a major role in calcium and phosphate homeostasis and functions as a regulator of proliferation and differentiation of normal and malignant cells. The presence of the nuclear vitamin D receptor (VDR), which is a ligand-activated gene transcription factor, determines cellular responsiveness to the anti-mitogenic action of the steroid hormone. In order to evaluate an interaction between the vitamin D system and calcium sensing we investigated the expression of the CaR in vitamin D receptor knockout (VDR-KO) mice which were generated by the group of Dr. Shigeaki Kato (University of Tokyo, Japan) using gene targeting to ablate exon 2 containing the Zn^{++}-finger region from the VDR gene (see, e.g. 5)

Methods DNA and RNA preparation: Genomic DNA was extracted from mouse tail tissue using standard proteinase K-SDS digestion. Briefly: 5 mm of the tail of a >10 days old mouse was resuspended in Tail buffer (50 mM Tris-HCl, pH 8.0, containing 0.1 M EDTA, 100 mM NaCl, 1% SDS, 20 µg/ml RNase, DNase-free, 0.5 mg/ml proteinase K). Samples were incubated for 3 h at 55°C with agitation. Proteins were precipitated by adding 170 µl saturated NaCl. Supernatant was removed to a fresh tube and an equal volume of isopropanol was added to precipitate DNA. The DNA was washed once in 70% isopropanol. It was allowed to air-dry for 10-15 min and dissolved in TE buffer. Total RNA was prepared with Trizol. 2 µg were used for synthesis of single stranded cDNA (SUPERSCRIPT^{TM}II kit).

PCR and RT-PCR was performed at a final concentration of 1x DyNAzyme buffer, 0.25 mM dNTP, 0.25 µM of forward and reverse primers and 1 U DyNAzyme II DNA polymerase. Conditions were: 33 cycles at 94°C for 15 sec, 59°C for 30 s, 72°C for 1 min, with a final extension at 72°C for 10 min.

Glyceraldehyde-3-phosphate dehydrogenase (GAPDH) was used as an internal control for the RT-PCR reaction. Primers were designed to span introns to ensure that the products were not the result of amplification of contaminating genomic DNA segments. To avoid differences among tubes, RT-PCR was performed in the same tube for amplification of the CaR mRNA and of GAPDH.

Western blotting: The mucosa of the large bowel was scraped into ice cold PBS containing 10 mM sodium pyrophosphate and 1 mM sodium orthovanadate. Excess PBS was drained and 1 ml lysis solution (50 mM Tris-HCl pH 7.4 , 150 mM NaCl, 2 mM sodium orthovanadate, 10 mM NaF, 4 mM EDTA, 10 mM sodium pyrophosphate, 10 µg/ml aprotinin, 10 mg/ml Pefabloc, 1% NP-40, 0.1% Na deoxycholate) was added. Samples were homogenized and centrifuged at 14,000 x g for 10 minutes at 4°C. Protein concentration was measured with the BCA method. Samples were run on 7.5% SDS-polyacrylamide gel. Proteins were transferred to a nitrocellulose membrane. After blocking in SuperBlock the membrane was incubated with a polyclonal antibody against the CaR (generously provided by Drs. Allan Spiegel and Paul Goldsmith) overnight at 4°C. The blot was washed in PBS containing 0.5% Tween 20 (PBS-T) and incubated with a secondary antibody conjugated to horseradish peroxidase. CaR protein was detected using the ECL detection kit followed by autoradiography.

Immunohistochemistry: Pieces of ascending and descending colon of wild type (WT) and VDR knock-out (KO) mice were deep frozen. Cryo-sections were stained according to the Histomouse-SP kit instructions (Zymed Laboratories Inc.). A rabbit polyclonal anti-CaR antibody directed against a synthetic peptide corresponding to amino acids 214-235 in the extracellular domain was used (generously provided by Drs. Allan Spiegel and Paul Goldsmith). Negative controls for CaR were carried out by incubation of the sections with anti-CaR antibody preabsorbed with 6 µg/ml of the immunogenic peptide.

Results The CaR gene is present unaltered in both wild type and in VDR-KO mice. This could be deduced from the results of the PCR reaction with primers designed to span two introns of the CaR gene. The sequences of these primers are based on the mouse calcium sensing receptor sequence (GenBank accession number NM 013803.) Using genomic DNA as template, the introns were amplified as well.

In order to determine whether the CaR mRNA is expressed in mouse kidney and colon we used the CaR specific primers designed on the basis of the reported cDNA in mouse keratinocytes (6). Total RNA from WT and VDR-KO mice was extracted. The mRNA was reverse-transcribed into single stranded cDNA. This cDNA was used as template for the PCR reactions. As negative control, samples without reverse transcriptase were used. The primers amplified a product with the expected size (972 bp). This demonstrated that the product was not amplified from contaminating genomic DNA. The product was identified as the expected fragment of the extracellular domain of the CaR by restriction enzyme analysis. The restriction enzyme Cla I cut the 962 bp product into the proper 295 bp and 677 bp fragments. In samples without reverse transcriptase no product was amplified demonstrating the purity of the RNA preparation.

GAPDH was used as an internal control. The ratios between the density of the fragments obtained for the CaR and GAPDH were similar in the WT and KO kidney, suggesting comparable expression levels in this organ (Fig. 1).

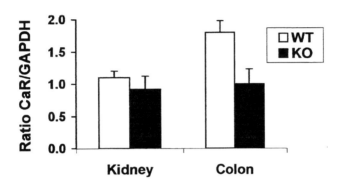

Fig. 1. RT-PCR amplification of CaR and GAPDH mRNA in the kidney and colon of WT and VDR-KO mice (n=3, data are mean ± SD)

Western blot analysis of the WT and VDR-KO mice kidney showed no significant difference in expression of the CaR protein.

However, there is a striking difference between WT and VDR-KO mice with respect to CaR expression in the colon at both the mRNA and protein level. When CaR mRNA from WT and VDR-KO animals was amplified together with GAPDH mRNA, a decreased expression of the CaR mRNA in the ascending colon of the VDR-KO mice was found (Fig. 1).

Ascending and descending segments of the colon were deep frozen, cut into 5 µm sections and stained with an antibody against the CaR. The immunohistochemical staining of large bowel mucosa indicated reduced expression of the CaR protein in VDR-KO animals both in ascending and descending segments of the colon (not shown).

Discussion Both 1,25-D_3 and calcium have an anti-proliferative and pro-differentiating effect on colonocytes and are suggested to inhibit tumor progression in the human colon. Decreased expression of the CaR in the colon of VDR-KO mice indicates an overlap of biological activity between the vitamin D/VDR system and the CaR. It also implies, that genomic action of 1,25-D_3

mediated by a functional VDR might be necessary to have normal CaR mRNA and protein expression. Therefore, the antimitotic effect of dietary calcium in the colon could in fact be enhanced by 1,25-D$_3$ due to VDR-mediated up-regulation of the CaR.

References

1.   Garland, C., Shekelle, R.B., Barrett-Connor, E., Criqui, M.H., Rossof, A.H. and Paul, O. (1985) Lancet 1, 307-309.

2.   Lipkin, M. and Newmark, H. (1985) N. Engl. J. Med. 313, 1381-84.

3.   Kállay, E., Kifor, O., Chattopadhyay, N., Brown, E.M., Bischof, M.G., Peterlik, M. and Cross, H.S. (1997) Biochem. Biophys. Res. Comm. 232, 80-83.

4.   Sheinin, Y., Kállay, E., Wrba, F., Kriwanek, S., Peterlik, M. and Cross, H.S. (2000) J. Histochem. Cytochem. 48, 595-601.

5.   Yoshizawa T., Handa Y., Uematsu Y., Takeda S., Sekine K., Yoshihara Y., Kawakami T., Arioka K., Sato H., Uchiyama Y., Masushige S., Fukamizu A., Matsumoto T., and Kato S. (1997) Nature Genetics 16, 391-396.

6.   Oda, Y., Tu, C. L., Chang, W., Crumrine, D., Komuves, L., Mauro, T., Elias, P.M. and Bikle, D.D. (2000) J. Biol. Chem. 275, 1183-1190.

STUDIES WITH CALBINDIN-D$_{28k}$ KNOCKOUT MICE PROVIDE DIRECT EVIDENCE FOR A ROLE FOR CALBINDIN IN RENAL CALCIUM REABSORPTION, INSULIN SECRETION, PROTECTION AGAINST NEURONAL CELL DEATH AND IN MEMORY FUNCTION

Karen Sooy[+], Jody Kohut[+], Michael Meyer[*], Teh-Li Huo[++], Devin Gary[**], Mark Mattson[**], Thomas Schermerhorn[#], Geoffrey W. Sharp[#], Meredith Kneavel[##], Victoria Luine[##] and Sylvia Christakos[+], [+]Dept. of Biochemistry and Molecular Biology, UMDNJ-New Jersey Medical School, Newark, NJ, [*]Dept. of Neurochemistry, Max-Planck Institute, Martinsried, Germany, [++]Dept. of Medicine, University of Arizona Health Science Center, Tucson, AZ, [**]Sanders Brown Center on Aging, Lexington, KY, [#]Dept. of Molecular Medicine, New York State College of Veterinary Medicine, Cornell University, Ithaca, NY, [##]Dept. of Psychology, Hunter College, New York, NY

Introduction: One of the most pronounced effects of 1,25dihydroxyvitamin D$_3$ known is the induction of the calcium binding protein, calbindin, the first known target of vitamin D action (1). There are two major subclasses of vitamin D dependent calcium binding proteins, calbindin-D$_{28k}$ (28,000Mr) which is highly conserved during evolution (present in avian intestine, mammalian and avian kidney, pancreas and bone and mammalian to molluskan brain) and calbindin-D$_{9k}$ (9,000Mr) which is present only in mammals and in highest concentrations in mammalian intestine as well as in murine kidney (2-4). The phylogenetic conservation of calbindin-D$_{28k}$ has suggested an important fundamental role for calbindin-D$_{28k}$ in mediating intracellular calcium dependent processes. To investigate the physiological role of calbindin, calbindin-D$_{28k}$ nullmutant mice were generated by targeted gene disruption (5).

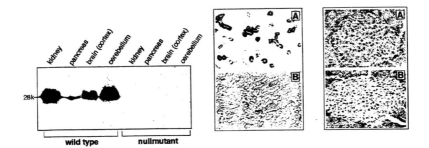

Figure 1: Calbindin-D$_{28k}$ protein is absent in calbindin-D$_{28k}$ knockout mice; analysis by Western blotting (left panel) and immunocytochemical analysis of wild type (A) and calbindin-D$_{28k}$ knockout (B) kidney (middle panel) and pancreatic islet (right panel) using calbindin-D$_{28k}$ antiserum.

Results: Male calbindin-D_{28k} knockout (KO) mice fed a high calcium (HC;1%) diet for 4 weeks were found to have a 2.3 fold increase in the urinary Ca/Cr ratio compared to wild type controls (n=12, *p<0.01; Table 1).

Table 1: Urinary Calcium

	Cr mg/dl	uCa^{2+} mg/dl	Ca^{2+}/Cr ratio	Na^+/Cr ratio
WT	26±3	7±2	0.3±0.1	7±1
KO	21±2	15±1*	0.7±0.1*	8±1

No significant differences in serum calcium or PTH or in serum and urinary Mg and P were observed between WT and KO mice fed the high calcium diet. Renal calbindin-D_{9k} levels are similar in both WT and KO mice, suggesting that changes in calbindin-D_{9k} are not compensating for the lack of calbindin-D_{28k}. Although previous studies provided correlative evidence between hypercalciuria and a decrease in renal calbindin-D_{28k} (6), these findings represent direct in vivo evidence for a role for calbindin-D_{28k} in renal calcium reabsorption.

Studies in the pancreas indicate a significant potentiation in potassium chloride induced insulin release and in the K^+ induced rise in $[Ca^{2+}]_i$ in islets isolated from KO mice compared to islets from WT mice (Fig. 2,3). Although further studies are needed to determine mechanisms involved, our findings using islets from KO mice are important because they define a role for calbindin in the β cell in calcium regulation and modulation of insulin release (7).

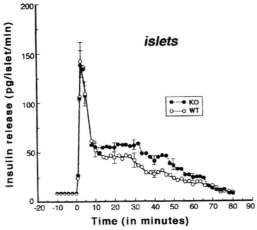

Figure 2: Potassium stimulated insulin release from WT and calbindin-D_{28k} KO islets under perifusion conditions. Significant potentiation in the sustained phase of insulin release in response to 45mM KCl was observed in islets isolated from KO mice.

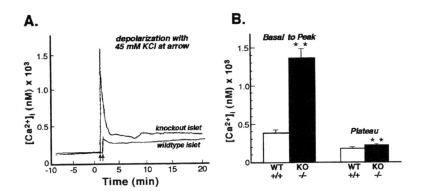

Figure 3: In response to 45mM KCl the peak $[Ca^{2+}]_i$ was markedly increased in islets from KO mice compared to those from WT mice (p<0.01). The plateau $[Ca^{2+}]_i$ was also significantly increased.

Studies of neuronal viability indicate a protective effect of calbindin-D_{28k} in response to the seizure inducing excitotoxin, kainic acid, specifically in CA1 neurons in the hippocampus. Neuronal viability was determined by quantitation of number of undamaged neurons and calcium/calpain dependent proteolysis in the brain was assessed by calpain-cleaved spectrin immunoreactivity. Since the CA1 region of the hippocampus is involved in memory function, nonspatial memory was tested in KO and WT mice using the object recognition test in the presence or absence of stress (4h/day/14 days of spatial restraint). Stressed KO mice had a significantly impaired ability to perform this task relative to stressed control mice (p<0.01; n=8). These findings suggest a role for calbindin in calcium signaling underlying memory function as previously suggested in studies in transgenic mice deficient in calbindin-D_{28k} (8).

In summary, these findings are important since they define for the first time, by direct in vivo evidence, a role for calbindin-D_{28k} in kidney, pancreas and brain.

References:

1.   Christakos, S., Raval-Pandya, M., Wernyj, R.P. and Yang, W. (1996) Biochem.J. **316**, 361-371.

668

2. Christakos,S., Gabrielides, C. and Rhoten, W.B. (1989) Endocr. Rev. **10**, 3-26.
3. Christakos, S. (1995) Endocr. Rev. Monogr. **4**, 108-110
4. Christakos, S., Beck, J.D., Hyllner, S.J. (1997) in Vitamin D (Feldman, D., Glorieux, F. and Pike,J.W. eds.) pp.209-221, Academic Press, San Francisco, CA
5. Airaksinen, M.S., Eilers, J., Garaschuk, O., Thoenen, H., Konnerth, A. and Meyer, M. (1997) Proc. Natl. Acad. Sci. U.S.A. **94**, 1488-1493.
6. Aicher, L., Meier, M., Norcross, A.J., Jakubowski, J., Varela, M.C., Cordier, A. and Steiner, S. (1997) Biochem. Pharmacol. **53**, 723-731
7. Sooy, K., Schermerhorn, T., Noda, M., Surana, M., Rhoten, W.B., Meyer, M., Fleischer, N., Sharp, G.W.G. and Christakos, S. (1999) J. Biol. Chem. **274**, 34343-34349
8. Molinari, S., Battini, R. Ferrari, S., Pozzi, L., Killcross, A.S., Robbins, T.W., Jouvenceau, A., Billard, J.M., Dutar, P., Lamour, Y., Baker, W.A., Cox, H. and Emson,P.C. (1996) Proc. Natl. Acad. Aci. U.S.A. **93**, 8028-8033

ALUMINUM-INDUCED REDUCTION OF DUODENAL CALBINDIN-D$_{9k}$ IS MEDIATED BY 1α,25(OH)$_2$D$_3$ IN OVARIECTOMIZED FEMALE RATS

Daniel Orihuela¶, Cristian Favre*, Cristina E. Carnovale* and María Cristina Carrillo*, ¶Cátedra de Fisiología Humana, Facultad de Bioquímica y Ciencias Biológicas, Universidad Nacional del Litoral, 3000 Santa Fe, Argentina. *Instituto de Fisiología Experimental, Facultad de Ciencias Bioquímicas y Farmacéuticas, Universidad Nacional de Rosario, 2000 Rosario, Argentina

<u>Introduction</u>   It is known that intestinal absorption of aluminum is dependent of vitamin D status and that aluminum and calcium share a common saturable vitamin D-dependent absorption pathway (1). Dietary aluminum chloride inhibits the vitamin D-dependent calcium transport in the intestine of chicks reducing the content of intestinal calbindin-D$_{28k}$ (2). The aluminum effect on rat intestinal calbindin-D$_{9k}$, showed a direct relationship with duodenal content of the protein, suggesting that aluminum could affect the synthesis of calbindin-D$_{9k}$ at the level of vitamin D-receptor in duodenal cells (3). On the other hand, the duodenal mucosal cells of rat present estrogen receptor immunoreactivity (4), express the mRNA for estrogen receptors (5), and respond directly to 17β-estradiol with enhanced calcium transport (6,7). This response can be suppressed by gene transcription and protein synthesis inhibitors. We previously reported that, in ovariectomized rats treated with estrogen, the sensitiveness to the effect of aluminum on *in vitro* mucosa-to-serosa calcium flux, in everted duodenal sacs, increased (lower IC$_{50}$) with increasing 17β-estradiol serum levels, with no changes in the I$_{max}$ value of the dose-response curves (8). The purpose of the present study was to analyze whether the influence of estrogen on inhibition produced by aluminum of duodenal calcium transport is related to vitamin D system in the enterocyte. We investigated the effect of *in vivo* aluminum gavage on calbindin-D$_{9k}$ content in duodenum of ovariectomized female rats.

<u>Methods</u>   In four-month old female Wistar rats, fed with vitamin D-containing diet, were performed a bilateral ovariectomy (Ox). Ten days later Ox rats were randomly divided in groups that received, respectively : 10 mg/kg b.w/day of ethane-1-hydroxi-1,1-diphosphonate (EHDP) s.c (1α,25(OH)$_2$D$_3$ synthesis

inhibitor) (9), 200 µg/kg b.w/day of estradiol valerate (E_2) s.c, EHDP plus E_2 (at same doses that above mentioned) or vehicles. A sham group was included. Animals of each group were divided in two subgroups that received via endogastric catheter, 60 mg of aluminum chloride/kg b.w. per day and double-distilled water, respectively. All treatments were carried out during a seven-day period. Duodenal content of calbindin-D_{9k} ($CaBP_{9k}$) was determined in all groups by Western blot technique based on the combination of a molecular weight of 9 kDa and the ability of protein to bind ^{45}Ca with high affinity (2,10).

Measurement of intestinal calbindin-D_{9k} : Briefly, duodenal mucosa scrapings of three animals from each group were pooled, homogenized 50 % w/w with 20 mM Tris–HCl, 1 mM EGTA and 0.5 ml/L β-mercaptoethanol, pH 8, and centrifuged at 20,000 *xg* for 20 min at 4°C. 120 µg of supernatant protein were separated with a discontinuous SDS-PAGE system, using aprotinin (6.5 kDa) as molecular weight marker. Gels were equilibrated for 20 min in transfer buffer (200 ml/L methanol, 25 mM Tris–HCl, 129 mM glycine, pH 8.5) and transferred onto 0.45-µm nitrocellulose membranes. The membranes were incubated in a buffer of 60 mM KCl, 5 mM $MgCl_2$ and 10 mM imidazole-HCl, pH 6.8, containing 50 µCi/ml [^{45}Ca]Cl_2 , rinsed and exposed to X-ray film (Kodak). Quantitation of protein bands were expressed in densitometric arbitrary units (a.u) of the scanned image of autoradiography. *Statistics:* Means of two groups were compared by grouped Student's *t*-test. Multiple means were compared by one-way analysis of variance followed by Newman-Keuls test. Significance level was set at 0.05.

Results and Discussion   We have examined the effects of aluminum on the major protein that is expression of genomic action of $1\alpha,25(OH)_2D_3$ in the enterocyte, in rats depleted of estrogen by mean of ovariectomy. To reduce the circulating level of $1\alpha,25(OH)_2D_3$, disodium etidronate was used since it is demonstrated that at large doses (like administered in this study) inhibits the synthesis of vitamin D_3 active metabolite (9). We designed four experimental conditions in which $1\alpha,25(OH)_2D_3$ and 17β-estradiol hormones reached very different serum levels. In ovariectomized rats treated with E_2, are found high levels of 17β-estradiol together with $1\alpha,25(OH)_2D_3$ in physiological range. In ovariectomized rats treated with EHDP plus E_2, are found   high levels of 17β-estradiol   together with

$1\alpha,25(OH)_2D_3$ in a sub-physiological range. In ovariectomized rats without treatment, are found a physiological level of $1\alpha,25(OH)_2D_3$ together with a very low level of 17β-estradiol, and in ovariectomized rats treated with EHDP, are found a very low level for both hormones.

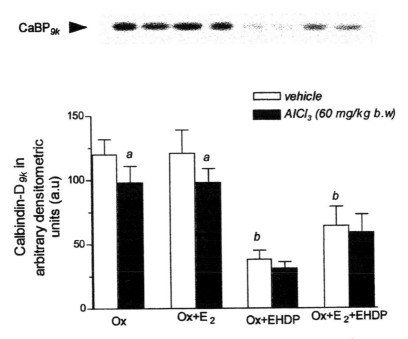

Figure 1: Bands corresponding to duodenal calbindin-D_{9k} protein in the autoradiography (*upper panel*) of ovariectomized female rats (Ox) injected with estradiol (E_2) and/or disodium etidronate (EHDP), treated with aluminum chloride (Al) or vehicle. Densitometry of bands is expressed as arbitrary units (a.u). Data are mean ± S.D (*lower panel*). Vehicle is double-distilled water. [a]$P < 0.05$ significant difference between Al-treated subgroup compared to respective vehicle-treated subgroup. [b]$P < 0.05$ vs. vehicle-treated Ox rats.

As seen in the Figure 1, the duodenal calbindin-D_{9k} protein level was significantly diminished in Ox groups injected with EHDP (30 ± 8 a.u) or EHDP plus E_2 (53 ± 16 a.u), as compared to Ox rats (120 ± 22 a.u, $P < 0.05$), but the aluminum had no effect on CaBP_{9k}. The administration of aluminum chloride significantly reduced the CaBP_{9k} duodenal content in both Ox and E_2-treated Ox rats.

672

Aluminum overload produced a significant reduction of $CaBP_{9k}$ only in groups with a physiological level of $1\alpha,25(OH)_2D_3$. When circulating $1\alpha,25(OH)_2D_3$ was reduced by EHDP administration, aluminum had no effect on $CaBP_{9k}$.

Conclusion   In summary, the inhibitory effect of aluminum on calbindin-D_{9k} was not modified by the circulating estrogen level, suggesting that the influence of estradiol on inhibition of calcium intestinal transport produced by aluminum in female rats is not exerted through an effect on this protein. Instead, the aluminum-induced calbindin-D_{9k} duodenal content drop showed a high dependence of $1\alpha,25(OH)_2D_3$ in ovariectomized rats.

References

(1) Boudey, M., Bureau, F., Placé, C., Neuville, D., Drosdowsky, M., Arhan, P. And Bouglé, D. (1997) J.Pediatr. Gastroenterol. Nutr. 24, 124-127
(2) Dunn, M.A., Saw Leng Too and Ishizaki, A.S. (1995) J.Nutr. 125, 2916-2924
(3) Orihuela, D., Favre, C., Monti, J.A., Carnovale, C. and Carrillo, M.C. (1999) Toxicol. Lett. 104, 211-219
(4) Arjmandi, B.H., Salih, M.A., Herbert, D.C., Sims, S.H. and Kalu, D.N. (1993) Bone Miner. 21, 63-74
(5) Arjmandi, B.H., Hollis, B.W. and Kalu, D.N. (1994) Bone Miner. 26, 181-189
(6) Criddle, R.A., Zheng, M.H., Dick, I.M., Callus, B. and Prince,R.L. (1997) J.Cell.Biochem. 65, 340-348
(7) Brommage, R., Binacua, C. And Carrie, A.L. (1993) Biol. Reprod. 49, 544-548
(8) Orihuela, D., Carnovale, C., Monti, J.A. and Carrillo, M.C. (1996) Toxicol. Lett. 85, 165-171
(9) Bonjour, J.P., Fleisch, H. and Trechsel, U. (1977) J.Physiol. 264(1), 125-139
(10) Maruyama, K., Mikawa, T. And Ebashi, S. (1984) J.Biochem. 95, 511-519

RENAL CALCIUM HANDLING AND VITAMIN D METABOLISM IN DIABETIC RATS

Andrew P Mee, Donald T Ward, S Kam Yau, Christopher A Miller, Hugh O Garland, Daniella Riccardi and E Barbara Mawer, Musculoskeletal Research Group, University Department of Medicine, Manchester Royal Infirmary, Manchester M13 9WL, UK.

Introduction

Altered divalent cation homeostasis with bone mineral loss, hypercalciuria and hypomagnesemia are well recognised consequences of human diabetes mellitus. Delayed insulin treatment only partly restores the bone loss, suggesting that, in the early stages of the disease, some irreversible changes take place. Previous studies have shown that in the streptozotocin (STZ) model of type I diabetes mellitus, renal tubular Ca^{2+} excretion is raised, despite the maintenance of normal serum calcium concentration. We have used the STZ model to investigate renal function, biochemical parameters, renal expression of proteins involved in renal calcium and water transport, and markers of bone remodelling

Methods

Sprague-Dawley rats aged 8 weeks were rendered diabetic with STZ (60mg/kg IP in citrate buffer). Control rats received citrate buffer alone. Diabetes was confirmed by the development of glycosuria within 36h and hyperglycaemia. Rats were catheterised for servo-controlled fluid replacement as described previously (1). Urine samples were collected over three 30 minute intervals during the period 3-4.5h after t_0 (the start of the renal clearance experiments). Blood samples were taken at the midpoint of the urine collection periods (3, 3.75 and 4.5h). GFR was determined by [^{3}H] inulin clearance, urinary calcium and magnesium were analysed by atomic absorption spectrophotometry, and urinary glucose was determined using a kit (Ames Sera-Pak, Bayer Diagnostics). Calculations of renal function were performed as described previously (2). After 14 days, animals were killed and their kidneys were excised and used for immunoblotting, or were perfusion fixed with 4% paraformaldehyde and cryoprotected in sucrose solution, for immunohistochemistry. The antibodies used were affinity-purified anti-CaR (rabbit anti-rat) (Lofstrand Inc), monoclonal anti-calbindin-D_{28k} (Sigma-Aldrich), monoclonal anti-plasma membrane Ca^{2+} ATPase (PMCA) (Cambridge Bioscience), and affinity purified anti-rabbit polyclonal anti-thiazide-sensitive NaCl cotransporter (NCCT) (a gift of Dr Steven Hebert, Vanderbilt University, Nashville). Plasma $25D_3$ was measured by HPLC, and $1,25D_3$ by RIA; PTH, osteocalcin and deoxypyridinoline crosslinks were measured using commercially available kits (Metra Biosystems, USA). Data are presented as mean±SE, and statistical significance was determined by MANOVA (urine and plasma) or paired t-test (semi-quantitative immunoblots).

Results

STZ-treated rats exhibited marked hyperglycemia (34.3±3.1mM) compared with control and insulin-replaced STZ rats (6.6±0.6mM, and 4.9±0.4mM respectively). Urinary glucose was also significantly elevated in STZ rats (50.7±6.9mM/min, $p < 0.001$) compared with normal and insulin-replaced rats (0.02±0.01mM/min). STZ rats exhibited elevated urinary calcium output (+568%), GFR (+70%) and urinary flow rate (+296%) compared with control animals. The effect of diabetes on each parameter was corrected by insulin. CaR abundance in STZ-diabetic kidneys was reduced by 52±11% ($p < 0.05$), whilst renal NCCT expression was elevated by 192±46% of control ($p < 0.05$). These changes were confirmed by immunofluorescence.

The levels of calbindin D_{28k} and PMCA were unchanged by STZ treatment. Blood levels of $1,25D_3$ were reduced in diabetes (27.17±6.63pg/ml cf. 121±65.34 in controls, $p < 0.0001$), as were levels of osteocalcin (21.45±10.59ng/ml cf.

45.45±13.72 in controls, p<0.05). The levels of other biochemical markers were not significantly altered in the STZ-diabetic group.

Conclusions

Diabetic hypercalciuria in rats involves elevated GFR with raised urinary output, reduced renal Ca^{2+} reabsorption and impaired bone deposition. The reduced renal Ca^{2+} reabsorption could be due, at least in part, to the reduced levels of $1,25D_3$, which would also be expected to reduce intestinal absorption of calcium.

Changes in CaR and NCCT protein expression could also account for the altered divalent cation homeostasis seen during diabetes mellitus.

References

1 Burgess WJ, Shalmi M, Petersen JS, Plange-Rhule J, Balment RJ, Atherton JC (1993). Clin Sci 85:129-137.

2 Garland HO, Hamilton K, Freeman S, Burns C, Cusack M, Balment RJ (1999). Clin & Exper Pharmacol & Physiol 26:803-808.

IMMUNOCYTOCHEMICAL DETECTION OF CALBINDIN D$_{28K}$ IN THE CHICKEN TECTOFUGAL AND THALAMOFUGAL VISUAL PATHWAYS.

G. Díaz de Barboza[1], C. Beltramino[2], L. Britto[3], A. Alisio[1] and N. Tolosa de Talamoni[1]. [1] Cátedra de Química Biológica, Facultad de Ciencias Médicas, Universidad Nacional de Córdoba, Córdoba, Argentina, [2] Instituto Ferreyra, Córdoba, Argentina and [3] Instituto de Ciencias Biomédicas, Universidade de São Paulo, Brazil. E-mail: ntolosa@biomed.uncor.edu

Introduction Calbindin D$_{28k}$ is a high-affinity Ca^{2+}-binding protein found to be widely distributed in the central nervous system (1), abundant in neurons (2) but also present in some glial cells (3). Certain evidences indicate that calbindin acts as a buffer for cytoplasmic Ca^{2+}(4, 5) avoiding the deleterious effects of excessive Ca^{2+} accumulation. However, the physiological role of calbindin in the brain is not quite clear. It fails to protect hippocampal neurons against ischemia in spite of its calcium buffering properties as shown in calbindin knockout mice (6). On the contrary, the overexpression of the gene for calbindin, via herpes simplex virus amplicon vector, increases the survival of hippocampal neurons in vitro following energetic or excitotoxic insults (7). Christakos et al. have also reported a cytoprotective role of calbindin in astrocytes showing that the protein, by buffering calcium, can suppress apoptosis induced by calcium ionophore and amiloid β-peptide (8)

The distribution of calbindin in the central visual pathways has been extensively described in mammals and the effects of visual deprivation on the distribution of calbindin in retinorecipient structures of the brain have been also evaluated in several species (9,10). The aim of this study was to localize calbindin by immunocytochemistry in the structures of the tectofugal and thalamofugal systems, the two main visual pathways of the chick brain, and to compare the calbindin expression in the same pathways after monocular enucleation or retinal lesions.

Material and methods Cobb Harding chicks were subjected to retinal lesions or left eye enucleated in sterile conditions under anesthesia (5 mg of ketamine / 100 g of b.w. and 1 mg of xylazine / 100 g of b.w.). At different times, all experimental animals were deeply anesthetized and perfused through the ascending aorta with normal saline, followed by a fixative solution composed by 4% paraformaldehyde in PBS, pH 7.3. Brains were soaked 5 h in the same fixative and transferred to a 30% sucrose solution in buffer PBS. Transversal sections 30 μm thick were used for immunocytochemistry with a mouse anti-calbindin D_{28k} monoclonal antibody (Sigma, St. Louis, MO, USA). The immunocytochemical detection was accomplished by using the avidin-biotin complex staining technique. The primary antibody (dilution 1: 2,000) was incubated with the sections overnight at room temperature whereas the incubation with the biotinylated secondary antibody (1:200) lasted for 1.5 h at room temperature. Avidin-peroxidase conjugate was visualized employing 0.05% diaminobenzidine and 0.01% H_2O_2.

Results and Discussion All neural structures of the chick tectofugal visual pathway were positive for calbindin D_{28k} staining. In the optic tectum, characterized by an extensive lamination in birds, the positive staining was present in several layers but it was more intense in the stratum griseum et fibrosum superficiale (especially in Cajal's layer 5), mainly in dendrites and axons. However, some cells from the same lamina were positive stained in their somata and processes. An important number of large cells from the nucleus rotundus were also calbindin positive while in the ectostriatum only a few cells were positive. Nuclei from the pretectal region, such as the nucleus spiriformis lateralis and the nucleus spiriformis medialis were labeled by the anti-calbindin antibody. The thalamofugal visual system of the chicks also exhibited calbindin staining in cells of the nucleus opticus principalis thalami as well as in cells from the visual Wulst. The staining was positive in cells of the nucleus dorsolateralis anterior thalami and the nucleus dorsomedialis anterior thalami but the immunoreactivity with the anti-calbindin antibody was very poor in the hyperstriatum dorsale and accesorii. A clear reduction in the calbindin staining was noted in the stratum griseum et fibrosum superficiale from the contralateral optic tectum of the enucleated eye compared to the ipsilateral optic tectum. When retinal lesions were performed in one eye, a decrease in the expression of this protein was also observed 7 days later in the stratum et fibrosum superficiale of the contralateral optic tectum being this decrease more pronounced on the day 15th after the injury (Figure 1). A reduction in the calbindin staining was also shown in the contralateral nucleus rotundus. On the other hand, the thalamofugal visual pathway appears not to be altered either by deafferentation or retinal lesions. To our knowledge this is the first report describing directly the distribution of calbindin in the chicken tectofugal and

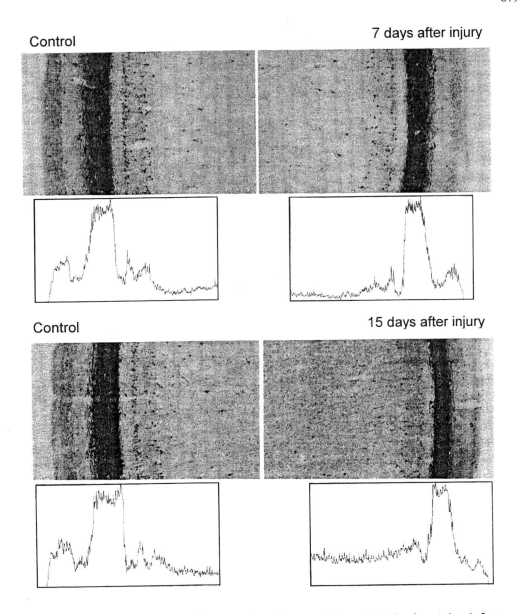

Figure 1: Digital images of coronal sections of the chick brain stained for calbindin D_{28K} showing a reduction in the immunolabeling of the contralateral optic tectum to the injured retina. Stained sections and optical density after 7 days of retinal lesion are shown on the upper panel. Sections and optical density after 15 days of injured retina are shown on the lower panel.

thalamofugal visual pathways. Different responses of calbindin expression have been observed after enucleation or deafferentation of visual pathways from other species (11,12). The depletion of calbindin immunoreactivity in the tectum and in the nucleus rotundus after enucleation or retinal lesions may indicate that the retinal input might control, at least partially, the expression of calbindin D_{28k} in the tectofugal visual pathway but probably not in the thalamofugal pathway.

Acknowledgments: This work was supported by FONCYT(BID 802/OC-AR 05-03126), SECYT(UNC) and CONICOR (Argentina, N. Tolosa de Talamoni), and FAPESP, CNPq, and Pronex/MCT (Brazil, L.R.G. Britto).

References

1. Baimbridge, K., Celio, M. and Rogers, J. (1992) Trends Neurosci. 15, 303-308.
2. Stuart, E. and Lephart, E. (1999) Mol. Brain Res. 73, 60-67.
3. Toyoshima T., Yamagami S., Ahmed, B., Jin, L., Miyamoto, O., Itano, T., Tokuda,M., Matsui, H. and Hatase, O. (1996) NeuroReport 7, 2087-2091.
4. Batini, C., Palestini, M., Thomasset, M. and Vigot, R. (1993) NeuroReport 4, 927-930.
5. Fierro, L. and Llano, I. (1996) J. Physiol. 496, 617-625.
6. Klapstein G., Vietla S., Lieberman, N., Gray, P., Airaksinen, Thoenen H., Meyer, M. and Mody, I. (1998) Neurosci. 85, 361-373.
7. Phillips, R., Meier, T., Giuli, L., McLaughlin, J., Ho, D. and Sapolsky, R. (1999) J. Neurochem. 73, 1200-1205.
8. Wernyj, R., Mattson, M. and Christakos, S. (1999) Mol. Brain Res. 64, 69-79.
9. Mize, R. and Luo, Q. (1992) Vis. Neurosci. 9, 157-168.
10. Britto, L., Gobersztejn, F., Karten, H. and Cox, K. (1994) Brain Res. 661, 289-292.
11. Hidalgo, M., Ito, H. and Lara, J. (1991) Cell Tissue Res. 265, 511-516.
12. Mize, R. and Luo, Q. (1992) Vis. Neurosci. 9, 471- 482.

RAPID ACTIONS
OF VITAMIN D STEROIDS

ARACHIDONIC ACID IS A PIVOTAL AUTOCOID MEDIATOR OF THE MEMBRANE EFFECT OF $1\alpha,25\text{-}(OH)_2D_3$ AND $24R,25\text{-}(OH)_2D_3$ ON GROWTH PLATE CHONDROCYTES

Barbara D. Boyan[1,2,3], David D. Dean[1], Victor L. Sylvia[1], and Zvi Schwartz[1,2,4], Departments of [1]Orthopaedics, [2]Periodontics, and [3]Biochemistry, University of Texas Health Science Center at San Antonio, San Antonio, TX, 78229-3900, USA. [4]Department of Periodontics, Hebrew University, Hadassah Faculty of Dental Medicine, Jerusalem, Israel 91010.

Introduction. $24R,25\text{-}(OH)_2D_3$ and $1\alpha,25\text{-}(OH)_2D_3$ regulate protein kinase C (PKC) (1) in costochondral growth plate chondrocytes in a cell maturation-dependent manner. $24,25\text{-}(OH)_2D_3$ causes an increase in PKC activity of resting zone (RC) cells, whereas $1,25\text{-}(OH)_2D_3$ stimulates PKC activity in cells from the prehypertrophic and upper hypertrophic zones (growth zone, GC). Not only are the effects of these vitamin D metabolites target cell-specific, but they also exert their effects over different time courses. The maximal effect of $24R,25\text{-}(OH)_2D_3$ on PKC in RC cells occurs at 90 minutes and involves both genomic and nongenomic mechanisms. In contrast, the maximal effect of $1\alpha,25\text{-}(OH)_2D_3$ on PKC in GC cells occurs at 9 minutes and involves only nongenomic mechanisms.

Studies in our lab indicate that these effects are mediated through specific membrane receptors. Studies using 1α-hydroxymethyl-3β,25-dihydroxyvitamin D_3, an analogue of $1,25\text{-}(OH)_2D_3$ that is anti-proliferative but exhibits less than 0.1% of the binding to the nuclear vitamin D receptor (nVDR) (2,3), indicated that PKC activity is stimulated in RC cells in a manner similar to $24,25\text{-}(OH)_2D_3$ and in GC cells in a manner similar to $1,25\text{-}(OH)_2D_3$ (4), suggesting that nontraditional receptors might be involved. The stereoisomer of this analogue, 1β-hydroxymethyl-3α,25-dihydroxyvitamin D_3, had no effect on PKC, demonstrating stereospecificity indicative of a receptor-mediated mechanism. This hypothesis was supported by the observation that $24S,25\text{-}(OH)_2D_3$, the stereoisomer of $24R,25\text{-}(OH)_2D_3$, also failed to cause an increase in PKC activity in RC cells (5). Moreover, PKC activity could be stimulated directly by incubating isolated plasma membranes directly with the two metabolites or with the active analogue (6,7). This suggested that if specific receptors were involved, they were associated with the membrane.

Parallel studies by Norman and Nemere (8) indicated that basal lateral membranes of chick intestinal epithelial cells had specific binding sites for $1\alpha,25\text{-}(OH)_2D_3$. An antibody generated to the protein responsible for the binding (Ab99) was shown to block the binding as well as inhibit Ca^{++} transcaltachia (9). In collaboration with Ilka Nemere (Utah State University, Logan, Utah), we determined whether similar $1,25\text{-}(OH)_2D_3$ binding sites were present in rat chondrocytes. When GC cells were treated with Ab99, PKC activity was inhibited (10), as were physiological responses of the cells to $1,25\text{-}(OH)_2D_3$ that had previously been shown to be mediated through PKC (4,10). To verify that the antibody was blocking a separate membrane receptor, matrix vesicles were isolated from the chondrocyte cultures and were incubated directly with $1,25\text{-}(OH)_2D_3 \pm$ Ab99. The antibody blocked the effect of $1,25\text{-}(OH)_2D_3$ on matrix vesicle PKC. Moreover, it recognized a single band on Western blots at an Mr of 66,000, essentially the same size as the chick intestinal basal lateral membrane $1,25\text{-}(OH)_2D_3$ binding protein. Analysis of binding to $[^3H]$-$1,25\text{-}(OH)_2D_3$ showed that GC matrix vesicles bound the seco-steroid with high specificity, exhibiting a Kd of 17.2 fmol/ml and a Bmax of 124 fmol/mg protein.

Similarly, matrix vesicles isolated from RC chondrocyte cultures exhibited specific binding for $[^3H]$-24,25-$(OH)_2D_3$ (4), with a Kd of 69.2 pmol and a Bmax of 52.6 fmol/mg protein. To show that this was not the 1,25-$(OH)_2D_3$ receptor, matrix vesicles were incubated directly with 1α-hydroxymethyl-3β,25-dihydroxyvitamin D_3 ± Ab99. The antibody failed to block the effect of the analogue on PKC activity.

While these data strongly suggested distinct membrane-associated VDRs for 1,25-$(OH)_2D_3$ (1,25-mVDR) and 24,25-$(OH)_2D_3$ (24,25-mVDR), they did not rule out the possibility that the nVDR was responsible for the response. Antibody to the traditional nVDR did not recognize the band detected by Ab99 on western blots of matrix vesicle proteins, however. In addition, matrix vesicles contain no RNA or DNA, so even if the traditional 1,25-$(OH)_2D_3$ nVDR was present, its mode of action could not be via genomic mechanisms.

Matrix vesicles are extracellular organelles produced by growth plate chondrocytes under genomic control, thereby regulating their composition. Once they are released into the matrix, however, the cells must modulate their activity through other methods. RC and GC chondrocytes produce and secrete 1,25-$(OH)_2D_3$ and 24,25-$(OH)_2D_3$ (11). The cells can then modify matrix vesicle behavior through direct action of the vitamin D metabolites on the matrix vesicle membrane. For both cell types, the PKC isoform that is responsive in the cell is PKCα, and the effect of the metabolite is to stimulate activity. However, in matrix vesicles, the responsive isoform is PKCζ, and the effect of the metabolite is to inhibit this enzyme activity. While this explains, in part, the differential effects of the metabolites on the cells and matrix vesicles, it does not explain the remarkable difference in metabolite specificity.

The Role of Phospholipase A_2 and Arachidonic Acid. Earlier studies had shown that 1,25-$(OH)_2D_3$ stimulates phospholipase A_2 (PLA_2) activity in GC cultures, but 24,25-$(OH)_2D_3$ inhibits this enzyme activity in RC cultures (12). The cell specificity of this effect was also noted in isolated plasma membranes and matrix vesicles incubated directly with the vitamin D metabolites (13). When purified PLA_2 was incubated with 1,25-$(OH)_2D_3$, its activity was increased, but when it was incubated with 24,25-$(OH)_2D_3$, activity was decreased (14). These observations suggested that PLA_2 might be a pivotal regulatory point in determining the specificity of the response of the target cells to their metabolite.

The experiments described above examined the effect of 1,25-$(OH)_2D_3$ and 24,25-$(OH)_2D_3$ on metabolism of one specific phospholipid class, phosphatidylethanolamine, which is enriched in matrix vesicles (15). To determine if either metabolite caused a change in the total pool of phospholipid, we examined arachidonic acid release from pre-labeled cells as a measure of PLA_2 activity (16). Indeed, 1,25-$(OH)_2D_3$ caused an increase in arachidonic acid release by GC cells that was evident within 1 minute, and 24,25-$(OH)_2D_3$ caused a rapid decrease in arachidonic acid release by RC cells that was evident within 1 minute and extended for up to 15 minutes.

These studies also examined whether either or both metabolite modulated phospholipid synthesis. Studies on the effects of 1,25-$(OH)_2D_3$ on liver and kidney phospholipid metabolism had demonstrated that the seco-steroid regulated turnover of fatty acids, resulting in altered membrane fluidity and calcium ion transport (17,18). 1,25-$(OH)_2D_3$ also affected re-incorporation of arachidonic acid by GC chondrocytes (14) and caused an increase in plasma membrane fluidity (19). In contrast, 24,25-$(OH)_2D_3$ affected re-incorporation of arachidonic acid by RC cells

(14), but fluidity of the plasma membrane was decreased (19). These two cell types exhibit differences in the phospholipid composition of their plasma membranes (15), and this is sensitive to the vitamin D metabolites (20), reinforcing the hypothesis that phospholipid metabolism differs between the cells in general and in response to $1,25\text{-}(OH)_2D_3$ and $24,25\text{-}(OH)_2D_3$ and that arachidonic acid plays a central role in the differential response.

To test this hypothesis, GC cells were treated with arachidonic acid $\pm$ $1\alpha,25\text{-}(OH)_2D_3$ and RC cells were treated with arachidonic acid $\pm$ $24R,25\text{-}(OH)_2D_3$ (21). The effect on PKC activity was determined in cell lysates. Arachidonic acid caused a small but significant increase in PKC activity of GC cells, but when it was added to the cultures together with $1\alpha,25\text{-}(OH)_2D_3$, PKC activity was increased in a synergistic manner (Figure 1A). In contrast, arachidonic acid caused a small but significant decrease in PKC activity in RC cultures and inhibited the $24R,25\text{-}(OH)_2D_3$-stimulated increase in enzyme activity by approximately 40% (Figure 1B).

Not only did arachidonic acid regulate PKC directly and modulate the effects of the vitamin D metabolite on its target cell, but it also affected the physiological responses of the cells to $1,25\text{-}(OH)_2D_3$ and $24,25\text{-}(OH)_2D_3$ (22,23). Arachidonic acid caused a dose-dependent increase in $[^3H]$-thymidine incorporation by RC cells and abolished the inhibition of $[^3H]$-thymidine incorporation due to $24,25\text{-}(OH)_2D_3$ (Figure 2A). The fatty acid had no effect on $[^{35}S]$-sulfate incorporation by RC cells, but it caused a dose-dependent decrease in the stimulatory effect of $24,25\text{-}(OH)_2D_3$ on this parameter (Figure 2B).

Arachidonic acid has recently been shown to have its own RXR receptors in the nucleus of responding cells, suggesting that part of its effects on the chondrocytes might include genomic mechanisms. To assess whether the effect of arachidonic acid on PKC activity in the growth plate chondrocytes was at least in part through direct action on the membrane, we incubated isolated plasma membranes and matrix vesicles isolated from RC cell cultures with the fatty acid (22). Arachidonic acid caused a decrease in basal PKC activity of plasma membranes and completely blocked the stimulatory effect of $24,25\text{-}(OH)_2D_3$ on this enzyme (Figure 3A). In contrast, arachidonic acid stimulated PKC activity in matrix vesicles, whereas $24,25\text{-}(OH)_2D_3$ caused a decrease in basal activity and also decreased the stimulatory effect of arachidonic acid (Figure 3B). Since PKCα is lipid-dependent (22), it is probable that arachidonic acid affects primarily this isoform in both membrane preparations, but it is clear that any increase in PKCζ in matrix vesicles is abolished by $24,25\text{-}(OH)_2D_3$.

The Role of Arachidonic Acid Metabolism in Cell Response. Arachidonic acid metabolism is also affected by the vitamin D metabolites in a target cell-specific manner, suggesting that the metabolites of this fatty acid also play a role in cell response. Basal levels of prostaglandin E_2 (PGE_2) production are different, with higher levels being produced by RC cells than by GC cells (24). Whereas $1,25\text{-}(OH)_2D_3$ causes an increase in PGE_2 production by GC cells, $24,25\text{-}(OH)_2D_3$ causes a decrease in PGE_2 production by RC cells. Both cell types are sensitive to PGE_2 and express EP1 and EP2 receptors for this prostaglandin, as well as a variant of EP1, EP1v (25). In GC cells, PGE_2 stimulates PKC, but in RC cells PGE_2 causes a decrease in PKC activity. Studies using agonists and antagonists to the EP1 and EP2 receptors demonstrated that both PGE_2 and $1,25\text{-}(OH)_2D_3$ exert their effects on PKC activity in GC cells through EP1 only, and the stimulatory effect on

686

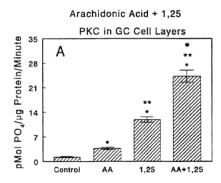

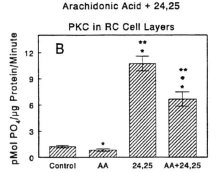

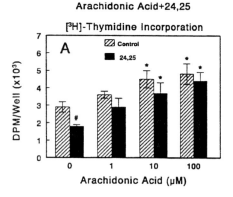

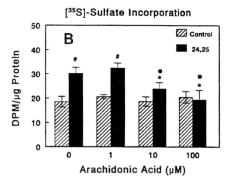

Figure 1: Regulation of PKC activity in GC and RC cell layers by arachidonic acid (AA) and vitamin D metabolites. Top Panel: GC cultures were treated for 9 mins. with vehicle, 100 µM AA, 10^{-8} M 1,25-$(OH)_2D_3$ (1,25), or both mediators together. Lower Panel: RC cultures were treated for 90 mins. with vehicle, 100 µM AA, 10^{-7} M 24,25-$(OH)_2D_3$ (24,25), or both mediators together. For both panels, PKC activity in the cell layer was determined at harvest. Values are the mean ± S.E.M. for n = 6 cultures in a representative experiment; the experiment was repeated three times with nearly identical results. *P < 0.05, vs. control; **P < 0.05, vs. AA alone; •P < 0.05, vs. 1,25, 24,25, or AA alone.

Figure 2: Effect of arachidonic acid (AA) and 24,25-$(OH)_2D_3$ (24,25) on [^{3}H]-thymidine incorporation and [^{35}S]-sulfate incorporation by resting zone chondrocytes. Top Panel: RC cultures were treated for 24 hours with vehicle or 10^{-7} M 24,25 in the presence and absence of 1, 10, and 100 µM AA. At harvest, [^{3}H]-thymidine incorporation by the cultures was determined. Lower Panel: RC cultures were treated for 24 hours with vehicle or 10^{-7} M 24,25 in the presence and absence of 1, 10, and 100 µM AA. At harvest, [^{35}S]-sulfate incorporation by the cultures was determined. Values are the mean ± S.E.M. for n = 6 cultures in a representative experiment; the experiment was repeated three times with nearly identical results. *P < 0.05, vs. cultures not treated with AA; #P < 0.05, vs. cultures not treated with 24,25; •P < 0.05, vs. cultures treated with 1 µM AA.

PKC is mediated through PKA. In contrast, in RC cells, both PGE_2 and 24,25-$(OH)_2D_3$ regulate PKC through both EP1 and EP2. While this may appear contradictory, it is important to remember that the primary effect of 24,25-$(OH)_2D_3$ is to decrease substrate for PGE_2 production. Thus, the inhibitory effect of PGE_2 on PKC activity in RC cells is reduced.

These observations raised the question of whether production of arachidonic acid is the critical regulatory point in control of PKC or if metabolism of arachidonic acid is the critical point. Arachidonic acid is metabolized to prostaglandins and leukotrienes through a complex series of intermediates. The enzyme that controls the entry into the prostaglandin pathway is cyclooxygenase (Cox). Cox-1 is constitutively expressed, and Cox-2, normally associated with inflammation, is inducible. RC and GC cells express mRNAs for both isoforms (5). Neither 1,25-$(OH)_2D_3$ nor 24,25-$(OH)_2D_3$ regulates mRNA levels for either enzyme, nor is activity of either enzyme altered. Moreover, studies using specific activators and inhibitors of Cox-1 and Cox-2 demonstrated that the isoform that is sensitive to the vitamin D metabolites is Cox-1 since only when Cox-1 is inhibited or stimulated is PKC affected. Thus, the rate-limiting step is the production of substrate via the action of the vitamin D metabolites on PLA_2.

Role of Phospholipase C and Phospholipase D. $PKC\alpha$ is regulated by a number of factors that are also sensitive to 1,25-$(OH)_2D_3$ and 24,25-$(OH)_2D_3$ in a cell maturation-specific manner. 1,25-$(OH)_2D_3$ causes translocation of existing $PKC\alpha$ to the plasma membrane of GC cells (26), accounting for some of the increase in plasma membrane activity. There is a rapid change in Ca^{++} flux in response to 1,25-$(OH)_2D_3$ (27) that may also play a role since $PKC\alpha$ is Ca^{++} sensitive. Inositol 1,4,5 tris-phosphate production is increased (26), as is the production of diacylglycerol (DAG). The enzyme responsible for the increase in DAG is phosphatidylinositol-specific phospholipase C (PI-PLC) (26).

The situation in RC cells is very different. Ca^{++} flux is also altered by 24,25-$(OH)_2D_3$, but in a manner that is opposite to that of the effect of 1,25-$(OH)_2D_3$ on GC cells. 24,25-$(OH)_2D_3$ has no effect on IP3 production, but DAG is increased. The mechanism involved in DAG production is not via either PI-PLC or via phosphatidylcholine-specific PLC. DAG can also be produced by the action of phospholipase D (PLD) on phosphatidylcholine. To test if this was the case in response to 24,25-$(OH)_2D_3$, we first determined whether the growth plate chondrocytes expressed PLD. Both RC and GC cells express mRNAs for PLD1 and PLD2 and have PLD activity (unpublished data). However, levels are 5-fold higher in RC cells. 24,25-$(OH)_2D_3$ activated PLD2 in RC cells and had no effect on PLD in GC cells. This effect was receptor-mediated, since 24R,25-$(OH)_2D_3$, but not 24S,25-$(OH)_2D_3$, elicited the effect. 1,25-$(OH)_2D_3$ had no effect on PLD in either cell type.

Differential Mechanisms of 1,25-$(OH)_2D_3$ and 24,25-$(OH)_2D_3$ Action. These studies clearly demonstrate that 1,25-$(OH)_2D_3$ and 24,25-$(OH)_2D_3$ exert their effects in a cell maturation-dependent manner in growth plate chondrocytes, suggesting that cell maturation may be a determinant in the sensitivity of other cell types to these metabolites as well. The differences in response, shown in Figure 4, result from phenotypic differences in the two cell maturation states, including the numbers of membrane receptors for each metabolite, the phospholipid composition of the membranes, and the activity of enzymes involved in the production of co-factors needed for activity.

688

Arachidonic Acid + 24,25

PKC in RC Plasma Membranes

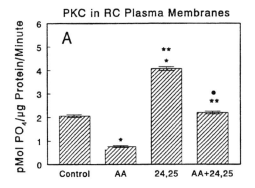

Arachidonic Acid + 24,25

PKC in RC Matrix vesicles

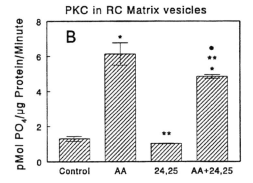

Mechanism of Action of $1\alpha,25\text{-(OH)}_2D_3$ in Growth Zone Chondrocytes

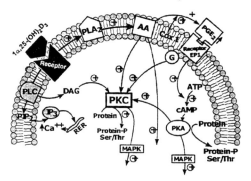

Mechanism of Action of $24R,25\text{-(OH)}_2D_3$ in Resting Zone Chondrocytes

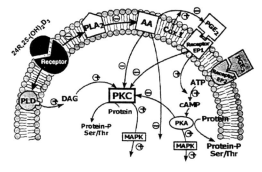

○ Different between RC /24R, 25 from GC /1α, 25

Figure 3: Regulation of PKC activity in RC plasma membranes and matrix vesicles treated with $24,25\text{-(OH)}_2D_3$ (24,25) or arachidonic acid (AA). RC plasma membranes (top panel) or matrix vesicles (lower panel) were treated for 90 mins. with vehicle, 100 μM AA, 10^{-7} M 24,25, or both mediators together and then assayed for PKC activity. Values are the mean ± S.E.M. for n = 6 membrane preparations; the experiment was repeated three times with nearly identical results. *P < 0.05, vs. control; **P < 0.05, vs. AA alone; *P < 0.05, vs. 24,25 or AA alone.

Figure 4: Schematic showing proposed mechanism of action for $1\alpha,25\text{-(OH)}_2D_3$ in growth zone chondrocytes (top panel) and $24R,25\text{-(OH)}_2D_3$ in resting zone chondrocytes (lower panel). Note that differences in the pathways activated by the two vitamin D metabolites are shaded

$1\alpha,25\text{-(OH)}_2D_3$ acts on its mVDR to increase PLC activity, resulting in increased production of IP3 and DAG, and movement of Ca^{++} from the rough endoplasmic reticulum to the cytoplasm of the cells. DAG directly activates PKC. PKC translocates to the plasma membrane. At the same time PLA_2 activity is increased, resulting in an increase in production of arachidonic acid. The increase in substrate results in an increase in prostaglandin production via the action of Cox-1. PGE_2 acts back on its EP-1 receptor to activate PKC through production of cAMP and activation of PKA. Both the PKC pathway and the PKA pathway converge at MAP kinase (28), resulting in phosphorylation of transcription factors and new gene expression.

24R,25-$(OH)_2D_3$ acts on its mVDR in RC cells to activate PLD, resulting in DAG production and activation of existing membrane PKC. At the same time, PLA_2 is inhibited, resulting in decreased production of arachidonic acid and, therefore, a decrease in substrate for Cox-1 action. Production of PGE_2 is decreased, reducing autocrine binding to the EP-1 and EP-2 receptors. This reduces PGE_2's inhibition of PKC. PGE_2 binding also activates PKA. The PKC and PKA pathways converge at MAP kinase, leading to new gene expression, including production of new PKC. As a result, 24,25-$(OH)_2D_3$ increases existing PKC within 3 minutes and has a delayed effect that is maximal at 90 minutes.

Acknowledgments. We would like to thank Sandra Messier for her help in the preparation of the manuscript. We also thank our students, fellows and collaborators that made this research possible. Particular acknowledgements are due to Drs. Ilka Nemere, Gary Posner, and Tony Norman. This research was supported by US PHS grants DE-05937 and DE-08603 and the Center for the Enhancement of the Biology/Biomaterials Interface.

References

1. Sylvia, V.L., Schwartz, Z., Schuman, L., Morgan, R.T., Mackey, S., Gomez, R., and Boyan, B.D. (1993) *J. Cell. Physiol.* **157**, 271-278

2. Posner, G.H., Nelson, T.D., Guyton, K.Z., and Kensler, T.W. (1992) *J. Med. Chem.* **35**, 3280-3287

3. Posner, G.H., Lee, J.K., White, M.C., Hutchings, R.H., Dai, H., Kachinski, J.C., Dolan, D., and Kensler, T.W. (1997) *J. Org. Chem.* **62**, 3299-3314

4. Pedrozo, H.A., Schwartz, Z., Rimes, S., Sylvia, V.L., Nemere, I., Posner, G.H., Dean, D.D., and Boyan, B.D. (1999) *J. Bone Miner. Res.* **14**, 856-867

5. Schwartz, Z., Sylvia, V.L., Del Toro, F., Hardin, R.R., Dean, D.D., and Boyan, B.D. (2000) *J. Cell. Physiol.* **182**, 390-401

6. Sylvia, V.L., Schwartz, Z., Ellis, E.B., Helm, S.H., Gomez, R., Dean, D.D., and Boyan, B.D. (1996) *J. Cell. Physiol.* **167**, 380-393

7. Greising, D.M., Boyan, B.D., Posner, G.H., Campos, J., Sylvia, V.L., Dean, D.D., and Schwartz, Z. (1996) *J. Dent. Res.* **75**, 351

8. Nemere, I., Dormanen, M.C., Hammond, M.W., Okamura, W.H., and Norman, A.W. (1994) *J. Biol. Chem.* **269**, 23750-23756

9. Nemere, I., Ray, R., and Jia, Z. (1996) *J. Bone Miner. Res.* **11**, S312

10. Nemere, I., Schwartz, Z., Pedrozo, H., Sylvia, V.L., Dean, D.D., and Boyan, B.D. (1998) *J. Bone Miner. Res.* **13**, 1353-1359

690

11. Schwartz, Z., Brooks, B.P., Swain, L.D., Del Toro, F., Norman, A.W., and Boyan, B.D. (1992) *Endocrinology* **130**, 2495-2504

12. Schwartz, Z. and Boyan, B.D. (1988) *Endocrinology* **122**, 2191-2198

13. Schwartz, Z., Schlader, D.L., Swain, L.D., and Boyan, B.D. (1988) *Endocrinology* **123**, 2878-2884

14. Swain, L.D., Schwartz, Z., and Boyan, B.D. (1992) *Biochim. Biophys. Acta* **1136**, 45-51

15. Boyan, B.D., Schwartz, Z., Swain, L.D., Carnes, D.L., Jr., and Zislis, T. (1988) *Bone* **9**, 185-194

16. Schwartz, Z., Swain, L.D., Ramirez, V., and Boyan, B.D. (1990) *Biochim. Biophys. Acta* **1027**, 278-286

17. Rasmussen, H., Matsumoto, T., Fontaine, O., and Goodman, D.B. (1982) *Fed. Proc.* **41**, 72-77

18. Matsumoto, T., Fontaine, O., and Rasmussen, H. (1981) *J. Biol. Chem.* **256**, 3354-3360

19. Swain, L.D., Schwartz, Z., Caulfield, K., Brooks, B.P., and Boyan, B.D. (1993) *Bone* **14**, 609-617

20. Boyan, B.D., Schwartz, Z., Carnes, D.L., Jr., and Ramirez, V. (1988) *Endocrinology* **122**, 2851-2860

21. Boyan, B.D., Sylvia, V.L., Curry, D., Chang, Z., Dean, D.D., and Schwartz, Z. (1998) *J. Cell. Physiol.* **176**, 516-524

22. Schwartz, Z., Sylvia, V.L., Curry, D., Luna, M., Dean, D.D., and Boyan, B.D. (1999) *Endocrinology* **140**, 2991-3002

23. Boyan, B.D., Sylvia, V.L., Dean, D.D., Pedrozo, H., Del Toro, F., Nemere, I., Posner, G.H., and Schwartz, Z. (1999) *Steroids* **64**, 129-136

24. Schwartz, Z., Swain, L.D., Kelly, D.W., Brooks, B.P., and Boyan, B.D. (1992) *Bone* **13**, 395-401

25. Del Toro, F., Jr., Sylvia, V.L., Schubkegel, S.R., Campos, R., Dean, D.D., Boyan, B.D., and Schwartz, Z. (2000) *J. Cell. Physiol.* **182**, 196-208

26. Sylvia, V.L., Schwartz, Z., Curry, D.B., Chang, Z., Dean, D.D., and Boyan, B.D. (1998) *J. Bone Miner. Res.* **13**, 559-569

27. Langston, G.G., Swain, L.D., Schwartz, Z., Del Toro, F., Gomez, R., and Boyan, B.D. (1990) *Calcif. Tissue Int.* **47**, 230-236

28. Cobb, M.H. (1999) *Prog. Biophys. Molec. Biol.* **71**, 479-500

1α,25(OH)$_2$-vitamin D$_3$ mediated
rapid and genomic responses in NB4 cells:
Evidence for cross-talk from rapid responses to genomic effects

Anthony W. Norman[1], Xin-De Song[1], June E. Bishop[1], William H. Okamura[2], and
Seiichi Ishizuka[3]

Departments of Biochemistry[1] & Chemistry[2], University of California, Riverside, CA
92521 and Department of Bone and Calcium Metabolism[3], Teijin Institute for
Bio-Medical Research, 4-3-2 Asahigaoka, Hino, Tokyo 191-8512, Japan.

1α,25(OH)$_2$-Vitamin D$_3$ [1α,25(OH)$_2$D$_3$] is the major hormonally active product of the vitamin D endocrine system (1). This seco steroid is able to generate biological effects both by genomic and rapid, nongenomic mechanisms. The genomic effects, which have been studied in great detail by many laboratories, are dependent upon the interaction of 1α,25(OH)$_2$D$_3$ with a cytosolic/nuclear receptor protein [VDR$_{nuc}$] followed by interaction of the steroid receptor complex in the nucleus with selective regions of the promoter of genes which are either to be activated or repressed (2). The stimulation of rapid responses by 1α,25(OH)$_2$D$_3$ has been postulated to result as the consequence of interaction of the ligand with a putative cell membrane receptor [VDR$_{mem}$] for 1α,25(OH)$_2$D$_3$ (3) so as to activate a variety of signal transduction systems that include the following: G-protein coupled activation of protein kinase C, phospholipase C, opening of Ca^{2+} or Cl$^-$ channels, adenyl cyclase, increases in intracellular [Ca^{2+}], and activation of both the Raf and MAP-kinase pathways; reviewed in (4;5).

One of the hallmarks of 1α,25(OH)$_2$D$_3$ as a steroid hormone is that it is conformationally flexible and is capable of generating a wide array of shapes (Fig. 1). This has apparently, over evolutionary time, allowed generation of more than one general type of receptor which can selectively bind different shapes of 1α,25(OH)$_2$D$_3$ as a ligand (6). Our laboratory has conducted structure-function studies utilizing a wide variety of analogs of 1α,25(OH)$_2$D$_3$ which are locked in a variety of conformational shapes (7). We have presented evidence that the preferred shape for the VDR$_{mem}$, which is linked to rapid responses, is that represented by the 6-s-*cis* locked planar 1α,25(OH)$_2$-lumisterol (JN; see Fig. 2). Further, as a consequence of developing a molecular model of the ligand binding domain (LBD) of the VDR$_{nuc}$ (8), and the recent publication of the x-ray crystal structure of the VDR$_{nuc}$-LBD (9), it is now established that the preferred agonist shape of VDR$_{nuc}$ is that represented by a twisted 6-s-*trans* bowl shape (see Fig. 1). Thus, the VDR$_{nuc}$ and VDR$_{mem}$, indeed, utilize different shapes of 1α,25(OH)$_2$D$_3$ as their preferred ligands.

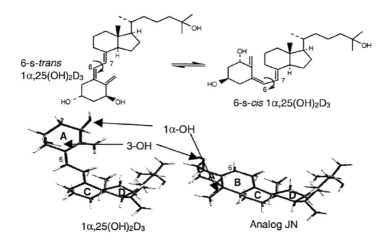

Figure 1:   Preferred conformation of the agonist ligands for the VDR$_{mem}$ (rapid responses) and the VDR$_{nuc}$ (genomic responses).   As shown in the top row, 1α,25(OH)$_2$D$_3$ can rotate 360° about the single 6,7 carbon bond to generate a multitude of different shapes; in the limit, the 6-s-*trans* and 6-s-*cis* conformers are generated. The bottom row emphasizes the difference in ligand shape for the VDR$_{nuc}$ (twisted 6-s-*trans*) versus that for the VDR$_{mem}$ (6-s-*cis*).

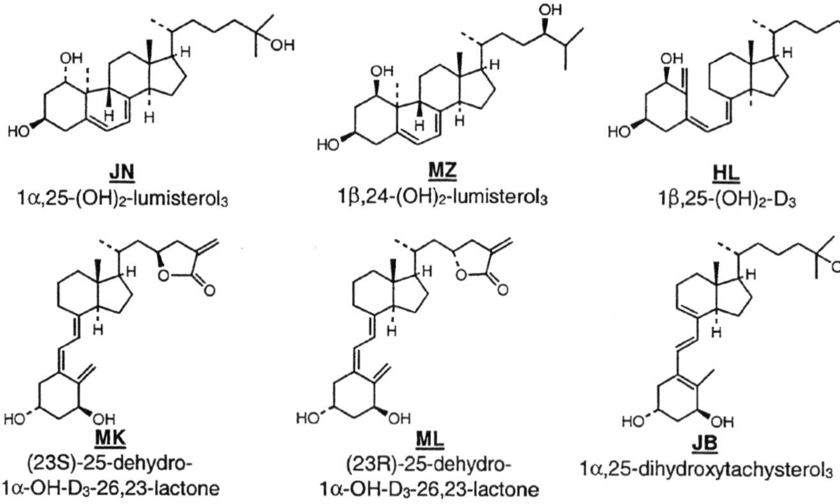

JN
1α,25-(OH)$_2$-lumisterol$_3$

MZ
1β,24-(OH)$_2$-lumisterol$_3$

HL
1β,25-(OH)$_2$-D$_3$

MK
(23S)-25-dehydro-
1α-OH-D$_3$-26,23-lactone

ML
(23R)-25-dehydro-
1α-OH-D$_3$-26,23-lactone

JB
1α,25-dihydroxytachysterol$_3$

Figure 2:   Structures of analogs of 1α,25(OH)$_2$D$_3$ utilized in the research described in this report. The structure of 1α,25(OH)$_2$D$_3$ is presented in the top row of Fig. 1. **JN** [1α,25(OH)$_2$-lumisterol] and **MZ** [1β,24R(OH)$_2$-lumisterol] are both 6-s-*cis* locked analogs; **JN** is an agonist of rapid responses. Both **HL** [1β,25(OH)$_2$D$_3$] and **MZ** are antagonists of rapid responses. **MK**, also known as TEI-9647 [(23S)-25-dehydro-1α-OH-vitamin D$_3$-26,23-lactone] and **ML** also known as TEI-9648 [(23R)-25-dehydro-1α-OH-vitamin D$_3$-26,23-lactone] are both antagonists of VDR$_{nuc}$-mediated genomic responses. **JB** [1α,25(OH)-dihydrotachysterol$_3$] is a 6-s-*trans* locked analog that is neither an agonist nor antagonist for either the VDR$_{nuc}$ or VDR$_{mem}$.

One interesting possibility concerning rapid responses is that one aspect of their activation by the conformationally flexible $1\alpha,25(OH)_2D_3$ is their cross-talk with the nucleus so as to modulate VDR_{nuc}-mediated genomic responses. Both PKC and MAP-kinase are present in the human promyelocytic leukemia NB4 cells and have been implicated in the process of cell differentiation stimulated by $1\alpha,25(OH)_2D_3$ (10;11). This communication reports our recent studies in NB4 cells where we have utilized 6-s-*cis* locked analogs as a tool to study cross-talk between rapid responses and nuclear response signal transduction pathways.

Figure 3 contrasts the responses of human promyelocytic NB4 cells with those of the HL-60 human promyelocytic cells to $1\alpha,25(OH)_2D_3$ to various antagonists of

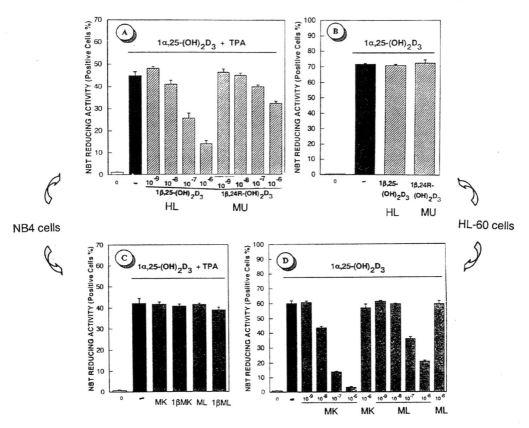

NB4 cells

HL-60 cells

Figure 3: Comparison of the effects of antagonists of rapid responses and genomic responses on $1\alpha,25(OH)_2D_3$ induced cell differentiation in NB4 cells and HL-60 cells. (A) NB4 cells (10^5 cells/ml) were exposed to $1\alpha,25(OH)_2D_3$, 10^{-8} M, **HL** 10^{-8} M, or **MU**, 10^{-8} M, for 8 hrs. The cells were washed and TPA, 2×10^{-9} M, was added for the next 64 hrs. (B) HL-60 cells, (10^5 cells/ml), were exposed to $1\alpha,25(OH)_2D_3$, 10^{-8} M, $\pm$ **HL**, 10^{-8} M, or **MU**, 10^{-8} M, for 72 hrs. The resulting extent of cell differentiation, as judged by NBT-reducing activity, was determined as described by (16). The protocol for the results shown in panels C and D were as described for panels A and B respectively.

the VDR$_{nuc}$ and VDR$_{mem}$. HL-60 cells have been shown to be a good system to study the genomic cell differentiation actions 1α,25(OH)$_2$D$_3$ that convert these cells to macrophages (12). In contrast, NB4 cells are an *in vitro* model for study of the rapid membrane actions of 1α,25(OH)$_2$D$_3$ or 6-s-*cis* locked analogs (13) which contribute to their differentiation into macrophages. 1α,25(OH)$_2$D$_3$ is required during the first 8 hours priming phase of NB4 cell differentiation and tyrosine phosphorylation was reported to be involved in this priming phase process (13-15). In NB4 cells, the cell differentiation responses of 1α,25(OH)$_2$D$_3$ are blocked by the rapid response antagonist 1ß,25(OH)$_2$D$_3$ (HL), but not by the VDR$_{nuc}$ antagonists MK, whereas in HL-60 cells the reverse is this case; see also (16). Thus, cell differentiation of NB4 cells is dependent on activation of a first phase rapid response signal transduction event that is subsequently required for the traditional cell differentiation genomic response(s).

Figure 4 presents a summary of our previous results indicating that MAP-kinase phosphorylation can be regulated in NB4 cells by 1α,25(OH)$_2$D$_3$ (17). MAP-kinase belongs to the family of serine/threonine protein kinases and can be activated by phosphorylation on a tyrosine residue induced by mitogens or cytodifferentiating agents (18). MAP-kinase activation integrates multiple intracellular signals transmitted by various second messengers and regulates many

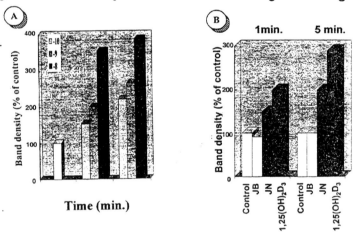

Figure 4:   Dose- and time-dependent effects of 1α,25(OH)$_2$D$_3$ (panel A), and 6-s-*cis* locked analog **JN** and 6-s-*trans* locked **JB** (panel B) on the phosphorylation of MAP-kinase in NB4 acute promyelocytic leukemia cells. This data was abstracted from (17). In panel B the NB4 cells were treated with the indicated analog at 10^{-8} M for 1 and 5 minutes at 37^0 C. Vehicle and 1α,25(OH)$_2$D$_3$ at 10^{-8} M were used as negative and positive controls. The cells were collected after 1 and 5 minutes. The MAP-kinase phosphorylation was assayed as described in (17).

cellular functions by phosphorylation of numbers of cytoplasm kinases and nuclear transcription factors including the EGF receptor, c-Myc and c-Jun (19;20). These rapid actions of 1α,25(OH)$_2$D$_3$ have been postulated to regulate cell biological function and potentially to interact with other membrane-mediated kinase cascades or to cross-talk with the cell nucleus to control genomic responses associated with cell differentiation and proliferation (21). Panel 4A reports the $1\alpha,25(OH)_2D_3$ time- and dose-dependent effects on MAP-kinase activation, while panel 3B compares the effects of the 6-s-*cis* locked JN and the 6-s-*trans* locked JB in relation to the conformationally flexible $1\alpha,25(OH)_2D_3$. Only $1\alpha,25(OH)_2D_3$ and JN, but not JB, were able to activate the MAP-kinase. This was the first report that MAP-kinase phosphorylation can be related to rapid membrane effect(s) of $1\alpha,25(OH)_2D_3$ (17;21).

One of the hallmarks of cell differentiation of NB4 cells is the slow appearance of alkaline phosphatase (22). Induction of alkaline phosphatase is known to be dependent upon the presence of the VDR_{nuc} and its ligand $1\alpha,25(OH)_2D_3$ (23;24). Figure 5 documents the ability of the 6-s-*cis* locked JN [$1\alpha,25(OH)_2$-lumisterol] with Bryostatin present after 8 hrs to stimulate in NB4 cells the appearance over 72 hrs of a 3500% increase in alkaline phosphatase activity. Further, the actions of three antagonists on the JN stimulation of alkaline phosphatase are presented. While the VDR_{nuc} antagonist MK was without any significant effect, the rapid response inhibitor, HL, mediated a dose-dependent inhibition of alkaline phosphatase induction. Intriguingly, the presence of the MAP-kinase activation inhibitor, PD-98059 (25), also achieved an effective and significant inhibition of the induction of alkaline phosphatase. Our results substantiate the suggestion that in NB4 cells, the 6-s-*cis* shaped agonist ligands for the VDR_{mem} are able to modulate genomic events, such as the induction of alkaline phosphatase. Further, the inhibition by PD-98059 suggests that MAP-kinase activation results in second messengers that achieve cross-talk with nuclear genomic events.

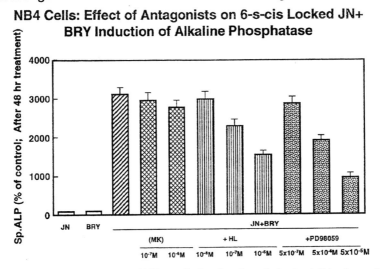

Figure 5: Stimulation of NB4 cells by the 6-s-*cis* locked JN, via rapid response initiated signal transduction pathways, of the genomic response of induction of alkaline phosphatase. NB4 cells (10^5 cells/ml) were exposed to JN, 10^{-8} M $\pm$ MK, HL, or PD-98059, followed by the addition at 8 hrs of Bryostatin, 7.5×10^{-9} M, for a total of 72 hrs. Alkaline phosphatase, as a measure of a genomic response, was determined as described by (22).

A further test of the cross-talk hypothesis is presented in Fig. 6 where it is shown that $1\alpha,25(OH)_2D_3$ + TPA can achieve transactivation of the $25(OH)D_3$-24-hydroxylase promoter that has been transfected into NB4 cells. Again, the MAP-kinase activation inhibitor, PD-98059 (25), achieved a significant reduction in the transactivation of the 24-hydroxylase gene.

NB4 Cells: PD98059 Inhibits $1\alpha,25(OH)_2D_3$ Activation of Transfected $25(OH)D$-24-hydroxylase Reporter

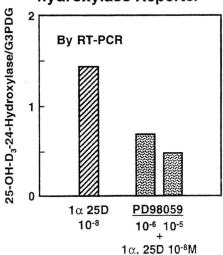

Figure 6: $25(OH)D_3$-24-hydroxylase gene expression induction by $1\alpha,25(OH)_2D_3$ in NB4 cells and its inhibition by the MAP-kinase activation inhibitor, PD-98059. The $25(OH)D_3$-24-hydroxylase promoter was transfected into NB4 cells. After 24 hrs the cells were then exposed to $1\alpha,25(OH)_2D_3$, 10^{-8} M, $\pm$ PD-98059 for 24 hrs. The total RNA was isolated and the amount of the $25(OH)D_3$-24-hydroxylase and G3PDH mRNA determined via quantitative reverse transcriptase-PCR (RT-PCR) as described in (28). The PCR products were analyzed by 2% agarose gel electrophoresis, followed by densitometry.

Figure 7 presents a schematic model summarizing in NB4 cells our current understanding of the signal transduction processes by which $1\alpha,25(OH)_2D_3$ mediated rapid responses can, under appropriate circumstances, engage in cross-talk so as to modulate selected genomic responses. It is well established that the MAP-kinase pathway sequentially links cell surface receptor mediated signals to the nucleus and regulates the expression of selected genes by phosphorylation of nuclear transcription factors (20;26). In this report and elsewhere, we have shown that $1\alpha,25(OH)_2D_3$ or the 6-s-*cis* locked JN can stimulate the genomic responses of cell differentiation, induction of alkaline phosphatase and transactivation of a transfected promoter bearing a VDRE response element. Since the MAP-kinase activation inhibitor, PD-98059, diminished all three of these genomic responses, this suggests that the MAP-kinase signaling pathway, under appropriate circumstances, can, via cross-talk, modulate genomic events. It is not yet known what are the targets of the MAP-kinase species engaging in cross-talk with the nucleus. One possible target might be the VDR_{nuc} which is known to have a number of phosphorylation sites (27). Alternatively, other transcription factors may be phosphorylated as a consequence of 6-s-*cis* activation of the MAP-kinase pathway. These possibilities are currently under investigation.

$1\alpha,25(OH)_2D_3$ and SIGNAL TRANSDUCTION IN NB4 CELLS: RAPID RESPONSE "CROSS-TALK" WITH GENOMIC RESPONSES

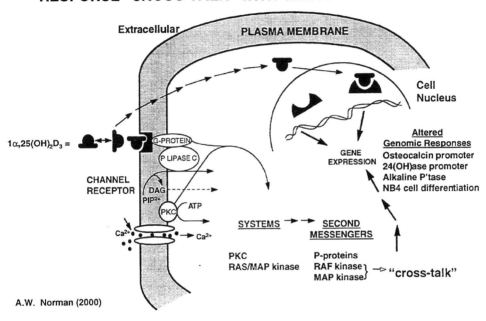

A.W. Norman (2000)

Figure 7: $1\alpha,25(OH)_2D_3$-mediated signal transduction in NB4 cells. $1\alpha,25(OH)_2D_3$ can initiate biological responses via both its nuclear receptor and a putative cell membrane receptor which generates rapidly the appearance of selected second messengers, including PKC, phospho-proteins, and activated MAP-kinase, that in NB4 cells can act via "cross-talk" to the nucleus so as to modulate selected genomic events.

A key aspect of this model is that $1\alpha,25(OH)_2D_3$ as a conformationally flexible hormone is capable of generating a wide array shapes. This has apparently over evolutionary time allowed the generation of more than one general type of receptor [VDR_{nuc} and VDR_{mem}] which can bind $1\alpha,25(OH)_2D_3$ as a ligand.   It remains to the future to define further details of this model and to identify what are the cellular circumstances that can invoke cross-talk from the VDR_{mem} receptor to the VDR_{nuc} receptor.

698

References

1. Bouillon, R., Okamura, W.H., and Norman, A.W. (1995) Endocr. Rev. 16, 200-257.
2. Haussler, M.R., Whitfield, G.K., Haussler, C.A., Hsieh, J.C., Thompson, P.D., Selznick, S.H., Dominguez, C.E., and Jurutka, P.W. (1998) J. Bone Miner. Res. 13, 325-349.
3. Nemere, I., Dormanen, M.C., Hammond, M.W., Okamura, W.H., and Norman, A.W. (1994) J. Biol. Chem. 269, 23750-23756.
4. Norman, A.W. (1997) in: Vitamin D (Feldman, D., Glorieux, F.H., and Pike, J.W., Eds.), pp. 233-256 Academic Press, San Diego, CA.
5. Norman, A.W., Song, X-D., Zanello, L.P., Bula, C.M., and Okamura, W.H. (1999) Steriods 64 , 120-128.
6. Norman, A.W. (1998) J. Bone Miner. Res. 13, 1360-1369.
7. Norman, A.W., Okamura, W.H., Hammond, M.W., Bishop, J.E., Dormanen, M.C., Bouillon, R., Van Baelen, H., Ridal, A.L., Daane, E., Khoury, R., and Farach-Carson, M.C. (1997) Molecular Endocrinology 11, 1518-1531.
8. Norman, A.W., Adams, D., Collins, E.D., Okamura, W.H., and Fletterick, R.J. (1999) J.Cell Biochem. 74, 323-333.
9. Rochel, N., Wurtz, J.M., Mitschler, A., Klahholz, B., and Moras, D. (2000) Molecular Cell 5, 173-179.
10. Berry, D.M., Antochi, R., Bhatia, M., and Meckling-Gill, K.A. (1996) J. Biol. Chem. 271, 16090-16096.
11. Kraft, A.S., Baker, V.V., and May, W.S. (1987) Oncogene 1, 111-118.
12. Mangelsdorf, D.J., Koeffler, H.P., Donaldson, C.A., Pike, J.W., and Haussler, M.R. (1984) J. Cell. Biol. 98, 391-398.
13. Bhatia, M., Kirkland, J.B., and Meckling-Gill, K.A. (1995) J. Biol. Chem. 270, 15962-15965.
14. Bhatia, M., Kirkland, J.B., and Meckling-Gill, K.A. (1996) Exp. Cell Res. 222, 61-69.
15. Berry, D.M. and Meckling-Gill, K.A. (1999) Endocrinology 140, 4779-4788.
16. Miura, D., Manabe, K., Gao, Q., Norman, A.W., and Ishizuka, S. (1999) FEBS Lett. 460, 297-302.
17. Song, X., Bishop, .E., Okamura, W.H., and Norman, A.W. (1998) Endocrinology 139, 457-465.
18. Pelech, S.L. and Sanghera, J.S. (1992) Trends Biochem Sci 17, 233-238.
19. Elion, E.A. (1998) Science 281, 1625-1626.
20. Roberts, J.R., Nelson, B., Marton, M.J., Stoughton, R., Meyer, M.R., Bennett, H.A., He, Y.D., Dai, H., Walker, W.L., Hughes, T.R., Tyers, M., Boone, C., and Friend, S.H. (2000) Science 287, 873-880.
21. Norman, A.W., Zanello, L.P., Song, X-D., de Boland, A.R., Farach-Carson, M.C., Bouillon, R., and Okamura, W.H. (1997) in: Vitamin D: Chemistry, Biology and Clinical Applications of the Steroid Hormone (Norman, A.W., Bouillon, R., and Thomasset, M., Eds.), p. 331-338, University of California, Riverside, Riverside, CA.
22. Song, X-D. and Norman, A.W. (1998) Leuk. Res. 22, 69-76.
23. Kyeyune-Nyombi, E., Lau, K.-H.W., Baylink, D.J., and Strong, D.D. (1991) Arch. Biochem. Biophys. 291, 316-325.
24. Kyeyune-Nyombi, E., Lau, K.-H.W., Baylink, D.J., and Strong, D.D. (1989) Arch. Biochem. Biophys. 275, 363-370.
25. Pang, L., Sawada, T., Decker, S.J., and Saltiel, A.R. (1995) J. Biol. Chem. 270, 13585-13588.
26. Gniadecki, R., Gajkowska, B., and Hansen, M. (1997) Endocrinology 138, 2241-2248.
27. Jurutka, P.W., Hsieh, J.-C., and Haussler, M.R. (1993) Biochem. Biophys. Res. Commun. 191 , 1089-1096.
28. Miura, D., Manabe, K., Ozono, K., Saito, M., Gao, Q., Norman, A.W., and Ishizuka, S. (1999) J. Biol. Chem. 274, 16392-16399.

1,25-DIHYDROXYVITAMIN D₃ STIMULATES PHOSPHORYLATION OF IκBα AND PROMOTES ITS DEGRADATION TO RELEASE THE TRANSCRIPTION FACTOR NFκB, DURING MONOCYTIC DIFFERENTIATION OF NB4 LEUKEMIA CELLS

Christina S. Clark, Donna Berry and Kelly A. Meckling-Gill, Department of Human Biology and Nutritional Science, University of Guelph, Guelph, ON Canada N1G 2W1

Introduction Nuclear factor κB (NFκB) is a family of transcription factors expressed in a wide variety of cell types (1). The NFκB transcription factor is a known regulator of immune and inflammatory responses, apoptosis and cell differentiation (1). Known gene targets of NFκB include cytokines and their receptors, cell adhesion molecules, inducible nitric oxide synthase (iNOS), growth regulatory factors and other transcription factors (1). Extracellular stimuli capable of activating the NFκB pathway include TNF-α, IL-1, phorbol esters, UV radiation, viral DNA and lipopolysaccharide (2).

NFκB is kept inactive in the cytoplasm by inhibitory factor kappa B (IκB) proteins (3). Degradation of IκB requires phosphorylation of two specific serine residues (S32 and S36 in IκBα) (4). Phosphorylation targets IκB for ubiquitination and degradation by the 26S proteasome (5, 6). IκB degradation releases NFκB, allowing it to translocate to the nucleus and activate transcription of specific target genes.

IκB phosphorylation was shown to be necessary, but not sufficient for, nuclear translocation of NFκB (7). Recently, the kinase responsible for phosphorylating IκB, the IκB kinase (IKK) signalsome, was identified (6, 8). Although the specific kinase responsible for activating IKK has not yet been elucidated, upstream activators of IKK, including mitogen-activated protein kinase kinase kinase 1 (MEKK-1) and NFκB inducing kinase (NIK) have been implicated (9, 8).

The role of the NFκB signaling pathway in cell differentiation is poorly defined. Rearrangements and amplifications of NFκB and IκB genes have been reported in many types of cancer and leukemia (10). Increases in NFκB expression and DNA binding activity have been demonstrated during monocyte/macrophage maturation of other cells lines (11, 12). Inhibition of NFκB using anti-sense oligonucleotides was shown to enhance monocytic differentiation in the HL-60 myeloblastic leukemia cell line (13). Our laboratory has previously shown that NB4 cells, the most appropriate model for studying acute promyelocytic leukemia *in vitro*, differ from HL-60 cells in their response to agents which induce monocytic differentiation (14-16). Previous findings from our laboratory have shown that 1α,25-dihydroxyvitamin D₃ (1α,25-(OH)₂D₃ primes cells for monocytic differentiation in response to the phorbol ester 12-O-tetradecanoyl-13-phorbol-acetate (TPA) through non-genomic signaling pathways (14-17).

Berry et al found that $1\alpha,25$-$(OH)_2D_3$ together with TPA lead to a reduction in $I\kappa B\alpha$ expression and increased NFκB nuclear localization in NB4 cells after a 12 hour treatment (unpublished). In addition, they showed that $1\alpha,25$-$(OH)_2D_3$ alone or in combination with TPA induces rapid phosphorylation of serine residue(s). Non-genomic signaling, cytosolic calcium and calpain activity were also shown to be required for NFκB activation. In this report, we have focussed on identifying signaling molecules in the NFκB pathway involved in $1\alpha,25$-$(OH)_2D_3$-mediated phosphorylation of $I\kappa B\alpha$ in NB4 cells.

Results

A detailed time course of $1\alpha,25$-$(OH)_2D_3$ action was carried out to determine if $1\alpha,25$-$(OH)_2D_3$ affects $I\kappa B\alpha$ expression at times earlier than 12 hours. NB4 cells were treated with 200 nM $1\alpha,25$-$(OH)_2D_3$ or vehicle (ethanol) for 10 min, 30 min, 1 h, 2 h, 4 h, 8 h and 12 h. Whole cell lysates were prepared in PBS + Complete™ protease inhibitors (Boehringer Mannheim) and phosphatase inhibitors (100 µM sodium orthovanadate and 2 mM sodium fluoride). Cells were resuspended in SDS buffer, sonicated and boiled for 5 min before electrophoresis on 12% acrylamide gels. Proteins were transferred to nitrocellulose membranes and probed with either an anti-$I\kappa B\alpha$ antibody (0.025 µg/mL; Santa Cruz) or a phospho-specific $I\kappa B\alpha$ antibody (1:2,500; New England Biolabs). Polypeptides were detected using the ECL kit (Amersham-Pharmacia) and quantified by autoradiography and densitometry.

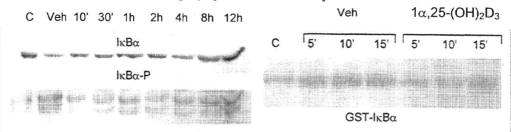

Figure 1: NB4 cells treated with 200 nM $1\alpha,25$-$(OH)_2D_3$ show no change in $I\kappa B\alpha$ expression over a 12 h time course (upper). A more slowly migrating $I\kappa B\alpha$ species appears at later time points, as shown with a phospho-specific IkBa antibody (lower).

Figure 2: Stimulation with 200 nM $1\alpha,25$-$(OH)_2D_3$ does not change IKK kinase activity compared with vehicle-treated samples, as determined by a $^{\gamma-32}P$ kinase assay using a full-length GST-$I\kappa B\alpha$ (1-317) fusion protein as substrate.

As shown in <u>Figure 1</u> (upper panel) the expression of IκBα in NB4 cells treated with 1α,25-(OH)$_2$D$_3$ does not significantly change over a 12 h treatment. However, a shift in IκBα mobility to a slower migrating species appeared at later time points. This slowly migrating form of IκBα was shown to be phosphorylated IκBα, as shown in the lower panel of <u>Figure 1</u>.

To determine if the IKK signalsome is responsible for the rapid phosphorylation of IκBα following 1α,25-(OH)$_2$D$_3$ stimulation, a $^{\gamma\text{-}32}$P kinase assay was performed using a full-length GST-fusion protein (1-317) (Santa Cruz) as substrate, following a method previously described (18). NB4 cells were incubated with vehicle (ethanol) or 200 nM 1α,25-(OH)$_2$D$_3$ for 5, 10 and 15 min, and collected for immunoprecipitation with an IKK-α antibody (Santa Cruz). Samples were analyzed by SDS-PAGE on 10% acrylamide gels. Autoradiography was performed (<u>Figure 2</u>). IKK kinase activity does not change following 1α,25-(OH)$_2$D$_3$ treatment compared to control or vehicle-treated samples.

Discussion

Studies have shown that phosphorylation of IκBα is necessary, but not sufficient for, degradation and release of NFκB (7). This regulated step in activation of the NFκB signaling pathway occurs rapidly and targets IκBα for subsequent degradation by the 26S proteasome or calpain (5, 6). Here we examined the early effects of 1α,25-(OH)$_2$D$_3$ on the expression of IκBα and the activity of the IKK signalsome. Treatment of NB4 cells with 1α,25-(OH)$_2$D$_3$ over a 12 h time course resulted in an apparent shift in IκBα mobility towards a more slowly migrating species. This mobility shift is consistent with a change in IκBα phosphorylation state (10) and was demonstrated here using a phospho-specific IκBα antibody.

Recently, the IKK signalsome was identified as the kinase responsible for phosphorylating IκBα in response to extracellular (9, 11). Berry et al reported a rapid phosphorylation of IκBα at serine residue(s) following stimulation with 1α,25-(OH)$_2$D$_3$ (unpublished). Here we studied IKK kinase activity to determine if this signalsome is responsible for 1α,25-(OH)$_2$D$_3$ -mediated IκBα phosphorylation. Our results show no change in IKK activity. This negative result could be due to an induced IKK activity that occurs earlier than at 5 min. Alternatively, the full-length GST-IκBα (1-317) fusion protein substrate may sterically hinder the kinase reaction. Other research groups have reported other problems using the full-length substrate (Ed Harhaj personal communication). Further studies using shorter substrates (1-55 and 1-54) will be performed. Mutant substrates in which the inducible phosphorylation sites (S32 and S36 in IκBα) have been replaced with either alanines or threonines will be used as control.

702

References

1. Verma, I.M., Stevenson, J.K., Schwarz, E.M., Van Antwerp, D. and Miyamoto, S. (1995) Genes and Dev. 9, 2723-2735.
2. Miyamoto, S. and Verma, I.M. (1995) Adv. Cancer Res. 66, 255-292.
3. Beg, A.A. and Baldwin Jr., A.S. (1993) Genes and Dev. 7, 2064-2070.
4. DiDonato, J. Mercurio, F., Rosette, C., Wu-Li, J., Suyang, H., Ghoshi, S. and Karin, M. (1996) Mol. Cell. Biol. 16, 1295-1304.
5. Li, J., Peet, G.W., Pullen, S.S., Schembri-King, J., Warren, T.C., Marcu, K.B., Kehry, M.R., Barton, R. and Jakes, S. (1998) J. Biol. Chem. 273, 30736-30741.
6. DiDonato, J.A., Hayakawa, M., Rothwarf, D.M., Zandi, E. and Karin, M. (1997) Nature 388, 548-554.
7. DiDonato, J.A., Mercurio, F. and Karin, M. (1995) Mol. Cell. Biol. 15, 1302-1311.
8. Regnier, C.H., Yeoung Song, H., Gao, X., Goeddel, D.V., Cao, Z. and Rothe, M. (1997) Cell 90, 373-383.
9. Nakano, H., Masahisa, S., Sakon, S., Nishinaka, S., Mihara, M., Yagita, H. and Okumura, K. (1998) Proc. Natl. Acad. Sci. USA 95, 3537-3542.
10. Rayet, B. and Gelinas, C. (1999) Oncogene 18, 6938-6947.
11. Conti, L., Hiscott, J., Papacchini, M., Roulston, A., Wainberg, M.A., Belardelli, F. and Gessani, S. (1997) Cell. Growth. Diff. 8, 435-442.
12. Griffin, G.E., Leung, K., Folks, T.M., Kunkel, S. and Nabel, G.J. (1991) Res. Virol. 142, 233-238.
13. Sokoloski, J.A., Narayanan, R. and Sartorelli, A.C. (1998) Cancer Lett. 125, 157-164.
14. Bhatia, M., Kirkland, J.B. and Meckling-Gill, K.A. (1994) Leukemia 8, 1744-1749.
15. Bhatia, M., Kirkland, J.B. and Meckling-Gill, K.A. (1995) J. Biol. Chem. 270, 15962-15965.
16. Bhatia, M., Kirkland, J.B and Meckling-Gill, K.A. (1995) Biochem. J. 308, 131-137.
17. Berry, D.M. and Meckling-Gill, K.A. (1999) Endocrinology 140, 4779-4788.
18. Devalaraja, M., Wang, D.Z., Ballard, D.W. and Richmond, A. (1999) Cancer Res. 59, 1372-1377.

RAPID STIMULATION OF NON-RECEPTOR TYROSINE KINASE SRC IN MUSCLE CELLS BY 1,25(OH)$_2$-VITAMIN D$_3$ INVOLVES TYROSINE PHOSPHORYLATION OF THE VITAMIN D RECEPTOR (VDR) AND ITS ASSOCIATION TO SRC.

C. Buitrago, G. Vazquez, A. R. de Boland and R. L. Boland. Dpto de Biologia, Bioquímica y Farmacia, Universidad Nacional del Sur.
E-mail: rboland@criba.edu.ar.

INTRODUCTION

The steroid hormone 1α,25-dihydroxy-vitamin-D$_3$ [1α,25(OH)$_2$D$_3$] modulates calcium homeostasis in skeletal muscle cells by both a genomic action which elicits control of gene expression through interaction with a specific intracellular receptor (VDR: vitamin D receptor) (1), and a non-genomic mechanism implying direct membrane effects of the sterol mediated by a complex array of signalling systems (2, 3). Recent data indicates that tyrosine kinase phosphorylation of cellular proteins plays a key role in 1α,25(OH)$_2$D$_3$– dependent modulation of non-genomic responses, such as fast increases in cytosolic Ca^{2+} and mitogen-activated protein kinase (MAPK) stimulation (4). In the present study we investigated wether the cytosolic non-receptor tyrosine kinase Src is involved in 1α,25(OH)$_2$-vitamin D$_3$ signalling in these cells. Moreover, the existence of an association between VDR and Src was also evaluated.

METHODS

Undifferentiated, myogenic chick skeletal muscle cells (myoblasts) were isolated from the breast muscle of 13-day-old chick embryos essentially as described before (3), and cultured until confluence (4-6 days after plating). Immunoprecipitation of cell lysates were performed with either anti-Src, anti-phosphotyrosine or anti-VDR antibodies, followed by precipitation of the immunocomplexes with protein A-Sepharose. Co-immunoprecipitation assays were performed under native conditions in order to preserve protein-protein associations, and were conducted essentially as described (5). Src activity was assayed using $[\gamma^{32}\text{-P}]$ATP and enolase as Src substrate, essentially as described by Kapus et al. (6).

RESULTS AND DISCUSSION

Exposure of cultured myotubes to $1,25(OH)_2D_3$ caused a time-dependent increase in Src activity of cell lysate immunoprecipitates (Fig.1), which was evident at 1 min (1-fold) and reached a maximum at 5 min (15-fold). Immunoblotting with anti-phosphotyrosine antibody of immunoprecipitated Src showed that the hormone decreased Src tyrosine phosphorylation state with maximal effects at 5 min. Using a database for protein consensus motifs we found a putative tyrosine phosphorylation site (aminoacids 164-170: KTFDTTY) within the primary sequence of the chick VDR.

Fig.1 *Time course of 1,25(OH)₂D₃*
   -stimulation of Src kinase activity

Fig.2 *Tyrosine phosphorylation of VDR*

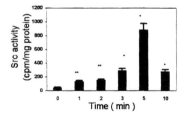

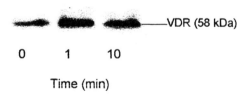

As shown in Fig. 2, when the myotube VDR was immunoprecipitated it appeared onto SDS-PAGE gels as a single band of 58 kDa recognized by an anti-phosphotyrosine antibody. Prior treatment of cells with $1,25(OH)_2D_3$ significantly increased tyrosine phosphorylation of the VDR (3-fold above basal levels). As only one consensus motif for tyrosine-phosphorylation was found within the avian VDR sequence, we hypothesize that the increased amount of cellular tyrosine-phosphorylated VDR observed upon 1,25-dihydroxyvitamin D_3 treatment occurs at the expense of an increase in the number of VDR molecules that become tyrosine-phosphorylated. Although a total of seven tyrosine residues exist within Gallus gallus VDR sequence, only one of them (Y170) fits the requirements of a consensus motif for tyrosine phosphorylation; however, the lack of consensus environment in the remaining six tyrosines does not allow us to rule out the possibility that, under the present conditions, more than one tyrosine residue becomes phosphorylated within a VDR molecule. In either case, the present finding represents the first evidence to

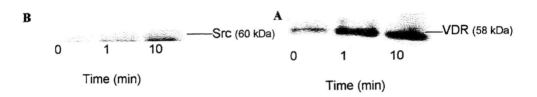

Fig. 3 *Association of VDR with the non-receptor tyrosine kinase Src.*

A)Muscle cells were exposed to 1 nM $1,25(OH)_2D_3$ or vehicle (ethanol<0.1%) for the indicated times. Cell lysates were obtained, VDR was immunoprecipitated with anti-VDR monoclonal antibody under native conditions, resolved onto 10% SDS-PAGE gels and then immunoblotted with anti-Src monoclonal antibody. **B)** As in panel A, but immunoprecipitation was performed with anti-Src monoclonal antibody and immunoblotting with the anti-VDR antibody.

date for tyrosine phosphorylation of the VDR. In agreement with Src being a SH2-domain containing protein involved in recognition of tyrosine-phosphorylated targets, by immunoprecipitating with anti-Src antibody under native conditions followed by blotting with anti-VDR it was found that the VDR co-precipitates with Src, thus indicating the existence of a VDR/Src complex (Fig.3). Similar results were obtained by using the antibodies in inverse order. Stimulation with the cognate VDR ligand significantly increased formation of the complex with respect to basal conditions.

These results altogether provide the first evidence to date for $1,25(OH)_2D_3$ stimulation of Src activity mediated by tyrosine phosphorylation of the VDR and its association to Src.

REFERENCES

1. Boland R, De Boland AR, Marinissen M, Santillan G, Vazquez G, Zanello S. (1995) Mol. Cell. Endocrinol. 114, 1-8.
2. De Boland AR, Boland R. (1994) Cell. Signal. 6, 717-724.
3. Morelli S, De Boland AR, Boland R. (1993) Biochem. J. 289, 675-679.
4. De Boland AR, Vazquez G, Morelli S, Boland R. (1998) First International Meeting on Rapid Responses to Steroid Hormones. Mannheim, Germany, p. 90
5. Xu XS, Li HS, Guggino S, Montell C. (1997) Cell 89, 1155-1164.
6. Kapus A, Szászi K, Sun J, Rizoli S, Rotstein OD. (1999) J. Biol. Chem. 274, 8093-8102.

IMMUNOLOCALIZATION OF MEMBRANE VITAMIN D RECEPTOR IN HUMAN TOOTH GERM.

M. Mesbah[1], P. Papagerakis[1], C. Teillaud[1], I. Nemere[2] and A. Berdal[1].
[1]Univ. Paris 7, EA 2380, Cordeliers Institute, Paris, France and [2]Utah State Univ., Dpt Nutrition and Food Sciences, Logan, Utah, USA.

Introduction Tooth morphogenesis and differentiation are controled by a cascade of epithelial-mesenchymal interactions. Differentiated dental cells secrete extracellular matrix proteins - ameloblasts for enamel and odontoblasts for dentin - (1) that provides a gel scaffold which supports apatitic crystal growth (2). Vitamin D regulates gene expression of proteins involved in the formation of mineralized tissues (3). Several of these proteins, jointly present in teeth and bone appear to be the target of $1,25(OH)_2$ vitamin D_3 in teeth (4). They may also coordinate the influx of calcium and phosphate ions required for growth of crystals (5) through the action of vitamin D-dependant calciprotein, calbindins (4) and alkaline phosphatase (6). The nuclear VDR has been shown to be expressed and functional in osteoblasts, odontoblasts and ameloblasts in rodents (4, 7) and humans (8). In addition, tooth- specific matrix proteins have been shown to be also controlled by $1,25(OH)_2$ vitamin D_3 in the ameloblasts (7). However, there exist some discrepancies between the large distribution of the vitamin D nuclear receptor and a cell-specific up-regulation of this vitamin D receptor by vitamin D in the ameloblasts (4). Therefore, our hypothesis is that another pathway for vitamin D action may contribute to this ameloblast-specific sensivity. In the present study, we investigate in detail the temporal relationships of the membrane vitamin D receptor in epithelial and mesenchymal cells of developping human teeth from embryonic weeks 4 to weeks 27.

Materials and Methods Immunoperoxidase in human samples was performed as follows.

Tissue collection and preparation. A restricted collection of craniofacial samples (n = 16) from human embryos and fetuses were obtained under the approval of the National Ethics Committee. The fetuses studied ranged from 4 to 27 weeks of pregnancy. For immunodetection, human samples were fixed in 10% formalin for several days at 4°C, decalcified or not, deshydrated, and embedded in paraffin.

Immunolocalization. For these studies, serial dilutions of Ab99 antibody (from 1:25 to 1:100) were used. Ab99 is a rabbit polyclonal antisera generated against the $1,25(OH)_2$ D_3 binding protein isolated from the basolateral membrane of chick duodenal cells (9).

Results Immunolabelling was first tested in several control tissues which are suspected to express the membrane vitamin D receptor. Cells were immunopositive in the buccal mucosa, the nasal epithelium and the border epithelium (Figure 1). Furthermore, osteoblasts were differentiated and secreting the bone matrix proteins in several foci. The expression of the membrane vitamin D receptor was related to the terminal differentiation of this osteogenic cells. In the other hand, the chondrocytes of Meckel's cartilage appeared also to be immunopositive.

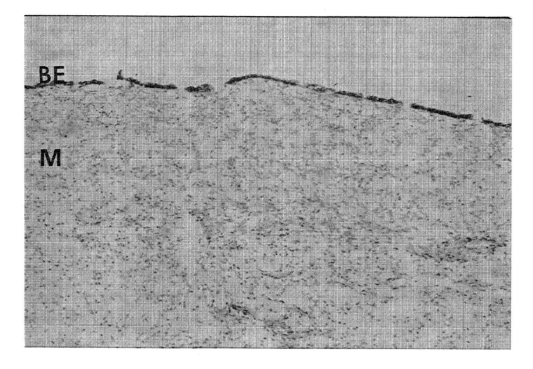

Figure 1. BE : Border epithelium and M : mesenchyme

Immunolabelling during tooth development allowed to show specific up- and down-regulation of this receptor. More specifically, the terminal differentiation of ameloblasts was associated with a prominent expression of the receptor in these cells which secrete enamel matrix (Figure 2).

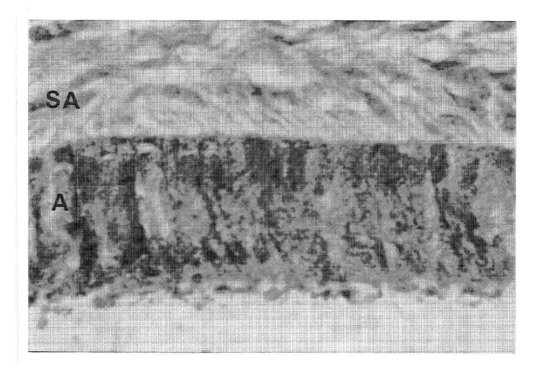

Figure 2. A : Ameloblasts and SA : Supra-ameloblastic cells

Immunocontrols were realised by using a rabbit normal serum using the same dilution.

Discussion   The present data show for the first time the expression of membrane vitamin D receptor in human teeth, suggesting that the action of 1,25(OH)$_2$ vitamin D$_3$ may act through both the genomic (8) and non-genomic (this study) pathways.

Two striking features emerge from the developmental pattern of expression :

1 - Characteristic up- and down-regulation of the membrane VDR in the epithelial and mesenchymal dental cells which may be related to the epigenetic cascades involved in cell differentiation where human Msx and Dlx homeogenes play a key-role (10).

2 - An ameloblast specific expression of the membrane receptor which suggests that the up-regulation of the nuclear receptor by 1,25(OH)$_2$ vitamin D$_3$ is secondary to a cell-specific effect of the non-genomic pathway.

In conclusion, 1,25(OH)$_2$ vitamin D$_3$ may act specifically on enamel and dentin formation through a complex network of both the non-genomic and genomic pathways.

References

1. Deutsch, D., Catalano-Sherman, J., Dafni, L., David, S. and Palmon, A. (1995) Connect Tissue Res. 32(1-4), 97-107.
2. Fincham, A. G. and Simmer, J. P. (1997) Dental enamel. Wiley, Chichester, Ciba Foundation Symposium, 205, 118-130.
3. Yoshizawa, T., Handa, Y., Uematsu, Y., Takeda, S., Sekine, K., Yoshihara, Y., Kawakami, T., Arioka, K., Sato, H., Uchiyama, Y., Masushige, S., Fukamizu, A., Matsumoto, T. and Kato, S. (1997) Nature Genet. 16, 391-396.
4. Berdal, A., Hotton, D., Pike, J.W., Mathieu, H. and Dupret, J.M. (1993) Dev. Biol. 155, 172-179.
5. Robinson, C., Brookes, S.J., Shore, R.C. and Kirkham, J. (1998) Eur. J. Oral Sci. 106(suppl 1) , 282-291.
6. Hotton, D., Mauro, N., Lézot, F., Forest, N. and Berdal A. (1997) J. Histochem. Cytochem. (4), 822-830.
7. Papagerakis, P., Hotton, D., Lézo,t F., Brookes, S., Bonass, W., Robinson, C., Forest, N. and Berdal A (1999) J. Cell Biochem. 76, 194-205.
8. Bailleul-Forestier, I., Davideau, J.L., Papagerakis, P., Noble, I., Nesmann, C., Peuchmaur, M. and Berdal A. (1996) Pediatr. Res. 39, 636-642.
9. Nemere, I., Dormanen, M.C., Hammond, M.W., Okamura, W.H. and Norman, A.W. (1994) J. Biol. Chem. 269, 23750-23756.
10. Davideau, J.L., Demri, P., Gu, T.-T., Simmons, D., Nessman, C., Forest, N., MacDougall, M. and Berdal, A. (1999) Mech Dev. 81, 183-186, 1999.

EXPRESSION OF 1α,25-(OH)$_2$D$_3$ MEMBRANE RECEPTOR IN MURINE DENTAL CELLS

Christophe Teillaud*, Ilka Nemere°, Mary MacDougall#, Mohand Mesbah*, Nadine Forest*, Ariane Berdal*.
*Laboratoire de Biologie-Odontologie. Institut Biomédical des Cordeliers. Université Paris VII. EA 2380, 15-21, rue de l'Ecole de Médecine. Paris, France.
°Department of Nutrition and Food Sciences, Logan, Utah State University, USA.
#UTHSC, Department of Pediatric Dentistry, San-Antonio, Texas, USA.

Introduction The genomic responses to 1α,25-dihydroxyvitamin D$_3$ (1α,25-(OH)$_2$D$_3$ in dental cells are related, at least in part, to the nuclear high affinity receptor for 1α,25-(OH)$_2$D$_3$ resulting in the modulation of gene expression such as calbindins and amelogenin genes (1, 2, 3). Rapid/nongenomic actions of 1α,25-(OH)$_2$D$_3$ have been described *in vitro* including changes in membrane fluidity (4), turnover of phospholipids (5), increase of intracellular calcium uptake (6), and the activation of protein kinase C (7, 8) in various cells such as chondrocytes, rat and chick epithelial intestinal cells (7, 9, 10, 11). These direct and rapid effects have been related to a protein membrane receptor for 1α,25-(OH)$_2$D$_3$ (mVDR) with a molecular weight of 65 kDa (7, 9, 11). It has been characterized at biochemical and functional levels from chick epithelial intestinal cells and from rat chondrocytes using a rabbit polyclonal antibody (Ab99) (7, 9, 11). Currently, no information is avaible concerning the nongenomic pathway of 1α,25-(OH)$_2$D$_3$ in dental tissues. The aim of our study was to analyse the expression of the 1α,25-(OH)$_2$D$_3$ membrane receptor in murine dental cells and in the stable mouse odontoblast-like cell line MO6G3 (12) for further biochemical and functional investigations.

Results
Western-blotting analysis
Total protein extract from dental mesenchyme of rat incisors was analysed by Western-blotting, with Ab99, for the expression of mVDR. 10 μg of total protein were applied to 10% polyacrylamide gels in a minislab gel system (Mini-Protean II Electrophoresis cell ; Bio-Rad, Richmond, VA). SDS-PAGE was performed under reducing conditions. Proteins were transferred onto nitrocellulose membranes (Hybond ECL, Amersham, England) using a semi dry transblot apparatus (Bio Trans Midi, An Arbor, MI). After washing, membranes were incubated with Ab99 diluted at 1/4000 and then incubated with horse radish peroxidase-F(ab')$_2$ goat anti-rabbit IgG diluted at 1/40000. Membranes were incubated with the Super

Signal Substrate (WB, Pierce, Rockford, IL) and chemiluminescence was detected by exposure of the membranes to an Hyperfilm ECL (Amersham, Life Science, England) for 5 minutes. Western-blotting analysis of the dental mesenchyme of rat incisors with Ab99, showed a 65-66 kDa band (Figure 1a). No signal was seen with normal rabbit IgGs ascertaining the specificity of the detection (Figure 1b).

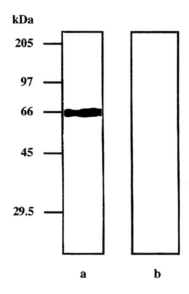

Figure 1 (a, b)
(a) 10 µg of dental mesenchyme of rat incisor incubated with Ab99 (1/4000)(b) 20 µg of dental mesenchyme of rat incisor incubated with control IgG (1 µg/mL).

Surface expression of mVDR by mouse odontoblast-like cell line MO6G3
The expression of mVDR by MO6G3 cells was investigated by means of indirect immunofluorescence. MO6G3 cells were cultured in α-MEM supplemented with 10% FCS, 100 Units/mL penicillin/streptomycin, 50 µg/mL ascorbic acid, and 10 mM Na-β-glycerophosphate (Sigma, France) at 33°C. Before analysis, MO6G3 cells were treated with 0.25% trypsin, and washed twice in phosphate-buffered saline (PBS)-0.5% BSA (Bovine Serum Albumin). Viability of cells was checked by trypan blue exclusion test, the number of dead cells was always below 5%. 5.10^5 cells were incubated with different dilutions of Ab99 at +4°C during 30 minutes. After two washing in PBS-0.5% BSA, cells were incubated with fluorescein isothiocyanate (FITC)-labeled F(ab')2 goat anti-rabbit IgG(H+L) diluted at 1/50 (Southern Biotechnology, USA) during 30 minutes at +4°C. Cells were then washed twice in PBS-0.5% BSA and analysis was performed on a FACSCalibur flow cytometer (Becton Dickinson). Relative cell number is plotted against a

logarithmic scale of fluorescence intensity, measured by flow cytometry. Our results showed that mVDR is specifically expressed by MO6G3 cells : 60% at 1/10 (Figure 2a). No signal was seen with control rabbit IgGs at 1 µg/mL (Figure 2b).

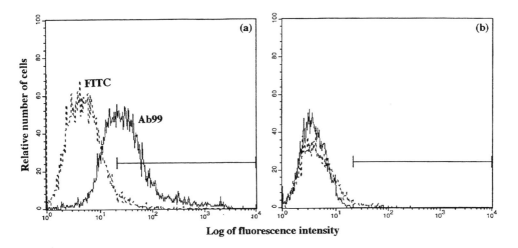

Figure 2 (a, b)
(a) MO6G3 cells incubated with Ab99 (1/10) and FITC-F(ab')2 goat anti-rabbit (1/50).
(b) MO6G3 cells incubated control rabbit IgGs (1 µg/mL) and FITC-F(ab')2 goat anti-rabbit (1/50).

Discussion Altogether, these results indicates that murine dental cells express mVDR, corresponding to that previously described in others tissues and species (7, 9, 11). We have shown, for the first time, by Western-blotting, that the dental mesenchyme of rat incisor and that the mouse odontoblast-like cell line MO6G3 expressed specifically the membrane receptor for $1\alpha,25\text{-}(OH)_2D_3$ with a molecular weight of 65-66 kDa. Flow cytometric analysis confirms the constitutive expression of mVDR by MO6G3 cells. Furthermore histochemistry analysis realized on mouse incisor showed that ameloblasts and odontoblasts express the mVDR (data not shown). The genomic responses in dental cells are related to the nuclear high affinity receptor for $1\alpha,25\text{-}(OH)_2D_3$ resulting in the regulation of calbindins and amelogenin genes (1, 2, 3). In addition, the rapid and non/genomic responses to $1\alpha,25\text{-}(OH)_2D_3$ in dental cells have not been investigated. The functions of mVDR have been described in rat chondrocytes ; its includes the activation of PKC and the regulation of chondrocyte proliferation (11). In others cells such as intestinal epithelial cells, this receptor is involved in calcium transport (9). Currently, no information is available concerning the role of mVDR in dental cells. This receptor could be involved in some rapid/nongenomic responses to $1\alpha,25\text{-}(OH)_2D_3$ such as the regulation of intracellular calcium uptake. In addition to the genomic response to $1\alpha,25\text{-}(OH)_2D_3$ these rapid effects could play indirectly a role in the dentinogenesis or in the differentiation of dental cells. These hypothesis remain to be investigated. MO6G3 cells could be used for a better understanding of the nongenomic response to $1\alpha,25\text{-}(OH)_2D_3$ in dental tissues.

References

1. Berdal, A., Hotton, D., Pike, J.W., Mathieu, H. and Dupret, J.M. (1993) Dev. Biol. 155, 172-179.
2. Berdal, A. (1997). In : Vitamin D. Feldman D., Glorieux F.H., Pike J.W., (Eds). Academic Press, pp. 423-435.
3. Papagerakis, P., Hotton, D., Lézard, F., Brookes, S., Bonass, W. and Robinson, C. (1999) J. Cell. Biochem. 76, 194-205.
4. Swain, L.D., Schwartz, Z., Caulfield, K., Brooks, B.P. and Boyan, B.D. (1993) Bone. 14, 609-617.
5. Swain, L.D., Schwartz, Z. and Boyan, B.D. (1992) Biochim. Biophys. Acta. 1136, 45-51.
6. Langston, G.G., Swain, L.D., Schwartz, Z., Del Toro, F., Gomez, R. and Boyan, B.D. (1990) Calcif. Tissue Int. 47, 230-236.
7. Nemere, I, Schwartz, Z., Pedrozo, H., Sylvia V.L., Dean, D.D. and Boyan B.D. (1998) J. Bone Miner. Res. 13, 1353-1359.
8. Sylvia, V.L., Schwartz, Z., Curry, D.B., Chang, Z., Dean, D.D. and Boyan, B.D. 1998) J. Bone. Miner. Res. 13, 559-569.
9. Nemere, I., Dormanen, M.C., Hammond, M.W., Okamura, W.H. and Norman, A.W. (1994) J. Biol. Chem. 269, 23750-23756.
10. Lieberherr, M., Grosse, B., Duchambon, P. and Drüeke, T. (1989) J. Biol. Chem. 264, 20403-20406.
11. Pedrozo, H.A., Schwartz, Z., Rimes, S., Sylvia, V.L., Nemere, I., Posner, G.H., Dean, D.D. and Boyan, B.D. (1999) J. Bone. Miner. Res. 6, 856-867.
12. MacDougall, M., Thiemann, F., Ta, H., Hsu, P., Chen, L.S. and Snead, M.L. (1995) Conn. Tissue. Res. 33, 97-103.

1,25-DIHYDROXYVITAMIN D₃ AND CALCIUM SIGNALING

Igor N. Sergeev and Anthony W. Norman

Department of Chemistry and Biochemistry, South Dakota State University, Brookings, SD 57007, and Department of Biochemistry, University of California, Riverside, CA 92521, USA

The vitamin D hormone, $1,25(OH)_2D_3$, generates a wide array of biological responses both by classical regulation of gene expression and rapid signal transduction pathways involving a putative membrane receptor (1, 2). The major thesis of biochemical and mechanistic studies, presented here, is that Ca^{2+} is an intracellular messenger involved in signal transduction of rapid actions of $1,25(OH)_2D_3$. The hormone rapidly (within seconds) triggers oscillations of intracellular Ca^{2+}. Mechanism of the oscillations includes entry of Ca^{2+} from the extracellular space through voltage-insensitive and voltage-dependent Ca^{2+} channels, which is coordinated with mobilization of Ca^{2+} from intracellular stores via Ca^{2+} release channels (ryanodine and inositol 1,4,5-trisphosphate receptors). Shape (i.e., amplitude, frequency and/or duration of oscillations) and spatial distribution of the $1,25(OH)_2D_3$-induced Ca^{2+} signal are important in regulation of cellular processes (e.g., insulin secretion in pancreatic β-cells, induction of programmed cell death (apoptosis) in cancer cells and cellular responses to microgravity in space flight).

This communication presents a summary of our studies conducted over the past several years concerning the $1,25(OH)_2D_3$-activated intracellular Ca^{2+} signaling pathway. These include the following: (i) regulation of intracellular Ca^{2+} in pancreatic β-cells, (ii) calbindin-D_{28k} and cytosolic Ca^{2+} buffering, (iii) Ca^{2+} signaling and apoptosis in breast cancer cells, and (iv) Ca^{2+} signaling and calbindins in microgravity and space flight. In our research, we utilize cellular biochemical approaches, including high-resolution digital and confocal imaging of intracellular Ca^{2+}, vitamin D receptors, and Ca^{2+} channels.

$\underline{Ca^{2+}\text{ oscillations in pancreatic β-cells.}}$ $1,25(OH)_2D_3$ rapidly, within 5-10 s, triggered synchronous Ca^{2+} oscillations in pancreatic β-cells (see figure below) (3). Amplitude of the Ca^{2+} oscillations depended on $1,25(OH)_2D_3$ concentration, but the oscillations were independent of glucose. Removal of extracellular Ca^{2+} blocked the $1,25(OH)_2D_3$-induced Ca^{2+} oscillations.

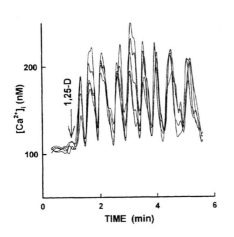

Addition of La^{3+}, an antagonist of Ca^{2+} channels, also blocked the oscillations, but they were restored after La^{3+} removal and addition of Ca^{2+}. Nifedepine, an antagonist of voltage-dependent Ca^{2+} channels, did not block the oscillations, but decreased their amplitude. These observations imply that $1,25(OH)_2D_3$ D stimulates Ca^{2+} influx mainly through voltage-insensitive Ca^{2+} channels. To directly evaluate this, we used Mn^{2+} quench technique. Mn^{2+} ions enter the cell via voltage-insensitive Ca^{2+} channels and quench fluorescence of the Ca^{2+} probe. We found that β-cells express voltage-insensitive Ca^{2+} channels, and that $1,25(OH)_2D_3$ increases the slope of the quench traces, i.e. Ca^{2+} influx. These findings indicate that Ca^{2+} influx is required for the $1,25(OH)_2D_3$-induced Ca^{2+} oscillations in β-cells.

We also investigated the role of intracellular Ca^{2+} stores and found that endoplasmic reticulum Ca^{2+} stores must be filled for $1,25(OH)_2D_3$ to evoke Ca^{2+} oscillations. When the stores were depleted with thapsigargin, $1,25(OH)_2D_3$ failed to induce oscillations. Further analysis revealed, that $1,25(OH)_2D_3$ activates oscillatory release of Ca^{2+} via the ryanodine receptor/Ca^{2+} channel, but not through the IP_3 receptor/Ca^{2+} channel. We concluded that $1,25(OH)_2D_3$ induces Ca^{2+} oscillations via coordinative regulation of Ca^{2+} entry and Ca^{2+} release pathways.

Calbindin-D_{28k} and cytosolic Ca^{2+} buffering. Intracellular Ca^{2+} buffering is critical for shaping the Ca^{2+} signal. Over 90% of Ca^{2+} in cytosol is in bound form, and the Ca^{2+} signal represents an increase in free Ca^{2+}, which transiently exceeds the cytosolic Ca^{2+} buffering capacity. Cytosolic Ca^{2+} buffers with fast binding kinetics are critical in Ca^{2+} signaling (2). We investigated how Ca^{2+} buffering capacity, increased with the vitamin D-dependent Ca^{2+} binding protein calbindin-D_{28k}, affects Ca^{2+} signaling in pancreatic β-cells.

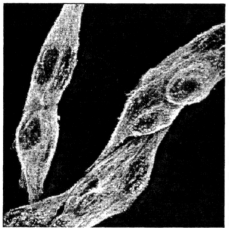

Ca^{2+} signaling in β-cells overexpressing calbindin-D_{28k} was dramatically altered (4). There were no Ca^{2+} responses in those cells to agents which were effective in cells with basal levels of calbindin-D_{28k}. Ca^{2+} released from endoplasmic reticulum stores was also effectively buffered by calbindin-D_{28k}. Cells loaded with cytosolic Ca^{2+} buffer BAPTA (its affinity to Ca^{2+} is comparable to that of calbindin-D_{28k}) demonstrated absence of Ca^{2+} responses as well.

The figure on the left shows three-dimensional confocal image of β-cells labeled for calbindin-D_{28k} and microtubules (β-tubulin). This is a merged image, so that association of calbindin-D_{28k} with microtubules can be appreciated (on the original image, superimposed red and green colors indicate co-localization of calbindin-D_{28k} and microtubules).

These findings show how important cytosolic Ca^{2+} buffering is for Ca^{2+} signaling and how precisely Ca^{2+} signal is organized. Even a moderate increase in calbindin-D_{28k} dramatically disrupts, essentially eliminates, the Ca^{2+} signal. These results also imply that propagation of the Ca^{2+} signal along microtubules depends on the level and distribution of calbindin-D_{28k}.

Ca^{2+} and vitamin D signaling in breast cancer cells. Regulation of intracellular Ca^{2+} in breast cancer may be important in modulating cell proliferation, differentiation, apoptosis, and cytotoxicity, as well as contributing to mechanisms of action of anticancer agents, including $1,25(OH)_2D_3$ and its analogs. We investigated Ca^{2+} regulatory pathways in human breast cancer cell lines BT-20 and MCF-7 and the role of $1,25(OH)_2D_3$ in modulating these pathways (5, 6). We found that breast cancer cells express voltage-insensitive Ca^{2+} channels, as indicated by their permeability to Mn^{2+}, increase in Ca^{2+} conductance with increasing extracellular Ca^{2+}, blockage by La^{3+} and Ni^{2+}, response to depolarization with decrease in Ca^{2+} influx. However, there was no evidence for voltage-dependent Ca^{2+} channels. Endoplasmic reticulum was a major Ca^{2+} storage compartment. After application of a Ca^{2+} ionophore ionomycine in Ca^{2+}-free buffer to cells with depleted Ca^{2+} stores, there was only small additional Ca^{2+} release. Mobilization of Ca^{2+} from the endoplasmic reticulum stores occurred through IP_3 receptor, while ryanodine receptor was not expressed.

Two major effects of 1,25(OH)₂D₃ on intracellular Ca²⁺ in breast cancer cells were observed. First, 1,25(OH)₂D₃ D rapidly increased Ca²⁺influx through voltage-insensitive Ca²⁺ channels (see fig.below). Second, treatment of the cells with 1,25(OH)₂D₃ significantly increased basal levels of cytosolic Ca²⁺. Importantly, those cells had depleted endoplasmic reticulum Ca²⁺ stores. Thus, breast cancer cells demonstrate early and late changes in Ca²⁺ in response to 1,25(OH)₂D₃. Early changes are due to Ca²⁺ influx, and late changes result from mobilization of endoplasmic reticulum Ca²⁺ stores.

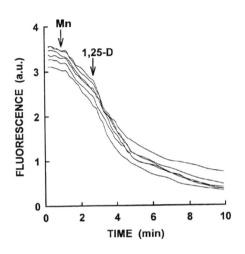

How does 1,25(OH)₂D₃-evoked increase in intracellular Ca²⁺ relate to cell fate in breast cancer? We (2, 6) have shown that early and late changes in intracellular Ca²⁺ levels occur in programmed cell death (apoptosis). Mechanisms of action of intracellular Ca²⁺ in apoptotic pathways are not known and apoptosis related Ca²⁺ targets have not been identified. With respect directly to intracellular Ca²⁺, our hypothesis is that a sustained increase in intracellular Ca²⁺, not reaching cytotoxic levels, signals the cell to enter an apoptotic pathway.

We detected apoptosis in individual cell nuclei by fluorescent labeling of internucleosomal DNA fragments generated by an apoptotic endonuclease. Additionally, we used standard morphological criteria of apoptosis: nuclear and chromatin condensation, and formation of apoptotic bodies.

Increase in intracellular Ca²⁺ with 1,25(OH)₂D₃ did trigger apoptosis in breast cancer cells. Confocal imaging of the nuclei of cells at the early stage of apoptosis showed scattered pattern of DNA fragmentation. Double-labeling of nuclei for total and fragmented DNA at later stage of apoptosis revealed characteristic peripheral areas of fragmented and condensed DNA. Compact DNA-containing apoptotic bodies were observed at the final stage of cell death, induced by 1,25(OH)₂D₃. Importantly, increase in intracellular Ca²⁺ preceded an onset of the early stage apoptosis. Breast cancer cells loaded with cytosolic Ca²⁺ buffer BAPTA did not undergo apoptosis in response to 1,25(OH)₂D₃. On the other hand, treatment of the cells with a Ca²⁺ ionophore ionomycine similarly induced apoptosis.

These results show that 1,25(OH)₂D₃ triggers apoptosis in breast cancer cells by cauising an increase in Ca²⁺ entry through voltage-insensitive Ca²⁺ channels and depletion of endoplasmic reticulum calcium stores. The resulting elevated cytosolic Ca²⁺ seems sufficient to elicit apoptosis.

Ca²⁺ signaling in microgravity and space flight. Earlier we demonstrated changes in Ca²⁺ metabolism and the Ca²⁺ regulatory vitamin D endocrine system in human and animal models for microgravity and after space flight (7, 8). Signaling mechanisms triggering these changes involve intracellular Ca²⁺. We found that Ca²⁺ oscillations are desynchronized and that coupling of the of the Ca²⁺ signal is impaired in cells exposed to simulated microgravity. Importantly, calbindin-D₂₈ₖ and calbindin-D₉ₖ were decreased and the rate of apoptosis was increased in the intestine and kidneys of rats after space flight (7).

718

Conclusions

1,25(OH)$_2$D$_3$ evokes Ca^{2+} oscillations in pancreatic β-cells. Mechanism of the oscillations includes coordinative regulation of Ca^{2+} entry and Ca^{2+} release channels by the hormone. Ca^{2+} oscillations are desynchronized in cells grown in microgravity.

1,25(OH)$_2$D$_3$ triggers apoptosis in breast cancer cells via activation of intracellular Ca^{2+} signaling pathways.

Calbindin-D$_{28k}$, associated with microtubules, regulates Ca^{2+} signaling by buffering cytosolic Ca^{2+}.

Taken together, our results clearly show that 1,25(OH)$_2$D$_3$ regulates cell function and determines cell fate via interactions with Ca^{2+} signaling pathways.

1,25(OH)$_2$D$_3$-mediated Ca^{2+} signaling

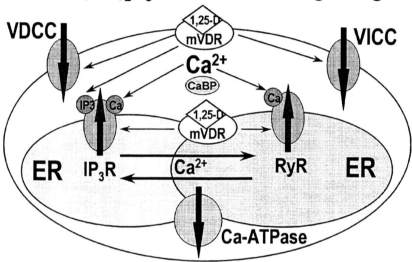

Abbreviations: VDCC, voltage-dependent Ca^{2+} channels; VICC, voltage-insensitive Ca^{2+} channels; IP$_3$R, inositol 1,4,5-trisphosphate receptor; RyR, ryanodine receptor; mVDR, membrane VDR; CaBP, calbindin-D$_{28k}$; ER, endoplasmic reticulum.

Acknowledgments

This work was supported in part by NIH/NCI CA-67317 (INS) and USDA SD00179-H (INS).

References

1. Norman, A.W. (1997). In: *Vitamin D* (Feldman, D., Glorieux, F.H., and Pike, J.W., eds), pp. 223-256, Academic Press, San Diego, CA.
2. Sergeev, I.N., Rhoten, W.B. and Spirichev, V.B. (1998). In: *Subcellular Biochemistry: Fat-Soluble Vitamins.* vol. 30, (Quinn, P and Kagan, V., eds.), Plenum Press: N.Y., p.271-297.
3. Sergeev, I.N. and Rhoten, W.B. (1995). *Endocrinology* 136: 2852-2861.
4. Rhoten, W.B. and Sergeev, I.N. (1994). *Endocrine* 2: 989-995.
5. Sergeev, I.N. and Rhoten, W.B. (1998). *Endocrine* 9: 321-327.
6. Sergeev, I.N., Rhoten, W.B. and Norman, A.W. (1997). In: *Vitamin D: Chemistry, Biology and Clinical Applications of the Steroid Hormone* (Norman, A.W., Bouillon, R., and Thomasset, M., eds.), Univ. California Printing: Riverside, p. 473-474.
7. Sergeev, I.N., Rhoten, W.B., and Carney, M.D. (1996). *Endocrine* 5: 335-340; Cover Illustration.
8. Spirichev, V.B. and Sergeev, I.N. (1988). In: *Aspects Nutr. Physiol.* (Bourne, G.H., ed.) Karger: Basel, pp. 173-216.

REGULATION OF INTRACELLULAR CALCIUM IN SIMULATED MICROGRAVITY

I.N. Sergeev, W.B. Rhoten*, M.A. Chaudhry* and A.W. Norman**

*Department of Chemistry and Biochemistry, South Dakota State University, Brookings, SD 57007, *Department of Anatomy, Cell and Neurobiology, Marshall University School of Medicine, Huntington, WV 25704 and **Department of Biochemistry, University of California, Riverside, CA 92521*

Microcarrier rotating culture is analogous to some aspects of a microgravity environment and is used as a model to simulate in the laboratory some of the effects of spaceflight on cells. We hypothesized that Ca^{2+} signaling, which depends on the vitamin D hormone (1,25$(OH)_2D_3$), may underlie the mechanism of gravity-induced signal transduction (1).

Pancreatic anchorage-dependent β-cell line RIN 1046-38 (RIN), which we earlier have characterized in detail with respect to cellular Ca^{2+} homeostasis and signaling (2), was cultivated in incubator-compatible horizontally rotating vessels on collagen-coated microcarriers (Fig. 1). The system provided a low-turbulence, high mass transfer, low-shear cell culture environment. After a lag attachment phase of nearly 24 hrs, the cells grew rapidly on the microcarriers and reached confluence after 3 days. The microcarrier cultures were stable for at least an additional 3-4 days. During this period, an enhanced bridging resulted in formation of aggregates incorporating several microcarriers. Portions of peripheral confluent cell layers in a later stage of cultivation (> 7 days) often shed from the microcarriers, resulting in free spheroidal clusters.

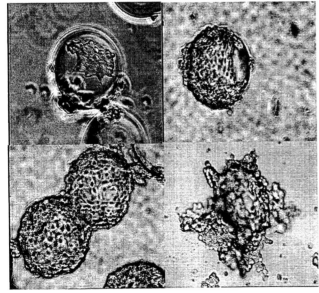

FIG. 1. RIN cells cultured on microcarriers in a high aspect ratio vessel (HARV) bioreactor for 1, 3, 5, and 7 days. Note cell attachment and spreading at 1st day *(upper left panel)*; round morphology and confluency of the cells at 3rd day *(upper right panel)*; multilayer growth and formation of bridges between the microcarriers at 5th day *(lower left)*; shedding of the cells from the microcarriers in a later stage of cultivation (7th day) *(lower right)*. Phase-contrast images were captured using a Nikon Diaphot inverted microscope (20X objective) equipped for video imaging.

For measurements of intracellular Ca^{2+} ($[Ca^{2+}]_i$) the cells grown for 3-4 days in rotating culture were loaded with fura-2/AM for 40 min in stationary conditions and analyzed using the fluorescence digital imaging system (2). Because coated microcarrier beads produced weak fluorescence after loading with fura-2, the cells grown on the lateral surface of the beads and detached cell clusters were used.

720

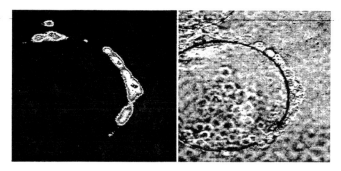

FIG. 2. Pseudo-color (gray-scale) [Ca²⁺]ᵢ and phase-contrast images of RIN cells grown on microcarriers and loaded with the Ca²⁺ probe fura-2/AM. Identical fluorescence ratio*(left panel)* and phase-contrast *(right panel)* images were captured using a Nikon Diaphot inverted microscope (Fluor 40X objective) equipped for video imaging. Hexagonal patterned background in phase-contrast image is from the image intensifier.

RIN cells expressed typical Ca²⁺ responses to modulators of Ca²⁺ influx from the extracellular space and Ca²⁺ mobilization from intracellular stores (KCl, carbachol, thapsigargin, ionomycin), as compared with our previous results(Fig. 3-5) (1). The noticeable differences were de-synchronization of Ca²⁺ oscillations evoked by the Ca²⁺-regulating hormone 1,25(OH)₂D₃ and the L-type voltage-gated Ca²⁺ channel agonist Bay K8644 (see Fig. 3), as well as decreased release of Ca²⁺ through the ryanodine receptor/Ca²⁺ channel (as evaluated with caffeine; see Fig. 5).Confocal microscopy of RIN cells grown on microcarriers in rotating culture revealed characteristic cytosolic distribution of the Ca²⁺-binding protein calbindin-D₂₈ₖ (Fig. 6).

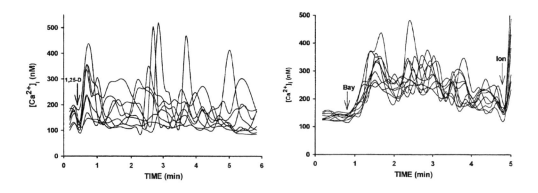

FIG. 3. The steroid hormone 1,25(OH)₂D₃ evokes asynchronous [Ca²⁺]ᵢ oscillations in RIN cells cultivated in an HARV bioreactor *(left panel)*. 1,25(OH)₂D₃ induced highly synchronized oscillations in RIN cells grown in a stationary culture *(not shown)*.The L-type Ca²⁺ channel agonist Bay K8644 triggers slow, irregular [Ca²⁺]ᵢ oscillations in RIN cells cultivated in an HARV bioreactor *(right panel)*. The oscillations in RIN cells grown in a stationary culture, were synchronized *(not shown)*.Here and in Figs. 4-5, addition of chemicals and drugs is indicated by *arrows*.

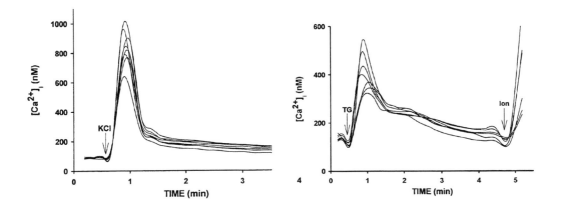

FIG. 4. RIN cells cultivated in an HARV bioreactor, show typical $[Ca^{2+}]_i$ responses to K^+ depolarization (70 mM KCl) *(left panel)*, a mobilizer of the endoplasmic reticulum Ca^{2+} stores thapsigargin (2 µM), and Ca^{2+} ionophore ionomycin (5 µM) *(right panel)*.

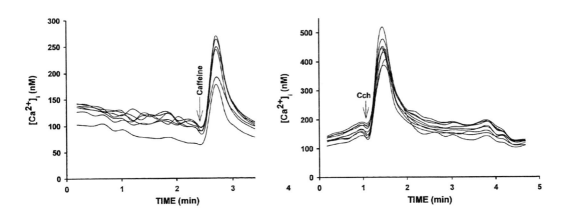

FIG. 5. Caffeine (40 mM), an agonist of ryanodine receptor/Ca^{2+} release channel, *(left panel)* and carbachol (0.1 mM), an activator of inositol trisphosphate receptor/Ca^{2+} release channel, *(right panel)* induce typical Ca^{2+} mobilization responses. Magnitude of the caffeine-induced Ca^{2+} response was somewhat lower in RIN cells exposed to simulated microgravity, as compared with cells in a stationary cultur. Because endoplasmic reticulum Ca^{2+} stores appear to be not depleted in most cells (see Fig. 4, right panel), it may imply that regulation of the ryanodine receptor (e.g., its mechanical activation) is affected in simulated microgravity.

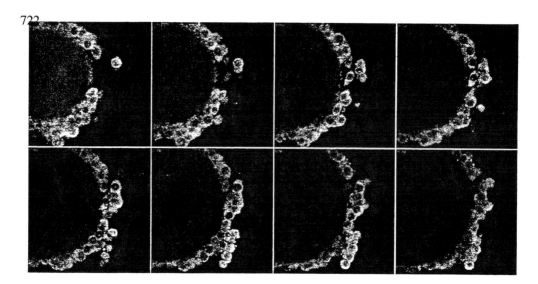

FIG. 6. Confocal imaging of calbindin-D_{28k} in RIN cells cultivated in an HARV bioreactor. For fluorescence labeling of calbindin-D_{28k}, mouse monoclonal antibody (clone CL300; Sigma) and FITC-conjugated anti-mouse IgG (Sigma) were used. Images from optical sections 0.5 µm thick were obtained using BioRad MRC-1024 laser scanning confocal microscope.

Conclusion. The results obtained indicate that cellular Ca^{2+} responses, requiring intercellular communication (synchronization of Ca^{2+} oscillations) and signal transduction via the ryanodine receptor (Ca^{2+}-induced Ca^{2+} release and/or mechanical coupling), are altered in microgravity environment. Dysregulation of intracellular Ca^{2+} in simulated microgravity may be related to decreased levels of cytosolic vitamin D-dependent Ca^{2+} buffers, calbindins, which we observed in rats after space flight (3).

References
1.   Sergeev, I.N., Rhoten, W.B., and Spirichev, V.B. (1998). In: *Subcellular Biochemistry: Fat-soluble Vitamins,* vol. 30, (Quin, P and Kagan, V., eds), Plenum Press: N.Y., p. 271-279.
2.   Sergeev, I.N. and Rhoten, W.B. (1995). *Endocrinology* 136: 2852-2861.
3.   Sergeev, I.N., Rhoten, W.B., and Carney, M.D. (1996). *Endocrine* 5: 335-340; Cover Illustration.

KINETICS OF CALCIUM SUPPLEMENTATION IN CALCIUM DEFICIENCY: *IN VIVO* AND *IN VITRO* STUDIES

Geneviève Mailhot[1-2], Jean-Luc Petit[1], Christian Demers[1], Marielle Gascon-Barré[1-3], [1]Centre de recherche, Hôpital Saint-Luc, Department of [2]Nutrition and [3]Pharmacology, Université de Montréal, Montréal, Québec, Canada.

Introduction Ca^{2+} is an important second messenger molecule involved in several cellular signaling pathways. Interactions between hormones, neurotransmitters, cytokines, growth factors or pharmacological agents and their respective membrane receptors lead to increases in the cytoplasmic Ca^{2+} concentration ($[Ca^{2+}]_c$) in a spontaneous, sustained or oscillatory manner. $[Ca^{2+}]_c$ elevation leads subsequently to the activation of Ca^{2+}-dependent cellular responses which lead to the achievement of specific biological functions.

Chronic hypocalcemia (Ca-D-) is a pathological condition often observed in humans at all ages. Alterations of the Ca^{2+} status is observed in several situations such as rickets, osteoporosis and hypoparathyroidism. Chronic hypocalcemia is also associated with perturbations of the Ca^{2+} signaling pathway leading to cellular defects in many tissues and organs (1-3).

We had previously shown that chronic hypocalcemia coupled to vitamin D deficiency is associated with a reduction in the: 1) resting $[Ca^{2+}]_c$, 2) mobilization of the IP_3-sensitive Ca^{2+} pools by several agonists and 3) level of the gene transcript of the major endoplasmic reticulum (ER) Ca^{2+} binding protein, calreticulin (4,5,7).

Aims The aim of the studies was to investigate the kinetics of dietary Ca^{2+} supplementation in Ca-D- rats on intracellular Ca^{2+} homeostasis. *In vitro* studies were also carried out in VDR-positive *ROS 17/2.8* cells to probe the influence of extracellular Ca^{2+} on the regulation of intracellular Ca^{2+}.

Materials and methods *In vivo studies*: Sprague Dawley Ca-D- rats [induced by a functional Ca^{2+} depletion through vitamin D deficiency as previously described (2,6)] were repleted with dietary Ca^{2+} for a period of 14 days with a 3% Ca^{2+} gluconate solution as drinking water. Hepatocytes were isolated and kept in short term primary culture in a William's E medium adjusted at a Ca^{2+} concentration similar to that prevailing *in vivo* (1,1 to 1,35 mM).

In vitro studies: VDR-positive *ROS 17/2.8* cells were 1) cultured for 24 hours in a Ca^{2+}-free DMEM/F12 (1:1) medium and then 2) another seven days in the medium mentioned above adjusted at 3 mM of Ca^{2+} in order to achieve Ca^{2+} repletion.

Intracellular Ca^{2+} measurements. The intracellular Ca^{2+} signal was analysed using the fluorescent probe FURA-2 AM in both cellular models. Ca^{2+} ionophore and agonists acting through the Ca^{2+} mobilizing pathway were used to achieve the Ca^{2+} mobilization of cellular pools.

Results and discussion

1. *Resting cytoplasmic Ca²⁺ and Ca²⁺ mobilization of the intracellular Ca²⁺ pools in rat hepatocytes*

Figure 1-A illustrates the resting $[Ca^{2+}]_c$ in hepatocytes isolated from rats Ca-D- and after seven days of Ca^{2+} repletion. As shown, the resting $[Ca^{2+}]_c$ is significantly higher in Ca^{2+}-repleted cells compared to that observed in Ca-D- cells demonstrating a sensitivity of the cytoplasmic Ca^{2+} compartment to dietary Ca^{2+} supplementation. In order to investigate the state of the cellular pools following Ca^{2+} supplementation, we achieved Ca^{2+} mobilization of the cellular pools with the α_1-adrenergic agent, phenylephrine in combination with the Ca^{2+} ionophore, ionomycin. Phenylephrine mobilized the IP_3-sensitive Ca^{2+} pools while ionomycin mobilized particularly the mitochondrial Ca^{2+} pool. As illustrated in figure 1-B Ca^{2+} mobilization by those two agents showed a trend similar to that observed for the resting $[Ca^{2+}]_c$ where Ca^{2+} repletion increased the Ca^{2+} mobilization of the cellular pools when compared to Ca^{2+} mobilization in hepatocytes obtained from Ca-D- animals. The data illustrate that intracellular Ca^{2+} homeostasis is highly regulated by the *in vivo* Ca^{2+} status in a cell type well characterized for its cellular Ca^{2+} response. The mechanisms involved in the regulation process associated with the cellular Ca^{2+} repletion are currently unknown but the main ER Ca^{2+}-binding protein, calreticulin seems to act as a regulator of the size of the hormone-sensitive Ca^{2+} pools as already proposed (8).

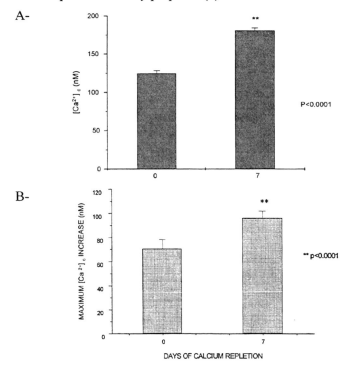

Figure 1. Resting cytoplasmic Ca²⁺ (A) and Ca²⁺ mobilization by the α₁-adrenergic agonist, phenylephrine and the Ca²⁺ ionophore, ionomycin in rat hepatocytes (B)

2. Ca²⁺ mobilization by 1,25(OH)₂D₃ and ionomycin in ROS 17/2.8 cells

In vitro studies were carried out in a cell model known to be modulated by the Ca^{2+}/vitamin D endocrine system. Figure 3 illustrates the pattern of $[Ca^{2+}]_c$ response to ionomycin and the vitamin D hormone, 1,25(OH)₂D₃ in cells cultured in a Ca^{2+}-free medium (—) and in a medium adjusted at 3 mM Ca^{2+} (...) . The data clearly demonstrate that cells cultured in the highest Ca^{2+} concentration show a greater Ca^{2+} mobilization in response to both compounds than the cells cultured in the Ca^{2+}-free medium. The data, obtained in a cell model responsive to the hormone 1,25(OH)₂D₃ , indicate that the extracellular Ca^{2+} concentration strongly influences intracellular Ca^{2+} homeostasis.

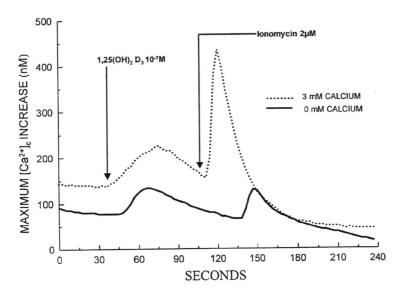

Figure 2. Ca²⁺ mobilization by 1,25(OH)₂ D₃ and ionomycin in ROS 17/2.8 cells

<u>Conclusion</u> Our data demonstrate in an *in vivo* model (rat hepatocytes), and in an *in vitro* model (ROS 17/2.8 cells) that extracellular Ca^{2+} is an important determinant of cellular Ca^{2+} homeostasis. These observations may help understand the influence of dietary Ca^{2+} supplementation on cellular Ca^{2+} homeostasis in the context of several pathological conditions associated with a suboptimal Ca^{2+} status.

References

1) Bilodeau M., Provencher S., Néron S., Haddad P., Vallières S.,Gascon-Barré M.(1995). Hepatology. 21, 1576-1584.

2) Éthier C., Kestekian R., Beaulieu C., Dubé C., Havrankova J., Gascon-Barré M. (1990). Endocrinology. 126, 2947-2959.

3) Demers C., Lemay J., Hendy GN., Gascon-Barré M. (1997). J Mol Endocrinol.18, 37-48.

4) Gascon-Barré M., Petit J.L., Éthier C., Bilodeau S. (1997). Cell Calcium. 22, 343-356.

5) Mailhot G., Petit J.-L., Demers C., Gascon-Barré M. (2000). Endocrinology. 141, 891-900.

6) Haddad P., Gascon-Barré M., Brault G., Plourde V. (1986). J Clin Invest. 78, 1529-1537.

7) Gascon-Barré M., Haddad P., Provencher S.J., Bilodeau S., Pecker F., Lotersztajn S., Vallières S. (1994). J Clin Invest. 93, 2159-2167.

8) Liu N., Fine R.E., Simons E., Johnson R.J. (1994). J Biol Chem. 269, 28635-28639.

MEMBRANE-INITIATED EFFECTS OF 1,25(OH)₂D₃: MODULATION BY VITAMIN D SATUS AND 24,25(OH)₂D₃

MEMBRANE-INITIATED EFFECTS OF $1,25(OH)_2D_3$: MODULATION BY VITAMIN D SATUS AND $24,25(OH)_2D_3$

Ilka Nemere, Department of Nutrition and Food Sciences and the Biotechnology Center, Utah State University, Logan, UT.

Effects of vitamin D status. Previous studies have described the immunological characterization of an antibody (Ab 099) generated toward the putative plasma membrane receptor for $1,25(OH)_2D_3$ (pmVDR) in chick intestine [1], kidney, and brain [2]. The antibody was found to be monospecific for a 64.5 kD protein and to be largely localized to the plasmalemmas of the three tissues tested [1,2]. In the current report, Western analyses with Ab 099, in conjunction with binding assays, were used to investigate the effect of vitamin D status on pmVDR levels in the three tissues. In intestine, exposure to ligand results in an apparent translocation of pmVDR to the nucleus [1]; thus in vitamin D-deficient (−D) chicks, basal lateral membranes might be postulated to have higher levels of the putative receptor. Also in intestine, differences in vitamin D status were further compared to the ability of $1,25(OH)_2D_3$ to activate signal transduction pathways.

Figure 1 demonstrates the effects of vitamin D status on intestine and kidney: in intestine, both specific binding and protein levels are highest in −D tissue, and decreasing with repletion (+D). In kidney, vitamin D repletion resulted in higher levels of both specific binding and protein levels. In brain, no vitamin D difference was found (data not shown).

Intestine

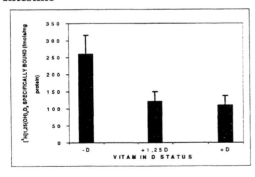
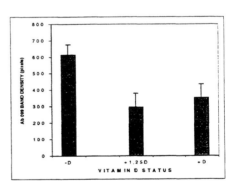

Kidney

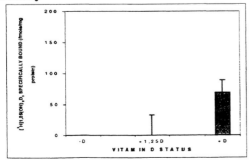
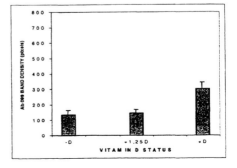

Fig. 1. Plasma membranes were prepared from intestine (top panels) or kidney (bottom panels) by a combination of density and Percoll-gradient sedimentation, and identified by the marker enzyme activity Na^+,K^+-ATPase. Membranes were removed from Percoll and analyzed for specific binding of $[^3H]1,25(OH)_2D_3$, or resolved on SDS-PAGE for Western blotting and subsequent incubation with Ab 099 followed by alkaline phosphatase-conjugated secondary antibody.

Since isolated intestinal cells from –D chicks exhibited an apparent increase in ^{45}Ca extrusion when exposed to 130 pM $1,25(OH)_2D_3$ in vitro, the effect of seco-steroid on various signal transduction pathways was assessed. As shown in Fig. 2, intestinal cells isolated from vitamin D-replete birds and loaded with fura-2 responded to exogenous seco-steroid with rapid oscillations in intracellular calcium. In contrast, cells isolated from –D chicks failed to respond to hormone in a similar fashion.

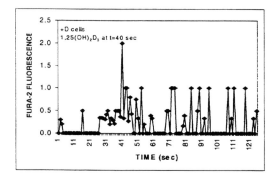 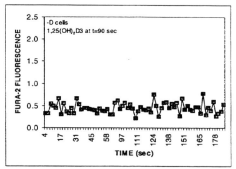

Fig. 2. Intestinal cells were isolated by chelation from +D (left panel) or –D (right panel) chicks, resuspended in PBS-BSA and loaded with fura-2 for 20 min on ice (3). Two hundred μl aliquots were placed in wells on microscope slides and monitored for basal fluorescence. At the indicated times, 130 pM $1,25(OH)_2D_3$ was added and fluorescence monitoring continued.

The activities of protein kinases C and A were also tested. Isolated intestinal cells from +D or –D chicks were incubated with vehicle or 130 pM hormone for either 5 min (PK C) or 7 min (PK A), centrifuged, and the cell pellets extracted. The extracts were tested for the ability to phosphorylate exogenous substrate (4). The results, presented in Fig. 3, indicate that $1,25(OH)_2D_3$ elicited a two-fold increase in PK C activity relative to corresponding vehicle controls, in cells isolated from either +D or –D chicks. In comparison, the hormone elicited an increase in PK A activity only in cells from +D chicks, but not from –D birds. The observation that PK A activity is not activated by seco-steroid in enterocytes of –D chicks compliments the earlier observations that $1,25(OH)_2D_3$ stimulates synthesis of adenylate cyclase in rachitic animals (5-7).

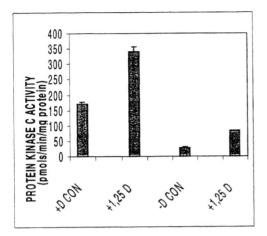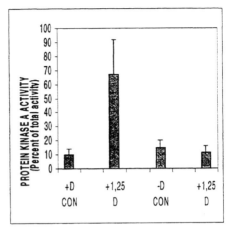

Fig. 3. Effect of vitamin D status on PK C and PK A specific activity in isolated cells treated with vehicle (CON) or 130 pM 1,25(OH)$_2$D$_3$. Enterocytes were prepared by chelation from vitamin D replete chicks (+D), or vitamin D-deficient chicks (-D), resuspended in Gey's balanced salt solution lacking bicarbonate, and incubated with the indicated additions for either 5 min (PK C) or 7 min (PK A) prior to extraction of cell pellets for enzyme analyses.

Effect of 24,25(OH)$_2$D$_3$. The metabolite 24,25(OH)$_2$D$_3$ is produced *in vivo* when 1,25(OH)$_2$D$_3$, calcium, and phosphate are sufficient. We therefore investigated whether 24,25(OH)$_2$D$_3$ production might represent an endocrine feedback loop to inhibit the rapid stimulatory action of 1,25(OH)$_2$D$_3$ on calcium (4) and phosphate transport in intestine. In the perfused duodenal loop system, vascular exposure to control media resulted in a calcium transport ratio (treated/average basal) of 1.07 ± 0.06 at t=40 min, while perfusion with 65, 130, 300, or 650 pm 1,25(OH)$_2$D$_3$ yielded ratios of 1.92 ± 0.23, 2.6 ± 0.4, 2.8 ± 0.08, and 3.34 ± 0.37, respectively. Simultaneous perfusion with each of these doses and 6.5 nM 24,25(OH)$_2$D$_3$ reduced t=40 min calcium transport ratios to ~1.4.

In phosphate transport studies, control media yielded a ratio of 1.00 ± 0.09 at t=40 min, while perfusion with 65, 130, 300, or 650 pm 1,25(OH)$_2$D$_3$ yielded ratios of 1.36 ± 0.13, 1.44 ± 0.06, 2.15 ± 0.21, and 1.14 ± 0.10, respectively. Simultaneous perfusion with each of these doses and 6.5 nM 24,25(OH)$_2$D$_3$ reduced t=40 min phosphate transport ratios to ~1.07. The combined observations may explain why rapid effects of 1,25(OH)$_2$D$_3$ are difficult to observe in vivo, as well as the observation that many 24-hydroxylase knockout mice are hypercalcemic (8).

Activation of both protein kinases C and A were observed with $1,25(OH)_2D_3$, and $24,25(OH)_2D_3$ suppressed activation of both protein kinases. However, forskolin (a PKA activator) failed to stimulate phosphate transport (in the absence of lumenal calcium), whereas perfusion with phorbol ester (a PKC activator) increased phosphate transport ratios to 3.47 ± 1.21 at t= 40 min. Thus, $24,25(OH)_2$ may suppress $1,25(OH)_2D_3$-stimulated calcium transport by inhibiting either PKC or PKA, whereas phosphate transport is mediated through PKC. Supported by NRICGP/USDA 98-35200-6466.

References

1. Nemere, I., Ray, R., McManus, W. (2000) Immunochemical studies on the putative plasmalemmal receptor for 1,25-dihydroxyvitamin D_3: I. chick intestine. *Am J Physiol* (in press)

2. Zhiheng, J. and Nemere, I. (1999) Immunochemical studies on the putative plasmalemmal receptor for 1,25-dihydroxyvitamin D_3: II. chick kidney and brain. *Steroids* 64: 541-550.

3. Nemere, I., and Campbell, K. (2000) Immunochemical studies on the plasmalemmal membrane receptor for 1,25-dihydroxyvitamin D_3: Effect of vitamin D status. *Steroids* (in press)

4. Nemere, I. (1999) 24,25-dihydroxyvitamin D_3 suppresses the rapid actions of 1,25-dihydroxyvitamin D_3 and parathyroid hormone in chick intestine. *J. Bone Mineral Res* 14:1543-1549.

5. Neville, E., and Holdsworth, E.S. (1969) A 'second messenger' for vitamin D. *FEBS Lett* 2: 313-15.

6. Walling, M.W., Brasitus, T.A., and Kimberg, D.V. (1967) Elevation of cyclic AMP levels and adenylate cyclase activity in duodenal mucosa from vitamin D-deficient rats by $1\alpha,25$-dihydroxycholecalciferol. *Endocr Res Commun* 3: 83-6.

7. Corradino, R.A. (1979) Embryonic chick intestine in organ culture: hydrocortisone and vitamin D-mediated processes. *Archs Biochem Biophys* 192: 302-10.

8. Jones, G., Strugnell, S.A., and DeLuca, H.F. (1998) Current understanding of the molecular actions of vitamin D. *Physiol. Rev.* 78: 1193-1231.

PROTEIN KINASE C α MODULATES THE 1,25(OH)$_2$-VITAMIN D$_3$-DEPENDENT Ca^{2+} RESPONSE AND PROLIFERATION OF SKELETAL MUSCLE CELLS

Daniela A. Capiati*†, Guillermo Vazquez*, María T. Tellez Iñón† and Ricardo L. Boland*‡

* Departamento de Biología, Bioquímica y Farmacia, Universidad Nacional del Sur. San Juan 670, 8000 Bahía Blanca, Argentina.
† Instituto de Investigaciones en Ingeniería Genética y Biología Molecular,CONICET. Vuelta de Obligado 2490, 1428 Buenos Aires, Argentina.

INTRODUCTION

Stimulation of chick skeletal muscle cells with 1α,25-dihydroxy-vitamin D$_3$ [1α,25(OH)$_2$D$_3$] triggers a rapid and sustained increase in cytosolic Ca^{2+} which depends upon Ca^{2+} mobilization from inner stores and extracellular Ca^{2+} influx (1-3). The role of individual protein kinase C (PKC) isoforms in the regulation of intracellular Ca^{2+} levels ([Ca^{2+}]$_i$) by the hormone was investigated in cultured proliferating (myoblasts) and differentiated (myotubes) chick skeletal muscle cells as well as their function in myoblast proliferation.

METHODS

Myoblasts were obtained from the breast muscle of 12-day-old chick embryos. Changes in intracellular Ca^{2+} concentration ([Ca^{2+}]$_i$) were monitored by using the Ca^{2+}-sensitive fluorescent dye Fura-2. Measurements were carried out on cell monolayers or individual cells. Western blot analysis were performed using antibodies against PKC isozymes. Treatment of muscle cells with anti-PKCα antibodies was carried out using saponin as membrane permeant. Antisense oligodeoxynucleotides against PKCα (5'-ATGGTPCCCCCCAACCACC-3', P=T or C) were incorpored into the cells by transfection using lipofectin (Gibco) or by nuclear microinjection. The rate of DNA synthesis was determined by [^{3}H]thymidine incorporation into DNA.

RESULTS AND DISCUSSION

1α,25(OH)$_2$D$_3$ (10^{-9} M) rapidly increased [Ca^{2+}]$_i$ in myoblasts and myotubes, an effect which was suppressed by the PKC inhibitor calphostin C (fig. 1A-D). The calcium response was greater in myotubes than in myoblasts. These effects were correlated to the translocation of the PKCα isoform from cytosol to the particulate fraction, which was more pronounced in differentiated cells (fig. 1E). No significant increase in the fraction associated to the particulate compartment was observed for PKC β, δ, ε and ζ (not shown).

Experiments were then carried out to corroborate the role of PKCα in the [Ca^{2+}]$_i$ response induced by the hormone. Specific inhibition of PKCα activity or expression using antibodies or antisense oligodeoxynucleotides against this isoform decreased the 1α,25(OH)$_2$D$_3$-induced [Ca^{2+}]$_i$ response associated to the Ca^{2+} influx phase (fig. 2 A and B), without affecting the early mobilization of the cation from inner stores.

732

The phospholipase C inhibitor neomycin was used to study the participation of phosphoinositide breakdown in the hormone activation of PKCα. Neomycin blocked $1\alpha,25(OH)_2D_3$ effects on $[Ca^{2+}]_i$, and translocation of PKCα (fig. 3 A and B). Besides, exposure of myotubes to the syntetic diacylglycerol, 1,2-dioleyl-rac-glycerol (1,2-diolein), increased $[Ca^{2+}]_i$ and the amount of PKCα associated to the particulate fraction (fig. 4 A and B), mimicking the effects of the hormone owed to the activation of phospholipase C. The effect on $[Ca^{2+}]_i$ was specific as it could not be triggered by the inactive derivate 1,3-diolein (not shown).

On the other hand, treatment of myoblasts with antisense oligodeoxynucleotides against PKCα reduced cell density and inhibited [³H]thymidine incorporation into DNA (fig. 4 A-C).

In conclusion, the present results indicate that in skeletal muscle cells $1\alpha,25(OH)_2D_3$ activates PKCα through the PLC pathway and that this isoenzyme is involved in both up-regulation of Ca^{2+} entry and in the signalling pathways mediating the sterol-dependent muscle cell proliferation.

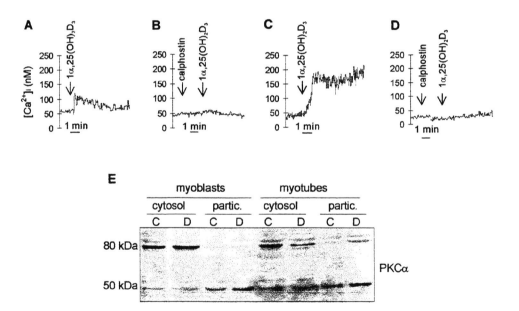

Figure 1. *Changes in intracellular Ca^{2+} levels ($[Ca^{2+}]_i$) and PKCα subcellular distribution induced by $1\alpha,25(OH)_2D_3$ in myoblasts and myotubes.* Cultured chick embryo myoblasts (**A** and **B**) and myotubes (**C** and **D**) were treated with 10^{-9} M $1\alpha,25(OH)_2D_3$ (arrow in **A** and **C**, right arrow in **B** and **D**) in the absence or presence of 100 nM calphostin (left arrow in **B** and **D**). ($[Ca^{2+}]_i$) was determined fluorimetrically. (**E**) Myoblasts and myotubes were treated with 10^{-9} M $1\alpha,25(OH)_2D_3$ for 5 min. The cytosolic and particulate fractions were isolated by differential centrifugation followed by Western blot analysis of PKCα.
C: control; D: $1\alpha,25(OH)_2D_3$.

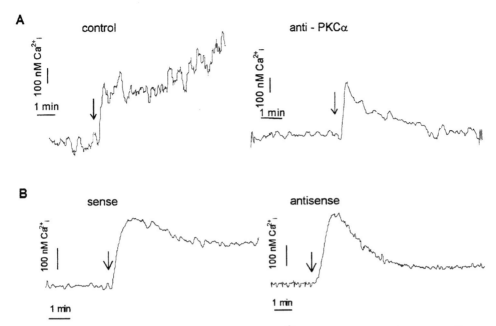

Figure 2. *Inhibition of 1α,25(OH)₂D₃-induced Ca²⁺ influx by antibodies or antisense oligonucleotides against PKCα.* Myotubes were treated with 25 µg/mL of anti-PKCα antibodies or normal rabbit serum (control) (**A**) or microinjected with antisense or sense oligodeoxynucleotides (**B**), loaded with Fura-2 and [Ca²⁺]ᵢ was measured fluorimetrically after treatment with 1α,25(OH)₂D₃ 10⁻⁸ M (arrow).

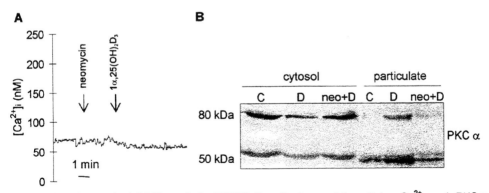

Figure 3. *Neomycin inhibition of 1α,25(OH)₂D₃ effects on intracellular Ca²⁺ and PKCα translocation in myotubes.* (**A**) Myotubes loaded with Fura-2 were treated with 500 µM neomycin (left arrowhead) for 3 min before addition of 10⁻⁹ M 1α,25(OH)₂D₃ (right arrowhead). (**B**) Myotubes were treated for 5 min with 10⁻⁹ M 1α,25(OH)₂D₃ in the absence and presence of 500 µM neomycin which was added 3 min prior to hormone treatment. Subcellular fractions were isolated and Western blot analysis of PKCα was performed. A representative time trace(**A**) and immunoblot (**B**) from 3 independent experiments are shown. C: control; D: 1α,25(OH)₂D₃; neo: neomycin.

734

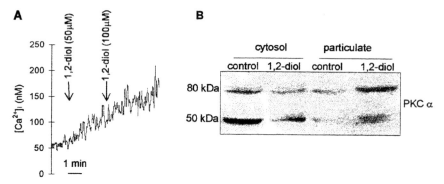

Figure 4. *Effects of diolein on intracellular Ca²⁺ and translocation of PKCα in myotubes.* (A) Myotubes loaded with Fura-2 were treated successively with 50 μM (left arrowhead) and 100 μM (right arrowhead) 1,2diolein (1,2-diol). [Ca²⁺]ᵢ was determined fluorimetrically. (B) Myotubes were incubated with 50 μM 1,2-diolein for 5 min. Subcellular fractions were isolated and Western blot analysis of PKCα was performed. Representative time trace recordings (A) and immunoblot (B) from 3 independent experiments are shown.

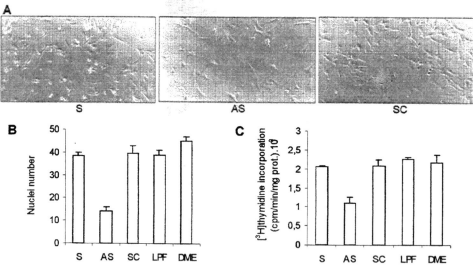

Figure 5. *Effect of inhibition of PKCα expression on myoblast proliferation.* 24 h-cultured chick embryo myoblasts were transfected with antisense-PKC α (AS), sense (S) or scrambled (SC) olideoxynucleotides. Treatments with Lipofectin (LPF) or DME medium (DME) only were carried out as controls. 48 h after transfection monolayers were photographed with a 10 X objective lens (A), the nuclei present in 40X fields were counted (B) and [³H]thymidine incorporation into DNA was determined (C). Results are the means ± S.D. from 3 independent experiments; p<0.005 for AS vs. S and AS vs. SC in **B** and **C**.

REFERENCES
(1) Morelli, S., De Boland, A. and Boland R. (1993) Biochem. J. 285, 675-679.
(2) Vazquez, G. and De Boland, A. (1996) Biochim. Biophys. Acta 1310, 157-162.
(3) Vazquez, G., de Boland A.R. and Boland, R. (1997) Biochem. Biophys. Res. Commun. 239, 562-565

CALCITRIOL-REGULATION OF IP$_3$ PRODUCTION IN SKELETAL MUSCLE AND INTESTINE FROM YOUNG AND AGED RATS.

M.M.Facchinetti and A.R. de Boland. Depto. Biologia, Bioquimica & Farmacia, Universidad Nacional del Sur. 8000 Bahia Blanca, Argentina. E-mail: aboland@criba.edu.ar

INTRODUCTION

Calcitriol [1,25-dihydroxyvitamin D$_3$], the major biologically active metabolite of Vitamin D$_3$, has a central role in the regulation of mineral metabolism. The mechanisms by which the signals provided by the hormone binding to the membrane putative VDR are transduced are not completely elucidated. However, the involvement of G proteins in calcitriol signal transduction has been evidenced (1). In a variety of cell types, including rat intestinal and skeletal muscle cells, calcitriol stimulates phosphoinositide hydrolysis resulting in the production of the second messengers inositol trisphosphate (IP$_3$, a Ca^{2+} mobilizer) and diacylglycerol (DAG, the endogenous activator of protein kinase C (PKC). Furthermore, in muscle and duodenal cells, as a consequence of DAG generation, the hormone rapidly activates PKC (2,3). Age-related alterations of calcitriol-signal transduction have been recently reported. In enterocytes and skeletal muscle isolated from aged rats, the transient production of IP$_3$ and DAG generated by the hormone decreased significantly (4,5). In addition, the stimulation of cAMP/protein kinase A-dependent calcium uptake by calcitriol in these cells is severely impaired with senescence. Moreover, age-related alterations of calcitriol-induced duodenal protein phosphorylation has been recently reported (6). In the present work we further examined age-related changes in the mechanism by which calcitriol stimulates IP$_3$ production in rat skeletal muscle and duodenum.

METHODS

Duodenal mucosae and back leg skeletal muscle were isolated from Wistar rats aged 3 and 24 months old (4,5), and the postmitochondrial fraction was obtained by centrifugation (15 min at 12,000 x g) and exposed to GTPγS (100 µM) or calcitriol (1 nM) in the presence or abscence of GDPβS (100 µM) for 15 s. To test the effects of Bordetella pertussis toxin (PTX) on calcitriol-induced IP$_3$ release, the samples were preincubated with PTX (100 ng/ml) for 30 min before treatment. When anti Gαi (1:200) and anti Gαq (1:200) antibodies were used, they were added to the samples together with 30 nM LiCl$_3$, and incubated for 10 min on ice, followed by hormone treatment. IP_3 was measured with a commercial radioreceptor kit (7). $G\alpha i$ and $G\alpha q$ protein levels were assayed in cells lysates using anti-$G\alpha i$ and $G\alpha q$ antibodies on a Western blot.

RESULTS AND DISCUSSION

In the present study we have further examined the effects of aging on calcitriol-induced IP_3 production in skeletal muscle and duodenum isolated from 3 and 24 month-old rats. The non-hydrolyzable analogue of GTP, GTPγS (100 μM, 15 s), known to lead to a permanent activation of G proteins, increased IP_3 from young rats to the same extent than 1 nM calcitriol (100 % over basal values). Similarly to calcitriol, the GTPγS response was diminished in the aged tissues. When GTPγS and calcitriol were added simultaneously, release of IP_3 was the same than with either agent alone . GDPβS (100 μM), a non-hydrolyzable GDP analogue suppressed calcitriol-dependent IP_3 release at 15 s without significant effects on basal values both in young and aged animals tissues. In rat duodenum, calcitriol-dependent IP_3 production was insensitive to Bordetella pertussis toxin (PTX), while in rat muscle, hormone effect is sensible to PTX. PTX catalyzes ADP-ribosylation of the α subunit of certain GTP-binding proteins including Gi and Go, and causes uncoupling of receptor from these GTP-binding proteins. Generally, receptor-induced stimulation of PLC has been shown to occur via PTX-insensitive $G\alpha q/11$ or via Gβγ from activated PTX-sensitive Gi. Since PLC-β isoforms are activated by G proteins, therefore, it is likely that in rat duodenum as in skeletal muscle, calcitriol activates a PLC-β, although a detailed characterization of PLC isoforms

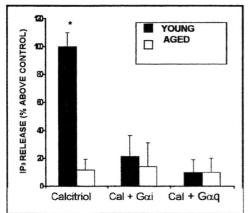 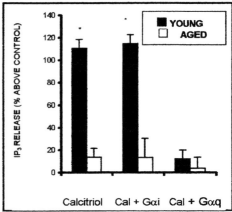

Effects of anti Gαi and anti Gαq antibodies on calcitriol-induced IP3 production

Fig. 1 *rat skeletal muscle.*   **Fig. 2** *rat duodenum*

involved is under current investigation. We then look for the specific G proteins that might be involved in calcitriol signalling. As shown in Fig. 1, in muscle form 3 month old rats, preincubation with anti Gαq or anti Gαi$_{1,2,3}$ antibodies inhibited calcitriol (1nM, 15 sec.)- induced IP$_3$ release.

Since antibodies against any Gα subunit could coimmunoprecipitate with the G$\beta\gamma$ subunits, our results suggest the involvement of the α subunit of Gq and the $\beta\gamma$ subunits of Gi in calcitriol stimulation of PLCβ in rat muscle. In the aged muscle the hormone response is mediated by Gαq, this is in agreement with a loss of calcitriol sensitivity to PTX and impaired activation of a Gi/Go protein coupled to PLC with ageing. In duodenum, only anti Gαq abolished calcitriol-induced IP$_3$ release, both in young and aged animals (Fig. 2). The efficiency of interaction between G-protein coupled receptors and heterotrimeric G proteins is greatly influenced by the absolute and relative amounts of these proteins in the plasma membrane. Changes in heterotrimeric G protein expression in rat muscle and duodenum with ageing, have not been previously described. Therefore, the amounts of immuno detectable Gαi and Gαq was determined with the use of specific antisera. Both antibodies recognized a major peptide band at 40 KDa. As shown in Fig. 3, at 3 months of age relative Gαq proteins levels were signifincantly greater in both skeletal muscle (+90%) and duodenum (+ 40%), as compared to 24 months old rats. Gαi protein expression was also reduced with ageing in both tissues (-50% and –25% in muscle and duodenum, respectively).

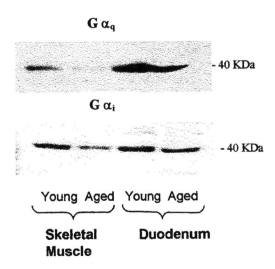

Fig. 3 *Gi and Gq protein levels in skeletal muscle and duodenum from young (3 months) and aged (24 months) rats.*

Therefore, a deficiency in G protein expression with ageing may have important consequences for correct receptor/effector coupling in the ageing tissues and may explain age-related declines in the function of second messenger systems linked to G proteins. Age-related decline changes in calcitriol receptor levels and occupancy status have been shown (8). These alterations, coupled with G-protein changes found with ageing, may combine to produce an impairment of PLC activity with advance age.

REFERENCES

1. Boland A.R. de, Flawia M., Coso O. And Boland R. (1991) Biochim. Biophys. Acta 1094, 238-242.
2. Facchinetti M.M. and Boland A.R. de. (1999) Cell. Signal. 11, 39-44.
3. Balogh, G; de Boland, A.R; Boland, R.(1997) Molec. and Cell. Endocrinology 129, 127-133.
4. Boland AR de, Facchinetti MM, Balogh G, Massheimer V and Boland R. (1996). Cell. Signal. 8, 153-157.
5. Facchinetti M.M., Boland R. and Boland A.R. de. (1998) Mol. Cell. Endocrinol. 136, 131-138.
6. Balogh GA and Boland AR de. (1999) Experimental Gerontology 34, 983-996.
7. Bredt DS, Mourey RJ, Snyder SH. (1989) Biochem Biophys Res Commun 159,76-82.
8. Takamoto S., Seino Y, Saktor B. And Liang CT. (1990) Biochim. Biophys. Acta 1034, 22-28.

PARATHYROID HORMONE ACTIVATES EXTRACELLULAR REGULATED KINASES (ERK1/2) IN RAT ENTEROCYTES.

C. Gentili, R. Boland and A.R. de Boland. Depto. Biologia, Bioquimica & Farmacia, Universidad Nacional del Sur. 8000 Bahia Blanca, Argentina. E-mail; aboland@criba.edu.ar

INTRODUCTION:

In rat duodenal cells, we have recently shown that parathyroid hormone (PTH) stimulates Ca^{2+} influx through the activation of dihydropyridine-sensitive calcium channels and activation of the adenylyl cyclase/cAMP and PLC/IP$_3$/DAG second messenger pathways (1,2) and that the the transient and biphasic production of IP$_3$ and DAG generated by PTH, is severely altered with ageing (2). Tyrosine phosphorylation of cellular proteins, controlled coordinately by tyrosine kinases and phosphatases, is a crucial event in signal transduction mechanisms linked to the mitogen-activated protein kinase (MAPK) cascade or extracellular regulated kinases (ERK1 and ERK2), underlying the regulation of cell proliferation and differentiation (3). Modulation of protein tyrosine phosphorylation in rat enterocytes by PTH and the influence of ageing thereupon have not been investigated yet. In the present work we study the effect of the N-terminal PTH-like region PTHrP (1-34) on protein tyrosine phosphorylation and ERK activation in enterocytes isolated from 3 and 24-months old rats.

METHODS:

Duodenal cells were isolated from Wistar rats aged 3 and 24 months old (1), and exposed to 10^{-11}-10^{-7} M PTH for 0.5-5 min. ERK1/2 phosphorylation was assayed in cells lysates using anti-active ERK1/2 antibodies on a Western blot as previously described (4). Src was immunoprecipitated with a specific anti-Src antibody, following by immunoblotting with anti-phosphotyrosine antibody.

RESULTS AND DISCUSSION:

As shown in Fig. 1, brief exposure of enterocytes from young rats (3 months) to 10^{-9} M PTH rapidly increased ERK1/2 phosphorylation (+3 fold, 1 min), but in aged animals (24 months) the response was greatly reduced (+ 0.5 fold). This age-related decline was observed within 0.5-5 min of hormone treatment. The PTH response was dose-dependent (10^{-11} M-10^{-7} M) with maximal stimulation achieved at 10^{-9} M. Hormone-induced ERK1/2 phosphorylation was effectively suppressed by the tyrosine-kinase inhibitors, genistein (100 μM) and herbimycin (2 μM) in both young and aged enterocytes. Moreover, the tyrosine phosphorylation and activation of ERK was dependent on the cytosolic Src kinase, since PP1 (10 and 20 μM), a specific Src family tyrosine-kinase inhibitor, blocked PTH action (Fig.2).

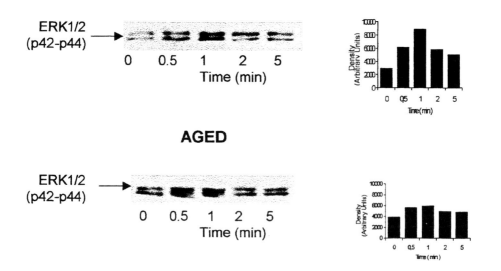

Fig.1 *Time course of PTH-induced ERK1 and ERK2 phosphorylation in rat enterocytes form young and aged rats. A representative immunoblot and its quantitation is shown*

Immunoblotting with anti-phosphotyrosine antibody of immunoprecipitated Src showed that the hormone activates Src decreasing its tyrosine phosphorylation state. With ageing, the response to PTH decreased signifincantly. However, the amount of basal protein expression determined by Western blot analysis for ERK was not different in the enterocytes from young and aged rats. The physiological significance of decreased MAPK tyrosine phosphorylation by PTH and its interrelationship to $1,25(OH)_2D_3$ in aged enterocytes remains to be determined.

In conclusion, the results obtained in this work expand our knowledge on the mechanism of action of PTH in duodenal cells, revealing that protein tyrosine phosphorylation is linked to PTH regulation of enterocyte ERK activation, and that this mechanism is impaired with ageing. Understanding the molecular mechanisms for the age-ralated differences in PTH signalling will require more information about the subtle mechanisms that modulate PTH receptor-ERK signaling pathway.

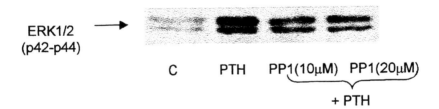

ERK1/2 (p42-p44)

C   PTH   PP1(10μM)   PP1(20μM)

\+ PTH

Fig.2 *PTH-dependent* ERK1 and ERK2 *phosphorylation Is suppressed by the specific cSrc inhibitor PP1.*

REFERENCES

1. Picotto G., Massheimer V., Boland R. (1997). Am. J. Physiol. 273, C1349-C1353.

2. Massheimer V., Picotto G. Boland R., de Boland A.R. (2000). J. Cell. Physiol. 182, 429-437.

3. Marshall CJ (1995). Cell 80, 179-185.

4. Boland AR de and Norman AW (1998) J. Cell. Biochem 69, 470-482.

INVOLVEMENT OF VITAMIN D RECEPTOR (VDR)-CONTAINING SUPRAMOLECULAR SIGNALING COMPLEXES IN 1,25(OH)$_2$D$_3$ REGULATION OF SOC INFLUX IN MUSCLE CELLS.

Graciela Santillán, Carolina Baldi, Guillermo Vazquez, Ana R. De Boland and Ricardo L. Boland. Depto. Biología, Bioquímica y Farmacia, Universidad Nacional del Sur. San Juan 670 (8000) Bahía Blanca, Argentina. (rboland@criba.edu.ar)

INTRODUCTION

Modulation of calcium homeostasis in skeletal muscle cells by the secosteroid hormone 1α,25-dihydroxy-vitamin-D$_3$ (1α,25(OH)$_2$D$_3$) is now a well established fact (1,2). This occurs by both a genomic action (long-term responses) which involves control of gene expression, and a non-genomic mechanism (rapid responses) implying direct membrane effects of the hormone through activation of diverse signaling systems (3). In avian (Gallus gallus) skeletal muscle cells the steroid exerts a fast regulation of Ca^{2+} influx by G-protein-dependent activation of both phospholipase C (PLC) and adenylyl cyclase, thus driving the activation of PKC, PKA, release of Ca^{2+} from intracellular stores and activation of voltage-dependent Ca^{2+} channels (VDCC) from the L-type. Examination of the action of 1,25(OH)$_2$D$_3$ on cytosolic Ca^{2+} ([Ca^{2+}]$_i$) levels in these cells shows that the cytosolic Ca^{2+} response to the hormone involves an initial rapid sterol-induced Ca^{2+} mobilization from IP$_3$/thapsigargin-sensitive stores, followed by cation influx from the outside accounting for a sustained Ca^{2+} phase. This Ca^{2+} influx pathway has been shown to be composed by both an L-type VDCC-mediated Ca^{2+} influx and a store operated Ca^{2+} entry (SOC) process (4, 5). Demonstration of the existence of such a SOC entry pathway introduced a novel feature into the mechanism of 1,25(OH)$_2$D$_3$ -induced Ca^{2+} influx across the plasma membrane of animal cells. In various mammalian cell types TRP proteins have been shown to function as channels mediating SOC influx. In the present work the presence of TRP and INAD proteins in avian muscle cells as well as their possible involvement in 1,25(OH)$_2$D$_3$ regulation of SOC influx was evaluated.

METHODS

Skeletal muscle cell culture, intracelluar Ca^{2+} measurements and immunoblotings were performed essentially as described in refs. 4 and 5. Molecular biology techniques were performed according to conventional protocols.

RESULTS

We recently reported functional evidence on the existence of a SOCE pathway in avian skeletal muscle cells and its modulation by 1,25(OH)$_2$D$_3$ (4). In agreement with these observations, a single band of 76 kDa was detected on lysates from chick (Gallus gallus) cultured muscle cells by using a specific anti-TRP antibody, suggesting that a TRP-like protein was expressed by these cells. In order to specifically address the involvement of such a TRP-like protein in the sterol-dependent SOC influx, an antisense oligonucleotide directed against a highly conserved region among all TRP proteins was microinjected in subconfluent muscle cells and the 1,25(OH)$_2$D$_3$-induced SOC influx was fluorimetrically monitored. As shown in Figure 1, the sterol-dependent SOC entry was inhibited by 60% respect to control, uninjected cells; moreover, a scrambled oligonucleotide was devoided of effect. By applying RT-PCR to total muscle cell RNA, four fragments of expected size were isolated, sharing more than 90% sequence homology respect to human

A 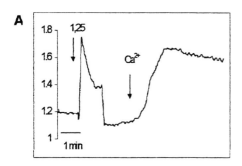   **B**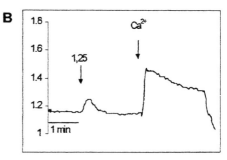

Figure 1:
Effect of anti-TRP antisense oligonucleotides on the 1,25(OH)$_2$D$_3$-dependent SOC influx in avian skeletal muscle cells. Cells were loaded with Fura-2 and [Ca]$_i$ was monitored in Ca^{2+} free medium. 1,25(OH)$_2$D$_3$ (10^{-8} M) stimulation and Ca^{2+} re-addition are indicated by arrows. A) Control, uninjected cells; B) Cells microinjected with an anti-TRP antisense oligonucleotide.

TRP3 mRNA (Santillán G. and Boland R., manuscript in preparation). In both invertebrate photoreceptor cells as well as some vertebrate systems, TRP proteins have been shown to interact with PDZ domain-containing proteins with adaptor function, from which INAD constitutes the best characterized one. Such interactions result in formation of supramolecular signaling complexes (signalplexes) which allow for a very fast and coordinated signal transduction process. When chick skeletal muscle cells were saponin-permeabilized in the presence of a specific anti-INAD antibody, the thapsigargin-dependent SOC influx was almost completely abolished, whereas permeabilization in the presence of normal rabbit IgG was without effect on the SOC entry pathway (Figure 2).

The nature of the non-genomic actions of $1\alpha,25(OH)_2D_3$, has led to the proposal that a putative cell surface receptor for the sterol is involved in the activation of signaling systems in muscle cells (2) as postulated for this and other steroids in various cell types. Up to date, the existence of such novel membrane receptor has been not conclusively demonstrated. Other lines of evidence have alternatively pointed to a role of the VDR itself in mediating some of the rapid, non-genomic effects of the hormone (6), with VDR oftenly forming part of signaling protein complexes. We found here that when muscle cell lysates are immunoprecipitated with either anti-TRP or anti-VDR antibodies under non-denaturing conditions, either VDR or TRP, respectively, coimmunoprecipitated, thus suggesting the existence of an association between these two proteins. Moreover, exposure of the cells to $1\alpha,25(OH)_2D_3$ significantly increased complex formation, indicating that such association could be playing a role into the mechanism by which the sterol modulates SOC entry into skeletal muscle cells.

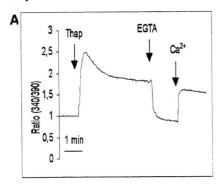
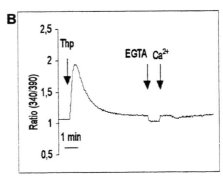

Figure2 :
Effect of an anti-INAD antibody on the thapsigargin-dependent SOC influx in avian skeletal muscle cells. Cells were permeabilized with saponin in the presence of either normal rabbit IgG (A) or anti-INAD antibody (B). The SOC influx dependent upon store depletion by thapsigargin, was fluorimetrically measured by the Ca^{2+}-readition protocol as in Figure 1.

CONCLUSION
In the present work we provide evidence for the existence of TRP-like proteins mediating $1,25(OH)_2D_3$ dependent SOC influx in avian skeletal muscle cells, sharing high homology with known mammalian TRP counterparts. The

association between TRP and VDR suggests the involvement of signaling complexes in the mechanism by which the sterol modulates Ca^{2+} entry, as is the case for several invertebrate and vertebrate cell types. In this context, preliminar evidence indicates that INAD-like proteins could be involved as putative adaptors within such signaling complexes.

REFERENCES
1. Boland, R. (1986) Endocr. Rev. 7, 434-448.
2. Boland, R., de Boland, A.R., Marinissen, M., Santillan, G., Vazquez, G., and Zanello, S. (1995) Mol. Cell. Endocrinol. 114, 1-8.
3. de Boland, A.R., and Boland, R. (1994) Cell. Signal. 6, 717-724.
4. Vazquez G., Boland A.R. de and Boland R. (1998) J. Biol. Chem 273, 33954-33960.
5. Vazquez G., Boland A.R. de and Boland R. (2000) J. Biol. Chem. 275, 16134-16138.
6. Buitrago C., Vazquez G., Boland A.R. de and Boland R. J. Cell. Biochem. (in press).

NON-GENOMIC REGULATION OF THE Ca^{2+} MESSENGER SYSTEM IN RAT DUODENAL CELLS BY 17ß-ESTRADIOL: POTENTIATION OF $1,25\alpha(OH)_2D_3$ ACTIONS AND EVIDENCE ON THE PRESENCE OF MEMBRANE-BOUND ESTROGEN RECEPTOR (ER)-LIKE PROTEINS

Gabriela Picotto, Paula Monje and Ricardo Boland, Departamento de Biología, Bioquímica y Farmacia, Universidad Nacional del Sur. 8000 Bahía Blanca, Argentina (rboland@criba.edu.ar)

Introduction:

It has been previously shown a rapid and direct modulation of Ca^{2+} influx in rat duodenal cells mediated by $1,25(OH)_2D_3$ [1] and 17ß-estradiol [2], through the activation of the cAMP [1,2] and the PLC [3,4] cascades and involving voltage-dependent calcium channels (VDCC). Either steroid also increases intracellular calcium concentration ($[Ca^{2+}]_i$) in fura-2 loaded enterocytes. The response pattern is characterized by an initial fast rise followed by a sustained phase [4]. In the present study experiments were designed to further determine whether the actions of $1,25(OH)_2D_3$ and 17ß-estradiol were due to Ca^{2+} mobilization from intracellular stores and/or to an influx of the cation from the extracellular medium, and to investigate differences between the hormones on the regulation of these pathways.

The existence of the classical estrogen receptor (ER) in the gastrointestinal tract has been reported [5]. The rapid and specific nature with which 17ß-estradiol exerts its action has led to hypothesize the existence of cell-surface resident ER (ERm) acting in membrane-linked events. This work also provides preliminary evidence of the presence of ERm-like proteins in rat duodenal epithelial cells.

Methods:

Rat duodenal cells were isolated from Wistar female rats (3-6 months) as previously described [2] and $[Ca^{2+}]_i$ was measured according to Grynkiewicz et al. [6]. For Western immunoblotting, microsomal membranes were obtained [7] and resolved on 8% SDS-PAGE. Proteins were then electroblotted onto PVDF membranes and incubated with anti-ER monoclonal antibody (12 h; 1:50). Antimouse horseradish peroxidase-conjugated was used as secondary antibody and proteins were visualized as previously described [8].

748

Results and Discussion:

Spectrofluorimetric analysis of rat enterocytes loaded with fura-2 using selective inhibitors (neomycin, U-73122, nitrendipine, EGTA) confirmed the activation by

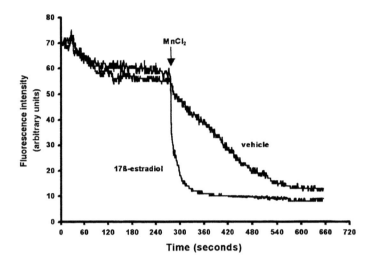

Figure 1: 17ß-estradiol-induced Mn^{2+} influx into rat duodenal cells.
Fura-2 loaded cells were treated with vehicle (ethanol<0.1%, control) or 17ß-estradiol (0.1 nM) in a Ca^{2+}-free extracellular medium. When [Ca^{2+}]$_i$ was stabilized, Mn^{2+} influx was initiated by addition of 1 mM MnCl$_2$ to the medium. Mn^{2+} quenching of fura-2 was determined at the Ca^{2+}-insensitive isosbestic point of the dye (360 nm excitation wavelength). After 5 min, maximal quenching (100%) at each condition was obtained by lysing the cells with 0.1% (v/v) Triton X100. Time-traces representative from 3 independent recordings are shown.

either steroid of both Ca^{2+} inner store mobilization and influx pathways previously reported (4). However, 17ß-estradiol stimulates, in addition to VDCC, Ca^{2+} influx through store-operated calcium (SOC) channels as evidenced by the inhibitory effects of Ni^{2+} and La^{3+}, selective blockers of SOC channels (not shown) and the increased permeability to Mn^{2+} detected measuring fura-2 fluorescence quenching (Fig. 1). 1,25(OH)$_2$D$_3$ did not stimulate Ca^{2+} influx through SOC channels in rat enterocytes (data not given). In agreement with these observations, sequential addition of 17ß-estradiol and 1,25(OH)$_2$D$_3$ to

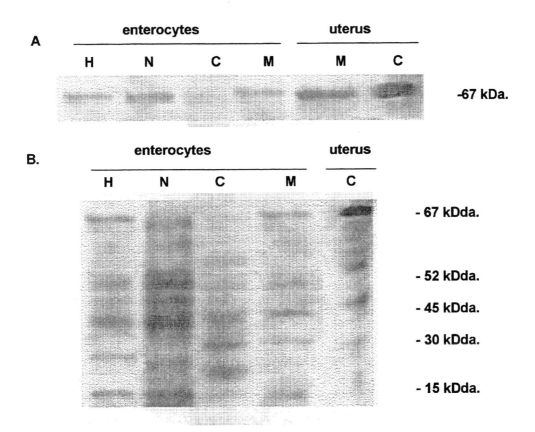

Figure 2: Comparison of western blot profiles from subcellular fractions using ER antibodies

Equal protein samples were treated as described in Methods. The antibody is directed to linear aminoacid sequences localized in the steroid binding domain. (Ab-10) **A**. Detection of the protein of 67 kDa. **B**. Detection of additional protein bands with lower molecular weight. (H: total fraction; N: nuclear fraction; C: cytosolic fraction; M: microsomal fraction). Uterus was included as control (9).

duodenal cells revealed additive effects (+60%) on the Ca^{2+} influx phase, confirming SOC influx activation as an alternative mechanism for 17ß-estradiol non-genomic regulation of Ca^{2+} entry in duodenal cells.

Preliminary evidences on the existence of ERm-like proteins acting as primary loci of these estrogen membrane-linked events were also obtained. As shown in Fig. 2, western blotting analysis using specific monoclonal antibodies against classic ER domains showed the presence of various immunoreactive proteins in the microsomal membrane, corresponding to the ER (67 kDa) and lower molecular weight (57 to 11 kDa). The participation of one or more of these proteins in the non-genomic effects of 17ß-estradiol on rat enterocytes was supported by the fact that the estrogen covalently linked to BSA induced an increase of intracellular Ca^{2+} concentration similar to the free hormone (not shown).

Conclusions:

17ß-estradiol and $1,25(OH)_2D_3$ increase $[Ca^{2+}]_i$ in rat duodenal cells through both intracellular Ca^{2+} release and VDCC Ca^{2+} influx. SOC channels also mediate the non-genomic actions of 17ß-estradiol. Estrogen effects on rat duodenal cells are possibly related to ER-like proteins residing at the cell surface.

References:

1) Massheimer, V., Boland, A.R. and Boland, R. (1994) Cell. Sign. 6, 299-304.
2) Picotto, G., Massheimer, V. and Boland, R. (1994) Mol. Cell. Endocrinol. 119, 129-134.
3) Boland, A.R., Facchinetti, M.M., Balogh, G. and Boland, R. (1996) Cell. Sign. 8, 153-157.
4) Picotto, G., Massheimer, V., Boland, A.R. and Boland, R. (1997) In: Vitamin D: Chemistry, Biology and Clinical Applications of the Steroid hormone (Norman, A.W., Bouillion, R. and Thomasset, M., eds.), pp 375-376.
5) Arjmandi, B.H., Salih, M.A., Damon, H.C., Sims, S.H. and Kalu, D.N. (1993) Bone Miner. 21, 63-74.
6) Grynkiewicz, G., Poenie, M. and Tsien, R. (1985) J. Biol. Chem. 260, 3440-3450.
7) Picotto, G, Massheimer, V. and Boland, R. (1997) Am. J. Physiol. 273, C1349-C1353.
8) Monje, P. and Boland, R. (1999) Mol. Cell. Endocrinol. 147, 75-84

BONE / CARTILAGE

THE MOLECULAR MECHANISM OF BONE RESORPRION BY VITAMIN D

Tatsuo Suda, Nobuyuki Udagawa, Toshimasa Shinki, Eijiro Jimi, Kanichiro Kobayashi, and Naoyuki Takahashi, Department of Biochemistry, School of Dentistry, Showa University, Hatanodai, Shinagawa-ku, Tokyo 142-8555, JAPAN

Introduction

It is well known that, in healthy humans and animals, serum calcium levels are tightly regulated from 9 to 10 mg/dl. Intestine, bone and kidney are the three major organs responsible for this calcium homeostasis. Vitamin D plays a major role in regulating serum calcium homeostasis together with parathyroid hormone and calcitonin. Physiological doses of vitamin D preferentially stimulate intestinal calcium absorption, which in turn stimulates bone mineralization. Whether vitamin D is directly involved in osteoblastic bone mineralization is still a matter of controversy, but the recent findings of VDR knockout mice suggest that the stimulating effect of vitamin D on bone mineralization is an indirect one through stimulation of intestinal absorption of calcium by this vitamin.

It appears to be paradoxical, but vitamin D functions in the process of calcium mobilization from calcified bone, making calcium available to the extracellular fluid upon demand by the calcium homeostatic system. It is now well established that $1\alpha,25$-dihydroxyvitamin D3 [$1\alpha,25(OH)_2D_3$] stimulates bone resorption, but the role of the vitamin in bone resorption was not known until quite recently.

In 1981, Abe et al. (1) discovered so-called cell differentiation-inducing activity of $1\alpha,25(OH)_2D_3$ using mouse and human myeloid leukemia cells. HL-60 is a promyelocytic leukemia cell line established from a leukemic patient, and it can be induced to differentiate into granulocytes by retinoic acid or monocyte-macrophages by $1\alpha,25(OH)_2D_3$. $1\alpha,25(OH)_2D_3$ was a potent and selective inducer of differentiation of HL-60 cells into macrophages (2). Furthermore, $1\alpha,25(OH)_2D_3$ directly induced fusion of macrophages at a very high rate (3). About 80% of the alveolar macrophages fused to form multinucleated giant cells within 3 days. From these results, we speculated that $1\alpha,25(OH)_2D_3$ is involved in osteoclast formation by stimulating differentiation and fusion of osteoclast progenitors. However, these multinucleated giant cells formed from alveolar macrophages were not osteoclasts, since they did not form any resorption pits on bone slices. We wanted to make multinucleated cells in vitro, which satisfy major criteria of osteoclasts.

Establishment of mouse co-culture system to examine osteoclastogenesis

It is well recognized that osteoclasts are derived from hemopoietic cells of the monocyte-macrophage lineage. We were interested in the phenomenon that hemopoietic monocytic cells are present in almost all tissues, whereas osteoclasts are present only in bone. This led us to speculate that some local factors or local mechanisms are involved in this tissue-specific localization of osteoclasts in bone. We paid special attention to the role of osteoblasts in osteoclast development, since osteoblasts are present only in bone. The process of osteoclast development consists of several steps: they are proliferation, differentiation, fusion, and activation of osteoclasts. We attempted to develop assay systems to examine each step of osteoclast development in vitro.

In 1988, we established an efficient mouse co-culture system to recruit osteoclasts (4). Osteoblastic cells were isolated from mouse calvaria, and spleen cells were used as osteoclast progenitors. They were either separately cultured or co-cultured together with or without $1\alpha,25(OH)_2D_3$. When osteoblastic cells alone or spleen cells alone were cultured, no osteoclasts were formed even in the presence of $1\alpha,25(OH)_2D_3$. Multinucleated osteoclasts were formed only when mouse spleen cells and osteoblastic cells were co-cultured in the presence of $1\alpha,25(OH)_2D_3$. Cell-cell contact between spleen cells and osteoblastic cells appeared important for osteoclast formation, since no osteoclasts were formed when spleen cells and osteoblastic cells were co-cultured but separated by a membrane filter even in the presence of $1\alpha,25(OH)_2D_3$. From these results, we hypothesized that the direct contact of spleen cells and osteoblastic cells is essential for osteoclast differentiation, suggesting the requirement of a membrane-associated factor for osteoclast formation. This is the key point of our strategy for osteoclast differentiation. Spleen cells represent osteoclast progenitors, in other words **"seeds"**, and osteoblastic cells represent supporting cells to provide a suitable microenvironment for osteoclast formation in bone, in other words **"farm"**. This hypothesis appeared to explain why osteoclasts are present only in bone.

After extensive studies, we found that not only $1\alpha,25(OH)_2D_3$ but also PTH, IL-1, PGE_2, IL-6, and IL-11 similarly stimulated osteoclast formation in mouse co-cultures (5). The target cells of these bone-resorbing factors were osteoblastic cells, but not hemopoietic osteoclast precursors. These three diverse signals appeared to stimulate osteoclast differentiation independently, since osteoclasts were present both in VDR-knockout mice and in gp130-knockout mice. In other words, there is redundancy in bone-resorbing factors to recruit osteoclasts. We proposed that osteoclast differentiation factor (**ODF**) is commonly induced on the plasma membrane of osteoblastic cells in response to these bone-resorbing factors (5). Osteoclast precursors having ODF receptor recognize ODF by cell-cell contact and differentiate into osteoclasts (**Fig. 1**). M-CSF appeared to play an important role in the proliferation and differentiation of osteoclast progenitors, since M-CSF deficient op/op mutant mice showed severe osteopetrosis with no bone marrow cavity.

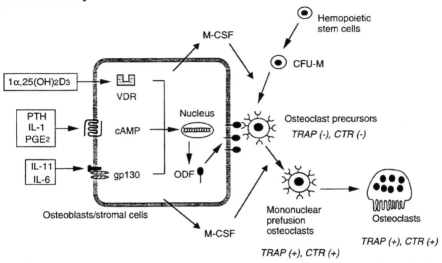

Figure 1: A hypothetical concept of osteoclast differentiation, proposing the requirement of a membrane-associated factor, ODF, in osteoblasts/stromal cells for osteoclastogenesis.

The molecular mechanisms of osteoclast formation and activation

In 1998, we finally succeeded in the molecular cloning of such a membrane-associated factor responsible for osteoclastogenesis (6). The Amgen group also succeeded in the molecular cloning of such a factor (7). Amgen named it OPG ligand (OPGL), which was identical to our ODF. All bone-resorbing factors like 1α,25(OH)2D3, PGE2, PTH, and IL-11 act on osteoblastic cells to induce ODF. ODF recognizes osteoclast progenitors having ODF receptor by a mechanism involving cell-cell contact. M-CSF is also an essential soluble factor for osteoclast differentiation which is produced by osteoblastic cells. Osteoclast progenitors differentiate into osteoclasts by binding to ODF. When OPG/OCIF (osteoprotegerin/osteoclastogenesis inhibitory factor) covers ODF, osteoclast progenitors having ODF receptor are unable to bind ODF, thus osteoclast formation is inhibited (**Fig. 2**) (6, 8).

The molecular cloning of ODF revealed that this molecule was identical to RANKL

(RANK ligand), TRANCE (TNF-related activation-induced cytokine) and OPGL (OPG ligand), all of which were independently identified by different research groups as a novel member of the TNF ligand family. TRANCE was cloned from a cDNA library of murine T cell hybridomas. RANK ligand (RANKL) was cloned from a cDNA library of human dendritic cells. OPG ligand (OPGL) was cloned from an expression vector of the murine myelomonocytic cell line 32D. Thus, ODF, OPGL, TRANCE and RANKL are the same molecule important for the development of T cells and dendritic cells as well as the development of osteoclasts. RANK which has been cloned as a receptor of RANK ligand (RANKL) is the transmembrane signaling receptor for ODF as well. OCIF/OPG is a soluble receptor for ODF and it appears to function as a decoy receptor **(Fig. 2)**. Standardization of nomenclature for new TNF receptor-ligand family members is needed, and it is now in progress at the ASBMR ad hoc committee chaired by Dr. Larry Riggs.

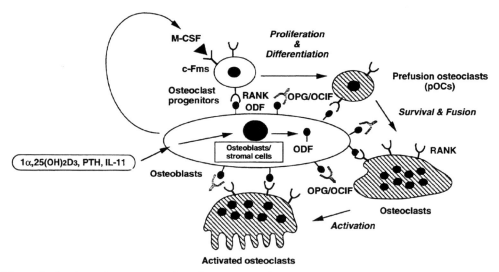

Figure 2: A schematic representation of osteoclast differentiation and activation supported by osteoblasts/stromal cells

ODF is involved not only in osteoclast differentiation but also in osteoclast activation. The lifetime of osteoclasts can be divided into three steps: the first step is proliferation and differentiation, the second step survival and fusion, and the third activation of osteoclasts. Proliferation and differentiation of osteoclasts essentially require ODF together with M-CSF. Survival and fusion of osteoclasts are induced by either ODF or M-CSF. Activation of osteoclasts is induced by ODF but not by M-CSF. Thus, ODF appears to be involved in the entire lifetime of osteoclasts **(Fig. 2)** (8).

Signaling system of ODF/RANK, TNFα and IL-1

The next question was to examine whether the ODF/RANK signaling system is also involved in inflammatory bone diseases such as periodontal diseases and rheumatoid arthritis. Two inflammatory cytokines, IL-1 and TNFα, appeared important in considering the pathogenesis of such inflammatory bone resorption. Recent studies have indicated that the cytoplasmic tail of ODF receptor (RANK) interacts with several TNF receptor-associated factors (TRAFs), TRAF 1, 2, 3, 5 and 6. Mapping of the structural requirement for TRAF/RANK interaction revealed that selective TRAF binding sites are clustered in two distinct domains in the RANK cytoplasmic tail. TRAF 6 interacts with the proximal domain of the cytoplasmic tail distinct from the binding sites for TRAF 1, 2, 3 and 5. TNFα induces its biological response through two cell surface receptors called TNF receptor type 1 and type 2. Both TNF receptor type 1 and type 2 bind TRAF 2. In contrast, IL-1 receptor binds TRAF6, but not TRAF2. The Amgen group reported that TRAF 6 knockout mice have many osteoclasts in bone tissues, but they are not capable of resorbing bone (9). Thus, TRAF 6 appears essential for osteoclast activation, but not for osteoclast differentiation. These results led us to examine if IL-1 directly acts on mature osteoclasts to induce bone resorption.

It has been reported that IL-1 induces its biological response through activation of nuclear factor kappa B (NFkB) in many types of cells. We have proved that mature osteoclasts possess both ODF receptor (RANK) and IL-1 receptor type 1. TRAF 6 appears to be a common signaling molecule for IL-1- and ODF-induced osteoclast activation. Treatment of purified osteoclasts with either IL-1 or ODF similarly and strongly activated NF-kB within 30 min (8). IL-1 receptor antagonist (IL-1ra) inhibited IL-1-induced NF-kB activation, but it did not inhibit ODF-induced NF-kB activation. In contrast, OPG/OCIF inhibited ODF-induced NF-kB activation, but it did not inhibit IL-1-induced NF-kB activation (8). Thus, it is concluded that the direct action of IL-1 on osteoclast activation occurs by a mechanism independent of the ODF-RANK interaction (8). It is also likely that ODF and IL-1 share a common intracellular signaling pathway for NF-kB activation via TRAF 6 in mature osteoclasts. How NF-kB induces ruffled border formation is not known at present.

In order to examine the role of TNFα in osteoclastogenesis, we prepared M-CSF-dependent bone marrow macrophages, which did not contain any appreciable amounts of stromal cells (10). These bone marrow Mφ were cultured for 3 days with bone-resorbing hormones or cytokines to examine osteoclast formation in the presence of M-CSF. Many TRAP-positive mononuclear and multinucleated cells were formed in response to mouse TNFα as well as ODF (10). Morphology of TRAP-positive cells induced by mouse TNFα was quite similar to that induced by ODF. Human TNFα induced only a small number of TRAP-positive mononuclear cells even at a high concentration of TNFα. This indicates the importance of both TNF receptor type 1 and type 2 for TNFα-induced osteoclastogenesis, since mouse TNFα binds both mouse TNF receptor type 1 and 2, but human TNFα binds only mouse TNF receptor type 1. Neither IL-1 nor 1α,25(OH)2D3 induced TRAP-positive cell formation in bone marrow Mφ cultures. This is due to the lack of osteoblastic stromal cells in this bone marrow macrophage preparation. These results show that, unlike IL-1 and 1α,25(OH)2D3, mouse TNFα directly acts on bone marrow macrophages to induce osteoclast differentiation via TNF receptor type 1 and 2, but not ODF receptor (RANK). Very recently, the Amgen group reported that ODF receptor (RANK) knockout mice showed severe osteopetrosis without any osteoclasts in bone. Administration of 1α,25(OH)2D3, PTH and IL-11 into RANK knockout mice did not induce osteoclasts at all, but TNFα did induce some osteoclasts. These in vivo results confirm that TNFα-induced osteoclast formation does not occur through RANK. Figure 3 summarizes schematic representation of the ligand-receptor systems for osteoclast differentiation and activation by TNFα, ODF/RANKL and IL-1.

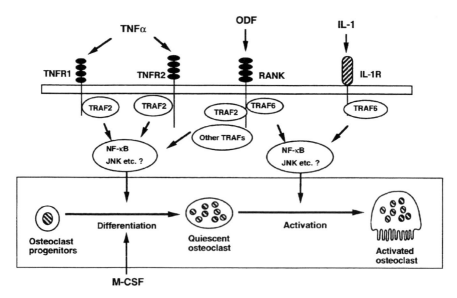

Figure 3: Schematic representation of the ligand-receptor systems in osteoclast differentiation and activation by TNFα, ODF/RANKL and IL-1. TNFα and IL-1 stimulate osteoclast differentiation and activation, respectively, by a mechanism independent of the ODF/RANKL-RANK interaction.

ODF-RANK dependent and independent pathways

These results indicate that there are two signalling pathways for osteoclast development. One is the ODF-RANK-dependent pathway, and the other is an independent pathway. Under physiological conditions, the ODF-RANK dependent pathway appears to play a major role in osteoclast differentiation and activation in the presence of M-CSF. In contrast, in pathological conditions such as rheumatoid arthritis, LPS-induced periodontitis and possibly postmenopausal osteoporosis, TNFα and IL-1 also appear to play a role in osteoclast differentiation and activation in the presence of M-CSF, which is independent of the ODF-RANK interaction. Thus, TNFα and IL-1 can be substituted for ODF in the whole processes of osteoclastic bone resorption. However, we do not know, at present, quantitative contribution of the ODF-independent pathway in pathological bone resorption. The cross-talk of the ODF-RANK-dependent and - independent pathways is also likely.

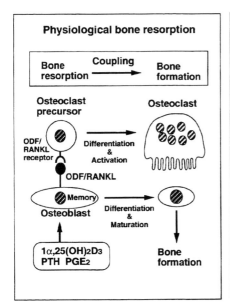
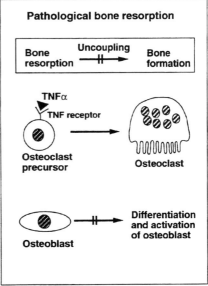

Figure 4: The biological significance of the involvement of osteoblasts in physiological bone resorption.

Under physiological conditions, osteoclast formation requires cell-cell contact with osteoblasts/stromal cells, which generates ODF/RANKL as a membrane-bound factor in response to several bone-resorbing factors. In normal bone remodeling, bone formation by osteoblasts always occurs in a programmed manner accurately and quantitatively just after bone resorption by osteoclasts. In contrast, in pathological bone resorption like in periodontitis and postmenopausal osteoporosis, cytokines such as TNFα directly act on osteoclast progenitors without cell-cell contact, which leads to an extensive bone loss with no new bone formation. Thus, it is attractive to speculate that cell-cell contact between osteoclast progenitors and osteoblasts/stromal cells may leave some memories for bone formation in osteoblasts/stromal cells **(Fig. 4)**. This possibility is currently under investigation in our laboratory.

The present study was undertaken in our laboratory in collaboration with the research groups of Snow Brand Milk Products in Japan headed by Dr. Higashio and of St. Vincent's Institute of Medical Research in Melbourne headed by Dr. T. John Martin.

References
1. Abe, E., Miyaura, C., Sakagami, H., Takeda, M., Konno, K., Yamazaki, Y., Yoshiki, S. and Suda, T. (1981) Proc. Natl. Acad. Sci. USA 78, 4990-4994.
2. Miyaura, C., Abe, E., Kuribayashi, T., Tanaka, H., Konno, K., Nishii, Y., and Suda, T. (1981) Biochem. Biophys. Res. Commun. 102, 937-943.
3. Abe, E., Miyaura, C., Tanaka, H., Shiina, Y., Kuribayashi, T., Suda, S., Nishii, Y., DeLuca, H.F. and Suda, T. (1983) Proc. Natl. Acad. Sci. USA 80, 5583-5587.
4. Takahashi, N., Akatsu, T., Udagawa, N., Sasaki, T., Yamaguchi, A., Moseley, J.M., Martin, T.J. and Suda, T. (1988) Endocrinology 123, 2600-2602.
5. Suda, T., Takahashi, N. and Martin, T.J. (1992) Endocri. Rev. 13, 66-80.
6. Yasuda, H., Shima, N., Nakagawa, N., Yamaguchi, K., Kinosaki, M., Mochizuki, S., Tomoyasu, A., Yano, K., Goto, M., Murakami, A., Tsuda, E., Morinaga, T., Higashio, K., Udagawa, N., Takahashi, N. and Suda, T. (1998) Proc. Natl. Acad. Sci. USA 95, 3597-3602.
7. Lacey, D.L., Timms, E., Tan, H.L., Kelley, M.J., Dunstan, C.R., Burgess, T., Elliott, R., Colombero, A., Elliott, G. and Scully, S. (1998) Cell 93, 165-176.
8. Suda, T., Takahashi, N., Udagawa, N., Jimi, E., Gillespie, M.T. and Martin, T.J. (1999) Endocrine Rev. 20, 345-357.
9. Lomaga, M.A., Yeh, W.C., Sarosi, I., Duncan, G.S., Furlonger, C., Ho, A., Morony, S., Capparelli, C., Van, G. and Kaufman, S. (1999) Genes Dev. 13, 1015-1024.
10. Kobayashi, K., Takahashi, N., Jimi, E., Udagawa, N., Takami, M., Kotake, S., Nakagawa, T., Higashio, K., Martin, T.J. and Suda, T. (2000) J. Exp. Med. 191, 275-285.

ACTIONS OF 1,25(OH)$_2$D$_3$ ON CALCIUM HOMEOSTASIS IN BONE CELLS

Wei Li and Mary C. Farach-Carson, Department of Biological Sciences, University of Delaware, Newark, DE, 19716 USA

Introduction Acting together, 1,25-dihydroxyvitamin D$_3$ (1,25(OH)$_2$D$_3$) and parathyroid hormone (PTH) serve as calcitropic hormones that regulate bone remodeling and systemic Ca^{2+} homeostasis. The osteoblast is an important target cell for calcitropic hormones, and expresses functional receptors for both PTH and 1,25(OH)$_2$D$_3$ (1). As shown in osteoblastic cell lines including ROS 17/2.8, 1,25(OH)$_2$D$_3$ activates rapid, plasma membrane-initiated and longer term nuclear receptor-mediated pathways via separate receptor systems (2). Activation of the plasma membrane signal transduction system by 1,25(OH)$_2$D$_3$ produces a number of measurable effects including activation of voltage sensitive calcium channels (VSCCs); electrophysiological studies have revealed that 1,25(OH)$_2$D$_3$ increases plasma membrane permeability to Ca^{2+} by shifting the threshold of activation toward the resting potential and prolonging the channel mean open time of L-type VSCCs present in osteoblastic cells within milliseconds (3). This "left shift" can be simulated by an analog of 1,25(OH)$_2$D$_3$ called AT (25-hydroxy-16-ene-23-yne-D$_3$) that lacks the 1-α-hydroxyl group considered to be essential for binding to the nuclear receptor (4). Analog AT, like 1,25(OH)$_2$D$_3$, also can enhance PTH-induced Ca^{2+} transients in osteoblastic cells by activating L-type VSCCs (5). Another analog, BT (1,24-dihydroxy-22-ene-24-cyclopropyl D$_3$ also known as MC 903 or calcipotriol) has vastly diminished ability to mobilize Ca^{2+} but binds well to the nuclear receptor and up-regulates expression of bone matrix proteins including osteopontin and osteocalcin (6). Based upon these observations, we proposed that these readily distinguishable activities of 1,25(OH)$_2$D$_3$ reflect a pharmacological distinction between the two classes of receptors for 1,25(OH)$_2$D$_3$, one nuclear and one in the plasma membrane (7).

A clinically important aspect of seco-steroid drug design lies in the potential to develop non-calcemic analogs of 1,25(OH)$_2$D$_3$ for replacement therapy. The availability of such compounds provides a novel means to deliver vitamin D-related compounds without producing hypercalcemia (8). *In vivo* studies have demonstrated the ability of at least two analogs, BT and another compound 22-oxacalcitriol or OCT, to replace 1,25(OH)$_2$D$_3$ and lower circulating PTH levels without elevating serum Ca^{2+} (9,10). Interestingly, both of these analogs bind well to nuclear receptors but do not mobilize intracellular Ca^{2+}. In this study, we used a cultured calvarial model to examine the mechanism by which 1,25(OH)$_2$D$_3$ analogs and 1,25(OH)$_2$D$_3$ interact with PTH to regulate Ca^{2+} release from bone. The results suggest a model in which the plasma membrane-initiated actions of 1,25(OH)$_2$D$_3$ are those associated with the tendency to induce hypercalcemia by stimulation of Ca^{2+} release from bone.

Materials and Methods

Materials

Timed pregnant rats (Sprague-Dawley) were purchased and delivered on days fourteen to sixteen of gestation. Bovine PTH (1-34) and other chemicals were purchased from Sigma Chemical (St. Louis, MO). 1,25(OH)$_2$D$_3$ was from Biomol Research Laboratories, Inc. (Plymouth Meeting, PA) and structural analogs AT and BT were kindly provided by Dr. Tony Norman (University of California at Riverside, Riverside, CA). 24 well plates were purchased from Corning, Inc. (Corning, N.Y.) and tissue culture medium was from Life Technologies, Inc. (Rockville, MD).

Labeling of calvaria in utero, calvarial culture and measurement of ^{45}Ca^{2+} release

All procedures were in accordance with IACUC approved procedures for animal care and use. On day 19 of gestation, timed pregnant rats were injected with 500 μCi of ^{45}Ca^{2+}. One day later, the female rat was sacrificed and fetuses (usually 12-15 per litter) harvested from uteri. Radiolabeled calvarial bones were dissected out, then cleaned free of blood and excess tissue. Pre-labeled rat calvaria were cut into approximately equal sized pieces, then weighed and individual calvarial pieces were cultured in 24-well dishes on a partially floating piece of Millipore filter near the surface in 0.5 ml of serum-free medium containing various combinations of reagents including 1,25(OH)$_2$D$_3$, analogs AT or BT, and PTH. The calvarial culture protocol was modified from earlier published techniques (11). Bone resorption was measured as the amount of ^{45}Ca^{2+} released into the incubation medium after various times of culture. Aliquots of medium were removed, counted and the dpm's released to the medium corrected for tissue weight in that well. All assays were performed in triplicate after which mean and standard deviations were calculated. Each table shown represents a complete series run in parallel with calvarial samples obtained from pups from one litter. Statistical significance was determined by ANOVA followed by a Tukey-Kramer multiple comparisons test using the InStat program (GraphPad, San Diego, CA). P values of >0.05 were considered not significant; p values <0.05 were considered significant; p values of <0.001 were considered extremely significant.

1,25(OH)$_2$D$_3$ and structural analogs

1,25(OH)$_2$D$_3$ and structural analogs AT and BT were stored as stock solutions in absolute ethanol in the dark at -20° C until use. The structural integrity and concentrations of the compounds were routinely monitored from the absorption spectra and by comparison of the absorbency ratio at 264/228 nm as described previously (12). Solutions with a ratio less than 1.6 were discarded.

Other Methods

Bovine PTH (1-34) was dissolved in distilled water and stored frozen in aliquots until use. All above reagents were stored at $-20°$ C. The delivery vehicle was used as a control in all experiments.

Results

Release of $^{45}Ca^{2+}$ from calvarial cultures requires co-stimulation with 1,25(OH)$_2$D$_3$ and PTH. Calvaria cultured over a 72 hr period remained viable. As reported in table 1, addition of PTH alone (0.2 μM) or 1,25(OH)$_2$D$_3$ alone (10 nM) had no significant effect on the amount of $^{45}Ca^{2+}$ release at 48 hr compared to control. A slight increase was observed in both treatment groups at 72 hr. In contrast, co-stimulation with 1,25(OH)$_2$D$_3$ and PTH significantly increased $^{45}Ca^{2+}$ release to the medium, an index of bone resorption (p<0.001 at both 48 and 72 hr). This increase was first detected at the 48 hr time point, and persisted through the 72 hr time point.

Table 1: *1,25(OH)$_2$D$_3$ and PTH together stimulate $^{45}Ca^{2+}$ release.* Pre-labeled rat calvarial samples were cultured as described in 0.5 ml of serum-free medium containing reagents as indicated. Bone resorption was measured as the dpm of $^{45}Ca^{2+}$ released (50 μl counted of 0.5 ml incubation medium) at various times of culture. As shown, the greatest amount of resorption ($^{45}Ca^{2+}$ release) occurred in the presence of both PTH and 1,25(OH)$_2$D$_3$ (10 nM). All values are the average of three individually cultured calvarial pieces.

Treatment\Time	0	24 hr	48 hr	72 hr
Control	230	370	360	360
PTH (0.2 μM)	240	360	350	500
1,25(OH)$_2$D$_3$ (10 nM)	240	370	380	470
PTH (0.2 μM) + 1,25(OH)$_2$D$_3$ (10 nM)	230	360	700	1020

Analog AT, but not analog BT, can augment PTH-induced $^{45}Ca^{2+}$ release from cultured calvaria. We next tested the ability of two classes of 1,25(OH)$_2$D$_3$ analogs to augment PTH-induced $^{45}Ca^{2+}$ release from pre-labeled bone in culture. These analogs were selected because they selectively activate either nuclear receptor-mediated (BT) or membrane-initiated Ca^{2+} mobilizing pathways (AT) in osteoblastic cells. As shown in table 2, neither analog AT nor BT alone stimulated $^{45}Ca^{2+}$ release beyond control levels at any time point (p>0.05 compared to control). In this experiment, PTH alone had no significant effect relative to vehicle control at either 24 or 48 hrs (p>0.05), but did have a modest but significant effect at the 72 hr time point (p<0.05). Addition of analog AT along with PTH consistently produced a statistically significant (p<0.001) stimulation of $^{45}Ca^{2+}$ release that occurred 24 hr earlier than that seen previously with $1,25(OH)_2D_3$. Comparison of the 24 hr time points for $1,25(OH)_2D_3$/PTH and AT/PTH in tables 1 and 2 demonstrates this accelerated $^{45}Ca^{2+}$ release. Analog BT did not produce this co-stimulatory effect when added with PTH (p>0.05). In neither case was the stimulation with analog as great as seen with $1,25(OH)_2D_3$ (table 1).

Table 2. *Analog AT, but not BT, co-stimulates PTH-induced $^{45}Ca^{2+}$ release.* Pre-labeled rat calvarial pieces were cultured as described in the text with the reagents added to the medium as indicated. Assessed by release of $^{45}Ca^{2+}$ as in table 1, the greatest stimulation of bone resorption occurred when analog AT and PTH were both present. When compared to release induced by $1,25(OH)_2D_3$ and PTH (table 1), release was faster in the presence of AT/PTH than $1,25(OH)_2D_3$/PTH. This is illustrated best by comparing the stimulation of release at 24 hr by AT/PTH but not until 48 hr by $1,25(OH)_2D_3$/PTH (compare tables 1 and 2). Analog BT did not stimulate release of $^{45}Ca^{2+}$. All values are the average of triplicate wells. Conclusions were based upon a multiple comparisons test.

Treatment\Time	0	24 hr	48 hr	72 hr
Control	230	390	380	300
Analog AT (10 nM)	210	300	300	270
Analog BT (10 nM)	220	320	310	280
PTH (0.2 μM)	230	400	420	410
AT (10 nM) + PTH (0.2 μM)	230	570	560	450
BT (10 nM) + PTH (0.2 μM)	220	310	300	250

Discussion

Addition of PTH to primary cultures of osteoblasts (13) or to clonal osteoblast-like osteosarcoma cell lines including ROS 17/2.8 and MC3T3-E1 (5,14) elicits a rapid, but transient, elevation of intracellular Ca^{2+} that appears to be generated by influx of Ca^{2+} through the plasma membrane. It has also been shown that $1,25(OH)_2D_3$ at low nM concentrations shifts the threshold of activation of inward calcium currents to more negative and physiological potentials and at same time leads to prolonged open time of individual channels (3). Interestingly, pretreatment with $1,25(OH)_2D_3$ for only 10 minutes can dramatically enhance the PTH-induced Ca^{2+} transient measured with fura-2 fluorescence (5). These data were interpreted to mean that $1,25(OH)_2D_3$ "primed" (i.e. left shifted) VSCCs are much more sensitive to depolarizing signals such as those initiated by PTH. This cooperativity between $1,25(OH)_2D_3$ and PTH at the membrane level occurs in addition to downstream coordinate regulation of osteoblastic gene expression (15).

Our laboratory and others have spent considerable effort to measure the ability of structural analogs of 1,25 $(OH)_2D_3$ to stimulate various aspects of target cell activation, including both nuclear receptor-mediated and plasma membrane-initiated events (2,16,17). It is clear that 1,25$(OH)_2D_3$ functions as the natural ligand for initiation of both long-term nuclear receptor-mediated and rapid membrane-initiated Ca^{2+} responses in osteoblastic cells. We developed *in vitro* assays to classify structural analogs of 1,25$(OH)_2D_3$ that are either "calcemic" (activate plasma membrane Ca^{2+} signaling events and may or may not be genomically active) or non-calcemic (do not stimulate Ca^{2+} influx). Analog AT activates plasma membrane VSCCs without binding to nuclear receptors, while analog BT binds to nuclear receptors for 1,25 $(OH)_2D_3$ without left shifting VSCCs or triggering Ca^{2+} influx (4,6).

In this study, we used a calvarial culture model to examine the interactions of 1,25$(OH)_2D_3$, analog AT, analog BT and PTH on one parameter of systemic Ca^{2+} homeostasis, namely Ca^{2+} release from bone. An advantage of this approach was the ability to examine mechanism in a more natural model system containing both bone- forming osteoblasts and bone-resorbing osteoclasts. The results indicated that 1,25$(OH)_2D_3$ and the Ca^{2+}-mobilizing analog, AT, enhanced PTH-stimulated bone resorption in organ culture. 1,25$(OH)_2D_3$ along with PTH produced a greater level of stimulation than did analog AT along with PTH (compare tables 1 and 2). In contrast to previous findings (18), little stimulation of Ca^{2+} release was seen following addition of 1,25$(OH)_2D_3$ in the absence of PTH. The nuclear receptor-activating analog, BT, did not enhance the rate of Ca^{2+} release alone or with PTH. A final observation was that the purely Ca^{2+}-mobilizing analog AT actually accelerated release of $^{45}Ca^{2+}$ from bone compared to 1,25$(OH)_2D_3$, a finding that was unexpected. Taken together, a logical interpretation of these findings is that the Ca^{2+}-mobilizing activity of 1,25$(OH)_2D_3$, not its nuclear receptor binding properties, may be responsible for the co-activation of bone resorption by 1,25$(OH)_2D_3$/PTH. The majority of the available data indicates that this occurs through signaling in the osteoblast where receptors for both hormones clearly reside. These data provide a rationale for the notion that therapeutic analogs of 1,25$(OH)_2D_3$ that lack calcium mobilizing activity might not produce hypercalcemia during long term use.

Acknowledgements This work was supported by a grant from the NIDCR RO1 DE12641 (to MCF-C).

References

1. Marks, Jr. S. C. and S.N. Popoff. (1988) Am. J. Anat. 183: 1-44.

2. Farach-Carson, M.C. and A.L. Ridall. (1998) Am. J. Kidney Disease 31(4): 729-742.
3. Caffrey, J.M. and M.C. Farach-Carson. (1989) J. Biol. Chem. 264: 20265-74.
4. Yukihiro, S., G.H. Posner and S.E. Guggino. (1994) J. Biol. Chem. 269: 23889-93.
5. Li W., R. L. Duncan, N. J. Karin and M.C. Farach-Carson. (1997) Am. J. Physiol. 273: (Endocrin. Metab. 36) E599-E605
6. Khoury, R., A.L. Ridall, A.W. Norman and M.C. Farach-Carson. (1994) Endocrinol. 135(6): 2446-2453.
7. Farach-Carson, M.C. and R.E. Devoll. (1995) NIPS 10: 198-204.
8. Jones, G., D.B. Hogan, E. Yendt and D.A. Hanley. (1996) CMAJ 155(7): 955-961.
9. Abe, J., T. Nakano, Y. Nishii, T. Matsumoto, E. Ogata, and K. Ikeda. (1991) Endocrinol. 129(2): 832-837.
10. Binderup, L. and E. Bramm. (1988) Biochem. Pharmacol. 37(5): 889-895.
11. Raisz, L. G. (1963) Nature 197: 1015-1016.
12. Farach-Carson, M.C., I. Sergeev and A.W. Norman. (1991) Endocrinol. 139: 1876-1884.
13. Wiltink, A. and M.P. Bos. (1995) Cell Calcium 17(4): 270-278.
14. Donahue, H.J., E.F. Fryer, E.F. Eriksen and H. Heath. (1988) J. Biol. Chem. 263: 13533-13527.
15. Segaert S. and R. Bouillon. (1998) Curr. Opin. Clin. Nutr. Metab. Care 1(4): 347-54.
16. Bouillon, R., W.H. Okamura and A.W. Norman. (1995) Endocrine Rev. 16: 200-257.
17. Slatopolsky, E., A. Dusso and A. Brown. (1999) Kidney Int. Suppl. 73: S46-51.
18. Raisz, L.G., B.E. Kream, M.D. Smith and H.A. Simmons. (1980) Calcif. Tissue Int. 32(2): 135-138.

DEFICIENT MINERALIZATION OF INTRAMEMBRANOUS BONE IN CYP24-K.O. MICE IS DUE TO ELEVATED $1\alpha,25(OH)_2D_3$ AND NOT TO THE ABSENCE OF $24,25(OH)_2D_3$

René St-Arnaud, Alice Arabian, Chantal Mathieu*, Marie B. Demay† and Francis H. Glorieux, Genetics Unit, Shriners Hospital, Montreal (Quebec) H3G 1A6
*Laboratorium voor experimentele geneeskunde en endocrinologie, Catholic University of Leuven, B-3000 Leuven, Belgium
†Endocrine Unit, Massachusetts General Hospital, Harvard Medical School, Boston, MA 02114

Introduction The maintenance of calcium homeostasis is critical for mammals. The primary endocrine system regulating circulating calcium concentrations involves vitamin D and parathyroid hormone (PTH). The active metabolite of vitamin D_3, $1\alpha,25(OH)_2D_3$, is responsible for intestinal calcium and phosphorus absorption, mobilization of calcium from bone, and renal reabsorption of calcium and phosphorus (1). To maintain mineral homeostasis, both the production and degradation of $1\alpha,25(OH)_2D_3$ need to be tightly regulated. While PTH increases the transcription of the enzyme 25-hydroxyvitamin D-1α-hydroxylase (1α-hydroxylase), $1\alpha,25(OH)_2D_3$ suppresses PTH release and inhibits 1α-hydroxylase mRNA production in a classic negative feedback loop (1). To provide even greater control, the $1\alpha,25(OH)_2D_3$ hormone induces the expression of the gene involved in its catabolic breakdown: 25-hydroxyvitamin D-24-hydroxylase (CYP24) (2).

CYP24 acts on the $1\alpha,25(OH)_2D_3$ substrate to produce 1,24,25-trihydroxyvitamin D_3, the initial reactant in the 24-oxidation pathway that leads to metabolite inactivation (3). When CYP24 utilizes 25-hydroxyvitamin D_3 as a substrate, $24,25(OH)_2D_3$ is produced. Synthesis of $24,25(OH)_2D_3$ may be viewed as a mechanism to inactivate circulating 25-hydroxyvitamin D_3 and thus regulate production of $1\alpha,25(OH)_2D_3$. In this view, $24,25(OH)_2D_3$ is considered a catabolite of 25-hydroxyvitamin D_3. Support for the notion that the $24,25(OH)_2D_3$ molecule has little biological function came primarily from experiments utilizing analogs of vitamin D fluorinated at position 24 (thus preventing further hydroxylation at that position). When these analogs were used as the sole source of vitamin D, they produced the same biological responses as those resulting from 25-hydroxyvitamim D_3 with respect to intestinal calcium transport, mobilization of calcium from bone, and mineralization of vitamin D-deficient bone (4,5).

An extensive literature challenges this view. The development of vitamin D-deficient chick embryos is impaired, and normal development and egg hatchability requires both $1\alpha,25(OH)_2D_3$ and $24,25(OH)_2D_3$ (6). Growth plate chondrocytes respond to $24,25(OH)_2D_3$ in a cell maturation-dependent fashion (7). Treatment with high doses of $24,25(OH)_2D_3$ increases bone mass in vitamin D-replete rats, rabbits, and dogs (8). Finally, recent results support a role of physiological concentrations of $24,25(OH)_2D_3$ as an essential vitamin D metabolite for fracture repair (9,10).

We have inactivated the CYP24 gene in mice to examine the physiological role of the CYP24 enzyme and address the putative role of $24,25(OH)_2D_3$. Our results confirm the role of CYP24 in the regulation of vitamin D_3 homeostasis. The survival of some CYP24 mutant animals to adulthood has also allowed us to breed them and study the effect of perturbing vitamin D metabolism during development. Bone development is abnormal in homozygous mutants born of homozygous females. Crossing the CYP24-deficient animals with mice carrying an inactivating mutation of the vitamin D receptor gene (VDR) (11) rescued the bone phenotype, providing genetic evidence that expression of the VDR is necessary for the manifestation of the impaired mineralization phenotype of the CYP24-deficient mice. These results show that elevated $1\alpha,25(OH)_2D$ levels during gestation affect mineralization and reveal that impaired vitamin D metabolism during development perturbs bone mineralization.

Results The CYP24 gene was mutated by homologous recombination in embryonic stem cells. The targeting vector was constructed by inserting the

PGK-neo selection cassette in place of exons 9 and 10, effectively removing the heme binding domain of the cytochrome P450 molecule and generating a null allele. In mice homozygous for the engineered mutation, no CYP24 mRNA or circulating $24,25(OH)_2D_3$ could be detected (12).

Genotyping of live animals around the time of weaning demonstrated that 50% of homozygous mutant animals died before 3 weeks of age (Table 1).

Table 1: incomplete penetrance of the perinatal lethality phenotype in CYP24-null mice

Number of -/-	Alive at weaning	Dead at weaning
578	274	304
	(47%)	(53%)

Somewhat surprisingly, baseline circulating levels of $1\alpha,25(OH)_2D_3$ were lower in CYP24 mutant animals that survived past weaning than in wild-type controls (Fig.1).

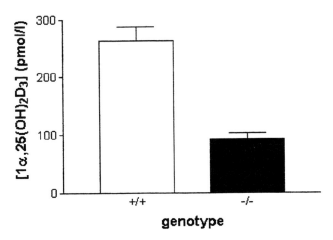

Figure 1: steady-state circulating levels of $1\alpha,25(OH)_2D_3$ in CYP24-deficient mice. $1\alpha,25(OH)_2D_3$ concentrations were measured from serum or plasma samples using a specific radioimmunoassay (ImmunoDiagnostic Systems Ltd., Boldon, UK). Results are expressed as mean ± SEM, n=10.

The perinatal lethality is most likely a consequence of hypercalcemia secondary to hypervitaminosis as the inactivation of the CYP24 gene in mice impaired the ability of the animals to maintain $1\alpha,25(OH)_2D_3$ homeostasis (12). We have also measured the clearance and metabolism of labeled $1\alpha,25(OH)_2D_3$ in CYP24 mutant mice and heterozygote controls. These experiments have shown that CYP24-null mice have a greatly reduced ability to clear a bolus of $1\alpha,25(OH)_2D_3$ from their body and convert it to water-soluble catabolites. Surprisingly, CYP24-null mice appear to lack 24-hydroxylated metabolites but also $1\alpha,25(OH)_2D$-26,23-lactone, supporting the view that the CYP24 enzyme is also responsible for hydroxylating $1\alpha,25(OH)_2D_3$ at C-23 and C-26 (13,14).

Since the antimicrobial action of macrophages can be modulated by vitamin D metabolites (15), we also examined macrophage function to determine if impaired responses to infection could be responsible for perinatal death. No abnormalities in macrophage function were detected in CYP24 mice (Table 2). Both markers for chemotaxis were present in comparable levels between homozygote mutant and wild-type mice. Phagocytosis ability, measured as capacity to ingest Zymosan particles, was also normal in CYP24 -/- mice.

Table 2: macrophage function in CYP24-mutant mice

	+/-	-/-
phagocytosis	64 ± 9	62 ± 7
chemotaxis: casein	22 ± 9	20 ± 8
chemotaxis: FNLPNTL	70 ± 21	65 ± 12

peritoneal macrophages were tested for phagocytosis using fluorescein-labeled Zymosan particles and for chemotaxis using fluorescein-labeled casein or formyl-Nle-Leu-Phe-Nle-Tyr-Lys (FNLPNTL). Results are expressed as percent fluorescein positive cells.

Fifty percent of homozygote mutant animals survived to adulthood and were fertile, which has allowed us to breed them and examine the effect of a complete lack of CYP24 activity during development. Bone development is abnormal in homozygous mutants born of homozygous females (12). Histological examination of the bones from these animals revealed an accumulation of osteoid at sites of intramembranous ossification. Control heterozygote littermates showed normal bone structure (12). Pregnant CYP24-deficient females showed elevated circulating levels of $1\alpha,25(OH)_2D_3$ (12), leading to hypercalcemia and hypercalciuria (Fig. 2). Although $1\alpha,25(OH)_2D_3$ does not readily cross the placenta (16,17), it is likely that very high maternal circulating levels would lead to increased fetal $1\alpha,25(OH)_2D_3$ concentrations.

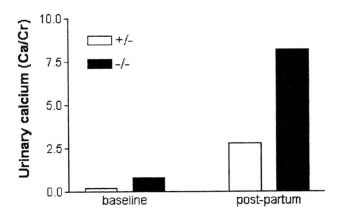

Figure 2: calciuria in gestating CYP24-deficient dams. Urine was collected from homozygote mutant and heterozygote control littermates prior to gestation, and after delivery. Urinary calcium levels were quantified using a Monarch automated system.

To examine the possible contribution of the elevated levels of $1\alpha,25(OH)_2D_3$ measured during gestation (12) to the abnormal bone phenotype, we crossed the CYP24-deficient animals with mice carrying an inactivating mutation of the vitamin D receptor gene (11). If elevated $1\alpha,25(OH)_2D_3$ levels, acting through the VDR, were responsible for the observed phenotype, then mice lacking the VDR and the CYP24 gene should not show the aberrant intramembranous bone development. Compound mutant homozygotes (CYP24 -/- and VDR -/-) showed normal intramembranous bone formation at all sites examined (ref. (12) and data not shown). Thus expression of the VDR is necessary for the manifestation of the impaired mineralization phenotype of the CYP24-deficient animals and that elevated $1\alpha,25(OH)_2D_3$ levels during gestation affect mineralization.

Discussion The role of the CYP24 enzyme in the catabolism of $1\alpha,25(OH)_2D_3$ had already been demonstrated in tissue culture (18). Our results confirm the function of the CYP24 protein as an effector of $1\alpha,25(OH)_2D_3$ breakdown in vivo. Unexpectedly, baseline circulating levels of $1\alpha,25(OH)_2D_3$ were lower in CYP24 mutant animals that survived past weaning than in wild-type controls, but CYP24-null mice have a reduced ability to clear a bolus of $1\alpha,25(OH)_2D_3$ from their body and convert it to water-soluble catabolites (12). These surprising findings suggest that the CYP24-null survivors adapt to the impaired vitamin D catabolism not by using an alternative catabolic route, but by limiting the synthesis of the active compound. We will test this hypothesis by measuring the expression of the 1α-hydroxylase gene in -/- mutants and +/- controls using RT-PCR.

CYP24-deficient pups born from CYP24 mutant females have impaired bone mineralization (12), showing that the complete absence of CYP24 activity during development leads to abnormal bone structure. Crossing the CYP24-deficient animals to VDR-ablated mice totally rescued the bone phenotype, confirming that the elevated $1\alpha,25(OH)_2D_3$ levels, acting through the VDR, were responsible for the observed accumulation of osteoid. Chronic treatment of rats with high doses of $1\alpha,25(OH)_2D_3$ perturbs mineralization, leading to accumulation of osteoid at the endosteal surface of long bones as well as in bone trabeculae (19,20). These sites are mostly normal in CYP24 mutant animals (12), but the differences may reflect variations in pre- versus post-natal responses. At any rate, our results demonstrate the need for controlled $1\alpha,25(OH)_2D_3$ homeostasis during intramembranous bone formation and suggest that $1\alpha,25(OH)_2D_3$ may have a different role in intramembranous versus endochondral bone.

References

1. Heany, R. P. (1997) in *vitamin D* (Feldman, D., Glorieux, F. H., and Pike, J. W., eds), pp. 485-498, Academic Press, SanDiego

2. Omdahl, J., and May, B. (1997) in *vitamin D* (Feldman, D., Glorieux, F. H., and Pike, J. W., eds), pp. 69-86, Academic Press, SanDiego

3. Makin, G., Lohnes, D., Byford, V., Ray, R., and Jones, G. (1989) *Biochem J* **262**(1), 173-80

4. Jarnagin, K., Brommage, R., DeLuca, H. F., Yamada, S., and Takayama, H. (1983) *Am J Physiol* **244**(3), E290-7

5. Parfitt, A. M., Mathews, C. H., Brommage, R., Jarnagin, K., and DeLuca, H. F. (1984) *J Clin Invest* **73**(2), 576-86

6. Henry, H. L., and Norman, A. W. (1978) *Science* **201**(4358), 835-7

7. Boyan, B. D., Dean, D. D., Sylvia, V. L., and Schwartz, Z. (1997) in *vitamin D* (Feldman, D., Glorieux, F. H., and Pike, J. W., eds), pp. 395-422, Academic Press, SanDiego

8. Tanaka, H., and Seino, Y. (1997) in *vitamin D* (Feldman, D., Glorieux, F. H., and Pike, J. W., eds), pp. 305-312, Academic Press, SanDiego

9. Seo, E. G., Einhorn, T. A., and Norman, A. W. (1997) *Endocrinology* **138**(9), 3864-72

10. Seo, E. G., and Norman, A. W. (1997) *J Bone Miner Res* **12**(4), 598-606

11. Li, Y. C., Pirro, A. E., Amling, M., Delling, G., Baron, R., Bronson, R., and Demay, M. B. (1997) *Proc Natl Acad Sci U S A* **94**(18), 9831-5

12. St-Arnaud, R., Arabian, A., Travers, R., Barletta, F., Raval-Pandya, M., Chapin, K., Depovere, J., Mathieu, C., Christakos, S., Demay, M. B., and Glorieux, F. H. (2000) *Endocrinology* **141,** in press

13. Miyamoto, Y., Shinki, T., Yamamoto, K., Ohyama, Y., Iwasaki, H., Hosotani, R., Kasama, T., Takayama, H., Yamada, S., and Suda, T. (1997) *J Biol Chem* **272**(22), 14115-9

14. Beckman, M. J., Tadikonda, P., Werner, E., Prahl, J., Yamada, S., and DeLuca, H. F. (1996) *Biochemistry* **35**(25), 8465-72

15. Rook, G. A., Taverne, J., Leveton, C., and Steele, J. (1987) *Immunology* **62**(2), 229-34

16. Noff, D., and Edelstein, S. (1978) *Horm Res* **9**(5), 292-300

17. Kovacs, C. S., and Kronenberg, H. M. (1997) *Endocr Rev* **18**(6), 832-72

18. Reinhardt, T. A., and Horst, R. L. (1989) *Arch Biochem Biophys* **272**(2), 459-65

19. Hock, J. M., Kream, B. E., and Raisz, L. G. (1982) *Calcif Tissue Int* **34**(4), 347-51

20. Hock, J. M., Gunness-Hey, M., Poser, J., Olson, H., Bell, N. H., and Raisz, L. G. (1986) *Calcif Tissue Int* **38**(2), 79-86

THE EFFECT OF 24,25-DIHYDROXYVITAMIN D$_3$ TO VITAMIN D RECEPTOR GENE KNOCKOUT MICE.

KEIKO KINUTA, HIROYUKI TANAKA, MAYU SHINOHARA, SHIGEAKI KATO and YOSHIKI SEINO

Department of Pediatrics, Okayama University Medical School, Okayama, 700-8558, Japan and Institute of Molecular and Cellular Biosciences, The University of Tokyo, Tokyo, 113-0032, Japan.

Introduction

Many investigators including us have suggested the unique actions and unique signal transduction systems of 24,25-dihydroxyvitain D$_3$ [24,25(OH)$_2$D$_3$]. We have previously reported that 24,25(OH)$_2$D$_3$ had unique bone forming activity in hypophosphatemic (Hyp) mice, a murine model for familial X-linked hypophosphatemic rickets (1,2). However, the unique biological actions of 24,25(OH)$_2$D$_3$ are still controversial. For the solution of this controversy, we need to identify unique signal transductin systems such as 24,25(OH)$_2$D$_3$ specific receptor or to identify the action of the 24,25(OH)$_2$D$_3$ without vitamin D receptor (VDR). Using vitamin D receptor knockout mice (VDRKO), we investigated the bone forming ability of 24,25(OH)$_2$D$_3$.

Methods

VDRKO were generated by gene targeting as described previously (3). Mice were weaned at 3 weeks of age, and were then fed a chow diet, MF (Ca, 11.1 mg/g; P, 8.3 mg/g; vitamin D$_3$, 1.08 IU/g). The mice were administrated doses of 10,100,1000 µg/kg day of 24,25(OH)$_2$D$_3$ or 10 µg/kg day of 1,25(OH)$_2$D$_3$ for two weeks. Assay for serum calcium and phosphorous concentration were determined by the o-cresol-phthalein comlexone method and the p-methyl-aminophenol reduction method. Bone histomorphometry was measured by micro CT analysis. Bone mineral density was measured by soft X ray and the image was analyzed by a computerized image analyzing system.

Results

The serum levels of calcium and phosphorous in the VDRKO are shown in Figure1. Untreated VDRKO reveals severe hypocalcemia (5.36±0.25mg/dl vs.

The Effect of 24,25(OH)2D3 to Serum Ca and Pi in VDRKO

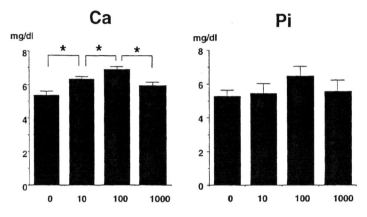

Figure 1. Left ; Serum calcium levels in VDRKO with administrated with $24,25(OH)_2D_3$ 1-1000µg/kg day. Right ; Serum phosphorous levels in VDRKO with administrated with $24,25(OH)_2D_3$ 1-1000µg/kg day. * $p < 0.05$

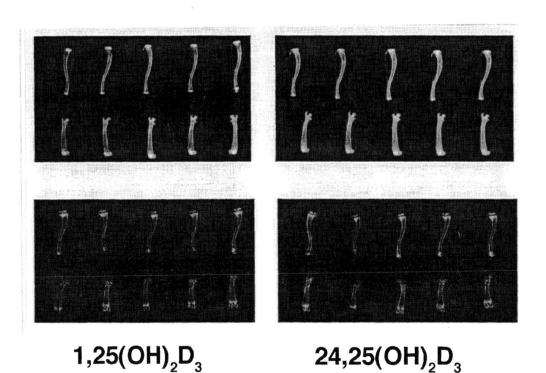

$1,25(OH)_2D_3$ $24,25(OH)_2D_3$

Figure 2. Bone mineral density analysis by soft X-ray. There was significantly difference between 1,25(OH)$_2$D$_3$ and 24,25(OH)$_2$D$_3$ in VDR+/- (p< 0.01). In VDRKO, there was no positive effect on bone mineral density.

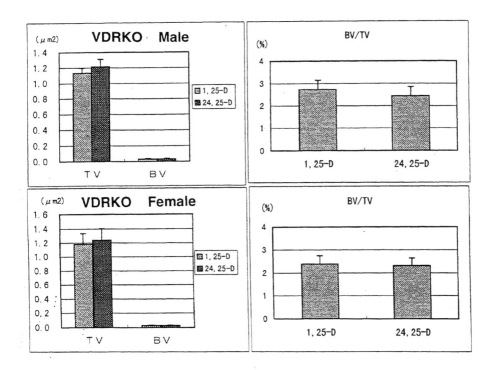

Figure 3. Bone histomorphometry analysis by micro focus CT (TV,BV,BV/TV). There was no significant difference between 1,25(OH)$_2$D$_3$ and 24,25(OH)$_2$D$_3$ in VDRKO.

8.30±0.26 mg/dl in the wild type). In VDRKO, two weeks treatment of 24,25(OH)$_2$D$_3$ increased serum levels of calcium (6.35±0.16 mg/dl at 10 µg/kg day, 6.93±0.18 mg/dl at 100 µg/kg day) significantly and phosphorous (5.47±0.48 mg/dl at 10 µg/kg day, 6.49±0.57 mg/dl at 100 µg/kg day) slightly. Bone mineral density analysis by soft X-ray (Figure2) revealed that there was no positive effect on bone mineral density in VDRKO. However, there was significant difference between the effect of 1,25(OH)$_2$D$_3$ and 24,25(OH)$_2$D$_3$ in VDR+/- (p< 0.01). Bone histomorphometry analysis by micro focus CT (TV,BV,BV/TV), there was no significant difference between the effect of 1,25(OH)$_2$D$_3$ and 24,25(OH)$_2$D$_3$ in VDRKO (Figure3).

Discussion

Previous studies suggested that 24,25(OH)$_2$D$_3$ has unique bone forming activities. 24,25(OH)$_2$D$_3$ at doses of 1-1000 µg/kg day had dose-dependent effects in increasing bone formation and bone mineralization in hypophosphatemic (Hyp) mouse, a murine model for familial X-linked hypophosphatemic rickets (1,2). The histologic findings of the calvariae in 24-hydroxylase gene knockout mouse have suggested that 24,25(OH)$_2$D$_3$ has the unique action in membranous ossification (4). In this study, two weeks treatment with 24,25(OH)$_2$D$_3$ increased serum calcium and phosphorous, however, not increased in bone mineral density and histomorphometric parametors in VDRKO. From the present study, we could not obtain any evidences of the action of 24,25(OH)$_2$D$_3$ on membranous ossification. However, we could not exclude the possibility of unknown signal transduction of the vitamin D other than VDR in calcium and phosphorous homeostasis.

References

1. Yamate T., Tanaka H., Nagai Y., Yamato H., Taniguchi N., Nakamura T., and Seino Y. (1994) *J. Bone and Mineral Res.* 9:1967-1974.
2. Ono, K., Tanaka H., Yamate T., Nagai Y., Nakamura T., and Seino Y. (1996) *Endocrinology.* 137:2633-2637.
3. Yoshizawa, T., Handa, Y., Uematsu, Y., Takeda, S., Sekine, K., Yoshihara, Y., Kawakami ,T., Arioka, K., Soto, H., Uchiyama, Y., Masushige, S., Fukamizu, A., Matsumoto, T., Kato, S (1997) *Nature genetics.* 16:391-396.
4. St-Arnaud R., and Glorieux F.H. (1998) *Endocrinology.* 139:3371-3374.

MSX1 INVOLVEMENT IN BONE FORMATION DURING DEVELOPMENT AND POST-NATAL GROWTH

S. Orestes-Cardoso[1], B. Robert [2], F. Lézot[1], D. Hotton[1], A. Berdal[1],
[1]EA 2380, Cordeliers Institute, University Paris 7 and [2]CNRS URA 1947, Institut Pasteur, Paris, France.

Introduction The cranio-facial skeleton is formed through a multi-step process involving neural crest-derived cells, in contrast to the axial and appendicular skeleton, which is of mesodermal origin (1). Homeobox genes are key-factors in patterning and morphogenesis, as shown in the axial and appendicular skeleton for the Hom/Hox homeogene family. These genes constitute a particular subset of regulatory genes encoding nuclear proteins which act as transcription factors which contain the highly conserved homeodomain. Among the 170 different homeobox genes identified, the classical Hom/Hox genes are not expressed in the developing head and facial primordia. Therefore, divergent homeogenes have been proposed as alternative candidates for the patterning of cranio-facial skeleton. These genes include Msx1 and Msx2, Dlx1-6, Barx1, 2, Otx2, GH6 ; Bicoid-homologues such as Gsc1 and Rieg (also called Otlx2 or Pitx2) ; the paired-box homologues Pax3,6,7, Cart1 and paired-related genes such as Ptx1, Prx1 (also called Mhox), Prx2 (also called S8) and Uncx4.1. The present study is devoted to the analysis of the role of one of these divergent homeogenes, Msx1, in the late formation and biomineralization of the cranio-facial skeleton.

Experimental strategy and methods The experimental strategy (2) was to insert LacZ gene inside the Msx1 gene homeobox resulting in : 1) reporter constructs to study Msx1 gene activity in heterozygous Msx1+/- mice, and 2) Msx1 null mutation in homozygous Msx1 -/- mice until birth as they die (C57BL6J controls). Mice (n = 252) were genotyped by PCR. The phenotypic Msx1 -/- traits were palatal clefting and early inhibition of odontogenesis. Msx1 +/- and Msx1 -/- genotypes were supported by ß-galactosidase staining. Whole-mount ß-galactosidase histoenzymology was followed by histological procedures and uncoupled to immunolabelling (type I collagen and tartrate-resistant acid phosphatase). Microradiographic and electron-microscopic investigations were made without decalcification.

Results Msx1 territories appeared related to the odontogenic units and mandibular basis. Functional disruption of Msx1 induced a general flattening related to selective growth inhibition of Msx1 territories.

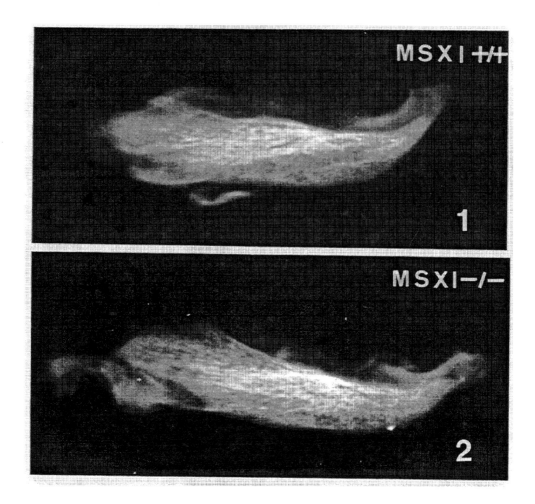

Microradiographs of half-mandibles in Msx1 +/+ (Figure 1) and Msx1 -/- (Figure 2) mice.

At the ultrastructural level, osteoblasts activity and bone matrix were not affected. Msx1 +/- mice allowed to show the post-natal Msx-1 expression maintained with the same anatomical pattern. It involved several populations of bone cells and corresponded to the sites of bone growth affected in Msx1 -/- mice. A distinct pattern characterized bone surfaces : periosteum osteoblast differentiation was related to Msx1 down-regulation while in the endosteum differentiated cells could express the homeoprotein.

Discussion By using a variety of approaches, the molecular basis of a number of hereditary disorders affecting skeletal patterning in both humans and mice have been identified. More specifically, several mutations involving divergent homeogenes have been documented, showing major cranio-facial defects, for instance tricho-dento-osseous syndrome and Dlx3 (3), craniosynostosis and Msx2 (4) and finally hypodontia, palate cleft and Msx1 (5, 6). Transgenic mice have proven useful models for the understanding of disturbed patterning during early development. The upstream and downstream positions of encoded homeoproteins were consequently identified inside the involved signalling cascades. However, the physiology of specialized tissues in the null mutants has not been analyzed. The present study supports that the functions of homeobox genes is not restricted to early development but that they play also a major role during skeletal growth and homeostasis, as previously shown for Dlx2 and enamel formation (7). Interestingly, these homeogenes appeared to be disturbed in rachitic mice (Berdal et al., this proceeding), suggetsing the existence of cross-talks between vitamin D pathway and epigenetic signalling cascade.

References

1. Francis-West, P., Ladher, R., Barlow A. and Graveson, A. (1998) Mech. Dev. 75, 3-28.
2. Houzelstein, D., Cohen, A., Buckingham, M.E. and Robert, B. (1997) Mech. Dev. 65,123-133.
3. Price, J.A., Bowden, D.W., Wright, J.T., Pettenati, M.J. and Hart, T.C. (1998) Hum .Mol. Genet. 7, 563-569.
4. Jabs, E.W., Müller, U., Li, X., Ma, L., Luo, W., Haworth, IS, Klisak, I., Sparkes, R., Warman, M.L., Mulliken, J.B., Snead, M.L. and Maxson, R. (1993) Cell 75, 443-450.
5. Vastardis, H., Karimbux, N., Guthua, S.W., Seidman, J.G. and Seidman, C.E. (1996) Nature Genet. 13, 417-421.
6. van Den Boorgaard, M.-J., Dorland, M., Beemer, F.A. and van Amstel, H.K.P. (2000). Nature Genet. 24, 342-343.
7. Lézot, F., Thomas, B., Hotton, D., Forest, N., Orestes-Cardoso, S., Robert, B., Sharpe, P. and Berdal, A. (2000) J. Bone Min. Res. 15, 430-441.

REGULATION OF CONECTIVE TISSUE GROWTH FACTOR IN PRIMARY RAT OSTEOBLAST CULTURES BY 1,25(OH)₂D₃

S.N. Popoff[1], J. Xu[1], V. Zakhaleva[1], M. Mendis[1], S.L. Smock[2], S.C. Marks, Jr.[3], T.A. Owen[2] and F.F. Safadi[1]
[1]Department of Anatomy and Cell Biology, Temple University School of Medicine, Philadelphia, PA, 19140; [2]Department of Cardiovascular and Metabolic Diseases, Pfizer, Inc., Central Research Division, Groton, CT 06340; [3]Department of Cell Biology, University of Massachusetts Medical School, Worcester, MA, 01655.

Introduction Connective Tissue Growth Factor (CTGF) is a cysteine-rich protein first discovered by screening a human umbilical vein endothelial cell cDNA expression library using a polyclonal anti-PDGF antibody (1). Since that time, CTGF has been isolated, cloned and sequenced in several other species including the rat (2). The CTGF gene belongs to a larger CCN gene family that also includes Cyr61, *nov* and the more recent additions ELM-1 (WISP-1), WISP-3 and COP-1 (WISP-2) (3,4). With the exception of *nov*, CTGF family members are immediate early growth-responsive genes that regulate the proliferation and differentiation of various connective tissue cell types (3). All members of the CCN family share from 30-50% amino acid sequence identity, possess a secretory signal peptide at the N-terminus, and contain 38 cysteine residues that are largely conserved (4). The CCN proteins are organized into discrete structural domains each encoded by a separate exon (4).

CTGF is a secreted protein that regulates diverse cellular functions including proliferation/differentiation, adhesion, migration, matrix production and survival (3). CTGF is expressed in many tissues with highest levels in the kidney and brain (5); CTGF mRNA and/or protein expression has been demonstrated in fibroblasts, endothelial cells, vascular smooth muscle cells and chondrocytes (6,7). In a recent study using the *osteopetrotic* (*op*) mutation in the rat as a model to examine differential gene expression between normal and *op* bone, we discovered that CTGF mRNA was expressed in bone (2). Although it was highly over-expressed in *op* mutant bone, its expression in normal bone (albeit at lower levels) was not previously reported. Western blot analyses using anti-CTGF antibodies showed a similar pattern of expression for the protein. Subsequent immunohistochemical analyses clearly demonstrated CTGF expression in osteoblasts *in situ*. *In situ* hybridization and immunolocalization studies in primary cultures demonstrated CTGF mRNA and protein in osteoblasts. CTGF mRNA demonstrated a temporal pattern of expression during osteoblast development in primary cultures, with highest levels of expression at earlier (proliferation commitment) stages with a progressive decrease during terminal stages of differentiation. The purpose of this study was two-fold. First, we utilized an affinity-purified anti-CTGF neutralizing antibody to block the activity of CTGF that is constitutively produced by osteoblasts *in vitro*. Using primary osteoblast cultures derived from normal neonatal rat calvaria, we examined the dose-dependent effects of anti-CTGF treatment on nodule formation and mineralization to establish a functional link between CTGF production and osteoblast function. Second, since serum levels of 1,25(OH)₂D₃ are markedly elevated in *op* mutants (8) and CTGF is markedly over-expressed in mutant bone (2), we examined the effects of 1,25(OH)₂D₃ on CTGF

784

mRNA and protein expression in primary osteoblast cultures at different stages of differentiation. In addition, we examined CTGF expression and its regulation by 1,25(OH)$_2$D$_3$ in osteoblast cultures derived from *op* mutant calvaria.

Results Primary osteoblast cultures were established using calvaria from normal neonatal rats as previously described (2). Cultures were treated with either non-immune IgY (control) or anti-CTGF IgY at concentrations ranging from 25-250 μg/ml beginning at three days and with every medium change thereafter until termination of the cultures at 2 or 3 weeks. The anti-CTGF antibody used in these experiments was raised in chicken against a peptide representing a 13 amino acid sequence located at the end of domain III and the beginning of domain IV. This peptide was selected because of its high antigenicity and was screened against the protein database to assure lack of homology with any known protein sequences. The antibody was tested for its specificity by Western blot analysis of protein isolated from bone. Cultures treated with the neutralizing antibody demonstrated a dose-dependent inhibition of nodule formation and mineralization, with maximal effects at 100 μg/ml. As shown in figure 1, bone nodules formed in the antibody-treated cultures were significantly smaller in size compared with those in the control (non-immune IgY) cultures at 2 weeks. At 3 weeks there was no evidence of mineralization in the treated cultures (data not shown). Results were similar for control and untreated cultures.

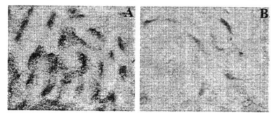

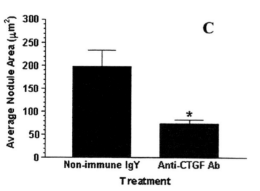

Figure 1 – Effects of anti-CTGF antibody on nodule formation by osteoblasts in culture. A neutralizing anti-CTGF antibody (Ab-243) was used to block constitutive CTGF production in primary osteoblast cultures. **A** and **B** – Photomicrographs of control (non-immune IgY) and treated (100 μg/ml anti-CTGF) cultures at 2 weeks stained with von Kossa and counterstained with light green; X15. **C** – Graph of the average size of bone nodules in control and treated cultures. Data expressed as the mean + SEM with greater than 100 nodules measured in each group. *p < 0.01 evaluated by Student *t*-test.

We examined the effects of 1,25(OH)$_2$D$_3$ on CTGF mRNA and protein expression in primary osteoblast cultures at different stages of development. Osteoblast cultures were established from normal or *op* mutant neonatal rat calvaria and maintained for one (proliferation/commitment), two (matrix production/maturation) or three (matrix mineralization) weeks. Cultures were treated with either 10^{-8}M 1,25(OH)$_2$D$_3$ or vehicle (ethanol) for 48 hours prior to cell collection and either total RNA or protein was isolated for Northern or Western blot analysis. The CTGF cDNA used as a probe for Northern analysis was a 717 bp fragment of the 3' UTR. All blots were stripped and reprobed with an 18S cDNA probe used as a control to normalize for differences in loading and transfer. For Western analysis, the primary anti-CTGF antibody used was the same as described above and the secondary antibody was HRP-donkey anti-chicken; signal was visualized by ECL. As shown in figure 2A and B, $1,25(OH)_2D_3$ treatment caused a significant (2 to 3-fold) increase of CTGF mRNA in both normal and mutant osteoblast cultures. Furthermore, CTGF mRNA expression was similar in untreated normal versus mutant osteoblast cultures at all time points examined. CTGF protein levels were also increased in $1,25(OH)_2D_3$-treated cultures, as shown by the Western blot in figure 2C.

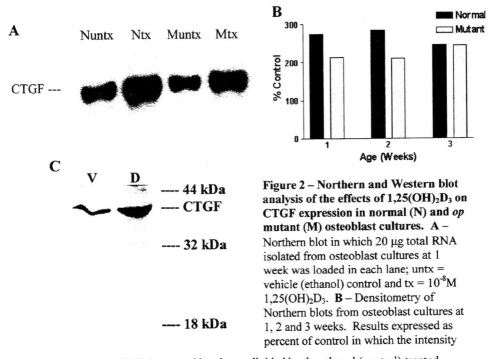

Figure 2 – Northern and Western blot analysis of the effects of $1,25(OH)_2D_3$ on CTGF expression in normal (N) and *op* mutant (M) osteoblast cultures. A – Northern blot in which 20 µg total RNA isolated from osteoblast cultures at 1 week was loaded in each lane; untx = vehicle (ethanol) control and tx = 10^{-8}M $1,25(OH)_2D_3$. B – Densitometry of Northern blots from osteoblast cultures at 1, 2 and 3 weeks. Results expressed as percent of control in which the intensity of the $1,25(OH)_2D_3$-treated bands are divided by the ethanol (control)-treated bands after correction with the corresponding 18S RNA for each sample. C – Western blot analysis in which 20 µg total protein isolated from normal osteoblast cultures at 2 weeks was loaded in each lane and probed using an anti-CTGF antibody; V = vehicle (ethanol) control and D = 10^{-8}M $1,25(OH)_2D_3$.

Discussion The antibody neutralization experiments effectively blocked the CTGF that is constitutively produced and secreted by osteoblasts in culture in a dose-dependent fashion with maximal effectiveness at 100 µg/ml. The inhibitory effects of neutralizing anti-CTGF antibody on nodule formation and mineralization establish a functional link between CTGF and osteoblasts, thereby supporting the hypothesis that CTGF is a novel bone anabolic factor. We propose that CTGF is synthesized and secreted by osteoblasts, where it acts as either an ECM-associated signaling molecule and/or a soluble factor to regulate osteoblast development and function in an autocrine fashion. Additional experiments examining the effects of anti-CTGF treatment on other parameters such as cell proliferation, matrix production and gene expression are currently being pursued. Furthermore, a baculovirus expression system is being employed to generate purified recombinant rat CTGF. Once available, the recombinant protein will allow us to directly examine the effects of CTGF on osteoblasts *in vitro* and bone *in vivo*.

There are no previous reports concerning the effect of $1,25(OH)_2D_3$ on CTGF expression in any cell or tissue. Treatment of osteoblast cultures with $1,25(OH)_2D_3$ resulted in significant up-regulation of CTGF mRNA and protein in both normal and *op* mutant cultures. It is important to note that CTGF expression in the control (vehicle-treated) cultures was similar in both normal and mutant osteoblasts, despite the markedly increased expression of CTGF by *op* osteoblasts *in vivo*. It is likely that CTGF expression in *op* bone is up-regulated by some other factor(s), and $1,25(OH)_2D_3$ is a potential candidate. Serum $1,25(OH)_2D_3$ levels are elevated in *op* mutants (8) and CTGF is also over-expressed in *op* kidney, another target tissue for $1,25(OH)_2D_3$, but not in other *op* tissues (2). Previous studies analyzing portions of the mouse and human CTGF gene promoters have identified various regulatory elements including a novel TGF-β response element (3,9), but a VDRE has not been identified. Additional studies are required to; 1) analyze the rat CTGF gene promoter for a VDRE, 2) evaluate the kinetic requirements for $1,25(OH)_2D_3$-mediated induction of CTGF expression, 3) examine the role of CTGF in mediating the effects of $1,25(OH)_2D_3$ on osteoblasts, and 4) determine whether $1,25(OH)_2D_3$ treatment increases the secretion of CTGF into the conditioned medium, and 5) define the role played by $1,25(OH)_2D_3$ in up-regulating CTGF expression in *op* mutants.

Acknowledgements This study was supported by grants AR39876 (to SNP) and DE07444 (to SCM) from the NIH and a research grant from Pfizer Central Research, Inc.

References
1. Bradham, D.M., Igarashi, A., Potter, R.L. and Grotendorst, G.R. (1991) J. Cell Biol. 114, 1285-1294.
2. Xu, J., Smock, S.L., Safadi, F.F., Rosenzweig, A.B., Odgren, P.R., Marks, S.C., Jr., Owen, T.A. and Popoff, S.N. (2000) J. Cell. Biochem. 77, 103-115.
3. Brigstock, D.R., Steffen, C.L., Kim, G.Y., Vegunta, R.K., Diehl, J.R. and Harding, P.A. (1997) J. Biol. Chem. 272, 20275-20282.
4. Lau, L.F. and Lam, S.C.T. (1999) Exper. Cell Res. 248, 44-57.
5. Oemar, B.S. and Luscher, T.F. (1997) Arterioscler. Thromb. Vasc. Biol. 17, 1483-1489.
6. Lin, J., Liliensiek, B., Kanitz, M., Schimansk,U., Bohrer, H., Waldherr, R., Martin, E., Kauffmann, G., Ziegler, R. and Nawroth, P.P. (1998) Cardiovasc. Res. 38, 802-813.
7. Nakanishi, T., Kimura, Y., Tamura, T., Ichikawa, H., Yamaai, Y., Sugimoto, T. and Takigawa, M. (1997) Biochem. Biophys. Res. Comm. 234, 206-210.
8. Hermey, D.C., Ireland, R.A., Zerwekh, J.E. and Popoff, S.N. (1995) Amer. J. Physiol. 268 (Endocrinol. Metab. 31), E312-E317.
9. Gortendorst, G.R., Okochi, H. and Hayashi, N. (1996) Cell Growth Differ. 7, 469-480.

COMPARISON OF THE NATURAL HORMONE $1\alpha,25(OH)_2D_3$ AND THE HYBRID ANALOG 1β-HYDROXYMETHYL-3,20-epi-22-OXA-26-HYDROXY-27,28-BISHOMO-VITAMIN D_3 (MCW-YB) IN TERMS OF INHIBITORY ACTIVITY ON MINERALIZED BONE NODULE FORMATION (MBNF) IN LONG-TERM CULTURES OF SaOS-2 CELLS.

L.G. Rao, LJ-F Liu, T.M. Murray and G.H. Posner.[*] Calcium Research Laboratory, St. Michael's Hospital and Dept of Medicine, University of Toronto, Toronto, Ontario M5B 1A6 and [*]Chemistry Department, School of Arts and Sciences, The Johns Hopkins University, Baltimore, Maryland USA 21218.

Introduction - The active vitamin D hormone, $1\alpha,25$-dihydroxyvitamin D_3 $[1\alpha,25(OH)_2D_3]$, has been considered for clinical treatment of osteoporosis (1). However, the effective doses required were associated with toxicity due to hypercalcemia and hypercalciuria (2). A large number of analogs of $1\alpha,25(OH)_2D_3$ with low calcemic activity have therefore been developed in different laboratories in an effort to make them more suitable for clinical use (3). One such analog, MCW-YB, was shown to be 200-300 times less calcemic than $1\alpha,25(OH)_2D_3$ (4) and to have greater growth-inhibitory activity in malignant cells and increased vitamin D receptor (VDR)-mediated transcriptional activity without change in the affinity for VDR (5).

$1\alpha,25(OH)_2D_3$ has been shown to have direct effects on osteoblasts (6). In order to assess the effectiveness of $1\alpha,25(OH)_2D_3$ and its analogs on these cells, we have been studying their actions using the osteoblast-like osteosarcoma SaOS-2 cell models representing two stages of diffferentiation (7,8). We have shown that the analogs with a 23-yne,16-ene (7) and 16-ene (8) substitutions were more potent than the parent compound in their effects on alkaline phosphatase activity depending on the stage of cell differentiation. In the present study, we have compared the effects of MCW-YB with that of $1\alpha,25(OH)_2D_3$ on mineralized bone formation and alkaline phosphatase activity (ALP) in SaOS-2 cells that form bone when cultured in the presence of dexamethasone, ascorbic acid and β-glycerophosphate.

Methods - SaOS-2 cells were cultured in HAM's F-12 supplemented with 10% fetal calf serum, 50 μg/ml ascorbic acid, and 10 nM dexamethasone. At day 8, and at every medium change thereafter, 10 mM β-glycerophosphate and increasing doses of $1\alpha,25(OH)_2D_3$ or MCW-YB were added. At day 15, the cells were fixed with neutral buffered formalin, stained with von Kossa and mineralized bone nodule number and area analyzed by image analysis. Parallel experiments were conducted for ALP assay as we have previously described (7) The data were analyzed using the one-way ANOVA followed by the Dunnett multiple comparison test (Instat, v 2.02, GraphPad Software, San Diego, CA). Graphs were drawn using Prism (version 1, GraphPad Software).

788

Results A photomicrograph shown in Fig. 1 demonstrates some representative nodules stained with von Kossa indicating mineralization. Examination of some of these nodules by electron microscopy revealed that the nodules had bone-like structure with active osteoblasts, entrapped osteocytes, extracellular collagen fibrils and deposited hydroxyapatite crystals (data not shown). Thus the system is ideal for studying and comparing the effects of $1\alpha,25(OH)_2D_3$ and the analog MCW-YB on bone formation.

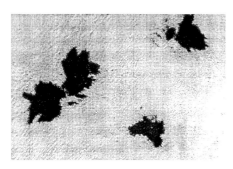

Fig. 1. Photomicrograph of representative mineralized bone nodules made visible by von Kossa stain (100 x magnification).

The effects of $1\alpha,25(OH)_2D_3$ on mineralized nodule number and area, as well as the ALP activity are illustrated in Fig. 2. Statistical analyses of the data revealed the following results: a dose-dependent inhibition of **(i)** mineralized nodule number ($p < 0.001$, F=82.36, n=9). The inhibition was observed at $1\alpha,25(OH)_2D_3$ concentrations of 10^{-10} M ($p < 0.01$) and 10^{-8} M ($p < 0.01$) (Fig. 2A). **(ii)** mineralized nodule area ($p < 0.0001$, F=162.1, n=9), with a pattern of inhibition similar to that for nodule number (Fig.2B) and **(iii)** ALP which was maximal at a concentration of 1 x 10^{-12}M and remained similarly inhibited up to 1 x 10^{-8} M ($p < 0.001$, F=19.83, n=9) (Fig 2. C).

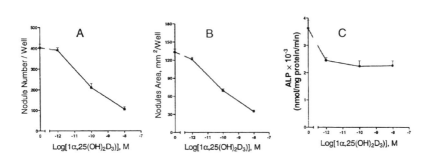

Fig 2. Dose-dependent effects of $1\alpha,25(OH)_2D_3$ on bone nodule (A) number and (B) area and (C) ALP in 15-day cultures of SaOS-2 cells cultured as described under Methods.

On the other hand, although MCW-YB also inhibited the mineralized nodule number (3A) and area (3B), as well as the ALP activity (3C), the inhibition (p<0.01) of all three parameters was not observed until an MCW-YB concentration of 1×10^{-8} M was reached.

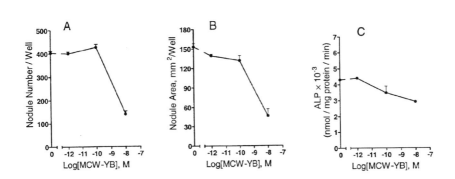

Fig. 3. Dose-dependent effects of MCW-YB on mineralized bone nodule (A) number and (B) area and (C) ALP in 15-day cultures of SaOS-2 cells cultured as described under Methods.

Discusssion: The results of this study clearly showed that $1\alpha,25(OH)_2D_3$ and the analog MCW-YB differed in their effects on mineralized bone nodule formation and ALP. While both compounds inhibited these parameters, the analog MCW-YB was found to have an inhibitory property that is 100-fold less than that of the parent compound. The reason for this observed difference in their action is presently unclear, but we can speculate that it maybe a result of the differences in their affinity for the vitamin D receptor (VDR) (4), nature of their chemical structures (5) or in the metabolites produced in SaOS-2 cells. It is clear, however, that the hybrid analog MCW-YB, which was shown to be non-calcemic in an in vivo assay (4), is still quite potent in our bone-forming SaOS-2 cell model despite its lack of the natural 1-α-OH group considered essential in eliciting strong biological responses (5).

$1\alpha,25(OH)_2D_3$ has been shown to have complex and dual effects on bone formation in vitro. Thus, it has been shown to stimulate in vitro mineralization by osteoblast-like MC3T3-E1 (9), either inhibitory or stimulatory effects in two human cell lines E6 and E10 (10) and inhibitory or no effect (11) in rat calvarial cells depending on the mode and time of addition. It appears that the inhibitory effect of $1\alpha,25(OH)_2D_3$ on mineralization is due to inhibition of osteoprogenitor cells (11). Since in our study the $1\alpha,25(OH)_2D_3$ and MCW-YB were added when cells were still actively dividing at day 8, it would seem to indicate that the effect we observed is inhibition of osteoprogenitor cells. This is the first study which showed that the analog MCW-YB also has an effect on mineralized bone nodule formation. The dual inhibitory and stimulatory effects of $1\alpha,25(OH)_2D_3$ maybe related to its action in maintaining the level of calcium and phosphate in circulation in an in vivo situation. The lower inhibitory property of MCW-YB may be of advantage in its application as treatment for abnormalities in calcium homeostasis.

References

1) Kanis J.A., McCloskey E.V., deTakats D., et al. (1997) Osteoporosis Int 7 (suppl 3):S140-S146.
2) Schwartzman M.S. and Franck W.A. (1984) Am J Med 82:224-230.
3) Bouillon R., Okamura W.H., Norman A.W. (1995) Endocrine Reviews 16:200-257.
4) Posner G.H., Lee J.K., Li Z., et al. (1995) Bioorg Med Chem Letter 5:2163 - 2168.
5) Peleg S., Liu Y.-Y., Reddy S., et al. (1996) J Cell Biochem 63:149.
6) Lian J.B. and Stein G.S. In: Berdanier CD and Hargrove IL, Eds, Nutrition and Gene Expression. Baton Roca:CRCP, 1993; 391-429.
7) Rao L.G., Sutherland M.K., Reddy G.S., et al. (1996) Bone 19:621-627.
8) Rao L.G., Sutherland M.K.,Liu L. J.-F.. et al. In: Norman A., Bouillon R. and Thomasset M. Eds, Vitamin D: Chemistry, Biology and Clinical Applications of the Steroid Hormone. Vitamin D Workshop Inc., Riverdale, Ca, 1997; 501-502.
9) Matsumoto T., Igarashi C., Takeuchi Y. et al. (1991) Bone 12:27-32.
10) Bodine R., Henderson R., Green J., et al. In: Norman A., Bouillon R., and Thomasset M. Eds, Vitamin D: Chemistry, Biology and Clinical Applications of the Steroid Hormone. Vitamin D Workshop Inc., Riverdale, Ca, 1997; 665-666.
11) Ishida H., Bellows C.G., Aubin J.E., et al. (1993) Endocrinology 132:61-66.

ASSAYS FOR VITAMIN D STEROIDS

QUALITY ASSURANCE OF 25-HYDROXYVITAMIN D ASSAYS: VIGILANCE IN THE PURSUIT OF EXCELLENCE.

G.D. Carter*, J. Nolan, D.J.H. Trafford and H.L.J. Makin *Endocrine Laboratory, Charing Cross Hospital, London W6 8RF, UK and Department of Clinical Biochemistry, St. Bartholomew's and the Royal London School of Medicine & Dentistry, London E1 2AD, UK.

Quality assurance for laboratory assays is achieved by the introduction of properly organised quality assessment (QA) schemes **(1)**. Prior to the introduction of the international vitamin D external quality assessment scheme (DEQAS) in 1989, there was no QA scheme available for vitamin D assays. Initially DEQAS operated only in the UK and monitored the performance of assays of 25-hydroxyvitamin D (25-OHD) but it was extended to cover participants throughout the world. It now has 75 subscribing laboratories in 13 countries. In 1997 the scheme was extended to include assays of calcitriol (1,25(OH)$_2$D). The majority of participants (73) are sent samples for 25-OHD and a further 27 participants are also sent samples for 1,25(OH)$_2$D. Each quarter 5 serum samples for each metabolite are distributed to all participating laboratories and results, which must be returned within 4 weeks, are collated and compared to the all laboratory trimmed mean (ALTM) which we have previously shown, for 25-OHD, to be very close to the target value obtained by gas chromatography-mass spectrometry **(2)**. In 1999 an Advisory Committee was set up to monitor the scheme's performance and it was decided that a proficiency certificate would be awarded to those laboratories and/or individuals who reached the required standard which is set every year by the Advisory Committee. Figure 1 shows a pie chart showing the country of origin of the participants in the DEQAS scheme.

Figure 1 - *Country of origin of participants in the DEQAS. Countries are identified by the International Vehicle Mark. Countries are listed in clockwise order starting at the line indicated (-AR : Argentina)*

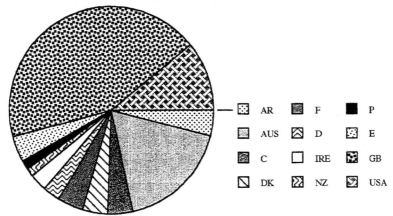

Laboratories are required to be both accurate and precise and in deciding the performance targets the Advisory Committee took as a measure of accuracy, % bias which is defined as being the difference between the reported result and the ALTM as a % of the ALTM. In order to meet the performance target the % bias must be consistently low. In the 1999/2000 distribution cycle, the target required at least 80% of the results to be within ± 33% of the ALTM. All laboratories achieving this were issued with a certificate. It is considered likely that in future years the performance targets will be tightened and consistently lower bias values will be required. Figure 2 shows a histogram indicating the performance of individual participants in the 1999/2000 round. The y axis plots the highest % bias among 'the best' 80% of results from individual laboratory (Bmax). The horizontal line at 33% bias indicates the highest acceptable % bias and it can be seen that a significant minority (approximately 28%) of participants fell outside the acceptable limits. This graph does not include participants who returned results on less than 16 of the circulated samples.

Figure 2 - *Performance of individual participants in the DEQAS 1999/2000 distribution round.*

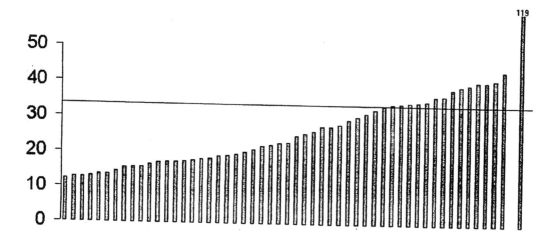

A wide variety of methods for the assay of 25-OHD are used by participants. However there has been increasing use of simple immunoassay methods and Figure 3 shows the distribution of methods which are used by participants in the 1999/2000 round. During 1999 serum samples to which 40.7nmol/L of 25-OHD$_2$ had been added were included in a distribution together with a sample of the serum to which no 25-OHD$_2$ had been added. The 25-OHD$_2$ was added as an ethanolic solution directly to the plasma. The concentration was measured by UV absorbance assuming a molar extinction coefficient at 264nm of 19,400. In the UK very little 25-OHD$_2$ is seen in serum samples but in countries consuming foods fortified with vitamin D_2 the contribution of 25-OHD$_2$ to the total 25-OHD value may be considerable. It was therefore considered necessary to evaluate the performance of the different methods used when substantial quantities of 25-OHD$_2$ was present in the serum. The results returned for this experiment were disappointing. The mean recovery for all methods was 59.3% with a wide range from individual laboratories (14.9-133). The best recoveries were obtained by a small group of laboratories using in-house ligand binding assay or HPLC. The 2 commercial immunoassay kits gave widely differing results (66.1% recovery in one case and 24.2% recovery in the other). The design of this simple experiment has been criticised and will be repeated in the 2000/2001 distribution round using freshly synthesised and characterised 25-OHD$_2$ (by courtesy of Professor A. Mourino).

Figure 3 - *Distribution of methods for 25-OHD assay by DEQAS participants. Methods are listed in clockwise order starting at the line indicated (- Other. CLBA indicates ligand binding assay with chromatography)*

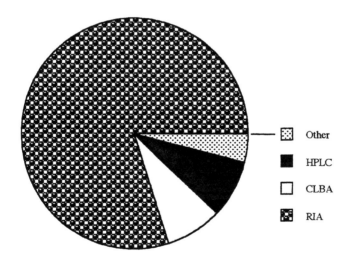

As the purpose of the DEQAS is to improve individual and general laboratory performance, we asked ourselves the question whether the performance of 25-OHD assay had improved since the last Vitamin D Workshop in 1997. Performance was assessed in the same way as illustrated in Figure 1 using Bmax and comparing the Bmax values for each participant in 1996/97 with that in 1999/2000. These data are plotted in Figure 4. While some participants have dramatically improved their results, there are a number whose performance has deteriorated rather than improved and this is disappointing. The reason for this is not clear but efforts will continue to persuade participants to improve performance

796

and where laboratories under perform consistently, it is hoped that advice will be sought to establish what is going wrong.

Figure 4 - *Improvement of 25-OHD assay performance between 1997 and 2000.*

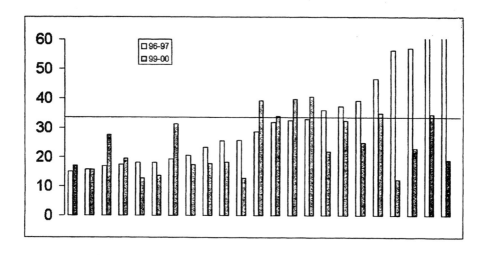

In the coming year, performance targets for 25-OHD will be reviewed by the Advisory Committee, and a new performance target for 1,25(OH)$_2$D will be introduced. At a meeting of the Advisory Committee in 1999 it was agreed to set up a DEQAS website. This site would provide detailed information about the organisation and processes used by DEQAS and would also permit participants to submit results electronically. Such a website would allow faster return of results to participants and would encourage more interaction between the DEQAS organiser and individual participants. All delegates to the 2000 Vitamin D Workshop were encouraged to visit the website, which can be found at http://www.deqas.org and constructive comments on this site would be welcomed by the organiser Graham Carter by e-mail (g.carter@cxwms.ac.uk or organiser@deqas.org) or by post.

References

(1) Healey, M.J.R. (1979) Clin. Chem. 25, 675-677.

(2) Carter, G.D., Nolan, J., Trafford, D.J.H., and Makin, H.L.J. (1997) in Vitamin D: Chemistry, Biology and Clinical Application of the Steroid Hormone (eds. Norman A.W., Bouillon, R., Thomasset, M), University of California, Riverside, USA, pp.737-738.

25-HYDROXYVITAMIN D ASSAY KITS: SPEED AT THE EXPENSE OF ACCURACY?

Jacqueline L. Berry, Julie Martin and E. Barbara Mawer
Musculoskeletal Research Group, School of Medicine, Manchester Royal Infirmary, Manchester, M13 9WL, U.K.

Introduction

Vitamin D is metabolised in the liver to form 25-hydroxyvitamin D (25OHD) which is the major circulating metabolite of vitamin D in the normal population. Measurement of the serum concentration of 25OHD is considered to be the most reliable index of vitamin D status. Recently new assay kits for the measurement of 25OHD have been developed that speed up the assay process by using iodinated tracer. We have used two of these ^{125}I RIA kits and compared the results with our in-house, straight phase HPLC method.

Materials and Methods

Assays: Kit 1 was obtained from ImmunoDiagnostic Systems Ltd (Boldon, Tyne and Wear, UK) and kit 2 was from DiaSorin Inc (Stillwater, MN, USA). Each kit assay was performed exactly according to the manufacturers' instructions.

The in-house method has been described in detail previously (1). Briefly, samples (2ml) were extracted using acetonitrile and applied to C18 silica Sep-paks. Initial separation of metabolites was by straight phase HPLC (Waters Associates, Milford, MA) using a Hewlett Packard Zorbax-Sil column (4.6x250mm, 5-µ) (Hicrom Ltd, Reading, Berkshire UK), eluted with hexane:propan-2-ol: methanol (92:4:4). 25OHD$_2$ and 25OHD$_3$ were collected together between 4 and 6 min and assayed by PBA using ^{3}H-25OHD$_3$ as tracer or applied to a second Zorbax-Sil column (6.2x80mm, 3-µ), eluted with hexane:propan-2-ol (98:2). 25OHD$_2$ and 25OHD$_3$ were measured separately by UV absorbance at 265 nm and the results corrected for recovery.

Serum samples: Serum was obtained from patients at the Manchester Royal Infirmary, some of whom had been treated with vitamin D$_2$, and frozen at -20°C until use. The samples were divided into three groups on the basis of the results for 25OHD$_2$ and 25OHD$_3$ obtained using the in-house HPLC assay. The groups were:

low 25OHD$_2$, low 25OHD$_3$	(A)
low 25OHD$_2$, high/normal 25OHD$_3$	(B)
high 25OHD$_2$, low 25OHD$_3$	(C)

Five control pools of serum were used to test the kits against the in-house HPLC method. Control pools 16 and 17 contained 25OHD$_2$ present from endogenous production by patients treated with vitamin D_2. Pool 16 contained approximately two-thirds as $25OHD_2$; pool 17 was virtually all $25OHD_2$. Control pools 18-20 were supplemented with synthetic, crystalline $25OHD_2$ (>98% pure, Fluka Chemie AG, Switzerland) at the following levels: pool 18: 20 nmol/L; pool 19: 50 nmol/L; pool 20: 100 nmol/L.

Results

The chromatographic method: Retention times of reference standards were established to ensure that the fractions assayed for $25OHD_2$ and $25OHD_3$ did not include other known metabolites: Retention times (min) were:

$$24OHD_2: \quad 7.7\pm0.1$$
$$25OHD_2: \quad 10.8\pm0.2$$
$$25OHD_3: \quad 14.8\pm0.2$$
$$24,25(OH)_2D_3: \quad 60.8\pm0.4$$

The fractions assayed were not contaminated with known 24-hydroxylated metabolites (2).

Assays: The results showed a good correlation (figure 1) between both kit 1 and kit 2 and the HPLC method with all samples tested (n=91), but only kit 2 showed equivalence (figure 1).

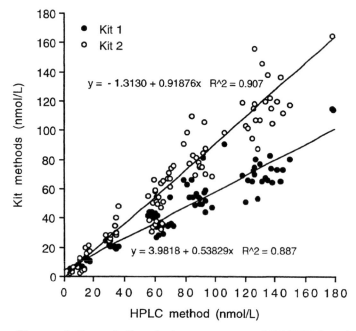

Figure 1 Correlation between assayed 25OHD levels

Serum samples: In serum from severely vitamin D deficient patients (group A) there were no significant differences in assayed values between the methods (table 1). However, when serum levels of 25OHD were higher (group B), kit 1 significantly (p<0.01) under-estimated 25OHD levels, especially when 25OHD was in the D_2 form (group C) compared to both HPLC and kit 2.

Table 1: 25OHD (mean±sem, nmol/L) in serum samples

Pool	n	HPLC	Kit 1 (%HPLC)	Kit 2 (%HPLC)
A	9	8.5±1.2	7.2±0.6 (84)	5.6±1.1 (66)
B	8	88.7±4.0	60.2±4.9 (68)	80.8±5.7 (91)
C	10	109.2±9.9	58.2±5.5 (53)	94.4±6.6 (87)

Control samples: In the control samples with a high proportion of the 25OHD as D_2 (pools 16, 17, 19, 20) kit 1 consistently underestimated 25OHD in comparison to the HPLC method or kit 2 (table 2). In control 18 with a relatively low D_2 content, kit 1 performed better but was still low at 72% of HPLC values.

Table 2: 25OHD (mean±sem, nmol/L) in control samples

Pool	n	HPLC	Kit 1 (%HPLC)	Kit 2 (%HPLC)
Natural D_2				
C16	11	63.7±0.6	33.2±1.0 (52)	51.3±3.6 (81)
C17	10	127.7±2.8	72.0±1.8 (56)	115.8±5.8 (91)
Synthetic D_2				
C18	9	58.5±0.9	42.0±0.5 (72)	53.9±1.8 (92)
C19	5	88.8±1.3	53.1±0.9 (60)	76.6±2.0 (86)
C20	5	136.1±1.7	67.6±1.5 (50)	125.8±7.3 (92)

Assay performance: Double dilutions of control sera C16, 17 and 18 showed good linear responses for all methods. 50% and 25% dilutions gave mean responses of 53.9±0.7 and 26.6±0.5 % for HPLC; 50.0±0.8 and 28.2±0.2 % for kit 1 and 52.6±3.4 and 30.8±2.0 % for kit 2.

Intra-assay variation measured using control samples was significantly lower when using HPLC (3.0±0.2%) and kit 1 (4.6±0.6%) than kit 2 (10.1±1.3%). This was also true for the inter-assay variation (HPLC: 4.2%, Kit 1: 10.4%, Kit 2: 17.3%). A possible explanation for the greater variation with kit 2 is the critical nature of the extraction procedure, which is acknowledged by the manufacturers, with the instruction to perform this step SLOWLY.

Conclusions

Kit 1 had good precision but accuracy was poor. Serum 25OHD was significantly and consistently under-estimated, compared to our HPLC method, especially when present as $25OHD_2$, and will result in substantial under-estimation in vitamin D_2-treated patients.

Kit 2 had lower precision but much greater accuracy compared to the reference HPLC method. We found no significant differences between 25OHD measured by HPLC and kit 2.

Both kits were faster than our in-house method and required smaller serum volumes.

References

1. Mawer EB, Hann JT, Berry JL and Davies M (1985) Clin. Sci. 68, 35-141.
2. Mawer EB, Jones G, Davies M, Still PE, Byford V, Schroeder NJ, Makin HLJ, Bishop CW and Knutson JC (1998) J Clin Endocrinol Metab 83:2156-2166.

A SENSITIVE AND PRECISE ENZYME IMMUNOASSAY (EIA) FOR THE MEASUREMENT OF 25-HYDROXYVITAMIN D.

M.J. Gardner, D. Laurie, A.K. Barnes, J. Browbank and R.T. Duggan.
IDS Ltd . Boldon Business Park, Boldon, Tyne and Wear, U.K. NE35 9PD.

Introduction The major circulating form of vitamin D is 25-Hydroxyvitamin D (25-OH D) and its measurement is widely used as an index of vitamin D status (1). There are currently several commercially available 25-OH D assays which use solvent for sample extraction and radioisotope tracers for detection. Increasingly, laboratories prefer to avoid the hazards associated with handling radioactive materials and we have embarked on development of a non-isotopic assay.

There are fewer non isotopic microtitre plate 25-OH D assays available mainly as a result of increased technical difficulties in producing a low volume final assay format. Problems encountered are mainly due to the hydrophobicity of 25-OH D. One major difficulty is keeping the 25-OH D molecule available in the assay mixture whilst preventing absorption to surfaces. This is particularly difficult in EIA compared to RIA methods, where plastic microtitre plate rather than glass tube surfaces are used.

In a previous assay format, sample extract was directly added to a buffer mixture giving a final concentration of solvent in the microtitre plate of 20%. (2) However, this assay was plagued by drift problems across the plate. It was considered that this was a result of the solvent stripping off antibody from the plate.

We have developed the assay further so that the solvent concentration is low (5%) on addition to the wells. The new method uses an intermediate dilution of the sample extract in conjugate reagent to reduce the final concentration of the solvent in the assay mixture. Although this method has an additional dilution step, improvement of other reagents has enabled us to maintain excellent precision and sensitivity in the assay.

Results with this assay show that a suitable standard curve can be obtained in a microtitre plate format. Precision and sensitivity data are comparable with the RIA without drift problems encountered in the original assay. Results from patient samples also show excellent correlation between the 2 methods.

Materials Microtitre plates (NUNC Maxisorp F8 modules) were coated by passive adsorption with donkey anti-sheep IgG capture antibody. Plates were washed 3 times and coated with sheep anti-25-OH D IgG overnight at room temperature. Plates were washed again, treated with a plate coat stabiliser, dried overnight and stored desiccated at 4°C. The conjugate reagent was 25-OH D linked to biotin diluted in 50mL phosphate buffered saline (PBS) containing polypep and detergent. Avidin HRP Detection Reagent was Avidin HRP (Vector) diluted to 250ng/mL in PBS containing BSA. The TMB peroxidase substrate was a ready to use, single component TMB reagent (Moss Inc.) and the Stop reagent used was 0.5M HCl.

Assay Method The 25-OH D assay employs a simple, 2 step extraction procedure followed by an enzyme immunoassay. The extraction procedure is the same as that as used in the IDS Gamma-B RIA.

Calibrators and samples were added to disposable glass tubes. Addition of Extraction Reagent 1 and Extraction Reagent 2 causes precipitation of serum proteins and extraction of 25-OH D. Centrifugation allows separation of the liquid extract containing 25-OH D and solid sample debris.

Extract (50µL) was added to 1mL of the 25D-biotin conjugate in a separate glass tube. 200µL of the mixture was added to the anti-25D antibody coated microtitre plate. The assay mixture was incubated for 2hr after which the plate was washed.

Detection of bound tracer was accomplished by addition of 200µL Avidin HRP for 30min after which the plate was washed.

TMB substrate was added, incubated for 30min and the reaction stopped with acid. The absorbance is inversely proportional to the concentration of 25-OH D. The calibration curve gives serum 25-OH D values for unknowns directly.

Results The assay has a range of 0-400nM. The sensitivity defined as the concentration corresponding to the mean minus 2 standard deviations of 10 replicates of the zero calibrator was 3.8 nmol/L (1.5 ng/mL).

Within assay variation, determined from 5 extraction replicates of each sample (giving 10 assay replicates), were 5.5%, 3.7% and 3.8% CV for samples of 21.4nM, 50.6nM & 108.9nM levels. Between assay variation was 8.1-13.9% CV for 7 samples run in 14-33 separate assays (Table 1).

Sample	Mean (nmol/L)	%cv	N
A	19.5	9.8%	33
B	53.1	11.6%	33
C	132.7	11.5%	33
D	36.4	9.0%	14
E	183.0	13.9 %	14
F	32.6	8.1%	17
G	145.6	8.1%	17

Table 1. Within assay variation for 7 samples run in 14-33 assays.

Crossreactivity of the antibody was determined by spiking various concentrations of the metabolites into calibrator matrix to obtain standard curves. From these curves the concentration relating to 50% binding was determined and expressed as a % of the 50% binding concentration of the 25-OH D calibrator curve. Crossreactivities were 25-Hydroxyvitamin D_3, 100%; 25-Hydroxyvitamin D_2, 75%; 24,25 Dihydroxyvitamin D_3, >100%; Cholecalciferol (D_3), <0.01% and Ergocalciferol (D_2), <0.30%.

Linearity was determined by diluting samples with buffer prior to extraction and assay. The mean linearity of 5 samples was 113% (Range 96-135%, Table 2).

Sample	Observed (nmol/L)	Expected (nmol/L)	OBS/EXP%
A	23.7		
A/2	13.7	11.8	116%
A/4	8.0	5.9	135%
B	30.9		
B/2	16.1	15.4	104%
B/4	9.2	7.7	120%
C	45.8		
C/2	23.7	22.9	104%
C/4	11.0	11.4	96%
D	64.8		
D/2	35.4	32.4	109%
D/4	17.8	16.2	104%
E	190.0		
E/2	110.6	95.0	116%
E/4	55.3	47.5	116%
		Mean	113%

Table 2. Linearity of 5 samples diluted in buffer prior to extraction and assay.

Recovery was determined by spiking samples with calibrator buffer containing 25-OH D_3 (17.6nM & 39.9nM). The mean recovery of the 5 samples was 116% (Range 85-139%, Table 3).

Sample	Observed (nmol/L)	Increment (nmol/L)	Recovery
A	10.6		
+17.6	30.0	19.4	110%
+39.9	54.9	44.3	111%
B	16.2		
+17.6	36.0	19.8	113%
+39.9	63.6	47.4	119%
C	18.0		
+17.6	39.4	21.4	122%
+39.9	68.2	50.2	126%
D	21.8		
+17.6	44.4	22.6	128%
+39.9	63.4	41.6	104%
E	47.6		
+17.6	72.1	24.5	139%
+39.9	81.4	33.8	85%
		Mean	116%

Table 3. Recovery of 5 samples spiked with 25-OH D_3 (17.6nM & 39.9nM).

A range of patient samples were assayed by the EIA and by the IDS Gamma-B RIA kit. (Fig. 1). A good correlation between both assays was found. [EIA = 1.02 x RIA- 0.18nmol/L   (R^2 = 0.85)   n = 85].

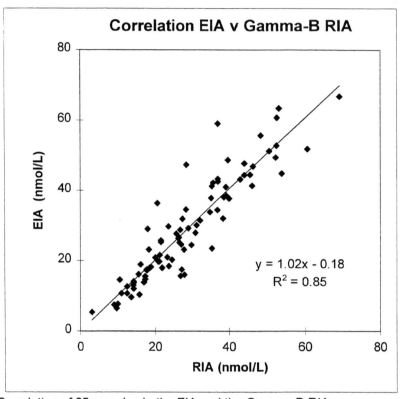

Fig1. Correlation of 85 samples in the EIA and the Gamma-B RIA.

Conclusions We have developed an EIA for measurement of 25-OH D with comparable assay performance to the best RIAs on the market.

The EIA method provides for the precise and sensitive measurement of 25-OH-D without the need for radioactive handling facilities. The method correlates well with the IDS Gamma B RIA kit and the assay is rapid, giving results within 3.5 hours.

All reagents used in this assay should be stable for at least 6 months prior to use and for at least 12 weeks after first use. This makes these reagents suitable for development into a commercially available diagnostic kit.

References
1. Schmidt-Gayk, H., Bouillon, R. and Roth, H.J. (1997) Scand. J. Clin. Lab. Invest. 57, (Suppl 227) 35-45
2. Gardner, M.J., Barnes, A.K., Laurie, D., Browbank, J., Duggan, R.T. (1999) J. Bone Miner. Res. 14, (Suppl 1, Abstract SU479) S551

POLYCLONAL ANTIBODIES TO EB1089, AN ANALOG OF 1α,25-DIHYDROXY-VITAMIN D₃ IN CLINICAL TRIALS

Lars K. A. Blæhr, Fredrik Björkling, Ernst Binderup, Martin J. Calverley, and Peter Kaastrup[a], Department of Medicinal Chemistry, Leo Pharmaceutical Products Ltd., DK-2750 Ballerup, Denmark and [a]Institute of Medical Microbiology and Immunology, University of Copenhagen, DK-2200 Copenhagen, Denmark.

Introduction. EB1089 (seocalcitol, **1**) is a synthetic, low-calcemic analog of the natural hormone 1α,25-dihydroxyvitamin D_3 (1,25(OH)$_2$D$_3$), that has recently been selected for clinical trials as a potential anti-cancer agent (1). The analog is 50-200 times more potent than 1,25(OH)$_2$D$_3$ in inhibiting cellular proliferation, but is only 50% as calcemic.

The evaluation of EB1089 as a potential anti-cancer agent in the clinic has demanded methods for quantifying the drug in biological samples. We describe herein the synthesis of an EB1089 hapten **2** and the characterization of polyclonal antibodies raised in 3 rabbits against the hapten conjugated to BSA.

Results And Discussion. The analysis of vitamin D related compounds in serum represents a challenge, due to low serum concentrations of the compounds, and because closely related, endogenous metabolites interfere. Recently, a sensitive mass spectrometric method has been developed for the quantification of EB1089 in serum samples (2), but the method requires preliminary extraction and isolation of EB1089 prior to analysis. In the present study, we set out to develop an immunoassay with specific antibodies that will allow direct measurement in serum of EB1089, and for this purpose we raised polyclonal antibodies to EB1089.

The hapten of EB1089 used for immunization was designed in such a way that only key structural features of the compound of interest were included, namely the CD-ring and the side-chain. This was done in order to avoid possible calcemic side effects that could result from long-time immunization with large doses of conjugates of EB1089 itself. The synthesis is outlined in scheme 1. Despite the missing A-ring in the hapten, the antibodies raised toward the hapten were expected to cross react with EB1089 to a high degree. The antibodies were characterized with respect to titer, avidity and specificity in an enzyme immunoassay (3).

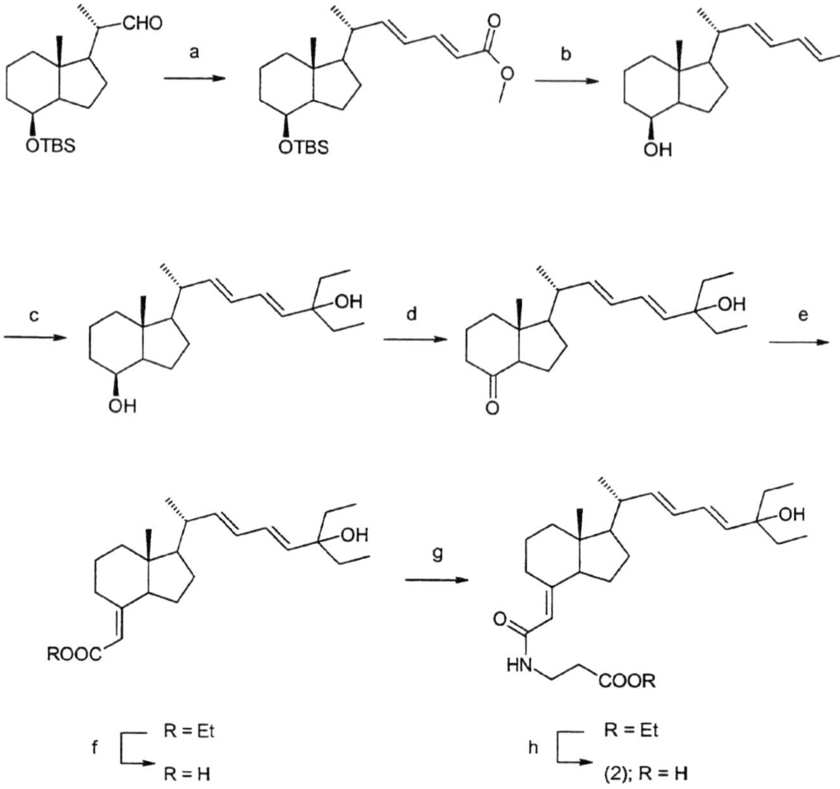

Scheme 1 Reagents, conditions, and yields: a) *Trans*-trimethyl 4-phosphonocrotonate, LHMDS, THF, -78 °C; 95%; b) 2,5% HF, CH$_3$CN-H$_2$O; 100%; c) EtLi (2 eq.), THF; 78%; d) Dess-Martin periodinane, CH$_2$Cl$_2$; 90%; e) Triethyl phosphonoacetate, NaH, THF; 76%; f) KOH, MeOH; 55%; g) ClH$_3$N(CH$_2$)$_2$COOEt, DCC, Et$_3$N, CH$_2$Cl$_2$; 58%; h) NaOH, dioxane/H$_2$O; 100%

Determination of titer. Antisera from three rabbits (As-1, As-2 and As-3) were obtained by immunizations with a BSA-conjugate of hapten 2 over a 6-month period. Antibody dilution curves were determined by measuring the binding of a series of concentrations of antiserum to covalently bound EB1089 hemisuccinate in Covalink™ microtiter plates (3). Bound antibody was detected with a swine anti-rabbit peroxidase labeled secondary antibody. The titer of all three antisera had increased 3-5 fold during the last three months of immunization, as measured by the lateral displacement of the absorption curves.

Avidity measurement. Measurement of avidity was performed using chaotropic ion elution (4). A chaotropic ion (thiocyanate) was added in serial dilutions to the antibody-hapten complex. The chaotropic ion decreases hydrophobic interactions, resulting in a dissociation of the complex. The avidity index was defined as the concentration of thiocyanate at which the maximal binding to immobilized EB1089 was reduced to 50%.

Figure 1 shows the development of avidity index as a function of time after immunization for the three antisera.

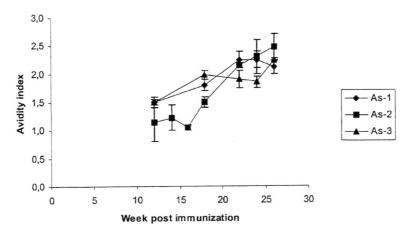

Figure 1. Avidity index vs. time post immunization of rabbit antisera. Apparently the avidity increased as a function of time for all antisera. As-1 and As-3 exhibited a similar, modest increase, while antiserum As-2 showed the most marked increase.

Cross-reactivity. To assess the specificity of the antisera we measured the cross-reactivity with various common vitamin D metabolites and with 4 metabolites of EB1089. The metabolites of EB1089 contain an additional hydroxyl group in the side chain and are shown to the right. The metabolite EB1446 has been identified as the major metabolite of EB1089 (5).

Antisera from week 26 diluted at a concentration of 1:4000 were preincubated with serial dilutions of metabolite overnight, and the resulting reaction to immobilized EB1089 in Covalink™ plates was determined. The IC_{50} value was measured as the concentration of metabolite that was necessary to reduce the maximal binding to 50%. The cross-reactivity with a metabolite was then calculated as the percentage of the IC_{50} value of EB1089 to that of the metabolite. The results are listed in table 1.

The specificity profiles of the three antibodies are similar. The antibodies all discriminated EB1089 from endogenous metabolites of vitamin D. In particular, the cross-reactivity with 25-hydroxyvitamin D_3 was 0.01% for the antibody As-3, which is excellent taking into account the large amounts of this metabolite in serum (up to 1 ng/mL in humans). The cross-reactivity with the active metabolite $1,25(OH)_2D_3$ was generally slightly higher, but this form is present in equimolar amounts in serum compared to the expected serum levels of EB1089. Cross-reactivities with vitamin D_2 and vitamin D_3 were negligible for the three antibodies.

Table 1. Percent cross-reactivity

Compound	Antibody (Week 26)		
	As-1	As-2	As-3
EB1089	100	100	100
$1,25(OH)_2D_3$	0.3	0.78	0.1
$25(OH)D_3$	0.09	0.16	<0.01
$24R,25(OH)_2D_3$	0.04	0.07	0.07
Vitamin D_2	<0.01	<0.01	<0.01
Vitamin D_3	<0.01	<0.01	<0.01
EB1446	26	35	40
EB1436	16	28	29
EB1445	26	78	44
EB1470	26	70	27

All three antisera showed relatively high cross-reactivities with the four metabolites of EB1089. Thus, additional hydroxylation of the EB1089 side chain did not affect binding to the antibodies significantly.

Conclusion. In conclusion, we successfully prepared antibodies specific to EB1089 by immunization of rabbits with a truncated form of the molecule. The antibodies were highly selective for EB1089 over endogenous vitamin D metabolites, enough to allow direct measurement in serum of the analog. Cross-reactivities with 25-hydroxyvitamin D_3, the most abundant vitamin D metabolite in serum, were in the range 0.01-0.2% relative to EB1089.The further development of an immunoassay with these antibodies could therefore obviate the need for preliminary isolation of EB1089, which is a requirement in existing methods.

References
1. Hansen, C.M., Hamberg, K.J., Binderup, E., Binderup, L. (2000) *Current Pharm. Design* 6, 881-906.
2. Kissmeyer, A.M., Sonne, K., Binderup, E. (2000) *J. Chromatogr. B.* 740, 117-128.
3. Lind, C., Chen, J., Byrjalsen, I. (1997) *Clin. Chem.* 43, 943-949.
4. Pullen, G.R., Fitzgerald, M.G., Hosking, C.S. *J. Immunol. Methods* **1986**, 86, 83-87.
5. Kissmeyer, A.M., Binderup, E., Binderup, L., Hansen, C.M., Andersen, N.R., Makin, H.L.J., Schroeder, N.J., Shankar, V.N., Jones, G. (1997) *Biochem. Pharmacol.* 53, 1087-1097.

SUPERCRITICAL FLUID EXTRACTION OF VITAMINS D_2 AND D_3 IN PHARMACEUTICALS

J.M. Quesada Gómez[+], L. Gámiz-Gracia[*] and M.D. Luque de Castro[*],
[+]Mineral Metabolism Unit, Hospital Reina Sofía, University of Córdoba, E-14004, Córdoba, Spain
[*]Analytical Chemistry Division, Faculty of Sciences, University of Córdoba, E-14004 Córdoba, Spain

Introduction. Vitamin D in pharmaceutical products has been determined most frequently by liquid chromatography, involving liquid-liquid or solid-liquid extraction, as previous steps for the preparation of the sample, with waste of both organic solvents and time, as a result. Supercritical fluid extraction (SFE), particularly using CO_2 as extractant, has proved to be one of the most significant techniques for solid sample pre-treatment in the last few years [1,2]. This technique has been applied in pharmaceutical analysis both for the extraction of the pharmaceuticals [3] and preparation of samples from tablets, animal feeds, creams, ointments and infusions, in which the analytes are currently non-polar compounds [4]. SFE has been applied to the removal of vitamins from different matrices, namely: vitamin E in white of egg [5], pharmaceutical preparations [6] and corn oil [7]; vitamin A in cereal products [8] and liver [9]; vitamins A and E in pharmaceutical preparations [10], cosmetics [11] and ointments [12]; vitamin K in infant formulas [13] and blood [14]; and also to sample preparation prior to the analysis of water-soluble vitamins in foods [15]. In this work, a method for the extraction and analysis of vitamin D in pharmaceutical products, based on SFE extraction and HPLC separation with photometric determination is proposed [16].

Results and Discussion

Pharmaceutical Samples Preparation. All the samples were multivitamin complexes, with different vitamins and minerals in their composition. When the sample was in a liquid form, no previous preparation was required. In this case, the sample was spiked directly on 0.5 g of diatomaceous earth contained in the extraction cell. The contact time before extraction was 10 min. In the case of solid samples, 5 dosages were accurately weighed and mixed in a mortar, and an appropriate amount of the powder was placed in the extraction cell. In all instances, 0.25 mL of ethyl ether was added, waiting for 10 min before the extraction.

Chromatographic Separation/Detection. The separation of the vitamins D_2 and D_3 was performed on an Ultrabase C_{18} column. The injection volume was 100 µL and the flow-rate of the mobile phase (methanol:acetonitrile, ratio 90:10) was 1.5 mL min^{-1}. The chromatograms were obtained at a wavelength of 266 nm.

Supercritical Fluid Extraction. The CO_2 was delivered from a cylinder supplied with a dip tube, at a flow-rate of 2.0 mLmin^{-1}, aspirated by a double-piston pump and passed through the cell that contained the sample. The extraction process started after the extraction vessel had attained the working conditions (temperature, 40 °C and pressure, 281 bar). After an equilibration time of 1 min, the supercritical fluid passed through the sample for 60 min, leached the analytes and drove them to a stainless-steal balls trap through a variable diameter restrictor which avoided plugging and provided a constant flow-rate during the extraction process. In a subsequent step, a syringe pump pumped a methanol stream at a flow-rate of 0.5 mL min-1 through the trap. The trap temperature during the rinsing step was set at 40 °C. The extract was finally collected into vials.

Features of the method. The features of the method were obtained from the data set of the calibration curve [17]. All the values where calculated using the Alamin program [18], and are shown in Table 1.

Table 1. Features of the analytical method obtained from the calibration data sets

	Vitamin D_2	Vitamin D_3
Equation *	Y = 1.0 + 5.8·C	Y = 1.1 + 4.8·C
r^2 (%)	99.29	99.29
Detection limit (µg)	1.3	1.3
Quantification limit (µg)	4.1	4.1
Precision (RSD%)	3.8	6.3

* Y denotes mAU and C µg of analyte;

Application of the method to pharmaceutical samples. The method was applied to different pharmaceutical samples, namely: two kinds of drops (0.5 mL and 0.250 mL of each, for samples 1 and 2, respectively), one powder (4.1 g of sample) and one granulated (3.5 g of sample). In all the cases, 0.250 mL of ethyl ether was added to the sample contained in the extraction cell, waiting for 10 min before starting the extraction. The analyses were carried out in triplicate. The results are shown in Table 2.

Table 2. Application of the method to pharmaceutical samples

Pharmaceuticals	Nominal value		Found value (n=3)[a]		R (%)[a]
	Vit D_2	Vit D_3	Vit D_2	Vit D_3	
Drops 1[b]		1667	92±5	1599±36	101±2 [d]
Drops 2[b]	900	-----	766±86	-----	85±12
Powder[c]	-----	40	-----	42.0±0.7	105±2
Granulated[c]	-----	400	-----	417±5	104±5

[a] Mean value ± standard deviation; [b] Values expressed in UI mL^{-1}. (1 UI=25 ng of cholecalciferol or ergocalciferol); [c] Values expressed in UI g^{-1}; [d] Calculated as $D_2 + D_3$ content

Figure 1 shows the chromatograms obtained from the analytes extracted from spiked diatomaceous earth and from a pharmaceutical sample.

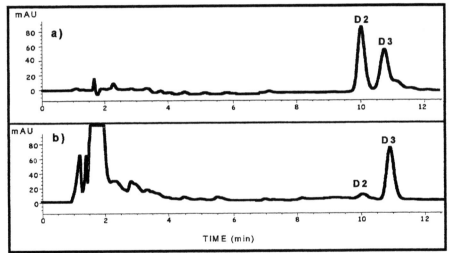

Fig. 1. Chromatograms obtained from 10 μg of vitamins D_2 and D_3 extracted from 0.5 g of diatomaceous earth (a) and 0.5 ml of pharmaceutical drops. (b)

Conclusions. A method for the supercritical fluid extraction of vitamins D_2 and D_3 and their HPLC determination has been proposed. This method has been applied to the analysis of different pharmaceutical preparations, providing recoveries close to 100% in all instances, with acceptable precision. The method avoids liquid-liquid extraction or solid-phase extraction, usually employed for this kind of matrices, reduces the waste of organic solvents and requires less human participation than the previous ones, by partial automation of the process.

812

References

[1]   Luque de Castro, M.D., Valcárcel M. and Tena M.T., (1994) Analytical Supercritical Fluid Extraction, Springer, Heidelberg.

[2]   Charpenter, B.A. and Sevenants, M.R. (1988) Supercritical Fluid Extraction and Chromatography. Techniques and Application. American Chemical Society, Washington, DC.

[3]   Dean, J.R. and Khunder, S. (1996) J. Pharm. and Biom. Anal. 15, 875-886.

[4]   Karlsson, L., Torstensson, A. and Taylor, L.T. (1997) J. Pharm. and Biom. Anal. 15, 601-611.

[5]   Colombo, M.L., Corsini, A., Mossa, A., Sala, L. and Stanca, M. (1998) Phytochem. Anal. 9, 192-195.

[6]   Salvador, A., Jaime, M.A., De la Guardia, M. and Becerra, G. (1998) Anal. Commun. 35, 53-55.

[7]   Li, K., Ong, C.P. and Li, S.F.Y. (1994) J. Chromatogr. Sci. 32, 53-56.

[8]   Schneiderman, M. A., Sharma, A.K. and Locke, D.C. (1997) J. Chromatogr. 765, 215-220.

[9]   Burri, B.J., Neidlinger, T.R., Lo, A.O., Kwan, C. and Wong, M.R. (1997) J. Chromatogr. 762, 201-206.

[10]   Scalia, S., Ruberto, G. and Bonina, F. (1995) J. Pharm. Sci. 84, 433-436.

[11]   Scalia, S., Renda, A., Ruberto, G., Bonina, F. and Menegatti, E. (1995) J. Pharm. Biomed. Anal. 13, 273-277.

[12]   Masuda, M., Koike, S., Handa, M., Sagara, K. and Mizutani, T. (1993) Anal. Sci. 9, 29-32.

[13]   Schneiman, M.A., Sharma, A.K., Mahanama, K.R.R. and Locke, D.C. (1988) J. Assoc. Off. Anal. Chem. 71, 815-817.

[14]   Hondo, T., Saito, M. and Senda, M. (1986) Bunseki Kagaku 35, 316-319.

[15]   Buskov, S., Moller, P., Sorensen, H., Sorensen, J.C. and Sorensen, S. (1998) J. Chromatogr. 802, 233-241.

[16]   Gámiz-Gracia, L., Jiménez-Carmona, M.M. and Luque de Castro, M.D. (2000) Chromatographia, 51, 428-432.

[17]   Cuadros Rodríguez, L., García Campaña, A.M., Jiménez Linares, C. and Román Ceba, M. (1993) Anal. Letters 26, 1243-1258.

[18]   García Campaña, A.M., Cuadros Rodríguez, L., Alés Barrero, F., Román Ceba, M. and Sierra Fernández, J.L. (1997) Trend in Anal. Chem. 16, 381-385.

THE CONCENTRATION OF VITAMIN D IN FORTIFIED MILK

Saleh H. Sedrani
King Saud University, College of Science, Biochemistry Department, P.O. Box 2455, Riyadh 11451, Saudi Arabia.

Introduction. Rickets and vitamin D deficiency diseases occur in Saudi Arabia despite of the abundance of sunshine throughout the year (1,2,3). Alternative source can be obtained by including vitamin D in the diet. Similar to the United States the chief food that is fortified with vitamin D in Saudi Arabia is milk (4). However, underfortification and overfortification can have deleterious consequences (4,5). It is therefore the objective of this study to determine, systematically, the vitamin D content of milk and liquid yogurt (laban) produced in Saudi Arabia by employing High Performance Liquid Chromatography technology.

Materials and Methods. Seven brands of milk and liquid yogurt (148 containers) from different milk processors fortified with vitamin D and 8 brands (34 containers) not fortified with the vitamin were purchased randomly from supermarkets. the brand names, date of purchase, expiration date, fat content, form of vitamin D added and concentration of vitamin D as claimed on the label were recorded. To 10 ml of milk samples, 6000 dpm tritiated vitamin D derivative were added. After overnight saponification at room temperature samples were extracted with diethyl ether. The extract was passed through an anhydrous sodium sulphate column to remove residual water. Then the fraction containing vitamin D was collected, concentrated and injected into normal phase HPLC and the fraction containing vitamin D was collected for determination of vitamin D. The quantification of D_2 and D_3 was performed by reverse phase HPLC using 10% methanol in acetonitrile as mobile phase and detected by spectrophotometer at 254 nm.

Results. Of the 148 milk and yogurt samples from 7 milk processors, only 5 percent contained 80% - 120% of the amount of vitamin D claimed on the label (400 IU/L). Eighteen percent contained 32% - 262% more than the amount stated on the label, and eighteen percent of the samples contained 51% - 65% less than the amount stated on the label. Whereas, 59% of the fortified milk samples contained vitamin D in the level of non-fortified milk. Table 1 shows the distribution of the percentage of samples within 80% - 120%, <80%, >120% of vitamin D claimed on the label. The vitamin D contents of the 34 non-fortified milk samples were ranging from undetectable level to 50 IU/L except for two samples where the level was 195±1.5 IU/L.

Table 1. The variation between vitamin D content stated on the label
(400 IU/L) and the measured vitamin D concentration

Brand	N	Percentage of Samples		
		80%-120%	< 80%	> 120%
Milk	102	8	76	16
Yogurt	46	0	78	22
Total Samples = 148				

Conclusion. Since only 8 percent of the 102 fortified milk samples and none
of the 46 liquid yogurt (Table 1) analyzed contained 80% - 120% of the
amount of vitamin D stated on the label and the rest of the samples
contained vitamin D in the level of non-fortified milk or were underfortified or
overfortified, it is concluded that milk and liquid yogurt preparations do not
contain the amount of vitamin D stated on the label.

REFERENCES

1. Elidrissy, A.T.H., Sedrani, S.H. and Lawson, D.E.M. (1984) Vitamin D
   Deficiency in Mothers of Rachitic Infants. Calcif. Tissue Int. 36: 266-268.
2. Sedrani, S.H., Al-Arabi, K.M. and Elidrissy, A. (1983) Are Saudis at Risk
   of Developing Vitamin D Deficiency? Saudi Medical Journal. 7: 427-433.
3. Sedrani, S.H., Al-Arabi, K.M., Abanmy, A. and Elidrissy, A. (1990)
   Study of Vitamin "D" Status and Factors Leading to its Deficiency in Saudi
   Arabia. KACTS p. 324.
4. Holick, M.F., Shao, Q., Liu, W.W., and Chen, T.T. (1992) The Vitamin
   D Content of Fortified Milk and Infant Formula. New Eng. J. Med. 326:
   1178-1181.
5. Jacobus, C.H., Holick, M.F., Shao, Q., Chen, T.C., et al. (1992)
   Hypervitaminosis D Associated with Drinking Milk. N. Engl. J. Med. 326:
   1173-1177.

VDR POLYMORPHISMS

ARE HUMAN VITAMIN D RECEPTOR GENE POLYMORPHISMS FUNCTIONALLY SIGNIFICANT?

G. Kerr Whitfield, Lenore S. Remus, Peter W. Jurutka, Heike Zitzer, Anish K. Oza, Hope T. L. Dang, Carol A. Haussler, Michael A. Galligan, Michelle L. Thatcher, Carlos Encinas Dominguez, Mark R. Haussler, Department of Biochemistry, The University of Arizona College of Medicine, Tucson, AZ, U.S.A. 85724.

Introduction: The biological actions of 1,25-dihydroxyvitamin D_3 (1,25$(OH)_2D_3$) are mediated largely, if not entirely, by the vitamin D receptor (VDR), a member of the superfamily of nuclear hormone receptors (1). This protein is found in tissues known to play a role in calcium homeostasis, and also in numerous other tissues, where it appears to regulate a variety of processes, including cell proliferation and differentiation (2). The significance of the nuclear VDR in calcium homeostasis, as well as in certain proliferation/differentiation processes in skin and uterus, has been confirmed by gene knockout studies in mice (3,4). Human (h)VDR mediates transcriptional activation by the 1,25$(OH)_2D_3$ hormone by the following mechanism: i) liganding of nuclear VDR by 1,25$(OH)_2D_3$, ii) recruitment by 1,25$(OH)_2D_3$-VDR of its retinoid X receptor (RXR) heteropartner that, in turn, facilitates high-affinity interaction of the dimeric complex with vitamin D responsive elements (VDREs) upstream of target genes, iii) attraction by VDR of basal transcription factor IIB (TFIIB) (5), the rate-limiting component of the transcription preinitiation complex, and iv) recruitment by the heterodimer of a number of transcription coactivators, some with histone acetyl transferase (HAT) activity to modify nucleosome/chromatin organization, such as SRC-1 (6), and others like the DRIPs (7) that target the VDR supercomplex to the TATA-box/TBP and RNA polymerase II transcription initiation machinery. The net result of this 1,25$(OH)_2D_3$-triggered response is the regulation of genes coding for proteins that carry out intestinal calcium absorption, bone remodeling, cell differentiation, etc. (8). Because transactivation is the ultimate biochemical action of the liganded VDR and depends on all of the other capabilities of the receptor (ligand binding, nuclear localization, heterodimerization and VDRE/DNA binding), the present study focuses on this parameter of receptor activity in order to probe for functional significance of hVDR gene polymorphisms.

The chromosomal gene for VDR has been cloned (9), and several common genetic variants have been described in humans, most of which are identified by a biallelic variation in a restriction endonuclease site (Fig. 1). Polymorphisms are observed in specific intronic sites for *Bsm I* (10) and *Apa I* (11), a silent *Taq I* site in exon IX (10), as well as in a singlet(A) repeat in the portion of exon IX encoding the 3' UTR (12) (see Fig. 1, right). All of these variations near the 3' end of the gene are in linkage disequilibrium (10,13), although this linkage is weaker in ethnic groups such as African-Americans (12). None of these polymorphisms affect the VDR protein, although the singlet(A) repeat in the 3' UTR is expressed in the mature mRNA for hVDR. Singlet(A) variants are classified according to length by the number of consecutive A's in the repeat, with ≥17 A's scored as "long" (*L*), and ≤15 A's considered "short" (*S*).

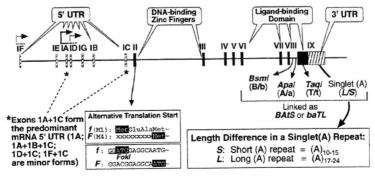

Fig. 1. Features of the human VDR gene relevant to polymorphic variation in VDR expression/activity.

Another polymorphic site has been found in exon II near the center of the hVDR gene (14). This site, which is genetically unlinked to the above *Bsm/Apa/Taq*/singlet(A) cluster, is the only currently known hVDR variant to result in an alteration of hVDR protein structure (Fig. 1, center left). Presence of the *Fok I* site (designated *f*) predicts a 427-residue VDR protein beginning at Met-1 (according to the numbering scheme of Baker *et al.* (15)), whereas absence of this site (denoted *F*) dictates translation from Met-4, producing a protein of 424 amino acids (16).

In an initial report (17), allelic variation in the chromosomal gene for the vitamin D receptor was proposed to represent a major part of the genetic predisposition for low bone mineral density (BMD), and perhaps for osteoporosis and/or skeletal fractures, although these associations have been disputed by other studies (reviewed in (18)). More recently, correlations have been reported between VDR allelic variants and risk of prostate cancer (19), breast cancer (20), and sarcoidosis (21). However, conflicting reports have appeared that minimize or even contradict these associations (19,22). Likewise, direct testing of hVDR alleles for activity has yielded somewhat variable results, although, when a difference is found, the *b* and *F* hVDR alleles appear to be more active than the *B* or *f* alleles (see Discussion).

A caveat in most of the above-cited studies is the fact that correlations were sought between a single polymorphism, or between the *Bsm-Apa-Taq* linkage group, and the physiological parameter of interest. Very few studies have attempted to control for hVDR genotype at both the *Bsm/Apa/Taq*/singlet(A) cluster and the *Fok I* site. In one example (23), a correlation between *Fok I* alleles and BMD could not be demonstrated, but "cross-genotyping" with *Bsm I* alleles revealed a potentially important positive association in prepubertal girls between the *ffBB* hVDR genotype and low BMD (23).

In the present communication, we report the evaluation of twenty human fibroblast lines, simultaneously considering hVDR genotypes at both the singlet(A) and the *Fok I* loci, which are then .correlated with the phenotypic activity of the endogenous VDR in the corresponding cell line. From these data, we conclude that: a) biallelic variants at both the *Fok I* and the singlet(A) sites affect transcriptional activation by the endogenous hVDR in the tested human fibroblasts, b) the singlet(A) *L* allele is more active than the *S* allele, and c) a third, unknown genetic variable appears to influence VDR activity.

Results: Genomic DNA samples were extracted from all twenty fibroblast cell lines, subjected to PCR, and analyzed for their genotype at the polymorphic *F/f* and the *L/S* sites. *F/f* genotypes were determined by digestion of the PCR products from each line with the restriction enzyme *Fok I* (24). The frequencies of the *F* and *f* alleles in the present sample group were 62.5% and 37.5%, respectively. This distribution of hVDR alleles is similar to that characterized for Caucasian populations in other studies (24-26).

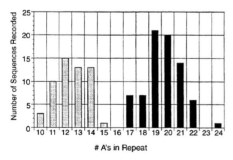

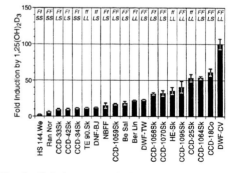

Fig. 2. Compilation of sequencing results from *L/S* genotyping (4-5 sequences per cell line).

Fig. 3. Relative transcriptional activity of endogenous VDR in 20 human fibroblast lines.

L/S genotypes were determined by sequencing of PCR products to determine the exact length of the singlet(A) repeat (27). As reported by others (12), we observed (Fig. 2) multiple alleles at this locus which segregate into a "long" (*L*) group with 17-24 A's in the repeat, and a "short" group (S) with 10-15 A's in the repeat. The frequencies of the L and S hVDR alleles in the present panel of cell lines were 60% and 40%, respectively, similar to that previously published for Caucasian populations (12).

Fig. 3 shows the hVDR-mediated transcription results from all 20 cell lines after transfection with a $1,25(OH)_2D_3$-responsive reporter plasmid $((CT4)_4TKGH$ (28)) and incubation for 48 h in the presence or absence of 10^{-8} M $1,25(OH)_2D_3$, expressed as fold-induction by the hormone. The assay conditions, including quantitative monitoring of transfection efficiency using a β-galactosidase vector, were designed to permit comparison of endogenous VDR activity between cell lines. The data (Fig. 3) reveal a striking spectrum of activities, ranging from only a 1.75-fold induction of the growth hormone reporter to a 100-fold effect of hormone, with a mean of 28 ± 24 (SD) fold induction.

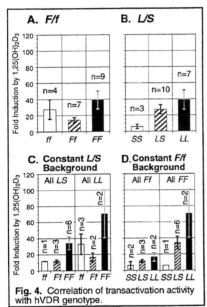

Fig. 4. Correlation of transactivation activity with hVDR genotype.

Correlations were next sought between the genotypes of each cell line at the Fok I and L/S loci and the relative activities of the corresponding endogenous VDRs. Accordingly, all twenty cell lines were grouped into ff (4 lines), Ff (7 lines) or FF (9 lines). The average fold-inductions by $1,25(OH)_2D_3$ for each group are displayed ± SEM in Fig. 4A. Although no clear trend is evident, it is notable that the FF group displays the highest average fold-induction. These F/f groupings were then subdivided into sets with the LS genotype (Fig. 4C, left panel) and the LL genotype (Fig. 4C, right panel), thereby controlling for the L/S genotype when evaluating the activity of endogenous F/f hVDR. Again, in both groups of data, the FF cells display the highest activity. However, none of the differences between sets in either Fig. 4A or 4C achieve statistical significance (at the 95% confidence interval). Nevertheless, it has previously been reported by our group (5) that F hVDR interacts more efficiently (approximately 2-fold) with TFIIB than does the f hVDR isoform, thus providing a plausible mechanism for the greater transactivation potency of the F hVDR. Whether this difference in activity reflects that occurring under in vivo conditions is not known; however, these results provide a reasonable mechanism by which to explain the enhanced transactivation ability of the F/M4 hVDR isoform, in vitro (5,16,29), and are consistent with a proposed bioactivity for F hVDR that is also greater than that of f hVDR, in vivo (16,24,25,29-32).

When $1,25(OH)_2D_3$-stimulated transcription activities in the twenty lines are grouped by L/S genotype (Fig. 4B), a much clearer, but still not statistically significant, trend emerges, with SS having the lowest fold-induction, LL possessing the highest, and the LS genotype exhibiting intermediate activity. This trend persists when the groupings are subdivided into Ff or FF genotypic backgrounds (Fig. 4D), leading to the tentative conclusion that the L hVDR allele is more active than the S allele. The SS and ff subsets were not included in Figs. 4C and 4D, because of the low number of samples of both SS and ff homozygotes (3 and 4, respectively), as well as the complete lack of the ffSS hVDR genotype in the current series.

Considering the lack of genetic linkage between the Fok I and L/S polymorphisms (23,24), plus the fact that both loci appear to affect function of endogenous hVDR, in vivo (Fig. 4), as well as evidence that F hVDR is more active than f, in vitro, we attempted next to correlate the combined genotypes at both loci with hVDR transactivation ability. In order to condense genotypic information from both sites into a single variable, an "allele score" was devised based on which allelic variants appear more active in the literature and in the present experiments. Since the F genotype is more active than f both in vivo and in vitro, each F hVDR allele was assigned a value of 1, while f alleles were scored as zero. Likewise, because the data in Fig. 4, panels B and D, indicate the L hVDR alleles to be more active than the *S* alleles, *L* and *S* alleles received scores of 1 and 0, respectively. Therefore, possible total allele scores for the hVDR autosomal gene range from 0 to 4 for both sexes. After grouping all twenty cell lines according to this formula, the average fold-induction by $1,25(OH)_2D_3$ was plotted vs. the allele score (Fig. 5A). A striking trend emerges from this analysis, with each increasing increment in allele score yielding a higher average fold-induction by $1,25(OH)_2D_3$. A qualitatively similar trend was seen if $1,25(OH)_2D_3$-stimulated values for reporter gene transcription were plotted instead of fold-induction values (data not shown). Thus, the dramatic escalation of hVDR functional activity appears to correlate with the combined hVDR genotypic allele score at the *F/f* and *L/S* loci. Importantly, the difference between the two groups with allele scores of 2 and 4 achieves statistical significance by the two-tailed Student's t-test ($P = 0.035$).

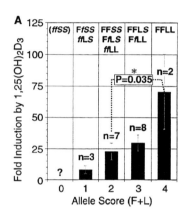 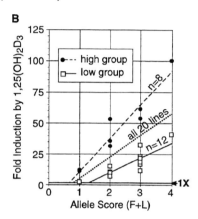

Fig. 5. Correlation of transcriptional activity with hVDR genotype at both *F/f* and *L/S* loci.

Fig. 5B depicts the identical data set analyzed in A, but with each cell line plotted as an individual point. When a linear regression line is calculated for all 20 lines, the allele score shows a moderately strong, and statistically significant, positive correlation with transactivation (correlation coefficient = 0.595; $P = 0.012$). If, however, the cell lines are divided into a high group (above the n=20 regression line) and low group (below the n=20 line), the respective correlation coefficients are markedly improved, to 0.958 for the high group (n=8, P <0.001) and 0.858 for the low group (n=12, P < 0.001). This apparent segregation of values into high and low groups argues for the existence of a new, third variable, other than the *FokI* or 3' cluster of polymorphisms containing *L/S*, in determining hVDR functional activity.

Discussion: A goal of the present study was to examine endogenous hVDR transcriptional activity in relation to hVDR genotype at unlinked polymorphic sites in both exons II and IX. The results reveal a strong correlation between genotype and VDR activity when both polymorphic sites are simultaneously considered (Fig. 5). Considering each site separately may not reveal significant effects. Thus, the current data may explain why many attempts to correlate hVDR activity with genotype at a single locus have been unsuccessful.

The assignment of *F* as the more active hVDR allele is based not only on the current analysis of fibroblast lines, but also on *in vitro* data collected with *F* and *f* proteins expressed in transfected cells (5,16). Another group (29) has also studied *F* vs. *f* hVDR proteins, and reported a lower ED_{50} for $1,25(OH)_2D_3$ with the *F* allele. These data indicating a more active *F* hVDR allele are consistent with a number of epidemiological studies which suggest that the *F* allele, when compared with the *f* allele, is associated with increased BMD (16,24,30,31,33,34), lower risk for primary hyperparathyroidism (35), lower risk for intervertebral disc degeneration (32) or lower incidence of vertebral fracture (25). However, it should be acknowledged that not all studies have found these associations. For instance, one group (26) did not observe a correlation between hVDR genotype and BMD in a large cohort of French women. Also, another group (36) was unable to correlate any hVDR-related functional parameter with *F/f* genotype in either cells transfected with vectors expressing *F* vs. *f* hVDRs, or in a small panel of human fibroblast lines. The fact that *only* the *F/f* genotype was considered in the above investigations implies, however, that the *L/S* genotype could have been a significant confounder in these studies.

The assignment of *L* hVDR as more active than *S* is based primarily on observations with the present panel of fibroblast cell lines. *L* and *S* hVDR alleles do not produce different proteins, and therefore cannot be tested in the same fashion as *F/f* isoforms. Since the *L/S* polymorphism occurs in exon IX, but is expressed only in the 3' UTR of hVDR mRNA, the working hypothesis presented herein states that the *L* allele may produce receptor mRNA that is more stable and/or is translated more efficiently into hVDR protein than the *S* allele.

Because several experiments indicate that mRNA stabilities are similar for hVDRs containing the *baTL* and *BAtS* polymorphic clusters (13,37,38), the more likely possibility is that the *L* allele produces more VDR protein from a given unit of mRNA. While there is a paucity of data relating to this hypothesis, it is notable that ligand binding assays (36) seem to indicate a trend toward higher VDR abundance (expressed as N_{max}) in *bb* vs. *BB* fibroblast lines, although these differences were not statistically significant. Should it be the case that *L* alleles (linked to *b*) produce more hVDR protein, what could be the mechanism for such an effect? Recent observations regarding mammalian and yeast poly(A) binding proteins (PABPs) indicate that binding of PABP to mRNA enhances translatability of mRNAs via an association with other proteins that interact with the 5' end of the message (39,40). Usually, multiple PABP monomers bind to poly(A)⁺ RNAs, with each monomer occupying approximately 27 adenylate residues (41). Intriguingly, further studies with human PABP suggest that as few as 11 consecutive A's can bind to PABP, with 25 A's giving maximum affinity (42). Thus, one could speculate that: a) PABP may be capable of binding to the singlet(A) repeat in the hVDR gene, and b) its ability to bind may be enhanced in long (*L*) alleles (17-24 A's) vs. short (*S*) alleles (10-15 A's). Greater association of PABP with *L* alleles would then lead to more efficacious translation via a more potent interaction with translation factors such as EF-4B (40).

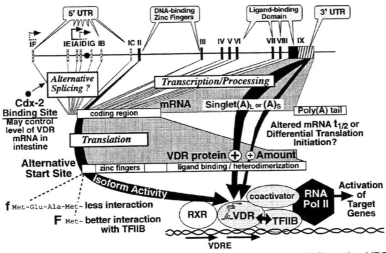

Fig. 6. Summary of common polymorphic variations in the hVDR gene influencing VDR activity.

Fig. 6 presents an illustration of how hVDR gene polymorphisms may affect VDR potency. The *F/f* allelic variation affects the quality of hVDR, with the *F* isoform possessing enhanced transcriptional potency by virtue of its stronger interaction with TFIIB. *L* may be more active than the S hVDR allele because the quantity of hVDR protein is augmented, perhaps via more efficacious translation of its mRNA. When considered together, the *F/f* and *L/S* alleles appear to significantly impact hVDR activity, but because the two polymorphisms are unlinked, the effect is likely an additive rather than synergistic one. A recent epidemiological study (43), in which a large cohort with malignant melanoma was genotyped at the *T/t* and *F/f* loci, supports this conclusion. It was found that *fftt* homozygotes (recall that *t* is often linked to *S*) had significantly thicker tumors (*P* = 0.001). These results intimate that the *fftt* allele combination might be associated with less active hVDR, as VDR has been reported to have antiproliferative effects that might be expected to counter the malignant phenotype (2).

Finally, the presence of two distinct groupings of hVDR activity vs. allele score in Fig. 5B argues in favor of the existence of another variable that influences innate hVDR activity, at least in fibroblasts. The hypothesis put forth in the present communication (Fig. 6) is that there exists one or more additional polymorphic variations in the hVDR gene beyond those at the *F/f* locus and in the 3' cluster (*Apa/Bsm/Taq* and *L/S*) that affect(s) hVDR activity. The coding exons of the hVDR gene have been studied rather extensively, and have yielded numerous point mutations causing hereditary vitamin D resistant rickets (2,44-46), but little evidence has been presented for the occurrence of common polymorphic sites other than the *Fok I* site in exon II and the linked cluster of sites in the exon VIII-IX region. Yet, recent investigations into the portion of the hVDR gene encoding the 5' untranslated region (5' UTR) have revealed a surprising complex of at least seven exons (denoted IA-IG, see Fig. 6, top left), with evidence for alternative splicing (9,47). It is possible that undiscovered common polymorphic sites may exist in this newly described complex of multiple exons at the 5' end of the gene. Such polymorphisms could even alter VDR protein structure b y introducing in-frame initiator methionine codons leading to the expression of VDRs with N-terminal extensions, as already proposed by one research group (47).

Still another possibility is that polymorphisms in the 5' region of the VDR gene might affect the activity of one of the three proposed hVDR promoters (47), leading to the expression of altered quantities of VDR proteins under physiologic conditions. Here again, a precedent exists from a recent report (48) that describes a polymorphism in a binding site for Cdx-2, a homeodomain protein related to *caudal* (position of Cdx binding site in the hVDR gene is shown in Fig. 6, top left). The importance of Cdx-2 for intestine-specific expression of hVDR was demonstrated previously (49). It is, of course, not possible to invoke this polymorphism to explain the present results in fibroblast lines, given the intestine-specific nature of Cdx-2 regulated expression (50). However, the existence of this polymorphism should certainly be considered in epidemiological studies relating VDR-mediated intestinal absorption of calcium and phosphate as they impact BMD and parathyroid gland function. Indeed, in a large cohort of Japanese women, the *A* allele at the Cdx-2 locus correlated with higher BMD in the lumbar spine, consistent with a slightly greater activity of a VDR promoter construct incorporating the Cdx-*A* type element (48).

Rather than evoking Cdx-2 or any other known polymorphism to explain the present results, we prefer the interpretation that a novel polymorphism exists, likely located in the incompletely characterized 5' region of the hVDR gene. A full recognition of the genetic complexity of VDR action in humans may eventually allow for accurate prediction of VDR activity in individual patients based on genotype, along with an enhanced ability to assess disease risk as well as response to pharmacologic agents related to VDR action.

Summary: Common polymorphisms in the hVDR gene have been associated in epidemiologic studies with BMD and several clinical disorders, although the data are often conflicting. We evaluated the functional roles of two unlinked hVDR polymorphisms, the first in a *Fok I (F/f)* restriction site at the start of translation, and the second in a singlet(A) repeat in the 3'-untranslated region. A panel of 20 human fibroblast cell lines was genotyped at both polymorphic sites, and evaluated for the relative transcription activities of endogenous receptor using a transfected $1,25(OH)_2D_3$-responsive reporter gene. A spectrum of hVDR activities was observed, ranging from approximately 2- to 100-fold induction of the reporter construct by $1,25(OH)_2D_3$. When *F/f* genotypes were segregated, there was a trend indicating *F* to be more active than *f*, although statistical significance was not achieved. Independent investigation of artificially constructed *F* and *f* hVDR isoforms, *in vitro*, has revealed that *F* is approximately 2-fold more active than *f*, and that *F* VDR interacts more efficiently with basal transcription factor IIB. When singlet(A) genotypes were examined in transfected fibroblast lines, the long *(L)* alleles, in general, produced more active endogenous

VDRs than the short *(S)* alleles, but again without statistical significance. However, when genotypes at both sites, expressed as an "allele score" (total number of *F* + *L* alleles), were plotted against fold induction by $1,25(OH)_2D_3$, a statistically significant correlation was seen between genotype and relative VDR activity, with response to $1,25(OH)_2D_3$ ranging from 8-fold with an allele score = 1, up to 70-fold with a score = 4. Interestingly, the 20 cell lines examined appeared to segregate further into two activity groups at each allele score, a high group (n = 8; correlation coefficient (r) = 0.96) and a low group (n = 12; r = 0.86). These preliminary results indicate functional relevance for both the *Fok* I and singlet(A) polymorphisms, and provide evidence for a third genetic variable. We conclude that hVDR genotype/clinical phenotype investigations must consider simultaneously the *F/f* and *L/S* polymorphisms, as well as an additional polymorphism(s) functionally significant to receptor activity. The observed differences in hVDR potency could, over a lifetime, have a major impact on intestinal calcium absorption, BMD, and the susceptibility to osteoporotic fractures, as well as the risk of hyperproliferative disorders.

Acknowledgements: Supported by National Institutes of Health grants to Mark R. Haussler.

References:

1. Whitfield, G. K., Jurutka, P. W., Haussler, C. A., and Haussler, M. R. (1999) *J. Cell. Biochem.* **Suppl. 32/33**, 110-122
2. Haussler, M. R., Whitfield, G. K., Haussler, C. A., Hsieh, J.-C., Thompson, P. D., Selznick, S. H., Encinas Dominguez, C., and Jurutka, P. W. (1998) *J. Bone Miner. Res.* **13**, 325-349
3. Kato, S., Takeyama, K., Kitanaka, S., Murayama, A., Sekine, K., and Yoshizawa, T. (1999) *J. Steroid Biochem. Molec. Biol.* **69**, 247-251
4. Li, Y. C., Amling, M., Pirro, A. E., Priemel, M., Meuse, J., Baron, R., Delling, G., and Demay, M. B. (1998) *Endocrinology* **139**, 4391-4396
5. Jurutka, P. W., Remus, L. S., Whitfield, G. K., Thompson, P. D., Hsieh, J. C., Zitzer, H., Tavakkoli, P., Galligan, M. A., Dang, H. T., Haussler, C. A., and Haussler, M. R. (2000) *Mol. Endocrinol.* **14**, 401-420
6. Gill, R. K., Atkins, L. M., Hollis, B. W., and Bell, N. H. (1998) *Mol. Endocrinol.* **12**, 57-65
7. Rachez, C., Lemon, B. D., Suldan, Z., Bromleigh, V., Gamble, M., Naar, A. M., Erdjument-Bromage, H., Tempst, P., and Freedman, L. P. (1999) *Nature* **398**, 824-828
8. Jurutka, P. W., Whitfield, G. K., Hsieh, J.-C., Thompson, P. D., Haussler, C. A., and Haussler, M. R. (2000) *Reviews in Endocrinology and Metabolic Disorders,* **in press**
9. Miyamoto, K.-i., Kesterson, R. A., Yamamoto, H., Taketani, Y., Nishiwaki, E., Tatsumi, S., Inoue, Y., Morita, K., Takeda, E., and Pike, J. W. (1997) *Mol. Endocrinol.* **11**, 1165-1179
10. Morrison, N., Yeoman, R., Kelly, P. J., and Eisman, J. A. (1992) *Proc. Natl. Acad. Sci. USA* **89**, 6665-6669
11. Faraco, J. H., Morrison, N. A., Baker, A., Shine, J., and Frossard, P. M. (1989) *Nucleic Acids Res.* **17**, 2150
12. Ingles, S. A., Haile, R. W., Henderson, B. E., Kolonel, L. N., Nakaichi, G., Shi, C. Y., Yu, M. C., Ross, R. K., and Coetzee, G. A. (1997) *Cancer Epidemiol. Biomarkers Prev.* **6**, 93-98
13. Verbeek, W., Gombart, A. F., Shiohara, M., Campbell, M., and Koeffler, H. P. (1997) *Biochem. Biophys. Res. Commun.* **238**, 77-80
14. Saijo, T., Ito, M., Takeda, E., Mahbubul Huq, A. H. M., Naito, E., Yokota, I., Sone, T., Pike, J. W., and Kuroda, Y. (1991) *Am. J. Hum. Genet.* **49**, 668-673
15. Baker, A. R., McDonnell, D. P., Hughes, M. R., Crisp, T. M., Mangelsdorf, D. J., Haussler, M. R., Pike, J. W., Shine, J., and O'Malley, B. W. (1988) *Proc. Natl. Acad. Sci. USA* **85**, 3294-3298
16. Arai, H., Miyamoto, K.-I., Taketani, Y., Yamamoto, H., Iemori, Y., Morita, K., Tonai, T., Nishisho, T., Mori, S., and Takeda, E. (1997) *J. Bone Miner. Res.* **12**, 915-921
17. Morrison, N. A., Qi, J. C., Tokita, A., Kelly, P. J., Crofts, L., Nguyen, T. V., Sambrook, P. N., and Eisman, J. A. (1994) *Nature* **367**, 284-287
18. Wood, R. J., and Fleet, J. C. (1998) *Ann. Rev. Nutr.* **18**, 233-258
19. Miller, G. J. (1998) *Cancer Metastasis Rev.* **17**, 353-360
20. Ingles, S. A., Garcia, D. G., Wang, W., Nieters, A., Henderson, B. E., Kolonel, L. N., Haile, R. W., and Coetzee, G. A. (2000) *Cancer Causes Control* **11**, 25-30
21. Niimi, T., Tomita, H., Sato, S., Kawaguchi, H., Akita, K., Maeda, H., Sugiura, Y., and Ueda, R. (1999) *Am. J. Respir. Crit. Care Med.* **160**, 1107-1109

22. Cheng, W. C., and Tsai, K. S. (1999) *Osteoporos. Int.* **9**, 545-549
23. Ferrari, S., Rizzoli, R., Manen, D., Slosman, D., and Bonjour, J. P. (1998) *J. Bone Miner. Res.* **13**, 925-930
24. Gross, C., Eccleshall, T. R., Malloy, P. J., Villa, M. L., Marcus, R., and Feldman, D. (1996) *J. Bone Miner. Res.* **11**, 1850-1855
25. Gennari, L., Becherini, L., Mansani, R., Masi, L., Falchetti, A., Morelli, A., Colli, E., Gonnelli, S., Cepollaro, C., and Brandi, M. L. (1999) *J. Bone Miner. Res.* **14**, 1379-1386
26. Eccleshall, T. R., Garnero, P., Gross, C., Delmas, P. D., and Feldman, D. (1998) *J. Bone Miner. Res.* **13**, 31-35
27. Ingles, S. A., Ross, R. K., Yu, M. C., Irvine, R. A., La Pera, G., Haile, R. W., and Coetzee, G. A. (1997) *J. Natl. Cancer Inst.* **89**, 166-170
28. Terpening, C. M., Haussler, C. A., Jurutka, P. W., Galligan, M. A., Komm, B. S., and Haussler, M. R. (1991) *Mol. Endocrinol.* **5**, 373-385
29. Colin, E. M., Weel, A. E., Uitterlinden, A. G., Buurman, C. J., Birkenhager, J. C., Pols, H. A., and Van Leeuwen, J. P. (2000) *Clin. Endocrinol. (Oxf)* **52**, 211-216
30. Lucotte, G., Mercier, G., and Burckel, A. (1999) *Clin. Genet.* **56**, 221-224
31. Harris, S. S., Eccleshall, T. R., Gross, C., Dawson-Hughes, B., and Feldman, D. (1997) *J. Bone Miner. Res.* **12**, 1043-1048
32. Videman, T., Leppavuori, J., Kaprio, J., Battie, M. C., Gibbons, L. E., Peltonen, L., and Koskenvuo, M. (1998) *Spine* **23**, 2477-2285
33. Tao, C., Yu, T., Garnett, S., Briody, J., Knight, J., Woodhead, H., and Cowell, C. T. (1998) *Arch. Dis. Child.* **79**, 488-493
34. Ferrari, S., Manen, D., Bonjour, J. P., Slosman, D., and Rizzoli, R. (1999) *J. Clin. Endocrinol. Metab.* **84**, 2043-2048
35. Sosa, M., Torres, A., Martin, N., Salido, E., Liminana, J. M., Barrios, Y., De Miguel, E., and Betancor, P. (2000) *J. Intern. Med.* **247**, 124-130
36. Gross, C., Krishnan, A. V., Malloy, P. J., Eccleshall, T. R., Zhao, X. Y., and Feldman, D. (1998) *J. Bone Miner. Res.* **13**, 1691-1699
37. Durrin, L. K., Haile, R. W., Ingles, S. A., and Coetzee, G. A. (1999) *Biochim. Biophys. Acta* **1453**, 311-320
38. Mocharla, H., Butch, A. W., Pappas, A. A., Flick, J. T., Weinstein, R. S., De Togni, P., Jilka, R. L., Roberson, P. K., Parfitt, A. M., and Manolagas, S. C. (1997) *J. Bone Miner. Res.* **12**, 726-733
39. Munroe, D., and Jacobson, A. (1990) *Gene* **91**, 151-158
40. Le, H., Tanguay, R. L., Balasta, M. L., Wei, C. C., Browning, K. S., Metz, A. M., Goss, D. J., and Gallie, D. R. (1997) *J. Biol. Chem.* **272**, 16247-16255
41. Baer, B. W., and Kornberg, R. D. (1980) *Proc. Natl. Acad. Sci. USA* **77**, 1890-1892
42. Deo, R. C., Bonanno, J. B., Sonenberg, N., and Burley, S. K. (1999) *Cell* **98**, 835-845
43. Hutchinson, P. E., Osborne, J. E., Lear, J. T., Smith, A. G., Bowers, P. W., Morris, P. N., Jones, P. W., York, C., Strange, R. C., and Fryer, A. A. (2000) *Clin. Cancer Res.* **6**, 498-504
44. Lin, N. U.-T., Malloy, P. J., Sakati, N., Al-Ashwal, A., and Feldman, D. (1996) *J. Clin. Endocrinol. Metab.* **81**, 2564-2569
45. Hawa, N. S., Cockerill, F. J., Vadher, S., Hewison, M., Rut, A. R., Pike, J. W., O'Riordan, J. L., and Farrow, S. M. (1996) *Clin. Endocrinol. (Oxf)* **45**, 85-92
46. Whitfield, G. K., Selznick, S. H., Haussler, C. A., Hsieh, J.-C., Galligan, M. A., Jurutka, P. W., Thompson, P. D., Lee, S. M., Zerwekh, J. E., and Haussler, M. R. (1996) *Mol. Endocrinol.* **10**, 1617-1631
47. Crofts, L. A., Hancock, M. S., Morrison, N. A., and Eisman, J. A. (1998) *Proc. Natl. Acad. Sci. USA* **95**, 10529-10534
48. Arai, H., Miyamoto, K., Yoshida, M., Kubota, M., Yamamoto, H., Taketani, Y., Yoshida, S., Ikeda, M., and Takeda, E. (1999) *J. Bone Miner. Res.* **14**, S191 (Abstract #T084)
49. Yamamoto, H., Miyamoto, K., Li, B., Taketani, Y., Kitano, M., Inoue, Y., Morita, K., Pike, J. W., and Takeda, E. (1999) *J. Bone Miner. Res.* **14**, 240-247
50. Suh, E., Chen, L., Taylor, J., and Traber, P. G. (1994) *Mol. Cell. Biol.* **14**, 7340-7351

VARIABILITY ON 5' AND 3' UTR POLYMORPHIC SITES OF VITAMIN-D RECEPTOR GENE AND PARATHYROID RESPONSE IN DIALYSIS PATIENTS.

Joan Fibla*, Maria P Marco+ , Yolanda Barber* , Àngels Betriu+, Xènia Triquell*, Jaume Mas* and Elvira Fernández+. * Department of Basic Medical Sciences and +Department of Medicine. University of Lleida, 25199 LLEIDA, Spain.

Introduction Variability on the FokI restriction site at the start codon of the vitamin D receptor (VDR) gene has been related to bone mineral density. In addition, allelic variations at the 3' untranslated region (UTR) of this gene (the BsmI restriction site and the Poly(A) microsatellite) has been associated with variations in bone mineralization and with risk of developing prostate cancer, respectively. In a previous work we found association between BB homozygous for the BsmI polymorphism and hypoparathyroidism in dialysis patients (1). In the present work we investigated the distribution of FokI and Poly(A) genotypes in patients with end-stage renal disease (ESRD) in dialysis. We also studied the haplotype distribution of these three polymorphic sites in patients and controls.

Table I.- Genotype distributions of Fok I and Poly (A) polymorphisms

Genotypes&Alleles		Controls no (%)	All patients no (%)	Low PTH no (%)	High PTH no (%)
		n=119	n=168	n=40	n=38
Fok I					
	FF	47 (39%	70 (42%)	20 (50%)	16 (42%)
	Ff	59 (50%	79 (47%)	17 (42%)	17 (45%)
	ff	13 (11%	19 (11%)	3 (8%)	5 (13%)
	allele (f)	85 (36%	117 (35%)	23 (29%)	27 (35%)
	allele (F)	153 (64%	219 (65%)	57 (71%)	49 (65%)
Poly(A)					
	SS	18 (15%	38 (23%)	14 (35%)#	10 (26%)
	SL	62 (52%	68 (40%)	17 (42%)	11 (29%)$
	LL	39 (33%	62 (37%)	9 (23%)	17 (45%)
	allele (L)	140 (59%	192 (57%)	35 (44%)	45 (59%)
	allele (S)	98 (41%	144 (43%)	45 (56%)#	31 (41%)

Association of genotype or allele distributions by contingency tables:
(#) "Low PTH" group compared with controls (genotypes, p=0,024, alleles p=0,019)
($) "High PTH" group compared with controls (genotypes, p=0,039)

Methods Patients on maintenance in dialysis (168) were divided in two groups: those with "low" serum PTH levels (<12 pmol/L) and those with "high" serum PTH levels (>60 pmol/L). A control population of 119 healthy individuals belonging to the same geographic area was used. Both, patients and controls were from Caucasian origin. Genotypes were determined by SSCP analysis or polyacrylamide gel electrophoresis of PCR amplified fragments. Hardy-Weinberg equilibrium was tested using a Chi-square test. Association was tested by contingency tables. Linkage disequilibrium was evaluated using standard log likelihood methods (2). The EM algorithm was used to obtain the maximum likelihood estimates of the haplotype frequencies and the standardized disequilibrium coefficient (D') was calculated (2). PTH, and other biochemical parameters were also determined. Differences of means of demographic and biochemical parameters in patient groups were compared across genotypes by unpaired t-test and ANOVA. Interaction between genotypes and PTH levels in all the patient population was tested by univariate analysis after adjusting for gender, serum calcium, phosphorous and aluminum levels, time on dialysis and ESRD ethiology.

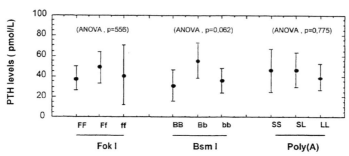

Figure 1.- PTH levels across VDR marker genotypes in the total dialysis population

Results Genotype frequencies of the markers analyzed were under Hardy-Weinberg equilibrium in controls. FokI genotypes were also in equilibrium in patients. However, significant departure from equilibrium was observed for Poly(A) genotypes (p=0,024). In the total dialysis population no differences on PTH levels were observed across FokI or Poly(A) genotypes (ANOVA, p=0,556 and p=0,775 respectively) (Figure 1). As we have previously described PTH levels of homozygous BB genotypes were lower than heterozygous Bb (ANOVA, p=0,062, t-test BB vs. Bb, p= 0,036). Univariate analysis reveals that phosphorous (p=0,017) and BsmI genotype (p=0,028), but not FokI (p=0,682) or Poly(A) (p=0,063), affect PTH levels. Following a case-control study genotype frequencies of patients, grouped according to PTH levels, were compared with genotype frequencies of control population. In contrast to the previously described association for BsmI polymorphism, no association was observed for FokI genotypes. On the contrary, Poly(A) genotype SS was overrepresented in the "low PTH" group (35% vs. 15% in controls, $X^2=7,47$, df=1, p= 0,024) and the S allele was overrepresented in the "low PTH" group (56% vs. 41% in controls, $X^2=5,49$, df=1, p= 0,019). Haplotype distribution for FokI, BsmI and Poly(A) sites show that FokI was in linkage equilibrium in relation to the other two sites. However, BsmI and Poly(A) were in linkage disequilibrium in controls (D'= 0,803, p<0,0001) and patients (D'= 0,966, p<0,0001) (Table II). BsmI/Poly(A) haplotypes were differentially distributed between the "low PTH" group and controls ($X^2=8,02$, df=3, p=0,045). SB haplotype was overrepresented in the "low PTH" group (52% vs. 39% in controls) and Lb haplotype was underrepresented in the "low PTH" group (39% vs. 57% in controls).

Discussion There is a wide variation in parathyroid cell function in ESRD patients. Whereas some patients develop severe and uncontrollable hyperparathyroidism, others show very low levels of PTH, which fail to promote adequate bone turnover and, finally, lead to adynamic bone disease. In our previous study we showed that BsmI polymorphism was related to parathyroid function in ESRD patients. In the present work we have extended the study to two additional polymorphic markers, one located in the 5' region of VDR locus (FokI polymorphism) and the other close to the Bsml polymorphism in the 3'UTR region of VDR locus (Poly(A) polymorphism). We have also studied the haplotype distribution of these three polymorphic markers in controls and patients. The distribution of FokI and Poly(A) genotypes found in our control population was consistent with that found in other Caucasian populations. We arranged the patients undergoing dialysis into two groups on the basis of their PTH levels. In order to minimize the effect of factors other than genetic background, additional selection criteria were applied (1). The "high PTH" group had PTH levels over than 60 pmol/L and less than 5 years on dialysis. The "low PTH" group had levels lower than 12 pmol/L and more than 2 years on dialysis. We also excluded patients having any of the risk factors previously described to favor the existence of secondary hyperparatiroidism or adynamic bone disease. Following the application of these selection criteria, 38 patients remained in the "high PTH" group and 40 patients remained in the "low PTH" group. The distribution of FokI genotypes and alleles in both groups were not different from that obtained in the control population (Table I). In contrary, differences in genotype and allele distribution for Poly(A) polymorphism were statistically significant when comparing low or high PTH groups with controls (p=0,024 and p=0,039, respectively). Using the EM algorithm we have determined the maximum likelihood estimates of haplotype frequencies for FokI/Poly(A), FokI/Bsml and Bsml/Poly(A) marker pairs. FokI/Poly(A) and FokI/Bsml were in linkage equilibrium in the control population as well as in the patient groups. Consequently, no association was observed in haplotype distribution for FokI/Bsml and for FokI/Poly(A) between control and patient groups. On the contrary, Bsml/Poly(A) haplotypes were in strong linkage disequilibrium in both, control and patient groups. This is in agreement with data reported by Ingles et al. (3). Haplotypes SB and Lb together represent 96% in controls and 93% in all patient population (expected values assuming linkage equilibrium 52% and 51% respectively). In the low PTH group the proportion of SB haplotype was higher than in controls, whereas for Lb haplotype the proportion was lower than in controls (Table II). We also compared serum PTH levels across genotypes in the total patient population (Figure 1). As previously described, serum PTH levels were lower in BB than in Bb or bb genotypes. Although, serum PTH levels were not statistically different across FokI or Poly(A) genotypes. Consistently, univariate analysis after adjusting for gender, serum calcium, phosphorous and aluminum levels, time on dialysis and ESRD ethiology only supports a significant interaction between Bsml genotype and serum PTH levels. In summary, these results seems to indicate that parathyroid function is influenced by Poly(A) polymorphism but not by FokI genotypes. Although the effect of Poly(A) polymorphism on PTH function could be explained by the observed linkage disequilibrium with the Bsml marker. As for Bsml polymorphism, FokI polymorphism has been related to bone mineralization in several populations. However controversial results have also been reported, indicating that the association detected should be population dependent, affected by environmental factors or related to other at-risk locus. FokI polymorphism defines two potential translation initiation codons in the VDR protein. Allele "F" produces a protein three aminoacids shorter than allele "f". How this structural difference does affect VDR function is controversial.

Table II.- Haplotype frequencies for BsmI/Poly(A) markers

	Haplotype frequencies				SB+Lb		Disequilibrium coeficient		
	SB	LB	Sb	Lb	Estimated	xpected+	D	D'=D/Dmax	p value
Controls	0,4	0	0,02	0,57	0,96	0,52	0,225	0,803	<0,001
All Dialysis	0,4	0	0,03	0,54	0,93	0,51	0,214	0,966	<0,001
Low PTH	0,52	0	0,04	0,39#	0,92	0,51	0,207	0,883	<0,001
High PTH	0,3	0	0,07	0,55	0,89	0,51	0,215	0,829	<0,001

* Maximum likelihood estimates based on observed genotype frequencies using the EM algorithm
+ Expected frequencies under the assumption of linkage equilibrium
\# Significant differences when compared whith controls

Data reported by Arai et al. (4) have proposed that FokI VDR variants have a different transactivation activity able to differentially modulate the expression of genes containing VDR responsive elements (VDREs), but this finding has not been confirmed by others (5). The lack of association between FokI genotypes and parathyroid function detected in our study is in agreement with the reported absence of association between FokI and primary hyperparathyroidism (6). According to Arai et al. (4), these results suggest that parathyroid hormone VDREs would not be influenced by the variability of the N-terminal portion of the VDR protein. Alternatively, if we consider FokI to be a marker for a putative at-risk locus, a linkage equilibrium between FokI and the at-risck locus in our control population could also explain the lack of association detected. This is what we find between FokI and BsmI and between FokI and Poly(A). If BsmI or Poly(A) were the at-risk locus, we would expect linkage disequilibrium between FokI and one of both polymorphisms, in those reports in which 5' and 3'UTR markers were disease associated. No data has been reported for FokI and Poly(A) polymorphisms that could be used to test this hypothesis. However, our results seems to indicate that BsmI polymorphism is a better marker for parathyroid function than Poly(A) polymorphism. This argues against considering the Poly(A) polymorphism as the at-risk locus. In addition, the controversial data relating BsmI polymorphism with some vitamin D metabolism disfunction do not allow to consider BsmI as the at-risk locus. Therefore, a third at-risk locus could be envisaged.

References

1. Fernandez, E., Fibla, J., Betriu, A., Piulats, J., Almirall, J., and Montoliu, J. (1997) *J Am Soc Nephrol* 8(10), 1546-1552
2. Weiss, K. (1993) *Genetic variation and human disease.* Cambridge Studies in Biological Anthropology (Lasker, G., Mascie-Taylor, C., Roberts, D., and Foley, R., Eds.), Cambridge University Press, Cambridge
3. Ingles, S. A., Haile, R. W., Henderson, B. E., Kolonel, L. N., Nakaichi, G., Shi, C. Y., Yu, M. C., Ross, R. K., and Coetzee, G. A. (1997) *Cancer Epidemiol Biomarkers Prev* 6(2), 93-98
4. Arai, H., Miyamoto, K., Taketani, Y., Yamamoto, H., Iemori, Y., Morita, K., Tonai, T., Nishisho, T., Mori, S., and Takeda, E. (1997) *J Bone Miner Res* 12(6), 915-921
5. Gross, C., Krishnan, A. V., Malloy, P. J., Eccleshall, T. R., Zhao, X. Y., and Feldman, D. (1998) *J Bone Miner Res* 13(11), 1691-1699
6. Correa, P., Rastad, J., Schwarz, P., Westin, G., Kindmark, A., Lundgren, E., Akerstrom, G., and Carling, T. (1999) *J Clin Endocrinol Metab* 84(5), 1690-1694

VITAMIN D RECEPTOR GENE POLYMORPHISMS AND INCREASED BREAST CANCER RISK

Deborah Bretherton-Watt, Rosalind Given-Wilson*, Janine L Mansi, Valerie Thomas[1], Nick Carter[2] and Kay W Colston. Dept. Oncology, Gastroenterology, Endocrinology and Metabolism, [1]Dept. Histopathology and [2]Medical Genetics Unit, St. George's Hospital Medical School, and *Duchess of Kent Breast Screening Unit, London, UK.

Introduction

There is increasing evidence that adequate vitamin D can help to protect against breast cancer. Vitamin D exerts its cellular actions by binding to a specific intracellular receptor, the vitamin D receptor (VDR). Activity and function of the VDR may therefore influence responses at a cellular level and alter breast cancer risk. The gene encoding the human VDR is known to contain a number of polymorphisms. A polymorphic start codon in the 5' end of the gene (identified by the restriction enzyme *FokI*) results in VDR proteins that differ in length by 3 amino acids. This polymorphism has been associated with increased breast cancer risk in African-American women (1). Three sequences in the 3' end of the gene (generating *BsmI*, *ApaI* and *TaqI* restriction sites) are thought to be linked to a further polymorphism, the variable length poly (A) sequence in the 3' untranslated region (3' UTR). An association between these 3' polymorphisms and bone mineral density has been widely reported (2,3).. They have also been related to a number of other diseases including prostatic and breast carcinoma: in separate US studies, increased risk of prostate cancer has been associated with a long poly (A) allele (4), absence of *TaqI* (5) and presence of *BsmI* (6) restriction sites. An association has also been reported between breast cancer risk and the *ApaI* polymorphism (7), breast cancer progression and absence of the *TaqI* polymorphism (8), and *BsmI* genotype and increased risk of breast metastases (9). The aim of the present study was to establish whether polymorphisms in the VDR gene are associated with breast cancer risk in a UK Caucasian population.

Methods

241 control, healthy Caucasian women (median age 55.2 years, range 51-79 years) were recruited through the Breast Screening Unit, St. George's Hospital. The UK National Breast Screening Programme offers screening mammograms to all women between the ages of 50-65 years at 3 yearly intervals. Women were included in the study following a routine mammogram that confirmed they did not have any detectable breast cancer or precancerous breast changes. 184 Caucasian women with a known breast carcinoma (median age 62.1 years, range 29-91 years) were recruited through the Combined Breast Clinic, St. George's Hospital. These women had a median time since diagnosis of 4.3 years, range 0.4-27.5 years. Blood samples were obtained and VDR polymorphisms *FokI* and *BsmI* were determined by PCR amplification of

genomic DNA followed by digestion with the appropriate restriction enzyme, as previously described (10,2). The presence of the restriction site was indicated as *b,f* for *Bsm*I and *Fok*I respectively. For poly (A) analysis, PCR product was separated by denaturing gel electrophoresis, as previously described (4). The poly (A) region resolves into two distinct populations, long (L, A_{18}-A_{24})and short (S, A_{13}-A_{17}).Differences in genotype frequencies were assessed by χ^2 test and risks associated with genotype by odds ratio.

Results
There was a significant difference in genotype frequencies between patients and controls, such that the *bb* genotype was significantly over-represented in the patient population (Table 1). The odds of breast cancer for a woman of genotype *bb* were therefore twice those for a woman of genotype *BB*. This *Bsm*I polymorphism was in strong linkage disequilibrium with the variable length poly (A) sequence, such that the *bb* genotype co-segregated with LL long poly (A) alleles. Analysis of poly (A) genotype thus revealed an identical association with breast cancer risk (Table 1). The *Fok*I polymorphism did not show any association with breast cancer risk. However, the *Fok*I polymorphism did modulate the risk associated with *Bsm*I/poly (A) genotype, such that the increased risk associated with genotype *bb*/LL was mitigated in the presence of the *FF* genotype (Table 2).

Table 1: VDR gene polymorphism frequencies

	Controls n(%)	Allele Frequency	Cases n(%)	Allele Frequency	Odds Ratio (95% confidence interval)
*Bsm*I					χ^2 test, p=0.0071*
bb	69 (28.6)	*b* 0.56	79 (42.9)	*b* 0.66	**2.23** (1.19-4.19)
Bb	133 (55.2)	*B* 0.44	85 (46.2)	*B* 0.34	**1.25** (0.68-2.28)
BB	39 (16.2)		20 (10.9)		**1.0**
Poly A					χ^2 test, p=0.0081*
LL	67 (28.2)	L 0.56	77 (41.8)	L 0.66	**2.36** (1.25-4.47)
LS	132 (55.5)	S 0.44	88 (47.8)	S 0.34	**1.37** (0.74-2.52)
SS	39 (16.4)		19 (10.3)		**1.0**
*Fok*I					χ^2 test, p=0.56
FF	86 (35.7)	*F* 0.60	75 (40.8)	*F* 0.63	**1.21** (0.68-2.16)
Ff	116 (48.1)	*f* 0.40	81 (44.0)	*f* 0.37	**0.97** (0.55-1.71)
ff	39 (16.2)		28 (15.2)		**1.0**

Table 2: Risks of breast cancer for *Bsm*I and poly (A) genotype in relation to *Fok*I genotype

	Controls (*n*)	Cases (*n*)	Odds Ratio (95% confidence interval)
FF genotype			
bb	24	32	**2.07** (0.77-5.89)
Bb	48	34	**1.1** (0.43-2.84)
BB	14	9	**1.0**
Ff/ff genotype			
bb	45	47	**2.37** (1.05-5.38)
Bb	85	51	**1.36** (0.62-3.00)
BB	25	11	**1.0**
FF genotype			
LL	23	29	**1.82** (0.66-5.00)
LS	49	37	**1.09** (0.42-2.82)
SS	13	9	**1.0**
Ff/ff genotype			
LL	44	48	**2.84** (1.22-6.55)
LS	83	51	**1.60** (0.71-3.59)
SS	26	10	**1.0**

Discussion

We have demonstrated a significant association between two polymorphisms of the VDR gene and breast cancer risk in a UK Caucasian population. The two 'at risk' polymorphisms, *Bsm*I and variable length poly (A) sequence, were found to be in strong linkage disequilibrium. This has been reported in other Caucasian populations (11), but this is the first confirmation in a UK population. The *Bsm*I polymorphism is an intronic polymorphism, with no apparent consequences for either the transcribed mRNA or translated protein, while the poly (A) sequence is found in the 3' UTR of the gene. Such sequences have been suggested as modulators of mRNA stability or processing pathways (12), although attempts to demonstrate such effects have to date been inconclusive (13).

The *Fok*I polymorphism, an alternative translational start codon, is the only variant known to alter the VDR protein. While we found no direct association between the *Fok*I polymorphism and breast cancer risk, the risk was found to be exacerbated in the presence of one or more *f* alleles. There is evidence that the longer *f* VDR protein is associated with decreased transcriptional activity (14). Such an effect may result in altered actions of vitamin D at the cellular level.

Further investigations into the mechanisms by which VDR polymorphisms interact with other environmental, nutritional and/or genetic factors to alter breast cancer risk may lead to a new understanding of the role of vitamin D in the control of cellular and developmental pathways.

References
(1) Ingles, S.A., Haile, R.W., Henderson, B. and Coetzee, G.A. (1997) Proc. 10th Vitamin D Workshop pp. 813-815.
(2) Morrison, N.A., Qi, J.C., Tokita, A., Kelly, P.J., Crofts, L., Nguyen, T.V., Sambrook, P.N. and Eisman, J.A. (1994) Nature, 367, 284 - 287.
(3) Cooper, G.S. and Umbach, D.M. (1996) J. Bone Min. Res. 11,1841-1849
(4) Ingles, S.A., Ross, R.K., Yu, M.C. Irvine, R.A., La Pera, G., Haile R.W. and Coetzee, G.A. (1997) J. Natl. Canc. Inst. 89, 166 – 170
(5) Taylor, J.A., Hirvonen, A., Watson, M., Pittman, G., Mohler J.L. and Bell, D.A. (1996) Cancer Res. 56, 4108 - 4110
(6) Ma, J., Stampfer, M.J., Gann, P.H., Hough, H.L., Giovannucci E., Kelsey, K.T., Hennekens, C.H. and Hunter D.J. (1998) Cancer Epidem. Biomark. Prev. 7, 385-390.
(7) Curran, J.E., Vaughn, T., Lea, R.A., Weinstein, S.R., Morrison, N.A. and Griffiths, L.R. (1999) Int. J. Cancer 83, 723-726.
(8) Lundin, A-C., Soderkvist, P., Eriksson, B., Bergman-Jungerstrom, M., Wingren, S., and South-east Sweden Breast Cancer Group (1999) Cancer Res. 59, 2332-2334
(9) Ruggiero, M., Pacini, S., Aterini, S., Falai, C., Ruggiero, C., and Pacini, P. (1998) Oncol. Res. 10, 43-46.
(10) Gross, C., Krishnan, A.V., Malloy, P.J., Eccleshall, T.R., Zhao, X-Y. and Feldman D. (1998) J. Bon. Min. Res. 13, 1691-1699.
(11) Ingles, S.A., Haile, R.W., Henderson, B.E., Kolonel, L., Nakaichi, G., Shi, C-Y., Yu, M.C., Ross, R.K. and Coetzee G.A. (1997) Cancer Epidem. Biomark. Prev. 6, 93-98
(12) Day, D.A. and Tuite, M.F. (1998) J. Endocrinol. 157, 361-371
(13) Durrin, L.K., Haile R.W, Ingles, S.A. and Goetzee G.A. (1999) Biochem. Biophys Acta 1453, 311-320
(14) Jurutka, P.W., Remus, L.S., Whitfield, G.K., Thompson, P.D., Hseih, J.C., Zitzer, H., Tavakkoli, P., Galligan, M.A., Dang, H.T., Haussler, C.A. and Haussler, M.R. (2000) Mol Endocrinol 14, 401-420.

DEVELOPMENTAL AND NEONATAL EFFECTS OF VITAMIN D

MAMMARY GLAND DEVELOPMENT IN VITAMIN D₃ RECEPTOR KNOCKOUT MICE

Glendon Zinser, Kathryn Packman, and JoEllen Welsh.
Department of Biological Sciences, University of Notre Dame, Notre Dame, Indiana 46556 USA

INTRODUCTION The traditional role of 1,25-dihydroxyvitamin D_3 (vitamin D_3), the biologically active form of vitamin D_3, is maintenance of calcium homeostasis through its interaction with the vitamin D_3 receptor (VDR). Additionally, the VDR has been found in tissues that are not associated with the maintenance of calcium homeostasis, like the breast. The VDR has been localized to both normal and malignant breast cells, including about 80% of breast cancer cell lines. Vitamin D_3, when bound to the VDR, has been shown to promote differentiation, cell cycle arrest, and apoptosis in several malignancies including the breast (1). Vitamin D_3 participates in growth inhibition, while also inhibiting metastases and opposing estrogen mediated growth stimulation (2). Furthermore, vitamin D_3 has been shown to directly inhibit the development of pre-neoplastic lesions in mouse mammary glands (3). Vitamin D_3's primary mechanism of growth inhibition is by inducing apoptosis in cancerous cells and may thus represent an important breast cancer therapy. Although the VDR is present in the normal mammary gland and is dynamically expressed during pregnancy and lactation, a time when there are extremely high levels of both proliferation and apoptosis (4), nothing is known about the developmental role for VDR in the normal breast.

The mammary gland is an organ that completes its development postnatally. Development proceeds in distinct stages and is regulated by the hormonal status of the animal. Mammary gland development begins in the mouse after the onset of puberty (4 weeks of age), and involves the processes of ductal elongation and branching (ductal morphogenesis). Coordinate regulation of cell proliferation and cell death in the terminal end buds (TEBs) accomplishes ductal morphogenesis and lumen formation (5). The highly proliferative and undifferentiated TEB structures contain stem cell (cap cell) populations, which differentiate and give rise to the intermediate, luminal, and myoepithelial cells of the advancing duct (6). Mitotically quiescent terminal end ducts (TEDs), which represent differentiated cells, permanently replace the TEB structures as they reach the outer limits of the mammary fat pad (7). Therefore, developmental progress of the mammary gland can be assessed based on TEB number, which peak between five and seven weeks in the mouse, and the extent of the ductal mass.

It has been shown that the mammary gland has a unique dependence on hormonal signals and the nuclear receptors, such as estrogen (8), progesterone (9), and prolactin (10), for pronounced ductal outgrowth and proper mammary gland development. However, the involvement of vitamin D_3 and its receptor in mammary gland development has not yet been studied. To elucidate the possible role of vitamin D_3 in mammary gland development, the VDR knockout mouse (11) was studied during the pre-pubertal and pubertal stages of mammary gland development (4-10 weeks of age).

VDR knockout mice (-/-) as well as their wild type (+/+) counter parts were fed a rescue diet, which contained high calcium and lactose, to prevent disturbances in calcium homeostasis and hormonal imbalances (12). Although the diet normalized growth, mice homozygous for the VDR mutation experienced a delay in the differentiation of the TEBs during the pubertal stage of development, thus suggesting that vitamin D_3 may play a role in the normal development of the mammary gland.

Results   Homozygous VDR (-/-) are capable of pregnancy and lactation, although when compared to the VDR (+/+) mice, there is a significant difference in litter size (Fig.1A).   However, the percentage of pup survival in each litter is statistically equivalent between VDR (-/-) and VDR (+/+) (Fig.1B).   In addition, VDR (+/+) and VDR (-/-) mice fed the rescue diet exhibited no significant differences in average body weights at any time point up to ten weeks of age (Fig.2).

Figure 1. Comparison of litter size (A) and pup survival rate (B). Litter size is significantly smaller in the VDR null (n=25) compared to wild type (n=10) mice (p<0.01) while pup survival rates are equivalent.

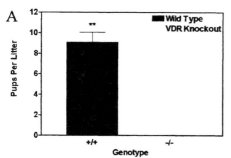

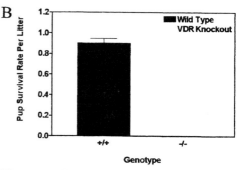

Figure 2. Comparison of body weights of wild type and VDR knockout mice from weaning to 10 weeks.   Average body weights were nearly identical in both genotypes.

Figure 3. Comparison of terminal end bud number in inguinal mammary glands from wild type and VDR knockout mice. A significant difference is observed between the wild type (n=8) and VDR knockout (n=6) at 6 weeks. *(p<0.05)

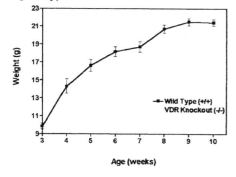

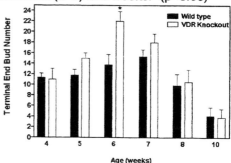

TEB numbers in inguinal mammary gland whole mounts from VDR (+/+) and VDR (-/-) mice were quantitated from weaning through ten weeks of age (Fig. 3). TEB number at the prepubertal (4 weeks) stage of development was equivalent for the two genotypes. By the end of prepubertal development and the beginning of pubertal (5-7 weeks) development the number of TEBs increases more rapidly in VDR (-/-) glands. By six weeks of age, compared to VDR (+/+) glands, glands from VDR (-/-) mice showed 30% more TEBs. However, by late pubertal (10 weeks) development, the TEB number was again equivalent (Fig. 3).

Although not quantitated, preliminary examination suggests that the number of secondary and tertiary branch points of mammary glands from (+/+) and (-/-) mice were approximately equivalent throughout development (Fig. 4). Histological comparisons at six and seven weeks of age in TEBs showed no significant difference in morphology between the VDR knockout and wild type glands (Fig.5 A&B). Thus, developmental variations seem to occur only during the pubertal (5-7 weeks) stage of development.

Figure 4. Whole mounts of inguinal mammary glands from 6 week old wild type (A) and VDR knockout (B) mice. Glands show similar branching, but increased TEB number in the knockout mice at 6 weeks of age.

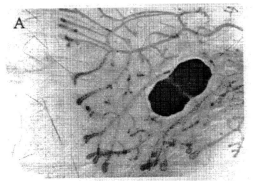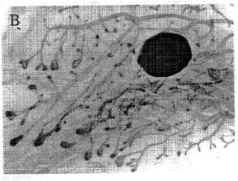

Figure 5. Morphological Comparison of TEBs. Hematoxylin and Eosin staining shows no morphological differences between the wild type (A) and the VDR knockout (B) TEBs.

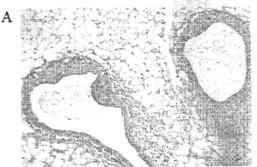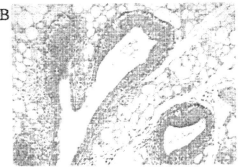

<u>Discussion</u> The effects of systemic hormones on mammary epithelial cells have been recognized for some time (13). However, only through the recent availability of knockout mice has it been possible to dissect the specific hormonal signals required for morphogenesis. In this study, we provide evidence of a role for the VDR in pubertal mammary gland development based on an increased number of undifferentiated TEBs in VDR null mice compared to their normal counterparts. This finding suggests that mammary gland differentiation is occurring at a slower rate in the VDR knockout mice. Since vitamin D_3 has been shown to play a role in cell differentiation (14), we speculate that increased TEB number reflects a delay in the differentiation of the cap cells (the stem cell population in mammary gland). It is well accepted that the TEBs are the targets for chemical carcinogens in mammary gland. The greater the number of highly proliferating undifferentiated cells (i.e. TEBs), the greater the susceptibility to carcinogens (15). Thus, the 30% increase in TEBs found in the glands of (-/-) mice suggests that mice lacking VDR may exhibit an enhanced susceptibility to mammary tumorigenesis. The results seen here are distinctly different from those found in the estrogen receptor knockout mice. Thus, vitamin D_3 and its receptor tend to have a distinct role in mammary gland differentiation. Future work will focus on quantitation of proliferation and apoptosis in the TEB structures of the developing gland to identify any functional differences between wild type and VDR null mammary glands.

<u>References</u>
1. Simboli-Campbell, M., Narvaez, C.J., Tenniswood, M., Welsh, J. (1996) J of Steroid Biochem Mol Biol. 58, 367-376.
2. Anzano, M.A., Smith, J.M., Uskokovic, M.R., Peer, C.W., Mullen, L.T., Letterio, J.J., Welsh, M.C., Schrader, M.W., Logsdon, J.L., Driver, C.L., Browh, C.C., Roberts, A.B., Sporn, M.B. (1994) Cancer Res. 54,1653-1656.
3. Mehta, R.G., Moriarty, R.M., Mehta, R.R., Penmasta, R., Lazzaro, G., Constantinou, A., Guo, L. (1997) Natl Cancer Inst. 89, 212-218.
4. Colston, K.W., Berger, U., Wilson, P., Hadcocks, L., Naeem, I., Earl, H.M., Coombes, R.C. (1988) Mol and Cell Endocrinol. 60,15-22.
5. Robinson, G.W. and Hennighausen, L. (1998) Genes Dev. 12, 449-455.
6. Williams, J.M. and Daniel, C.W. (1983) Dev Biol. 97, 274-290.
7. Topper, Y.J. and Freeman, C.S. (1980) Physiol Rev. 60, 1049-1097.
8. Zeps, N. (1997) J. Histochem Cytochem. 10,1323-1330.
9. Silberstein, G.B. (1996) Cell Growth Differ. 7, 945-952.
10. Horseman, N., Zhao, W., Montecino-Rodriquez, E., Tanaka, M., Nakashima, K., Engle, S., Smith, F., Markoff, E., Dorshkind, K. (1997) EMBO J. 16, 6926-6935.
11. Li, Y.C., Pirro, A.E., Demay, M.B. (1998) Endocrinology. 139, 847-851.
12. Amling, M., Priemel M., Holzmann, T., Chapin, K., Rueger, J.M., Baron, R., Demay, M.B. (1999) Endocrinology. 140, 4982-4987.
13. Sakakura, T., (1991) Int Rev Cytol. 125,165-202.
14. Bikle, D.D., Gee, E., Pillai, S. (1993) J Investig Dermatol. 101, 713-718.
15. Russo, I.H. and Russo, J. 1998 J Mam Gland Biol Neopl. 3, 49-61.

PREVENTION OF MATERNAL VITAMIN D DEFICIENCY (one oral dose of 2.5 mg vitamin D3 at the 6th and 8th month of pregnancy): EFFECTS ON NEONATAL CALCIUM HOMEOSTASIS AND INFANTILE GROWTH.

F Zeghoud,H Ben-Mekhbi*, M Garabédian. CNRS UPR 1524, Hôpital St-Vincent de Paul, 75014 Paris, France. * Department of Pediatrics, Ben-Badis Hospital, Constantine, Algeria.

Introduction In previous studies, we have frequently observed biological signs of vitamin D deficiency in pregnant women giving birth during the winter in France, as well as in some part of Algeria all year round, country where theoretically there is enough sunlight to supply adequate amounts of vitamin D (1,2). We have also shown that single dose vitamin D administration during the last trimester of pregnancy offers a logical approach to prevent maternal and neonatal vitamin D deficiency.

Few studies have evaluated the effects of maternal vitamin D supplementation on infantile growth during the first years of life (3-5). We therefore decided to carry out an interventional longitudinal study on 200 pregnant women and their neonates in Constantine, Algeria, to test the effects of maternal vitamin D supplementation on the calcium and vitamin D status of neonates, and on infantile growth from birth to 1 year of age.

One oral administration of 100 000 IU of vitamin D_3 at the 6th and 8th month of pregnancy was chosen as the maternal prophylaxis as regards the low vitamin D status of the pregnant women in this part of Algeria (2).

Subjects and methods: The survey included 200 healthy mothers and their healthy full-term neonates born from 1993 to 1996.These women were recruted at the Ben-Badis Hospital, Constantine (Algeria). The study protocol was approved by the local ethical committee and informed consent was obtained from all the mothers. Mean age of the women was 33.2 ± 7 years (range: 17 to 45). Mean parity was 3.2 ± 1.7 (range: 1 to 8).These women were included at their sixth month of pregnancy in a randomized placebo-controlled long-term trial. They were randomly assigned to one of 2 groups: 100 women received one oral dose of 100 000 IU (2.5 mg) cholecalciferol (Uvedose®; Crinex Laboratories, Montrouge, France) at the beginning of the 6th and 8th month of pregnancy (supplemented group), 100 women received no vitamin D supplementation (control group). All their neonates received an identical vitamin D prophylaxis from birth to 1 year of life (oral trimestrial doses of 100 000 IU of vitamin D_3, Uvedose®) (6).Venous blood samples were taken from the mothers at the 6th month of pregnancy before the start of vitamin D prophylaxis and at delivery, and from their neonates from birth to 1 year of life, for determination of serum levels of calcium, phosphate, alkaline phosphatase activities and 25-hydroxyvitamin D (25-(OH)D).

Anthropometric data (length, weight, head circumference) were recorded from birth to 1 year of life in all infants.

Serum 25-(OH)D concentration was determined with 50 µIL serum samples that were extracted with methanol-chloroform and chromatographed on Amprep minicolumns with 100mg C18 (Amersham, Buckinghamshire, UK) (7).

The metabolite was then measured by using a radiocompetitive protein-binding assay with rat serum. The assay detects both 25-hydroxyergocalciferol and 25-hydroxycholecalciferol.

Serum Ca, P and ALP were measured by standard methods.Statistical analysis was performed using the Mann-Whitney test for unpaired data and the Wilcoxon test for paired data. Data are given as the mean ± 1 SD.

Results: **At the 6th month of pregnancy,** most pregnant women (77 to 88%) had low serum 25-(OH)D concentrations, below 13 ng/ml.

At delivery, in the unsupplemented group, both mothers and neonates had low concentrations of 25-(OH)D; 69% of the neonates had 25-(OH)D concentrations below 13 ng/ml, the threshold for subclinical vitamin D deficiency at birth (8). Incidence of neonatal hypocalcemia (serum calcium below 8 mg/dl) was important in this group (48%).

In the supplemented group, maternal and newborn 25-(OH)D serum concentrations were significantly higher than in the control group (p<0.0001) and the incidence of neonatal hypocalcemia was much lower (8%).

	Control	Supplemented
Mothers at the 6th month of pregnancy	9.0 ± 7.0	9.8 ± 5.4
Percentage of women with 25-(OH)D < 13 ng/ml	88	77
Mothers at delivery	7.3 ± 5.1	36.3 ± 15.9***
Percentage of women with 25-(OH)D < 13 ng/ml	86.4	12.8
Neonates	11.9 ± 7.4	25.9 ± 15.7***
Percentage of neonates with 25-(OH)D < 13 ng/ml	69	27

p values (comparison between control and supplemented groups): ***: p<0.0001.

Table I. Effect of maternal vitamin D supplementation on maternal and neonate serum 25-(OH)D levels (ng/ml).

Maternal vitamin D supplementation had also clear beneficial effects **on fetal and post-natal growth**. Neonates in the vitamin D supplemented group had higher weights (p<0.0001), higher heights (p<0.001) and higher head circumferences (p< 0.0001). At the 6th month of life, infants born from vitamin D supplemented mothers still had higher weight, higher height, and higher head circumference (p<0.0001), despite the fact that all infants (even those born from unsupplemented vitamin D mothers) received the same vitamin D prophylaxis. Of interest, their body length remained 1 standard deviation over that measured in the control group up to the end of the first year of life (p<0.001).

	Maternal Treatment	Neonate at birth	6 months of age	12 months of age
Weight (kg)	0	2.8 ± 0.4	7.9 ± 1.0	11.5 ± 0.8
	D+	3.4 ± 0.6***	8.5 ± 0.6***	10.8 ± 0.9**
Height (cm)	0	49.5 ± 0.7	62.8 ± 1.5	71.9 ± 1.5
	D+	49.9 ± 0.8**	66.3 ± 1.4***	73.0 ± 1.3***
Head Circumference (cm)	0	34.8 ± 0.5	40.8 ± 0.6	44.5 ± 1.7
	D+	35.6 ± 1.5***	42.0 ± 1.0***	44.0 ± 2.0
Body Mass Index	0	11.4 ± 1.7	20.4 ± 2.6	22.7 ± 1.7
	D+	13.6 ± 2.3***	19.6 ± 1.5	20.0 ± 2.2***

p values (comparison between control and supplemented groups): ***: p<0.0001; **: p<0.001.
Table II. Long term effects of maternal vitamin D supplementation on anthropometric measurements in the infant from birth to 1 year of life.

In conclusion, our study confirms the high incidence of subclinical vitamin D deficiency in this area of Algeria with 48% of the neonates showing hypocalcemia. As expected, administration of single doses of vitamin D at the 6th and 8th month of pregnancy had benefic effects on the incidence of neonatal hypocalcemia.

Prevention of vitamin D deficiency during pregnancy had a significant impact on fetal growth (fetal birth weight, height, head circumference and body mass index). This effect on infantile growth was still found at the 6th month of age, and at 1 year of life for body lenght.

Prevention of maternal deficiency not only decreases the risk for neonatal hypocalcemia and vitamin D deficiency but also improves fetal and post-natal growth.

References:

1. Zeghoud, F., Garabedian, M., Jardel, A., Bernard, N., Melchior, J. (1988) J. Gynecol. Biol. Reprod. 17, 1099-105.

2. Ben-Mekhbi, H., Zeghoud, F., Guillozo, H., Garabedian, M. (1997) In: Norman AW, Bouillon R, Thomasset M, eds. Vitamin D, Chemistry, Biology and Clinical Applications of the Steroid Hormone. University of California, Riverside, 921-922.

3. Brooke, O.G., Brown, I.R., Bone, C.D., Carter, N.D., Cleeve, H.J., Maxwell, J.D., Robinson, V.P., Winder, S.M. (1980) Br. Med. J. 280, 751-754.

4. Brunvand, L.,Quigstad, E., Urdal,P., Haug, E. (1996) Early Human Development 45, 27-33.

5. Waiters, B., Godel, J.C., Basu, T.K. (1998) J. Am. Coll. Nutr. 18, 122-6.

6. Zeghoud, F., Ben-Mekhbi, H., Djeghri, N., Garabedian, M. (1994) Am. J. Clin. Nutr. 60, 393-396.

7. Zeghoud, F., Jardel , A., Guillozo, H., N'Guyen, T.M., Garabedian, M. (1991) In: Norman AW, Bouillon R, Thomasset M, eds. Vitamin D, Gene Regulation Structure-Function Analysis and Clinical Application. Berlin, New York: Walter de Gruyter & Co, 662-63.

8. Zeghoud, F., Vervel, C., Guillozo, H., Walrant-Debray, O., Boutignon, H., Garabedian, M. (1997) Am. J. Clin. Nutr. 65, 771-8.

EFFECT OF PRENATAL STEROIDS ON VITAMIN D AND CALCIUM METABOLISM IN NEONATAL RATS.

D. Williams, R Haidar, B. R Thomas. 'Science Dept., Philander Smith College. [2]Pediairics and Physiology, University of Arkansas for Medical Sciences, Little Rock, AR, 72205.

Antenatal steroids are routinely given to women at risk of preterm delivery (<34 weeks gestation) to decrease the incidence of respiratory distress syndrome, intraventricular hemorrhage and neonatal death (1). In both human and animal studies (either direct fetal or maternal treatment) these effects are more pronounced following repetitive doses (2). The effects of steroid are thought to be mediated through the activation of glucocorticoid receptors or via glucocorticoid-induced effects on paracrine cells. Although there is a dramatic improvement in postnatal lung function there are also unwanted effects such as reduced fetal weight, and perhaps alterations in neurodevelopmental outcome (2,3).

In vivo administration of glucocorticoid to both humans and animals decreases intestinal calcium absorption, and increase urinary calcium excretion resulting in a reduction in total body calcium (4). Ultimately leading to an increased risk of bone disease. Whether this effect is mediated by an alteration in the metabolism of vitamin D or through changes in vitamin D dependent proteins (calcium binding protein) remains unclear (5). Reports of the effects of glucocorticoids on vitamin D metabolism have been conflicting. Serum 25-hydroxyvitamin D [$25(OH)D_3$] is either decreased or unchanged (6). While serum 1,25-dihydroxyvitamin D [$1,25(OH)_2D_3$] levels are either decreased (6) or increased (7).

In view of the well documented effects of maternal steroids on fetal lung maturation the specific aim of this study was to evaluate whether the glucocorticoid dosage which is know to be effective in promoting fetal lung development also induces changes in fetal vitamin D and calcium homeostasis.

Materials and Methods

Materials: 25 hydroxyvitamin D_3 radioimmunoassay (RIA) & 1,25-dihydroxyvitamin D_3 radioreceptor assay (INSTAR). HPLC grade solvents (Fisher Scientific) Betamethasone ----6 mg/ml -(Schering).

Equipment: Packard 5650 scintillation counter & Packard Cobra II auto gamma counter (Packard Instrument Company). Corning 634 Calcium autoanalyzer .

Animals: Adult male and female Sprague-Dawley rats, SASCO (St. Louis MO) Acclimatized to a 12:12 light:dark cycle.

Methods: Animals were placed on a normal rodent diet (normal calcium and phosphorus, vitamin D replete), and water ad lib. Two males and one female were paired per cage. Date of conception was noted by the presence of a vaginal mucous plug.

Pregnant adult females were treated (Rx) with betamethasone (0.2 mg/kg/d) i.m. or normal saline, i.m. (Control) for 6 days. Animals were checked twice daily until time of delivery.

Newborns were randomly divided into 6 groups (table). Neonatal animals were sacrificed at 0,4,8,12,16 & 21days of age. Blood was collected. via cardiac puncture, pooled, heparinized and spun down for determination of serum ionized calcium, $25(OH)D_3$ and $1,25(OH)_2D_3$ by radioimmunoassay (8) and radioreceptor assay (9), respectively.

Results and Discussion:

Table: Plasma $25(OH)D_3$, $1,25(OH)_2D_3$ and ionized Ca^{++} levels (mean ± S.E.)

Age(d)	0	4	8	12	16	21
Ionized Calcium (mg/dl)						
Control	2.4 (5)	2.4 (4)	2.8 (4)	2.4 (5)	1.6 (5)	1.6 (4)
Rx	2.0 (6)	1.6 (4)	2.0 (4)	1.6 (6)	2.4 (5)	2.8 (5)
25-hydroxyvitamin D3 (ng/ml)						
Control	45.5 (5)	32.9 (4)	35.1 (4)	21.5 (5)	33.4 (5)	39.8 (4)
Rx	54.7 (6)	38.6 (4)	36.8 (4)	19.2 (6)	36.7 (5)	41.1 (5)
1,25-dihydroxyvitamin D3 (pg/ml)						
Control	51.8(5)	36.7(4))	64(4)	26.5(5)	38.9(5)	92.6(4)
Rx	49.2 (6)	37.7 (4)	63.4 (4	29.4 (6	41.4 (5)	137.0(5)

Due to the low blood volume of neonatal rats, blood samples were pooled in each age group. 25-hydroxyvitamin D_3 and 1,25-dihydroxyvitamin D_3 tended to be the same in treated vs control neonatal rats, at all ages studied. 1,25-dihydroxyvitamin D_3 tended to increase with increasing gestational age in treated and control animals while 25-hydroxyvitamin D_3 remained unchanged. There was no significant difference in serum ionized calcium in treated vs control animals (table, figure).

There is no difference in serum ionized calcium, 25-hydroxyvitamin D_3 and 1,25-dihydroxyvitamin D_3 levels in neonatal rats delivered to mothers treated with prenatal steroids vs non-treated (control) mothers (table & figure).

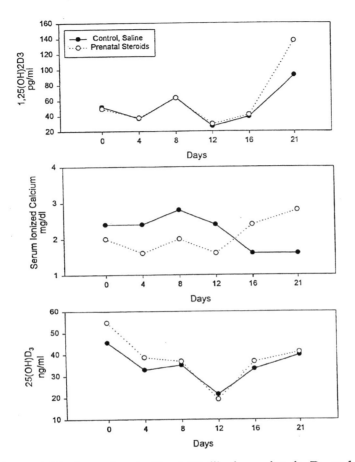

Figure: Plasma 25-hydroxyvitamin D₃, 1,25-dihydroxyvitamin D₃ and serum ionized calcium

Over the past decade improved perinatal and neonatal care has resulted in the increased survival of infants delivered between 24 and 25 weeks gestation. An important part of this care has been the growing practice of treating mothers at high risk for preterm delivery with glucocorticoids in an effort to promote fetal lung maturity. While there is the benefit of lung maturation there are also some undesired effects (reduced fetal body weight) of maternal glucocorticoid administration.(2,3)

Most preterm infants are in a relative state of negative calcium balance and are at an increased risk to develop bone disease (osteopenia). The administration of maternal glucocorticoids under these conditions may predispose the premature neonate to an even greater risk of osteopenia. In this study we evaluated the effect of repetitive maternal doses of glucocorticoids on neonatal vitamin D and calcium homeostasis. Our results show that serum levels of ionized calcium, 25-hydroxyvitamin D_3 and 1,25-dihydroxyvitamin D_3 tended to be the same in treated vs control neonatal rats, at all ages studied. Serum levels of 1,25-dihydroxyvitamin D_3 tended to increase with increasing postnatal age while 25-hydroxyvitamin D_3 remained unchanged. This finding is consistent with previous studies in the rat demonstrating that after weaning there is a marked increase in intestinal calcium transport and serum $1,25(OH)_2D_3$(10). The mechanism of these responses are not clear but may be due to developmental changes in vitamin D receptor number and function and/or changes in calcium binding protein (calbindin-D_{9k}).

Conclusion: In this study we have shown that there is no significant change in serum calcium, 25-hydroxyvitamin D_3 and 1,25-dihydroxyvitamin D_3 levels in neonatal rats delivered to mothers treated with prenatal steroids when compared to neonatal rats delivered to non-treated mothers. Although the results of this study show no difference in either 25-hydroxyvitamin D_3 or 1,25-dihydroxyvitamin D_3 in treated vs control animals, this maybe among the first reports of neonatal vitamin D levels in response to maternal glucocorticoid administration. Studies are in progress to evaluate the effect of maternal glucocorticoids on both the intestinal $1,25(OH)_2D_3$ receptor (VDR) and calcium binding protein (calbindin-D_{9k}) and their possible role in perinatal vitamin D and calcium homeostasis.

References:
1. National Institute of Health. JAMA. (1995);273:413-418.
2. Jobe, A.H. Newham, J. Willet K., Sly P., and Ikegami, M. Pediatrics (1998);102:1116-1125.
3. Sun, Bo. Jobe, A., Rider, E., and Ikegami, M. Pediatric Res 33:256-260, 1993.
4. Hahn, TJ, Halstead, LR, Baran, DT. J. Clin. Endocrinology Metab 52:111.
5. Korkor, A.B. Kuchibolta, J., Arrieh, M., Gray, R.W. and Gleason, W.A. (1985) Endocrinology 117:2267-3373,
6. Seeman, E., Kumar R., Hunder, GG, Scott, M., Heath, H., Riggs BL. J Clin Invest 66:664.
7. Braun, JJ., Juttmann, JR, Visser, TJ, Birkenhager, JC (1982)l Clin Endocrinology 17:21
8. Horst, R.L., Shepard, R.M., Jorgensen N.A., DeLuca H.F. (1979) Arch. Biochem. Biophys. 192:512.
9. Reinhardt, T.A., Horst, R.L., Orf, J.W. and Hollis, B.W. (1984) J Clin. Endo. And Metab. 58, 91-98.
10. Halloran, B.P and DeLuca, H.F. Am. J. Physiol. 239 (gastrointest. Liver Physiol. 2) (1980)G473-G479.

LOW CIRCULATING LEVELS OF 1,25-DIHYDROXYVITAMIN D AND INSULIN-LIKE GROWTH FACTOR-I IN SMALL FOR GESTATIONAL AGE INFANTS BORN FROM PREECLAMPTIC WOMEN

Ali Halhali[*], Armando R. Tovar[*], Nimbe Torres[*], Héctor Bourges[*], Michèle Garabédian[**], and Fernando Larrea[*]. [*]Instituto Nacional de la Nutrición Salvador Zubirán, México D.F., México, and [**]Unité CNRS UPR 1524, Hôpital Saint Vincent de Paul, Paris, France.

Introduction. Preeclampsia is a disorder of pregnancy characterized by reduced uteroplacental blood flow and fetal intrauterine growth retardation (1). Insulin-like growth factor I (IGF-I) is involved in fetal growth (2). During preeclampsia, maternal serum IGF-I concentrations are lower in comparison with those in normal pregnant women (3-5). In addition to its effects on fetal growth, IGF-I stimulates renal 1,25-dihydroxyvitamin D (1,25-$(OH)_2$D) synthesis in nonpregnant humans and rodents (6-15). Furthermore, we previously demonstrated that IGF-I stimulates human placental 1,25-$(OH)_2$D production (16). Interestingly, maternal serum 1,25-$(OH)_2$D concentrations are lower in preeclampsia than in normal pregnancy (3, 5, 17-19). Since preeclampsia is associated with low birth weight, and IGF-I may be involved in fetal growth and 1,25-$(OH)_2$D synthesis, the aim of the present work was to study circulating levels of these two hormones in small (SGA) and appropriate (AGA) for gestational age infants born from preeclamptic women. The study was done cross-sectionally at delivery in 24 preeclamptic women that delivered 8 newborns SGA (SGA PE group) and 16 AGA (AGA PE group). Diagnosis of preeclampsia was based on the simultaneous presence of hypertension (systolic blood pressure $\geq$140 mm Hg and/or diastolic blood pressure $\geq$90 mm Hg) and marked proteinuria (at least 2+ on depstick: > 100 mg/dL). Only women giving birth to a single product were included in the study. Newborns small for gestational age (below the 10th percentile) were classified according to the criteria of Lubchenco et al. (20).

Results and Discussion. Results are presented as the mean ± S.D. Analysis of statistical differences between the AGA and SGA PE groups was performed by unpaired Student's "t" test after logarithm transformation of the data, and associations between variables were tested using Spearman rank correlation. As shown in Table I, gestational age and blood pressure were similar in both groups. However, newborn birth weight and lenght were significantly (P < 0.001) lower in the SGA PE group than in the AGA PE group. Since blood pressure and proteinuria (data not show) were similar in both groups, the occurence of SGA infants may not be due to the severity of preeclampsia. However, an early development of the disease leading to a longer fetal nutritional deficit resulting from reduced uteroplacental blood flow may explain the low birth weight and lenght observed in the SGA PE group.

Table II summarizes maternal and umbilical serum levels of 1,25-(OH)2D, vitamin D binding protein (DBP), PTH and IGF-I. Maternal serum 1,25-(OH)2D, DBP and PTH concentrations did not show significant differences between SGA and AGA PE groups.

Table 1. Clinical characteristics of the AGA and SGA PE groups.

	AGA PE group (n=16)	SGA PE group (n=8)	P value
Gestational age (weeks)	39.7 ± 1.2	140.1 ± 0.9	NS
Sistolic blood pressure (mm Hg)	142 ± 5	143 ± 7	NS
Diastolic blood pressure (mm Hg)	96 ± 5	99 ± 6	NS
Newborn birth weight (kg)	3.18 ± 0.32	2.09 ± 0.37	<0.0001
Newborn birth lenght (cm)	50.3 ± 1.8	45.0 ± 3.5	<0.001

We previously reported that maternal serum 1,25-(OH)2D levels are significantly lower in preeclampsia than in normal pregnancy even when newborns are AGA (5). This observation may indicate that vitamin D metabolism alteration during preeclampsia is independent of birth weight. In contrast, small birth weight for gestational age was associated with a significant decrease ($P < 0.001$) in maternal serum IGF-I concentrations of the SGA PE.

Table 2. Maternal and umbilical cord serum concentrations of 1,25-(OH)2D, DBP, IGF-I, and PTH in the AGA and SGA PE groups.

	AGA PE group (n=16)	SGA PE group (n=8)	P value
Maternal 1,25-(OH)2D (pg/mL)	47 ± 11	47 ± 10	NS
Maternal DBP (mg/L)	412 ± 73	430 ± 54	NS
Maternal IGF-I (ng/mL)	298 ± 61	202 ± 56	<0.001
Maternal intact PTH (pg/mL)	28.8 ± 10.2	30.6 ± 8.3	NS
Cord 1,25-(OH)2D (pg/mL)	32 ± 6	26 ± 9	<0.05
Cord DBP (mg/L)	195 ± 28	209 ± 57	NS
Cord IGF-I (ng/mL)	84 ± 38	53 ± 24	<0.05
Cord intact PTH (pg/mL)	3.8 ± 2.7	3.5 ± 2.5	NS

In the umbilical compartment, serum 1,25-(OH)2D levels were significantly ($P <$ 0.05) lower in SGA PE group than in AGA PE group. This finding suggests a low synthesis of this hormone in the fetoplacental unit leading to reduced placental calcium transport and/or fetal bone mineralization. As previously mentioned, IGF-I stimulates renal and placental 1,25-(OH)2D synthesis (6-15). In the present study both maternal and umbilical compatments of the SGA PE group showed a significant reduction in serum IGF-I concentrations. However, the analysis of associations between 1,25-(OH)2D and IGF-I did not show significant correlations in maternal and umbilical cord compartments of the SGA PE group. In contarst, in the AGA PE group a significant association (Rho = 0.65, $P =$ 0.001)) between these two hormones was observed in the umbilical cord. This observation may suggest that fetal IGF-I action and/or 1,25-(OH)2D synthesis are altered in intrauterine growth retardation. In addition, low circulating IGF-I levels observed in the SGA PE group may explain restricted fetal growth. As show in table III, in the AGA PE group, only umbilical cord serum IGF-I levels correlated with newborn birth weight and lenght ($P < 0.05$).

Table 3. . Correlation between serum IGF-I concentrations and newborn birth weight and length in the indicated groups.

	AGA PE group (n=16)		SGA PE group (n=8)	
	Rho	P	Rho	P
Maternal IGF-I vs:				
- Birth weight	0.09	NS	0.83	<0.05
- Birth lenght	-0.32	NS	0.86	<0.05
Umbilical IGF-I vs:				
-Birth weight	0.62	<0.05	0.81	<0.05
-Birth lenght	0.54	<0.05	0.95	<0.05

In contrast, in the SGA PE group, both maternal and umbilical cord serum IGF-I concentrations were significantly ($P < 0.05$) associated with these anthropometrical parameters. These observations suggest that maternal IGF-I is required for fetal growth only in intrauterine growth retardation condition. In conclusion, low umbilical cord IGF-I and 1,25-(OH)$_2$D concentrations observed in the SGA PE group may be implicated in fetal growth retardation and abnormal skeletal mineralization.

Acknoledgment. This work was supported by grants from the National Council of Science and Technology (CONACYT, México; 26238-M) the Nord/Sud INSERM (France, 493 NS4), and the Special Program of Research, Development, and Research Training in Human reproduction of the WHO (Geneva, Switzerland).

References

1. Redman, C.W.G. (1991) Placenta. 12, 301-308.

2. Chard, T. (1994) Growth Regul. 4, 91-100.

3. Halhali, A., Bourges, H., Carrillo, A. and Garabédian, M. (1995) Rev. Invest. Clin. 47, 259-266.

4. Giudice, L.C., Martina, N.A., Crysta, R.A., Tazuke, S. and Druzin, M. (1997) Am. J. Obstet. Gynecol. 176, 751-758.

5. Halhali, A., Tovar, A.R., Torres, N., Bourges, H., Garabédian, M. and Larrea, F. (2000) J. Clin. Endocrinol. Metab. 85, 1828-1833.

6. Nesbitt, T. and Drezner, M.K. (1993) Endocrinilogy 132, 133-138.

7. Gray, R.W. (1987) Endocrinology 121, 504-512.

8. Halloran, B.P. and Spencer, E.M. (1988) Endocrinology 123, 1225-1229.

9. Caverzasio, J., Montessuit, C. and Bonjour, J.P. (1990) Endocrinology 127, 453-459.

10. Condamine, L., Vzovsnik, F., Friedlander, G., Menaa, C. and Garabédian, M. (1994) J. Clin. Invest. 94, 1673-1679.

11. Menaa, C., Vrtovsnik, F., Friedlander, G, Corvol, M. and Garabédian, M. (1995) J. Biol. Chem. 270, 25461-25467.

12. Wong, M.S., Sriusadaporm, S., Tembe, V.A. and Favus, M.J. (1997) Am. J. Physiol. 272, F698-F703.

13. Bianda, T., Hossain, M.A., Glatz, Y., Bouillon, R., Froesch, E.R. and Schmid, C. (1997) J. Intern. Med. 241, 143-150.

14. Bianda, T., Glatz, Y., Bouillon, R., Froesch, E.R. and Schmid, C. (1998) J. Clin. Endocrinol. Metab. 83, 81-87.

15. Wei, S., Tanaka, H. and seino, Y. (1998) Eur. J. Endocrinol. 139, 454-460.

16. Halhali, A., Díaz, L., Sánchez, I., Garabédian, M., Bourges, H. and Larrea, F. (1999) Mol. Hum. Reprod. 5, 771-776.

17. August, P., Marcaccio, B.G., Gertner, J.M., Druzin, M.L., Resnick, L.M. and Laragh, J.H. (1992) Am. J. Obstet. Gynecol. 166, 1295-1299.

18. Seely, E.W., Wood, R.J., Brown, E.M. and Graves, S.W. 1992 J. Clin. Endocrinol. Metab. 74, 1436-1440.

19. Tolaymat, A., Sanchez-Ramos, L., Yergey, A.L., Vieira, N.E., Abrams, S.A. and Edelstein, P. (1994) Obstet. Gynecol. 83, 239-243.

20. Lubchenco, L.O., Hansman, C., Dressler, M. and Boyde, E. (1963) Pediatrics 32, 793-800.

DOES "IMPRINTING" WITH PRENATAL VITAMIN D CONTRIBUTE TO THE RISK OF VARIOUS ADULT DISORDERS?

J McGrath, Queensland Centre for Schizophrenia Research, Wolston Park Hospital, Wacol, Queensland, Australia.

This paper presents a hypothesis linking low prenatal vitamin D and adverse adult health outcomes. It draws from recent advances in our understanding of the early origin of adult disease and proposes a "critical window" during which vitamin D levels may have a persisting impact on adult health outcomes. *The broad hypothesis proposes that low pre- and perinatal vitamin D levels imprint on the functional characteristics of various tissues throughout the body, leaving the affected individual at increased risk of developing a range of adult-onset disorders.* Specifically, it is proposed that low prenatal vitamin D increases the risk for multiple sclerosis, certain cancers (prostate, breast and colorectal), insulin-dependent diabetes and schizophrenia.

Pre- and perinatal exposures and metabolic imprinting

Hypovitaminosis D is still relatively common in developed countries (1,2). A large US survey reported that 12% of women aged 20 to 39 (peak ages for child-bearing) had serum 25-hydroxyvitamin D levels $\leq$ 15mg/ml (3). Pregnant women are at risk of hypovitaminosis D because of the increased needs of the fetus and potential decrease in outdoor activity (4,5).

The hypothesis that environmental factors may "imprint" on the fetus and contribute to adult health has been stimulated by the work of Barker and colleagues (6). Metabolic imprinting has two key features; (a) there is a critical window during fetal development or early life when the fetus is particularly sensitive to exposures; and (b) the exposure leads to changes that persist throughout adulthood. Waterland and Garza (7) have recently proposed several mechanisms for metabolic imprinting: (a) induced variations in organ structure (eg. vascularization and/or innervation during organogenesis); (b) alterations in cell numbers (eg. changes in neuronal count/density after prenatal malnutrition); (c) clonal selection. Nutritional or hormonal exposures may differentially advantage certain cell lines that could have persisting consequences for the adult organism; (d) metabolic differentiation, the process of cells acquiring a stable quantitative pattern of basal and inducible gene expression. These mechanisms may relate to enzymes, hormones and their receptors and other components of cellular molecular biology. Metabolic differentiation includes epigenetic mechanisms related to chromatin structure, DNA methylation, and autoregulatory patterns of DNA binding protein (e) hepatocyte polyploidization (a mechanism that creates diversity in hepatic metabolic activity).

With respect to the current hypothesis, mechanism related to alterations in cell numbers and type may be implicated in neurodevelopment disorders such as schizophrenia, while factors related to clonal selection and metabolic differentiation may be particularly important in the vitamin D-related cancers (breast, prostate, colorectal), multiple sclerosis and diabetes. These mechanisms have been supported by the demonstration of persisting alterations in cellular responsivity and organ differentiation after early life exposure to vitamin D (8,9).

Health and vitamin D: Clues from biology and epidemiology
The list of disorders that have links to vitamin D continues to grow. Evidence linking vitamin D and various disorders comes from research showing the presence of vitamin D receptors on cell lines, the response of cell cultures to vitamin D, and impact of vitamin D on animal models of certain diseases. In addition, epidemiology has also found links between certain diseases and variables related to vitamin D. None of these features in isolation would be sufficient "proof" that vitamin D is involved in causal pathways, however the coherence of the data suggests that low vitamin D is a candidate risk-modifying factor for a range of diseases other than rickets and osteoporosis. Some of these epidemiological features are listed below:

(1) Latitude gradients. Many diseases have gradients in incidence, prevalence and outcome that are correlated with latitude. Latitude acts as a risk indicator (or proxy) for the population distribution of serum vitamin D levels. A negative correlation between latitude and disease incidence is found for disorders such as multiple sclerosis (10,11), breast cancer (12), prostate cancer (13), colorectal cancer (14), insulin dependent diabetes (15,16) and schizophrenia (17,18).

(2) Ultraviolet B radiation (UVB). The geographical distribution of several diseases has been linked to measures related to the availability of UVB. This exposure is strongly correlated with latitude and vitamin D levels (19). Diseases that have been associated with measures related to sunshine include multiple sclerosis (10), breast cancer (20,21), prostrate cancer (13,22), colorectal cancer (12,22,23), and insulin dependent diabetes (24). The between-year fluctuations in schizophrenia birth rates have also been linked to measures of sunshine (25).

(3) Season of birth. The amount of ultraviolet radiation fluctuates across the seasons such that individuals born in winter and early spring tend to be exposed to lower levels of vitamin D than those born in other months. Disorders that have an excess of winter/spring births suggest that early life exposures to low vitamin D may be a risk-modifying exposure. There is robust evidence from the Northern Hemisphere showing that schizophrenia has seasonality of birth (26), and similar but weaker evidence for multiple sclerosis (27).

(4) Urban-rural gradient. Urban residence is associated with higher prevalence of hypovitaminosis D (19). Diseases that have an urban excess include breast cancer (28) and schizophrenia (29). Urban residence is also strongly linked to air pollution, a local factor that influences the availability of UVB. Colorectal and breast cancer (30) have been associated with air pollution.

(5) Migrant studies. The offspring of dark-skinned migrants to cold climates are prone to low vitamin D. Those with dark skin require slightly longer exposure to UVB in order to produce previtamin D, and their behaviour (eg. dress, outdoor activity, diet) may amplify the risk of hypovitaminosis D. Multiple sclerosis has a lower incidence in first generation Asian migrants to the United Kingdom than second generation migrants (those born in the in the United Kingdom) (31). There is a significantly higher rate of schizophrenia in the second but not the first generation of Afro-Caribbeans in the UK (18).

(6) Oral Vitamin D intake. Apart from sunshine exposure, Vitamin D can be derived from certain foods in the diet, cod liver oil intake and vitamin supplementation. Case-control and cohort studies have found links between oral vitamin D intake and prostate cancer, colorectal cancer (32,33) and insulin dependent diabetes (34).

Testing the hypothesis

One could measure vitamin D levels in a large cohort of pregnant women, and then follow-up their offspring for several decades in order to search for a dose-response relationship (a biological gradient) between low Vitamin D and increased risk of the candidate disorders. If sera from pregnant women and/or cord blood from their offspring were "banked down" during past decades, maternal vitamin D levels and rates of candidate disorders in the offspring could be examined. From an ecological perspective, "natural" and opportunistic experiments that impact on Vitamin D may provide exposed and nonexposed cohorts for birthrate comparisons (e.g. famine, clusters of rickets, the introduction of vitamin D supplementation). Between-year fluctuations in birth rates of candidate disorders could be examined for associations in duration of sunshine. For example, geographically-defined birth cohorts (born over several decades) could be divided according to quartiles of perinatal sunshine exposure, and then rates of diseases could be examined in these quartiles. It would be predicted, for example, that rates of schizophrenia, diabetes, multiple sclerosis, breast cancer, prostate cancer and colorectal cancer would be higher in those born in months with less sunshine. The hypothesis predicts that vitamin D related disorders will cosegregate in birth cohorts that have been exposed to low prenatal vitamin D. If possible, case-control studies of candidate disorders should ask mothers about prenatal sunshine behaviour, and vitamin D intake. If the hypothesis gains support, then a randomized controlled trial of vitamin D supplementation during pregnancy is indicated. The assessment of outcomes would require several decades of observations. Animal experiments could examine the impact on low prenatal vitamin D on a range of health outcomes, however not all human diseases have robust animal models. The hypothesis also suggests new directions for genetic research - as the hypothesis implicates a prenatal vitamin D deficiency, maternal genes related to vitamin D metabolism warrant consideration in addition to those of the affected offspring.

Implications for public health

Programs that aim to reduce the prevalence of hypovitaminosis D in pregnant women could translate into a lower incidence of candidate disorders in their offspring. Just as folate supplementation has been shown to reduce the incidence of neural tube defects, attention to vitamin D status (diet, sunlight exposure) could reduce the burden of a range of diseases. The population attributable fraction of a particular disease that could be linked to low prenatal vitamin D is not clear. In addition, the specificity of the outcomes is weak. However, this feature is a distinct advantage from the public health perspective. If an intervention designed to reduce one particular exposure translates into reduced incidence of several disorders, then these exposures are deemed more attractive candidates for preventive medicine (35).

References

1. Lawson, M. and Thomas, M. (1999) BMJ 318, 28.
2. Utiger, R. D. (1998) NEJM 338, 828-829.
3. Looker, A. C. and Gunter, E. W. (1998) NEJM 339, 344-345.
4. Hillman, L. S. and Haddad, J. G. (1976) Am.J.Obstet.Gynecol. 125, 196-200.
5. Markestad, T. (1983) Acta Paediatr.Scand. 72, 817-821.
6. Barker, D. J. P. (1992) Fetal and infant origins of adult disease, 1 Ed., British Medical Journal, London

7. Waterland, R. A. and Garza, C. (1999) Am J Clin Nutr 69, 179-197.
8. Konety, B. R., Nangia, A. K., Nguyen, T. T., Thomas, A., and Getzenberg, R. H. (1999) The Prostate 41, 181-189.
9. Mirzahoseeini, S., Karabélyos, C., Dobozy, O., and Csaba, G. (1996) Hum Exp Toxicology 15, 573-576.
10. Norman, J. E., Jr., Kurtzke, J. F., and Beebe, G. W. (1983) J.Chronic.Dis. 36, 551-559.
11. Weinshenker, B. G. (1996) Neurol.Clin. 14, 291-308.
12. Lipkin, M. and Newmark, H. L. (1999) J.Am.Coll.Nutr. 18, 392S-397S.
13. Hanchette, C. L. and Schwartz, G. G. (1992) Cancer 70, 2861-2869.
14. Wolfgram, F. (1975) Acta Neurol.Scand. 52, 294-302.
15. LaPorte, R. E., Tajima, N., Akerblom, H. K., Berlin, N., Brosseau, J., Christy, M., Drash, A. L., Fishbein, H., Green, A., and Hamman, R. (1985) Diabetes Care 8 Suppl 1, 101-107.
16. Akerblom, H. K. and Reunanen, A. (1985) Diabetes Care 8 Suppl 1, 10-16.
17. Welham, J., Davies, G., Auliciems, A., and McGrath, J. (2000) Int J Mental Health *in press*.
18. McGrath, J. (1999) Schizophr.Res. 40, 173-177.
19. Holick, M. F. (1995) Am.J.Clin.Nutr. 61, 638S-645S.
20. Garland, F. C., Garland, C. F., Gorham, E. D., and Young, J. F. (1990) Prev.Med. 19, 614-622.
21. Gorham, E. D., Garland, F. C., and Garland, C. F. (1990) Int.J.Epidemiol. 19, 820-824.
22. Emerson, J. C. and Weiss, N. S. (1992) Cancer Causes Control 3, 95-99.
23. Garland, C. F. and Garland, F. C. (1980) Int.J.Epidemiol. 9, 227-231.
24. Nystrom, L., Dahlquist, G., Ostman, J., Wall, S., Arnqvist, H., Blohme, G., Lithner, F., Littorin, B., Schersten, B., and Wibell, L. (1992) Int.J.Epidemiol. 21, 352-358.
25. McGrath, J., Welham, J., Davies, G., Chant, D., and Auliciems, A. (2000) Schizophr Res 41, 63.
26. Davies, G., Welham, J., Torrey, E. F., and McGrath, J. (2000) Schizophr Res 41, 62.
27. Templer, D. I., Trent, N. H., Spencer, D. A., Trent, A., Corgiat, M. D., Mortensen, P. B., and Gorton, M. (1992) Acta Neurol.Scand. 85, 107-109.
28. Doll, R. (1991) Int.J.Cancer 47, 803-810.
29. McGrath, J. (1999) Schizophr.Res. 40, 173-177.
30. Gorham, E. D., Garland, C. F., and Garland, F. C. (1989) Can.J.Public Health 80, 96-100.
31. Elian, M., Nightingale, S., and Dean, G. (1990) J.Neurol.Neurosurg.Psychiatry 53, 906-911.
32. Pritchard, R. S., Baron, J. A., and Gerhardsson, d., V (1996) Cancer Epidemiol.Biomarkers Prev. 5, 897-900.
33. Garland, C. F., Garland, F. C., and Gorham, E. D. (1991) Am.J.Clin.Nutr. 54, 193S-201S.
34. The EURODIAB Substudy 2 Study Group (1999) Diabetologia 42, 51-54.
35. Rose, G. (1992) *The Strategy of Preventive Medicine*, Oxford University Press, Oxford

RENAL OSTEODYSTROPHY

VITAMIN D IN RENAL OSTEODYSTROPHY

Adriana S. Dusso, Alex J. Brown and Eduardo A. Slatopolsky, Department of Internal Medicine, Renal Division. Washington University School of Medicine. St. Louis. MO.63110. USA

Introduction
Secondary hyperparathyroidism is a frequent complication in patients with chronic renal failure characterized by parathyroid hyperplasia and enhanced synthesis and secretion of parathyroid hormone (PTH). High circulating levels of parathyroid hormone cause osteitis fibrosa, bone loss and abnormal mineral metabolism known as renal osteodystrophy.

Hypocalcemia, hyperphosphatemia due to phosphate retention, and vitamin D deficiency are the main direct causes of hyperparathyroidism. Hyperphosphatemia and $1,25(OH)_2D_3$ deficiency also exert indirect effects on parathyroid function through lowering serum calcium. As renal disease progresses, a reduction in parathyroid levels of the vitamin D receptor (VDR) and calcium sensor renders the parathyroid gland resistant to the inhibitory effects of $1,25(OH)_2D_3$ and Ca on PTH synthesis (1). This review presents the current understanding of the mechanisms mediating the abnormalities in both vitamin D bioactivation to $1,25(OH)_2D_3$, and in $1,25(OH)_2D_3$-VDR action responsible for parathyroid hyperplasia and secondary hyperparathyroidism in renal failure patients.

Mechanisms for defective vitamin D bioactivation in renal failure.
We have known for many years that in renal failure, serum $1,25(OH)_2D_3$ decreases with the progressive reduction in glomerular filtration rate (GFR), as renal function deteriorates (2). This reduction in $1,25(OH)_2D_3$ results not only from limiting 1-hydroxylase, but also from inhibition of its activity by hyperphosphatemia, acidosis and accumulation of uremic toxins. However, in patients with a GFR below 25 ml/min, and therefore very limiting 1-hydroxylase activity, serum $1,25(OH)_2D_3$ is low only if serum 25(OH)D is in the normal range. $1,25(OH)_2D_3$ can be normalized in these severely uremic patients by increasing serum 25(OH)D to supraphysiological levels through oral 25(OH)D supplementation (3). This correlation between serum levels of substrate and product of renal 1-hydroxylase does not occur in normal individuals, and suggests impaired 25(OH)D availability to the renal enzyme in severe renal failure. Only recently, studies in the megalin knock out mouse (4) provided an explanation for both the abnormal correlation between serum 25(OH) D and $1,25(OH)_2D_3$, and the impaired substrate availability.

Nykjaer and collaborators demonstrated that most of renal 25(OH)D uptake by proximal tubular cells did not occur by simple diffusion of 25(OH)D through the basolateral membrane, after dissociating from its carrier, the vitamin D binding protein DBP. The simple diffusion model for renal 25(OH)D uptake could not explain impaired 25(OH)D availability. Instead, the 25(OH)D-bound to DBP in the circulation is filtered through the glomerulus and endocytosed into the proximal tubular cell via the apical membrane receptor megalin (4). In renal failure, the lower the GFR, the lower the amount of 25(OH)D-bound to DBP filtered thus limiting the amount of intracellular 25(OH)D available for conversion to $1,25(OH)_2D_3$. 25(OH)D administration to renal failure patients increases the proportion of 25(OH)D bound to DBP in blood, and consequently both the amount of bound 25(OH)D filtered and the intracellular 25(OH)D available for bioactivation to $1,25(OH)_2D_3$ by limiting 1-hydroxylase.

Mechanisms for impaired $1,25(OH)_2D_3$-VDR action in renal failure.
In addition to low serum $1,25(OH)_2D_3$, parathyroid VDR content is also reduced in the parathyroid glands of uremic humans, especially in areas of more aggressive nodular growth, as demonstrated in the immunohistochemical studies by Fukuda and collaborators in nodular and diffuse hyperplastic human parathyroid glands (5). One reason for reduced VDR levels is the low serum$1,25(OH)_2D_3$, since $1,25(OH)_2D_3$ is known to up-regulate VDR content. Studies in parathyroid glands from uremic rats demonstrate a strong correlation between serum levels of $1,25(OH)_2D_3$ and parathyroid VDR content, suggesting the potential for $1,25(OH)_2D_3$ therapy to correct the reduced parathyroid-VDR content in renal failure patients. In fact, the reduced VDR content in the parathyroid glands of uremic rats can be increased to normal levels by administration of $1,25(OH)_2D_3$ (6).
In addition to the impaired formation of the $1,25(OH)_2D_3$-VDR complex resulting from a combination of decreases in $1,25(OH)_2D_3$ synthesis as well as in parathyroid VDR content, abnormalities in steps downstream from ligand binding to the VDR also contribute to further impair $1,25(OH)_2D_3$-VDR inhibition of parathyroid gene transcription. Additional contributors to impairing $1,25(OH)_2D_3$-VDR control of parathyroid function in renal failure include: (a) *Reduced retinoid X receptor(RXR)*. Studies in unilaterally nephectomized rats demonstrated a reduction in kidney content of a 50 KDa RXR isoform, which impairs the binding of endogenous VDR/RXR complex to the Vitamin D Responsive Element (VDRE) of the mouse osteopontin gene promoter, despite no changes in serum $1,25(OH)_2D_3$ or VDR. A similar reduction in RXR in the parathyroids could explain the enhanced serum PTH levels in these rats, in the absence hypocalcemia or hyperphosphatemia (7); (b) *Accumulation of uremic toxins.* Ultrafiltrate from uremic plasma caused a dose dependent inhibition of VDR/RXR binding to VDRE and $1,25(OH)_2D_3$-VDR transactivating function (8); (c) *Increases in parathyroid calreticulin.* Calreticulin is a cytosolic protein that binds integrins in the plasma membrane and the zinc finger domain of nuclear receptors, including the VDR, thus interfering with receptor mediated transactivation (9). Hypocalcemia, commonly present in renal failure, and caused by both low $1,25(OH)_2D_3$ or hyperphosphatemia, enhances nuclear levels of calreticulin in parathyroid glands (10). In vitro studies demonstrate that increases in calreticulin inhibit VDR/RXR binding to VDRE in a dose-dependent manner, and totally abolish $1,25(OH)_2D_3$ suppression of PTH gene transcription (10).

Efficacy of $1,25(OH)_2D_3$ therapy in the control of parathyroid function.
1,25(OH)_2D_3 control of PTH gene transcription.
Despite the multiple defects in $1,25(OH)_2D_3$-VDR action in uremia, we demonstrated in 1984 that intravenous administration of calcitriol to hemodialysis patients is effective in suppressing serum PTH levels by 70% (11). More recent long-term studies demonstrated that if serum phosphorus is controlled, intravenous $1,25(OH)_2D_3$ given three times a week, suppressed PTH by 60% without any changes in ionized calcium for up to 12 weeks. Subsequently, a mild elevation in ionized calcium further suppressed serum PTH (84% reduction) by week 35. Most importantly, bone biopsies in these patients showed a marked improvement of bone

histology (12). The goal of 1,25(OH)$_2$D$_3$ therapy is to maintain serum PTH at levels 2 to 3 fold above normal levels to prevent adynamic bone disease. Avoiding hypercalcemia and hyperphosphatemia is crucial for the efficacy of 1,25(OH)$_2$D$_3$ treatment. Hypercalcemia will lead to excessive PTH suppression and adynamic bone disease whereas hyperphosphatemia renders the parathyroids insensitive to 1,25(OH)$_2$D$_3$. Today, patients in the USA and Japan benefit from the use of Vitamin D analogs that retain the ability to suppress PTH with much less calcemic and phosphatemic activity (13).

1,25(OH)$_2$D$_3$ control of parathyroid hyperplasia.

The mechanisms responsible for parathyroid hyperplasia in renal failure are poorly understood.

Studies in our laboratory on parathyroid hyperplasia in uremic rats, demonstrated that most of the enlargement of the parathyroid gland is caused by enhanced parathyroid cell growth and occurs within 4-6 days of the onset of renal failure (6,14). Recent studies on the mitogenic and antimitogenic signals triggered by uremia in parathyroid cells demonstrated that uremia-induced parathyroid cell growth correlates with enhanced expression of the growth promoter transforming growth factor alpha (TGFα) (15). We also demonstrated that parathyroid-growth arrest in renal failure is associated with increased expression of the cyclin-dependent kinase inhibitor p21 (16). Several laboratories demonstrated a role for 1,25(OH)$_2$D$_3$ in the control of parathyroid cell proliferation. 1,25(OH)$_2$D$_3$ was shown to suppress parathyroid cell growth in vitro, and also uremia-induced parathyroid hyperplasia in 5/6 nephrectomized rats (18, 19). In cells of the monocyte-macrophage lineage, 1,25(OH)$_2$D$_3$ was shown to suppress proliferation through transcriptional activation of p21 (20). Based on these reports and our demonstration of a role of induction of p21 in the control of uremia induced parathyroid growth, we examined whether 1,25(OH)$_2$D$_3$ treatment could counteract the growth-promoting effect of enhanced TGFα in early renal failure. 5/6 nephrectomized rats were fed a high phosphorus diet to further induce parathyroid hyperplasia over the signal triggered by the onset of renal failure. 1,25(OH)$_2$D$_3$ (4 ng daily) and and the vitamin D analog 19 nor-1,25(OH)$_2$D$_2$ (30ng/daily) was administered intraperitoneally. Seven days after the onset of renal failure, immunohystochemical assessment of parathyroid expression of the marker of mitosis PCNA, TGFα, and p21 demonstrated that 1,25(OH)$_2$D$_3$ and 19-nor 1,25(OH)$_2$D$_2$ were equally effective in preventing parathyroid hyperplasia and enlargement of parathyroid gland size induced by high P. The antiproliferative properties of both vitamin D metabolites involved two distinct mechanisms. As expected, both compounds induced parathyroid p21 expression. Interestingly, vitamin D therapy also prevented the enhancement of parathyroid TGFα induced by high phosphorus (Unpublished data). These results suggest that, in addition to induction of p21, 1,25(OH)$_2$D$_3$-inhibition of TGFα expression could also contribute to the antiproliferative properties of the sterol.

1,25(OH)$_2$D$_3$ regulation of calcium-control of parathyroid function.

It is well known that 1,25(OH)$_2$D$_3$ controls serum calcium and that calcium controls PTH synthesis through the calcium sensor. Similar to the VDR, the calcium sensor is markedly reduced in hyperplastic parathyroid glands from renal failure patients (21). We examined whether 1,25(OH)$_2$D$_3$ deficiency itself affected parathyroid expression of the calcium sensor. Studies in vitamin D deficient rats demonstrated that similar to renal failure patients, vitamin

D deficiency results in enlargement of the parathyroid glands and a marked reduction in calcium sensor expression (22). These results suggest an additional mechanism for $1,25(OH)_2D_3$ deficiency to worsen secondary hyperparathyroidism

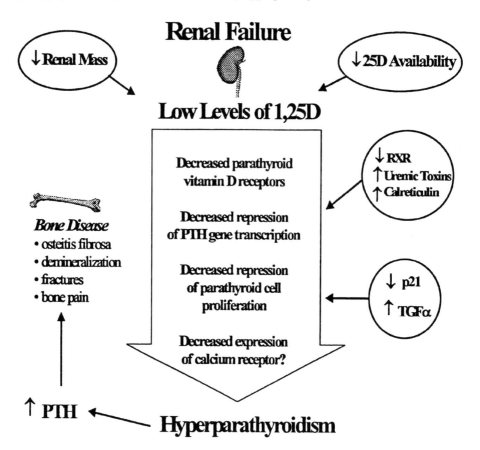

In summary, in chronic renal failure, impaired 25(OH)D availability adds to limiting 1-hydroxylase activity causing $1,25(OH)_2D_3$ deficiency, which in turn reduces parathyroid VDR content. The resultant decreased $1,25(OH)_2D_3$-VDR complex formation, together with decreased RXR and increases in uremic toxins and calreticulin, contribute to impair both $1,25(OH)_2D_3$-VDR suppression of parathyroid gene transcription and 1,25D-VDR transcriptional activation of p21. $1,25(OH)_2D_3$-inhibition of TGFα expression will also be impaired further contributing to the defective suppression of parathyroid cell proliferation. A reduction of parathyroid expression of the calcium sensor by $1,25(OH)_2D_3$ deficiency in uremia may also contribute to worsen hyperparathyroidism and bone disease.

References
1. Slatopolsky, E., Delmez, J. (1995) Min. Electrolyte Metab. 21, 91-96.
2. Martinez, I., Saracho, R., Montenegro, J., Llach, F. (1996) Nephrol. Dial. Transplant. 11,22-28.
3. Halloran, B.P., Schaeffer, P., Lifschitz, M., Levens, M., Goldsmith R.S.(1984) J.Clin. Endocrinol. Metab.59,1063-1069.
4. Nykjaer, A., Dragun, D., Walther, D., Vorum, H., Jacobsen, C., Herz, J., Melsen, F., Christensen, E.I., Willnow, T.E. (1999) Cell 96,507-515.
5. Fukuda, N., Tanaka H., TominagaY.,Fukagawa, M., Kurokawa, K, SeinoY. (1993) J. Clin. Invest. 92, 1436-1443.
6. Denda, M., Finch, J., Brown, A.J. Nishii, Y, Kubodera, N, Slatopolsky, E. (1996) Kidney Int. 50, 34-39.
7. Sawaya B.P., Koszewski N.J., Qi, Q., Chris Langub, M. Monier-Faulgere M.C., Malluche, H.H.(1997) J.Am. Soc. Nephrol.8, 271-278.
8. Patel, S.R., Ke, H.Q., Vanholder, R., Koenig, R.J., Hsu, C.H. (1995) J. Clin. Invest. 96, 50-59.
9. Dehdar, S., Rennie, P.S., Shago, M, Leung-Hagestein, C., Yang, H., Hilmus, J., Hawley R.G., Bruchovsky, N., Cheng, H., Matusik, R.J., Giguere, V. (1994) Nature 367, 480-483.
10. Sela-Brown, A., Russell, J., Koszewski, N.J., Michalak, M., Naveh-Many, T., Silver, J. (1998) Molec. Endocrinol.12, 1193-1200.
11. Slatopolsky, E., Weerts, C., Theilan, J., Horst., R., Harter, H., Martin, K.J. (1984) J. Clin. Invest. 74, 2136-2143.
12. Cannella, G., Bonucci, E., Rolla, D., Ballanti P., Moriero E., De Grandi, R., Augeri, C., Claudian, F., Di Maio, G. (1994) Kidney Int.46, 1124-1132.
13. Brown, A.J. (1998) Am. J. Kidney Dis. 32, S35-S39.
14. Slatopolsky, E., Brown, A.J., Dusso, A.S. (1999) Kidney Int. 56, S14-S19.
15. Dusso, A.S., Lu, Y., Pavlopoulos, T., Slatopolsky, E.(1999) J. Am. Soc. Nephrol. 10, 617A
16. Dusso, A.S., Naumovich, L., Pavlopoulos, T., Finch, J., Morrissey, J, Slatopolsky, E.(1998) J. Am. Soc. Nephrol. 9, 564A
17. Kremer, R., Bolivar, I., Goltzman, D., Hendy, G.N. (1989)Endocrinology 125, 935-941.
18. Szabo, A., Merke, J., Beier, E., Mall, G., Ritz,E. (1989) Kidney Intern. 35, 1049-1056.
19. Liu, M., Lee, M.H., Cohen, M., Bommakanti, M., Freedman, L.P. (1996) Genes Dev. 10142-153.
20. Liu, M., Lee, M.H., Cohen, M., Bommakanti, M., Freedman, L.P. (1996) Genes Dev. 10142-153.
21. Gogusev, J., Duchambon, P., Hory, B., Giovannini, M., Goureau, Y., Sarfati, E., Drueke, T.B. (1997) Kidney Int. 51, 328-336.
22. Brown, A.J., Zhong, M., Finch, J., Ritter, C., Mc-Craken R., Morrisey, J., Slatopolsky, E. (1996) Am. J. Physiol. 270, F454-F460.

AN UPDATE ON DOXERCALCIFEROL ($1\alpha D_2$): THE "NEW PLAYER" FOR THE MANAGEMENT OF MODERATE TO SEVERE 2° HYPERPARATHYROIDISM IN RENAL FAILURE.

J.W. Coburn,[1,2] H.M. Maung,[1] J.M. Frazão,[1,2] L. Elangovan,[1] R.W. Chesney,[4] S.R. Acchiardo,[5] J.D. Bower,[6] B.J. Kelley,[5] H.J. Rodriguez,[2] K.C. Norris,[3] J.A. Robertson,[1] B.S. Levine,[1,2] W.G. Goodman,[2] D. Gentile,[2*] R.B. Mazess,[7] D.M. Kyllo,[7] L.L. Douglass,[7] and C.W. Bishop.[7]   *Deceased

[1]Medical and Research Services, Greater Los Angeles V.A. Healthcare Center and [2]Dept. Medicine, UCLA School of Medicine and [3]Charles R. Drew Univ., Los Angeles, CA; Dept. [4]Pediatrics and [5]Medicine, Univ. Tennessee at Memphis, Memphis, TN; [6]Nephrol. Division, Univ. Mississippi, Jackson, MS; and [7]Bone Care International, Inc., Madison WI, USA.

Introduction: The search for a vitamin D that effectively suppresses PTH in patients with 2° hyperparathyroidism but has limited calcemic and phosphatemic effects has led to the introduction of several analogs, including maxicalcitol (oxacalcitriol) (1), falecalcitriol (26,27-hexafluorocalcitriol) (2), paricalcitol (19-nor-1,25-dihydroxyvitamin D_2) (3), and doxercalciferol (1α-hydroxyvitamin D_2 or $1\alpha D_2$) (4). Doxercalciferol ($1\alpha D_2$) largely undergoes hepatic conversion to 1,25-dihydroxyvitamin D_2; thus, it is a prohormone that bypasses the need for renal 1α-hydroxylation. In preliminary trials, $1\alpha D_2$, in oral doses of 10 µg given thrice weekly, effectively suppressed PTH levels in hemodialysis patients without significant hypercalcemia or hyperphosphatemia (5,6). Therefore, a large number of hemodialysis patients with moderate-to-severe 2° hyperparathyroidism (pretreatment intact PTH [iPTH], 442 to 4706 pg/ml) were entered into the present 32 week study; it consisted of 8 weeks of Washout, 16-weeks of open label $1\alpha D_2$ treatment, and 8 weeks of double blinded crossover to Placebo or continued $1\alpha D_2$ treatment. The open label treatment was undertaken first because it was considered unethical to withhold vitamin D for up to 32 weeks in those with severe 2° hyperparathyroidism. The $1\alpha D_2$ treatment was started at a "high" dose of 10 µg with each dialysis and then adjusted to keep the iPTH within a preselected range of 150 to 300 pg/ml. This differs from the usual method of treating 2° hyperparathyroidism with calcitriol or alfacalcidol, wherein doses are cautiously low and adjusted according to changes in serum Ca. The primary goal was to evaluate the efficacy and safety of intermittent high oral doses of $1\alpha D_2$ to treat moderate-to-severe 2° hyperparathyroidism. The secondary goal was to identify the doses required to treat hyperparathyroidism of differing severity and to characterize the therapeutic responses.

Materials and methods: This randomized, double blinded, placebo-controlled trial enrolled hemodialysis patients with moderate-to-severe 2° hyperparathyroidism from 18 hemodialysis units in southern California and western Tennessee/eastern Arkansas/Mississippi. Protocols were approved by the institutional review board at each center, with informed consent obtained from each patient. The design was to enroll patients with 2° hyperparathyroidism of unlimited severity as determined from entry PTH levels, with safety limitations for the degree of hypercalcemia or hyperphos-phatemia at entry. Entry criteria, described in detail elsewhere (7) included an iPTH above 400 pg/ml with no calcitriol, a mean serum P of 2.5 to 6.9 mg/dl over 2 recent months, no use of aluminum-containing phosphate-binders for 1 year, and no parathyroid surgery within 1 year. Patients were excluded from open label treatment if during washout they did not fulfill the same entry criteria noted above or if they had a mean serum Ca above 10.5 mg/dl or a mean serum Ca X P product > 70.

The 10 μg oral dose of $1\alpha D_2$ was given after each hemodialysis with dose adjust-ments to keep the iPTH in a target range of 150 to 300 pg/ml, values associated with normal or near normal bone formation and minimal features of 2° hyperparathyroidism in hemodialysis patients (8). When the patients switched from open label treatment to double blinded treatment, the dose was continued with 50% of the patients changing to Placebo, according to blinded assignment made at entry into Washout. Only $CaCO_3$ or Ca-acetate were used as phosphate binders, with doses adjusted to keep the serum P below 6.9 mg/dl. Serum Ca and P and plasma iPTH were drawn weekly before dialysis, and treatment was adjusted according to a specific protocol (7) to keep iPTH in the target range. For safety, treatment was stopped for hypercalcemia (Ca > 11.2 mg/dl), significant hyperphosphatemia (P > 8.0 mg/dl) or a serum Ca X P product > 75.0. Later, $1\alpha D_2$ was resumed at a dose lowered by 2.5 μg; such reductions were repeated as needed. At Week 8 and then at 8-weekly intervals, the dose could be increased by 2.5 to 5.0 μg if iPTH did not fall into the target range and it was not lowered from Baseline by 50%; the maximum dose was 20 μg thrice weekly. The biochemical methods utilized and statistical methods employed are described in detail elsewhere (7).

Results: Of the 138 patients who qualified to enter open treatment, 99 completed the study per protocol. The most common reasons for disqualification included protocol violations with the inadvertent administration of intravenous calcitriol or aluminum hydroxide (n=13) or the mean serum P exceeding the allowable level of < 6.9 mg/dl (n=9); 19 patients withdrew or were disqualified during open label treatment and 20 during double-blinded treatment, 13 of the latter receiving $1\alpha D_2$ and 7, placebo (n.s.). The demographic data and Baseline biochemical data did not differ between those assigned to $1\alpha D_2$ or placebo.

From the Baseline value of 897 ± 52 pg/ml, iPTH levels fell to 80.2 ± 3.43% of Baseline by 1 week of $1\alpha D_2$ treatment (p < 0.001); they continued to fall reaching 44.7 ± 2.87% of Baseline at Week 16 (p < 0.001) [Figure]. During double blinded treatment, the iPTH levels remained suppressed in patients continuing on $1\alpha D_2$. In contrast, the median plasma iPTH rose 28.7% (25:75 percentiles, +1.3%:+100.5%) in those assigned to placebo by week 17 (p < 0.001); thereafter, iPTH levels continued to rise reaching a value no different from Baseline by 4 weeks after $1\alpha D_2$ withdrawal. The extent of PTH suppression differed significantly between the Placebo and $1\alpha D_2$ groups during weeks 17 through 24 (p < 0.05). In a comparison of 138 intent to treat (ITT) patients with the 99 per protocol (PP) patients, there were no differences between the Baseline iPTH levels nor the degree of suppression between the two groups at any time during therapy. Among the 99 patients completing the study PP, 91.9% had iPTH suppression by more than 50%, and 83% reached the target range.

The effect of $1\alpha D_2$ on iPTH changes in patients divided according to varying severity of 2° hyperparathyroidism was examined by grouping patients into those with Baseline iPTH < 600 pg/ml (Group A, n = 33), Baseline iPTH, 600 - 1200 pg/ml (Group B, n = 48), and Group C, Baseline iPTH > 1200 pg/ml (n = 18). Patients randomized to placebo were excluded for Weeks 16 through 24, leaving 16, 22, and 10 $1\alpha D_2$-treated patients in Groups A, B, and C, respectively [Figure]. Plasma iPTH levels fell quickly in Group A, reaching the target after two weeks. In Group B, 10 to 11 weeks were needed before iPTH leveled off in the target range. In Group C, iPTH levels decreased more slowly over the entire 24 weeks. Since the groups were separated according to the Baseline iPTH, the mean iPTH levels of each group differed from the other two at Weeks 1 - 4; subsequently, iPTH levels of Groups A and B were not different. For Group C, iPTH values were significantly greater than Groups A and B from Weeks 2-24 with the exception of Week 17.

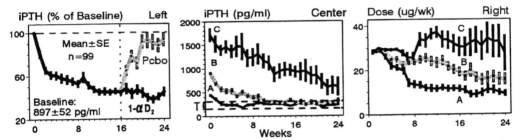

Figure: <u>Left</u>: Changes of plasma iPTH as percent of baseline value. All received $1\alpha D_2$ during open label treatment; at Week 16, half were randomized to double-blinded treatment with Placebo (Shaded line) and half continued $1\alpha D_2$ (Dark line). <u>Center</u>: Patients divided into 3 groups according to baseline iPTH levels: A < 600 pg/ml; B, 600-1200; and C, > 1200. The dotted lines show the target range (T) for iPTH (150-300 pg/ml). <u>Right</u>: Weekly doses of $1\alpha D_2$ given to 3 groups (A,B and C) stratified according to baseline iPTH levels. [Modified from reference (7)]

During the first few weeks of open label treatment, serum Ca rose slightly and reached significance by Week 2; subsequently, serum Ca remained above Baseline, with mean values ranging from 9.23 ± 0.84 to 9.74 ± 1.05 mg/dl (±SD). Serum Ca fell slightly in the Placebo group during randomized treatment and differed from the $1\alpha D_2$ group at each week except 19 (p <0.05). During open label treatment, serum P levels rose slightly from Baseline and were higher than Baseline at Weeks 1-16; mean serum P ranged from 5.42 ± 1.10 to 5.86 ± 1.55 mg/dl (±SD). With double blinded treatment, serum P fell slightly in the Placebo group and differed significantly between the Placebo and $1\alpha D_2$-treated groups only at Weeks 18 and 19. Mean serum Ca and P levels did not differ between the three PTH groups at any time during the 24 treatment-weeks, despite the differences in dosage of $1\alpha D_2$ given to the three groups [Figure].

The prevalence of hypercalcemia and of hyperphosphatemia, defined as serum Ca > 11.2 mg/dl and serum P > 8.0 mg/dl, respectively, was evaluated in 138 ITT patients. Elevations of serum Ca > 11.2 mg/dl occurred in 0.19% of measurements during Washout and 3.84% during open label treatment (p < 0.001). During double blinded treatment, the incidence of such hypercalcemia was 0.46 and 3.26% in Placebo and $1\alpha D_2$-treated patients, respectively (p < 0.01). Serum Ca exceeded 13.0 mg/dl in only two patients, representing 0.08% of the 2,398 calcium determinations during therapy, and no-one had any symptoms attributable to hypercalcemia. After $1\alpha D_2$ treatment was interrupted because of hypercalcemia, serum Ca fell below 11.2 mg/dl within seven days in all but one instance. Throughout the 32 weeks of observation, 46 patients among the 138 ITT patients accounted for all episodes of serum Ca > 11.2 mg/dl.

Significant hyperphosphatemia (Serum P > 8.0 mg/dl) occurred in 1.14% of measurements during Washout and 6.37% during open label treatment (p < 0.001). During double blinded treatment, the percentages were 2.32 and 7.14 of measurements in Placebo and $1\alpha D_2$ patients, respectively (p = < 0.01).

From week 1 to week 16, the dose of $1\alpha D_2$ fell from 28.7 ± 0.34 µg/week to 17.5 ± 1.51 µg/week; doses remained low in $1\alpha D_2$-treated patients during randomized double-blinded therapy. Plasma levels of $1\alpha,25$-$(OH)_2D_3$ were near detection limits and remained unchanged throughout. Plasma levels of $1\alpha,25$-$(OH)_2D_2$ correlated with the $1\alpha D_2$ dose given during the preceding week. An analysis of plasma $1,25(OH)_2D_2$ levels in 45 patients receiving constant weekly doses of $1\alpha D_2$ revealed no change in serum $1,25(OH)_2D_2$ levels with the length of therapy, a finding indicating no accumulation of plasma $1,25(OH)_2D_2$ levels with time.

Evaluation of weekly doses of $1\alpha D_2$ in the 3 PTH groups described above revealed that the doses for Group A were lower than Group C during Weeks 3-8; after Week 8, when the dose could be adjusted upwards, the doses in Group C rose and exceeded those of both Groups A and B except at Week 17 [Figure]. Of interest, the doses of Groups A and B differed from Weeks 9 - 16 despite the lack of difference between the mean iPTH levels.

Discussion: These studies show that intermittent oral doxercalciferol (1α-hydroxyvitamin D_2 or $1\alpha D_2$) suppresses iPTH levels effectively in hemodialysis patients, even those with severe 2° hyperparathyroidism, observations confirming results of pilot studies (5,6). Serum Ca levels rose slightly but generally remained within the normal range. There were marked differences in PTH suppression with $1\alpha D_2$ compared to placebo in the controlled double-blinded phase.

Vitamin D_2, which differs from vitamin D_3 only in its side-chain structure, was widely used in the past because of its lower cost; vitamin D_2 and D_3 were believed to be equally potent in humans and certain other mammals (9). However, data reviewed elsewhere (5,10) indicate that vitamin D_2 has 1/5th to 1/8th the toxicity of vitamin D_3 in several animal models. The toxicity of $1\alpha D_2$ and alfacalcidol (1α-hydroxyvitamin D_3 or $1\alpha D_3$) show similar differences. Such observations prompted the present trials with $1\alpha D_2$ in 2° hyperparathyroidism. The reasons for different potencies of certain sterols having a D_2-side chain compared to a D_3-side chain are uncertain, but it could relate to hepatic 24-hydroxylation of the D_2-side chain, a conversion that does not occur with D_3 (11,12). A demonstration that $1\alpha D_2$ is less calcemic than $1\alpha D_3$ or calcitriol in clinical trials awaits clinical trials that directly compare these sterols.

Our data show that the time required for suppression of plasma iPTH levels increases with the severity of the 2° hyperparathyroidism; they show that higher doses of $1\alpha D_2$ are needed for patients with severe 2° hyperparathyroidism compared to those with mild-to-moderate hyperparathyroidism. In patients with iPTH levels < 1200 pg/ml, PTH was suppressed into the target range within 12 weeks or less. Patients with iPTH levels > 1200 pg/ml had a slow, progressive reduction of iPTH over the entire 24 weeks of $1\alpha D_2$-treatment. Our observations that considerable time must elapse before iPTH levels fall substantially in patients with severe 2° hyperparathyroidism are consistent with reports on use of intravenous calcitriol (13,14). The responsible mechanism is unclear, but it may relate to the slow up-regulation of vitamin D receptors, which are reduced in the large, nodular parathyroid glands found in patients with severe 2° hyperparathyroidism (15). The administration of large doses of $1\alpha D_2$ effectively and safely lowered iPTH levels in those with very severe 2° hyperparathyroidism.

Our study shows that iPTH levels rise promptly to reach values no different from baseline values when $1\alpha D_2$ was replaced with placebo after 16 weeks of $1\alpha D_2$-treatment. This rapid increase of iPTH after withdrawal of $1\alpha D_2$ suggests there is little or no reduction of parathyroid gland size after 4 months of treatment. Other data, reported elsewhere in this volume (16), indicate that treatment with $1\alpha D_2$ for approximately 6 months did induce long-lasting effects consistent with regression of gland size or a reduced ability to increase PTH secretion.

There was a small but statistically significant effect of $1\alpha D_2$-treatment to elevate serum Ca levels, although most were well within normal limits. The higher incidence of mild hypercalcemia was easily managed by lowering $1\alpha D_2$-dose or by reducing the intake of calcium-containing, phosphate-binders. The number of hypercalcemic episodes did not increase as the $1\alpha D_2$-dose was raised to 60 µg/week, in comparison to the largest dose of 30 µg/week in earlier trials (5,6), providing evidence of the favorable safety profile of $1\alpha D_2$. Also, serum levels of $1,25(OH)_2D_2$ showed no tendency to rise, indicating the lack of accumulation of the active sterol during long-term $1\alpha D_2$-treatment.

It was recently recognized that hyperphosphatemia impacts negatively on the mortality of dialysis patients (17) and correlates with several abnormalities of cardiovascular function (18). This may have far-reaching implications about the ideal approach to management of mineral metabolism in ESRD patients. Whether vitamin D therapy of any kind is totally safe in the presence of increments of serum P above 6.0 mg/dl must await further long-term studies. Clearly, greater attention must be given to the control of serum P with phosphate-binding agents when vitamin D sterols are to be used treat dialysis patients with 2° hyperparathyroidism. The potential safety issue would seem to preclude long term vitamin D treatment in such patients. However, the prevalence of serum P elevation to values above 6.9 mg/dl during both open label and blinded therapy with $1\alpha D_2$ is considerably lower than the substantial prevalence of 31 to 32% reported among 6400 U.S. hemodialysis patients (17).

The design of our trials with $1\alpha D_2$ (5-7) differ from clinical trials using vitamin D sterols to manage 2° hyperparathyroidism in that dose adjustments were targeted to lower the iPTH levels to a specific range of 150 to 300 pg/ml, values associated with bone turnover that is close to normal and histologic features of 2° hyperparathyroidism are either absent or mild in hemodialysis patients (8). This iPTH target range was chosen to minimize the risk of inducing a state of low bone turnover, which may develop in the face of iPTH levels < 100-150 pg/ml following therapy with vitamin D (19,20). It remains to be determined whether the greater cost of measuring iPTH levels compared to serum Ca will be cost-effective to reduce the incidence of states with low bone turnover.

There is growing evidence that nutritional vitamin D-deficiency, identified by low serum 25(OH)-vitamin D levels may be common in the United States (21); such hypovitaminosis D can contribute to the severity of 2° hyperparathyroidism (22). Plasma levels of 25-hydroxy-vitamin D were not determined in the present study, but such observations would have no impact on the present successful results of therapy with $1\alpha D_2$.

Whether $1\alpha D_2$ has a more favorable therapeutic index compared with calcitriol, alfacalcidol ($1\alpha D_3$), and paricalcitol cannot be answered without direct comparisons with these sterols. These data compare favorably to our earlier pilot study (5); those results with $1\alpha D_2$ were compared with prospective studies using calcitriol or alfacalcidol in patients with moderate to severe hyperparathyroidism (5). Both the present multicenter study and our earlier studies (5,6) achieved suppression of intact PTH similar to the "best" results of trials done in single centers, using pulse intravenous calcitriol or $1\alpha D_3$, and giving only calcium-based phosphate-binders (14,23). Moreover, the incidence of hyperphosphatemia and hypercalcemia were acceptable despite the "high" doses of $1\alpha D_2$ utilized and the exclusive use of calcium-containing, phosphate-binders in large doses.

The mechanism by which $1\alpha D_2$ suppresses iPTH is unknown; $1\alpha D_2$, an inactive prodrug, is hydroxylated in the liver primarily to $1\alpha,25\text{-}(OH)_2D_2$ and secondarily to $1\alpha,24(S)\text{-}(OH)_2D_2$; one or both of these may act in a manner similar to calcitriol, although with greater safety. Both could act directly on the parathyroid gland to suppress the secretion of PTH. The small rise in serum calcium observed in the present study, which likely arises from enhanced intestinal calcium absorption, undoubtedly contributes to the PTH suppression. However, there was a poor correlation between the changes in the levels of serum Ca and those of iPTH. Further studies are needed to determine the precise mechanism of action of this vitamin D analog.

The present large trial demonstrates unequivocally that doxercalciferol (1α-hydroxyvitamin D_2 or $1\alpha D_2$), when given at the dosage regimens studied, is efficacious for the treatment of hemodialysis patients with moderate-to-severe 2° hyperparathyroidism. One-α-hydroxyvitamin D_2 is safe in uremic patients with 2° hyperparathyroidism. In the future, studies that directly compare doxercalciferol with other vitamin D sterols will be needed to provide proof of its relative safety.

Acknowledgements: Supported by a Grant from Bone Care International, Inc.; Dr Norris is supported, in part, by Grant 1 P20 RR11145-01 (NIH/NCRR).

References:

1. Kurokawa, K., Akizawa, T., Suzuki, M., Akiba, T., Ogata, E., and Slatopolsky, E. (1996) Nephrol. Dial. Transplant. **11 [Suppl 3]**, 121-124

2. Akiba, T., Marumo, F., Owada, A., Kurihara, S., Inoue, A., Chida, Y., Ando, R., Shinoda, T., Ishida, Y., and Ohashi, Y. (1998) Am J Kidney Dis. **32**, 238-246

3. Martin, K. J., González, E. A., Gellens, M., Hamm, L. L., Abboud, H., and Lindberg, J. (1998) J. Am. Soc. Nephrol. **9**, 1427-1432

4. Coburn, J. W., Tan, A. U.,Jr., Levine, B. S., Mazess, R. B., Kyllo, D. M., Knutson, J. C., and Bishop, C. W. (1996) Nephrol. Dial. Transplant. **11 (Suppl 3)**, 153-157

5. Tan, A. U.,Jr., Levine, B. S., Mazess, R. B., Kyllo, D. M., Bishop, C. W., Knutson, J. C., Kleinman, K. S., and Coburn, J. W. (1997) Kidney Int. **51**, 317-323

6. Frazao, J. M., Levine, B. S., Tan, A. U.,Jr., Mazess, R. B., Kyllo, D. M., Knutson, J. C., Bishop, C. W., and Coburn, J. W. (1997) Dial. Transplant. **26**, 583-595

7. Frazao, J. M., Elangovan, L., Maung, H. M., Chesney, R. B., Acchiardo, S. R., Bower, J. D., Kelley, B. J., Rodriguez, H. J., Norris, K. C., Robertson, J. A., Levine, B. S., Goodman, W. G., Gentile, D., Mazess, R. B., Kyllo, D. M., Douglass, L. L., Bishop, C. W., and Coburn, J. W. (2000) Am. J. Kidney. Dis. (in press)

8. Sherrard, D. J., Hercz, G., Pei, Y., Maloney, N. A., Greenwood, C., Manuel, A., Saiphoo, C., Fenton, S. S., and Segre, G. V. (1993) Kidney Int. **43**, 436-435

9. Hunt, R. D., Garcia, F. G., Hegsted, D. M., and Kaplinsky, N. (1967) Science **158**, 943-947

10. Hunt, R. D., Garcia, F. G., and Hegsted, D. M. (1969) Am. J. Clin. Nutr. **22**, 358-366

11. Mawer, E. B., Jones, G., Davies, M., Still, P. E., Byford, V., Schroeder, N. J., Makin, H. L. J., Bishop, C. W., and Knutson, J. C. (1998) J. Clin. Endocrinol. Metab. **83**, 2156-2166

12. Strugnell, S., Byford, V., Makin, H. L. J., Moriarty, R. M., Gilardi, R., Levan, L. W., Knutson, J. C., Bishop, C. W., and Jones, G. (1995) Biochem. J. **310**, 233-241

13. Sprague, S. M. and Moe, S. M. (1992) Am. J. Kidney Dis. **19**, 532-539

14. Llach, F., Hervas, J., and Cerezo, S. (1995) Am. J. Kidney Dis. **26**, 845-851

15. Fukuda, N., Tanaka, H., Tominaga, Y., Fukagawa, M., Kurokawa, K., and Seino, Y. (1993) J. Clin. Invest. **92**, 1436-1443

16. Maung, H. M., Chesney, R. W., Coburn, J. W., and 1αD2-Study Group, (2000) in Vitamin D [this volume] (Norman, A. W., Bouillon, R., and Thomasset, M., eds) Walter de Gruyter, Berlin

17. Block, G. A., Hulbert-Shearon, T. E., Levin, N. W., and Port, F. K. (1998) Am. J. Kidney Dis. **31**, 607-617

18. Marchais, S. J., Metivier, F., Guerin, A. P., and London, G. M. (1999) Nephrol. Dial. Transplant. **14**, 2178-2183

19. Andress, D. L., Norris, K. C., Coburn, J. W., Slatopolsky, E. A., and Sherrard, D. J. (1989) N. Engl. J. Med. **321**, 274-279

20. Kuizon, B. D., Goodman, W. G., Jüppner, H., Boechat, I., Nelson, P., Gales, B., and Salusky, I. B. (1998) Kidney Int. **53**, 205-211

21. Thomas, M. K., Lloyd-Jones, D. M., Thadhani, R. I., Shaw, A. C., Deraska, D. J., Kitch, B. T., Dick, I. M., Prince, R. L., and Finkelstein, J. S. (1998) N. Engl. J. Med. **338**, 777-783

22. Ghazali, A., Fardellone, P., Pruna, A., Atik, A., Achard, J. -M., Oprisiu, R., Brazier, M., Remond, A., Moriniere, P., Garabedian, M., Eastwood, J., and Fournier, A. (1999) Kidney Int. **55**, 2169-2177

23. Moriniere, P., Esper, N. E., Viron, B., Judith, D., Bourgeon, B., Farquet, C., Gheerbrandt, J. D., Chapuy, M. C., Orshoven, A. V., Pamphile, R., and Fournier, A. (1993) Kidney Int. **43 (Suppl 41)**, S121-S124

PARATHYROID REGRESSION WITH DOXERCALCIFEROL ($1\alpha D_2$) THERAPY: IMPORTANCE OF THE DURATION OF TREATMENT.

H.M. Maung,[1] R.W. Chesney,[2] J.W. Coburn[1] and the $1\alpha D_2$-Study Group.[1,2,3]

[1]Medical and Research Services, Greater Los Angeles V.A. Healthcare System and UCLA School of Medicine, Los Angeles CA, [2]Department of Pediatrics, University of Tennessee School of Medicine, Memphis TN and [3]Bone Care Int. Madison WI, USA.

Introduction: Calcitriol has been in use for more than 20 years in the management of secondary hyperparathyroidism in end-stage renal disease (ESRD), and the levels of parathyroid hormone (PTH) are often reduced by such therapy (1-3). In the few available studies that have addressed the subject, PTH levels returned to pre-treatment levels soon after treatment with calcitriol was discontinued (1,4); such data suggest that calcitriol produced little or no reduction of the size of the hyperplastic parathyroid glands. In contrast, other data obtained utilizing ultrasonography or isotopic imaging of the parathyroids suggest that the mass of the parathyroid glands is reduced after prolonged therapy with calcitriol (5,6); however, this may not occur, particularly in patients with severe secondary hyperparathyroidism (7,8). There are data indicating that the basal intact PTH (iPTH) levels reflect parathyroid gland mass in patients with secondary hyperparathyroidism (9,10). In a group of hemodialysis patients with moderate to severe secondary hyperparathyroidism, we had the opportunity to compare the baseline iPTH levels on two occasions following the total withdrawal of vitamin D treatment for at least 8 weeks. Between the two basal iPTH measurements, the patients received treatment with doxercalciferol ($1\alpha D_2$) for 16 to 24 weeks. This sterol, $1\alpha D_2$, exhibits a low prevalence of hypercalcemia and hyperphosphatemia during treatment of uremic secondary hyperparathyroidism (11,12). The factors that contributed to a lower basal iPTH after the second withdrawal of treatment were evaluated retrospectively. The major factor was the duration of earlier treatment with doxercalciferol.

Materials and methods: Seventy ESRD patients with moderate-to-severe secondary hyperparathyroidism and with mean initial basal iPTH levels of 926.4 ± 63.3 pg/ml (mean $\pm$ SE) (range, 289 to 3643 pg/ml) were studied on two occasions after all vitamin D treatment had been withdrawn for ≥ 8 weeks. The criteria for entering the first 8-weeks of Washout included an iPTH value above 400 pg/ml when calcitriol therapy was not utilized, a mean serum phosphorus of 2.5 to 6.9 mg/dl over two months, and no intake of aluminum-containing phosphate-binders for 12 months. After the first basal PTH (B_1), the patients entered into 16 weeks of open label treatment with oral $1\alpha D_2$, with the dosage adjusted to achieve iPTH levels in a target range of 150-300 pg/ml (12). After 16 weeks of open label treatment, the patients were randomly assigned in a double blinded fashion to either placebo or continued $1\alpha D_2$ therapy for 8 weeks. At variable times, ranging from 30 weeks to 3 days after completion of this 24 week study, the patients had vitamin D withdrawn again for 8 weeks for determination of the second basal iPTH level (B_2). During the interval between completion of the first study and beginning the second 8-week washout, 47

% of the patients were given intravenous calcitriol in varying doses at the discretion of their own nephrologist. After 16-weeks of open-label treatment with $1\alpha D_2$, mean iPTH levels, which had been suppressed by $53.0\pm4.5\%$ from B_1, rose quickly and reached values no different from B_1 by four weeks after conversion of half of the patients to placebo (12). In contrast, the mean iPTH levels of all 70 patients at B_2 were significantly lower than they had been at B_1. To clarify the reasons for the difference, we determined the $B_2{:}B_1$ ratio of iPTH in the forty-eight patients with B_1 iPTH levels between 600-2000 pg/ml. We compared the quartile of patients with the highest B_2/B_1 ratios (**Least** suppressed) with the quartile having the lowest B_2/B_1 ratio (**Most** suppressed).

Results: There were no differences between the **Most** and **Least** suppressed quartiles with regard to demographic data for age, sex, race distribution, body weight, or the duration of hemodialysis. Mean basal iPTH levels at B_1 for the **Most** and **Least** suppressed quartiles were 1073 ± 82 and 876 ± 63 pg/ml, respectively (n.s.). The ratios of B_2/B_1, the criteria for separation into the quartiles, averaged 0.41 ± 0.02 and 1.08 ± 0.10, respectively. in the **Most** and **Least** quartiles. The mean basal B_2 iPTH of 430 ± 28 pg/ml in the **Most** quartile was much lower than the mean B_1 value of 973 ± 78 pg/ml in the **Least** quartile (p <0.0001); the other significant differences between the **Most** and **Least** quartiles are shown in the table.

Table: Quartiles with Most and Least Suppressed Basal PTH after $1\alpha D_2$ Treatment:

Quartile (±SE)	B_1PTH pg/ml	B_2PTH pg/ml	Lowest PTH	Duration $1\alpha D_2$-Rx Weeks	Wk-16 PTH Suppression % of B_1	Average $1\alpha D_2$-Dose ug/wk
Most	1073 ± 82	430 ± 28	81 ± 11	23 ± 0.7	29.7 ± 3.8	25 ± 2.5
Least	876 ± 63	973 ± 78	150 ± 24	17 ± 0.9	39.0 ± 5.8	26 ± 2.5
p values	ns	<0.0001	<0.02	<0.0001	ns	ns

Among the 12 patients in **Most** quartile, 11 had been randomly assigned to receive $1\alpha D_2$ during the 8 week double blinded study, while 10 of the 12 patients in the **Least** quartile had been randomly converted to placebo. Thus, a major difference between the quartiles was the random assignment to a longer duration of treatment with $1\alpha D_2$ of 23 ± 0.7 weeks in the **Most** quartile, compared to 17 ± 0.9 weeks in the **Least** quartile (p < 0.0001). The lowest iPTH level achieved at any time during treatment with $1\alpha D_2$ was slightly but significantly lower in the **Most** quartile. However, the percent reduction of PTH from B_1 produced by $1\alpha D_2$ was not different between the two quartiles during 14 of the 16 weeks of open label therapy with $1\alpha D_2$, the exceptions being Treatment-weeks 6 and 15, when the **Least** quartile exhibited less suppression than the **Most** quartile (p < 0.05 and <0.01, respectively). The average weekly dose of $1\alpha D_2$ and the doses of calcium based phosphate binder used did not differ between the two quartiles. Serum levels of calcium and phosphorus did not differ between the quartiles at B$_1$, Week 16 of open label 1αD$_2$ treatment or at B$_2$. In the **Most** quartile, 7 of 12 patients received intravenous calcitriol for a variable period after completion of the 1αD$_2$ trial, while 5 of 12 in the **Least** quartile received intravenous calcitriol during this period (n.s.). There were no differences between the quartiles with regard to the time lapse between B$_1$ and B$_2$ nor the total interval between B$_1$ and B$_2$ without any vitamin D treatment.

Discussion: The present observations, based on basal iPTH levels after Washout from vitamin D sterol, indicate that treatment with 1αD$_2$ for up to 24 weeks leads to lower basal PTH levels, which suggests greater parathyroid regression, than does similar treatment lasting for only 16 weeks. The degree of "long term" lowering of basal iPTH levels did not depend on the magnitude of entry iPTH ranging from 600 to 2000 pg/ml, but the magnitude of maximal iPTH suppression during 1aD$_2$ treatment was associated with lower basal iPTH levels at the time of the second measurement. The question of whether vitamin D therapy can produce regression of parathyroid gland mass in patients with secondary hyperparathyroidism is controversial. The observations showing reduced gland mass by ultrasonography (5) were not confirmed in the study of most patients, particularly those with more markedly elevated PTH levels (8). In experimental animals, various forms of treatment may prevent parathyroid gland hyperplasia, but there are no data showing regression of established hyperplasia (13,14). Whether the lowering of the basal PTH levels actually reflects a reduction of the size of the parathyroid glands cannot be determined from the present observations. It is possible that prolonged 1αD$_2$ therapy affects parathyroid cells so there is less release of PTH at a given level of extracellular calcium, i.e., there is a change in "set point" for PTH secretion (15). No measurements were made in the present study to evaluate the Ca^{++}-PTH relationship. It has been suggested that a deficiency of calcitriol may act to regulate the expression of the calcium-sensing receptor (CaSR), which is of major importance in leading to PTH secretion in relation to changes in extracellular calcium (16), but others have found no effect of calcitriol on regulation of the CaSR (17). Further studies are needed to identify this relationship between prolonged therapy with 1αD$_2$ and parathyroid gland size and function.

Acknowledgments: Members of the 1αD$_2$-study group include D. Gentile, (deceased), W.G. Goodman, A.U. Tan, J.M. Frazão, L. Elangovan, B.S. Levine, K.C. Norris, H.J.Rodriguez, J.A. Robertson, S.R. Acchiardo, B.J. Kelley, J.D. Bower, L.L. Douglass, D.M. Kyllo, R.B. Mazess, and C.W. Bishop. Supported by a Grant from Bone Care International.

References:

1. Slatopolsky, E., Weerts, C., Thielan, J., Horst, R. L., Harter, H., and Martin, K. J. (1984) J. Clin. Invest. **74**, 2136-2143

2. Coburn, J. W. (1990) Kidney Int. **38 (Suppl. 29)**, S54-S61
3. Sprague, S. M. and Moe, S. M. (1992) Am. J. Kidney Dis. **19**, 532-539

874

4. Klaus, G., Mehls, O., Hinderer, J., and Ritz, E. (1991) Lancet **337**, 800-801

5. Fukagawa, M., Orazaki, R., Takano, K., Kaname, S. -Y., Ogata, E., Kitoaka, M., Karada, S. -I., Sekine, N., Matsumoto, T., and Kurokawa, K. (1990) N. Engl. J. Med. **323**, 421-422

6. Cannella, G., Bonucci, E., Rolla, D., Ballanti, P., Moriero, E., De Grandi, R., Augeri, C., Claudiani, F., and Di Maio, G. (1994) Kidney Int. **46**, 1124-1132

7. Quarles, L. D., Yohay, D. A., Carroll, B. A., Spritzer, C. E., Minda, S. A., Bartholomay, D., and Lobaugh, B. A. (1994) Kidney Int. **45**, 1710-1721

8. Fukagawa, M., Kitaoka, M., Yi, H., Fukuda, N., Matsumoto, T., Ogata, E., and Kurokawa, K. (1994) Nephron **68**, 221-228

9. Johnson, W. J., McCarthy, J. T., Van Heerden, J. A., Sterioff, S., Grant, C. S., and Kao, P. C. (1988) Am. J. Med. **84**, 23-32

10. Malberti, F., Farina, M., and Imbasciati, E. (1999) Nephrol. Dial. Transplant. **14**, 2398-2406

11. Tan, A. U.,Jr., Levine, B. S., Mazess, R. B., Kyllo, D. M., Bishop, C. W., Knutson, J. C., Kleinman, K. S., and Coburn, J. W. (1997) Kidney Int. **51**, 317-323

12. Frazao, J. M., Elangovan, L., Maung, H. M., Chesney, R. B., Acchiardo, S. R., Bower, J. D., Kelley, B. J., Rodriguez, H. J., Norris, K. C., Robertson, J. A., Levine, B. S., Goodman, W. G., Gentile, D., Mazess, R. B., Kyllo, D. M., Douglass, L. L., Bishop, C. W., and Coburn, J. W. (2000) Am. J. Kidney. Dis. (in press)

13. Szabo, A., Merke, J., Beier, E., Mall, G., and Ritz, E. (1989) Kidney Int. **35**, 1049-1056

14. Takahashi, F., Finch, J. L., Denda, M., Dusso, A. S., Brown, A. J., and Slatopolsky, E. (1997) Am. J. Kidney Dis. **30**, 105-112

15. Brown, E. M., Wilson, R. E., Eastmen, R. C., Pallotta, J., and Marynick, S. (1982) J. Clin. Endocrinol. Metab. **54**, 172-179

16. Brown, A. J., Zhong, M., Finch, J., Ritter, C., McCracken, R., Morrisey, J., and Slatopolsky, E. (1996) Am. J. Physiol. **270**, F454-F460

17. Rogers, K. V., Dunn, C. K., Conklin, R. L., Hadfield, S., Petty, B. A., Brown, E. A., Hebert, S. C., Nemeth, E. F., and Fox, J. (1995) Endocrinol. **136**, 499-504

LONG-TERM EFFECT OF 22-OXACALCITRIOL (OCT) ON OSTEITIS FIBROSA AND PARATHYROID HYPERPLASIA IN RATS WITH SLOWLY PROGRESSIVE RENAL FAILURE.

Michinori Hirata, K Katsumata, T Masaki, N Koike, F Ichikawa, K Endo, K Tsunemi, N Kubodera, H Ohkawa, K Kurokawa*, & M Fukagawa#
Chugai Pharmaceutical Co., Ltd., Shizuoka, Tokai University, Kanagawa*, Kobe University School of Medicine#, Kobe, Japan

Introduction 22-oxacalcitriol (OCT) is a unique vitamin D analogue with less-calcemic activity than calcitriol[1]. It has already been confirmed that OCT reduces PTH in chronic dialysis patients[2] and experimental model animals such as 5/6 nephrectomized rats[3] without hypercalcemia. Nevertheless the effects of OCT have been discussed only in terms of PTH suppression. Long-term effects of OCT on high turnover bone disease should also be clarified. Therefore, we examined the effects of long term intravenous OCT therapy on bone metabolism and parathyroid hyperplasia in slowly progressive nephritis model rats.

Methods Rats with slowly progressive renal failure (glycopeptide-induced nephritis rats: GN rats) were prepared by injection of nephritogenic glycopeptide isolated from rat renal cortical tissues by the method of Shibata et al[4]. At 250 days after injection of the glycopeptide, GN rats were divided into three groups with the same degree of serum N-PTH concentration. The treatment groups were as follows: Group 1, Age-matched control (Control); Group 2, GN-vehicle (Vehicle); Group 3, GN-OCT 0.03μg/kg body wt; Group 4, GN-OCT 0.15μg/kg body wt. OCT and vehicle were administered intravenously three times per week for 15 weeks. At sacrifice, serum PTH levels and ionized calcium were measured and bone histmorphometry of the 3rd vertebral body and parathyroid hyperplasia were also evaluated.

Results At sacrifice, serum PTH levels were significantly elevated in vehicle-treated rats compared with those of age-matched control rats (Fig.1). According to bone histmorphometry, bone formation rate (BFR/BS), bone resorption rate (Rs.R), and fibrosis (Fb.V/TV), suggesting the development of high turnover bone disease with osteitis fibrosa, were significantly elevated in vehicle-treated rats compared with those of age-matched control rats (Fig.1). In contrast, in the GN-OCT 0.15 μg/kg group, serum PTH levels, BFR/BS and Fb.V/TV were significantly prevented compared with those of vehicle-treated GN rats (Fig.1). OCT also prevented the marked parathyroid hyperplasia which were observed in vehicle-treated GN rats (Fig.2). Such amelioration of bone abnormalities by OCT was not accompanied by hypercalcemia.

Discussion In this study, long-term intravenous administration of OCT not only suppressed PTH hypersecretion and parathyroid hyperplasia, but also ameliorated bone abnormalities in uremia. Such effects of OCT on bone turnover were mainly achieved through the suppression of PTH, though direct actions of OCT on bone cells may have played a role, as suggested by several controversial reports [5-7].
In conclusion, these data indicate that OCT is a useful and safe agent not only for the suppression of PTH and parathyroid hyperplasia, but also for the amelioration of osteitis fibrosa and high turnover bone disease with less risk of hypercalcemia in chronic dialysis patients.

Fig.1

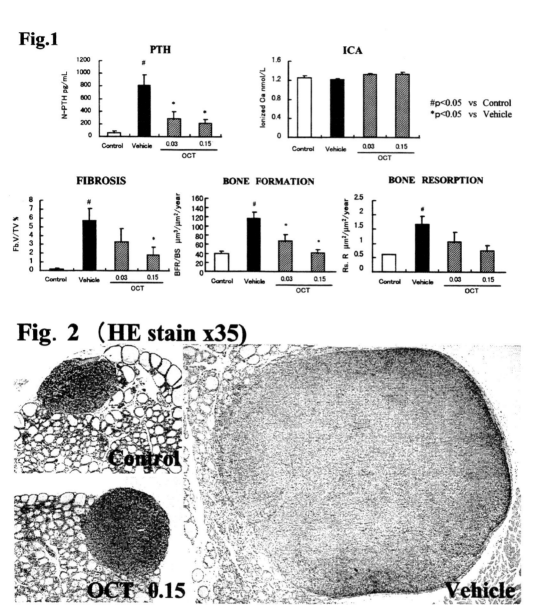

Fig. 2　(HE stain x35)

References

1.ABE J, SUDA T, NISHII Y (1989) *Endocrinology* 124: 2645-2647.
2.KUROKAWA K, OGATA E, SLATOPOLSKY E (1996) *Nephrol Dial Tranplant* 11: 121-124.
3.DENDA M, FINCH J, YASUHO N, NOBORU K, SLATOPOLSKY E(1996) *Kidney Int* 50: 34-39.
4.SHIBATA S, NARUSE T: Nephritogenic Glycoprotein (1972) *Lab Invest.* 27: 457-465.
5.PERNALETE N, NISHII Y, SLATOPOLSKY E, BROWN AJ (1991) *Endocrinology* 129: 778-784.
6.KANATANI M, SUGIMOTO T, KANO J, CHIHARA K (1995) *Eur J Endocrinol* 1133; 618-625.
7.MCINTYRE CW, SCHROEDER NJ, BURRIN JM, CUNNINGHAM J (1999) *Kidney Int* 55:500-511.

OSTEOPOROSIS

PROSPECTS FOR NEW THERAPIES IN BONE DISEASES

Gregory R. Mundy, Medicine/Endocrinology, University of Texas Health Science Center, San Antonio, Texas, USA.

The most demanding need in bone research is better therapies for patients with established osteoporosis. Currently, no available treatment is either totally satisfactory or universally acceptable. This is the reason that the pharmaceutical industry is now spending billions of dollars in the search for better modalities of treatment than those currently available. One of the major issues which interferes with advances in this area is incomplete understanding of the complexities of the normal bone remodeling sequence, which in turn prevents full understanding of the pathophysiology of bone loss responsible for osteoporosis. Moreover, there remains a lack of reliable in vitro and in vivo models for evaluating new potential drug therapies, and the animal models currently available are less than optimal for studying new treatment regimens. At the present time, the major need is clearly in the area of development of new agents for stimulating bone formation, or so called "anabolic agents". In contrast, there are a number of available agents which effectively inhibit bone resorption (estrogens, calcitonin, bisphosphonates).

Ideal therapy for patients with established osteoporosis would be an agent which inhibits osteoclastic bone resorption and stimulates new bone formation. There is no currently available therapeutic agent which convincingly achieves both resorption inhibition and significantly increased formation. The currently available resorption inhibitors (estrogen, bisphosphonates, calcitonin) are effective and successful agents, but have negligible to very modest effects on bone formation over prolonged periods. As a consequence, they may prevent further bone loss and stabilize bone mass, but do not substantially increase bone mass. There is currently no acceptable formation stimulator which is widely available.

Stimulators of Bone Formation   In aging patients with osteoporosis there is a decrease in osteoblast function characterized by a decrease in the capacity of osteoblasts to completely replace the defects left by osteoclastic resorption with new bone. This is referred to by bone histomorphometrists as decreased mean wall thickness (1). What is needed for patients with decreased mean wall thickness is an agent that stimulates osteoblasts to increase their bone forming activity. The agents which are known to have a stimulatory effect on new bone formation are fluoride, low-dose intermittent parathyroid hormone and the peptide growth factors. However, none of these agents fit the criteria of oral bioavailability combined with acceptable toxicity.

Vitamin D Analogs   A large amount of data has accumulated on the potential for vitamin D and its analogs as treatments for postmenopausal osteoporosis. Although there is a considerable body of supporting information on the role of the vitamin D-endocrine system in calcium metabolism and bone loss in the aging postmenopausal person, as yet neither 1,25 dihydroxyvitamin D nor its closely related analogs have been approved for treatment in the United States. In spite of this, they are widely used in many countries, and particularly in Japan. There is clear evidence that there is impaired calcium absorption in aging, associated with decreased circulating 25-hydroxyvitamin D concentrations (2) a renal calcium leak which is due to a decrease in glomerular filtration rate. This leads to a negative calcium balance of approximately 50 mg/day, more than enough to cause progressive bone loss. This negative calcium balance is associated with an increase in circulating concentrations of PTH which can be reversed by increasing calcium absorption. This negative calcium balance is almost certainly related to the vitamin D-endocrine system. In the first place, nutritional vitamin D deficiency is common in the elderly population who have limited calcium absorption from the gut. The major transport form of vitamin D, serum 25 dihydroxyvitamin D, varies with food fortification, the season and latitude, as well as with aging (2). There is also evidence that there is impaired renal 1,25 dihydroxyvitamin D production in the elderly, particularly those with hip fractures in response to parathyroid hormone. It is also possible there may be other factors that impair responsivity to 1,25 dihydroxyvitamin D, including decreases in vitamin D receptor levels in the intestine of the aging population, and the superimposed effect of estrogen deficiency which may also impair vitamin D metabolism (3). It is not surprising therefore that there have been a number of studies to determine the effects of vitamin D and its analogs on bone mineral density and fracture risk. In Japan, studies with 1α (OH)D_3 have shown beneficial effects on fracture rates (4,5). A widely reported study by Tilyard et al (6) showed beneficial effects of calcitriol on fracture rates. In the United States, vitamin D metabolites have fallen out of favor on the basis of American studies, which have shown that there are at best small increases in bone mineral density and marginal effects on fractures in the doses that have been used (7-10). This has been coupled with the problem that there is a narrow therapeutic window between toxicity and beneficial effects, with the potential for hypercalcemia and hypercalciuria as administered doses reach the range that produces more favorable skeletal effects.

On the other hand, there is considerable potential for the development of vitamin D analogs which have the beneficial effects of 1,25 dihydroxyvitamin D on the skeleton but avoid the toxic effects. There are multiple mechanisms whereby this may happen, including changes in metabolism and pharmacokinetics, but also the effects of certain analogs to cause specific changes in the vitamin D receptor and its association with co-activators or co-repressors in much the same way as has been shown for estrogen-related compounds. There is certainly evidence for differences in biological properties of some vitamin D analogs, and this is an area of very active research.

Statins Recently we have found that inhibitors of the enzyme 3-hydroxy-3-methylglutaryl coenzyme A (HMG Co-A) reductase stimulate bone formation both in vitro and in vivo in animal models of osteoporosis. This effect is associated with an increased expression of the bone morphogenetic protein-2 (BMP-2) gene in bone cells. These compounds, called statins, are widely-used agents for lowering cholesterol and reducing heart attacks. They have been used for many years and have acceptable toxicity profiles. If these results can be confirmed in randomized clinical trials in humans with osteoporosis, these drugs may have a place as anabolic agents in the treatment of this condition.

In attempts to identify small molecular weight compounds which are anabolic for bone and stimulate new bone formation, we focused on the growth regulatory factors that are responsible for the control of normal bone remodeling. Growth factors which are incorporated into the bone matrix are released in active form during resorption and are thereby locally available to control all of the subsequent events involved in the formation of bone locally to complete the normal remodeling cascade (11). These growth factors include the transforming growth factor beta superfamily, the insulin-like growth factor family, the fibroblast growth factor family, and platelet-derived growth factors. These growth factors are responsible for enhancing osteoclast apoptosis, cause chemotaxis of osteoblast precursors to sites of resorption defects, and stimulate the proliferation of osteoblast precursors to lead to a sufficient number of osteoblasts to ensure that normal bone formation can take place. The bone morphogenetic proteins, in contrast, are responsible for enhancing osteoblast differentiation, including stimulation of expression of the structural proteins of bone such as type I collagen and the mineralization of the bone matrix. We have found that when BMP-2 stimulates bone formation on bone surfaces in vivo, there is a powerful enhancement of new bone formation. We have hypothesized that BMP-2 is an autocrine factor involved in osteoblast differentiation, is expressed by osteoblasts as they differentiate and further enhances mineralization (12). We have characterized the BMP-2 promoter, and, based on the properties of BMP-2, we have utilized the promoter as a target to identify new compounds that stimulate its transcription and subsequent osteoblast differentiation.

We approached this task of identifying small molecules that enhance BMP-2 transcription by using a cell-based screening assay in which we utilized an osteoblast cell line which was derived from transgenic mice where the transgene was targeted to the osteoblast lineage and comprised SV40 large T-antigen (13). The osteoblast response was monitored in immortalized cells derived from these transgenic mice and which were transfected with the BMP-2 promoter operatively linked to the firefly luciferase reporter.

We screened a natural products collection, and identified a single extract that specifically stimulated the BMP-2 promoter. This extract was purified and found to contain the HMG Co-A reductase inhibitor Lovastatin. We then used commercially available lovastatin in the same assay and found that it increased BMP-2 transcription in doses of 1-5 uM. Other statins, namely simvastatin, mevastatin, fluvastatin and cerivastatin, had identical effects (14). Cerivastatin however was found to be several orders of magnitude more potent than the other statins.

These data suggested that the statins stimulate BMP-2 transcription. We next determined their effects on endogenous BMP-2 messenger RNA expression and BMP-2 protein production. We incubated human MG63 osteoblastic cells with simvastatin (1-5uM) and there was a 2-fold increase in BMP-2 messenger RNA. There was no effect on BMP-4 messenger RNA. In parallel, we noted that statins increase BMP-2 protein expression by cultured calvarial osteoblasts.

Since these experiments indicated that the statins stimulate BMP-2 transcription and increase protein expression, we wished to determine if this was accompanied by a parallel biologic effect, namely the stimulation of bone formation. We first cultured the statins with explants of murine calvarial bones. We found that each of the statins caused a marked increase in osteoblast accumulation and new bone formation in doses of 1-5 uM over 4-7 days of culture. The effect of the statins was even more obvious when there was transient exposure of the bones to the statins for only 24 hours and the cultures were examined 12 days later. We found a marked increase in new bone formation and osteoblast stimulation compared to correspond control bones.

We then tested the effects of the statins in vivo by local injections over the murine calvaria. We found that there was a 30-60% increase in cortical bone width after 5 days exposure to lovastatin and simvastatin, similar to the effects we have previously found when we have applied BMP-2 in this assay.

Since these data indicate that statins increase new bone formation in vitro and when applied locally in vivo, we next determined if they produced a similar effect when administered systemically. These experiments were performed in intact rats, or rats that had been ovariectomized. Following 35 days of administration of lovastatin or simvastatin by oral gavage in doses of 5-10 mg/kg body weight/day, there was a marked increase in trabecular bone area in both intact and ovariectomized rats associated with increases in bone formation and mineral apposition rate. We found similar effects whether rats were ovariectomized and statins given by oral gavage for the following 35 days, or were ovariectomized for several months previously then the statins administered. There was also a decrease in osteoclast numbers, suggesting that the statins may have been also reducing bone resorption.

These data show therefore that the statins are capable of stimulating new bone formation, and suggests this effect may be mediated by stimulation of the BMP-2 promoter leading to enhanced BMP-2 production and subsequent osteoblast differentiation. They are also interesting in light of the current notion of mechanism of action of the N2 -containing bisphosphonates on the cholesterol biosynthesis pathway. Recent experiments by Rogers and colleagues suggest that the bisphosphonates affect the cholesterol biosynthesis pathway by inhibiting enzymes responsible for converting precursors to geranylgeranylpyrophosphate, a step lower in the cholesterol pathway that the step controlled by HMG Co-A reductase. Our data show that the statins increase bone formation by inhibiting the enzyme HMG Co-A reductase, the rate-limiting enzyme in cholesterol biosynthesis. This was confirmed by reversing the effects on bone formation in organ cultures of calvaria and BMP-2 transcription in cultured bone cells when mevalonate, the immediate downstream metabolite of HMG Co-A reductase, was added back to the cultures.

The current available statins have all been selected as drugs to lower serum cholesterol because they are extracted by the liver and decrease hepatic cholesterol biosynthesis. Moreover, most are subject to first-pass metabolism in the liver by cytochrome p-450 enzymes. As a consequence, only very low concentrations of active metabolites get beyond the liver to peripheral tissues such as bone. To avoid liver extraction and first-pass metabolism, we have applied lovastatin topically to rats and found markedly enhanced biologic effects on trabecular bone volume and bone formation rates with only 5 days of dermal application, suggesting an alternative approach to avoiding this problem of poor peripheral availability of these drugs when administered by mouth.

Since our data suggest that the statins increase bone mass, it is of interest to know if statins have any observable protective effect on risk of fracture or bone mineral density in patients who have received them over a number of years. Bauer and Cummings recently examined data bases from the SOF, FIT and HERS trials, which comprised more than 18,000 people (15). Although relatively small numbers of these patients were taking statins (approximately 500), the results of this retrospective survey suggest that these patients tend to be associated with greater hip bone mineral density and reduced fracture risk.

In conclusion, our data show that statins are capable of increasing bone formation and bone mass in rodents. They suggest a potential new action for the statins which may be beneficial in patients with established osteoporosis. However, their precise place can only be determined by appropriate randomized clinical trials which demonstrate their efficacy in this regard in patients.

Conclusions Pharmaceutical companies attempting to develop new drugs in the bone field have to face some unpleasant realities. These include the enormous costs of bringing a new drug to the market, which are particularly severe in the osteoporosis field because of the FDA requirements to show beneficial effects on fracture rates, at least for drugs to be used in the United States. These issues are compounded somewhat by the current financial problems of the pharmaceutical industry and the decline in research and development budgets associated with the threat of reduced profits due to managed care. Establishing practice guidelines for osteoporosis may limit use of drugs, particularly those which are either expensive, or require treatment in many patients to see benefits in one. In the European community, price controls on drugs already exist. An additional important point for industry is the size of the available therapeutic market, and the potential that any drug can expect to have. For example, it seems likely that the bisphosphonate market will eventually be shared by a number of similar compounds, and the same appears likely for the estrogen/anti-estrogen market. The great need in the field is for stimulators of bone formation which will correct deficits in bone mass rather than simply stabilize it. Since the lag time from discovering a new lead for the bone field to the introduction of a drug in the clinic may be ten or more years, it seems likely that resorption inhibitors will be the mainstay for treatment for the next ten years. Hopefully, following that time, there will be acceptable drugs which will effectively and substantially stimulate bone formation.

References

1. Darby, A.J., and Meunier, P.J. (1981) *Calcif. Tissue Int.* **33**, 199-204

2. Francis, R.M., Peacock, M., Storer, J.H., Davies, A.E., Brown, W.B., and Nordin, B.E. (1983) *Eur. J. Clin. Invest.* **13,** 391-396

3. Slovik, D.M., Adams, J.S., Neer, R.M., Holick, M.F., and Potts, J.T. (1981) *N. Engl. J. Med.* **305,** 372-374

4. Hayashi, Y., Fugita, T., and Inoue, T. (1992) *Jap. Bone Min. Res.* **10**, 1984-1988

5. Orimo, H., Shiraki, M., Hayashi, T., and Nakamura, T. (1987) *Bone Miner.* **3**, 47-52

6. Tilyard, M.W., Spears, G.F., Thomson, J., and Dovey, S. (1992) *N. Engl. J. Med.* **326**, 357-362

7. Aloia, J.F., Vaswani, A., Yeh, J.K., Ellis, K., Yasumura, S., and Cohn S.H. (1988) *Am. J. Med.* **84**, 401-408

8. Gallagher, J.C., and Goldgar, D. (1990) *Ann. Intern. Med.* **113**, 649-655

9. Falch, J.A., Odegaard, O.R., Finnanger, A.M., Matheson, I. (1987) *Acta Med. Scand.* **221**, 199-204

10. Ott, S.M., and Chesnut, C.H. (1989). *Ann. Intern. Med.* **110**, 267-274

11. Mundy, G.R., Boyce, B., Hughes, D., Wright, K., Bonewald, L., Dallas, S., Harris, S., Ghosh-Choudhury, N., Chen, D., Dunstan, C., Izbicka, E., and Yoneda, T (1995) *Bone* **17**,71S-75S

12. Harris, S.E., Bonewald, L.F., Harris, M.A., Sabatini, M., Dallas, S., Feng, J., Ghosh-Choudhury, N., Wozney, J., and Mundy, GR. (1994) *J. Bone Miner. Res.* **9**,855-863

13. Ghosh-Choudhury, N., Windle, J.J., Koop, B.A., Harris, M.A., Guerrero, D.L., Wozney, J.M., Mundy, G.R., and Harris, S.E. (1996) *Endocrinology* **137,** 331-339

14. Mundy, G.R., Garrett, R., Harris, S., Chan, J., Chen, D., Rossini, G., Boyce, B., Zhao, M., and Gutierrez, G. (1999) *Science* **286**, 1946-1949.

15. Bauer, D.C., Mundy, G.R., Jamal, S.A., Black, D.M., Cauley, J.A., Harris, F., Duong, T., and Cummings, S.R. (1999) *J. Bone Min. Res.* **14**, (Suppl) #1188

A NOVEL TISSUE-SELECTIVE VITAMIN D RECEPTOR MODULATOR.

Brian H. Vickery[1], Zafrira Avnur[1], Milan Uskokovic[1] and Sara Peleg[2], [1]Musculoskeletal Research, Roche Bioscience, Palo Alto, CA 94304, [2] The University of Texas, M. D. Anderson Cancer Center, Houston, TX 77030.

Introduction

The active metabolite of $1\alpha,25$-dihydroxyvitamin D_3 ($1\alpha,25(OH)_2D_3$) is a calcium regulating pluripotent steroid-like hormone with effects on many organs, including those that regulate calcium homeostasis. Unfortunately, the pharmacological effects of $1\alpha,25(OH)_2D_3$ on many organ systems are accompanied by dose-limiting toxicity due to intolerable hypercalcemia. An approach to increase the therapeutic potential of $1\alpha,25(OH)_2D_3$ is to design or identify analogs of $1\alpha,25(OH)_2D_3$ that are tissue selective. Then, an appropriate profile of target tissues for individual analogs could be chosen for therapy of various diseases. Such an approach has been applied in the area of estrogens, and has progressed to include ligands for other members of the steroid receptor family including progestins and androgens [1,2].

The steroidal estrogens, which are gonadal in origin, are acting through their cognate receptor to mediate effects on the reproductive tract from ovulation to pregnancy, parturition and nursing. Their effects on both reproductive and non-reproductive tissues are dramatically revealed at the time of the menopause when cessation of ovarian function leads to deterioration in the skeleton, cardiovascular system and atrophic changes in the reproductive tract, including mammary tissue. Estrogen replacement therapy (**ERT**) has been capitalized on the ability to increase quality of life post-menopause by combating osteoporosis, the atrophic changes in the reproductive tract, and hot flushes, as well as onset of colorectal cancer and of Alzheimer's disease. Unfortunately, perceived adverse effects on the development of breast and uterine cancer counterbalance these beneficial effects. Serendipitous observations with tamoxifen, designed as antiestrogen, first suggested that this agent could also act as an estrogen in some tissues [3]. This has led to the generation of a whole series of non-steroidal **S**elective **E**strogen **R**eceptor **M**odulators (**SERMs**) with varying tissue selectivity; estrogenic in some tissues (bone, cardiovascular system) and inactive or antiestrogenic (breast, uterus) in others. In light of these findings, we explored whether vitamin D analogs with appropriate structural modifications may also possess tissue selective properties. In the study presented here we examined whether the principle of selective receptor modulation could be applicable to separate toxic hypercalcemia from therapeutic effects on bone in osteopenic rats.

Results and discussion

There has been an immense effort over the last 2 decades assessing structure-activity relationships (SAR) of vitamin D analogs focusing on the ability to divorce beneficial effects on bone from induction of hypercalcemia [4-6]. A survey of the published SAR data has led to the design and synthesis of a new structure, 1α-F, 25-hydroxy, 16,23-diene, 20-epi, 26,27-bishomo-cholecalciferol (RS-980400) which might have this desired profile (Figure 1). In the studies presented here, we used ovariectomized rats (a model of osteoporosis) to compare the effects of RS-980400 and 1α,25(OH)$_2$D$_3$, and to determine whether the efficacy of RS-980400 to protect against the bone loss from estrogen deprivation occurred at doses not inducing either hypercalcemia or hyeprcalciurea.

Figure 1. Structures of 1α, 25(OH)$_2$ D$_3$ and RS-980400

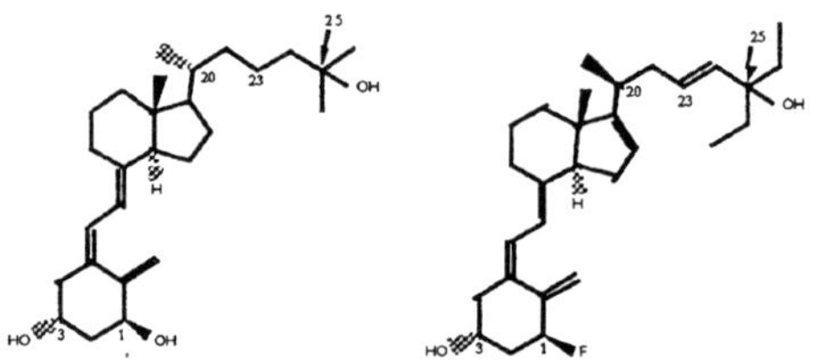

1α,25(OH) $_2$D$_3$ RS-980400

In vivo studies in rats

The in vivo studies were performed with osteopenic, ovariectomized (ovx) young adult rats. The first set of experiments compared the effects RS 980400 and its parent molecule 1α,25(OH)$_2$D$_3$. Compounds were administered orally once daily to 3 months old rats starting 3 weeks after ovx and continuing for 3 weeks. RS-980400 was effective in restoring trabecular bone mineral density (BMD) to the levels observed in controls (sham-operated rats) at 1-3 µg/kg/day, while inducing hypercalcmia only at doses higher than 17 µg/kg (Table 1).

In contrast, treatment of rats with 1α,25(OH)$_2$D$_3$ restored trabecular bone to sham levels with a narrow therapeutic window (Table 1). These effects of RS-980400 and 1α,25(OH)$_2$D$_3$ on BMD were associated with decreased urinary pyridinoline excretion, suggesting that both compounds have an anti-resorbing activity.

Table 1. Short Term Treatment of Osteopenic Rats

Compound	Minimal Dose (μg/kg/day) to Produce Significant ($p<0.05$) Response	
	BMD Response	Hypercalcemic Response
RS-980400	1-3	>17 < 27
$1\alpha,25(OH)_2 D_3$	0.05-0.1	0.1-0.2

Figure 2. A six weeks treatment of 3 month old rats strating at the time of ovariectomy (BMD of femur diapysis by DEXA)

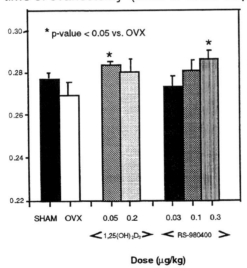

Dose (μg/kg)

To study the effects of RS-980400 or $1\alpha,25(OH)_2D_3$ in the prevention of bone loss, young adult rats were administered these compounds at the time of ovx and the treatment continued for 6 weeks. Treatment with 0.3 μg/ kg/day of RS-980400 resulted in a significant increase in BMD of the whole femur and femur diaphysis (Figure 2) compared to that of ovx controls. At this dose of RS-980400, the mean BMD was equal to, or above that of sham levels at all sites measured. Urine calcium levels were in the normal range through doses of 1 μg/kg/day of RS-980400 while serum calcium levels were in the normal range through doses as high as 27 μg/ kg/day.

In this experimental model of prevention, doses of $1\alpha,25(OH)_2 D_3$ that achieved mean increments in BMD approaching those induced by the highest dose of

RS-980400 did so at the expense of substantial hypercalcemia. Only the lowest dose of 1α,25(OH)₂D₃ (0.05 µg/kg/day) was both tolerated and effective.

Figure 3. Histomorphometry of trabecular bone from 3 month old OVX rats, three weeks after daily treatment with 1α,25(OH)₂D₃ or RS-980400

Cell Surface/ Bone Surface

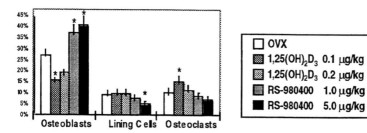

To further examine the effect of RS-980400 or 1α,25(OH)₂D₃ on bone turnover, 3-month old ovx rats were administered either RS-980400 or 1α,25(OH)₂D₃ for 3 weeks. For histomorphometric analysis, bones were labeled with bone-seeking dyes. The retention throughout the dosing period of mineral seeking fluorochrome label administered at baseline suggested an antiresorptive effect of the two compounds (data not shown). Further analysis of the cellular components in bone from these animals has revealed qualitative differences in the action of the two compounds (Figure 3), suggesting opposite effects on osteoblasts recruitment to the bone surface.

Ex vivo studies

Studies were conducted to compare the effects of 1α,25(OH)₂D₃ and RS-980400 on gene expression in calcium-regulating tissues: bone, kidney and duodenum. Both 1α,25(OH)₂D₃ and RS-980400 produced significant upregulation of mRNA encoding the osteoblast-specific gene products osteocalcin and osteopontin (data not shown) and of transforming growth factor β1 (TGF-β1) and TGF-β2 (Figure 4). 1α,25(OH)₂D₃ but not RS-980400 upregulated mRNAs encoding the bone resorbing cytokines interleukin-1β and interleukin 6 (data not shown). In the kidney and duodenum, mRNA of the vitamin D responsive gene, 24-hydroxylase was induced by 1α,25(OH)₂D₃ (Figure 4), whereas RS-980400 had no inductive effect in kidney and was less effective than 1α,25(OH)₂D₃ in the duodenum. These findings suggest that the unique properties of RS-980400 include: 1) a profile of tissue preference different from that 1α,25(OH)₂ D₃, 2) a potent transcriptional upregulation of gene products associated with bone matrix formation, and 3) an effective upregulation of gene products encoding growth factors without upregulation of bone resorbing cytokines.

Figure 4. Effect of 7 hours treatment on gene expression in duodenum and tibia from 3 month old OVX rats

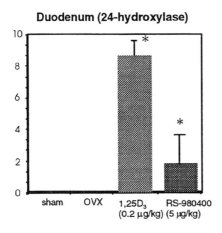 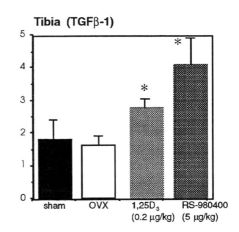

Conclusions

The vitamin D analog RS-980400 may be a representative of a new class of selective modulators of the vitamin D receptor. We have shown that it has tissue- and gene-specificity different from those of $1\alpha,25(OH)_2D_3$. Because the mRNAs examined are products of vitamin D receptor responsive genes (osteopontin, osteocalcin, 24-hydroxylase and TGF-β) we propose that RS-980400 induces VDR-mediated transcription preferentially in bone, while it has poor transcriptional potency in intestine or kidney. This profile translates, in osteopenic rats into a wide therapeutic window between doses protecting against bone loss and doses inducing intolerable hypercalcemia. Studies to elucidate the mechanism of the tissue selective effects of this and related compounds are ongoing.

References

1   McDonnell D.P., (2000) Selective Estrogen Receptor Modulators (SERMs): A First Step in the Development of Perfect Hormone Replacement Therapy. J Soc Gynecol Investig. **7**(1) Suppl., S11-S15.

2   Negro-Vilar A., (2000) New Progestins and Potential Actions. J Soc Gynecol Investig. **7**(1) Suppl., S53-S54.

3   Love R.R., Mazess R.B., Barden H.S., et al., (1991) Effects of Tamoxifen on Bone Mineral Density in Postmenopausal Women. Ann Int Med., **115**, 860-864.

4   Bouillon R., Okamura W.H., and Norman A., (1995) Structure-Function Relationship in the Vitamin D Endocrine System. Endocrine Reviews. 16(2), 200-256.

5   Drezner, M. K. and Nesbitt, T., (1990) Role of Calcitriol in Prevention of Osteoporosis: Part I. Metabolism Clinical and Experimental **39** (4), Suppl. 1, 18-23.

6   Malluche, H. H. and Faugere, M.-C., (1990) Role of Calcitriol in the Management of Osteoporosis. Metabolism Clinical and Experimental **39** (4), Suppl. 1, 24-26.

VITAMIN D DEPLETION AND REPLACEMENT IN PATIENTS WITH CYSTIC FIBROSIS

David A. Ontjes*, Robert K. Lark**, Gayle E. Lester**, Bruce W. Hollis***, Margaret M. Hensler* and Robert M. Aris*, *Department of Medicine and **Department of Orthopedics, University of North Carolina, Chapel Hill, NC, and ***Department of Pediatrics, Medical University of South Carolina, Charleston, SC, USA.

Introduction. Cystic fibrosis (CF) is the most common lethal autosomal recessive genetic disease in the Caucasian population, affecting approximately 60,000 individuals worldwide. Although respiratory disease is still the most common cause of death in CF, improvements in therapy have led to progressive increases in life expectancy and the recognition of other problems, including bone disease. Osteoporosis and fractures are common in the adult CF population (1,2). The pathogenesis of CF-associated osteoporosis is probably multifactorial, but is likely to include inadequate absorption of calcium and vitamin D in the ≥85% of patients who have pancreatic insufficiency. Our aims in the current studies have been to 1) delineate the adequacy of vitamin D and calcium absorption in young adults with CF and pancreatic insufficiency and 2) to examine the short term effects of vitamin D repletion with either ergocalciferol or calcitriol.

Results of Calcium Absorption Measurements. Twelve young adults with CF and pancreatic insufficiency were compared with 11 controls of similar age. Following baseline fasting measurements, all subjects were given a standardized high calcium breakfast containing 8-10 μCi ^{45}Ca. Timed urine and serum samples were collected following the meal. Fractional absorption of ^{45}Ca was estimated by the method of Marshall and Nordin (3). The CF subjects were studied with the same meal protocol on two different occasions, once without and once with the administration of pancreatic enzymes containing 80,000 units of lipase and 240,000 units each of amylase and protease. Baseline measurements showed that serum 25OH-D levels were lower in CF subjects than in controls (15.7 ± 5.8 vs 25.6 ±4.3 ng/ml; p<0.03), but 1,25(OH)2-D levels did not differ. PTH levels were higher in CF subjects (31.7 ± 17.4 vs 19.9 ± 10.7 pg/ml), although the difference was not significant (p=0.10) (4). Both control and CF subjects showed progressive increases in mean fractional absorption of ^{45}Ca after the meal, as well as increased urinary excretion of calcium, as shown in Figure 1. However, when group comparisons were made with repeated measures ANOVA, the fractional absorption of calcium was significantly higher for control subjects than for CF subjects (p=0.02). Postprandial urinary calcium excretion also increased more in the controls (p=0.025). There was no difference in either fractional absorption or urinary excretion of calcium attributable to pancreatic enzymes within the CF group.

894

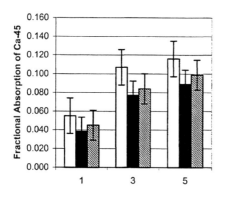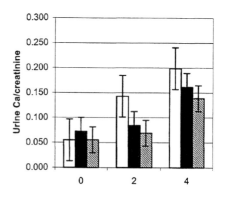

Hours after Meal

Figure 1. Fractional absorption of calcium (left) and urinary calcium excretion (right) following a test meal containing ^{45}Ca. Open bars indicate controls; solid bars indicate CF subjects without enzymes; and hatched bars indicate CF subjects with enzymes.

Results of Vitamin D Administration. We compared the absorption of oral ergocalciferol (D_2) and the consequent response of 25OH-D in 10 young adults with CF and 10 controls matched for age, sex and body mass index. Serum D2 and 25OH-D levels were measured for 36 hours following the ingestion of 100,000 IU of D_2 with food, and in the case of the CF subjects, pancreatic enzymes.

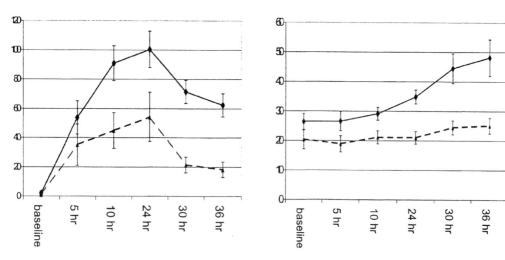

Figure 2. Serum D2 (left panel, ng/ml) and 25OH-D (right panel, ng/ml) after oral administration of 100,000 IU D2. Solid lines indicate controls; dashed lines indicate CF subjects.

Average D_2 absorption for CF subjects, as determined by area under the curve analysis was 55% lower than that of controls (P < 0.001). In controls, serum 25OH-D levels rose from 27 ng/ml at baseline to 48 ng/ml at 36 hours. In CF subjects, 25OH-D levels failed to rise significantly at any time after D_2 administration. Among individual CF subjects only two, both having baseline 25OH-D levels < 10 mg/ml, showed significant improvement in serum 25OH-D. These findings suggest that, in addition to impaired absorption of D_2, CF subjects might have a defect in the conversion of D_2 to 25OH-D or an accelerated clearance of 25OH-D from the serum.

In further studies we have compared the effects of a single intramuscular injection of D_2 (500,000 IU) and oral 1,25(OH)$_2$-D (1.0 mcg/day for two weeks) on fractional absorption of ^{45}Ca and urinary calcium excretion in both CF subjects and controls Our results, shown below, indicate that oral 1,25(OH)-D had a more positive effect after two weeks than intramuscular D_2 .

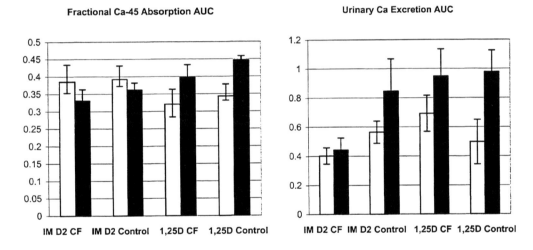

Figure 3. Fractional absorption of ^{45}Ca and urinary excretion of calcium in response to the test meal after administration of intramuscular D_2 or oral 1,25(OH)$_2$-D. Open bars indicate the AUC value in the baseline study and solid bars indicate the comparable response after treatment with either intramuscular D_2 or oral 1,25(OH)$_2$-D. Values for fractional absorption of ^{45}Ca represent areas under the curve based on serum measurements at 1, 3 and 5 hours after the test meal. Values for urinary calcium excretion represent areas under the curve based on timed urine collections at baseline, 0-2 hrs and 2-4 hrs following the meal.

After receiving oral 1,25(OH)$_2$-D, control subjects showed a significant increase in both fractional calcium absorption (p=0.043) and urinary calcium excretion (p=0.002). CF subjects showed a statistically significant increase in calcium absorption (p=0.046) but not urinary calcium excretion (p=0.16). CF subjects also showed a significant decrease in basal serum PTH after two weeks of receiving 1,25(OH)$_2$-D (15.3 pg/ml compared with an initial level of 24.8 pg/ml, p=0.044). Neither CF subjects nor controls showed significant improvement in calcium absorption two weeks following the intramuscular injection of D$_2$.

Summary and Conclusions. Young adults with CF and pancreatic insufficiency have lower mean serum levels of 25OH-D and higher levels of PTH than control subjects, in spite of receiving routine daily supplements of ADEK vitamins containing 400 to 800 IU of cholecalciferol. After a calcium-containing meal, CF subjects demonstrate a significant deficiency in the absorption of both calcium and vitamin D that is not corrected by pancreatic enzymes. After a single large oral dose of vitamin D$_2$, CF subjects showed significantly lower serum levels of D$_2$ than controls, and failed to increase their serum levels of 25OH-D. A large intramuscular dose of D$_2$ also failed to increase serum levels of 25OH-D or fractional absorption of [45]Ca in CF subjects. These findings clearly demonstrate a defect in vitamin D absorption and suggest that there may be further alterations in the formation or clearance of 25OH-D. Oral 1,25(OH)$_2$-D, under the conditions we have tested, appears to be more effective than either oral or intramuscular D$_2$ in increasing calcium absorption and reducing serum PTH in CF subjects. Long term administration of 1,25(OH)$_2$-D together with a calcium supplement may enable younger patients with CF to achieve a more positive calcium balance and a higher peak bone mass.

Acknowledgements. This research was funded, in part, by the Cystic Fibrosis Foundation (A936) and the Verne S. Caviness General Center for Clinical Research (NIH RR00046).

References.
1. Aris, R.M., Neuringer, I.P., Weiner, M.A., Egan, T.M., and Ontjes, D.A. (1996) Chest 109, 1176-1183.
2. Ott, S.M. and Aitken, M.L. (1998) Clinics in Chest Medicine 19, 555-567.
3. Marshall, D.H. and Nordin, B.E.C. (1981) Clinical Science 61, 477-481.
4. Aris, R.M., Lester, G.M., Dingman, S., and Ontjes, D.A. (1999) Osteoporosis International 10, 102-108.

SUPPLEMENTATION WITH 2000 I.U. VITAMIN D WITH OR WITHOUT 1 GM CALCIUM IN CHILDREN WITH CYSTIC FIBROSIS (CF) OR JUVENILE RHEUMATOID ARTHRITIS (JRA)

Laura Hillman, M.D., Giulio Barbero, M.D., Mihaela Popescu, M.S., and Florence Chanesta, PhD., Michelle Bergfeld, Ding Lee, M.D. James Cassidy,M.D. Department of Child Health, University of Missouri, Columbia, MO, USA

Introduction: Children with Cystic Fibrosis (CF) and children with Juvenile Rheumatoid Arthritis (JRA) both have decreased bone mineralization which falls further off of the normal curve as they go through puberty. Both diseases are associated with 1) decreased physical activity 2) marginal nutrition 3) increased inflammation and 4) delayed puberty. CF has the additional theoretical problems associated with pancreatic insufficiency; 1) fat malabsorption 2) fat soluble vitamin (including vitamin D) malabsorption and 3) calcium malabsorption secondary to fat malabsorption, however neither vitamin D malabsorption or calcium malabsorption have been documented by research in children. In both of our study populations calcium and vitamin D intakes are already at recommended levels and serum 25-OHD and $1,25(OH)_2D$ are within normal range. In both these groups we sought to establish the safety and efficacy of supplementation with 2,000 I.U. vitamin D/day, 1 gm calcium/day, and 2,000 I.U. vitamin D plus 1gm calcium/day.

Background: In a group of 30 children with JRA reported in 1994, we showed suboptimal bone mineralization by single photon absorption and demonstrated values of osteocalcin, bone alkaline phosphatase, TRAP, and urine Ca/Cr ratio lower than controls suggesting that bone turnover was decreased. Serum calcium and serum PTH were low and $1,25(OH)_2D$ was normal. (1) In 1996 this study was repeated in an additional 41 children with JRA confirming the bone findings by whole body DEXA and essentially repeating the laboratory finding. (2) In this study bone mineral content was inversely correlated with a number of clinical scales of disease severity suggesting that severity of the underlying disease was related to the degree of osteopenia. Further markers of bone formation (bone alkaline phosphatase, osteocalcin and procollagen I carboxy-terminal propeptides) were correlated with laboratory markers of inflammation (sedimentation rate, platelet count, serum albumin, hemoglobin, and copper) such that the worse the markers of inflammation the lower the bone formation markers.

A number of studies have now shown significant osteopenia in adults with Cystic Fibrosis (CF) (3,4,). A recent study showed that 38% of adults with CF had a serum 25-OHD <15 mg/ml on 900 I. U. vitamin D (4). However, osteopenia can occur even when 25-OHD is normal. Most studies have found 1,25(OH)$_2$D and PTH to be in normal ranges and markers of bone turnover have been normal or high normal (4). The high use of steroid in the population to treat lung disease may add an element of bone resorption to the underlying problems of growth. We reported 19 children in 1994 who were D sufficient with normal values of 25-OHD, 1,25(OH)$_2$ D and PTH. In these children particularly those who were prepubertal, markers of bone formation (bone alkaline phosphatase, osteocalcin and PICP) were all significantly lower than controls (5). We suggested that factors in addition to vitamin D which effect bone formation needed to be studied. The effect of supplemental Ca and/or Vitamin D has not been systematically studied in either CF or JRA.

Methods: Children with CF (n=15, 10M/5F, 9.1± 2.3 yrs, 10/15 Tanner 1) and JRA (n=16, 5M/11F, 10.4± 2.6 yr, 8/16 Tanner 1) were studied in two parallel studies using the same study protocol. Children were randomized to one of four study groups which differed in the order in which treatments were given. All subjects were given all four treatments. 6 month treatment periods were separated by a 3 month washout. Laboratory measurements were made before and after the washout. Ca and Mg measured by AA; TRAP, Albumin, and P by calorimetric assays; and 25-OHD, 1,25(OH)$_2$D, and PTH by RIA. Bone mineral content was measured using an Hollogic 1000 W for whole body, lumbar spine (LS) and hip after 9 months (treatment plus washout). All subjects were on additional vitamins containing 400 I.U. D.
Treatments were:
A) Placebo Ca, Placebo vitamins
B) 1000 mg Ca, Placebo vitamins
C) Placebo Ca, 1600 I.U. D containing vitamin
D) 1000 Ca, 1600 I.U. D containing vitamin

Results:

	Baseline data		
	JRA (n=16)	CF (n=15)	Normal (n=31)
Serum Ca mg/dl	9.12±0.3 +	8.99±0.25 +	10.1±0.6
Mg mg/dl	1.91±0.08	1.80±0.19 +**	2.06±0.15
P mg/dl	4.58±1.36 +	5.47±0.54*	5.6±0.9
25-OHD ng/ml	22.3±6.1	37.7±12.6 +**	22.0±8.5
1,25(OH)$_2$D pg/ml	36.1±11.7	49.6±10 +**	30.4±9.3
Albumin mg/dl	4.27±0.55 +	4.96±0.38**	~ 5.0
PTH pg/ml	22.8±8.7	26.2± 10.8	26.3±9.4
TRAP IU/L	13.5±3.2	19.4± 6.6**	14.4±5.8
LS Z score	-0.84±0.59	1.21±0.74	0

*JRA different from CF P<.05   ** P<.01   + different from normal

Serum calcium was low in both groups and magnesium was low in CF. Albumin was low in JRA as expected. Both 25-OHD and 1,25(OH)$_2$ D were higher in CF. PTH was normal in CF and slightly lower in JRA. TRAP was lower in JRA than CF.

Laboratory and BMC values after 6 months of treatment can be seen in the tables below. No differences by treatment can be seen in CF by ANOVA. In JRA both serum calcium and magnesium increased with vitamin D alone and vitamin D plus calcium. Comparison of end minus start of treatment periods also showed significant increase in serum albumin with vitamin D treatment in JRA but not CF. In all treatments 25-OHD increased in JRA and decreased in CF suggesting incomplete washout. In neither group were differences in bone mineral content seen.

CF

Means of measured parameters and ANOVA between groups after six months of treatment.					
	Treatment A	Treatment B	Treatment C	Treatment D	ANOVA
	n = 7	n = 9	n = 10	n = 10	
Serum Ca, mg/dl	8.95 ± 0.28	8.93 ± 0.17	9 ± 03	9.01 ± 0.32	NS
Serum Mg, mg/dl	1.75 ± 0.13	1.72 ± 0.14	1.77 ± 0.12	1.79 ± 0.15	NS
Serum P, mg/dl	5.43 ± 0.82	4.97 ± 1.46	4.83 ± 0.51	5.49 ± 1.27	NS
25(OH)D, ng/ml	25.32 ± 7.73	26.42 ± 8.72	26.33 ± 6.21	27.42 ± 13.3	NS
1,25(OH)2D, pg/ml	42.04 ± 15.97	46.73 ± 14.19	35.6 ± 15.53	38.19 ± 12.72	NS
Albumin, g/dl	4.89 ± 0.38	4.86 ± 0.60	4.68 ± 0.23	5.14 ± 1.17	NS
Whole Body BMC, g	1370.1 ± 443.3	1123.1 ± 422.0	1038.3 ± 395.9	1141.5 ± 571.9	NS
Whole Body BMD, g/cm2	0.91 ± 0.1	0.85 ± 0.09	0.83 ± 0.08	0.85± 0.12	NS
Lumbar Spine BMC, g	31.42 ± 13.03	25.47 ± 8.31	22.8 ± 6.77	26.34 ± 14.18	NS
Lumbar Spine Z score	-0.67 ± 0.79	-0.81 ± 0.64	-1.07 ± 0.89	-0.84 ± 0.96	NS
Hip BMC, g	20.25 ± 8.00	18.96 ± 7.61	14.37 ± 4.76	17.00 ± 6.02	NS

JRA

Means of measured parameters and ANOVA between groups after six months of treatment.					
	Treatment A	Treatment B	Treatment C	Treatment D	ANOVA
	n = 12	n = 12	n = 11	n = 13	
Serum Ca, mg/dl	8.87 ± 0.4[c]	9.15 ± 0.72[b, c]	9.56 ± 0.75[a, b]	10.04 ± 0.77[a]	P < 0.001
Serum Mg, mg/dl	1.79 ± 0.18[b]	1.88 ± 0.2[a, b]	2.00 ± 0.17[a]	1.99 ± 0.27[a]	P = 0.05
Serum P, mg/dl	5.01 ± 0.86	5.3 ± 1.00	5.34 ± 1.26	4.93 ± 0.79	NS
25(OH)D, ng/ml	39.28 ± 17.20	32.81 ± 16.24	40.98 ± 19.46	43.55 ± 24.26	NS
1,25(OH)2D, pg/ml	39.42 ± 11.25	30.82 ± 8.44	34.02 ± 12.96	31.83 ± 12.06	NS
Albumin, g/dl	4.82 ± 0.29	4.66 ± 0.46	4.65 ± 0.45	4.79 ± 0.59	NS
Whole Body BMC, g	1369.1 ± 597.7	1271.9 ± 519.5	1360.8 ± 377.8	1469.2 ± 585.9	NS
Whole Body BMD, g/cm2	0.88 ± 0.1	0.86 ± 0.09	0.89 ± 0.06	0.9 ± 0.09	NS
Lumbar Spine BMC, g	30.66 ± 14.39	28.75 ± 12.17	31.81 ± 10.94	34.57 ± 13.18	NS
Lumbar Spine Z score	-0.83 ± 1.10	-0.93 ± 1.18	-0.51 ± 1.03	-0.71 ± 0.92	NS
Hip BMC, g	20.91 ± 8.45	19.29 ± 8.53	20.94 ± 7.52	19.61 ± 9.07	NS

Conclusions: 2,000 I.U. vitamins D/day is a safe dose for children with diseases such as JRA where intestinal absorption is presumed to be normal resulting in modest increases in 25-OHD without effect on 1,25(OH)$_2$ D. Treatment with 2,000 I.U. vitamin D with or without calcium supplementation corrected low serum calcium values into the normal range in children with JRA. Treatment with 2,000 I.U. vitamin D corrected low values of serum albumin into the normal range in children with JRA. This may reflect an effect of vitamin D in suppressing immune responses involved in JRA. Vitamin D, in spite of increasing serum calcium, did not improve bone mineralization in JRA.

2,000 I.U. vitamin D/day is not an adequate dose to increase serum 25-OHD further in children with conditions associated with malabsorption such as CF. However much lower daily intakes can be associated with normal serum 25-OHD probably reflecting sun exposure. In CF, treatment with vitamin D did not alter serum calcium or albumin possibly because changes in vitamin D status did not occur. It is unknown whether higher doses would be effective. In CF, treatment with vitamin D, calcium, or both did not effect bone mineralization.

The failure to gain bone adequately in chronic diseases such as CF and JRA is primarily due to non-nutritional factors. Although adequate intakes of vitamin D and calcium need to be assured and children should be screened with serum 25-OHD to detect unsuspected deficiency, additional vitamin D and/or calcium will probably not alter bone mineralization. Treatment needs to focus on the underlying disease and effects on puberty. As a last resort, drugs which alter mineral metabolism may need to be used. Unfortunately only drugs which block resorption are currently available. Safe anabolic drugs are needed.

1) Hillman LS, Cassidy JT, Johnson L, Lee D, and Allen SH. Vitamin D metabolism and bone mineralization in children with Juvenile Rheumatoid Arthritis. J or Ped. 124:910-916, 1994
2) Pepmueller PH, Cassidy JT, Allen SH, and Hillman LS. Bone mineralization and bone mineral metabolism in children with Juvenile Rheumatoid Arthritis. Arthritis and Rheumatism 19:746-757, 1996
3) Bachrach LK, Loutit CW, Moss RB, et al. Osteopenia in adults with Cystic Fibrosis. Am. J, Med 96:27-34, 1994
4) Haworth CS, Selby PL, Webb AK, Dodd ME, Musson H, McL Niven R, Economou G, Horrocks AW, Freemont AJ, Mawer EB, Adams JE. Low bone mineral density in adults with Cystic Fibrosis.Thorax 54:961-7,1999.
5) Hillman LS, Allen S, Schlotzhaus D, Kline R, and Barbara G. Decreased bone mineralization in vitamin D sufficient children with Cystic Fibrosis. J. of Bone and Mineral Research. 9:5228, 1994

NUTRITION

WHAT IS THE OPTIMAL 25(OH)D LEVEL FOR BONE IN CHILDREN?

John M Pettifor, MRC Mineral Metabolism Research Unit and the Department of Paediatrics, University of the Witwatersrand and Chris Hani Baragwanath Hospital, Johannesburg, South Africa

Unlike adults, in whom a zero total body calcium balance is the goal for maintaining bone health, children require a positive calcium balance to allow for net bone accretion and skeletal growth. The amount of calcium accreted on a daily basis is not constant throughout childhood; values falling from the first year of life to reach a nadir between 3 and 5 years of age and then rising slowly until puberty when they rise sharply during the adolescent growth spurt.

In order to achieve this positive calcium balance and to optimise bone growth and mineralization, intestinal calcium absorption must be optimal. This is achieved mainly through the control of intestinal absorption by 1,25-dihydroxyvitamin D (1,25(OH)$_2$D), whose serum levels are dependent on the availability of substrate, 25-hydroxyvitamin D (25(OH)D), and the activity of the renal 1α-hydroxylase enzyme. A further key factor is the calcium content of the diet and its bioavailability. The importance of this latter factor in influencing bone health in children has only recently been fully realised, despite it being recognised for many years as being important in helping to maintain bone health in the elderly. Because of the close functional relationships between dietary calcium content, intestinal calcium absorption and the vitamin D endocrine system, it is difficult to determine an optimal serum 25(OH)D concentration for bone health without considering these other variables at the same time.

A further critical issue in determining optimal 25(OH)D levels is the criteria we choose to use to assess bone health in children. In adults a major emphasis of preventive health is to minimise bone loss and thus the development of osteoporosis and minimal trauma fractures in later life. With the advent of accurate methods to determine bone mass in adults, it is possible to assess the influence of vitamin D status on bone mass and the prevalence of osteoporosis relatively easily. In children, vitamin D deficiency has classically been considered synonymous with the development of rickets, which is readily detected by both biochemical and radiological techniques. Thus should the prevention of rickets be considered the goal in ensuring bone health in children? If we maintain a 25(OH)D level above a certain threshold concentration, and are be able to prevent rickets, are we optimizing bone health in the child?

The answer to the above question is probably no. Recently a retrospective cohort study in prepubertal girls provided suggestive evidence that vitamin D supplementation during infancy of those being breast-fed might improve bone mass at the hip and distal radius [1]. The results of this study need to be confirmed, but they do raise interesting questions around the relevance of improving bone mineral density in prepubertal children. Rickets obviously needs to be prevented to eradicate the risk of bone deformities and to optimise growth potential. Further, bone density and strength need to be sufficient to prevent an increased risk of minimal trauma fractures, but the evidence that an improvement in bone mass of prepubertal children will necessarily result in an improved peak bone mass in early adulthood, which is one of the factors reducing the risk of osteoporosis in later life, is limited.

Serum 25(OH)D levels in vitamin D deficiency rickets: Over the last 30 years a number of studies have documented serum 25(OH)D concentrations in children with untreated rickets. The majority of studies have reported 25(OH)D levels of <12 ng/ml (<30 nmol/l) in children with florid rickets [2-5] and subclinical rickets [6], although Arnaud and coworkers reported concentrations above this value in a study of rickets in the United States of America [7]. Children with subclinical rickets (very mild radiological changes) have also been reported to have values above 12 ng/ml [3], however a number of these children had healed spontaneously at follow-up 6 weeks later, suggesting that the values of 25(OH)D might not have reflected the values at which rickets had developed.

25(OH)D levels associated with biochemical perturbations in calcium homeostasis: The use of clinical criteria, eg. the presence or absence of clinical or radiological rickets, to determine vitamin D sufficiency is an insensitive approach, as detectable rickets may take several months to develop depending on the growth rate of the child, the dietary calcium intake and the degree of vitamin D deficiency. In countries, where marked seasonal variations in 25(OH)D levels occur, periods of impaired calcium absorption and disturbed calcium homeostasis may occur during winter and early spring without the development of radiological rickets. The biochemical abnormalities respond rapidly to an improvement in vitamin D status associated with the onset on summer [8]. A more sensitive method of assessing vitamin D sufficiency and thus optimal 25(OH)D concentrations is to determine the level of 25(OH)D below which perturbations of calcium homeostasis occur [9]. Alterations in serum parathyroid hormone (PTH) and/or $1,25(OH)_2D$ concentrations associated with changes in 25(OH)D have been used as indicators of vitamin D insufficiency [10-13]. In several studies, the seasonal decline in 25(OH)D concentrations during winter was accompanied by an increase in PTH values. However $1,25(OH)_2D$ values remained constant [12,8], suggesting that an increase in 1α-hydroxylase activity was necessary to maintain circulating $1,25(OH)_2D$ concentrations in the face of a reduced substrate level. It should be noted, however, that even though PTH values rose during winter and early spring, they still remained within the normal reference range. Thus the clinical relevance of this significant but small rise in PTH must be questioned. In adults, it is suggested that this marginal elevation of PTH might be detrimental to bone health through causing an increase in bone turnover [11]. Whether such concerns are warranted in children is unclear [14].

Zeghoud and coworkers used the biochemical criteria of disturbed calcium homeostasis to assess vitamin D sufficiency in the neonate [10]. They found an association between 25(OH)D levels <30 nmol/l (<12 ng/ml) and secondary hyperparathyroidism and hypocalcaemia. This value of <30 nmol/l is similar to that found in most children with radiological rickets.

Using the criteria and recommendations of Peacock et al [15], Docio and coworkers studied the level of 25(OH)D which could be defined as indicative of vitamin D deficiency in children [13]. Using an increase in 1,25(OH)$_2$D levels and/or a decrease in PTH values following 25(OH)D administration as the criteria for vitamin D deficiency, they arrived at a threshold 25(OH)D value of between 12 - 20 ng/ml (30 - 50 nmol/l) as the value below which children become vitamin D deficient. The lower threshold value of 12 ng/ml appears to be similar to the value Peacock et al derived in adults [15].

The effect of dietary calcium intake on optimal 25(OH)D levels in children: Although nutritional rickets is often considered to be synonymous with vitamin D deficiency, recent studies in several developing countries have highlighted the role of low dietary calcium intakes in the pathogenesis of the disease [16-19]. Dietary calcium intakes of affected children are remarkably similar in the various studies, being about 200 mg/day.

In a randomized controlled trial of the efficacy of vitamin D or calcium in the treatment of Nigerian children with rickets, calcium supplements with or without vitamin D were more effective than vitamin D alone [20]. At commencement of the trial, the mean 25(OH)D was 13.9 ± 10.2 ng/ml (34.7 ± 25.5 nmol/l), thus it could be argued that many of the children were actually vitamin D deficient. Yet despite this, calcium supplements alone were more effective than vitamin D, which increased mean levels of 25(OH)D to 26 ng/ml at 3 months and 35 ng/ml at 6 months, in healing the rickets as judged by both radiographic and biochemical improvement over a 6 month period. Of more relevance to the present discussion is the fact that two-thirds of the children with active rickets on entry into the study had normal 25(OH)D concentrations (>12 ng/ml), and of those treated with vitamin D alone only 19% had evidence of marked healing after 6 months compared with nearly 60% in the calcium treated groups.

These studies highlight the need to consider calcium intakes when discussing optimal 25(OH)D levels for bone health, as it is apparent that in situations of vitamin D sufficiency, rickets may occur if calcium intakes and intestinal absorption do not meet the requirements of the growing skeleton [21]. Thus the pathogenesis of nutritional rickets may be viewed as ranging from pure vitamin D deficiency at one end of the spectrum to pure dietary calcium deficiency at the other. In between these two extremes a variable mix of vitamin D insufficiency and poor dietary calcium intakes may precipitate the development of rickets.

Conclusions: In the majority of studies in children, vitamin D deficiency rickets is associated with 25(OH)D levels of <12 ng/ml (<30 nmol/l). Further the value of 12 ng/ml appears to be the threshold value below which a mild but significant rise in PTH values occurs in otherwise healthy children. In the neonatal period a similar threshold value was found to separate those neonates at risk of developing hypocalcaemia and secondary hyperparathyroidism from those who had normal calcium homeostasis.

The only study which has suggested a higher 25(OH)D threshold value for vitamin D sufficiency in children is that by Docio et al [13], who found that oral supplements of

25(OH)D given to children with basal 25(OH)D values of between 12 and 20 ng/ml resulted in a rise in $1,25(OH)_2D$ concentrations. Thus these authors argue that 20 ng/ml appears to be the minimum desirable level for circulating 25(OH)D in children.

Acting on such a recommendation would result in many children requiring vitamin D supplements as over 80% of children in the above study (Spain) had 25(OH)D values <20 ng/ml during winter. Similar high proportions of children would be found in many countries in Europe and other parts of the world. The public health and economic costs of such a recommendation need to be considered, before being implemented nationally. Although heed should be taken of the findings, further studies need to be undertaken to document the beneficial effects on bone health of maintaining serum concentrations of 25(OH)D above 20 ng/ml (50 nmol/l). However, there is now a considerable body of evidence to suggest that prolonged periods with 25(OH)D levels <12 ng/ml are detrimental to bone health and calcium homeostasis in children, thus measures should be taken to prevent such occurrences.

Further studies need to be conducted to determine whether the threshold of 12 ng/ml (30 nmol/l) holds for all paediatric age groups. The strongly positive calcium balance required during the pubertal growth spurt could conceivably require higher concentrations of 25(OH)D to achieve the $1,25(OH)_2D$ values needed to ensure adequate intestinal calcium absorption.

Finally, the effects of vitamin D insufficiency are probably more pronounced in children on low dietary calcium intakes or whose diets are high in phytates and oxalates.

References:

1. Zamora, S. A., Rizzoli, R., Belli, D. C., Slosman, D. O., and Bonjour, J. P. (1999) *J.Clin.Endocrinol.Metab* **84,** 4541-4544

2. Markestad, T., Aksnes, L., Ulstein, M., and Aarskog, D. (1984) *Am.J.Clin.Nutr.* **40,** 1057-1063

3. Goel, K. M., Sweet, E. M., Logan, R. W., Warren, J. M., Arneil, G. C., and Shanks, R. A. (1976) *Lancet* **i,** 1141-1145

4. Garabedian, M., Vainsel, M., Mallet, E., Guillozo, H., Toppet, M., Grimberg, R., NGuyen, T. M., and Balsan, S. (1983) *J.Pediatr.* **103,** 381-386

5. Specker, B. L., Ho, M. L., Oestreich, A., Yin, T., Shui, Q., Chen, X., and Tsang, R. C. (1992) *J.Pediatr.* **120,** 733-739

6. Pettifor, J. M., Isdale, J. M., Sahakian, J., and Hansen, J. D. L. (1980) *Arch.Dis.Child.* **55,** 155-157

7. Arnaud, S. B., Stickler, G. B., and Haworth, J. C. (1976) *Pediatrics* **57,** 221-225

8. Olivieri, M. B., Ladizesky, M., Mautalen, C. A., Alonso, A., and Martinez, L. (1993) *Bone Miner.* **20,** 99-108

9. Dawson-Hughes, B., Harris, S. S., and Dallal, G. E. (1997) *Am.J.Clin.Nutr.* **65,** 67-71

10. Zeghoud, F., Vervel, C., Guillozo, H., Walrant-Debray, O., Boutignon, H., and Garabedian, M. (1997) *Am.J.Clin.Nutr.* **65,** 771-778

11. Harris, S. S. and Dawson-Hughes, B. (1998) *Am.J.Clin.Nutr.* **67,** 1232-1236

12. Guillemant, J., Cabrol, S., Allemandou, A., Peres, G., and Guillemant, S. (1995) *Bone* **17,** 513-516

13. Docio, S., Riancho, J. A., Perez, A., Olmos, J. M., Amado, J. A., and Gonzales-Macias, J. (1998) *J.Bone Miner.Res.* **13,** 544-548

14. Slemenda, C. W., Peacock, M., Hui, S., Zhou, L., and Johnston, C. C. (1997) *J.Bone Miner.Res.* **12,** 676-682

15. Peacock, M., Selby, P. L., Francis, R. M., Brown, W. B., and Hordon, L. (1985) In: Norman, A. W. (ed.) Vitamin D. A Chemical, Biochemical and Clinical Update. Walter de Gruyter, Berlin, pp 569-570

16. Pettifor, J. M., Ross, P., Wang, J., Moodley, G., and Couper-Smith, J. (1978) *J.Pediatr.* **92,** 320-324

17. Oginni, L. M., Worsfold, M., Oyelami, O. A., Sharp, C. A., Powell, D. E., and Davie, M. W. (1996) *J.Pediatr.* **128,** 692-694

18. Thacher, T. D., Ighogboja, S. I., and Fischer, P. R. (1997) *Ambulatory Child Health* **3,** 56-64

19. Fischer, P. R., Rahman, A., Cimma, J. P., Kyaw-Myint, T. O., Kabir, A. R., Talukder, K., Hassan, N., Manaster, B. J., Staab, D. B., Duxbury, J. M., Welch, R. M., Meisner, C. A., Haque, S., and Combs, G. F., Jr. (1999) *J.Trop.Pediatr.* **45,** 291-293

20. Thacher, T. D., Fischer, P. R., Pettifor, J. M., Lawson, J. O., Isichei, C. O., Reading, J. C., and Chan, G. M. (1999) *N.Engl.J.Med.* **341,** 563-568

21. Pettifor, J. M. (1994) *J.Roy.Soc.Med.* **87,** 723-725

DEFINITION OF THE OPTIMAL 25OHD STATUS FOR BONE

Bess Dawson-Hughes and Susan S. Harris, Calcium and Bone Metabolism Laboratory at the Jean Mayer USDA Human Nutrition Research Center on Aging at Tufts University, Boston, MA, USA.

Introduction

Extreme vitamin D deficiency causes osteomalacia and lesser degrees of deficiency have been associated with osteoporosis. The prevalence of vitamin D insufficiency is perhaps greater than is generally appreciated. In studies conducted in the local Boston area, 80% of patients residing in nursing homes had 25OHD levels below 37 nmol/L in the wintertime (1), over half of the patients admitted to a local hospital with hip fractures had 25OHD levels under 30 nmol/L (2), and over half of the patients admitted to the medical service of another hospital had 25OHD levels of 37 nmol/L or below (3). Low vitamin D levels are even more common in Europe (4,5), because of its higher latitude and lower mean intake of the vitamin. Currently it is difficult to compare the prevalence of vitamin D insufficiency across populations because there is no standard definition of the term.

In this chapter, we will 1) consider the factors that influence the circulating 25OHD concentration, 2) propose a definition based on the association between serum concentrations of 25OHD and PTH, and then 3) address the impact of supplementation with vitamin D on 25OHD levels in healthy older men and women.

Factors that influence 25OHD concentrations

Parent vitamin D, from which 25OHD is derived, is produced when the skin is exposed to ultraviolet B (UVB) light, and is also obtained from dietary sources. Nursing home residents and others who spend little time outside generally have low 25OHD concentrations (6), but there is considerable variability in 25OHD levels among individuals who have regular sunlight exposure. The amount of UVB light that penetrates the atmosphere is reduced at northern latitudes relative to southern latitudes and reduced in the winter relative to the summer. In areas as far north as New England, little or no cholecalciferol is produced during sun exposure in winter (7) and there is marked seasonal variation in 25OHD concentrations (8). Skin pigmentation reduces the effectiveness of UVB exposure, and 25OHD concentrations in African-Americans are lower than those of Caucasians at all times of the year (9). Sunscreens block access of the UVB rays to the epidermal layer of skin, where most vitamin D is produced and thus limit the 25OHD response to sun exposure.

Aging influences the 25OHD concentration in several ways. Older individuals have reduced skin synthesis of cholecalciferol, apparently due to reductions in skin thickness (10) and skin concentrations of the precursor, 7-dehydrocholesterol (11). In a pilot study, we recently observed that older men had smaller increases in serum 25OHD concentrations than young men after three weeks of supplementation with 1800 IU/d of vitamin D (12). We are now exploring possible explanations for that finding including an age-related decline in vitamin D absorption, differences in metabolism of parent vitamin D to 25OHD, and differences in metabolism of 25OHD to 1,25-dihydroxyvitamin D and 24,25-dihydroxyvitamin D, the principal kidney metabolites.

Calcium intake may influence the 25OHD concentration achieved after a given sun exposure or dietary intake. We and other investigators have found that increasing calcium intake lowers blood concentrations of $1,25(OH)_2D$ in healthy postmenopausal women (13,14). This might be expected to have a sparing effect on the substrate, 25OHD. In patients with primary hyperparathyroidism, for instance, the half life of serum 25OHD was inversely correlated with serum $1,25(OH)_2D$ (15), indicating that a high serum $1,25(OH)_2D$ is associated with higher turnover of 25OHD. In contrast, in the calcium deficient state, synthesis of $1,25(OH)_2D$ is stimulated by the lower ionized calcium and the higher PTH concentrations, and so more 25OHD substrate would be metabolized. The extent to which the increased utilization of 25OHD would actually challenge the reserve is unknown. Normally, the serum concentration of 25OHD is 1000-fold higher that the $1,25(OH)_2D$ concentration. We examined this question indirectly in 321 healthy postmenopausal women who had self-reported usual calcium intakes of under 650 mg/d. The women were recruited to participate in a 2-year controlled calcium supplement trial (13). One third of the women were treated with placebo and two thirds with 500 mg/d of elemental calcium as either carbonate or citrate malate. The initial 25OHD and $1,25(OH)_2D$ levels of the women in the two treatment groups and their changes over the first year of the study are shown in Table 1. The women on placebo maintained their initial $1,25(OH)_2D$ level and had a 10 nmol/L decline in 25OHD at the end of one year. In contrast, the women taking calcium supplements had a significant decline in their mean $1,25(OH)_2D$ level and a more modest decline in their mean 25OHD level. While these findings are consistent with a 25OHD-sparing effect of supplemental calcium, the observation depends upon self-reports of vitamin D intake. Even if true, the finding may be of limited clinical significance because of the small magnitude of the effect.

Additional factors appear to affect 25OHD concentrations through mechanisms that are independent of parent vitamin D synthesis and consumption. For example, 25OHD concentrations are reduced in individuals with severe liver disease and certain malabsorption disorders (16). It has been observed that 25OHD concentrations are positively associated with exogenous estrogen use in both premenopausal (17) and postmenopausal women (18), perhaps by affecting

Table 1. Impact of calcium supplementation on vitamin D levels in 321 postmenopausal women

Measure	Baseline	1-Year Change
25OHD, nmol/L		
Calcium Supplemented	79±30	-5±24
Placebo	81±27	-10±23
sig. of difference	0.658	0.088
1,25(OH)$_2$D, pmol/L		
Calcium Supplemented	84±21	-12±25
Placebo	87±19	0±27
sig. of difference	0.219	<0.001

levels of vitamin D binding protein (19). Both obesity (20) and smoking (21) are associated with reduced 25OHD concentrations, but the mechanisms for these effects are unclear.

Definition of vitamin D status sufficiency

Currently, there is no widely accepted operational definition of vitamin D sufficiency. Subtle degrees of vitamin D deficiency, often referred to as vitamin D insufficiency, are associated with small decreases in circulating ionized calcium concentrations and accompanying small increases in serum concentrations of PTH (usually within the normal range). Small tonic increases in circulating PTH concentration increase bone resorption, and this is undesirable because a higher turnover rate not only increases bone loss, it is also an independent predictor of fracture (22). The increase in PTH need not be sustained for long periods in order to promote bone loss. It has been demonstrated that wintertime rises in serum PTH cause accelerated wintertime bone loss and that this can be reduced by supplementation with 10 mcg/d of vitamin D (23). In 1997, the National Academy of Sciences (NAS) selected the serum 25OHD level in conjunction with serum PTH as well as bone loss to be functional indicators of vitamin D adequacy in older adults (24).

Many investigators have observed an inverse association between serum 25OHD and PTH and noted that the association is hyperbolic, not linear. On the basis that a compensatory rise in circulating PTH is undesirable, several investigators have sought to identify the inflection point, or the 25OHD concentration below which PTH begins to rise. This is a rational approach to defining the optimal 25OHD level but one that has lead to a wide range of 25OHD threshold values. For example, in healthy postmenopausal women, mean age 58 years, we found that a 25OHD level of 90 nmol/L was needed to prevent wintertime rises in serum PTH (8). This value of 90 nmol/L is fairly close to the value of 80 nmol/L identified by Meunier (see accompanying chapter). In our STOP/IT population of healthy men and women, age 65 and older (mean age 71 years), a 25OHD level of 110 nmol/L was needed to maximally suppress serum PTH (25). This estimate was similar in the men and the women. It is notable however that the 95% confidence interval around the estimate of 110 nmol/L was quite broad (60 to 168 nmol/L), reflecting much biological variability in the association. In contrast, Lips *et al.* considers a 25OHD level of 30 nmol/L to be adequate because in his studies in the Netherlands, the associations between 25OHD and PTH were significant only when the 25OHD levels were less than 30 nmol/L (26). Additionally, at 25OHD levels over 30 nmol/L, Lips found that supplemental vitamin D did not increase the circulating level of $1,25(OH)_2D$. The explanation for why the threshold estimates vary so widely is not certain. Serum 25OHD assay differences between Boston, Lyon, and Amsterdam do not appear to account for the large differences in threshhold 25OHD values (27). Perhaps the serum PTH levels of the elderly subjects studied by Lips were already nearly maximally suppressed by the high calcium intakes of the participating men and women. At this time, the weight of the evidence suggests that a 25OHD level of 80 to 90 nmol/L be considered optimal. This means that 25OHD levels should be maintained in the upper half of the normal reference range (and that many people in the reference data base probably have a compensatory rise in their serum PTH levels).

Serum 25OHD response to vitamin D supplementation

Because many factors other than sun exposure and vitamin D intake influence serum concentrations of 25OHD, it is expected that the amount of sun exposure and/or intake needed to maintain a serum 25OHD of 80 to 90 nmol/L will vary among individuals and populations. For example, older individuals are expected to need higher intakes of vitamin D than young people. This was certainly the conclusion of the NAS in setting the Adequate Intakes (AIs) for vitamin D for adults (24). The Academy recommended intakes of 5 mcg/d (200 IU/d) for men and women aged 31-50, 10 mcg/d for those aged 51-70, and 15 mcg/d for those age 71 and older. These recommendations assume that no vitamin D is available from sun-mediated skin synthesis.

We recently examined the 25OHD levels achieved by older adults receiving vitamin D supplements. The 376 subjects in this analysis had completed a three-year randomized controlled calcium and vitamin D supplement trial (28). The men and women, mean age 71 years, consumed an average of 700 mg of calcium and 2.5 mcg of vitamin D/d in their diets. The subjects were enrolled and had 25OHD measurements at an even rate over a 12-month period. Half of these subjects were supplemented with 500 mg/d of elemental calcium, bringing their mean total intake up to the 1,200 mg/d (the amount recommended by the NAS) and with 17.5 mcg/d of supplemental vitamin D/d. Hence their total mean vitamin D intake exceeded 15 mcg/d, the amount recommended for men and women age 71 and older. In Table 2, we display the percentages of subjects who attained various levels of 25OHD after one year on the supplements. Ninety % of the men and 87% of the women reached the desired 25OHD threshold level of 80 nmol/L. Historically, recommended dietary allowances (RDAs) have been set sufficiently high to meet the needs of 97 or 98% of the population (24). Clearly, the intakes of vitamin D currently recommended by the NAS are insufficient to bring the desired proportion of elderly men and women to the threshold 25OHD level of 80 to 90 nmol/L. Table 2 also shows data for the group treated with placebo (total mean vitamin D intake estimated at 5 mcg/d). In this group, only 57% of the men and 28% of the women had 25OHD levels of 80 nmol/L. Thus this convenience sample of healthy older residents of the Boston area has a very high prevalence of undesirably low 25OHD levels. Furthermore, many of the people in this sample who had an adequate 25OHD level in the summer would have a 25OHD level below 80 nmol/L in the winter.

Table 2. Percentages of elderly men and women whose 25OHD concentrations reached selected levels after one year of supplementation with 700 IU/d of vitamin D and 500 mg/d calcium or placebo (N=376)

Group	25OHD, nmol/L	Men, %	Women, %
Vitamin D+Calcium	20	100.0	100.0
	40	100.0	99.0
	60	97.7	96.9
	80	89.8	86.6
	100	75.0	71.1
Placebo	20	100.0	95.1
	40	96.6	84.5
	60	77.3	58.3
	80	56.8	28.2
	100	35.2	15.5

In conclusion, based on the interrelationship between serum 25OHD and PTH levels, we believe that adults need to maintain their levels of 25OHD at 80 to 90 nmol/L or above, in order to minimize the compensatory rise in serum PTH that occurs at lower 25OHD levels and that is associated with increased bone loss. Further work is needed to elucidate why the threshold 25OHD value seems to vary widely from one study population to another. Work is also needed to identify how much vitamin D must be consumed by different segments of the population in order to reach and maintain the desired 25OHD level. Based on our recent study, men and women age 65 and older may need to have vitamin D intakes that are higher than those currently recommended by the NAS in order to reach and maintain the desired 25OHD levels.

Reference

1. Webb, A.R., Pilbeam C., Hanafin N., Holick M.F. (1990) Am J Clin Nutr 51:1075-81.

2. LeBoff M.S., Kohlmeier L, Hurwitz S., Franklin J., Wright J., Glowacki J (1999) JAMA 281:1505-11.

3. Thomas M.K., Lloyd-Jones D.M., Thadhani R.I., Shaw A.C., Deraska D. J., Kitch B.T. et al. (1998) New Engl J Med 338: 777-83.

4. van der Wielen R.P.J., Lowik M.R.H., van den Berg H., deGroot L., Haller J., Moreiras O., van Staveren W.A. (1995) Lancet 346:207-10.

5. McKenna M.J. (1992) Am J Med 93: 69-77.

6. Kinyamu, H.K., Gallagher, J.C., Balhorn, K.E., Petranick, K.M., Rafferty, K.A. (1997) Am J Clin Nutr 65:790-7.

7. Webb, A.R., Kline, L.W., Holick, M.F. (1988) J Clin Endocrinol Metab 67:337-338.

8. Krall E.A., Sahyoun N., Tannenbaum S., Dallal G.E., Dawson-Hughes B. (1989) New Engl J Med 321:1777-83.

9. Harris, S.S., Dawson-Hughes, B. (1998) Am J Clin Nutr 67:1232-6.

10. Need, A.G., Morris, H.A., Horowitz, M., Nordin, B.E.C. (1993) Am J Clin Nutr 58:882-5.

11. MacLaughlin, J., Holick, M.F. (1985) J Clin Invest 76:1536-8.

12. Harris, S.S., Dawson-Hughes, B. (1999). J Am Coll Nutr 18:470-4.

13. Dawson-Hughes B., Dallal G.E., Krall E.A., Sadowski L., Sahyoun N., Tannenbaum S. (1990) New Engl J Med 323: 878-83.

14. Elders P.J., Lips P., Netelenbos J.C., van Ginkel F.C., Khoe E., van der Vijgh W. J. F., van der Stelt P.F. (1994) J Bone Miner Res 9:963-70.

15. Clements M.R., Johnson L., Fraser D.R. (1987) Nature 325: 62-5.

16. Long, R.G., Meinhard, E., Skinner, R.K., Varghese, Z., Wills, M.R., Sherlock, S. (1978) Gut 19:85-90.

17. Harris, S.S., Dawson-Hughes, B. (1998). J Am Coll Nutr 17:282-4.

18. Sowers, M.F., Wallace, R.B., Hollis, B.W., Lemke, J.H. (1986) Am J Clin Nutr 43:621-628.

19. Bouillon, R.A., Auwerx, J.H., Lissens, W.D., Pelemans, W.K. (1987). Am J Clin Nutr 45:755-63.

20. Liel, Y., Ulmer, E., Shary, J., Hollis, B.W., Bell, N.H. (1988) Calcif Tissue Int 43:199-201.

21. Mellstrom, D., Rundgren, A., Jagenburg, R., Steen, B., Svanborg, A. (1982) Age and Ageing 11:45-58.

22. Garnero P. Somay-Rendu E., Chapuy M.C., Delmas P. (1996) J Bone Miner Res 11:337-49.

23. Dawson-Hughes B., Dallal G.E., Krall E.A., Harris S., Sokoll L.J., Falconer G (1991) Ann Int Med 115: 505-12.

24. Standing Committee on the Scientific Evaluation of Dietary Reference Intakes. Institute of Medicine (1997) Washington, DC: National Academy Press.

25. Dawson-Hughes B., Harris S.S., Dallal G.E. (1997) Am J Clin Nutr 65:67-71.

26. Lips P., Wiersinga A., van Ginkel F.C., Jongen M.J.M., Netelenbos J.C., Hackeng W.H.L. Delmas P. D., van der Vijgh W.J.F. (1988) J Clin Endocrinol Metab 67: 644-8.

27. Lips P., Chapuy, M.C., Dawson-Hughes B., Pols H.A.P., Holick M. (1999) Osteoporosis Intl 9:394-7.

28. Dawson-Hughes B., Harris S.S., Krall E.A., Dallal G.E. (1997) New Engl J Med 337: 670-76.

WHAT IS THE OPTIMAL SERUM 25(OH)D LEVEL APPROPRIATE FOR BONE ?

Pierre J. Meunier, Department of Rheumatology and Bone Diseases, INSERM Unit 403, Edouard Herriot Hospital, Lyon 69437, France.

Introduction It is well known that serum 25(OH)D is the best functional indicator of vitamin D status, but the threshold levels separating
- vitamin D *deficiency*, which induces a frank osteomalacia due to the inhibition of the primary mineralization of bone matrix, from
- vitamin D *insufficiency*, which induces a secondary hyperparathyroidism without mineralization defect and accelerates bone loss, and from
- vitamin D *sufficiency*

are still debated, and the aim of this review is to reappraise the definition of vitamin D insufficiency and of its bone consequences. This is not a theoretical issue but may have important practical consequences for the prevention of osteoporotic fractures, particularly in the elderly population. For a long time, secondary hyperparathyroidism induced by the combination of a vitamin D insufficiency and a low calcium intake has been suggested being a major determinant of bone loss and fracture risk in elderly subjects (1). In reality the role of this vitamin D insufficiency as a risk factor for osteoporotic fractures remained theoretical until it has been demonstrated that its correction, combined with a calcium supplement, was capable to prevent fractures through the normalization of both vitamin D and parathyroid status (2). This has been demonstrated now by the results from three randomized controlled trials which have provided evidence of the antifracture efficacy of vitamin D-calcium supplements, and it becomes important to better define the population which could benefit of these supplements. This implies a determination of the threshold level of serum 25(OH)D which triggers off the parathyroid response or reciprocally the level of 25(OH)D at which serum parathyroid hormone (PTH) concentration is minimized. This can be approached through the analysis of the relationship between serum PTH and 25(OH)D.

Influence of vitamin D supplements on fracture risk In Decalyos I study (3,4) a total of 3270 mobile elderly women (mean age 84 years) living in nursing homes were enrolled. Half the women received 1200 mg calcium daily in the form of tricalcium phosphate, together with 800 IU (20 µg) cholecalciferol ; the other half received a double placebo. All subjects were followed up every 6 months for 3 years ; biochemical variables were measured at baseline and every 6 months in a subgroup of 52 women. Hip fractures and all non vertebral fractures were separately analyzed using a log rank test and an actuarial method. The intention to treat analysis showed that 17% fewer subjects had one or more non vertebral fractures and 29% fewer subjects one hip fracture (p<0.02). This antifracture effect was combined with a normalization of serum 25(OH)D in the calcium-vitamin D group which increased from a low mean level of about 13 ng/ml (competitive-binding protein assay after extraction and purification) to 35-40 ng/ml from the 6th month. In parallel a high mean serum PTH concentration at baseline (about 55 pg/ml) returned after 6 months to the normal range (30-40 pg/ml) in the calcium-vitamin D group and significantly increased in the placebo group.

The antifracture effects of a calcium and vitamin D supplementation were confirmed in a population of 389 subjects living in the community (176 men and 213 women ; mean age 71 years) and receiving for 3 years either 500 mg of calcium plus 700 IU of vitamin D3 per day or placebo. Of 37 subjects who had non vertebral fractures, 26 were in the placebo group and 11 in the calcium-vitamin D group (p=0.02). In parallel an increase of the mean serum 25(Oh)D level from about 33 to 45 ng/ml and a significant decrease of serum PTH were noted (5).

In a recent study named Decalyos II and run in our Unit, we recruited 610 ambulatory women (mean age 85 years) living in 55 nursing homes who were randomized in 3 groups: 206 received a fixed combination containing 1200 mg calcium in the form of tricalcium phosphate and 800 IU of vitamin D3 ; 199 received a daily supplement of 1200 mg calcium and 800 IU of vitamin D3 (separately administrated) ; 205 received a double placebo. All women were followed up every 6 months for 2 years. In this population, the cumulative probability of hip fracture was reduced in the calcium-vitamin D groups with an odds ratio for hip fractures among women in the placebo group as compared with those in the vitamin D-calcium group was 1.69, almost similar to the odds ratio noted in Decalyos I study (1.70). The difference however did not reach the statistical significance (p value: 0.07), the study having not been powered to test an antifracture effect. As found in Decalyos I study, serum 25(OH)D increased from a mean level of about 9 ng/ml at baseline to about 35 ng/ml after 6 months. Serum PTH was also reduced of about 40% in both group supplemented with calcium and vitamin D, returning from a mean baseline level of 70 pg/ml to a mean normal level of 45 pg/ml after 6 months.

In contrast to these three studies which have provided evidence of an antifracture efficacy of vitamin D-calcium supplements through a complete normalization of both serum 25(OH)D and PTH, another study using a smaller dose of vitamin D (400 IU/day) and no calcium supplement in 2578 old subjects did not demonstrate any reduction in the incidence of hip fractures, did not induced a significant decrease in serum PTH concentration and did not increase the mean serum 25(OH)D level beyond 21.6 ng/ml (6).

<u>Relationship between serum 25(OH)D and serum PTH</u> We have analyzed first this relationship in an adult normal population of 1569 healthy volunteers living in 20 French cities and participating in the SUVIMAX study (765 men and 804 women ; mean age 50 years) (7). In this population we found 14% subjects with a serum 25(OH)D level lower than 12 ng/ml (30 nmol/l) which was considered 12 years ago as the "classical" threshold defining vitamin D insufficiency (8). A significant negative correlation was found between serum intact PTH and serum 25(OH)D values (p<0.01). Serum PTH held a stable plateau at about 36 pg/ml as long as serum 25(OH)D values were higher than 78 nmol/l (31 ng/ml). With this threshold of 31 ng/ml, 75% of the healthy volunteers recruited between November and April could be considered as having a suboptimal serum 25(OH)D level.

Using the same type of correlation between serum 25(OH)D and PTH, a similar threshold of 70-75 nmol/l (28-30 ng/ml) was found by Thomas in 290 medical in patients admitted to general medical wards at Massachusetts General Hospital in Boston (9). Identically, in comparing 45 published reports on untreated or vitamin D supplemented elderly people. M.J. McKenna found a threshold of 25(OH)D stimulating PTH response of 75 to 100 nmol/l (10). In our Decalyos II recent study we found from the relationship between serum 25(Oh)D and serum PTH measured in 583 elderly women living in nursing homes a threshold of 65-70 nmol/l (26-28 ng/ml) initiating the PTH response.

Another evidence of the fact that the serum 25(Oh)D level minimizing PTH secretion is much higher than the "classical" threshold of 30 nmol/l (12 ng/ml) was provided recently by Malabanan and Holick (11). In 35 patients having a serum 25(OH)D between 25 and 62 nmol/l at baseline, they gave 50.000 IU of vitamin D2 per week for 2 months and 1000-1500 mg calcium per day. On the total population they observed a 109% increase of serum 25(OH)D (from 42.5 to 87.5 nmol/l) and a 22% decrease in PTH values. When they divided their population in 3 groups in stratifying the pre-treatment 25(OH)D levels (27.5 to 39.9 ; 40 to 49.9 ; 50-60 nmol/l) they found a 35% decrease in PTH in the first group, a 26% decrease in the second one and no decrease in the third group having a serum 25(OH)D higher than 50 nmol/l at baseline.

<u>Table 1</u> summarizes the serum 25(OH)D levels at which serum PTH is minimized in the five studies described above. These data show that the lower limit of normal vitamin D status corresponds to values of serum 25(OH)D between 50 and 80 nmol/l. This range takes into account the differences existing between the assays used for the measurement of serum 25(OH)D (12).

Table 1

Serum 25(OH)D levels at which serum PTH is minimized

	nmol/l	ng/ml
. Suvimax study		
ref.7 – RIA	75-80	30-32
. Decalyos 2 study		
RIA	65-70	26-28
. Thomas		
ref 9 – CPBA	65-75	26-30
. Malabanan		
Ref 11 – CPBA	50	20
. Mc Kenna		
Ref 10	70-75	28-30

RIA: radio-immuno assay ; CPBA: competitive protein binding assay

With such thresholds, the percentage of subjects with vitamin D insufficiency is much greater than the one based on the old threshold of 12 ng/ml. This is of particular importance for the elderly population and, as an example, the distribution of serum 25(OH)D levels observed in 440 healthy elderly women from the Epidos study shows that the percentage of women with a vitamin D insufficiency increases form 39% to 82% when the threshold of the serum 25(OH)D is moved from 12 ng to 24 ng/ml (13). These results are also important to determine the optimal level of serum 25(OH)D to reach in persons receiving a vitamin D supplement. Interestingly the studies having demonstrated an antifracture effect are those where a significant reduction and a "normalization" of serum PTH has been obtained (3, 4, 5). It was not the case for Lip's study (12) where no reduction in hip fracture risk was observed.

In conclusion, the serum 25(OH)D level corresponding to the lower limit of vitamin D sufficiency is much higher than 30 nmol/l and is between 50 and 80 nmol/l. This reappraisal has two practical consequences :
-   vitamin D insufficiency is much more common than previously believed, and this is relevant to larger possibilities of vitamin D –or vitamin D and calcium-supplements for preventing osteoporotic fractures by minimizing serum PTH. This is of particular importance for the prevention of hip fractures in elderly people.

- It is important to ensure that serum 25(OH)D level obtained after vitamin D supplementation reaches this new threshold. This could lead to increase the supplement from 200 IU to 800 IU/day of vitamin D in patients with a vitamin D insufficiency identified from the new threshold.

References

1 – Riggs, B.L., Melton, L.J. (1983) Am. J. Med. 75, 899-901
2 – Meunier, P.J. (1998) Osteoporos. Int. 8, suppl. 2, 1-2.
3 - Chapuy, M.C., Arlot, M.E., Duboeuf, F. et al. (1992) N. Engl. J. Med. 327, 1637-1642
4 - Chapuy, M.C., Arlot, M.E., Delmas, P.D., and Meunier, P.J. (1994) B.M.J. 308, 1081-1082
5 - Dawson-Hughes, B., Harris, S.S., Krall, E.A. and Dallal, G.E. (1997) N. Engl. J. Med. 337, 670-676.
6 - Lips, P., Graafmans, W.C., Doms, M.E., Bezemer, P.D., Bouter, L.M. (1996) Ann. Intern. Med. 124, 400-406.
7 - Chapuy, M.C., Preziosi, P., Maamer, M. et al (1997) Osteoporos. Int. 7, 439-443.
8 - Lips, P., wierzinga, A., Van Ginkel, F.C., Jongen, M.J.M., Netelenbos, J.C. (1988) J. Clin. Endocrinol. Metab. 67, 644-650.
9 - Thomas, K.K., Lloyd Jones, D.M., Thadhani, R.I. et al (1998) N. Engl. J. Med. 398, 777-783.
10 - Mc Kenna, M.J., Freaney, R. (1998) Osteoporos. Int. 8, suppl 2, 3-6
11- Malabanan, A., Veronikis, I.E., Holick, M.F. (1998) Lancet 351, 805-806.
12- Lips, P., Chapuy, M.C., Dawson-Hughes, B., Pols, H.A.P., and Holick, M.F. (1999) Osteoporos. Int. 9, 394-397.
13- Chapuis, M.C., Schott, A.M., Garnero P. et al. (1996). J. Clin. Endocrinol. Metab. 81, 1129-1133

The D-lemma: How Much Vitamin D is Necessary for Bone and Cellular Health?

Michael F. Holick, Ph.D., M.D. Vitamin D, Skin, and Bone Research Laboratory; Department of Medicine, Section of Endocrinology, Diabetes, and Nutrition; Boston University School of Medicine, Boston, MA

Introduction For almost a century, as result of the pioneering work of Melanby, Hess, Steenbock, and McCollum, it has been appreciated that vitamin D is essential for the development and maintenance of the skeleton (1). In the 1940s, Carlsson was the first to demonstrate vitamin D's role in regulating intestinal calcium absorption and mobilizing calcium from the skeleton (2). In the late 1960s and early 70s, it was recognized that vitamin D required two successive hydroxylations first in the liver on carbon 25 to 25-hydroxyvitamin D [(25(OH)D)] and then in the kidney for a 1α-hydroxylation to form the biologically active form of vitamin D, 1,25-dihydroxyvitamin D_3 (1,25$(OH)_2$D) (1,3). In the late 1970s, it was appreciated that a wide variety of tissues not related to calcium metabolism had a nuclear receptor for 1,25$(OH)_2$D (4). A multitude of biologic functions have been attributed to 1,25$(OH)_2$D separate from its effects on calcium and bone metabolism. 1,25$(OH)_2D_3$ can modulate the immune system, inhibit cell proliferation and induce terminal differentiation, alter insulin secretion, and alter neurotransmission (5,6). With all of the biologic functions that vitamin D appears to play a role in, a reevaluation of the adequate daily intake of vitamin D is needed.

Sources of Vitamin D

Naturally, vitamin D is scarce in the diet. Fatty fish such as salmon and mackerel have vitamin D in the fat that is interspersed within their flesh. Cod liver oil and other oils from the liver of cartilaginous and bony fish contain variable amounts of vitamin D (7). Naturally, human and cow's milk has very little vitamin D. The appreciation that vitamin D was essential for bone health prompted the fortification of milk with vitamin D in the mid 1930s (8). This simple process eradicated rickets as a significant health problem in countries that practiced this fortification process. However, due to an outbreak of vitamin D intoxication in the 1950s in Great Britain, the fortification of milk with vitamin D has been prohibited in most European countries. Some breads and cereals are also fortified with vitamin D in the US, and, in Europe, margarine, and some cereals are fortified with vitamin D.

The major source of vitamin D for most vertebrates including humans is from exposure to sunlight (1). The skin has a very large capacity to produce a vitamin D_3. During exposure to sunlight, the 7-dehydrocholesterol in the epidermis and dermis absorbed ultraviolet B photons and undergo a ring opening to form previtamin D_3 (1). Since 7-dehydrocholesterol is in the plasma membrane, the formation of previtamin D_3 occurs in the same location. As a result, the previtamin D_3 is efficiently converted to vitamin D_3 within a few hours (9). As vitamin D_3 is being made, its change in conformation is the impetus for it to be free of the plasma membrane and enter into the extracellular fluid space to find its way into the dermal capillary bed. A wide variety of factors greatly influence the cutaneous production of vitamin D_3. Latitude, season, time of day, skin pigmentation, use of sunscreen, and aging can dramatically influence the cutaneous production of vitamin D_3 (1).

Recommended Adequate Intake for Vitamin D

In 1997, the Institute of Medicine released its recommendation for adequate intake of vitamin D (11). These recommendations were based on the available published literature regarding adequate vitamin D intake to prevent rickets in children and osteomalacia in adults. Based on the literature, the new recommendation for neonates, children, and adults up to the age of 50 years was 200 IU of vitamin D each day. For adults ages 51 to 70 and 71+ years, the new recommendations were 400 and 600 IU/day. However, in the absence of any exposure to sunlight, it is reasonable for children and adults up to the age of 50 years to receive 400-600 IU/d and for adults 51+ to receive 800 IU/d which would guarantee vitamin D sufficiency (10).

Is Vitamin D Deficiency a Health Problem Today?

It is well documented in the literature that adults over the age of 60 years are at risk for vitamin D deficiency in the United States and Europe (12-21). Most studies suggest that upwards to 50% of free-living adults, as well as institutionalized elders, are deficient in vitamin D (10-20). In 169 healthy adult Bostonians ages 49-83 years, 41% were found to be vitamin D deficient throughout the year (12). What is remarkable is that recent studies are now showing that vitamin D deficiency is also prevalent in young and middle-aged adults. We conducted a survey of medical students and residents in Boston at the end of this winter and found that 40% were vitamin D insufficient.

Consequences of Vitamin D Deficiency

Vitamin D deficiency results in a decrease in the efficiency of intestinal calcium absorption. This causes a decrease in ionized calcium, which is quickly recognized by the calcium sensor in the parathyroid glands resulting in an increase in the synthesis and secretion of parathyroid hormone (10,22,23). The function of parathyroid hormone is to interact with osteoblasts, which, in turn, stimulates the production of osteoclast differentiation factor (16). This receptor's signal interacts with preosteoclasts to induce them to become mature multinucleated osteoclasts whose function is to remove precious calcium stores for the bone in order to raise the blood ionized calcium into an acceptable physiologic range. The reason for this is that calcium became critically important early in evolution for a wide variety of metabolic activities and for neuromuscular function and neurotransmission. Thus, the body makes every effort to maintain the ionized calcium within a very finely tuned range.

In vitamin D deficiency, most often the serum calcium is normal because of secondary hyperparathyroidism (10). There are other consequences of the secondary hyperparathyroidism that results from vitamin D deficiency. PTH enhances tubular reabsorption of calcium in order to conserve the precious calcium stores. However, it also causes a phosphate wasting into the urine. It is the phosphate wasting that causes the serum phosphorus to be in the low normal or the below normal range in a fasting state. Thus, the calciumxphosphate product is no longer adequate for normal bone mineralization. As a result, the osteoid laid down by the osteoblasts can no longer be mineralized. The consequence in children is rickets and in adults osteomalacia. The increased PTH mediated bone destruction also exacerbates osteoporosis and increases risk of fracture (10,24,25). Since rickets is an extremely rare disease in children and osteomalacia often goes undiagnosed in adults, it is assumed by the general medical community that vitamin D deficiency is not a health problem in the 21st century.

Consequences of Vitamin D Supplementation

It has long been assumed that calcium and vitamin D supplementation is important for bone health of the elderly. Indeed, it was amply demonstrated by a multitude of studies that increasing calcium and vitamin D intake helped maintain and even marginally increase bone mineral density (10,12,16,18,19). In 1992, Chapuy et al. (24) reported in elderly French nursing home residents that they could substantially reduce hip and non-vertebral fractures by supplementing the residents with 800 mg of calcium and 800 IU of vitamin D. Dawson-Hughes et al. reported in the men and women over the age of 65 years a 116% decrease in risk of non-vertebral fractures for those who were maintained on their dietary intake of calcium which was estimated to be about 500 mg and who were supplemented with 700 IU of vitamin D (25).

How Do We Define Vitamin D Sufficiency?

The development of the assay for circulating concentrations of 25(OH)D heralded an accurate test for determining vitamin D status (26,27). The normal range is defined as the mean of a healthy population ± 2 standard deviations. Most assays report a normal range of 10-55 ng/ml. But is this really normal? We know that lifeguards have serum 25(OH)D levels that are 50 to 100 ng/ml and they do not suffer from any consequences that you would expect to see in vitamin D intoxication. Vitamin D intoxication is usually observed when the levels exceed 125-150 ng/ml. However, is the lower limit of 10 ng/ml normal? If you have a 25(OH)D of 11 ng/ml, do you have an adequate amount of vitamin D to satisfy the body's requirement? To answer this question, Malabanan et al. recruited 35 adults 49-83 years of age who had circulating concentrations of 25(OH)D of between 10 and 25 ng/ml (20). Each subject received 50,000 units of vitamin D once a week for eight weeks. Circulating concentrations of calcium, 25(OH)D, and PTH were determined before and at the end of the eight week trial. Overall, 22% of the otherwise healthy subjects had PTHs greater than the upper limit of normal of 65 pg/ml, and therefore, had secondary hyperparathyroidism. When the 25(OH)D were evaluated in quartiles, it was found that those subjects who had the lowest 25(OH)D had the highest risk of secondary hyperparathyroidism. Only when the 25(OH)D was greater than 20 ng/ml was there no effect on decreasing serum PTH values (Fig. 1). Thus, Malabanan et al. concluded that vitamin D insufficiency is physiologically relevant with serum 25(OH)D levels of less than 20 ng/ml in adults over the age of 49 years. Whether the same can be said for younger adults and children is not known at this time.

Figure 1. Relations between 25(OH)D and PTH before and after therapy with 50,000 IU of vitamin D, and calcium supplementation once a week for 8 weeks. Adapted with permission (21).

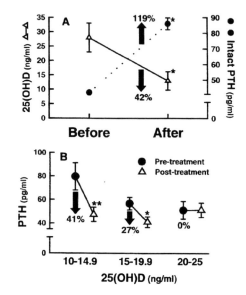

PTH and 1,25(OH)$_2$D are not good markers for vitamin D deficiency. 1,25(OH)$_2$D$_3$ levels have been reported to be low, normal, or elevated in vitamin D deficiency (28,29). This is, in part, due to the secondary hyperparathyroidism caused by vitamin D deficiency. PTH levels are elevated in patients with primary hyperparathyroidism which occurs in 0.1% of the adult population.

Vitamin D and the Cancer Connection

It is well known that a wide variety of cancer cells that possess a VDR decrease their proliferative activity and differentiate in the presence of 1,25(OH)$_2$D (30-32). There have been several reports that suggest that vitamin D deficiency and living at higher latitudes is associated with an increased risk or increased risk of dying from prostate cancer, colon cancer, breast cancer, and ovarian cancer (33-36). Initially, some investigators assumed that an increase of vitamin D intake or exposure to sunlight would result in an increase in the renal production of 1,25(OH)$_2$D. Thus, the increased circulating concentrations of 1,25(OH)$_2$D could be the hormonal signal to control and prevent abnormal cell growth of various tissues such as the colon, breast, prostate, etc. However, it was well known that the renal production of 1,25(OH)$_2$D was tightly feedback regulated and that an increase in exposure to sunlight or increase in vitamin D intake while increasing circulating concentrations of 25(OH)D would not result in any significant increase in circulating concentrations of 1,25(OH)$_2$D. Thus, it was unclear how increasing vitamin D intake or exposure to sunlight could be related to decreased risk of some of the more common cancers. It has been known for over a decade that some cells and tissues had the capacity to produce 1,25(OH)$_2$D. These included placenta (37), bone cells, and skin cells (38). The recent cloning of the 25-hydroxyvitamin D-1α-hydroxylase (1α-OHase) has provided the tool to unlock this mystery (39,40). We and others have now demonstrated that normal prostate cells, colon cells, and breast cells have 1α-OHase activity. Thus, a new function of vitamin D is finally being better appreciated. 25(OH)D can be metabolized to 1,25(OH)$_2$D in many different tissues to act as an autocrine hormone to prevent cellular hyperproliferation. It is possible that a higher circulating level of 25(OH)D is required for the extrarenal 1α-OHase to maximally function in the various tissues in the body for regulating cell growth.

Conclusion:

Vitamin D is critically important for maximal bone health and calcium metabolism. It is likely that circulating concentrations of 25(OH)D of greater than 20 ng/ml is required to satisfy the body's needs for optimally regulating intestinal calcium absorption. The newly appreciated function of vitamin D in cellular health may require higher circulating concentrations of 25(OH)D. These levels may be in the range of 30 ng/ml and above. Epidemiologic studies are required to better appreciate the consequences of vitamin D insufficiency for cellular health and cancer risk.

Acknowledgement: This work was supported in part by NIH Grants R01 AR36963 and M01RR 00533.

References:

1. Holick, M.F. McCollum Award Lecture (1994) Am. J. Clin. Nutr. 60, 619-630, 1994.
2. Carlsson, A. (1952) Acta Physiol. Scand 26, 212-220.
3. DeLuca, H. (1988) Fed. Proc. Am. Soc. Exper. Biol. 2, 224-236.
4. Stumpf, W.E., Sar, M., Reid, F.A., & et al. (1979) Science, 206, 1188-1190.
5. Holick, M.F. (1996) In: L.G. Raisz, G.A. Rodan, and J.P. Bilezikian (eds.) Principles of Bone Biology, chapter 32, pp. 447-460. Academic Press: San Diego.
6. Norman, A.W. (1994) Endocrinology, 134, 1601A-1601C.
7. Bills, C. E. (1927) Antiricketic Substances. VI. Research Laboratory, Mead Johnson and Company, Evansville, Indiana.
8. Steenbock, H. (1924) Science 60, 224-225.
9. Holick, M.F., Tian, X.Q., and Allen, M. (1995) Proc. Natl. Acad. Sci. 92, 3124-3126.
10. Holick, M.F. (1998) Osteoporos. Int. (Suppl.) 8, S24-S29.
11. Holick, M.F. (Contributor, Panel on Calcium and Related Nutrients) Calcium. (1999) In: Dietary Reference Intakes for Calcium, Phosphorus, Magnesium, Vitamin D, and Fluoride. Institute of Medicine. National Academy Press.
12. McGrath, N., Singh, V., Cundy, T. (1993) N. Zealand Med. J. 106, 524-526.
13. Villareal, D.T., Civitelli, R., Chines, A., Avioli, L. (1991) J. Clin. Endocrinol. Metab. 72, 628-634.
14. Chevalley, T., Rizzoli, R., Nydegger, V., Slosman, D., Rapin, C.H., Michel, J.P., Vasey, H., and Bonjour, J.P. (1994) Osteopor. Int. 4, 245-252.
15. Dawson-Hughes, B., Dallal, G.E., Krall, E.A., Harris, S., Sokoll, L.J., Falconer, G. (1991) Annals Int. Med. 115, 505-512.
16. Yasuda, H., Shima, N., Nakagawa, N., Yamaguchi, K., Kinosaki, M., Tsuda, E., Morinaga, T., Higashio, K., Udagawa, N., Takahashi, N., & Suda, T. (1998) Proc. Natl. Acad. Sci. 95, 3597-3602.
17. Ooms, R.E., Roos, J.C., Bezemer, P., Van Der Vijgh, W.J.F., et al. (1995) J. Clin. Endocrinol. Metab. 80, 1052-1058.

18. McKenna, M.J. (1992) Am. J. Med. 93, 69-77.

19. O'Dowd, K.J., Clemens, T.L., Kelsey, J.L., Lindsay, R. (1993) J. Am. Geriatr. Soc. 41, 414-421.

20. Lips, P., Graafmans, W.C., Ooms, M.E., Bezemer, D., Bouter, L.M. (1996) Ann. Intern. Med. 124, 400-406.

21. Malabanan, A., Veronikis, I.E., and Holick, M.F. Lancet 351, 805-806, 1998.

22. Brown, E. M., Gamba, G., Riccardl, D., Lombardi, M., Butters, R., Klfor, O., Sun, A., Hedlger, M. A., Lytton, J., and Hebert, S. C. (1993) Nature 366, 575-580.

23. Holick, M.F. (1998) In: M.F. Holick (ed) Vitamin D – Physiology, Molecular Biology and Clinical Applications, Chapter 1, pp. 1-16. Humana Press: New Jersey.

24. Chapuy, M.C., Arlot, M., Duboeuf, F., Brun, J., Crouzet, B., Arnaud, S., Delmas, P. (1992) N. Engl. J. Med. 327, 1637-1642.

25. Dawson-Hughes, B., Harris, S.S., Krall, E.A., Dallal, G.E. (1997) N. Eng. J. Med. 337, 701-702.

26. Belsey, R., Clark, M.B., Bernat, M., Glowacki, J., Holick, M.F., DeLuca, H.F., Potts, J.T. Jr. (1974) Am. J. Med. 57, 50-56.

27. Haddad, J. G. and Chuy, K. J. (1971) J Clin Endocrinol Metab 33, 992-995.

28. Adams, J. A., Clemens, T. L., Parrish, J. A., and Holick, M. F. (1981) N. Engl. J. Med. 306, 722-725.

29. Eastwood, J. B., De Wardener, H. E., Gray, R. W., and Lemann, J. L.,Jr. (1979) Lancet 1377-1378.

30. Tanaka, H., Abe, E., Miyaura, C., Kuribayashi, T., Konno, K., Nishi, Y., and Suda, T. (1982) Biochem. J. 204, 713-719.

31. Eisman, J. A., Suva, L. J., Sher, E., Pearce, P. J., Funder, J. W., and Martin, T. J. (1981) Cancer Res. 41, 5121-5124.

33. Garland, C., Shekelle, R. B., Barrett-Connor, E., Criqui, M. H., Rossof, A. H., and Oglesby, P. (1985) Lancet 9, February, 307-309.

34. Garland, C. F., Garland, F. C., Gorham, E. D., and Raffa, J. (1992) In: Biologic Effects of Light (Anonymous pp. 39-43, Walter de Gruyter & Co. New York.

35. Garland, F. C., Garland, C. F., Gorham, E. D., and Young, J. F. (1990) Preventive Med. 19, 614-622.

36. Hanchette, C. L. and Schwartz, G. G. (1992) Cancer 70, 2861-2869.

37. Gray, T. K., Lester, G. E., and Lorenc, R. S. (1979) Science 204, 1311-1313.

38. Bikle, D. D., Nemanic, M. K., Gee, E., and Elias, P. (1986) J. Clin. Invest. 78, 557-566.

39. Fu, G. K., Portale, A. A., and Miller, W. L. (1997) DNA Cell Biol. 16, 1499-1507.

40. Kong, X.F., Zhu, X.H., Pei, Y.L., Jackson, D.M., and Holick, M.F. (1999) Proc. Natl. Acad. Sci. USA 96, 6988-6993.

DEVELOPMENT OF A RATIONAL STRATEGY FOR THE TREATMENT OF HEREDITARY VITAMIN D RESISTANT RICKETS WITH ANALOGS OF 1,25 DIHYDROXYVITAMIN D$_3$.

Ali Gardezi, Cuong Nguyen, Peter J. Malloy *, David Feldman * and Sara Peleg
Department of Medical Specialties, The University of Texas, M.D Anderson Cancer Center. Houston, TX, USA 77030
* Endocrinology Division, Stanford University, School of Medicine, Stanford, California, USA 94305-5103.

INTRODUCTION: Hereditary Vitamin D Resistant Rickets (HVDRR) is an autosomal recessive disorder characterized by inactivating mutations in the vitamin D receptor (VDR) (1). Major clinical findings in patients with HVDRR include bone deformities, pain, muscle weakness, hypotonia, convulsions, alopecia, growth retardation and dental hypoplasia. Partially effective treatment modalities for this disorder have included calcium and high doses of active metabolites of vitamin D3. All patients that have mutations in the DNA binding domain of VDR thus far examined, are unresponsive to 1,25-dihydroxyvitamin D3 (1,25D3) treatment. However, in patients with mutations in the ligand-binding domain (LBD) of the VDR (1) there may be a limited response to high doses of vitamin D3. Previous studies from our laboratories have demonstrated that the 20-epi analogs of vitamin D3 interact differently with the VDR than 1,25D3 (2). These studies have also shown that the 20-epi analogs have transcriptional potency 100- to 1000-fold greater then 1,25D3 (2). These findings formed the rationale for the hypothesis that these analogs may be more effective than 1,25D3 in activating VDRs with mutations at their LBD. Results of experiments that examined the possibility that the analog 20-epi-1,25D3 (20E-1,25D3) has the potential to bind and restore transcriptional activity of VDR in HVDRR patients with LBD mutations are described below, and summarized in Table 1.

METHODS AND EXPERIMENTAL DESIGN: HVDRR patients selected for these studies have mutations that are restricted to the LBD of the VDR: arginine 274 to leucine (R274L), histidine 305 to glutamine (H305Q) and phenylalanine 251 to cysteine (F251C). The amino acid residues R274 and H305 are proposed contact points for 1,25D3 (3) whereas the residue F251 is in the E1 domain, which regulates dimerization and co-activator interaction (4). In each case we reproduced the mutation by site-directed mutagenesis and compared the mutant VDR to wild type with respect to ligand binding in COS-1 cells, ligand-induced transcription in CV1 cells and the ability to form ligand-dependent protease-resistant conformation *in vitro*.

In order to compare the relative affinities of 1,25D3 and 20E-1,25D3 for the mutant, homogenates from hVDR-transfected COS-1 cells were incubated with

[^{3}H]1,25D$_3$ with or without increasing amounts of unlabeled 1,25D$_3$ or the unlabeled 20E-1,25D$_3$. The free ligand was separated from bound by hydroxyapatite and specific binding of [^{3}H]1,25D$_3$ was measured by scintillation counting (2). Measurements of transcriptional activities were done using VDR-negative CV-1 cells cotransfected with a gene containing the osteocalcin vitamin D response element attached to the growth hormone reporter (ocVDRE-GH) and a VDR expression vector. 1,25D$_3$ or 20E-1,25D$_3$ was added to the culture medium and the reporter gene expression was examined 48h later. Results were expressed as percent of maximal reporter gene expression in 1,25D$_3$-treated cells (2).

An important aspect of ligand-receptor interaction is the ability of ligand to induce a transcriptionally active conformation in VDR. To compare the activity of the two ligands we performed protease sensitivity assays (2) with each of the three HVDRR mutants. In these assays, [^{35}S]-labeled VDR was incubated with increasing concentrations of ligand, then digested with trypsin, and the ligand-dependent protease-resistant fragments were visualized by SDS-PAGE and autoradiography. In these assays, the amount of ligand-dependent trypsin-resistant fragments reflects ligand-bound receptor complexes. The sizes of the trypsin-resistant fragments may indicate whether or not these VDR-ligand complexes are transcriptionally active.

To determine the effect of mutations on the potency of ligands to induce interaction with RXR or with the steroid receptor coactivator-1 (SRC-1), we used pull-down assays. In these assays a glutathione-S-transferase fused to either RXR (GST-RXR) or to SRC-1 (GST-SRC) was incubated with the [^{35}S]-labeled VDR in the absence or presence of ligand. The receptor-SRC-1 complexes were then isolated by chromatogrpahy on glutathione-sepharose beads, eluted and analyzed by SDS-PAGE and autoradiography.

RESULTS:
R274L: Ligand binding assays showed no detectable 1,25D$_3$ binding to this mutant VDR as previously reported (1). R274L had diminished 1,25D$_3$-mediated transcriptional activity, which was detectable only at 1 µM. In contrast, the 20E-1,25D$_3$ was able to induce transcriptional activity at 10 nM. The 20E-1,25D$_3$ induced a protease-resistant conformation of R274L at 10 nM while this activity was barely detectable in 1,25D$_3$ complexes with this mutant even at 1 µM. The results of the protease assay correlated with the ability of 20E-1,25D$_3$ to induce interaction of R274L with SRC-1, whereas no such activity was detected when the R274L was incubated with 1,25D$_3$.

H305Q: Ligand binding assays showed that there was no change in the affinity of either 1,25D$_3$ or its 20-epi analog for H305Q. The potency of 1,25D$_3$ to induce transcription in H305Q-transfected cells was decreased 100-fold. However, the potency of 20E-1,25D$_3$ to induce transcription in H305Q-transfected cells was

1000-fold greater then that of the natural hormone. These results correlated very well with the potencies of 1,25D3 and of 20E-1,25D3 to induce a protease-resistant conformation of H305Q VDR. Examination of SRC-1 interaction with H305Q showed that the 20E-1,25D3 was also a 1000-fold more potent in the induction of coactivator interaction with the mutant VDR than the natural hormone.

Table 1: 1,25D3- and 20E-1,25D3-mediated functions of mutant VDRs *

Function:	Binding affinity	Protease	Transcription	SRC-1 binding	Dimerization
WtVDR/ 1,25D$_3$	0.5 nM	0.7 nM	0.5 nM	0.7 nM	1.8 nM
WtVDR/20 E-1,25D$_3$	0.3 nM	0.8 nM	0.008 nM	1 nM	0.08 nM
H305Q/ 1,25D$_3$	1 nM	300 nM	40 nM	100 nM	Not done
H305Q/20 E-1,25D$_3$	0.4 nM	1 nM	0.03 nM	0.6 nM	Not done
R274L/ 1,25D$_3$	ND	NR	NR	ND	Not done
R274L/20 E-1,25D$_3$	ND	30 nM	20 nM	100 nM	Not done
F251C/ 1,25D$_3$	0.5 nM	0.6 nM	ND	ND	+/-
F251C/20 E-1,25D$_3$	0.4 nM	0.7 nM	ND	ND	+/-

* The data shown in this table are the effective doses required to reach 50% of maximal activity of wild-type (Wt)-VDR treated with 1,25D3. Binding affinity, competition assays with [^{3}H]1,25D3; Protease, protease sensitivity assays with [^{35}S]-VDR; Transcription, reporter gene expression in CV-1 cells trasfected with VDR; SRC-1 binding, binding assays of GST-SRC-1 fusion protein with [^{35}S]-VDR; Dimerization, binding assays of GST-RXR fusion protein with [^{35}S]-VDR. ND, not detectable; NR, not reached; +/-, a weak ligand-mediated dimerization was detected in the presence of 10 nM 1,25D3 or 20E-1,25D3

F251C: Ligand binding assays showed that the affinity of 1,25D3 or of 20E-1,25D3 for F251C was similar to their affinity for wild-type VDR. However, neither 1,25D3 nor 20E-1,25D3 induced any detectable transcription in cells transfected with this mutant VDR. Protease sensitivity assays showed the potency of the two compounds to stabilize the conformation of this mutant was identical to wild-type VDR. In coactivator interactions assays F251C had no detectable ability to interact with SRC-1, even in the presence of very high doses of either of the two ligands. However, F251C, was able to interact, though with a reduced efficacy, with RXR, in a ligand-dependent manner. These results suggest that diminished transcriptional activity of this mutant is due to a loss of coactivator binding site and not due to a loss of ligand binding activity.

DISCUSSION: The study presented here demonstrates the potential use of 20E-1,25D3 to treat a serious inherited disorder. The rationale for this study has two bases: 1) analogs that differently bind to VDR may alter the functional surface of the receptor, thereby providing alternative contact sites for interaction with transcriptional coactivators in mutant VDRs; 2) analogs that contact different amino acids within the LBD from those contacted by 1,25D3 may retain most, or all of their transcriptional activity if the mutated residue is not critical for their binding to the VDR. The results of this study suggest that vitamin D analogs may provide a useful alternative treatment in HVDRR if the mutation is at a binding site for the hormone and this site is not shared, or is only partially shared by the analog, as been demonstrated by the experiments with R274L and H305Q. In both cases the hormone lost a contact site that was essential for either inducing the functional conformation of the receptor (H305Q) or maintaining the affinity of the hormone for the receptor (R274L). Because the analog was able to interact with these mutant VDRs in a manner that induced a functional conformation, it was able to transactivate the mutant VDRs more effectively than the natural hormone. In contrast, mutations that directly alter the ability of the VDR to interact with proteins that are essential for its transcriptional activity probably cannot be restored by analogs, as been demonstrated by the inactivity of the mutant F251C. In this case, neither the affinity of the F251C for the ligands, nor its ability to form a functional conformation in response to the ligands were altered by the mutation. Therefore, we conclude that a loss of amino acid residues that are essential for protein-protein interaction cannot be restored by differential analog binding in the LBD. We propose that HVDRR patients with mutations that directly diminish 1,25D3 contact with the VDR, be considered for alternative treatment with vitamin D analogs.

REFERENCES:
1. Malloy, P. J., Pike, J. W., and Feldman, D. (1999) Endocr. Rev. 20, 156-158.
2. Liu, Y. Y., Collins, E. D., Norman, A. W., and Peleg, S. (1997) J. Biol. Chem, 272, 3336-3345
3. Rochel, N., Wurtz, J.M., Mitschler, A., Klaholz, B., and Moras, D. (2000) Molecular Cell. 5, 173-179
4. Haussler, M. R., Jurutka, P. W., Hsieh, J-C., Thompson, P.D., Haussler, C. A., Selznick, S. H., Remus, L. S., and Whitfield., G. K. (1997) In: Vitamin D, Feldman D., Glorieux FH, and Pike J. W. (eds). Academic Press, San Diego CA. pp. 149-177

DIET AND BONE HEALTH IN BRITISH WHITE AND ASIAN WOMEN

E. Barbara Mawer, Sarah Mylchreest, Michael Davies, Peter L. Selby, Judith E. Adams, Matthew G. Dunnigan* and Jacqueline L. Berry. Musculoskeletal Research Group, University School of Medicine, Manchester Royal Infirmary, Manchester, M13 9WL, and *University Dept of Human Nutrition, Glasgow Royal Infirmary, G31 2ER, U.K.

Introduction

Vitamin D deficiency leading to privational rickets and osteomalacia remains common in the British Asian population and in the housebound and institutionalised elderly in Britain.

Epidemiological evidence suggests that meat and meat products have a protective effect in the prevention and cure of rickets and that there is a strong association between vegetarianism and the severity of privational rickets and osteomalacia (1). The omnivore British western diet appears to provide complete protection against privational rickets at low levels of sunlight exposure – the principle source of vitamin D. This is most likely due to the relatively high intakes of meat and meat products which characterise this diet.

Recent detailed analyses (2), and our own studies (3), have defined the vitamin D content of meat and it is clear that the relatively low amounts of vitamin D metabolites in meat are unlikely to be responsible for its strong protective action.

We are now studying over two winters, groups of normal British women, white or Asian (from the Indian sub-continent) eating omnivorous or lacto-vegetarian diets. Following a dose of vitamin D, we aim to study whether the utilisation of vitamin D by lactovegetarian, low meat and normal meat consumption groups of white and Asian women differ. Here we present the first year baseline data up to April 1999.

Methods

Subjects: White and Asian volunteers were recruited from staff or outpatients at Glasgow and Manchester Royal Infirmaries or from local GP surgeries or day centres.

Analyses: Serum albumin, creatinine, calcium, phosphate and iron were analysed on a multichannel autoanalyser (American Monitor Co, IN). Serum calcium was corrected for changes in serum albumin.

Intact PTH was measured by IRMA, normal range 10-60 pg/ml (Manchester samples) or by mid-molecule IRMA, normal range 61-315 pg/ml (Nichols Institute, San Juan Capistrano, CA).

Bone specific alkaline phosphatase was measured using a Metra Biosystems Inc (Mountain View, CA) Alkphase-B® immunoassay kit, female normal ranges 25-44yrs 11-30 U/L, ≥45yrs 14-43 U/L.

Serum vitamin D metabolites were extracted with acetonitrile and applied to C18 silica cartridges. 25OHD was separated and quantified using successive straight phase HPLC (Waters Associates, Milford, MA). $1,25(OH)_2D$ was separated by HPLC and measured using an in-house RIA using a monoclonal antibody, normal range 20-50 pg/ml.

Bone density was measured using dual energy X-ray absorptiometry. In Manchester total hip and spine (L1-L4) were measured using a Hologic QDR 4500 Acclaim, with software version 8.17. In Glasgow femoral neck and spine (L1-L4) were measured by Lunar DPX-AP.

Results for Manchester and Glasgow samples were analysed separately and together by univariate analysis of variance, using a generalised linear model to control for confounders

Results

The measured serum and bone parameters are summarised in Table 1.

Results from the subjects in Glasgow and Manchester have been grouped for clarity since a similar pattern of results was found in each group. Note that results for PTH and total hip are from Manchester subjects only (n=8-26).

It was found that ethnicity was a significant factor for 25OHD (P=0.005), PTH (p=0.002), iron (p=0.031), bALP (p=0.050) and BMDs (p=0.002).

Diet was a significant factor for total hip BMD (p=0.030) and bALP (p=0.009).

Conclusions

The results expose the extent of vitamin D insufficiency in the Asian female population in Manchester and Glasgow. However, they reveal the efficiency of the homeostatic system in maintaining normocalcaemia, although at the cost of secondary hyperparathyroidism.

The hip BMD data suggest that within the Manchester Asian population, a meat-containing diet may improve bone health.

Table 1

	White meat eaters (n=39)	White vegetarians (n=26)	Asianmeat eaters (n=25)	Asian vegetarians (n=22)
Age (yrs)	43.3±2.0	35.2±1.8	38.9±2.6	50.9±3.0
Ht (m)	1.62±0.01	1.65±0.02	1.58±0.02	1.57±0.02
Wt (Kg)	68.1±2.0	65.2±2.6	67.0±2.9	64.4±2.5
Calcium (mmol/l)	2.35±0.01	2.35±0.01	2.35±0.02	2.37±0.02
Iron (μmol/l)	9.6±1.4	18.1±1.4	14.9±1.7	13.1±1.2
bALP (U/L)	13.7±0.9	11.8±1.4	16.4±1.3	14.1±0.7
25OHD (ng/ml)	13.8±1.7	14.6±1.6	7.1±0.9	10.1±1.6
1,25-D (pg/ml)	36±2	41±3	41±2	40±3
PTH_{1-84} (pg/ml)	32.3±2.9	28.4±3.1	54.9±12.8	69.5±12.7
BMD spine (g/cm^2)	1.11±0.03	1.02±0.02	1.05±0.04	1.00±0.05
BMD hip (g/cm^2)	0.93±0.03	0.93±0.02	0.96±0.02	0.78±0.04

References

1. Henderson, J.B., Dunnigan, M.G., McIntosh, W.B., Abdul Motaal, A. and Hole, D (1990) Quart J Med, 1990, 76 (281):923-933.
2. Chan, W., Brown, J., Lee, SM and Buss, D.H. (1995). *Supplement to McCance and Widdowson's The Composition of Foods:* London: Royal Society for Chemistry, and the Ministry of Agriculture Fisheries and Food.
3. Mawer E.B. and Gomes U.C.S. (1994). In *Vitamin D: A Pluripotent Steroid Hormone: Structural Studies, Molecular Endocrinology and Clinical Applications.* Eds. A.W. Norman, R. Bouillon, M. Thomasset, Walter de Gruyter, Berlin, New York pp 775-776.

Vitamin D deficiency in Asians in the U.K; An audit

Dr S J Iqbal, Dr P G Swift, Leicester Royal Infirmary, Leicester LE1 5WW, U.K.

Introduction

Although nutritional/deprivational vitamin D deficiency, osteomalacia and rickets had disappeared in the indigenous U.K. population post second world war, the latter half of the 20th century saw a resurgence of this condition in selected populations. Amongst the group affected included the very elderly housebound indigenous U.K. population and the Asian migrants to the U.K. Leicestershire has a total population of 865,133 and Leicester City a population of 266,473, of which 8.9% and 23.7% respectively are Asians. As in certain other parts of the U.K. the Asian population of Leicester had grown since the early 1960s following their migration from the Indian subcontinent directly or via East Africa. We have previously described a high prevalence of vitamin D deficiency, including some clinically severe cases. Although these patients present to medical specialties, quite a number of these come via the Metabolic Bone Disease Clinic and we now describe our audit.

Neonatal Hypocalcaemia and Maternal Vitamin D deficiency

Over the past five years we have seen a number of cases of neonates with hypocalcaemia who presented to hospital with fits. These neonates required the usual management of intravenous calcium and magnesium as required, and often anti-epileptic therapy which needed to be continued for months. Neonatal vitamin D status is entirely dependent on maternal vitamin D status and it was not surprising that in following up the mothers of these neonates almost all of these had vitamin D deficiency, some of some severity. These women were appropriately treated.

Infantile Rickets

Over this period we have seen a number of cases of infantile rickets presenting with difficult with walking or bowing of legs, all of the subjects subsequently turning out to have vitamin D deficiency. These infants presented between the ages of nine months to two years or so and the majority of these were breast fed by mothers who themselves had varying levels of vitamin D deficiency. Treatment resulted in the cure of mother and children.

Adolescent Rickets

We have seen a smaller number, largely girls, aged between 14 - 16, who were noticed to have difficulty with walking and PE at school who, on subsequent examination, were found to have severe vitamin D deficiency with clinical and biochemical features.

Presentation with Bone Fracture

Asian subjects presenting with bone fracture, some of whom were screened for possible vitamin D deficiency, turned out to have severe cases. A significant number of these patients presented with pseudofractures.

Adults with Bone Pain Myopathy

We have seen over 242 (184f and 58m) subjects with suspected vitamin D deficiency. On the basis of their biochemical measures, including adjusted calcium, phosphate, alkaline phosphatase, 25 hydroxy vitamin D (25(OH)VitD) (normal range 5-40 μg/L), parathyroid hormone levels (PTH) (norman range 0.8-5.4 pmol/l). We classified these patients. Those with normal vitamin D status, normal 25(OH)VitD and normal PTH, grade 1 vitamin D deficiency 25(OH)VitD <5 μg/L, normal PTH and grade 2 vitamin D deficiency, 25(OH)VitD <5 μg/L and/or PTH >5.4 pmol/l. In these subjects 42 had normal vitamin D status, 35 had grade 1 vitamin D deficiency and 136 grade 2 vitamin D deficiency. Symptoms included bone pain 29%, back pain 20%, muscle weakness 16%, difficulty with walking 25%, joint pain 20% and 79 patients had bone fracture or pseudofracture. All these patient were treated appropriately with Calciferol and calcium supplements and responded satisfactorily after a range of 3 - 18 months. Late complications of these included non compliance, recurrence in some subjects, unmasking underlying hyperparathyroidism (primary? Tertiary?) plus a small number of subjects who have been followed up with bone densitometry showed hyperostosis bone mineral density measurements.

Treatment and Prevention

The major issue which remains is a policy for the long term prevention, not only in patients who have presented with overt disease, but in this community as a large, as our former study has shown that one in two Asian subjects is likely to be vitamin D deficient, one in four is going to have this condition with some severity.

It is recognised that the two main natural sources of vitamin D are either by food or by photosynthesis in skin under the action of sunlight. The recent COMA Report (1998) confirms that the vitamin D content of British household food has not changed very much from around 3 - 5 µg per day over the last 2½ decades. Foods, especially rich in vitamin D source, such as oily fish and eggs, are not regularly eaten. Other natural foodstuffs, such as fortified margarine, flour, cereals, will not provide enough vitamin D. It is well recognised that the major determinant of vitamin D supply in the U.K. is the summer sunlight. Vitamin D deficiency in Asian subjects is due to a variety of factors; the social and cultural habits mean covering of the body. Dietary habits mean that many of the foods which are minimally fortified are often not eaten and it has been suggested that vegetarians are especially vulnerable.

Although preventative policies have been suggested, including fortification of chapati flour or annual injections of vitamin D , none of these have really been taken up. The recent COMA Report suggests that subjects such as these should be supplemented with vitamin D and that it is up to local Health Authorities to take this further. Although vitamin D defiency in the Asians has received social, clinical and political attention, as we have left the last century and millennium it is clear that this problem is very much an issue. For a condition which is simply preventable and treatable implementation of such a policy is long overdue.

(The author is very grateful for the support he has received from other consultant and junior

colleagues in these studies).

References

Dunnigan MG, Paton JPJ, Haase S, McNichol GW, Smith CM. Late Rickets and osteomalacia in Pakistani community in Glasgow. Scot Med J 1962; 7: 159-67.

Iqbal SJ, Kaddam I, Wassif W, Nichol F, Walls J. Continuing clinically severe vitamin D deficiency in Asians in the UK (Leicester). Postgrad Med J 1994; 70: 708-714.

Iqbal SJ, Garrick DP, Howl A. Evidence of continuing "deprivational" vitamin D deficiency in Asians in the UK. J Hum Nutr & Diet 1994; 7: 47-52.

Committee on Medical Aspects of Food and Nutritional Policy Sub Group on Bone Health. Nutrition and Bone Health: with particular reference to calcium and vitamin D. Department of Health 1998; 49. Stationery Office, London.

CLINICAL PRESENTATION OF VITAMIN D DEFICIENCY AMONG ADULTS AND CHILDREN

Henning Glerup*, Lene Rytter**, Erik Fink Eriksen*. *Department of Endocrinology, Aarhus Amtssygehus, DK-8000 C, Denmark, E-mail: h.glerup@dadlnet.dk, ** Department of Pediatric Dis., Aarhus University Hospital.

Introduction: We have studied the vitamin D status among adult and children immigrants of Palestinian origin living in Denmark. Due to cultural habits Palestinians use to avoid direct sunlight exposure of the skin. Moving to Denmark in more northern latitude (56°N) results in a high risk of development of vitamin D deficiency. The aims of our study were to evaluate the incidence of vitamin D deficiency among Palestinian immigrants in Denmark, and to describe their vitamin D deficiency related symptoms.

Methods and study group: We included 60 adult Palestinian women and 44 age matched ethnic Danish controls (Age: 32.2±1.4 vs 36.1±1.6 years, NS) randomly selected among patients coming to see the doctor in a primary health care centre. From the same primary health care centre 66 Palestinian children (0 – 16 years) were included and compared to 111 ethnic Danish controls. Blood tests for analysis of serum levels of 25-hydroxyvitamin D_{2+3} were used for estimation of vitamin D status. Further serum levels of 1,25-dihydroxyvitamin D, PTH(1-84), Calcium and alkaline phosphatase were measured. Hypovitaminosis D related symptoms were evaluated by the use of a standardised questionnaire. A DEXA scanner was used for estimation of bone mineral density. In adults muscle strength of the quadriceps muscle was estimated by an isometric dynamometer. In children "bone age" was estimated from analysis of a x-ray of the hand and forearm.

Results: Severe vitamin D deficiency was very common among adult Palestinian women with 88% having serum levels of 25-OHD < 10 nmol/l (mean 7.1±1.1 nmol/l) compared to 47.1±4.6 nmol/l ($p < 10^{-17}$) among Danish controls (1). Among Palestinian children s-25-OHD < 25 nmol/l was seen in 44% in the age 0 – 8 years and in 81% in the age 9 – 16 years, with secondary hyperparathyroidism seen in 15% and 44%. Mean levels among Palestinian girls were: 0 – 8 years 26.0±3.0 nmol/l, 9 – 16 years 11.7±2.7 nmol/l, Palestinian boys: 0 – 8 years 27.4±4.8 nmol/l, 9 –16 years 18.2±3.2 nmol/l compared to Danish controls 26.2 – 37.5 nmol/l (Winter values, 95% limits).
Hypovitaminosis D related symptoms were very common among adult Palestinians (2). 88% complained of diffuse muscle pain compared to 32% in Danish controls (p < 0.01), 26% experienced a change in gait vs 9% in controls (p < 0.03), 32% had difficulties in ascending a staircase or raising from a chair vs 14 % among controls (p < 0.04), 59% complained of acroparaesthesias compared to 0% in controls (3) (despite only 6% of the Palestinians had subnormal serum levels of calcium). Other common complaints were deep bone pain, fatigue,

muscle cramps and difficulties in carrying loads. All symptoms consequently improved during vitamin D treatment with bone pain being the longest lasting symptom. Among children hypovitaminosis D related symptoms were not very common, and was almost exclusively seen among the oldest children with closed growth zones.

DEXA-scan results showed that BMD of the lumbar spine and the hip was significantly reduced in adult Palestinians compared to controls: 0.92 ± 0.02 vs 1.03 ± 0.02 g/cm^2 ($p < 0.01$) and 0.78 ± 0.02 vs 0.83 ± 0.02 g/cm^2 ($p < 0.01$). High dose vitamin D and calcium treatment resulted in a 13.7% increase in lumbar BMD ($p < 10^{-4}$) and a 17.0% increase in hip BMD ($p < 10^{-3}$) (2). In children lumbar BMD tended to be lower in the age of maximal growth (11 – 14 years) but did not reach significance.

"Bone age" estimated from x-ray was reduced with sign of broadening of the growth zones in 26% of the Palestinian children.

Qudriceps muscle strength was found to be significantly reduced in vitamin D deficient adults compared to controls (259.4 ± 11.0 vs 392.6 ± 11.4 N, $p < 10^{-6}$) (4). Also muscle kinetics was disturbed, resulting in weaker and slower muscles. Based on the most commonly used biochemical marker for hypovitaminosis D related osteomalacia, vitamin deficient adults were divided into two groups: those with increased levels of alkaline phosphatase and those with alkaline phosphatase within the normal levels. Muscle strength was demonstrated to be equally reduced in the two groups compared to controls with normal levels of 25-OHD.

High dose vitamin D treatment (100.000 IU weekly for one month followed by 100.000 IU monthly) in six months resulted in significant improvement in quadriceps muscle power (320.7 ± 14.3 N, $p < 0.005$) and a complete normalisation of muscle kinetics.

Correlation analysis showed that both muscle power measurements and hypovitaminosis D related symptoms were significantly correlated to 25-OHD but not to 1,25-$(OH)_2$D.

Discussion: The clinical presentation of vitamin D deficiency seems to differ among adults and children. In adults with serum levels of 25-OHD < 25 nmol/l hypovitaminosis D related symptoms are very common, and knowledge of the typical clinical symptoms makes it easy to diagnose the disease. However, none of the symptoms are specific for hypovitaminosis D, and consequently rheumatic or even malignant diseases are often suspected instead. Hypovitaminosis D myopathy (HDM) is very common among adults with vitamin D deficiency. Our studies indicate that HDM is already maximal before biochemical signs of osteomalacic bone disease are present. This makes HDM an early clinical sign of vitamin D deficiency. It is important; however, to understand that the patient seldom will complain over muscle weakness before they lose the ability to do daily activities (ex. raising from a chair or ascending a staircase), their complaints would rather be fatigue. HDM is a reversible disease, - full normalisation of the muscle function can be expected 3 – 12 months after initiation of high dose vitamin D treatment. It is therefore of vital importance to measure s-25-OHD and eventually PTH on the suspicion of HDM, as these blood tests are the only reliable screening tests for HDM.

In children the hypovitaminosis D related symptoms seems to be less pronounced. We saw only complaints of bone and muscle pain among the elderly children. The mean values of 25-OHD were lower among Palestinian adults compared to children, but still we saw very low values of 25-OHD among children in all age groups. Muscle strength was not measured among children due to methodological problems, and consequently the presence of HDM among vitamin D deficient children can not be excluded, but the symptom seems to be less pronounced.

In adults we demonstrated significantly reduced BMD in both the hip and the lumbar spine. Treatment with vitamin D and calcium resulted in a significant increase in BMD in both locations, indicating that hypovitaminosis D osteopathy are very common among vitamin D deficient adults. In children we could only demonstrate a trend towards lower BMD in the age group with accelerated growth during puberty (11 – 14 years), but the difference did not reach significance. In the study of adults we have demonstrated severe osteomalacia also among very young girls (18 – 22 years) in whom we can demonstrate very low pretreatment BMD values. In the vitamin D deficient children we saw broadening of the growth zone in 26%. We suggests, that vitamin D deficiency in children with open growth zones primarily affects the length growth, whereas after the closure of the growth zone vitamin D deficiency leads to osteomalacia.

We demonstrated that muscle power measurement correlated to s-25-OHD (voluntary knee extension: $r = 0.34$, $p < 0.001$; electrical stimulated knee extension: $r = 0.42$, $p < 0.001$) and not to s-1,25$(OH)_2$D. The explanation of this phenomenon could be that 25-OHD has a direct effect on skeletal muscle. Alternatively 1,25$(OH)_2$D could be synthesised locally in the tissue, where it should be utilised. A local production of 1,25$(OH)_2$D will be dependent on the serum levels of the substrate 25-OHD.

Conclusions: The clinical presentation of vitamin D deficiency seems to differ among children and adults. In children the symptoms can be very few if the rickets is not severe. Broadening of the growth zones on x-ray can lead to the diagnosis. Reduced length growth in vitamin D deficiency is very likely. In adults the diagnosis can be suspected when the patient present symptoms as diffuse muscle pain, muscle cramps, acroparaesthesias, fatigue, muscle weakness, and deep bone pain. The diagnosis is confirmed by demonstration of low levels of 25-OHD and eventually secondary hyperparathyroidism. Treatment with ergocalciferol/cholecalciferol in megadosis (100.000 IU weekly) in combination with calcium (800 – 1200 mg daily) will often result in significant improvement within a month and complete normalisation within 3 – 12 months.

A daily supply of 1000 IU vitamin D to all risk groups will efficiently prevent vitamin D deficiency.

Reference List

1. Glerup, H., Thomsen, J., Mikkelsen, K., Poulsen, L., Hass, E., Overbeck, S., Charles, P., and Eriksen, E.F. (2000) *J.Intern.Med.* **247**, 260-268

2. Glerup, H. Investigations on the role of vitamin D in muscle function - A study of muscle function in vitamin D deficient humans and the effect of treatment with vitamin D. (1999) PhD-thesis;University of Aarhus, Denmark

3. Glerup, H. and Eriksen, E.F. (1999) *Br.J.Rheumatol.* **38**, 482-482

4. Glerup, H., Mikkelsen, K., Poulsen, L., Hass, E., Overbeck, S., Andersen, H., Charles, P., and Eriksen, E.F. (2000) *Calcif.Tissue Int.* , June issue, 2000.

PROGRESSIVE FAMILIAL INTRAHEPATIC CHOLESTASIS SYNDROME LEADING TO SEVERE RICKETS AND FRACTURES.

C.Tau*, V.Alvarez*, S.Lopez•, M.Cuarterolo•, M.Ciocca•, O.Brunetto# and MT García Davila∞.
*Laboratorio de Metabolismo Cálcico, Endocrinología, •Hepatology Section, Gastroenterología, ∞Patología, Hospital de Pediatría J.P.Garrahan and #Endocrinología, Hospital de Niños Pedro Elizalde, Buenos Aires, Argentina.

Introduction. Progressive Familial Intrahepatic Cholestasis(PFIC) is a group of inherited disorders in childhood characterized by severe cholestasis of hepatocellular origin, progressing to biliary cirrhosis and chronic liver failure usually during the first decade of life(1). There is heterogeneity in this group of clinical cholestasis suggesting the existence of different disorders affecting the hepatocytes and related to defects of bile acid secretion or bile acid metabolism (2). Clinical features include jaundice, hepatomegaly, growth retardation and sometimes severe pruritus. Bilirrubin and bile acids are increased in serum. Bile acids as ursodeoxycholic acid (UDCA) in some cases are an effective medical therapy for PFIC. Rickets has been reported in children with cholestasis as well as in biliary atresia, Alagille syndrome or inborn error of cholesterol and bile acid metabolism(3-6). We show a case of an infant with PFIC in whom rickets and fractures were the form of presentation.

Case Report. Caucasian girl born by cesarean, in Rio Grande, Argentina (52º southern latitude), fullterm, birth weight 3.2 kg. She developed jaundice since birth. When she was 5 months old (during spring), she had fractures on wrist, tibia and fibula. She received a unique dose of oral vitamin D 450,000 IU.

She was admitted when she was 10 months old with stunted growth (height Z-Score -3.79 and weight 7.9 kg), jaundice, hepatosplenomegaly, pale stools, dark urine, pruritus and bone pain. The laboratory showed: normal serum calcium(Ca) and reduced phosphate(P), increased alkaline phosphatases(AP), low 25-hydroxyvitamin D(25OHD) and calcitriol(1,25(OH)2D), and increased parathyroid hormone (PTH) with low tubular resorption of phosphate (TRP) indicating secondary hyperparathyroidism (Table 1). Serum bilirrubin(TBit/DBid) and transaminases(AST/ALT) were increased with normal gamma-glutamyl-transpeptidase (GGT), cholesterol, albumin and prothrombin time(PT). Vitamins A and E were both low(Table2).

A liver biopsy showed bile duct paucity with lobular and perisinusoidal fibrosis and hepato-canalicular cholestasis. X-rays showed evident and severe rickets in wrists, ankles and knees with signs of fractures and periostitis. Spine bone mineral density(BMD) showed severe osteopenia: 0.20 g/cm2, Z-Score: -4.03.

Inborn error of cholesterol and bile acid metabolism was excluded.The diagnosis of Progressive Familial Intrahepatic Cholestasis type Byler Syndrome was made by the cholestasis, pruritus, normal GGT and compatible biopsy.

Table 1: Biochemical parameters of bone metabolism:

Age(months)	10	14	16	19	21	normal value
Ca(mg/dl)	9.0	9.1	9.6	9.5	10.1	8.8-10.6
P(mg/dl)	2.5	1.6	2.5	4.8	4.4	4.1-5.8
ALK (IU/L)	3197	3980	2132	1193	987	150-550
Creat (mg/dl)	0.49	0.20	0.19	0.38	0.28	0.1-0.6
PTH (pg/ml)	301	528	-	27	-	12-72
25(OH)D (ng/ml)	9	8	-	5	4	10-40
1.25(OH)2D(pg/ml)	-	32	-	-		40-100
UCa (mg/mgCreat)	0.09	-	0.07	0.06	-	<0.21
TRP (%)	-47	-	-	-	-	80-95

Ca was measured by atomic absorption spectrophotometry. P, creatinin, liver function tests and AP by Autoanalyzer. PTH was measured by chemilluminiscence method and 25OHD by competitive protein binding assay. The detection of inborn errors in the cholesterol-bile acid biosynthetic pathway were analized in urine and serum in the Children Hospital of Cincinnati using fast atom bombardment ionization mass spectrometry. Lumbar Bone mineral density L1-L4, was measured by dual x-ray absorptiometry (DEXA Hologic 1000).

Table 2: Biochemical parameters of liver function:

Age(months)	10	14	16	19	21	normal value
AST (IU/L)	341	187	346	371	476	15-45
ALT (IU/L)	359	205	260	321	334	15-45
TBil (mg/dl)	4.6	2.1	-	-	12.2	0-1
DBil (mg/dl)	3.9	1.9	-	-	10.7	0-1
Cholesterol(mg/dl)	240	239	-	138	148	<200
GGT(U/L)	20	18	22	27	33	4-32
PT(%)	88	100	47	-	90	70-100
Retinol (ug/dl)	-	16	-	20	26.7	20-50
∂- tocopherol(ug/dl)	-	7	-	101	269	>600

Treatment. The patient was treated with UDCA 15 to 30 mg/day, vitamin A 100,000 IU/week, vitamin K 10 mg/ week, vitamin E 200 and vitamin D, 7,500 IU/day, calcium 500 mg/day(Table 3). After 9 months of treatment (19 months old), the patient had a good clinical bone response, beginning to walk and felling stronger. Height was (Z-Score) -3.28. Biochemical parameters of bone metabolism responded well to therapy: phosphate and PTH reached normal values, AP decreased but 25OHD remained low. Despite improved bone metabolism, liver function impaired, jaundice persisted, pruritus was intensive and prothrombin time began to be prolonged. Rickets improved on X-rays and deposition of bone mineral was present at the metaphyseal end of the bone. Bone mass increased 50%(BMD: 0.30 gr/cm2, Z-Score: -2.94).

Table 3. Treatment:

Age (months)	10	14	16	19	21
Vitamin D (IU)	450,000	770,000	1,247,500	1,327,500	1,597,500
UDCA (mg/k/d)		15-30		33	49
Calcium (mg/d)		500			
Vitamin A (IU/wk)			100,000		
Vitamin E (IU/d)			200		
Vitamin K (mg/wk)			10		

Comments. We present a case of an infant with Progressive Familial Intrahepatic Cholestasis related to a defect of bile acid secretion, with vitamin D deficient rickets resistant to large amounts of vitamin D. This infant presented jaundice very early in life, but, since it was intermitent, the diagnosis of cholestasis was initially omitted and fractures were the first sign of disease. The initial bone X-rays showed rickets that improved after large amounts of vitamin D. Hypocalcemia, osteopenia and rickets are often a complication in neonatal cholestasis (3-5,7). Recently, rickets in infancy has also been related to an inborn error of bile acid synthesis (6). Low levels of 25OHD without rickets on X-rays have also been described in several reports of children with chronic cholestasis(4).

Vitamin D deficiency in PFIC is probably due to impaired intestinal absorption of vitamin D secondary to low duodenal concentration of bile acid without effective solubilisation and absorption of lipids. Absorption and enterohepatic circulation of vitamin D are altered(8). Furthermore our patient had low serum concentration of vitamin D and other lipid soluble vitamins: A, E and K. A defect of 25-hydroxylation of vitamin D may also be a contributory factor.

An error in cholesterol-bile acid metabolism was ruled out in our patient. Liver biopsy with bile duct paucity , was indicative of intrahepatic cholestasis with loss of intralobular bile duct, a pathognomonic finding of biliary transport system dysfunction. All other causes of childhood cholestasis were excluded. Recent molecular and genetic studies have identified genes responsible for three types of PFIC (9): types 1 and 2 (Byler Disease and Byler Syndrome respectively) have low to normal GGT activity and cholesterol, whereas GGT activity is

950

increased in type 3. Bile acid replacement therapy was not effective in the management of this patient since liver function tests did not normalize. At present, the patient is waiting for external biliary diversion or liver transplantation as an attempt to reverse clinical symptomatology and improve liver function .

Our patient continued with severe vitamin D deficiency despite large amounts of vitamin D and improved biochemical bone metabolism parameters and X-rays. Rickets improved but severe osteopenia persisted despite the bone gain. Calcitriol level was low before treatment and could not be measured after therapy. Probably the 25OHD remained very low because its transformation in calcitriol was very fast and the dose of vitamin D, even it was large, was not enough to stock vitamin D. Finally, early diagnosis is essential in these patients to avoid nutritional and vitamin deficiencies, usually present in chronic cholestasis.

Summary. An infant with Progressive Familial Intrahepatic Cholestasis who developed evident early liver disease and resistant and severe rickets with osteopenia at infancy, is presented. Although liver alteration persisted, great quantities of vitamin D, calcium and stimulation of bile flow, resulted in considerable clinical, biochemical, radiologic and bone mass improvement.

References.
1-Bull I.N.,Carlton VEH, Stricker NL, Baharloo S, Deyoung JA, Freimer NB, Magid MS,Kahn E,Markowitz J, Dicarlo FJ, McLoughlin L, Boyle JT, Dahms BB,Faught PR,Fitzgerald JF,Piccoli DA, Witzleben CL, O'Connell NC, Setchell KDR,Agostini RM,Kocoshis SA,Reyes J andKnisely AS.(1997), Hepatology, 26,155-164.
2-Jaquemin E. (1999) J. Gastroenterol. Hepatol. 14, 594-599.
3- Kooh S,Jones G,Reilly B and Fraser D. (1979) J.Pediatr.94, 870-874.
4-Kobayashi Akio, Kawai Sakae, Ohkubo Michiko and Ohbe Yoshiro (1979) Arch Dis Child. 54, 367-370.
5-Harrison HE and Harrison HC in Disorders of calcium and phosphate metabolism in childhood and adolescence,Saunders (1979), p.169.
6-Akobeng A, Clayton P, Miller V, Super M. and Thomas A. (1999) Arch Dis Child,80, 463-465.
7- Heubi J, Hollis B,Specker B and Tsang R. (1989) Hepatology 9,258-264.
8-Sokol R, Farrell M,Heubi J,Tsang R and Balistreri W.(1983) J.Pediatr.103,712-717.
9-Jansen PL, Muller M.(2000) Can J Gastroenterol, 14, 233-238.

1α,25(OH)₂ VITAMIN D PLASMATIC LEVELS IN EXPERIMENTAL ANIMALS DOSED WITH AQUEOUS EXTRACTS OF *SOLANUM GLAUCOPHYLLUM*

María Elena Dallorso*, Sandra Eva Pawlak**, Susana Beatriz Gil**, Fabián Lema* and Adrián Gustavo Márquez***.

* Facultad de Ciencias Agrarias, Universidad Nacional de Lomas de Zamora. Ruta Nacional 4 Km 2 (1836), Buenos Aires, Argentina.

** Centro Atómico Ezeiza. Comisión Nacional de Energía Atómica. Argentina.

*** Facultad de Ciencias Veterinarias, Universidad de Buenos Aires. Argentina.

Introduction Enteque Seco is a disease of bovine grazing on low lands of the main breeding area of Argentina (1). The presence of *S. glaucophyllum* in enzootic areas and the experimental reproduction of the disease using dry leaves of the plant (2) led to the hypothesis that continuous ingestion of fallen leaves, during summer and fall, was the determinant cause of the syndrome (3). The 1α,25(OH)₂ vitamin D₃- glycoside was identified in this plant (4), in addition, glycosides containing vitamin D₃, 25(OH) vitamin D₃ and other aglycones without identification were encountered (5). Early augmentation of 1α,25(OH)₂ vitamin D plasmatic levels in chicks (6) and rats(7) dosed with *S. glaucophyllum* were reported in previous works employing vitamin D deficient animals. Based on these results it was hypothesized that 1α,25(OH)₂ vitamin D plasmatic concentration would be augmented in animals grazing in enzootic areas. Intoxication trials carried out to know 1α,25(OH)₂ vitamin D plasma concentration of bovines dosed with *S. glaucophyllum* showed higher levels in cows dosed with 50 g/week but failed to detect differences with control group in cows administered with 10 g/week. Both treatments led to clinical and biochemical signs of disease (8,9). The results mentioned above pointed out the fact that yet it is not known: the time evolution of the glycoside hydrolysis as a function of doses, the ulterior disappearance from blood of the liberated aglycone and, finally, details about the presence in blood of the other secosteroids present in *S. glaucophyllum.* With the aim to answer some of these questions and to compare ruminant and monogastric active principle metabolism, a series of experiments in ewes and rabbits administered with *S. glaucophyllum* by different routes, were conducted.

Materials and methods The *S. glaucophyllum* was harvested in Buenos Aires Province, Argentina, in February 1994, 1995, 1996 and 1999. Aqueous extracts (AE) were prepared incubating dry powdered leaves (DM) with distilled water during 1 hour at 38°C. The AE (0,33 g DM/ml) were filtered by cheese-cloth, by a Millipore filter (0.22 μm) and stored at -20°C in dark bottle closed under N₂. Animals were assigned at random to experimental groups and maintained in individual cages and fed dry standard diet (Cargill, Rabbits, Argentina), *ad-libitum.*. Heparinized blood samples obtained in the experiments were immediately centrifuged at 10.000 rpm for 10 min. and plasma separated and frozen until analysis. 1α,25(OH)₂ vitamin D plasma concentration was determined in the lipid extract of 1 ml aliquots. The supernatant obtained after lipid extraction was directly applied to octadecyl solid phase extraction cartridges (Bakerbond spe, 500 mg, Baker). The 1α,25(OH)₂ vitamin D fraction was dried under N₂ and diluted in ethanol for radioreceptor assay (RRA) (pg/ml) (10). The metabolite concentration was transformed to its decimal logarithm in order to normalize its frequency distribution. Differences were considered as significant at the 0.05 cut- off level of P value.

Experiment 1: Twelve New Zealand White (NZW) adult rabbits, body weight between 2 and 3 kg, were used. The dosed animals (n=7) were administered orally with an AE equivalent to 100 mg of DM/kg. of body weight, every day for 5, 7 or 9 days (Tr5, Tr7, Tr9). Control rabbits (n=5) were maintained with dosed animals during the experiment (C5, C7, C9). Animals were euthanized by complete bleeding under anesthesia with ether by cardiac puncture, 24 hours after 5- 7 or 9 doses according to the treatment, to collect the blood. Plasma $1\alpha,25(OH)_2$ vitamin D was studied by Student "t" Two Sample Test considering treatments (Tr, C) and by One Way Analysis of Variance (AOV), considering number of doses (0, 5, 7 and 9 doses). Linear regression analysis (LRA) of plasma $1\alpha,25(OH)_2$ vitamin D as a function of cumulative doses (CD) was practiced.

Experiment 2: Six NZW adult rabbits, body weight of 3,15±0.42 kg. were used. Group 1 (n=2): the animals were administered daily, by the oral route, with an AE equivalent to 100 mg of DM/kg. of body weight, during 17 days. Group 2 (n=2): the animals were administered daily, by the subcutaneous (s.c.) route, with an AE equivalent to 100 mg of DM/kg. of body weight, during 17 days. Group 3 (n=2): the animals remained as controls throughout the trial. At day 18 of the experiment animals were euthanized by complete bleeding under anesthesia with ether by cardiac puncture to collect the blood. Plasma $1\alpha,25(OH)_2$ vitamin D was studied by One Way AOV among groups of treatments.

Experiment 3: Six NZW adult rabbits, body weight of 2,81± 0,39 kg. were used. Group 1 (n=2): the animals were administered daily, by the oral route, with an AE equivalent to 200 mg of DM/kg. of body weight, during 5 days. Group 2 (n=2): the animals were administered daily, by the oral route, with an AE equivalent to 400 mg of DM/kg. of body weight, during 5 days. Group 3 (n=2): the animals remained as controls throughout the trial. At day 6th of the experiment animals were euthanized by complete bleeding under anesthesia with ether by cardiac puncture to collect the blood. Plasma $1\alpha,25(OH)_2$ vitamin D was studied by One Way AOV among groups of treatments. LRA between plasma concentration of $1\alpha,25(OH)_2$ vitamin D as a function of CD was practiced.

Experiment 4: Four cross-breed adult ewes weighing 54±18 kg. were used. Group 1 (n=2): the animals were administered with a single oral dose of an AE equivalent to 3,00 g of DM. Group 2 (n=2): the animals were administered with a single s.c. dose of an AE equivalent to 3,00 g of DM. Blood samples were obtained by jugular puncture immediately before the administration and 0,5 - 2 - 4 - 6 - 8 - 29 and 31 hours after it. It was assumed that basal values of $1\alpha,25(OH)_2$ vitamin D were normal (11,12), considered as population parameters and compared with values obtained after dosing in Group 1 (n=14) and Group 2 (n=14) separately, by the Student "t" One Sample Test. The values at the peak of the plasma concentration of $1\alpha,25(OH)_2$ vitamin D of each ewe along the trial were obtained, and compared between routes of administration (n=2) by the Student "t" Two Sample Test.

Experiment 5: Six NZW adult rabbits weighing 2,51±0,21 kg. were used. Group 1 (n=2): the animals were administered with a single oral dose of an AE equivalent to 1,00 g of DM. Group 2 (n=2): the animals were administered with a single s.c. dose of an AE equivalent to 1,00 g of DM. Group 3 (n=2): the animals remained as controls throughout the experiment. Blood samples were obtained from the marginal veins of the ears immediately before the administration and 1 - 4 - 6 - 8 – 24- 48- 72- 96- 120 and 168 hours after it. Plasma $1\alpha,25(OH)_2$ vitamin D levels among times after administration were compared by Kruskal Wallis non parametric AOV, within each group.

<u>Results</u> *Experiment 1:* Mean value of plasma concentration of $1\alpha,25(OH)_2$ vitamin D of control group was 41±7 pg/ ml. Treatment led to five to eight fold increments from basal values, being statistically significant considering treatment (p=0.0016) and number of doses (p=0.0097). There was significant LRA of plasma $1\alpha,25(OH)_2$ vitamin D ([1,25]) as a function of CD, between 0 and 900 mg of DM/kg. of body weight: [1,25]=43.44+0.12*CD (p=0.0002; R^2=0.87)   (1)

Experiment 2:.Basal mean value was 15±14 pg/ml. There were significant differences among groups (p=0.04). Rabbits dosed by either route showed up to eighteen fold increments in the plasmatic concentration of the metabolite over control rabbits.

Experiment 3: Mean value of control group was 26±5 pg/ml. There were significant differences among groups (p=0.02) and also significant LRA of [1,25] as a function of CD, between 0 and 2000 mg of DM/kg. of body weight: [1,25]=14.75+0.64*CD (p=0.03; R^2=0.85) (2)

Experiment 4: The 1α,25(OH)$_2$ vitamin D values of plasma samples taken before dosing and during the first 31 hours after dosing, in each ewe, are showed in Figure 1. Values obtained after dosing were higher than basal ones (p=0.0000) in orally dosed ewes. Plasma 1α,25(OH)$_2$ vitamin D of animals dosed by s.c. route did not show any increment (p=0.262). The peaks of the aglycone plasma concentration of each ewe were different comparing s.c. and oral routes (p=0.04).

Experiment 5: The metabolite levels of rabbits dosed by a single oral dose increased (p=0,05) from the first hour to the 24th hour (the peak occurred during the 6th hour). Animals dosed by the s.c. route showed augmented levels (p=0,05) from the 6th hour to the 24th hour (the highest value appeared during the 8th hour) post administration (see Figure 2). At this time (24th hour) the metabolite levels were equal in rabbits dosed by either route.

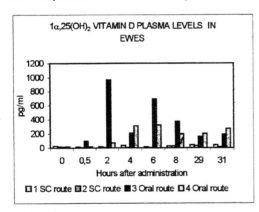

Figure 1

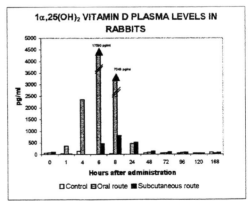

Figure 2

<u>Discussion</u> Plasma levels of the active metabolite of vitamin D have been previously measured in normal adult rabbits (11,12) and ewes (13,14) giving results comparable with ours. Calcinotic lesions and soft tissue calcium accumulation (data not shown) were seen simultaneously with augmented plasma levels of 1α25(OH)$_2$ vitamin D, in the rabbits dosed by both routes with *S. glaucophyllum* (15,16). Intoxication trials in ewes dosed by the s.c. route have not been conducted.

Conclusions Rabbits dosed with *S. glaucophyllum* showed higher $1\alpha,25(OH)_2$ vitamin D plasma levels than control in a dose related manner.

Rabbits and ewes dosed with *S. glaucophyllum* by the oral route showed higher plasma levels of the metabolite since the first hour after administration.

$1\alpha,25(OH)_2$ vitamin D plasma levels of ewes dosed with *S. glaucophyllum* by the oral route remained higher than control group up to 31 hours after administration. Ewes dosed by the subcutaneous route did not show any augmentation of the metabolite plasma levels up to 31 hours after administration.

Rabbits dosed by both routes showed increments of the plasma metabolite although those administered by the oral route reached the highest values before than those rabbits subcutaneously dosed.

References

1- Carrillo BJ, Worker NA. (1967) Rev Invest Agrop INTA,S4 Patol Anim, VI, 9-30

2- Carrillo BJ, Tilley NE, Gaggino P, Ruksan B, et al.(1971) Gaceta Veterinaria 33, 468-484

3- Gimeno E. (1977) Rev Med Vet 58, 149-161

4- Haussler MR, Wasserman RH, MC Cain TA, et al. (1976) Life Sci 18, 1049-1056

5- Esparza M, Vega M, Boland R. (1982) Biochem et Biophys Acta 719, 633-640

6- Peterlik M, Bursac K, Haussler MR, et al. (1976) Biochemical and Biophysical Research Communications 70, 797-804

7- Nápoli JL, Reeve LE, Eisman JA, et al. (1977) The Journal of Biological Chemistry 252, 2580-2583

8- Dallorso ME, Bozzo J, Benassati S, et al. (1994b) VII Congreso Argentino de Ciencias Veterinarias, Bs As, Noviembre-Diciembre.

9- Dallorso ME, Bozzo JA, Picardi H, et al. (1994a) Rev Med Vet 75,187-192

10- Reinhart T, Horst R, Orf J, et al. (1984) J. Clin Endocr and Metab 58, 91-98

11- Kubota M, Ohno J, Shiina Y and Suda T(1982) Endocrinology 110, 1950-1956

12- Fairham J and Harcourt-Brown F (1999) Vet. Rec. 145, 452-454

13- Maunder E, Pillay A and Care A (1986) Q. J. Exp. Physiol.71, 391-399

14- Paulson S and Langman C (1990) Comp. Biochem. Physiol. A 96, 347-349

15- Dallorso, M.E.;Lema, F.;Picardi, H.; Carou, N.;Gil, S y Márquez, A.(1998) Rev. Veterinaria e Zootecnia. UNESP, Sao Paulo, Brasil. (in Press)

16- Dallorso M, Gil S, Pawlak E, Lema F and Márquez A (2000) Austr. Vet. J. (sent to Editorial Comittee)

OTHER TOPICS

The function of vitamin D receptor in transcriptional repression.

Ken-ichi Takeyama, Akiko Murayama, Takafumi Asahina, Masayo Sindo, Junn Yanagisawa, Shigeaki Kato, Institute of Molecular and Cellular Biosciences, The University of Tokyo, Bunkyo-ku, Tokyo, and CREST, Japan Science and Technology Corporation, Kawaguchisi, Saitama, Japan

Introduction Vitamin D has roles in a variety of biological actions such as calcium homeostasis, cell proliferation and cell differentiation to many target tissues. Most of such biological actions of vitamin D are now considered to be exerted through nuclear vitamin D receptor(VDR)-mediated control of target genes. VDR belongs to the nuclear hormone receptor superfamily and acts as a ligand-inducible transcription factor. For the ligand-induced transctivation of VDR, the coactivator complexes have been recently shown essential(1). In addition of the target genes induced by vitamin D, there is a particular set of target genes, whose expressions are repressed by vitamin D(2). We have cloned the cDNA of 25-hydroxyvitamin D_3 1α -hydroxylase[1α(OH)ase] from the VDR gene knock-out mice(3). We showed that the gene expression of this enzyme is under negative control of vitamin D in intact animals(3). We furtheromore delineated a negative regulatory element by vitamin D(negative Vitamin D response element; nVDRE) in this gene promoter. We are currently characterizing the newly identified factor bound to the nVDRE in the human 1α(OH)ase gene promoter in terms of transcripional control of the vitamin D target genes.

Result & Discussion A hormonal form of vitamin D, $1\alpha,25$(OH)$_2$D$_3$, is metabolically formed through two steps of hydroxylation at the final stage(4). First, vitamin D is hydroxylated in the liver to 25-dihydroxyvitamin D_3 (25(OH)D$_3$), which is subsequently hydroxylated in the kidney to $1\alpha,25$(OH)$_2$D$_3$. For metabolic inactivation of 25(OH)D$_3$, or $1\alpha,25$(OH)$_2$D$_3$, the 24-hydroxylation to form 24,25(OH)$_2$D$_3$ or $1\alpha,24,25$(OH)$_3$D$_3$, is the first step in degradation of vitamin D.

The serum level of 1 α,25(OH)$_2$D$_3$ is kept constant in the normal state, and is strictly regulated in response to factors controlling calcium homeostasis. The regulation of 1α,25(OH)$_2$D$_3$ and 24, 25(OH)$_2$D$_3$ production by these factors is conducted by altering the activities of the enzymes that hydroxylate vitamin D derivatives. Vitamin D$_3$-25-hydroxylase(CYP27) catalyzes hepatic 25-hydroxylation, and renal 1α-hydroxylation is catalyzed by 25-hydroxyvitamin D$_3$ 1α - hydroxylase[1α(OH)ase]. The serum level of 1α, 25(OH)$_2$D$_3$ is strictly regulated in response to calcium requirement in body. Several enzymes, which are regulated by several factors including 1 α, 25(OH)$_2$D$_3$, are involved in synthesis and metabolism of 1α, 25(OH)$_2$D$_3$. The activities of 25(OH)D 1α-hydroxylase and 24-hydroxylase are regulated negatively and positively by 1α, 25(OH)$_2$D$_3$(4). In the VDR null mutant mice, a marked increase in serum 1 α, 25(OH)$_2$D, and a clear reduction in serum 24, 25(OH)$_2$D were seen, suggesting increased activity of 1α(OH)ase and reduced activity of 24-hydroxylase(5). Thus, it is clear that the expression of this enzyme is under a negative control of 1 α, 25(OH)$_2$D-bound VDR. Indeed, from the VDR KO mice, we for the first time reported to clone the cDNA encoding mouse 25(OH)D 1α-hydroxylase by a newly developed expression cloning method(3). This method is based on a principle that only 1α, 25(OH)$_2$D$_3$, but not any precursor and metabolite, can activate the transactivation function of VDR by its direct binding(Fig. 1). Therefore, when the 25(OH)D$_3$ is added to the medium, VDR is activated only in the cells expressing 1α(OH)ase. The predicted amino acid sequences revealed that 1α(OH)ase proteins harbor a mitochondrial target signal and two conserved regions(the sterol-binding domain and the heme -binding domain) , and significant homology throughout the entire amino acid sequence is found among the p450 enzymes. Mouse 1α(OH)ase exhibits most significant homologies to the vitamin D hydoxylases : 41.7 % homologous to the rat vitamin D$_3$-25-hydroxylase(CYP27), and 31.6 % homologous to the mouse 25(OH)D$_3$-24-hydroxylase (CYP24). The organization of the human 1α(OH)ase gene is composed of nine exons extending over 5 Kbp(6), and resembles those of the other p450 enzymes that hydroxylate steroids.

Cloning method for 1α-hydroxylase cDNA

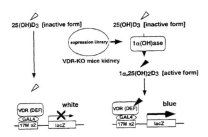

Figure 1.Illustration of the novel expression cloning method for mouse 25-hydroxyvitamin D3 1α-hydroxylase cDNA.

The reporter plasmid containing the β-galactosidase(LacZ) was co-transfected in Cos cells with the expression vector encoding the VDR ligand binding DEF region fused to the GAL4 DNA binding doamin. Precursor form of vitamin D[25(OH)D3] is converted into an active form of vitamin D, $1\alpha,25(OH)_2D_3$ to activate the VDR transactivation fuction only when the transfected cells with the cDNA libraly of the VDR KO mice express 25-hydroxyvitamin D3 1α-hydroxylase[1α(OH)ase].

The activity of 1α(OH)ase was first identified in kidney homogenates, and kidney was thought to be the sole tissue expressing 1α(OH)ase. Indeed the proximal convoluted tubule cells were mapped as its location in kidney(7). By Northern blot analysis with the cloned cDNA, it was shown that this gene abundantly expresses in kidney, while in the extra-renal tissues of mice and humans, the expressions appeared at almost undetectable levels. Analyses with a quantitative RT-PCR analysis suggests that the 1α(OH)ase gene expresses in many extrarenal tissues at very low levels(8). As $1\alpha,25(OH)_2D_3$ plays a primary role in calcium homeostasis, the renal activity of 1α(OH)ase is positively regulated by calcitropic hormones, responding to serum calcium levels(9). $1,25(OH)_2D_3$ has been well characterized as a negative regulator for the renal activity of 1α(OH)ase(10). Our study using VDR knock-out mice showed that $1\alpha,25(OH)_2D_3$ acts at the transcriptional level, and this negative regulation requires the liganded-VDR, since the gene expression of the mouse 1α(OH)ase was remarkably up-regulated in the VDR KO mice(3)(Fig. 2). In contrast, calcitropic hormones such as calcitonin and PTH are known to induce the activity of 1α(OH)ase, and cAMP was demonstrated to be mediatd this positive regulation by PTH, suggesting a possible involvment of the protein kinase A signaling pathway in the positive regulations. These findings are further supported by the recent obseravtions that the proximal promoters of the human and mouse 1α(OH)ase genes confer positve responses to PTH and calcitonine(11, 12). Moreover, in the human promoter we identified a kidney cell -specifc negative regulatory element to 1α,25(OH)2D3 in the MCT cell line(Fig. 3), though there is neither consensus negative VDREs nor siginificantly related sequences(see table I)(13,14). Overexpression of VDR along with RXR potentiated this negative regulation by 1α,25(OH)2D3. Together with the findings in the negative regulation

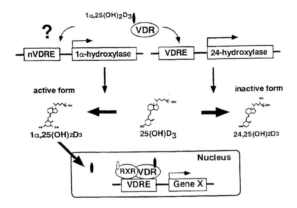

Figure 2. A proposed molecular mechanism of regulations of 1α,25(OH)2D3 biosynthesis by 25-hydroxyvitamin D3 1α-hydroxylase and 25(OH)D3-24-hydroxylase. The negative reguation of 1α(OH)ase gene expression by 1α,25(OH)2D3 did not occur in the mice lacking VDR(VDR knock-out mice), raises a possibility that a negative VDRE is present in the promoter of the 1α(OH)ase gene. The positive VDRE has been identified in the promoter of the 25(OH)D3-24-hydroxylase gene. The levels of serum 1α,25(OH)2D3 is positively and negatively regulated through these VDREs binding linganded VDR.

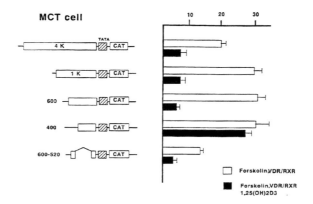

Figure 3. The delineationm of negative vitamin D response element(nVDRE) in 25-hydroxyvitamin D₃ 1α-hydroxylase gene promoter in the MCT cells.

negative VDRE

Gene	Response element		
Avian PTH	GGGTCA	GGA	GGGTGT
Human PTH	GGTTCA	AAG	CAGACA
Mouse osteocalcin	GGGCAA	ATG	AGGACA
Rat bone sialoprotein	AGGGTT	TAT	AGGTCA
PKA inhibitor	ATGTTG	CTG	AGGTCA
Rat PTHrP-proximal	AGGTTA	CTC	AGTGAA
Rat PTHrP-distal	GGGTGG	AGA	GGGGTG

Table 1. DNA sequences of negative vitamin D response elements(nVDREs).

The previously reported nVDREs are shown except the 1α(OH)ase nVDRE, which has not yet been delinerated to a core nVDRE motif.

in VDR KO mice, these obseravtions clearly indicate that VDR is esseential for the negative regulation of the 1α(OH)ase gene by $1\alpha,25$(OH)$_2$D$_3$. However, gel-shift analysis with nulear extracts and recombinant receptor proteins showed that this negative VDRE does not directly bind VDR or VDR-RXR hetrodimer, but binds unknown nulear factor(s) which is expressed in a tissue-specific manne. We further cloned the cDNA of a factor bound to the negative VDRE in human 1α(OH)ase gene promoter, and this clone encodes a basic helix-loop-helix(bHLH) type transcripton factor. We are currently characterizing this factor. Collecting these observations together, it is most likely that the transctivation function of this cloned bHLP factor, probably associating with the other factors, bound this negative VDRE is indirectly suppressed by ligand-bound VDR, probably through coactivators and/or repressors(1).

References

1) Freedman L.P, 1999. Increasing the complexity of coactivation in nuclear receptor signalinCell 97, 5-8.

2) Haussler, M. R., Whitfield, G. K., Haussler, C. A., Hsieh, J. C., Thompson, P. D., Selznick, S. H., C. E. Dominguez, and P. W. Jurutka. 1998. The nuclear vitamin D receptor: biological and molecular regulatory properties revealed. J. Bone Miner. Res. 13, 325-349.

4) Kato , S., Yanagisawa, J., Murayama, A., Kitanaka, S., Takeyama, K., 1998. The importance of 25-hydroxyvitamin D3 1a-hydroxylase gene in vitamin D-dependent rickets. Curr. Opi. Nephrol. Hypertention. 7, 377-383.

5) Yoshizawa T, Handa Y, Uemasu Y, Takeda S, Sekine K, Yoshihara Y, Kawakami T, Arioka K, Sato H, Uchiyama Y, Masushige S, Fukamizu A, Matsumoto T, Kato A, 1997. Impaired bone formation and uterine hypoplasia with growth retardation after weaning in mice lacking the vitamin D receptor. Nat. Genet. 16, 391-396.

6) Kitanaka S, Takeyama K, Murayama A, Sato T, Okumura K, Nogami M, Hasegawa Y, Niimi H, Yanagisawa J, Tanaka T, Kato S. 1998. Inactivating mutations in the human 25-hydroxyvitamin D3 1a-hydroxlase gene in patients with pseudovitamin D-deficient rickets. N. Engl.J. Med. 338, 653-661.

7) Kawashima H., Torikai S, Kurokawa K. 1981 Localization of 25-hydroxyvitamin D3-1a-hydroxylase along the rat nephron. Proc.Natl.Acad. Sci. USA, 78, 1199-1203.

8) Murayama, A., Takeyama, K., Kitanaka, S., Kodera, Y., Kawaguchi, Y., Hosoya, T., Kato, S. 1999 Positive and negative regulations of the renal 25-hydroxyvitamin D3 1a-hydroxylase gene by parathyroid hormone, calcitonin, and 1a, 25(OH)2D3 in intact animals. Endocrinology, 140, 2224-2231.

9) Henry HL, 1979. Regulation of the hydroxylation of 25-hydroxvitamin D3-1α-hydroxlase *in vivo* and in primary cultures of chick kidney cells. J. Biol. Chem., 254, 2722-2729.

10) Henry HL,1985. Parathyroid hormone modulation of 25-hydroxvitamin D3 metabolism by cultured chick kidney cells is mimicked and enhanced by forskolin. Endocrinology 116, 503-507.

11) Murayama A., Takeyama K., Kitanaka S., Kodera Y., Hosoya T., Kato S., 1998.The promoter of the human 25-hydorxyvitamin D3 1α-hydroxylase gene confers positive and negative responsiveness to PTH, calcitonin, and 1α,25(OH)2 D3. Biochem. Biophys. Res. Commun., 249, 121-16.

12) Brenza H., Kimmel-Jehan C., Jehan F., Shinki T., Wakino S., Anazawa M., Suda T., DeLuca H. F., 1998. Parathyroid hormone activation of the rat 25-hydroxyvitamin D3-1a-hydroxylase gene promoter. Proc.Natl.Acad. Sci. USA, 95, 1387-1391.

13) Demay M B., Kiernan M S., DeLuca HF, Kronenberg HM., 1992. Sequences in the human parathyroid hormone gene that bind the 1,25-dihydroxyvitamin D receptor and mediate transcriptional response to 1,25-dihydroxyvitamin D. Proc.Natl.Acad. Sci.USA, 89, 8097-8101.

14) Mackey, S L., Heymont JL., Kronenberg HM., Demay MB 1996 Vitamin D receptor binding to the negative human prathyroid hormone vitamin D response element does not require the retioind X receptor. Mol. Endocrinol. 10, 298-305.

NATURAL METABOLITES OF 1α,25-DIHYDROXYVITAMIN D₃ AND ITS ANALOGS

G. Satyanarayana Reddy, D. Sunita Rao, and M-L. Siu-Caldera
Women & Infants' Hospital, Brown Univ. School of Medicine, Providence, RI, U.S.A.

During the past two decades, several natural metabolites of 1α,25(OH)₂D₃ were identified. The natural metabolites are formed as a result of modifications of both the side chain and the A-ring of 1α,25(OH)₂D₃. At present, it is the general belief that the only function of 1α,25(OH)₂D₃ metabolism in its target tissues is to inactivate the hormone and the metabolites formed during the process of its inactivation are only catabolites. However, the possibility of the natural metabolites producing biological activities of their own has been considered. During the past decade, the main goal of our research has been to evaluate carefully the biological activities of the various natural metabolites of 1α,25(OH)₂D₃ and its analogs. The results of these studies are summarized below.

I. Metabolism of 1α,25(OH)₂D₃ via modifications of side chain and A-ring

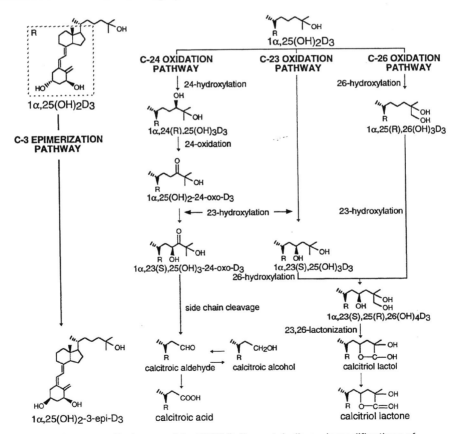

Figure 1. Pathways of 1α,25(OH)2D3 metabolism via modifications of both the side chain and the A-ring

By 1989, the full details of the pathways of $1\alpha,25(OH)_2D_3$ metabolism through side chain modification are described (Figure 1). The C-24 oxidation pathway, initiated by hydroxylation at C-24 is the major side chain modification pathway which leads to the formation of the final product, calcitroic acid (1-4). The C-23 and C-26 oxidation pathways, initiated by hydroxylations at C-23 and C-26 are the minor side chain modification pathways which lead to the formation of the final product, $1\alpha,25(OH)_2D_3$-23,26-lactone (4,5). It was found that the enzyme 24-hydroxylase, CYP24 was capable of performing various steps in the C-24 oxidation pathway, suggesting that the enzyme has multicatalytic functions (6-9). Relatively little is known regarding the enzymology of the C-23 and C-26 oxidation pathways. During our studies investigating the metabolism of the $1\alpha,25(OH)_2D_3$ in primary cultures of neonatal human keratinocytes, we identified for the first time $1\alpha,25(OH)_2$-3-epi-D_3 as one of the major metablites of $1\alpha,25(OH)_2D_3$ (10,11). $1\alpha,25(OH)_2$-3-epi-D_3, a novel A-ring modified metabolite is formed as a result of the change in the orientation of the hydroxyl group at the C-3 position from β to α. The formation of $1\alpha,25(OH)_2$-3-epi-D_3 was not inhibited by ketoconazole indicating that the enzyme(s) responsible for the C-3 epimerization do not belong to the cytochrome P450 class (12).

II. Tissue specific metabolism of $1\alpha,25(OH)_2D_3$

Tissues and Cell lines	Species	C-3 epimerization pathway	C-24 oxidation pathway
Keratinocytes (primary)	Human	Yes	Yes
HaCaT (Immortalized keratinocytes)	Human	Yes	Yes
Intestinal Cells (Caco-2)-Confluent	Human	Yes	No
Intestinal Cells (Caco-2)-Subconfluent	Human	No	Yes
Breast Cancer Cells (SKBR 3)	Human	No	Yes
Osteosarcoma Cells (U2-OS)	Human	Yes	Yes
Osteosarcoma Cells (Sa-OS)	Human	Yes	No
Myeloid Leukemic Cells (HL-60)	Human	No	Yes
Myeloid Leukemic Cells (RWLeU-4)	Human	No	Yes
Monocytic Leukemic Cells (U 937)	Human	No	Yes
Placenta (Explants)	Human	No	Yes
Osteosarcoma Cells (UMR-106)	Rat	Yes	Yes
Osteosarcoma Cells (ROS 17/2.8)	Rat	Yes	No
Vascular Smooth Muscle Cells (primary)	Rat	Yes	No
Aortic Rings (Explants)	Rat	Yes	No
Perfused Kidney	Rat	No	Yes
Parathyroid Cells (primary)	Bovine	Yes	Yes

Following the discovery of $1\alpha,25(OH)_2$-3-epi-D_3 production in human keratinocytes, we examined the metabolism of $1\alpha,25(OH)_2D_3$ into $1\alpha,25(OH)_2$-3-epi-D_3 in several other tissues which include both normal as well as cancer cell lines (table shown above). From these results it becomes obvious that while some tissues express only the C-24 oxidation pathway [eg. SKBR3, HL-60 (13), RWLeU-4 and U937 cells, placenta and perfused rat kidney (14)], most of the other tissues express both the C-24 oxidation and the C-3 epimerization pathways [eg. Caco-2 (15), keratinocytes (10,11), U2-0S, UMR 106 (14) and parathyroid cells (16)]. **Furthermore, from our studies it became apparent that the C-24 oxidation pathway like the C-3 epimerization pathway is also tissue specific. For example vascular smooth muscle cells and ROS 17/2.8 cells express only the C-3 epimerization pathway but not the C-24 oxidation pathway** (14,17).

III. Biological activities of the natural intermediary metabolites

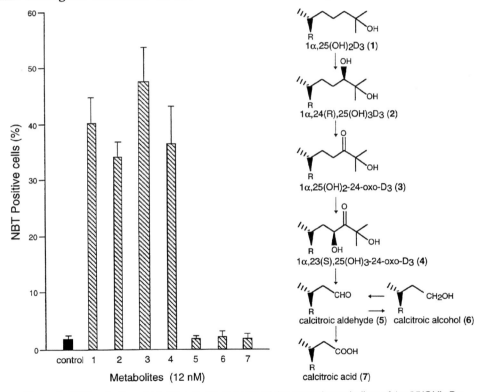

Figure 2. NBT reduction of HL-60 cells treated with all the natural metabolites of $1\alpha,25(OH)_2D_3$ produced *via* the C-24 oxidation pathway (13)

Biological activity of side chain modified metabolites: The various intermediary metabolites formed through the C-24 and C-23 oxidation pathways are found to be less active in generating the classical vitamin D hormone actions such as intestinal calcium absorption and bone calcium mobilization (18). Based on their calcemic activities, the natural intermediary metabolites were initially considered to be catabolites. However, the discovery that $1\alpha,25(OH)_2D_3$ generates not only calcemic actions but also noncalcemic actions such as modulation of cell growth and differentiation of a variety of cell types (19,20) raised the possibility that some of the natural intermediary metabolites of $1\alpha,25(OH)_2D_3$ (previously shown to be less calcemic) may still retain the noncalcemic actions of their parent. During the past decade, we studied carefully the noncalcemic actions of the various natural metabolites of $1\alpha,25(OH)_2D_3$ and its analogs. Our studies provide evidence to indicate that some of the natural metabolites can generate potent noncalcemic actions (21, 22). The 24-oxo metabolites are almost as potent as their parent, $1\alpha,25(OH)_2D_3$ in terms of their ability to differentiate HL-60 cells into monocyte macrophages (13) (Figure 2) and in suppressing parathyroid hormone secretion in bovine parathyroid cells (23). **Thus, the 24-oxo metabolites appear to play an important role in generating some of the noncalcemic actions of $1\alpha,25(OH)_2D_3$ in various cell types.**

Biological activity of A-ring modified metabolite: $1\alpha,25(OH)_2$-3-epi-D_3 when compared to $1\alpha,25(OH)_2D_3$ binds to vitamin D receptor (VDR) with less affinity (16,24). As a result, $1\alpha,25(OH)_2$-3-epi-D_3 was found to possess minimal activity in generating *in vivo* intestinal calcium transport and bone calcium mobilization (24). On the contrary, $1\alpha,25(OH)_2$-3-epi-D_3 was found to be almost equipotent to $1\alpha,25(OH)_2D_3$ in suppressing parathyroid hormone secretion in bovine parathyroid cells (16) and in inhibiting keratinocyte proliferation (24,25). At present, the possible mechanisms responsible for the high *in vitro* activity of $1\alpha,25(OH)_2$-3-epi-D_3 in parathyroid cells and keratinocytes are not fully understood.

IV. Metabolism of synthetic vitamin D analogs $[1\alpha,25(OH)_2$-16-ene-D_3 and $1\alpha,25(OH)_2$-20-epi-$D_3]$ into stable biologically active 24-oxo metabolites.

Further proof for the importance of the 24-oxo metabolites was obtained through our studies of the target tissue metabolism of 16-ene and 20-epi analogs. We have shown that in rat kidney (26), leukemic cells (27) and keratinocytes, $1\alpha,25(OH)_2$-16-ene-D_3 [which has a double bond between carbons 16 and 17 when compared to $1\alpha,25(OH)_2D_3$ (Figure 3)] is metabolized differently from $1\alpha,25(OH)_2D_3$. The '16-ene' modification decreases the rate of further metabolism of the 24-oxo metabolite $[1\alpha,25(OH)_2$-16-ene-24-oxo-$D_3]$ and therefore the 24-oxo metabolite accumulates in significant amounts. In some instances the amount of accumulated 24-oxo metabolite exceeds the amount of the remaining unmetabolized substrate (Figure 3). The stable 24-oxo metabolite is found to be almost as active as its parent compound in inhibiting proliferation and inducing differentiation of cancer cells, transactivating a VDRE reporter construct *in vitro* (27,28) and in exerting immunosuppressive activity *in vivo* without causing hypercalcemia (29).

Like $1\alpha,25(OH)_2$-16-ene-D_3, $1\alpha,25(OH)_2$-20-epi-D_3 [which differs from $1\alpha,25(OH)_2D_3$ by a simple modification in the stereochemistry of the methyl group at C-20 on the side chain (Figure 4)] is also metabolized into the stable bioactive 24-oxo metabolite $[1\alpha,25(OH)_2$-20-epi-24-oxo-$D_3]$ (30,31). **Thus, the block in the side chain metabolism of the 16-ene and 20-epi analogs (Figure 4) results in the accumulation of the corresponding stable bioactive 24-oxo intermediary metabolite which contributes significantly to the final expression of the enhanced biological activities ascribed to the parent analog.**

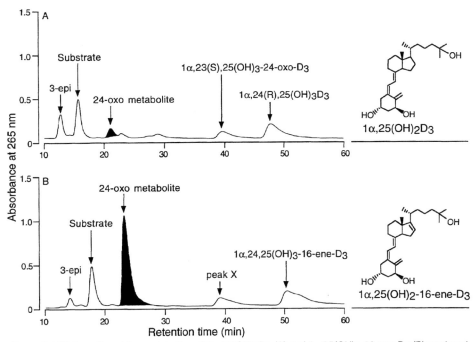

Figure 3. HPLC profiles of the metabolites of 1α,25(OH)2D3 (A) and 1α,25(OH)2-16-ene-D3 (B) produced by human keratinocytes incubated with 1 μM substrate concentrations. Lipid extracts of both cells and media were analyzed on a Zorbax-SIL column eluted with 6% isopropanol in hexane at a flow rate of 2 ml/min. The metabolites were identified by comigration with synthetic standards and through mass spectrometry. The identity of peak X is unknown.

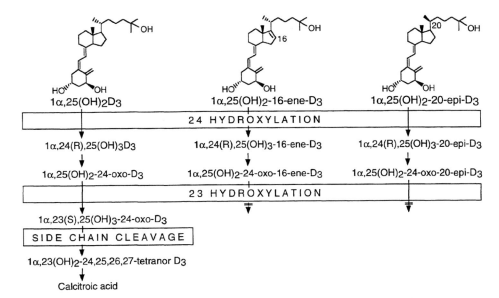

Figure 4. Metabolic Pathways of 1α,25(OH)2D3 and its 16-ene and 20-epi analogs
via C-24 oxidation pathway

V. Tissue specific metabolism of $1\alpha,25(OH)_2$-20-epi-D_3

In a recent study we investigated the metabolism of $1\alpha,25(OH)_2$-20-epi-D_3 in rat kidney and indicated that two metabolites of $1\alpha,25(OH)_2$-20-epi-D_3 namely, $1\alpha,25(OH)_2$-20-epi-24-oxo-D_3 and its precursor $1\alpha,24,25(OH)_3$-20-epi-D_3 are biologically active (31). We then embarked on a new study to identify other possible active intermediary metabolites of $1\alpha,25(OH)_2$-20-epi-D_3. For example, the conversion of $1\alpha,25(OH)_2$-20-epi-D_3 into its C-3 epimer has not been studied. Therefore, we studied the metabolism of $1\alpha,25(OH)_2$-20-epi-D_3 in UMR 106 cells which are known to express the C-3 epimerization pathway. Our results indicated that $1\alpha,25(OH)_2$-20-epi-D_3 is metabolized in UMR 106 cells into several metabolites derived *via* both the C-24 oxidation and the C-3 epimerization pathways. Along with these aforementioned metabolites, a novel less polar metabolite (LPM) is also produced

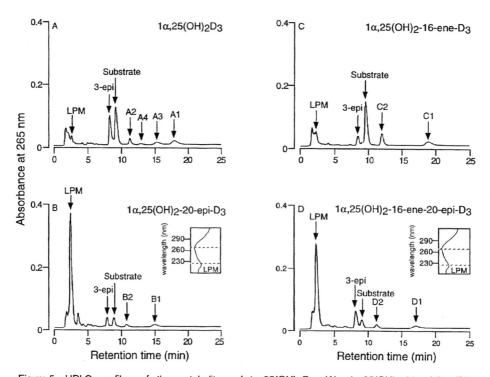

Figure 5. HPLC profiles of the metabolites of $1\alpha,25(OH)_2D_3$ (A), $1\alpha,25(OH)_2$-20-epi-D_3 (B), $1\alpha,25(OH)_2$-16-ene-D_3 (C), and $1\alpha,25(OH)_2$-16-ene-20-epi-D_3 (D) produced by UMR 106 cells incubated with 1 µM substrate concentrations. Lipid extracts of both cells and media were analyzed on Zorbax-SIL column eluted with 10% isopropanol in hexane at a flow rate of 2 ml/min. A1, A2, A3,A4; B1,B2; C1,C2; D1,D2: Metabolites formed *via* the C-24 oxidation pathway.

(Figure 5, panel B). Studies, determining the structure of the LPM are in progress. We also found that the analog $1\alpha,25(OH)_2$-16-ene-20-epi-D_3 was metabolized into LPM indicating that the formation of LPM is not affected by insertion of a double bond between carbons 16 and 17 (Figure 5, panel D). However, the formation of LPM was not significant when $1\alpha,25(OH)_2D_3$ (Figure 5, panel A) or $1\alpha,25(OH)_2$-16-ene-D_3 (Figure 5, panel C) are used as substrates. Thus, the 20-epi modification appears to enhance the rate of formation of LPM (Figure 5, panels B and D). We observed that this novel LPM pathway is also expressed in other tissues such as ROS 17/2.8 cells and primary rat vascular smooth muscle cells, but not in the isolated perfused rat kidney indicating that the LPM pathway is tissue specific. Furthermore, we also observed that all the natural metabolites of $1\alpha,25(OH)_2$-20-epi-D_3 including LPM retained significant activity in terms of their ability to induce VDR-mediated transcription in ROS 17/2.8 cells transfected with a growth hormone (GH) reporter gene containing a VDRE from the human osteocalcin gene (data not shown).

Thus, we report for the first time that unlike in rat kidney (31), $1\alpha,25(OH)_2$-20-epi-D_3 in UMR 106 cells is metabolized into several intermediary metabolites formed not only *via* the previously established C-24 oxidation and the C-3 epimerization pathways, but also *via* a novel LPM pathway. All the intermediary metabolites produced *via* the three aforementioned metabolic pathways are biologically active and thus contribute significantly to the final expression of the enhanced biological activities attributed to their parent, $1\alpha,25(OH)_2$-20-epi-D_3.

Conclusions

1. The studies from our laboratory indicate that the natural metabolites of $1\alpha,25(OH)_2D_3$ and its analogs play a significant role in the expression of some of the specific biological activities that are attributed to their parent.
2. The tissue specific metabolism and accumulation of the intermediary metabolites in significant amounts in specific tissues is one of the important mechanisms responsible for the tissue specific actions of some vitamin D analogs such as $1\alpha,25(OH)_2$-20-epi-D_3.

Acknowledgments

The concepts and the work presented here became possible due to the active collaborations and intellectually stimulating discussions with the following scientists: Dr. MR Uskokovic (Hoffmann-La Roche, Nutley, NJ, U.S.A), Drs. AW Norman and WH Okamura (Univ. of CA, Riverside, CA, U.S.A), Dr. P Koeffler (UCLA Sch. of Med., Los Angeles, CA, U.S.A), Dr. AJ Brown (Washington Univ. Sch. of Med., St. Louis, MI, U.S.A), Dr. K-Y Tserng (Case Western Reserve Univ., Cleveland, OH, U.S.A), Drs. I Schuster, HS Cross and M Peterlik (Univ. Vienna, Austria), Dr. S Peleg (M.D. Anderson Cancer Center, Houston, TX, U.S.A), Dr. JM Lemire (Univ. of California, San Diego, CA, U.S.A), Dr. MJ Campbell (Univ. Birmingham, U.K), Dr. P Williard (Brown Univ. Providence, RI, U.S.A), Dr. S Ishizuka (Teijin Inst. Bio-Med. Res, Tokyo, Japan), Dr. T Okano (Kobe Pharm. Univ., Japan), Drs. GH Posner and SE Guggino (The Johns Hopkins Univ., Baltimore, MD, U.S.A), Dr. G. Jones (Queen's Univ., Canada), Dr. P Vouros (Northeastern Univ. Boston, MA, U.S.A), Dr. H Takayama (Teikyo Univ., Japan), Drs. MF Holick and R Ray (Boston Univ. Sch. of Med., Boston, U.S.A), Dr. RL Horst (Natl. Animal Dis. Cen., Ames, IA, U.S.A), Dr. JW Clark (Harvard Medical Sch., Boston, MA, U.S.A) and Drs. H Harant and IJD Lindley (Novartis Res. Inst., Vienna, Austria). This work was supported by a research grant (DK 52488) from the National Institutes of Health.

References

1. Reddy GS, Tserng K-Y, Thomas BR, Dayal R, Norman, AW (1987) Biochem 26, 324-331.
2. Reddy GS, Tserng K-Y (1989) Biochem 28, 1763-1769.
3. Makin G, Lohnes D, Byford V, Ray R, Jones G (1989) Biochem J 262, 173-180.
4. Bouillon R, Okamura WH, Norman AW (1995) Endocrine Rev 16, 200-257.
5. Ishizuka S, Norman AW (1987) J Biol Chem 262, 7165-7170.
6. Ohyama Y, Okuda K (1991) J Biol Chem 266, 8690-8695.
7. Ohyama Y, Noshiro M, Okuda K (1991) FEBS Lett 278, 195-198.
8. Akiyoshi-Shibata M, Sakaki T, Ohyama Y, Noshiro M, Okuda K, Yabusaki Y (1994) Eur J Biochem 224, 335-343.
9. Beckman MJ, Tadikonda P, Werner E, Prahl J, Yamada S, DeLuca HF (1996) Biochem 35, 8465-8472.
10. Reddy GS, Muralidharan KR, Okamura WH, Tserng K-Y, McLane JA (1994) In: Vitamin D a pluripotent steroid hormone: structural studies, molecular endocrinology and clinical applications. (Norman AW, Bouillon R, Thomasset M Eds). New York, NY Walter de Gruyter pp. 172-173.
11. Reddy GS, Siu-Caldera M-L, Schuster I, Astecker N, Tserng K-Y, Muralidharan KR, Okamura WH, McLane JA, Uskokovic MR (1997) In: Vitamin D, chemistry, biology and clinical applications of the steroid hormone. (Norman AW, Bouillon R, Thomasset M Eds.) pp. 139-146. Univ. of California, Riverside, USA.
12. Masuda S, Kamao M, Schroeder NJ, Makin HL, Jones G, Kremer R, Rhim J, Okano T (2000) Biol Pharm Bull 23(2), 133-139.
13. Sunita Rao D, Campbell MJ, Koeffler HP, Ishizuka S, Uskokovic MR, Reddy GS (2000) Steroids (in press).
14. Siu-Caldera M-L, Sekimoto H, Weiskopf A, Vouros P, Muralidharan KR, Okamura WH, Bishop J, Norman AW, Uskokovic MR, Schuster I, Reddy GS (1999) Bone 24(5), 457-463.
15. Bischof MG, Siu-Caldera M-L, Weiskopf A, Vouros P, Cross HS, Peterlik M, Reddy GS (1998) Exp Cell Res 241, 194-201.
16. Brown AJ, Ritter C, Slatopolsky E, Muralidharan KR, Okamura WH, Reddy GS (1999) J Cell Biochem 73(1), 106-113.
17. Siu-Caldera M-L, Sekimoto H, Brem AS, Bina RB, Reddy GS (1998) J Bone Min Res 23 (Suppl), S426.
18. Mayer E, Bishop JE, Ohnuma N, Norman AW (1983)Arch Biochem Biophys 224, 671-676.
19. Abe E, Miyaura C, Sakagami H, Takeda M, Konno K, Yamazaki T, Yochiki S, Suda T (1981) Proc Natl Acad Sci USA 78, 4990-4994.
20. Van Leeuwen JPTM, Pols HAP (1997) In: Vitamin D. (Feldman D, Glorieux FH, Pike JW Eds.) pp. 1089-1105. Academic Press, CA, USA.
21. Harant H, Andrew PJ, Reddy GS, Foglar E, Lindley IJD (1997) Eur J Biochem 250, 63-71.
22. Harant H, Spinner D, Reddy GS, Lindley IJD (2000) J Cell Physiology 78, 112-120.
23. Lee NE, Reddy GS, Brown AJ, Williard PG (1997) Biochem. 36, 9429-9437.
24. Norman AW, Bouillon R, Farach-Carson MC, Bishop JE, Zhou L-X, Nemere I, Zhao J, Muralidharan KR, Okamura WH (1993) J Biol Chem 268, 20022-20030.
25. Schuster I, Astecker N, Egger H, Herzig G, Reddy GS, Schmid J, Vorisek G (1997) In: Vitamin D, chemistry, biology and clinical applications of the steroid hormone (Norman AW, Bouillon R, Thomasset M Eds.) pp. 551-558. Univ. of California, Riverside, USA.
26. Reddy GS, Clark JW, Tserng K-Y, Uskokovic MR, McLane JA (1993) Bioorg Med Chem Lett 3(9), 1879-1884.
27. Siu-Caldera M-L, Clark JF, Santos-Moore A, Peleg S, Liu YY, Uskokovic MR, Sharma S, Reddy GS (1996) J Steroid Biochem Mol Biol 59(5/6), 405-412.
28. Campbell MJ, Reddy GS, Koeffler HP (1997) J Cell Biochem 66, 413-425.
29. Lemire JM, Archer DC, Reddy GS (1994) Endocrinol 136(6), 2818-2821.
30. Dilworth FJ, Calverley MJ, Makin HJL, Jones G (1994) Biochem Pharmacol 47, 987-993.
31. Siu-Caldera M-L, Sekimoto H, Peleg S, Nguyen C, Kissmeyer AM, Binderup L, Weiskopf A, Vouros P, Uskokovic MR, Reddy GS (1999) J Steroid Biochem Mol Biol 71, 111-121.

REGULATION OF VITAMIN D₃ METABOLITE SYNTHESIS IN CULTURED *SOLANUM GLAUCOPHYLLUM*

A. Curino, L. Milanesi, M. Skliar, S. Benassati, R. Boland. Departamento de Biología, Bioquímica y Farmacia. Universidad Nacional del Sur. 8000 Bahía Blanca. Argentina. E-mail: rboland@criba.edu.ar

Introduction:

Solanum glaucophyllum (Sg) is a plant which causes calcinosis in animals (1). This property has been correlated to the existence of the hormonally active form of vitamin D_3, 1,25-dihydroxy-vitamin D_3 [1,25(OH)$_2$D$_3$; calcitriol] (2). It has been reported that Sg also contains vitamin D_3 and 25(OH)D$_3$ (3). There is controversial evidence regarding the native structure and the tissue distribution of 1,25(OH)$_2$D$_3$ and related metabolites in Sg. It has been reported that vitamin D_3 derivatives are mainly found as glycoconjugates (2,3). Other lines of evidence are indicative of the presence of free vitamin D_3 sterols (4). Also, in contradiction to the initial belief that 1,25(OH)$_2$D$_3$ was exclusively localized in the leaves, the application of more sensitive assays has allowed detection of this metabolite in all plant organs (5). Recent studies have shown the presence of 7-dehydrocholesterol, vitamin D_3, 25(OH)D$_3$ and 1,25(OH)$_2$D$_3$ in Sg callus and cell cultures (6). Calcitriol formation in Sg grown in vitro under strict conditions of darkness could be shown, suggesting that a synthetic metabolic route independent of light is also operative (6). As UV irradiation of cultures increased slightly the concentration of 1,25(OH)$_2$D$_3$ the question arose on whether photolytic cleavage of 7-dehydrocholesterol or the following hydroxylations would be limiting the efficiency of the light-dependent synthetic pathway of 1,25(OH)$_2$D$_3$ in culture systems. The identification of medium constituents influencing calcitriol synthesis in vitro may help to optimize conditions for its biotechnological production. In this work we investigate these still not clarified subjects and the influence of medium concentration of Ca^{2+} and plant growth factors on calcitriol production.

Results and Discussion:

Distribution of free and conjugated forms of 1,25(OH)$_2$D$_3$ in calli and plant tissues from different organs of Solanum glaucophyllum.

The distribution of free and conjugated forms of 1,25(OH)$_2$D$_3$ in calli growing in darkness as described Curino et al. (6) and plant tissue from different organs of Sg were evaluated using a radioreceptor assay (7). The amounts of metabolite in calli derived from stem and leaves were more elevated than in calli originated from fruits. However, fruits from Sg grown in the field contained higher concentrations than stems, roots and leaves. The differences in calcitriol levels observed between in vitro and in vivo conditions are in accordance with observations made with other plant secondary products and may be explained by cell transformation occurring upon culture. The free form of the metabolite was predominant in tissues obtained from plants and calli. Our data is in agreement with

form of the metabolite was predominant in tissues obtained from plants and calli. Our data is in agreement with various lines of evidence supporting the existence of free secosterols in the plant. It was found that the lipophilic fraction of Sg exhibited vitamin D_3-like activity when given to animals (8). Other workers observed that non-hydrolyzed plant extracts by glycosidases had the ability to compete with [^{3}H]1,25(OH)$_2$D$_3$ for binding to the chick intestine VDR (4). It has been detected both 1,25(OH)$_2$D$_3$ and 1,25(OH)$_2$D$_3$-glycoside in Sg, the free form prevailing in some tissues (5). Greater amounts of 1,25(OH)$_2$D$_3$ than its glycoside counterpart have been also detected in several plant species, e.g. *Cestrum diurnum* (9), *Lycopersicon esculentum* (10), *Nicotiana glauca* (11) *S. tuberosum, S. melongena* and *Curcubita pepo* (12). As recently reported (6), using the highly specific in vitro radioreceptor assay we have detected lower levels of 1,25(OH)$_2$D$_3$ in field- and culture-grown Sg than those reported in other studies (13). Factors which may explain these differences are the distant geographic locations of the plants used for direct analysis or generation of cultures, the specifity/sensitivity of the assay procedures used to quantify the metabolite and the culture medium composition (Fig 1).

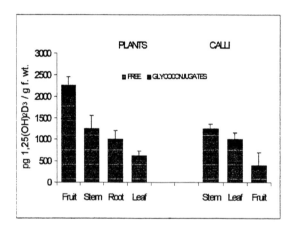

Fig. 1. Concentration of free and glycosidic 1,25(OH)$_2$D$_3$ in Sg tissues and calli from different primary explants. Lipids were extracted with chloroform-methanol (1:2) by the Bligh & Dyer (14) procedure. The remaining water soluble fraction was incubated with β-glucosidase to release sterols from their glyconjugated derivatives followed by organic solvent extraction. The 1,25(OH)$_2$D$_3$ content of extracts was measured by radioreceptor assays. Values are averages ± SD of 3 determinations.

Modulation by plant growth factors and calcium of 1,25(OH)$_2$D$_3$ production in cultured Solanum glaucophyllum.

It has been reported that Sg calli grown in Gamborg medium synthesize greater amounts of cholesterol, 7-dehydrocholesterol and vitamin D_3 sterols than in Murashige & Skoog medium (13). As both media have different content of plant growth factors and calcium, we investigated the effects of culturing Sg in the presence of varying concentrations of auxin (2,4-D), kinetin and Ca^{2+} on the formation of 1,25(OH)$_2$D$_3$. The studies with plant hormones comprised 4 different treatment conditions, as follows: A: 0.5 mg/L 2,4-D + 0.2 mg/L kinetin; B: 1.0 mg/L 2,4-D + 0.4 mg/L kinetin; C: 2.5 mg/L 2,4-D + 1.0 mg/L kinetin, and D: 0.5 mg/l 2,4-D + 2.0 mg/l kinetin. The concentrations of metabolite were determined by radioreceptor assays and the results were expressed relative to the standard condition A used in the other experiments. Increases of 1.7-, 4.2- and 17-fold in 1,25(OH)$_2$D$_3$ levels could be measured for treatments B, C and D, respectively. Less evident changes were detected when cell suspensions were used instead of calli, e.g. 1.3-fold for B, 1.4-fold for C and 3.1-fold for D. Similar relative increases were detected for calcitriol secreted into the culture medium. These results show a clear stimulation by the plant growth factor binary mixture on $1,25(OH)_2D_3$ synthesis in Sg. As suggested by data obtained with condition D, kinetin may play a major role in upregulating the production of the metabolite.

Regarding the influence of calcium concentration on calcitriol production by Sg in in vitro callus cultures, the studies performed with calli showed that media deprived of Ca^{2+} contained low levels of calcitriol. When using cation concentrations of 1mM, 8 mM and 13 mM the levels of metabolite detected by radioreceptor assays were increased 2.6-, 4.8- and 1.7-fold, respectively. When similar experiments were performed with cell suspensions, only at 13 mM Ca^{2+} a significant increase in $1,25(OH)_2D_3$ was observed (1.7-fold). Contrary to our observations, an inverse relationship between medium Ca^{2+} concentrations and $1,25(OH)_2D_3$ formation has been reported before (15), curiously homologated by these authors with Ca^{2+} regulation of calcitriol synthesis in animals which is known to be mediated by parathyroid hormone.

Effect of UV irradiation on the levels of vitamin D_3 and hydroxylated metabolites of Solanum glaucophyllum grown in vitro and in vivo.

The operation of the light-dependent pathway in the generation of vitamin D_3 sterols was reinvestigated measuring the effects of UV irradiation on the levels of $25(OH)D_3$ and vitamin D_3, in addition to $1,25(OH)_2D_3$, in view that the concentration of calcitriol could not be altered previously by this treatment (6). The concentrations of these metabolites isolated by Sephadex LH-20 chromatography (6) were measured by HPLC and compared to those of non-irradiated calli. (Table 1). The irradiation procedure induced marked increases in the levels of vitamin D_3 with respect to the tissue non-exposed to UV light; however, considerable less significant relative changes were observed for its mono and dihydroxylated derivatives. In contrast, UV irradiation of mature Sg plants markedly increased the amounts of $1,25(OH)_2D_3$ and less markedly the quantities of $25(OH)D_3$ and vitamin D_3, in comparison to non-irradiated plants. These results together with those obtained by UV exposure of calli suggest that in the less differentiated cultured cells low activity and/or expression of the vitamin D_3 and $25(OH)D_3$ hydroxylases and not the photolytic breakdown of 7-dehydrocholesterol hinder the production of $1,25(OH)_2D_3$ in vitro.

Table 1: Ultraviolet light irradiation of *Solanum glaucophyllum* calli stimulates vitamin D_3 formation without affecting $25(OH)D_3$ and $1,25(OH)_2D_3$ levels.

Irradiation Times (Days)	Vitamin D_3	$25(OH)D_3$	$1,25(OH)_2D_3$
	Percent	Increase Above	Control
5	350	28	32
10	556	5	37
15	280	0	22

Detection of 25(OH)D₃ -1α - hydroxylase activity in S. glaucophyllum cell suspensions.

25-vitamin D_3-1α-hydroxylase assays were performed by incubating Sg cells in culture medium containing [³H]25(OH)D₃ for 2-18 h followed by isolation of [³H]1,25(OH)₂D₃ by Bligh & Dyer, Sephadex LH-20 chromatography and HPLC. The conversion of [³H]25(OH)D₃ to [³H]1,25(OH)₂D₃ was time-dependent but as shown in Fig. 2, low 1α-hydroxylase levels were detected, supporting the interpretation in the conclusion above. Furthermore, when compared with Sg leaves (3) the activity of the enzyme was ca. 7 times lower (40 vs 6 pmol/mg prot./h, respectively).

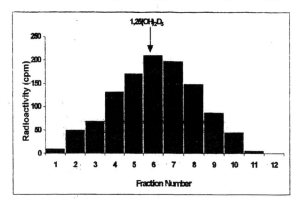

Fig. 2: 25-hydroxy-vitamin D₃-1α-hydroxylase activity of cultured Sg cells. Cells were incubated in culture medium containing [³H]25(OH)D₃ for 2 h followed by isolation of [³H]1,25(OH)₂D₃ produced. The radioactivity of the HPLC fraction coeluting with 1,25(OH)₂D₃ is shown.

References:

1) Worker N. A. and Carrillo B.J. (1967) Nature (London) 215, 72-74.

2) Wasserman R.H., Henion J.D., Haussler M.R. and McCain T.A. (1976) Science 194, 853-854.

3) Esparza, M.S., Vega, M. and Boland, R. (1982) Biochim. Biophys. Acta 719, 633-640.

4) Procsal, D.A., Henry, H.L., Hendrickson T. and Norman, A. W. (1976) Endocrinology 99, 437-444.

5) Weissenberg, M., Levy, A. and Wasserman, H. (1989) Phytochemistry 28: 795-798.

6) Curino, A., Skliar M. and Boland, R. (1998) Biochim. Biophys. Acta 1425: 485-492.

7) Wecksler, W.R. and Norman, A.W. (1979) Anal. Biochem. 92: 314-323.

8) Masselin, J.N., Abadie, G.J., Monesiglio, J.C. and Rossi, F.M. (1969) Rev. Invest. Agrop. INTA (Argentina) Serie 4, Patol. Anim. 8, 1-19.

9) Prema T.P. and Raghuramulu N. (1994) Free vitamin D₃ metabolites in *Cestrum diurnum* leaves. Phytochemistry 37, 677-681.

10) Prema, T.P. and Raghuramulu, N. (1996) Phytochemistry. 42, 617-620.

11) Skliar, M., Curino, A., Milanesi, L., Benassati, S. and Boland, R. (2000) Plant Sci. In press.

12) Aburjai, T., Al-Khalil, S. and Abuirjeie, M. (1998) Phytochemistry 49, 2497-2499.

13) Aburjai, T., Bernasconi, S., Manzocchi, L. and Pelizzoni, F., (1996) Phytochemistry 43, 773-776.

14) Bligh, E.G. and Dyer, W.J. (1959) Can. J. Biochem. Physiol. 37: 911-917.

15) Aburjai, T., Bernasconi, S., Manzocchi, L. and Pelizzoni, F., (1997) Phytochemistry 46, 1015-1018.

METABOLISM OF THE NONSTEROIDAL VITAMIN D ANALOGS, SL117 AND WU515 IN RAT OSTEOSARCOMA CELLS (UMR 106) AND KIDNEY

D. Sunita Rao[1], H. Sekimoto[1], M-L. Siu-Caldera[1], A. Verstuyf[2], Pierre De Clercq[3], M. Vandewalle[3], R. Bouillon[2], L.Gennaro[4], P. Vouros[4], and G. Satyanarayana Reddy[1]

[1]Women & Infants' Hosp,. Brown Univ, Providence, RI, U.S.A. [2]Lab. for Exptl. Med. & Endocrinol. (LEGENDO), Katholieke Univ., Leuven, Belgium. [3]Vakgroep voor Organische Chemie, Universiteit Gent, Gent, Belgium. [4]Northeastern Univ., Boston, MA, U.S.A.

Introduction: Recently, several nonsteroidal analogs (SL117 and WU515) of $1\alpha,25(OH)_2D_3$ were synthesized. The structures of $1\alpha,25(OH)_2D_3$ and the analogs which lack C-ring of the CD-ring skeleton are shown in the figure below. Biological activity studies indicated that SL117 [with the natural side chain of $1\alpha,25(OH)_2D_3$] is equipotent to $1\alpha,25(OH)_2D_3$ and WU515 [with a 23-yne side chain combined with hexafluorination at C-26 and C-27] is several fold more potent than $1\alpha,25(OH)_2D_3$ in modulating cell growth and differentiation *in vitro* with minimal calcemic actions *in vivo* (1). One of the mechanims for the unique biological activities of these analogs can be changes in their cellular metabolism and final inactivation. It is well established that $1\alpha,25(OH)_2D_3$ is metabolized *via* modifications of both the side chain (C-24 oxidation pathway) and A-ring (C-3 epimerization pathway) (2-5). We compared the metabolic fate of these analogs with that of $1\alpha,25(OH)_2D_3$ in rat osteosarcoma cells (UMR 106) and in the isolated perfused rat kidney. We hereby report the results of these findings.

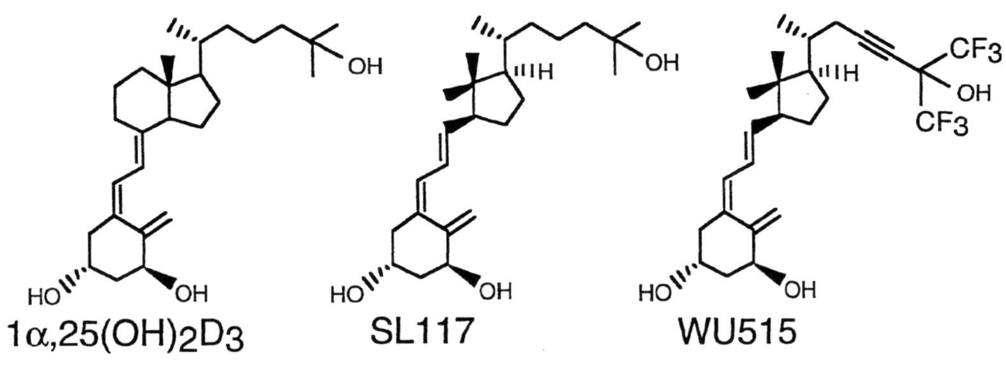

1α,25(OH)2D3   SL117   WU515

Chemical structures of 1α,25(OH)2D3 and the nonsteroidal analogs

Methods: **Metabolism studies:** Rats were pretreated with 2 µg of $1\alpha,25(OH)_2D_3$ 12 h before surgical removal of the right kidney. Three kidney perfusions were performed simultaneously in three separate perfusion systems for a period of 8 h using 200 µg of $1\alpha,25(OH)_2D_3$ or the analogs (SL117 or WU515) in 100 mL of perfusate (5 µM).

UMR 106 cells were maintained in McCoy's culture media supplemented with 10% FCS and antibiotics. Cultures of confluent UMR 106 cells were incubated with 1 μM concentrations of either $1\alpha,25(OH)_2D_3$ or the analogs in media containing 10% FCS in a humidified atmosphere under 5% CO_2 for 24 h. The lipid extraction was performed from both the kidney perfusate and the cells and media using a modified Bligh and Dyer method. The lipid extract was then subjected to HPLC directly for the separation of the various vitamin D metabolites.

Results: Comparative metabolism studies of $1\alpha,25(OH)_2D_3$ and the nonsteroidal analogs, SL117 and WU515 in the isolated perfused rat kidney indicate that SL117 [with the natural side chain of $1\alpha,25(OH)_2D_3$], like $1\alpha,25(OH)_2D_3$ is also metabolized into two polar metabolites derived *via* the C-24 oxidation pathway. One metabolite was identified as C-24 OH SL117 and the other metabolite was identified as C-24 oxo SL117 by GC/MS analysis (data not shown). WU515 (with altered side chain), unlike SL117 was not metabolized into polar metabolites indicating that this analog resists its metabolism *via* modifications of the side chain.

Comparative metabolism studies of $1\alpha,25(OH)_2D_3$ and the nonsteroidal analogs, SL117 and WU515 in UMR 106 cells indicated that like in the kidney, SL117 is also metabolized into polar metabolites derived *via* the C-24 oxidation pathway, while WU515 resists its metabolism *via* modifications of the side chain. [The GC/MS analysis of the metabolites produced in UMR 106 cells indicated that these metabolites are similar to the ones produced by rat kidney (data not shown)]. However, both SL117 and WU515 are metabolized into their corresponding less polar metabolites which were identified as the putative C-3 epimers of SL117 and WU515 by GC/MS analysis (data not shown).

Conclusion: Our results indicate that SL117 is metabolized *via* the same C-24 oxidation pathway like $1\alpha,25(OH)_2D_3$ in both UMR 106 cells and in rat kidney. WU515, unlike SL117 resists its metabolism *via* the C-24 oxidation pathway. However, both SL117 and WU515 are metabolized into their corresponding C-3 epimers in UMR 106 cells, which are known to express the C-3 epimerization pathway. In summary, we report for the first time that removal of the C-ring from the CD-ring skeleton of $1\alpha,25(OH)_2D_3$ does not affect its metabolism *via* the C-24 oxidation and C-3 epimerization pathways.

References:
1. Verstuyf, A., Verlinden, V., Van Etten, E., Shi, L., Wu, Y., D'Halleweyn, C., Van Haver, D., Zhu, G-D., Chen, Y-J., Zhou, X., Haussler, M.R., De Clercq, P., Vandewalle, M., Van Baelen, H., Mathieu, C. and Bouillon, R. (2000) J. Bone Min. Res. 15, 237-252.
2. Reddy, G.S. and Tserng, K-Y. (1989) Biochemistry 28, 1763-1769.
3. Bouillon, R., Okamura, W.H. and Norman, A.W. (1995) Endocrine Rev. 16, 200-257.
4. Makin, G., Lohnes, D., Byford, V., Ray, R., and Jones, G. (1989) Biochem. J. 262, 173-180.
5. Reddy, G.S., Muralidharan, K.R., Okamura, W.H., Tserng, K-Y. and McLane J.A. (1994) In: Vitamin D a pluripotent steroid hormone: structural studies, molecular endocrinology and clinical applications. (A.W. Norman, R. Bouillon, M. Thomasset Eds.) New York, NY: Walter de Gruyter; 172-173.

VASCULAR ENDOTHELIAL CELLS ARE SENSITIVE TARGETS OF 1,25-DIHYDROXYVITAMIN D$_3$

Sanjeev Puri*, Milan R Uskokovic** and Ronal R. MacGregor*, *Department of Anatomy & Cell Biology, Univ. of Kansas Medical Center, Kansas City KS. **Hofmann-La Roche Inc., Nutley, NJ

Introduction Vascular endothelial cells represent one of many cell types that contain a cytoplasmic/nuclear receptor for 1,25-dihydroxyvitamin D$_3$ (1,25D3) (1). We recently reported that rat heart cardiac microvascular cells in culture increased the rate of secretion of tissue plasminogen activator (tPA) in response to low concentrations of 1,25D3 and several of its synthetic analogs (2). The cells secreted more than their content of tPA in a 24 h period and there was no effect of 1,25D3 on cellular levels of tPA, indicating that 1,25D3 increased constitutive secretion of tPA by increasing its rate of synthesis. This conclusion is consonant with the presence of vitamin D-responsive elements in the tPA gene (3)

One of the notable aspects of the study on the effects of 1,25D3 on vascular cells was the high sensitivity of the cells to the hormone (2). In order to attain a higher level of sensitivity to the hormone than was expressed by the cells cultured in media containing fetal bovine serum (FBS), we cultured the cells initially in Leibovitz' L15 containing 20% FBS for several days, then cultured for two additional days in L15 containing 2% of a lipid-depleted, heat-treated, serum replacement (CPSR-1, Sigma). 24-hour test incubations were performed in L15 containing 0.2% of the serum substitute. Under these conditions maximal secretory responses to 10^{-10} to 10^{-14} M 1,25D3 were observed. The sensitivity of the microvascular cells to 1,25D3 was so high compared to that of other cell systems (reviewed in 4), that we decided to determine whether the supposedly inert hormone solvent 1,2-propanediol might somehow be increasing the cells' responsiveness to 1,25D3. We also began investigation of culture conditions that would preserve the high sensitivity to 1,25D3 but not require the use of lipid-depleted sera. In this report we demonstrate that under the culture conditions described above, 1,2-propanediol and similar compounds independently induce tPA secretion from rat microvascular cells. In addition, we report that human coronary artery endothelial cells (HCAECs) secrete increased amounts of tPA in response to 10^{-12} or 10^{-14} M 1,25D3 in a culture system that does not use lipid-depleted sera.

Results *Propanediols:* Rat heart microvascular cells were isolated (5) and cultured using the serum substitute as described above. During the 24-hour test incubations, they were treated with different concentrations of 1,2-propanediol, and samples of the conditioned media were assayed for tPA activity (6). The results (figure 1) showed that propanediol increased tPA secretion at concentrations as low as 2×10^{-8} M. By comparison, in the 1,25D3 studies described above (2), propanediol was present at 2×10^{-8} M when the concentration of 1,25D3 was 10^{-12} M.

In addition to 1,2-propanediol, we examined the effects on tPA secretion of 1,3-propanediol and glycerol (propanetriol). At concentrations of 2×10^{-8} and 2×10^{-6} M, 1,3-propanediol was equipotent to 1,2-propanediol and induced tPA secretion from rat heart microvascular cells approximately three-fold (n = six per group, p < 0.001). Glycerol at the same concentrations was less potent than the propanediols; it induced tPA secretion 1.7-fold at 2×10^{-6} M, and 1.2-fold at 2×10^{-8} M (both significant at p < 0.01).

1,25D3 in human endothelial cells: Human coronary artery endothelial cells (HCAECs) were purchased from Clonetics/Bio-Whittaker (San Diego, CA) and grown in their EGM2-MV medium.

980

Cells were split into 48-well plates coated with 2 ug/well of mouse laminin, and cultured initially in Leibovitz' L15 containing 20 % FBS, then for three days in Basal Clonetics medium containing either 2% or 5% FBS. The media were then changed (same compositions except FBS was heat-treated) and the effects of 1,25D3 on tPA secretion were examined during the next 24 h. The results of the assays for tPA activity (figure 2) indicated that compared to the diluent control groups, 10^{-12} M 1,25D3 increased secretion of PA activity in wells containing either 2% or 5% FBS. Samples of the media were subjected to gel electrophoresis followed by zymography. The zymograms (figure 3) showed that the type of PA increased by treatment with 1,25D3 was tPA;

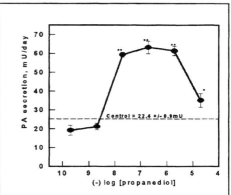

Figure 1 The effects of of 1,2-propanediol on secretion of tPA activity from rat heart microvascular cells during a 24 h incubation. Doses were 0.2, 2, 20, 200 nM and 2 and 20 uM. Control cells secreted 22.4± 0.9 (SEM) mU.

they showed further that both doses of 1,25D3 had increased tPA secretion. Interpretation of the zymograms suggested that 10^{-14} M 1,25D3 had increased tPA secretion but that the activity of the enzyme had not been expressed due to binding by an inhibitor, presumably PAI-1. This was shown by increased activity (at both concentrations of 1,25D3) at the migration position of a high molecular weight activity typical of tPA-PAI-1 complexes (the tPA in the complexes is activated by the presence of Triton X100 during the reaction). Only the zymogram representing 10^{-12} M 1,25D3 Lane 2), however, showed significantly increased activity in the position of authentic human tPA (compare the tPA standard in the left lane to corresponding activity in lane 2). The activity on the zymograms was not inhibited by incubation in the presence of EDTA, indicating that it represented plasminogen activators and not metalloproteinases (not shown).

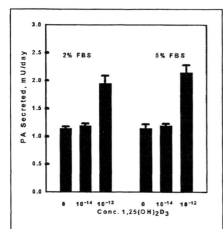

Figure 2. The effects of 1,25D3 on secretion of tPA from HCAECs. C = control, *, p < 0.001; n = 4 per group. 10^{-12} M significantly increased secretion.

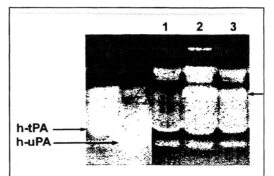

Figure 3: Migration of PA activity during electrophoresis on a gel containing plasminogen and fibrin. The white bands denote PA activity. Left lanes are human tPA and urokinase standards. Lane 1, control; lane 2, 10^{-12} M 1,25D3; lane 3, 10^{-14} M 1,25D3. The arrow on the right side denotes bands that migrated in a position typical of tPA-PAI-1 complexes.

Discussion In the present study we have illustrated a case in which an experimental manipulation designed to enhance the ability of endothelial cells to respond to 1,25D3 not only did so, but had additional effects that were not forseen, namely the observation of unexpected and potent biological effects of propanediols that have not been previously reported. The effect of propanediols was similar to the effect of 1,25D3 in this case. In biological research studies, 1,2-propanediol has been used as a solvent for lipid hormones both *in vivo* and *in vitro*. It is presumed to be nontoxic and without specific biological effects. In the commercial world, 1,2-propanediol is used as a food additive, a cryoprotectant for mammalian embryos, sperm and eggs, and in pharmaceutical and cosmetic preparations. The use of 1,2-propanediol is likely unimportant when used *in vivo* because it and similar compounds are already present in the tissues and circulation. Our study shows, however, that it may not be inert in *in vitro* studies with cultured cells; it may be particularly important under circumstances like those described herein when the culture system is depleted of lipids in order to study the action of a particular bioactive lipid like 1,25D3. Under these circumstances its possible effects on the system should be closely investigated or its use avoided.

The mechanism by which propanediol induces tPA secretion has not yet been investigated, but its structural similarity to glycerol permits it to undergo similar biochemical reactions. If it became acylated with fatty acids on both hydroxyls it would become an analog for diacylglycerols, and might activate the protein kinase C pathway, a known stimulus for tPA secretion (7). If it became acylated on one hydroxyl and the other were phosphorylated it would become an analog for lysophosphatidic acid or sphingosine-1-phosphate, potent mediators of growth, differentiation and cytoskeleton-dependent events including secretion (8).

In the case of possible synergy between 1,25D3 and 1,2-propanediol in our earlier study, our conclusion is that such an interaction is unlikely. This is based on the findings that *1)* 1,2-propanediol is inactive below 2×10^{-8} M, and *2)* 1,25D3 increases the secretion of tPA from rat heart microvascular cells at 10^{-15} M independent of the presence of 1,2-propanediol (unpublished results); hormone dissolved in ethanol or in dimethylsulfoxide is equipotent to that dissolved in 1,2-propanediol.

The second portion of this report describes the development of an *in vitro* cell culture system for the study of the effects of 1,25D3 on HCAECs. These cells are less stable to low serum concentrations than are the rat heart microvascular cells, probably because the latter may be stabilized by plating the vascular extracellular basement membrane along with the freshly isolated microvascular cells. In the HCAEC system, on the other hand, cells are plated directly in cultureware; this increases their dependence on added serum, and removal of serum leads to cell detachment and apoptosis. The cells did not tolerate culture in serum substitute or in ethanol-extracted FBS, but required native serum. In addition, the cells when plated directly on cultureware did not respond to 1,25D3 with increased tPA secretion; we found that laminin-coated cultureware was required. This may be connected to the activation of cell signalling systems or laminin/integrin-mediated increases in cytosolic $[Ca^{++}]$, but no data are yet available that bear on this question.

In spite of a requirement for serum, the HCAEC cultures were able to respond to physiological concentrations of 1,25D3 and to increase their secretion of tPA. Not only was tPA secretion increased, but in response to 10^{-12} M 1,25D3, it overcame the typically high PAI-1 levels in human endothelial cell cultures, and increased assayed enzyme activity. Possibly 1,25D3 and/or some of its synthetic analogs might be useful to increase circulating PA levels in patients, such as those at risk for initial or recurrent myocardial infarctions. In order to determine if this is a practical goal, it will be necessary to determine if the tPA synthetic and secretory system in humans can be stimulated by vitamin D-like compounds in addition to the numerous levels of control already exerted upon it.

This report points out that the sensitivity of an *in vitro* experimental system to a hormone or other bioactive agent depends to a great extent on the conditions under which that system is studied. In the case of tPA secretion by vascular cells, numerous agents and physiological conditions contribute to its regulation. In order to study the effects of only a single one of those hormones such as 1,25D3, it is necessary to avoid changing the levels of other agents that may normally regulate those effects by the same or by different signal transduction pathways. In the present case, it would be valuable to examine the sensitivity to 1,25D3 in a culture system where only 1,25D3 was removed from the culture system prior to the test incubations.

References

1. Merke J., Milde P., Lewicka S., Hugel U., Klause G., Mangelsdorf D.J., Haussler M.R., Rauterberg E.W. and Ritz E. (1989) J. Clin. Invest. 83, 1903-1915.
2. Puri S., Bansal D.D., Uskokovic M.R. and MacGregor R.R. (2000) Am. J. Physiol. Endocrinol. Metab. 278, E293-E301.
3. Merchiers, P., Bulens, F., Stockmans, I., De Vriese, A., Convents, R., Bouillon, R., Collen, D., Belayew, A., and Carmeliet, G. (1999) FEBS Lett. 460, 289-296.
4. Walters, M.R. (1992) Endocrine Rev. 13, 719-764.
5. Nishida, M., Carlyy, W.W., Gerritsen, M.E., Ellingsen O., Kelly R.A. and Smith T.W. (1993) Am. J. Physiol. 264, H639-H652.
6. Campbell, E.E., Shitman, M.A., Lewis, J.G., Pasqua, J.J. and Pizzo, S.V. (1982) Clin. Chem. 28, 1125-1128
7. Medh, R.D., Santell, L. and Levine, E.G. (1992) Blood 80, 981-987.
8. Goetzl, E.J. and An, S. (1998) FASEB J. 12, 1589-98.

METABOLISM OF THE ANTIPSORIATIC DRUG 1α,24(R)-DIHYDROXYVITAMIN D₃ IN HUMAN KERATINOCYTES

N. Astecker*, S. Ishizuka[+] and G.S. Reddy*; *Dept. of Pediatrics, Women & Infants' Hosp., Brown Univ. Sch. of Med., Providence, RI, U.S.A. [+]Teijin Institute for Bio-Medical Research, Tokyo, Japan.

Introduction: 1α,24(R)-Dihydroxyvitamin D_3 [1α,24(R)(OH)$_2$D$_3$], a synthetic analog of vitamin D_3, inhibits the growth of keratinocytes and promotes their differentiation as effectively as 1α,25-dihydroxyvitamin D_3 [1α,25(OH)$_2$D$_3$] (1). This in vitro activity of 1α,24(R)(OH)$_2$D$_3$ can be explained by the finding that both 1α,24(R)(OH)$_2$D$_3$ and 1α,25(OH)$_2$D$_3$ possess equal affinity to VDR (1). 1α,24(R)(OH)$_2$D$_3$ has been developed as a drug for the topical use in the treatment of psoriasis, since 1α,24(R)(OH)$_2$D$_3$ when compared to 1α,25(OH)$_2$D$_3$ induces less hypercalcemia (2). At present, the target tissue metabolism of this important vitamin D_3 analog is not completely understood. Previous metabolism studies in our laboratory revealed that rat kidney metabolizes 1α,24(R)(OH)$_2$D$_3$ via two metabolic pathways as shown in Figure 1 (3). The first pathway is initiated by 25-hydroxylation and proceeds further via the C-24 oxidation pathway. This leads to the production of metabolites

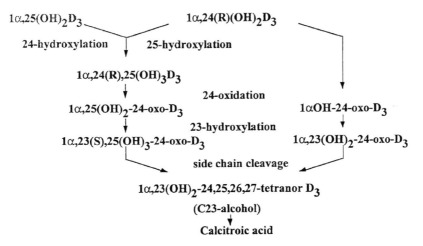

Figure 1: Metabolism of 1α,24(R)(OH)$_2$D3 in rat kidney

which are identical to those produced from 1α,25(OH)$_2$D$_3$. In the second pathway 1α,24(R)(OH)$_2$D$_3$ undergoes C-24 oxidation without prior 25-hydroxylation resulting in the production of metabolites which are unique for 1α,24(R)(OH)$_2$D$_3$. In the same study, we also noted that rat kidney does not convert 1αOHD$_3$ into 1α,25(OH)$_2$D$_3$. This finding led us to hypothesize that 24-hydroxylase (CYP24) is responsible for the C-25 hydroxylation of 1α,24(R)(OH)$_2$D$_3$. The present study investigates the metabolism of 1α,24(R)(OH)$_2$D$_3$ in primary human keratinocytes, which have been shown previously to possess not only 24-hydroxylase (CYP24) but also 25-hydroxylase (CYP27).

Methods: Confluent primary human keratinocytes were incubated with $1\alpha,24(R)(OH)_2D_3$ at 1 µM for 24 h. Lipids from both cells and media were extracted according to the procedure of Bligh and Dyer (4). Lipid extracts were subjected to HPLC-analysis. Metabolites of $1\alpha,24(R)(OH)_2D_3$ were purified using different HPLC-systems and their structures were established by GC/MS analysis. Similar experiments were performed with radiolabeled $1\alpha,24(R)(OH)_2[1\beta\text{-}^3H]D_3$ and $1\alpha,25(OH)_2[1\beta\text{-}^3H]D_3$ at nM concentrations. In these experiments cells were incubated with the respective substrates for 1 h and 3 h. Lipid extracts were spiked with authentic standards and analyzed by HPLC. Standards of the metabolites of $1\alpha,24(R)(OH)_2D_3$ and of $1\alpha,25(OH)_2D_3$ were synthesized biologically in the rat kidney perfusion system as described previously (5). $1\alpha,25(OH)_2\text{-}3\text{-epi-}D_3$ was a gift from Dr. Milan R. Uskokovic (Hoffmann-La Roche Inc. Nutley, NJ).

Results and discussion: Human keratinocytes convert $1\alpha,24(R)(OH)_2D_3$ into several side chain modified metabolites which are formed through the same metabolic pathways as described previously in rat kidney. In addition to these side chain modified metabolites $1\alpha,24(R)(OH)_2D_3$ is also converted into a less polar metabolite. This metabolite is identified as putative $1\alpha,24(R)(OH)_2\text{-}3\text{-epi-}D_3$ through mass spectrometry. Metabolism studies in which keratinocytes were incubated with $1\alpha,24(R)(OH)_2[1\beta\text{-}^3H]D_3$ and $1\alpha,25(OH)_2[1\beta\text{-}^3H]D_3$ for time periods ranging from 1 h to 3 h revealed that C-24 oxidation and C-25 hydroxylation of $1\alpha,24(R)(OH)_2D_3$ are detected only when CYP24 is induced. This finding strengthens our hypothesis that CYP24 is responsible not only for the C-24 oxidation but also for C-25 hydroxylation of $1\alpha,24(R)(OH)_2D_3$ even in human keratinocytes. At present studies examining the biological activities of the metabolites unique to $1\alpha,24(R)(OH)_2D_3$ are in progress. These studies will provide insight into our understanding of the mechanisms responsible for the ability of $1\alpha,24(R)(OH)_2D_3$ to generate in vitro cell differentiation activities equal to $1\alpha,25(OH)_2D_3$ without generating significant in vivo calcemic effects.

References:
1. Matsumoto, K., Hashimoto, K., Kiyoki, M., Yamamoto, M. and Yoshikawa, K. (1990) J. Dermatol. 17, 97-103.
2. Matsunaga, T., Yamamota, M., Mimura, H., Ohta, T., Kiyoki, M., Ohba, T., Naruchi, T., Hosoi, J. and Kuroki, T. (1990) J. Dermatol. 17, 135-142.
3. Weinstein, E.A., Rao, S.D., Siu-Caldera, M.-L., Tserng, K.-Y., Uskokovic, M.R., Ishizuka, S. and Reddy G.S. (1999) Biochem. Pharmacol. 58, 1965-73.
4. Bligh, E.G. and Dyer, W.J. (1958) Can. J. Biochem. Physiol. 37, 911-917.
5. Reddy, G.S., Jones, G., Kooh, S.W. and Fraser, D. (1982) Am. J. Physiol. 243, E265-E271.

1α,25-Dihydroxy-2β-(3-hydroxypropoxy)vitamin D3 (ED-71):

A Promising Candidate for the Treatment of Osteoporosis

Toshio Matsumoto[a], Noboru Kubodera[b] and The ED-71 Study Group

[a]First Department of Internal Medicine, University of Tokushima, Tokushima 770-0042, Japan

[b]Chugai Pharmaceutical Co., Ltd., Tokyo 104-8301, Japan

Summary

1α,25-Dihydroxy-2β-(3-hydroxypropoxy)vitamin D3 (ED-71) is a potent analog of active vitamin D, 1,25(OH)2D3, bearing a hydroxypropoxy substituent at the 2β-position. In ovariectomized rats, ED-71 prevented the reduction in bone mass and strength of not only lumbar spine and distal femur rich in trabecular bone, but also femoral diaphysis rich in cortical bone without causing hypercalcemia. From those results, it was suggested that ED-71 preferentially enhances bone formation with less effect on intestinal calcium absorption. Human studies in 40 healthy male volunteers revealed that daily oral administration of 0.1 to 1.0μg ED-71 for 15 days caused dose-dependent increase in urinary calcium excretion. However, none of the subjects showed sustained increase in urinary calcium over 400mg/day or hypercalcemia over 10.4mg/dl. ED-71 administration also caused a dose-dependent suppression of bone resorption markers such as urinary deoxypyridinoline without significant changes of bone formation markers including serum bone-specific alkaline phosphatase. Based upon these results, an open clinical trial was conducted in 109 osteoporotic patients. Interim results indicated that daily oral administration of ED-71 (0.25, 0.5, 0.75 and 1μg) for 6 months increased bone mineral density (BMD) at L2-4 in a dose-dependent manner. The effect on L2-4 BMD was better than that in estrogen-treated patients in previous studies. ED-71 also exhibited a dose-dependent suppression of urinary deoxypyridinoline with a slight increase in serum osteocalcin. ED-71 was well tolerated without causing any major adverse effects including sustained hypercalcemia or a reduction in renal function. These results demonstrate that ED-71 can effectively increase bone mass without causing hypercalcemia, and suggest that ED-71 can be a promising candidate for the treatment of osteoporosis with prominent effect on bone formation.

Introduction

Although 1α-hydroxyvitamin D3, a pro-drug of active vitamin D, has been widely prescribed for the treatment of osteoporosis in Japan and some other countries, the therapeutic efficacy of active vitamin D has yet to be approved in the US and many European countries. The controversy of active vitamin D as a therapeutic agent for osteoporosis comes from several reasons, *e.g.* the risk of causing hypercalcemia/hypercalciuria in vitamin D- and calcium-replete conditions, ambiguous mechanism of action in bone, and unestablished clinical efficacy in the management of osteoporotic patients.

Various analogs of 1,25(OH)2D3 have been synthesized in attempts to obtain tissue specific agonist of active vitamin D on bone in the last two decades. ED-71 was obtained during the course of these attempts[1,2,3] and has been shown to be a highly potent analog to act on bone with a long half-life in plasma due to its strong affinity to DBP.[4,5] The structure and characteristics of ED-71 are summarized in Fig. 1.

Based upon these characteristics of ED-71, preclinical as well as clinical studies have been performed to test its efficacy in the management of osteoporotic subjects. The results demonstrate that ED-71 potently inhibits bone resorption while slightly enhancing bone formation, and that it increases lumbar bone mineral density (BMD) in a dose-dependent manner with superior effect to estrogen. These observations suggest that ED-71 is a promising candidate for the treatment of osteoporosis.

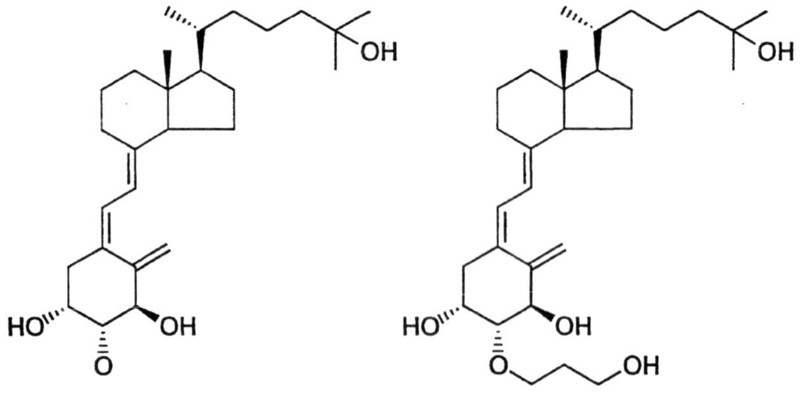

	1,25(OH)$_2$D$_3$	ED-71
VDR	1	1/8
DBP	1	2.7
T$_{1/2}$ in Plasma	short	long

Fig. 1 Structure and Characteristics of ED-71

Studies in ovariectomized (OVX) rats

It has been already demonstrated that ED-71 could completely suppress the reduction in bone mass of OVX rats.[6,7] Suppression of bone mass reduction by ED-71 is observed not only in the lumbar spine and the femoral metaphysis which are rich in cancellous bone but also in the femoral diaphysis which is rich in cortical bone. Accordingly, the administration of ED-71 could suppress the OVX-induced reduction in bone strength at both the lumbar spine and the middle femur. In the OVX rats, there is 20% decrease in bone mass 3 months after OVX compared to that in the sham rats. When ED-71 was administered to the OVX rats beginning 3 months after ovariectomy for 6 weeks, lumbar spine of these rats regained the bone mass to a level equivalent to that before ovariectomy. These results demonstrate that the reduction in bone mass and bone strength at post-menopausal phase can be recovered by the treatment with ED-71.[8] Table 1 summaries the effects of ED-71 and parathyroid hormone [rhPTH (1-84)] treatment for 12 weeks starting 3 months after ovariectomy at 9 months of age on bone markers (osteocalcin and deoxypyridinoline) and histomorphometry. The results are compared with those of estradiol treatment for 12 weeks starting after ovariectomy at 9 months of age. Low dose treatment of rhPTH (1-84) showed enhanced bone formation with little effect on bone resorption. High-dose treatment further enhanced bone formation with a slight increase in bone resorption with marked increase in BMD. Estradiol treatment reduced bone resorption, with less suppression in bone formation in both high and low doses, resulting in a small increase in BMD. In contrast, while the low-dose treatment with ED-71 strongly inhibited bone resorption without significant change in bone formation, the high-dose ED-71 stimulated bone formation with further inhibition of bone resorption, showing a marked increase in BMD comparable to that in rhPTH (1-84)-treated rats.

Table 1. Comparison of the effects of rhPTH (1-84) , estradiol and ED-71 in OVX rats.

	Osteocalcin		Deoxypyridinoline	
	low dose	high dose	low dose	high dose
rhPTH(1-84)	↑	↑ ↑	→	↑
Estradiol	↓	↓ ↓	↓ ↓	↓ ↓
ED-71	→	↑	↓ ↓	↓ ↓

	BFR/BS		Oc.S/BS	
	low dose	high dose	low dose	high dose
rhPTH(1-84)	↑ ↑	↑ ↑ ↑	↑	↑ ↑
Estradiol	↓ ↓	↓ ↓	↓	↓ ↓
ED-71	↓	↑	↓ ↓	↓ ↓

	BMD
	high dose
rhPTH(1-84)	↑ ↑
Estradiol	↑
ED-71	↑ ↑

988

Phase I clinical study

Based upon the preclinical studies in rats, we performed phase I clinical study in 40 healthy adult male volunteers. Repeated oral administration of ED-71 (0.1, 0.25, 0.5 and 1.0µg) for 15 days (once a day) showed efficient and dose-dependent absorption of dosed ED-71 (Fig. 2). As shown in Fig. 3, no significant changes in serum calcium levels were observed by the treatment with any doses of ED-71. Although urinary excretion of calcium was slightly increased (approximately 100mg/24 hours) at 1.0µg/day of ED-71, the increase was within the normal range. None of the subjects showed sustained increase in urinary calcium over 400mg/day or serum calcium over 10.4mg/dl. It is interesting to note that ED-71 at doses which caused a marked reduction in 1,25(OH)2D production did not significantly suppress PTH secretion (Fig. 4). ED-71 administration also caused a dose-dependent suppression of bone resorption markers without significant changes in bone formation markers (Fig. 5). These results demonstrate that ED-71 within this dose range can effectively suppress bone resorption without any significant reduction in bone formation, and that this dose range of ED-71 can be well tolerated without causing hypercalciuria or hypercalcemia.

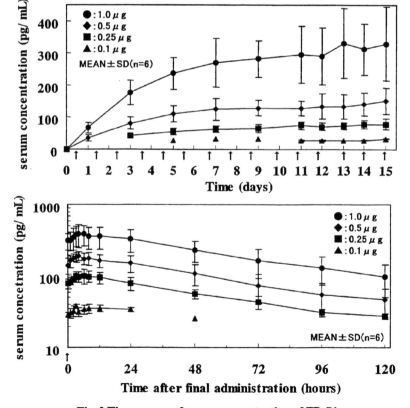

Fig. 2 Time course of serum concentration of ED-71

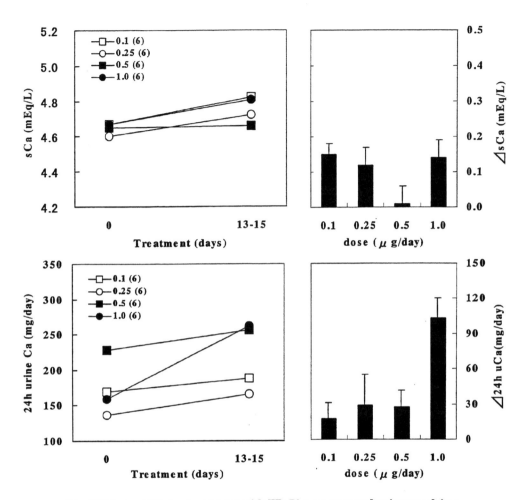

Fig. 3 Effects of 15-day treatment with ED-71 on serum and urinary calcium

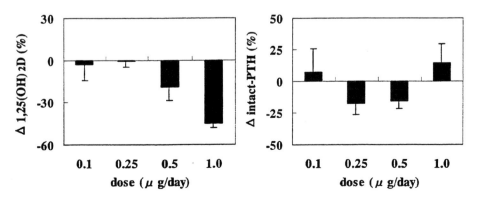

Fig. 4 Effects of 15-day treatment with ED-71 on changes in 1,25(OH)2D3 and intact PTH

990

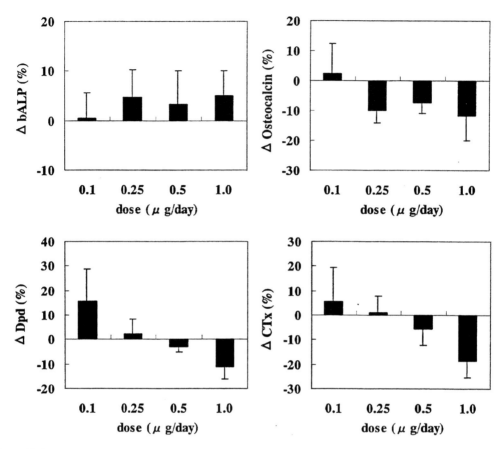

Fig. 5 Effects of 15-day treatment with ED-71 on changes in bone specific alkaline phosphatase, osteocalcin, deoxypyridinoline and type I collagen C-telopeptide

Phase II clinical study

The phase I study demonstrated that short-term treatment with up to 1.0 µg/day ED-71 did not cause hypercalciuria or hypercalcemia in normal volunteers, and that it effectively suppressed bone resorption without a reduction in bone formation. These observations prompted us to further evaluate the efficacy of treatment with ED-71 on the bone turnover and BMD of osteoporotic patients. Thus, phase II clinical studies of ED-71 were conducted under the protocol shown in Table. 2.

Table. 2 Design and end points of phase II clinical study

Subjects: Involutional osteoporosis
        109 patients (102 females and 7 males)
        49 to 81 years old

Design: Randomized controlled study

Dosages: 0.25µg/day, po (28 subjects)
        0.50µg/day, po (28 subjects)
        0.75µg/day, po (26 subjects)
        1.0µg/day, po (27 subjects)

Period: 24-week treatment
End points: Lumbar (L2 –L4) spine BMD at 24 weeks   Bone markers at 8, 16 and 24 weeks

The interim results demonstrated that ED-71 increased bone mass in a dose-dependent manner and the effect reached the peak at 0.75µg/day with approximately 2.5 % increase in the lumbar BMD.   The increase in bone mass was associated with a reduction in bone resorption markers with a slight increase in a late bone formation marker, osteocalcin.   The results of the 24-week clinical trial with ED-71 warrant a long-term clinical study to examine its effectiveness on bone mass and fracture prevention in osteoporotic patients especially with low bone turnover.   Detailed and finalized results will be reported elsewhere.   Taken together, these studies suggest that ED-71 is a promising candidate for the treatment of osteoporosis with unique effects on bone.

Conclusion

1. ED-71 substantially increases bone mass in osteoporotic subjects.
2. ED-71 has unique effects on bone turnover by inhibiting bone resorption while stimulating bone formation.
3. The effect to increase bone mass is dose-dependent and reaches the peak at 0.75µg/day.
4. ED-71 is well tolerated up to 1.0µg/day without causing hypercalcemia.
5. The results of the 24-week clinical trial warrant a long-term clinical study to examine the effectiveness on bone mass and fracture prevention in osteoporotic patients.

References

1. *Chem. Pharm. Bull.*, **1993**, *41*, 1111.
2. *Chem. Pharm. Bull.*, **1997**, *45*, 1626.
3. *Bioorg. Med. Chem.*, **1998**, *6*, 2517.
4. *Biol. Pharm. Bull.*, **2000**, *23*, 66.
5. *Biochem. Biophys. Res. Commun.*, **1989**, *163*, 1444.
6. *Calcif. Tissue Int.*, **1994**, *54*, 142.
7. *Bioorg. Med. Che. Lett.*, **1993**, *3*, 1815.
8. Further characters of ED-71 are shown in the following literatures: a) *Biochem. Biophys. Res. Commun.*, **1992**, *189*, 1231, b) *Bone*, **1993**, *14*, 47, c) *J. Bone Miner. Res.*, **1996**, *11*, 325, d) *Life Sci.*, **1998**, *62*, 453, e) *Bone*, **1999**, *24*, 187, f) *Mol. Cell. Biol.*, **1999**, *19*, 1049.

INDICES

Author Index

A

Acchiardo, S.R. 863,871
Achmatowicz, B. 81
Adams, J.A. 935
Adorini, L. 547
Alisio, A. 677
Alleva, D.G. 125
Alvarez, M.L. 239
Alvarez, V. 947
Amuchastegui, S. 547
Andersin, T. 255
Apolinário, D. 407
Arabian, A. 767
Aris, R.M. 893
Asahina, T. 957
Ashiwa, C. 163
Astecker, N. 983
Avila, E. 171
Avión, J. 97
Avnur, Z. 887

B

Bach, R.D. 111
Bailleul-Forestier, I. 365
Baldi, C. 743
Barber, Y. 825
Barbero, G. 897
Barbier, P. 615
Bareis, P. 495
Barletta, F. 313
Barley, N.F. 641
Barnes, A.K. 801
Barros, S.S. 435
Barsony, J. 379
Bartek, J. 411
Barto, R. 649
Bauer, F.W. 615
Bay, C. 485
Beckman, M.J. 155
Bell, N.H. 151
Bellido, T. 391
Beltramino, C. 677
Benassati, S. 973
Bendixen, A.C. 423
Ben-Mekhbi, H. 839
Berdal, A. 365,415,419,707,711,779
Bergfeld, M. 897
Bernardi, R.J. 461,469

Berry, D. 699
Berry, J.L. 797,935
Bertuzzi, F. 547
Betriu, A. 825
Bikle, D. 597,623
Bindels, R.J.M. 633
Binderup, E. 805
Binderup, L. 395,411,485,537
Bises, G. 495
Bishop, C.W. 135,863,871
Bishop, J.E. 263,691
Björkling, F. 35,805
Blæhr, L.K.A. 35,805
Bland, R. 159,167,301
Bleiberg, I. 423
Blin, C. 415
Blum, K.E. 461,469
Bogaerts, I. 117
Bohdanowicz, J. 431
Boland, R. 703,739,743,747,731,973
Bortman, P. 407
Bouillon, R. 23,57,117,129,507,
555,561,563,583,977
Bouizar, Z. 627
Bourges, H. 847
Bower, J.D. 863,871
Boyan, B.D. 683
Bradwell, A.R. 159
Brentani, M.M. 407,439
Bretherton-Watt, D. 829
Bretting, C. 35
Breves, G. 645
Britto, L. 677
Browbank, J. 801
Brown, A.J. 857
Brunetto, O. 947
Buitrago, C. 703
Bula, C.M. 263
Bunce, C. 301
Bury, Y. 69
Buurman, C.J. 179
Byford, V. 135
Byrne, I. 275

C

Cabral, A.L.B. 439
Calverley, M.J. 35,805
Capen, C.C. 537
Capiati, D.A. 731
Carlberg, C. 69,223,259,267,279,309

Subject Index

Cell Line Index

Workshop Zoo

C57/BL6 mouse   201
Chick (*Gallus gallus*)   369,677,703,727,731,743
Mouse   163,231,271,345,353,461,565,577,623,633,661,711,779,879,957
Mouse, C57BL/6   125
Mouse, Calbindin knockout   665
Mouse, CYP-24 knockout   135,767
Mouse, NCR-*nu*   515
Mouse, NMRI   507
Mouse, NOD   561
Mouse, nude, athymic   511
Mouse, nude, BNX 31
Mouse, VDR knockout   135,453,555,563,633,775,835,957
Pig   151,271
Pig, Hannover   175
Pig, newborn   645
Rabbit   435,633,805,953
Rat   129,271,345,461,649,657,711,747,761,783,843,879,887,957,979
Rat, male weanling   53
Rat, newborn   627
Rat, Sprague-Dawley   365,673
Rat, Wistar   431,573,669,735,739
Sheep   435,953